Oral and Oropharyngeal Cancer

Second Edition

Oral and Oropharyngeal Cancer

Second Edition

Jatin P. Shah, MD, MS (Surg), PhD (Hon), DSc (Hon), FACS, FRCS (Hon), FDSRCS (Hon), FRCSDS (Hon), FRCSI (Hon), FRACS (Hon)
Professor of Surgery, Weil Cornell Medical College
and
E W Strong Chair in Head and Neck Oncology
Memorial Sloan Kettering Cancer Center
New York, USA

Newell W. Johnson, CMG, FMedSci, MDSc, PhD, FDSRCS (Eng), FRACDS, FRCPath (UK), FFOP (RCPA), FOMAA, FHEA (UK), FICD
Honorary Professor of Dental Research, Menzies Health Institute Queensland
and
School of Dentistry and Oral Health, Griffith University
and
Emeritus Professor, Griffith Institute for Educational Research
Queensland, Australia
and
Emeritus Professor of Oral Health Sciences
King's College London
London, United Kingdom

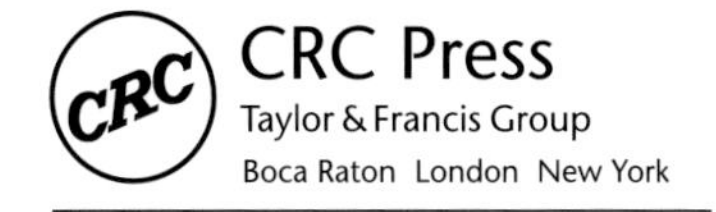
CRC Press
Taylor & Francis Group
Boca Raton London New York

CRC Press is an imprint of the
Taylor & Francis Group, an **informa** business

CRC Press
Taylor & Francis Group
6000 Broken Sound Parkway NW, Suite 300
Boca Raton, FL 33487-2742

Printed and bound in India by Replika Press Pvt. Ltd.

Printed on acid-free paper

International Standard Book Number-13: 978-1-4987-0008-5 (Hardback)

Library of Congress Cataloging-in-Publication Data

Names: Shah, Jatin P., editor. | Johnson, Newell W., editor.
Title: Oral and oropharyngeal cancer / [edited by] Jatin P. Shah, Newell W. Johnson.
Description: Second edition. | Boca Raton, FL : CRC Press, 2018. | Preceded by Oral cancer / edited by Jatin P. Shah, Newell W. Johnson, John G. Batsakis. 2003. | Includes bibliographical references.
Identifiers: LCCN 2017048943 (print) | LCCN 2017050075 (ebook) | ISBN 9781351138543 (eBook General) | ISBN 9781498700092 (eBook PDF) | ISBN 9781498715942 (eBook ePub3) | ISBN 9781498700085 (hardback : alk. paper)
Subjects: | MESH: Mouth Neoplasms | Oropharyngeal Neoplasms
Classification: LCC RC280.M6 (ebook) | LCC RC280.M6 (print) | NLM WU 280 | DDC 616.99/431--dc23
LC record available at https://lccn.loc.gov/2017048943

Visit the Taylor & Francis Web site at
http://www.taylorandfrancis.com

and the CRC Press Web site at
http://www.crcpress.com

Contents

Preface to the second edition

Since the first edition of this textbook was published in 2003, many changes in epidemiology and in management have occurred. Oral cancer—predominantly squamous cell carcinomas affecting the lips, intraoral tongue and the mucosae of the oral cavity—remains in the top ten malignancies that afflict humankind. Indeed, in many regions, such as south Asia and Melanesia, it can be *the* most common malignancy amongst males, perhaps sixth in women, often second overall. These remain predominantly due to tobacco use—both smoked and smokeless, the latter often in combination with areca (betel) nut, together with alcohol abuse, in a background of diets deficient in antioxidant vitamins and minerals. They are predominantly diseases of the deprived, though no socioeconomic group is immune. They continue to be a major public health and personal problem globally. Indeed, the burden of disease is rising, partly due to population growth and aging populations in the high-risk communities.

Management of oral cancer has improved considerably in terms of survival rates and quality of life over the decade and a half since we wrote the first edition, but this only applies to advanced multidisciplinary treatment centers, and most of these are in the developed countries. Many low- and middle-income countries still lack resources for early detection and effective treatment, though some are models of primary prevention through public education and sometimes screening programs.

Unfortunately, as the incidence rates of tobacco and alcohol-related cancers have begun to decline in some countries, the world has been swept by an epidemic of cancers of the oropharynx, and sometimes the mouth and hypopharynx, associated with oncogenic types of the human papillomavirus (HPV) family. These are the same viruses that cause over 90% of cancers of the uterine cervix and anal and penile cancers in men who have sex with men. These genital cancers and HPV-positive head and neck cancers are regarded today as sexually transmitted diseases. Fortunately, HPV-driven head and neck cancers respond relatively well to treatment, so that radiotherapeutic (with or without adjuvant chemotherapy) regimes can be de-escalated. Because of these dramatic changes, we have enlarged the book to cover cancers of the oropharynx as well as oral cancers.

Surgical approaches to the treatment of primary lesions and regional lymph node metastases, whether "conventional" open surgery or increasingly with robotics, have made great strides. Primary radiotherapy, adjuvant radiotherapy and/or cytotoxic chemotherapy regimens continue to be refined. Most strikingly, biologic therapies, particularly immunotherapeutic therapies, have blossomed. This has brought head and neck cancer treatment firmly into the age of personalized medicine. Many drugs and antibodies can diminish the effects of mutant genes in cancer cells and should be restricted to patients whose neoplasm expresses such mutations. Some neoplasms have molecular changes that block the body's natural defenses and agents are available that can reactivate the natural killer immune response of cell-mediated immunity. Many new drugs are becoming available and being licensed in many countries for a range of malignancies. Dramatic results are being shown, but most of these approaches remain not fully proven, so routine use should perhaps wait for the results of good-quality clinical trials.

Surgical ablation and reconstruction techniques have improved continuously. However, a high proportion of our patients still die with or of their cancer, so that we have again included a chapter on palliative care. Primary prevention through public education and health promotion, secondary prevention through screening where appropriate and early detection remain central to control of head and neck cancer. So this second edition has the same philosophical breadth as before, with extension to the oropharynx.

We wish to recognize the contributors to the first edition who are not represented this time. Especially we pay tribute to the late Professor John Batsakis, whose pre-eminence as a histopathologist contributed so much to the first edition. We welcome new authors who have filled the gaps he left so ably and who have added new depth to the chapters on diagnosis, pathology and molecular biology. Many of our colleagues have joined us in expanding and improving chapters for which we have remained primarily responsible. We thank them all for enhancing the quality of this edition.

Jatin P. Shah and Newell W. Johnson
New York, London and Brisbane, November 2017

Contributors

Nishant Agrawal, MD
Department of Surgery
University of Chicago
Chicago, Illinois

Nezar al-Hebshi, BDS, PhD
Kornberg School of Dentistry
Temple University
Philadelphia, Pennsylvania

Hemantha Amarasinghe, BDS, MSc, MD
Cancer Epidemiologist and Consultant in Community Dentistry
Institute of Oral health
Maharagama, Sri Lanka

George C Bohle III, DDS
The Dental Depot
Oklahoma

Jay O. Boyle, MD
Head and Neck Service
Memorial Sloan Kettering Cancer Center
New York City, New York

Pankaj Chaturvedi, MS, MNAMS, FICS, FAIS, FACS, PDCR
Department of Head Neck Surgery
Tata Memorial Hospital
Mumbai, India

Camile S. Farah, BDSc, MDSc, PhD, FRACDS (OralMed), FOMAA, FIAOO, FICD, FPFA
Australian Centre for Oral Oncology Research & Education
UWA Dental School
The University of Western Australia
Perth, Australia

Matthew G. Fury, MD PhD
Department of Medicine
Memorial Sloan Kettering Cancer Center
New York City, New York

Rachel A. Giese, MD
Department of Head and Neck Surgery
Memorial Sloan Kettering Cancer Center
New York City, New York

Ralph W. Gilbert, MD, FRCSC
Gullane/O'Neil Chair in Otolaryngology/H&N Surgery
University Health Network
University of Toronto
Toronto, Canada

Bhawna Gupta, PhD, MIPH, BDS
Menzies Health Institute
and
School of Dentistry and Oral Health
Griffith University
Queensland, Australia

Prakash C. Gupta, DSc
Healis–Sekhsaria Institute For Public Health
Navi Mumbai, India

Rifat Hasina, DDS, PhD
Department of Surgery
University of Chicago
Chicago, Illinois

Maryam Jessri, DDS, PhD
Australian Centre for Oral Oncology Research & Education
UWA Dental School
The University of Western Australia
Perth, Australia

Keziah John, BDSc, MPhil
Australian Centre for Oral Oncology Research & Education
UWA Dental School
The University of Western Australia
Perth, Australia

Newell W. Johnson, CMG, FMedSci, MDSc, PhD, FDSRCS (Eng), FRACDS, FRCPath (UK), FFOP (RCPA), FOMAA, FHEA (UK), FICD
Honorary Professor of Dental Research
Menzies Health Institute Queensland
and
School of Dentistry and Oral Health
Griffith University
and
Emeritus Professor
Griffith Institute for Educational Research
Queensland, Australia

and

Emeritus Professor of Oral Health Sciences
King's College London
London, United Kingdom

Allison J. Kobren, MS, CCC-SL
Department of Surgery
Speech-Language Pathology
NYU Langone Health at Bellvue Hospital Center
New York City, New York

Omar Kujan, DDS, PhD
Australian Centre for Oral Oncology Research & Education
UWA Dental School
The University of Western Australia
Perth, Australia

Yastira Lalla, BDSc, MPhil
Australian Centre for Oral Oncology Research & Education
UWA Dental School
The University of Western Australia
Perth, Australia

Mark W. Lingen, DDS, PhD, FRCPath
Department of Pathology
University of Chicago
Chicago, Illinois

Andres Lopez-Albaitero, MD
Ear Nose and Throat Associates of New York
and
Assistant Clinical Professor
Mount Sinai School of Medicine
New York City, New York

Evan Matros, MD, MMSc, MPH
Plastic and Reconstructive Surgical Service
Memorial Sloan Kettering Cancer Center
New York City, New York

Catriona R. Mayland, MBChB, MD, FRCPS (Glas)
Palliative Care Institute
University of Liverpool
and
Academic Department of Palliative and End-of-life Care
Royal Liverpool University Hospital
Liverpool, United Kingdom

Sean McBride, MD, MPH
Memorial Sloan Kettering Cancer Center
New York

Colleen McCarthy, MD, FRCS(C)
Memorial Sloan Kettering Cancer Center
New York

Nigel Alan John McMillan, BSc, PhD
Director, Understanding Chronic Conditions Program
Menzies Health Institute
and
School of Medical Sciences
Griffith University
Queensland, Australia

Jocelyn C. Migliacci
Department of Surgery
Head and Neck Service
Memorial Sloan Kettering Cancer Center
New York City, New York

Aviram Mizrachi, MD
Attending Surgeon
Department of Otorhinolaryngology Head and Neck Surgery
Rabin Medical Center
Director, Center for Translational Research in Head and Neck Cancer
Davidoff Cancer Center
Israel

Pablo H. Montero, MD
Research Associate, Head and Neck Service
Department of Surgery
Memorial Sloan Kettering Cancer Center
New York City, New York

and

Attending Surgeon, Head and Neck Surgery
Department of Surgery
Clínica Las Condes
Santiago, Chile

Snehal G. Patel, MD, FRCS
Department of Surgery
Head and Neck Service
Memorial Sloan Kettering Cancer Center
New York City, New York

Ivana Petrovic, MD, PhD
Memorial Sloan Kettering Cancer Center
New York

Cecily S. Ray, MPH
Healis–Sekhsaria Institute For Public Health
Navi Mumbai, India

Simon N. Rogers, MD, FRCS (Eng), FRCS (Maxfac)
Evidence-Based Practice Research Centre
Faculty of Health and Social Care
Edge Hill University
Omskirk, United Kingdom

and

Regional Maxillofacial Unit
Aintree University Hospitals NHS Trust
Liverpool, United Kingdom

Jatin P. Shah, MD, MS (Surg), PhD (Hon), DSc (Hon), FACS, FRCS (Hon), FDSRCS (Hon), FRCSDS (Hon), FRCSI (Hon), FRACS (Hon)
Professor of Surgery
Weil Cornell Medical College
and
E W Strong Chair in Head and Neck Oncology
Memorial Sloan Kettering Cancer Center
New York City, New York

Mushfiq Hassan Shaikh, BDS, MSc, PhD
Menzies Health Institute
and
School of Dentistry and Oral Health
Griffith University
Queensland, Australia

Bhuvanesh Singh, MD, PhD, FACS
Memorial Sloan Kettering Cancer Center
New York

Adrian Sjarif, MBBS (Hons), BSc, MS, FRACS
Department of Plastic and Reconstructive Surgery
St. George Hospital
Sydney, Australia

David J. Speicher
Menzies Health Institute
and
School of Dentistry and Oral Health
Griffith University
Queensland, Australia

Paul M. Speight, BDS, PhD, FDSRCPS, FDSRCS (Eng), FDSRCS(Ed), FRCPath
School of Clinical Dentistry
University of Sheffield
Sheffield, United Kingdom

An Vu, BDSc, MPhil
Australian Centre for Oral Oncology Research & Education
UWA Dental School
The University of Western Australia
Perth, Australia

Laura Wang, MBBS, MS
Liverpool Hospital
Sydney, Australia

Saman Warnakulasuriya, MDSc (Melb), PhD (Bristol), FDSRCS (Eng), FRACDS, FRCPath (UK), FFOP (RCPA), FICD, FILT, FMedSci
Dental Institute
King's College
London, United Kingdom

PART I

Pathology and biology

1

Global epidemiology

NEWELL W. JOHNSON AND HEMANTHA AMARASINGHE

DEFINITIONS OF ORAL CANCER

Malignant neoplasms are major causes of fear, morbidity and mortality all over the world. Cancer is one of the five main causes of death in all societies, with its relative position varying with age and sex. Figure 1.1 shows the main causes of death in England and Wales in 2014, as a typical example of Western industrialized countries (1). In developing countries the proportions will differ, with infectious diseases being a larger component and cardiovascular disease a smaller component. Cancer numbers are important, however. In England and Wales, for example, in the past 65 years infections have declined as a major cause (in spite of the HIV epidemic) so that diseases of the heart and circulatory system now dominate in men, with cancer second; however, cancer dominates in women, especially in the third to sixth decades of life. Globally, "oral cancer" is the sixth most common cause of cancer-related death, although many people are unaware of its existence.

This text deals with malignant neoplasms affecting the oral cavity, principally the oral mucosa, and the oropharynx. These diseases have much in common with squamous cell carcinomas arising elsewhere in the upper aerodigestive tract, which share common risk factors, so studies of "head and neck cancer" are frequently drawn upon when issues relevant to oral cancer are discussed. Of these cancers, the vast majority are squamous cell carcinomas arising in the mucous membranes of the mouth and the pharynx. Indeed, of all the oropharyngeal malignancies reported to the Surveillance, Epidemiology and End Results program of the National Cancer Institute of the United States Public Health Service (SEER) registries in the USA between 1975 and 2011, apart from lesions of the salivary glands, gingivae, nasopharynx, nasal cavity and sinuses, more than 95% were squamous cell carcinomas. The increasing number of cancers associated with Human Papillomaviruses, mostly in the oropharynx, have a more basaloid, non-keratinising morphology. Neverthless "upper aerodigestive tract alcohol- and tobacco-related oral squamous cell carcinomas" remain the major head and neck cancers. They represent a major global public health problem and constitute the major workload of head and neck oncologists worldwide. Our emphasis is thus on mucosal disease. Because cancers in these sites, especially in the mouth, often arise out of long-standing, potentially malignant disorders (earlier called lesions and conditions), these are given due consideration; less extensive coverage is given to other lesions.

Most of the international databases employ the International Classification of Diseases (ICD) coding system of the World Health Organization (WHO), and most of the data currently available are expressed according to the tenth revision of this system (ICD-10). It is particularly important to define these codes and to be clear how many of these precise anatomic sites are included in any particular dataset under study. Neoplasms of the major salivary glands clearly have quite distinct natural histories, ill-understood etiologies and distinct management protocols compared with mucosal cancers. Similarly, nasopharyngeal malignancies are usually Epstein–Barr virus-related carcinomas that differ distinctly from the more widespread alcohol- and tobacco-related squamous cell carcinomas of the rest of the upper aerodigestive tract. Datasets should be examined carefully to determine whether the major salivary glands and nasopharynx are included, as they so often are (ICD codes C07–08 and C11). Many datasets make a distinction

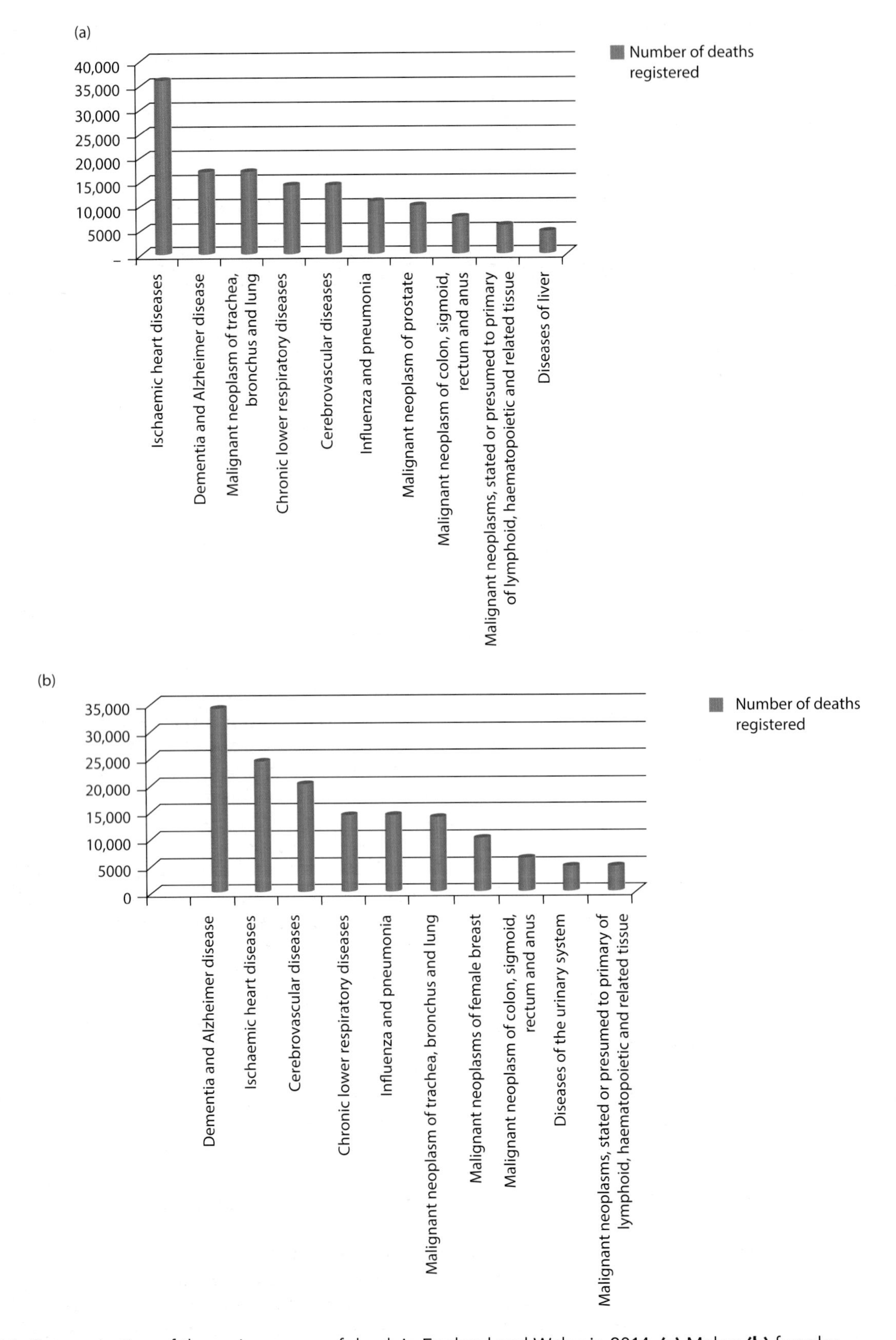

Figure 1.1 Categorization of the major causes of death in England and Wales in 2014. **(a)** Males; **(b)** females.

between lip and intraoral cancer and we have to be clear whether oral cancer is taken to include the oropharynx and hypopharynx in any given dataset. In this second edition we have added consideration of cancers of the oropharynx and of the hypopharynx, because of the global epidemic of Human Papillomavirus-related cancers of these sites (ICD-10 codes C01, C09, C10 and, less often, C12 and C13).

INCIDENCE RATES WORLDWIDE

The databases from which these estimates are derived are far from ideal: many parts of the world produce no data at all, in others (often among the most populous), the data may come from localized, atypical regions. Hospital-based cancer registries naturally gather biased information—those cases that present to hospital only; thus, in many developing countries, cases may not come to attention at all, either because of fear or the inability of poor people to access hospital services. This is certainly true of incidence data. Death rates may be even more unreliable because, in many developing countries, follow-up even of treated cases is impossible. Death certification is not always compulsory and there is limited international standardization in the categories of cause of death, let alone calibration of those signing death certificates.

Figure 1.2 plots the estimated numbers of new cases of most common cancers by anatomic site in male and in female patients. There are striking differences.

For 2012, GLOBOCAN estimates indicate that there were 9.1 million new cases of cancer and 4.4 million cancer deaths for those between the age of 0 and 69 years. Lung cancer is the leading cancer among men and breast cancer is the most common cancer among women (2).

According to the GLOBOCAN 2012 data, for both sexes, combined cancer of the lip and oral cavity (ICD-10 COO-CO6), excluding hypo-, oro-, and naso-pharynx) ranks ninth overall, behind lung, breast, colon and rectum, prostate, stomach, liver, cervix uteri and esophagus, in that order. When considering oral and pharyngeal cancer, the annual estimated incidence is around 300,373 cases for lip and oral cavity (ICD-10: C00–08) and 142,378 for "other" pharyngeal cancers (C09–C10, C12–14) i.e: *excluding the nasopharynx* because of its different aetiology and biology: two-thirds of these cases occurring in developing countries (2). Figure 1.3 shows the incidence and mortality due to cancer of the lip and oral cavity and "other pharynx" in the top 20 countries in the world.

There is wide geographical variation in the incidence of oral cancer and of "other pharynx" cancers (C09–C10) (Table 1.1). Figure 1.4 shows incidence rates for cancers of the lip and oral cavity, in quintiles, for the countries of the world. It has been apparent for decades that the global picture for head and neck cancer is dominated by the incidence of oral cancer in southern Asia and of oral cavity plus nasopharyngeal cancer in East Asia. In the 1980s, in India, Bangladesh, Pakistan and Sri Lanka, oral cancer was the most common site and accounted for about a third of all cancers; it is still the most common cancer among men in Sri Lanka (3–5). The proportion is falling, partly due to increased detection of other cancers by more extensive screening programs and improved techniques (5). Even within the subcontinent, there are striking differences in incidence rates. The highest rate for tongue and mouth cancers is reported for men living in South Karachi, Pakistan; the second highest is from Trivandrum city in Kerala, India. Extremely high rates for women are seen in the Tamil community in Malaysia—higher even than in Tamil Nadu itself: upper aerodigestive tract sites in Indian females in peninsular Malaysia are the second most common cancers, behind breast and above uterine cervix (6).

According to GLOBOCAN 2012 data, the highest incidence of oral cancers (ICD C00–C08) is found in Melanesia (astounding rates of 22.9 per 100,000 in men and 16.0 per 100,000 in women, though there are caveats about the quality of these data) (2). In India alone, over 100,000 cases of oral cancer are registered every year and the numbers are rising. Though men predominate overall, among females a very high incidence is found throughout south central Asia (4.7 per 100,000). In terms of countries, Maldives and Sri Lanka have the highest incidence of oral cancer in the south Asian region. Poor access to health services contributes to high mortality.

DIFFERENCES BY SEX

As already noted, worldwide, the incidence of oral and pharyngeal cancers overall is higher for males than females. According to the International Agency for Research on Cancer (2), the age-specific incidence of "oral cavity" and "other pharynx" cancers was 5.5 and 3.2 per 100,000 population for males in 2012 and 2.5 and 0.7 for females, respectively (see Table 1.1). This may be because of their greater indulgence in the most important risk factors, such as heavy alcohol and tobacco consumption for intra-oral cancer and sunlight for lip cancer in those who work outdoors. However, oral cancer in females is increasing in some parts of the world. For instance, a study from Argentina showed the male:female ratio to be 1.24:1 for the period 1992–2000 compared to 7.1:1 for the 1950–1970 period (7). The incidence of tongue and other intra-oral cancers for women can be greater than or equal to that for men in high-incidence areas such as India, where betel quid/areca nut chewing (and sometimes smoking) are common among women, although this varies considerably from region to region.

Early this century, within Europe, the incidence of oral cavity and pharyngeal cancers (C00–14) among males varied substantially between 5.9 (Finland) and 32 (France) per 100,000 per annum (8). Incidence rates among females were highest in northern and western Europe, but were consistently lower than those for males. The male-to-female ratio decreased during the last 10 years and recently varied between 1.5 and 2.5 in northern Europe to 7.7 in Lithuania. Between 1990 and 1999, the U.K. incidence rates for oral cancers rose in males of all ages from 6.5 to

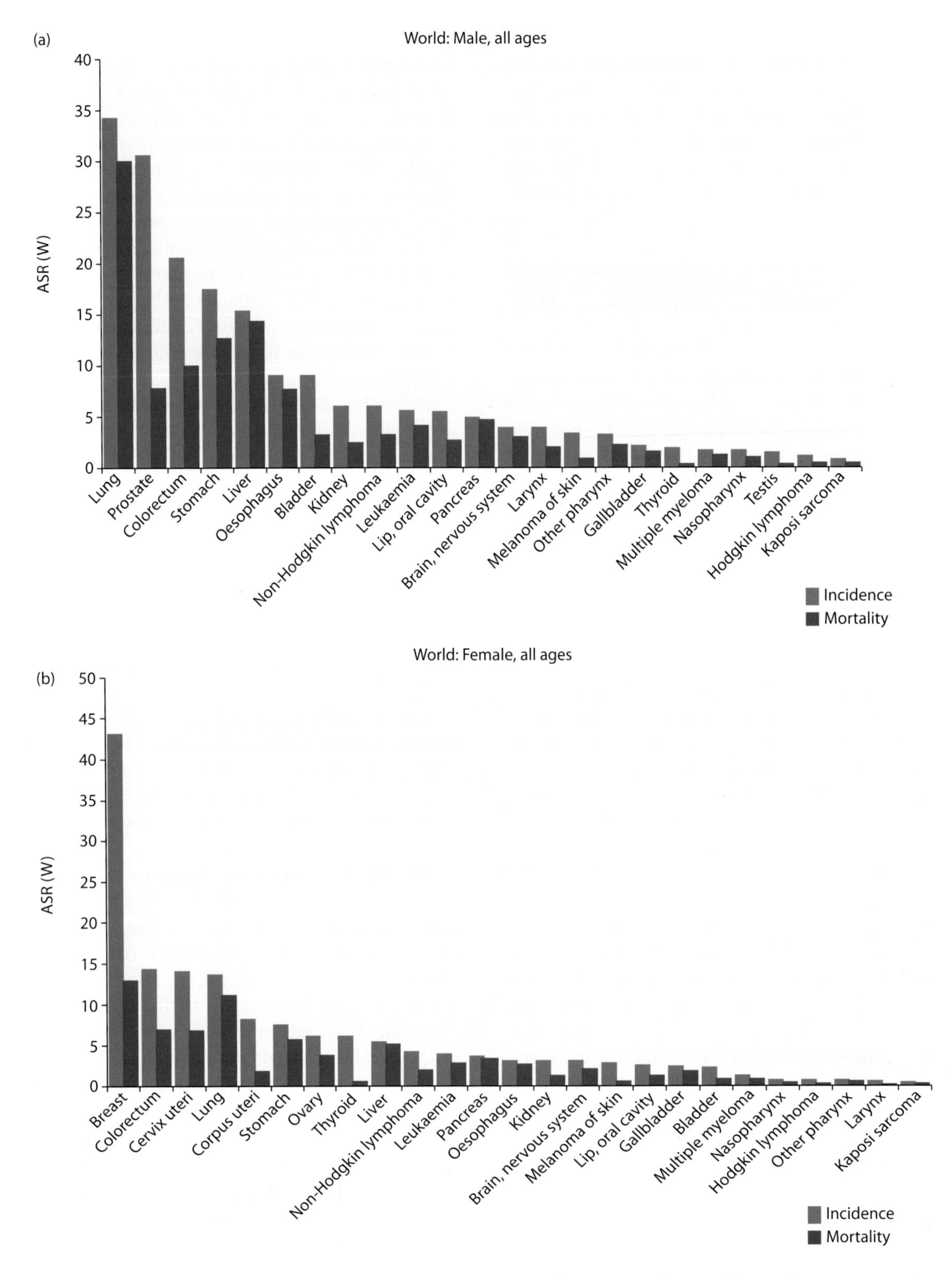

Figure 1.2 Global incidence rates for malignant neoplasms, age-standardized to the world population (ASR(W)), in both sexes. (Globocan 2012. http://gco.iarc.fr/today/.)

8.3 per 100,000 (an increase of 18%) and in females from 2.6 to 3.6 per 100,000 (an increase of 30%) and continues to be a concern (9).

In the USA, the death rate due to cancer of the oral cavity and pharynx per 100,000 population in 2007–2011 was 3.8 for males and 1.4 for females (10), down from 6.9 to 2.3, respectively, in 1975. This substantial improvement is not reflected in most of the rest of the world.

Apart from the traditional risk factors, it has been suggested that estrogen deficiency may influence susceptibility

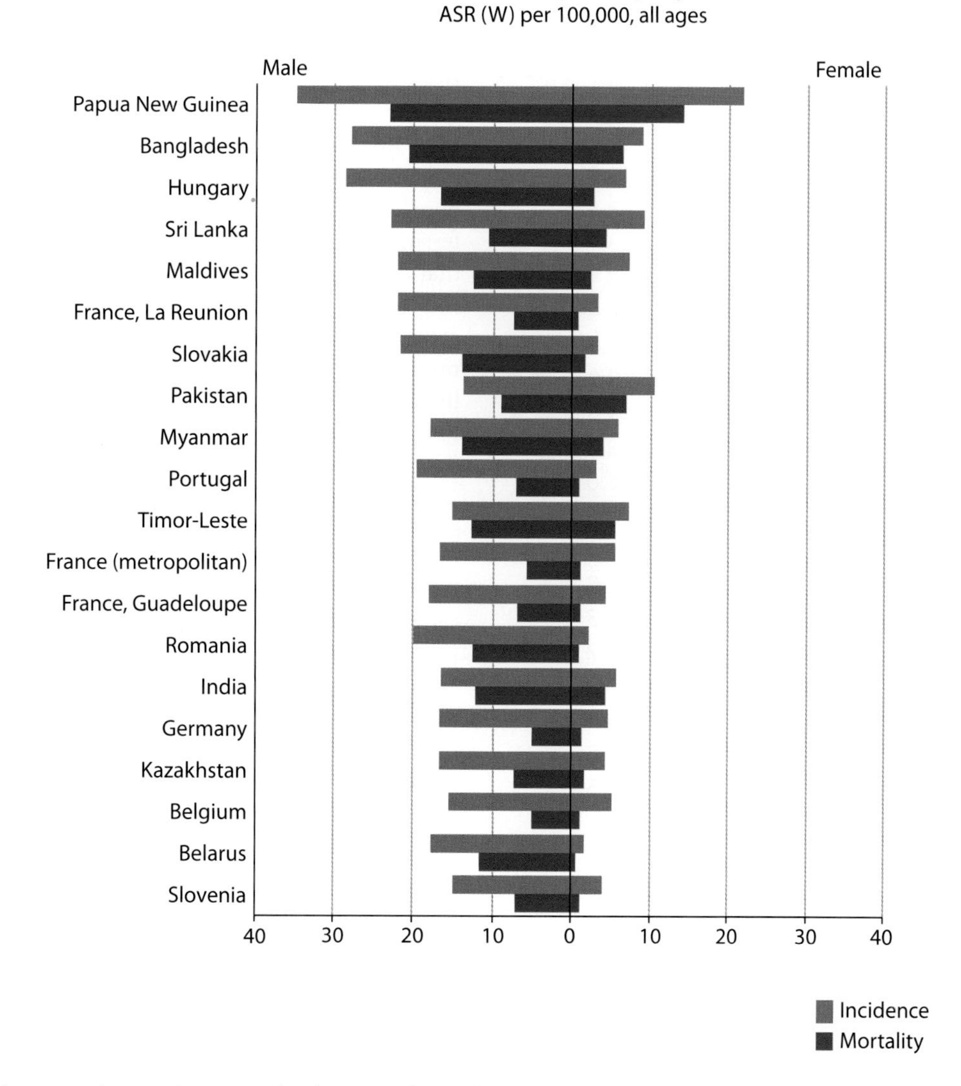

Figure 1.3 Incidence and mortality rates, both sexes, for malignant neoplasms of the lip, oral cavity and pharynx, excluding nasopharynx, in the 20 countries with the highest rates in the world. (Globocan 2012 http://gco.iarc.fr/today/.)

to oral cancer in women; significantly, a younger mean age at menopause and higher rates of hysterectomy may influence the higher rates of oral cancer seen among younger females (11). Data presented in this chapter are, whenever possible, separated by sex.

AGE DISTRIBUTIONS

Oral cancer is usually a disease that occurs in males after the fifth decade of life. The mean age at presentation is in the fifth and early sixth decades in Asian populations compared with the seventh and eighth decades in the North American population (12–17). Statistics in the USA for 1975–2011 show that the median age at diagnosis for cancer of the oral cavity and pharynx was 62 years (18).

Several studies suggest that 4%–6% of oral cancers now occur at ages younger than 40 years (19). An alarming increase in incidence of oral cancers among younger people has been reported from many parts of the world (20–23), a trend that appears to be continuing. There was a significant increase in the incidence of cancers in the tongue and tonsils among 20–40-year-olds in the USA between 1973 and 2001 (24).In Germany, Czechoslovakia and Hungary, there was an almost 10-fold rise in mortality from oral cancer in men aged 35–44 (25), within a single generation at the end of the last century. Robinson and Macfarlane showed a dramatic increase in incidence rates for younger males in Scotland from the 1980s to the 1990s (26). In the high-prevalence areas of the world, in many cases patients are less than 40 years old, probably owing to heavy use of various forms of tobacco from an early age, although some recent Indian data have not shown this (27).

It is also clear that a number of cases of squamous cell carcinoma occur in both young and old patients in the absence of traditional risk factors, in which the disease may pursue a particularly aggressive course, more so in the

Table 1.1 Estimated age-standardized incidence rate per 100,000 per annum (pa) for oral plus "other pharynx" cancers in 2012

Area	Male ASR (W)	Female ASR (W)
World	8.8	3.2
More developed	11.7	3.5
Less developed	7.7	3.1
Eastern Africa	5.5	3.4
Middle Africa	5.3	2.4
Northern Africa	3.6	2.5
Southern Africa	10.2	3.8
Western Africa	2.2	1.5
Caribbean	8.4	2.7
Central America	3.7	2.0
South America	8.2	3.0
Northern America	11.4	4.1
Eastern Asia: China	2.2	1.0
Eastern Asia: Japan	7.4	2.3
Eastern Asia: other	3.7	1.2
Southeastern Asia	6.2	3.2
South central Asia	16.2	6.1
Western Asia	3.5	2.0
Central and Eastern Europe	14.3	2.5
Northern Europe	9.3	4.1
Southern Europe	9.1	2.6
Western Europe	15.4	4.8
Australia/New Zealand	11.5	4.4
Melanesia	26.3	16.4
Micronesia/Polynesia	6.4	1.0

elderly. A study conducted in southern England concluded that a substantial proportion of cases of younger people diagnosed with oral cancer occur in the absence of known risk factors (28). This, together with the relatively short duration of exposure in users, suggests that factors other than tobacco and alcohol are implicated in the development of oral cancer in a significant minority of cases. Diets poor in fresh fruits and vegetables were identified as conferring significant risk. There is now substantial evidence that human papillomavirus (HPV) infections are driving this rise in younger adults but, fortunately, HPV-related oropharyngeal cancers respond well to radiotherapy, permitting treatment de-escalation and improved quality of life. It is also suggested that greater attention should be paid to familial antecedents of malignant neoplasms in younger patients with oral cancer (29).

Age distribution curves for the major oral and pharyngeal cancer sites are given for deliberately selected countries in Figures 1.5 and 1.6.

As shown in Figure 1.5, all oral and pharyngeal cancers show a similar distribution. Most cases occur in the fifth to seventh decades of life, presumably because decades of exposure to tobacco, alcohol and poor nutrition take time to synergize with other agents in triggering malignant transformation—or in allowing this to survive the host response! There are nevertheless a significant minority of cases appearing in the third and fourth decades of life. These attract much interest as, although associations with early commencement of smoking and with unsafe alcohol use can be demonstrated, a substantial minority of cases arise without exposure to traditional risk factors; here, dietary inadequacies and HPV infection are likely to be important, as may inherited predisposition.

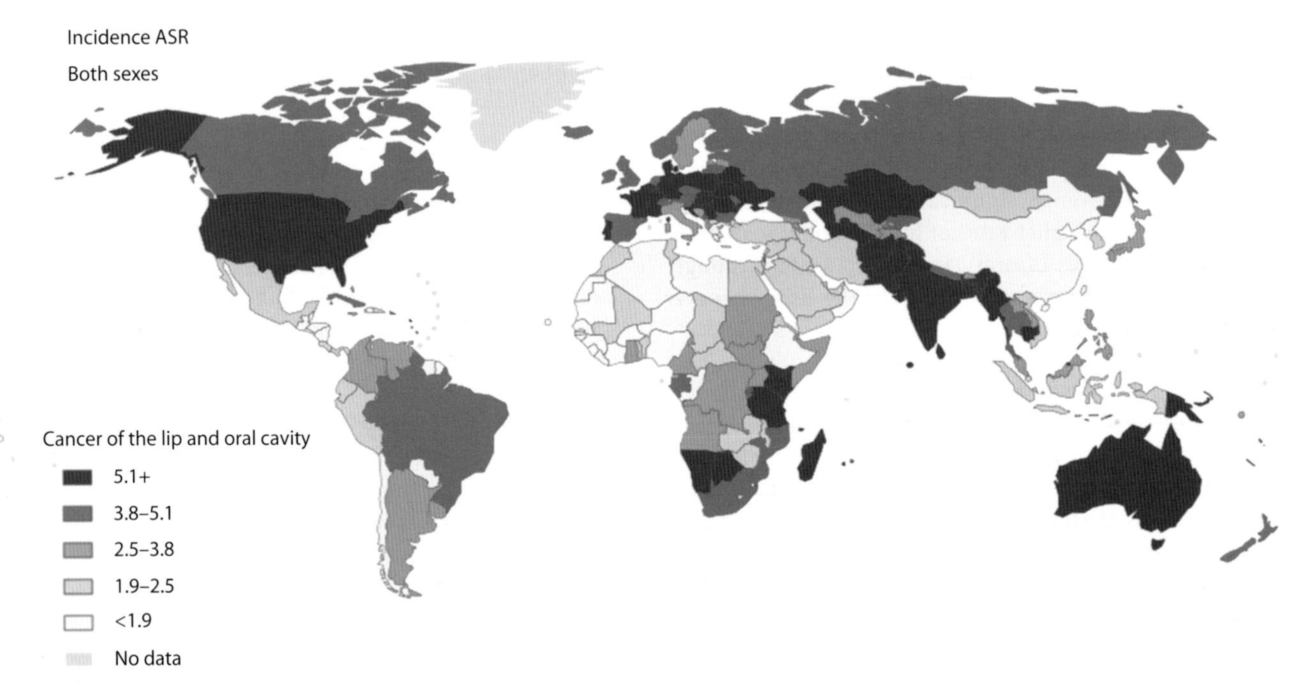

Figure 1.4 Age standardized incidence rates for cancers of the lip plus oral cavity, across the globe, presented in quintiles. (http://gco.iarc.fr/today/home; Accessed January 10, 2018.)

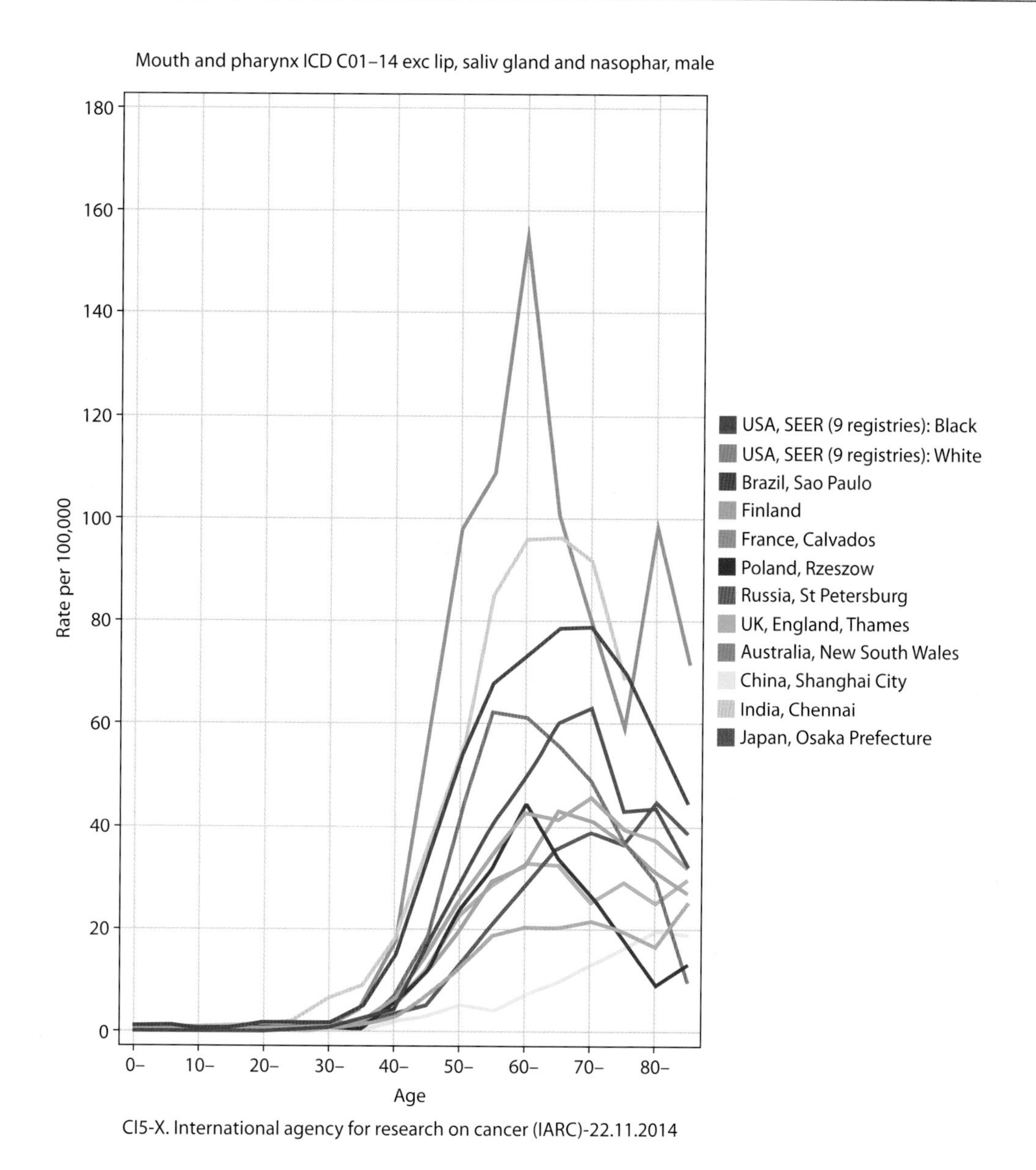

Figure 1.5 Male age-specific incidence curves for the mouth and pharynx for selected countries.

In the high-incidence age bands, there is an approximately 4–10-fold difference in incidence, with disturbingly high rates in northwest France, Brazil and south India among the countries selected here. Note the much worse situation in American blacks compared with whites, explained by a mixture of risk factor and socioeconomic reasons. Finland does comparatively well, which is not surprising in view of that nation's success in reducing the prevalence of smoking, though alcohol abuse remains a social problem. What is surprising are the low rates recorded for Shanghai, in spite of high smoking prevalence in this large city. China is currently developing a more comprehensive, nationwide cancer registry system so more cogent data will soon be available.

As shown in Figure 1.6, rates for females are lower and international differences are less marked. Women in south India stand out, and this is related to the use of betel quid and tobacco, together with low socioeconomic status

ETHNIC VARIATIONS

Variations by ethnicity are largely due to social and cultural practices and the influence of dietary and genetic factors, though the latter are less well quantified. Variations in outcome are also contributed to by differences in access to healthcare. Where cultural practices represent risk factors, their continuation by emigrants from high-incidence regions to other parts of the world results in comparatively high cancer incidence rates in immigrant communities. This can also affect the sub-sites of oral cancer most commonly affected, as shown in a study from California (30). The highest age-adjusted oral cancer rates in the USA are found among non-Hispanic men (17.5/100,000) followed by non-Hispanic women (6.6/100,000), with Asian and Hispanic populations showing lower incidence rates compared with white (Caucasian) ethnic groups. Tongue cancer was the

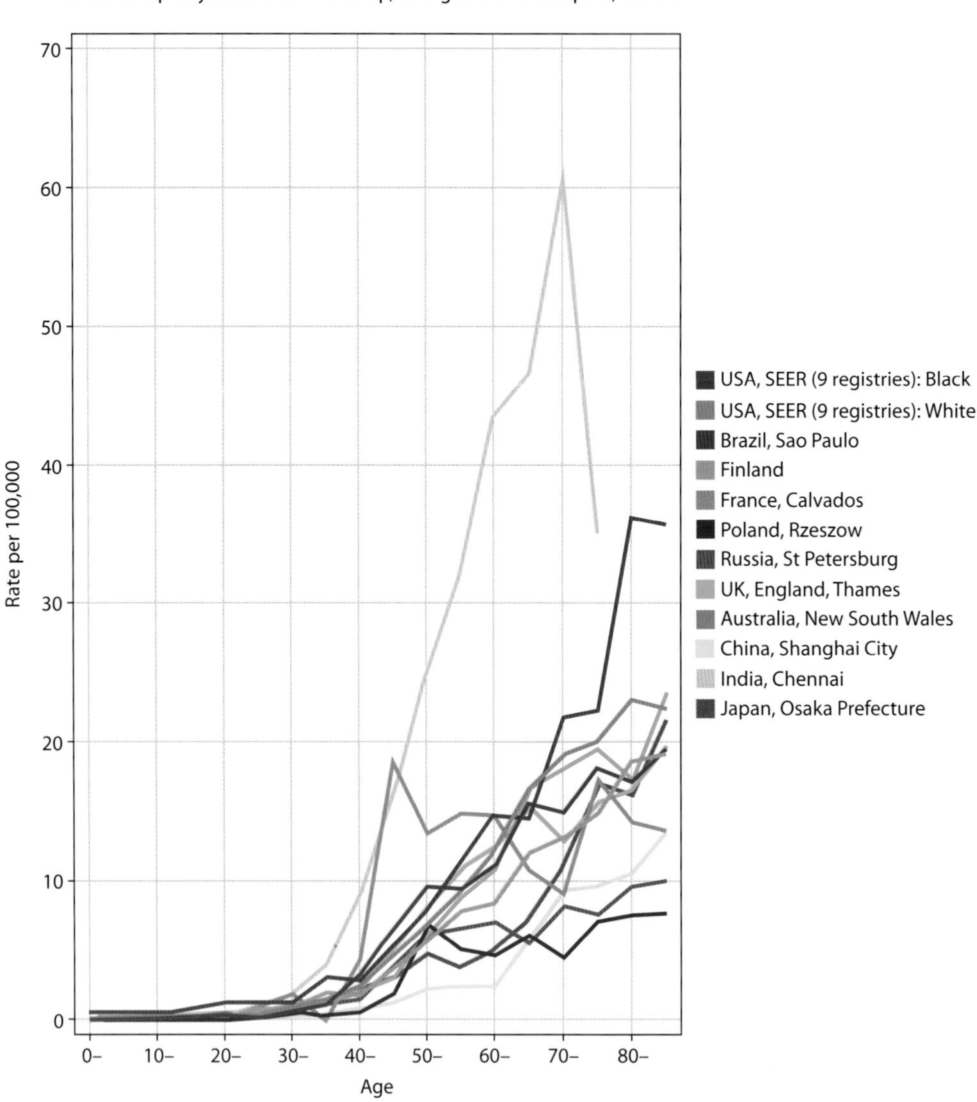

Figure 1.6 Female age-specific incidence curves for the mouth and pharynx for selected countries.

most common type of oral cancer among every ethnicity. Asians were more likely to develop their malignancy in the buccal mucosa, a reflection of continuing areca and tobacco chewing habits. Another study showed that American Indians and Alaskan Natives overall had significantly lower incidence rates than non-Hispanic whites (31). Several studies from the USA have demonstrated that black patients with oral cancer have poorer overall and disease-specific survival than whites, mainly because of their comparatively poor access to healthcare (32,33). This is especially concerning because the incidence of oral plus pharyngeal cancer for black men in the USA is so high and is the sixth most common site for malignant disease amongst this group (34).

In the Republic of South Africa, among Asian/Indian South Africans, oral and oropharyngeal cancer incidence rates were higher among females (Age-standardised incidence rate [ASIR] = 4.60) than among males (ASIR = 3.80). Excluding those involving the lip, these cancers were highest among coloreds (ASIR = 5.72) and lowest among blacks (ASIR = 3.16). Incidence rates increased significantly among colored South Africans over the period from 1992 to 2001 ($p < .05$), particularly for the oropharynx (available at http://repository.up.ac.za/bitstream/handle/2263/32412/AyoYusuf_Trends(2013).pdf?sequence=1).

The age-adjusted incidence rate for oral and pharyngeal cancers is higher for south Asians than for other residents in England, particularly among females (35). Interestingly, this study showed that British south Asian males have significantly better survival rates than their non-south Asian peers in the southeast of England, possibly a reflection of the more indolent progress of tobacco/areca nut-induced lesions (35).

According to the SEER statistics, incidence rates of oral cavity and pharynx cancers among black men and women

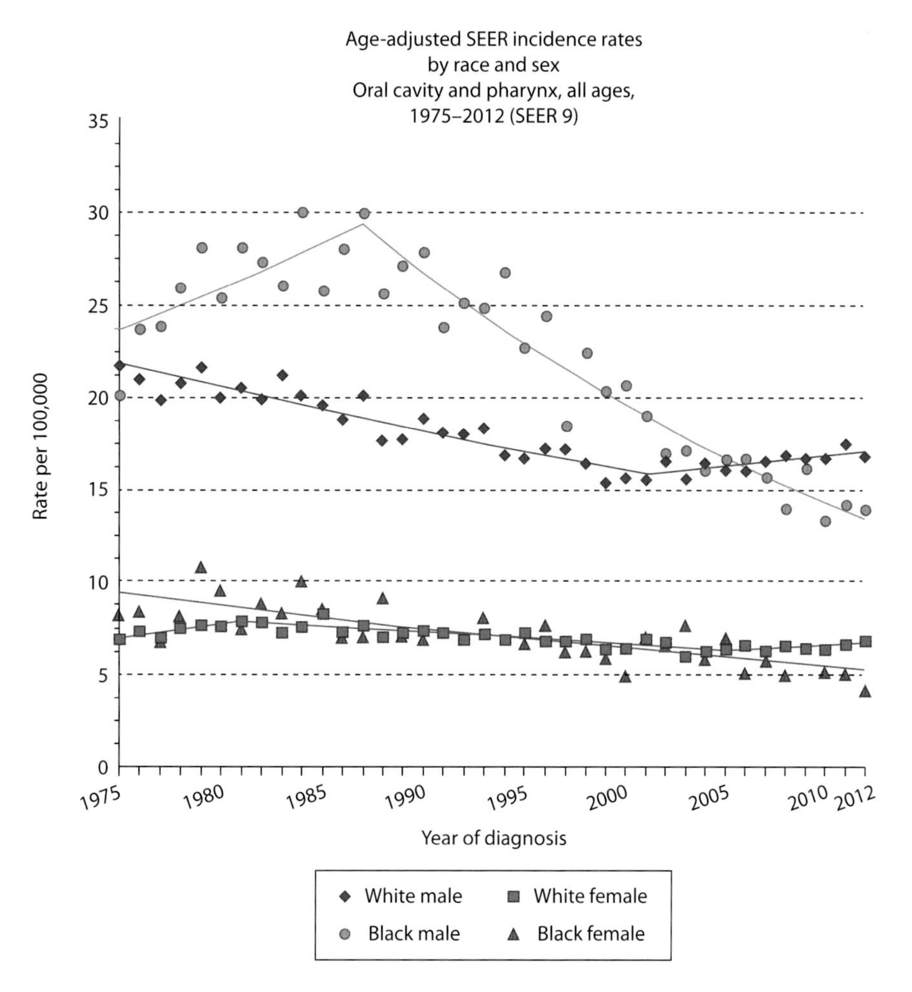

Figure 1.7 Incidence rates of cancer of the oral cavity and pharynx among black and white people in USA from 1975 to 2012.

declined dramatically throughout the period from 1975 to 2012 compared with white men and women. In 2012, incidence rates for black men and women were less than for white people (see Figure 1.7) (10).

MORTALITY RATES AND TRENDS

As with incidence rates and trends, there is much geographical variation. Figure 1.3 plots age-standardized mortality rates for lip, oral cavity and other pharynx cancers (ICD-10: C00–14 except C11) in the top 20 countries in the world in the year 2012. Mortality was highest in Papua New Guinea and countries in the southeast Asian region. Several European countries, namely France, Hungary and in the former Czechoslovakia, also have a high ranking. This is historically linked to heavy alcohol and tobacco use in these communities (Table 1.2).

Trends of age-standardized (world population) mortality rates for the lip, oral cavity and other pharynx cancer sites of interest within selected countries over the past three to six decades are presented in Figures 1.8 and 1.9, derived from the WHO mortality database (36).

Figure 1.8 shows that trends in mortality over time are important to track and to understand. Hungary is a disaster, though a declining trend is evident from the year 2003. Russia remains a concern. France demonstrates what can be achieved. The overall modest downward trend in the other countries illustrated is encouraging.

Figure 1.9 shows that, although only approximately a tenth of the male rate, Hungarian females remain a challenge.

Current male death rates for oral and pharyngeal cancer around the world are seen vividly in Figure 1.8. There was a steady rise in oral cancer mortality in men from the 1950s to late 1980s in most western European countries (37), but this trend has since declined in France, China and Hong Kong, which had exceedingly high rates in the past. Unfortunately, in most countries in central and Eastern Europe, oral cancer mortality in men continued to rise, reaching exceedingly high rates in Hungary, Slovakia, Slovenia and the Russian Federation at the end of the last century. Hungary, Ukraine, Estonia and Bulgaria showed more than a 100% increase in mortality rates for men during the 20-year period up to the turn of the millennium. Even though the rates of oral cancer are comparatively low among women (Figure 1.9), there was an increase in several countries in

Table 1.2 Mortality data extracted from the GLOBOCAN 2012 database for comparison with the incidence data in Table 1.1

Country	Mouth (ICD C00–08) Being lip, all of tongue, all of mouth and major salivary glands		Other pharynx (ICD C09–10, C12–14) Being tonsil, remainder of oropharynx, pyriform fossa, hypopharynx and sites not otherwise specified amongst C00–C13	
	Male	Female	Male	Female
World	2.7	1.2	2.2	0.5
More developed	2.3	0.6	2.2	0.3
Less developed	2.8	1.4	2.2	0.5
Africa	2.1	1.3	0.9	0.4
Eastern Africa	3.2	1.9	0.9	0.5
Middle Africa	2.9	1.4	1.6	0.6
Northern Africa	1.3	0.8	0.6	0.6
Southern Africa	2.8	1.0	2.2	0.6
Western Africa	1.2	1.0	0.5	0.1
Caribbean	2.0	0.6	2.4	0.6
Central America	0.8	0.5	0.7	0.2
South America	2.2	0.7	2.2	0.4
Northern America	1.2	0.5	1.2	0.3
Asia	3.0	1.4	2.4	0.5
Eastern Asia	1.1	0.5	0.7	0.1
Southeastern Asia	1.9	1.2	2.1	0.5
South central Asia	6.3	3.0	5.3	1.2
Western Asia	1.0	0.6	0.6	0.3
Europe	3.0	0.7	2.7	0.4
Central and Eastern Europe	5.1	0.7	3.8	0.3
Northern Europe	1.7	0.7	1.4	0.3
Southern Europe	1.9	0.6	1.8	0.3
Western Europe	2.0	0.6	2.7	0.5
Australia	1.3	0.6	1.2	0.3
New Zealand	1.4	0.7	1.0	0.2
Melanesia	14.4	10.2	2.8	0.4
Micronesia	2.0	0.0	0.0	0.0
Polynesia	1.4	0.0	2.0	0.3

Europe (notably Hungary, Belgium, Denmark and Slovakia) over this period. These disturbing rises are thought to have been related to high drinking and smoking patterns in these societies, together with poor diet in lower socioeconomic status groups. Fortunately, improvements are now evident.

The SEER program in the USA has reported an overall fall in the mortality from oral and pharyngeal cancer between 2002 and 2011 of 1.87% per annum Table 1.3.

Table 1.3 shows a fall in all mortality rates for oral and pharyngeal cancer in the USA between 2002 and 2011. There is a considerable fall in mortality among both black men and black women (Annual percentage change [APC] of −3.7 and −2.7, respectively). Furthermore, the SEER data show higher 5-year relative survival rates for whites (64.3%) and blacks (43.7%) who were diagnosed during the period 2004–2011 than rates for those who were diagnosed during the period 1974–1976 (when rates for whites and blacks were 55% and 36.3%, respectively) (38). The 5-year survival rates in the SEER registries range from a high of 72.1% for white women in Utah to a low of 24.8% for black men in metropolitan Atlanta. These striking differences are likely to be explained by a number of factors including socioeconomic condition, age, stage at diagnosis, continued presence or absence of environmental risk factors and access to hospital services. African–American patients have consistently poorer survival outcomes (See Figures 1.7 and 1.10) (39).

A study in Mumbai, India, indicated a decreasing trend in oral cancer incidence among Indian men, which was suggested may be due to a decrease in the use of betel quid/pan and associated oral smokeless tobaccos over this period (40). However, there continues to be a high prevalence of smokeless tobacco use among young adult men and women, especially in the form of Pan Parag/Gutka-type products, and cigarette smoking is increasing. Overall, cancer of the upper aerodigestive tract (UADT) will increase, as indicated earlier (12).

Population-based survival rates around the world show little evidence of improvement over recent decades, despite vast improvements in treatment modalities. Cure rates and survival rates have improved with advances in surgical and other techniques in highly specialized, high-volume treatment

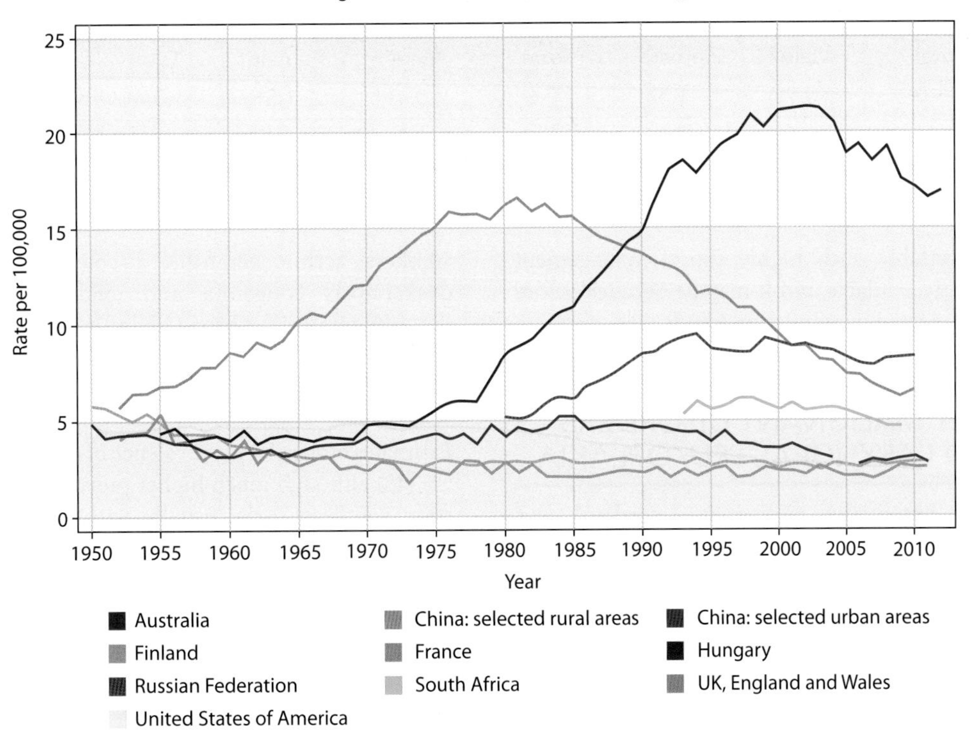

Figure 1.8 Mortality from cancer of the lip, oral cavity and pharynx: male.

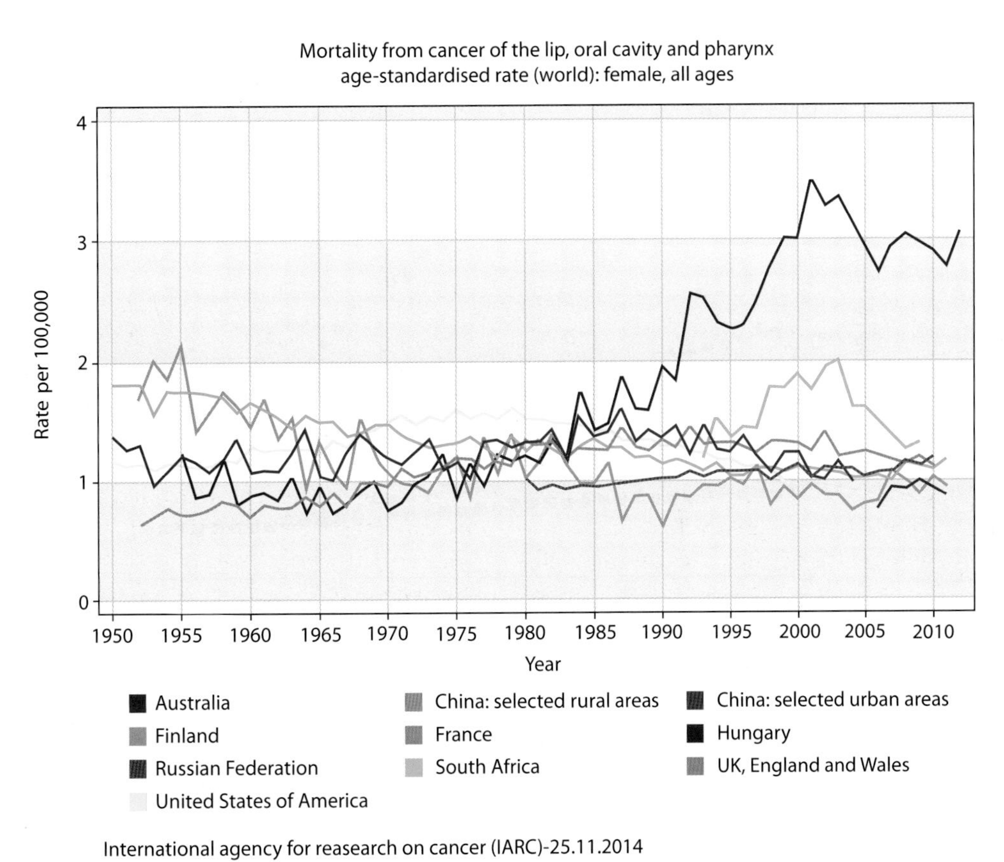

Figure 1.9 Mortality from cancer of the lip, oral cavity and pharynx: female.

Table 1.3 Mortality trends APC for oral and pharyngeal cancer in the USA between 2002 and 2011 by race and sex

	All races			White			Black		
	Total	Male	Female	Total	Male	Female	Total	Male	Female
All ages	−1.0[a]	−0.9[a]	−1.5[a]	−0.6[a]	−0.4[a]	−1.3[a]	−3.4[a]	−3.7[a]	−2.7[a]

Source: Howlader N et al. (eds). *SEER Cancer Statistics Review, 1975–2011*. Bethesda, MD: National Cancer Institute. Available from: http://seer.cancer.gov/csr/1975_2011/, based on November 2013 SEER data submission, posted to the SEER website, April 2014 (10).

[a] APC in rate is statistically significantly different from zero ($p < .05$).

institutions. Regrettably, such highly expert management is not yet uniformly available and it may be decades before these results are reflected in population trends.

GLOBAL SCENARIO OF ORAL POTENTIALLY MALIGNANT DISORDERS (OPMD) AND LARYNGEAL LEUKOPLAKIA

The term "oral potentially malignant disorders" was recommended by an international working group convened by the WHO Collaborating Centre for Oral Cancer and Precancer in London in 2005 (41). It conveys that not all disorders described under this umbrella will transform into invasive cancer—at least not within the lifespan of the affected individual. Leukoplakia, erythroplakia, oral submucous fibrosis, lichen planus, palatal lesions in reverse smokers, actinic keratosis, discoid lupus erythematosus, dyskeratosis congenita and epidermolysis bullosa are described under the broad definition of OPMD (41,42).

GLOBAL PREVALENCE OF OPMD

Estimates of the global prevalence of OPMD range from 1% to 5% (43) although much higher prevalence rates are reported from southeast Asia, usually with a male preponderance (e.g. in Sri Lanka [11.3%] (44), Taiwan [12.7%] (45) and Pacific countries like Papua New Guinea [11.7%] (46)). Wide geographical variations across countries and regions are mainly due to differences in sociodemographic characteristics, the type and pattern of tobacco use and clinical definitions of disease (see Table 1.4). In Western countries, the overall prevalence is low and a decreasing trend over time is observed.

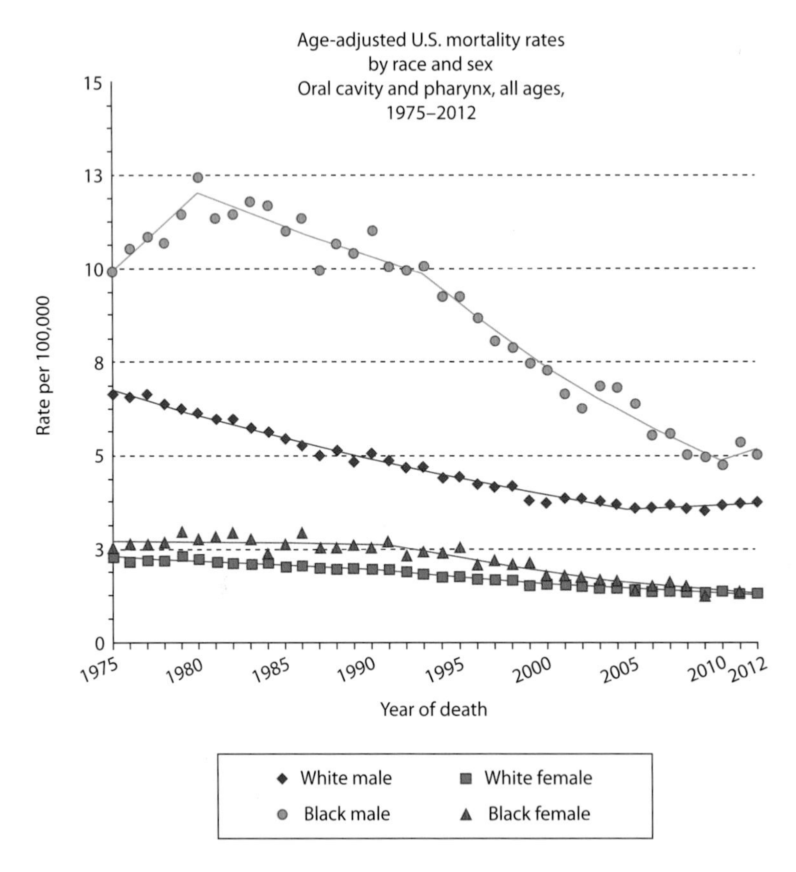

Figure 1.10 Cancer sites include invasive cases only unless otherwise noted. (Mortality source: US Mortality Files, National Center for Health Statistics, CDC. Rates are per 100,000 and are age-adjusted to the 2000 US Std Population (19 age groups—Census P25– 1130). Regression lines are calculated using the Joinpoint Regression Program Version 4.2.0, April 2015, National Cancer Institute.)

Table 1.4 Summary of the prevalence of OPMD reported in the literature

Ref.	Country (year)	Sampling method	Female/Male ratio	Age group (years)	Disease entity	Definition used	Prevalence (%)
–4	Sri Lanka (2008)	Multi-stage stratified cluster (MSSC)	0.6/1.0	≥30	OPMD	WHO 1994	11.3 weighted for gender and geographical location
17	Taiwan (2005)	Random	0.9/1.0	≥15	OPMD	Not given	12.7
					Leukoplakia		7.4
					Erythroplakia		1.9
					Lichen planus		2.9
					OSF		1.6
48	USA (2003)	MSSC	0.9/1.0	≥20	Leukoplakia	Kramer 1978 Kramer 1980	0.66 males and 0.21 females
49	Sri Lanka (2003)	MSSC	–	35–44 and 65–74	OPMD Leukoplakia/ erythoplakia	WHO 1994	4.1
							2.6
					OSF		0.4
50	Spain (2002)	Stratified, random	0.8/1.0	≥30	Leukoplakia	WHO 1978 Axell et al. 1984	1.6
51	Germany (2000)	Stratified, random	1.0/1.0	35–44	Leukoplakia	Axell 1976	1.6
			0.7/1.0	65–74	Leukoplakia	Zain 1995 WHO-ICD-DA	1.0
52	Japan (2000)	All invited	0.4/1.0	Male >40, female >20	Leukoplakia	WHO 1980	0.19
					Lichen planus		0.21
53	Malaysia (1997)	Stratified, random	0.7/1.0	≥25	Leukoplakia	WHO 1978	0.96
					Erythroplakia	Axell et al. 1984	0.01
					OSF		0.06
					Lichen planus		0.38
54	The Netherlands (1996)	Waiting room	0.9/1.0	13–93	Leukoplakia	Axell 1984 Axell 1996 Schepman 1995	0.6
55	Hungary (1991)	Random	0.7/1.0	All age groups	Leukoplakia	Axell 1984	1.3
					Lichen planus		0.1
56	Japan (1991)	Factory workers	0.5/1.0	18–63	Leukoplakia	Axell 1984	2.5
57	Sweden (1987)	Stratified random	Not found	≥15	Lichen planus	Axell 1976	1.9
58	Sweden (1987)	All-invited residents	0.9/1.0	≥15	Leukoplakia	Axell 1976	3.6

OSF = oral submucous fibrosis; WHO-ICD-DA = World Health Organisation-International Classification of Diseases-Dental Addendum.

Petti (59) conducted a meta-analysis of 23 primary studies on oral leukoplakia from international data published between 1986 and 2002. The point-prevalence estimates were 1.49% (95% confidence interval [CI] 1.42%–1.56%) and 2.6% (random effect, 95% CI 1.72%–2.74%). Leukoplakia was significantly more prevalent among males (prevalence ratio 3.22), but no difference was found between geographical areas and between younger and older adults. Using these data, Petti calculated that the crude annual oral cancer incidence rate attributable to leukoplakia would be between 6.2 and 29.1 per 100,000, thus suggesting that the global number of oral cancer cases is probably under-reported.

AGE AND GENDER DISTRIBUTION OF OPMD

This varies considerably, mainly being dependent on lifestyle and thus on ethnicity and geographical location. In the developed world, leukoplakia is usually found between the fourth and seventh decades of life; in the developing world, this occurs some 5–10 years earlier (60). Females are less commonly affected, largely reflecting greater use of relevant habits by men.

MALIGNANT TRANSFORMATION OF OPMD

Risk of malignant transformation varies from site to site within the mouth, from population to population and from study to study (61–63). A classic study conducted in the 1970s with follow-up over 7 years of over 30,000 Indian villagers showed transformation rates from 10–24 per 100,000 per year (62). Another classic study from the early 1980s, a hospital-based study in Californian patients with oral leukoplakia with a mean follow-up period of 7.2 years, revealed a malignant transformation rate of 17.5% (63). Rates for hospital-based studies are, unsurprisingly, consistently higher than community-based studies because of sampling bias.

Petti (59) has estimated a mean global prevalence of 2.6% for leukoplakia and a mean global transformation rate of 1.36% per year (95% CI 0.69–2.03). Extrapolating from these figures suggests that considerably more oral squamous cell carcinoma (OSCC) should have been reported in recent times, a possible reason being under-reporting of cases of oral cancer in the developing world. More recently, a careful study of 1,357 patients with an OPMD from the south of England revealed that 2.6% of cases transformed into invasive cancer for a total person follow-up time of 12,273 years (mean 9.04 years). The severity of epithelial dysplasia was a significant predictor for malignant transformation (64), especially if aneuploid (65). Similar findings come from a study of leukoplakia in Shanghai (66). A study from a dysplasia clinic in the north of England confirms the lateral tongue as a high-risk site and that non-smokers were 7.1-times more likely to undergo malignant transformation compared to heavy smokers (67).

Controversy continues as to whether or not oral lichen planus (OLP) should be considered an OPMD. Published studies give rates of transformation from 0% to 3.5% over varying time periods. A recent comprehensive systematic review evaluated 7806 patients with OLP, amongst which a mere 85 (1.09%) developed SCC in an average follow-up time of 51.4 months. Average age at onset of squamous cell carcinoma (SCC) was 60.8 years, with a slight female preponderance. The most common subsite of malignant transformation was the tongue (68). Size is also a critical determinant (69).

REFERENCES

1. Office for National Statistics. Death registered in England and Wales (series DR). *Stat Bull* 2014;109.
2. Ferlay J, Soerjomataram I, Ervik M, Dikshit R, Eser S, Mathers C, Rebelo M, Parkin DM, Forman D, Bray, F. *GLOBOCAN 2012 v1.0, Cancer Incidence and Mortality Worldwide: IARC Cancer Base No. 11 [Internet].* Lyon, France: International Agency for Research on Cancer; 2013. Available from: http://globocan.iarc.fr; Accessed on April 1, 2016.
3. Sankaranarayanan R. Oral cancer in India: an epidemiologic and clinical review. *Oral Surg Oral Med Oral Pathol* 1990;69(3):325–30.
4. World Health Organization. Control of oral cancer in developing countries. A WHO meeting. *Bull WHO* 1984;62(6):817–30.
5. National Cancer Control Programme Sri Lanka. *Cancer Incidence Data: Sri Lanka Year 2009.* Colombo: NCCP, 2015.
6. Ministry of Health Malaysia. Second report of the National Cancer Registry, Cancer Incidence in Malaysia 2003. Available from: ghdx.healthdata.org/organizations/national-cancer-registry-ministry-health-malaysia; Accessed January 10, 2018.
7. Brandizzi D, Chuchurru JA, Lanfranchi HE, Cabrini RL. Analysis of the epidemiological features of oral cancer in the city of Buenos Aires. *Acta Odontol Latinoam* 2005;18(1):31–5.
8. Karim-Kos HE, de Vries E, Soerjomataram I, Lemmens V, Siesling S, Coebergh JW. Recent trends of cancer in Europe: a combined approach of incidence, survival and mortality for 17 cancer sites since the 1990s. *Eur J Cancer* 2008;44(10):1345–89.
9. Conway DI, Stockton DL, Warnakulasuriya KA, Ogden G, Macpherson LM. Incidence of oral and oropharyngeal cancer in United Kingdom (1990–1999)—recent trends and regional variation. *Oral Oncol* 2006;42(6):586–92.
10. Howlader N, Noone AM, Krapcho M et al. (eds). *SEER Cancer Statistics Review, 1975–2011.* Bethesda, MD: National Cancer Institute. Available from: http://seer.cancer.gov/csr/1975_2011/, based on November 2013 SEER data submission, posted to the SEER website, April 2014.
11. Suba Z. Gender-related hormonal risk factors for oral cancer. *Pathol Oncol Res* 2007;13(3):195–202.

12. Chhetri DK, Rawnsley JD, Calcaterra TC. Carcinoma of the buccal mucosa. *Otolaryngol Head Neck Surg* 2000;123(5):566–71.
13. Diaz EM Jr, Holsinger FC, Zuniga ER, Roberts DB, Sorensen DM. Squamous cell carcinoma of the buccal mucosa: one institution's experience with 119 previously untreated patients. *Head Neck* 2003;25(4):267–73.
14. Iyer SG, Pradhan SA, Pai PS, Patil S. Surgical treatment outcomes of localized squamous carcinoma of buccal mucosa. *Head Neck* 2004;26(10):897–902.
15. Liao CT, Wang HM, Ng SH et al. Good tumor control and survivals of squamous cell carcinoma of buccal mucosa treated with radical surgery with or without neck dissection in Taiwan. *Oral Oncol* 2006;42(8):800–9.
16. Lin CS, Jen YM, Cheng MF et al. Squamous cell carcinoma of the buccal mucosa: an aggressive cancer requiring multimodality treatment. *Head Neck* 2006;28(2):150–7.
17. Sieczka E, Datta R, Singh A et al. Cancer of the buccal mucosa: are margins and T-stage accurate predictors of local control? *Am J Otolaryngol* 2001;22(6):395–9.
18. National Cancer Institute. Surveillance Epidemiology and End Results (SEER). SEER Cancer Statistic Review 1975–2004. Available from: http://seer.cancer.gov/statfacts/html/oralcav.html; Accessed on January 8, 2010.
19. Llewellyn CD, Johnson NW, Warnakulasuriya KA. Risk factors for squamous cell carcinoma of the oral cavity in young people—a comprehensive literature review. *Oral Oncol* 2001;37(5):401–18.
20. Warnakulasuriya S, Mak V, Moller H. Oral cancer survival in young people in south east England. *Oral Oncol* 2007;43(10):982–6.
21. Macfarlane GJ, Boyle P, Scully C. Rising mortality from cancer of the tongue in young Scottish males. *Lancet* 1987;2(8564):912.
22. Annertz K, Anderson H, Biorklund A et al. Incidence and survival of squamous cell carcinoma of the tongue in Scandinavia, with special reference to young adults. *Int J Cancer* 2002;101(1):95–9.
23. Schantz SP, Yu GP. Head and neck cancer incidence trends in young Americans, 1973–1997, with a special analysis for tongue cancer. *Arch Otolaryngol Head Neck Surg* 2002;128(3):268–74.
24. Shiboski CH, Schmidt BL, Jordan RC. Tongue and tonsil carcinoma: increasing trends in the U.S. population ages 20–44 years. *Cancer* 2005;103(9):1843–9.
25. Scully C, Bedi R. Ethnicity and oral cancer. *Lancet Oncol* 2000;1(1):37–42.
26. Robinson KL, Macfarlane GJ. Oropharyngeal cancer incidence and mortality in Scotland: are rates still increasing? *Oral Oncol* 2003;39(1):31–6.
27. Elango JK, Gangadharan P, Sumithra S, Kuriakose MA. Trends of head and neck cancers in urban and rural India. *Asian Pac J Cancer Prev* 2006;7(1):108–12.
28. Llewellyn CD, Johnson NW, Warnakulasuriya KA. Risk factors for oral cancer in newly diagnosed patients aged 45 years and younger: a case–control study in Southern England. *J Oral Pathol Med* 2004; 33(9):525–32.
29. Hirota SK, Braga FP, Penha SS, Sugaya NN, Migliari DA. Risk factors for oral squamous cell carcinoma in young and older Brazilian patients: a comparative analysis. *Med Oral Patol Oral Cir Bucal* 2008;13(4): E227–31.
30. Liu L, Kumar SK, Sedghizadeh PP, Jayakar AN, Shuler CF. Oral squamous cell carcinoma incidence by subsite among diverse racial and ethnic populations in California. *Oral Surg Oral Med Oral Pathol Oral Radiol Endod* 2008;105(4):470–80.
31. Reichman ME, Kelly JJ, Kosary CL, Coughlin SS, Jim MA, Lanier AP. Incidence of cancers of the oral cavity and pharynx among American Indians and Alaska Natives, 1999–2004. *Cancer* 2008;113(5 Suppl): 1256–65.
32. Nichols AC, Bhattacharyya N. Racial differences in stage and survival in head and neck squamous cell carcinoma. *Laryngoscope* 2007;117(5):770–5.
33. Gourin CG, Podolsky RH. Racial disparities in patients with head and neck squamous cell carcinoma. *Laryngoscope* 2006;116(7):1093–106.
34. Suarez E, Calo WA, Hernandez EY, Diaz EC, Figueroa NR, Ortiz AP. Age-standardized incidence and mortality rates of oral and pharyngeal cancer in Puerto Rico and among non-Hispanics whites, non-Hispanic blacks, and Hispanics in the USA. *BMC Cancer* 2009; 9:129.
35. Moles DR, Fedele S, Speight PM, Porter SR, dos S antos Silva I. Oral and pharyngeal cancer in south Asians and non-South Asians in relation to socioeconomic deprivation in south east England. *Br J Cancer* 2008;98(3):633–5.
36. World Health Organization. Mortality database. Available from: http://www.who.int/healthinfo/statistics/mortality_rawdata/en/index.html; Accessed on February 26, 2014.
37. La Vecchia C, Lucchini F, Negri E, Levi F. Trends in oral cancer mortality in Europe. *Oral Oncol* 2004; 40(4):433–9.
38. Morse DE, Kerr AR. Disparities in oral and pharyng eal cancer incidence, mortality and survival among black and white Americans. *J Am Dent Assoc* 2006; 137(2):203–12.
39. Moore RJ, Doherty DA, Do KA, Chamberlain RM, Khuri FR. Racial disparity in survival of patients with squamous cell carcinoma of the oral cavity and pharynx. *Ethn Health* 2001;6(3–4): 165–77.
40. Sunny L, Yeole BB, Hakama M et al. Oral cancers in Mumbai, India: a fifteen years perspective with respect to incidence trend and cumulative risk. *Asian Pac J Cancer Prev* 2004;5(3):294–300.

41. Warnakulasuriya S, Johnson NW, van der Waal I. Nomenclature and classification of potentially malignant disorders of the oral mucosa. *J Oral Pathol Med* 2007;36(10):575–80.
42. van der Waal I. Potentially malignant disorders of the oral and oropharyngeal mucosa; terminology, classification and present concepts of management. *Oral Oncol* 2009;45(4–5):317–23.
43. Napier SS, Cowan CG, Gregg TA, Stevenson M, Lamey PJ, Toner PG. Potentially malignant oral lesions in Northern Ireland: size (extent) matters. *Oral Dis* 2003;9(3):129–37.
44. Amarasinghe AAHK, Usgodaarachchi US, Johnson NW, Lalloo R, Warnakulasuriya S. Betel-quid chewing with or without tobacco is a major risk factor for oral potentially malignant disorders in Sri Lanka: a case–control study. *Oral Oncol* 2010;46(4):297–301.
45. Chung CH, Yang YH, Wang TY, Shieh TY, Warnakulasuriya S. Oral precancerous disorders associated with areca quid chewing, smoking, and alcohol drinking in Southern Taiwan. *J Oral Pathol Med* 2005;34:460–6.
46. Thomas SJ, Harris R, Ness AR et al. Betel quid not containing tobacco and oral leukoplakia: a report on a cross-sectional study in Papua New Guinea and a meta-analysis of current evidence. *Int J Cancer* 2008;123(8):1871–6.
47. Chung CH, Yang YH, Wang TY, Shieh TY, Warnakulasuriya S. Oral precancerous disorders associated with areca quid chewing, smoking, and alcohol drinking in southern Taiwan. *J Oral Pathol Med* 2005;34(8):460–6.
48. Scheifele C, Reichart PA, Dietrich T. Low prevalence of oral leukoplakia in a representative sample of the US population. *Oral Oncol* 2003;39(6):619–25.
49. Ministry of Health Sri Lanka. *National Oral Health Survey, Sri Lanka (2002/2003).* Colombo: 3rd publication, Ministry of Health, Sri Lanka, 2009.
50. Garcia-Pola Vallejo MJ, Martinez Diaz-Canel AI, Garcia Martin JM, Gonzalez Garcia M. Risk factors for oral soft tissue lesions in an adult Spanish population. *Community Dent Oral Epidemiol* 2002;30(4):277–85.
51. Reichart PA. Oral mucosal lesions in a representative cross-sectional study of aging Germans. *Community Dent Oral Epidemiol* 2000;28(5):390–8.
52. Nagao T, Ikeda N, Fukano H, Miyazaki H, Yano M, Warnakulasuriya S. Outcome following a population screening programme for oral cancer and precancer in Japan. *Oral Oncol* 2000;36(4):340–6.
53. Zain RB, Ikeda N, Razak IA et al. A national epidemiological survey of oral mucosal lesions in Malaysia. *Community Dent Oral Epidemiol* 1997;25(5):377–83.
54. Schepman KP, van der Meij EH, Smeele LE, van der Waal I. Prevalence study of oral white lesions with special reference to a new definition of oral leucoplakia. *Eur J Cancer B Oral Oncol* 1996;32B(6):416–9.
55. Banoczy J, Rigo O. Prevalence study of oral precancerous lesions within a complex screening system in Hungary. *Community Dent Oral Epidemiol* 1991;19(5):265–7.
56. Ikeda N, Ishii T, Iida S, Kawai T. Epidemiological study of oral leukoplakia based on mass screening for oral mucosal diseases in a selected Japanese population. *Community Dent Oral Epidemiol* 1991;19(3):160–3.
57. Axell T, Rundquist L. Oral lichen planus—a demographic study. *Community Dent Oral Epidemiol* 1987; 15:52–6.
58. Axell T. Occurrence of leukoplakia and some other oral white lesions among 20,333 adult Swedish people. *Community Dent Oral Epidemiol* 1987; 15(1):46–51.
59. Petti S. Pooled estimate of world leukoplakia prevalence: a systematic review. *Oral Oncol* 2003;39(8):770–80.
60. Napier SS, Speight PM. Natural history of potentially malignant oral lesions and conditions: an overview of the literature. *J Oral Pathol Med* 2008;37(1):1–10.
61. Reibel J. Prognosis of oral pre-malignant lesions: significance of clinical, histopathological, and molecular biological characteristics. *Crit Rev Oral Biol Med* 2003;14(1):47–62.
62. Pindborg JJ, Mehta FS, Daftary DK. Incidence of oral cancer among 30,000 villagers in India in a 7-year follow-up study of oral precancerous lesions. *Community Dent Oral Epidemiol* 1975;3(2):86–8.
63. Silverman S Jr, Gorsky M, Lozada F. Oral leukoplakia and malignant transformation. A follow-up study of 257 patients. *Cancer* 1984;53(3):563–8.
64. Warnakulasuriya S, Kovacevic T, Madden P et al. Factors predicting malignant transformation in oral potentially malignant disorders among patients accrued over a 10-year period in south east England. *J Oral Pathol Med* 2011;40(9):677–83.
65. Sperandio M, Brown AL, Lock C et al. Predictive value of dysplasia grading and DNA ploidy in malignant transformation of oral potentially malignant disorders. *Cancer Prev Res (Phila)* 2013;6(8):822–31.
66. Liu W, Shi LJ, Wu L et al. Oral cancer development in patients with leukoplakia—clinicopathological factors affecting outcome. *PLoS One* 2012;7(4):e34773.
67. Ho MW, Risk JM, Woolgar JA et al. The clinical determinants of malignant transformation in oral epithelial dysplasia. *Oral Oncol* 2012;48(10):969–76.
68. Fitzpatrick SG, Hirsch SA, Gordon SC. The malignant transformation of oral lichen planus and oral lichenoid lesions: a systematic review. *J Am Dent Assoc* 2014;145(1):45–56.
69. Brouns E, Baart J, Karagozoglu K, Aartman I, Bloemena E, van der Waal I. Malignant transformation of oral leukoplakia in a well-defined cohort of 144 patients. *Oral Dis* 2014;20(3):e19–24.

2

Etiology and risk factors

NEWELL W. JOHNSON, BHAWNA GUPTA, DAVID J. SPEICHER, CECILY S. RAY, MUSHFIQ HASSAN SHAIKH, NEZAR AL-HEBSHI, AND PRAKASH C. GUPTA

INTRODUCTION

Some definitions: *Etiology* (from Greek: *aitia* (cause) and *logos* (science) and late Latin) is that part of medical science that deals with the causes of disease. All diseases have predisposing and direct causes, the former setting the scene in which the latter is more likely to have an effect. Predisposition is always, to some extent, inherited; it is often a complex societal, cultural and environmental amalgam. For example, inheritance of a propensity to alcoholism, coupled with drunkenness, and the impairment of judgement and manual dexterity which follows, leads to a road traffic accident: trauma is the direct cause of the injuries sustained. Inheritance of the multiple polyposis coli gene increases the risk of colon cancer, but the more proximate causes related to diet are still influential.

The word *pathogenesis* (*pathos*, suffering or disease; *genein*, to produce) means production or development of disease, again from the Greek: it is used for the mechanisms involved. These are often difficult to separate, and causes and mechanisms are often described together as etiopathogenesis. Since most malignancies/cancers are multifactorial, and all mechanistic pathways complex, with perhaps several routes to a critical outcome such as malignant transformation of a single stem cell or clone of cells, care needs to be taken to ascribe proper weight to any factor under consideration.

We also need to be clear about the sense in which we refer to risk. Many terms are used in different senses by different authors. For the purposes of this discussion, we define a *risk factor* as an agent, attribute or behavior that is directly part of the causal chain of the disease (1). A *risk marker* or *risk indicator* is associated with the disease, and may or may not be causal: it will have power to predict the presence or likely future occurrence of disease, but may not explain the mechanisms. Socioeconomic status is an example of the latter: it is associated with many diseases, certainly with head and neck cancer (HNC), but is not of itself causal; the higher prevalence of smoking, alcohol abuse and poorer nutrition are the relevant factors. Social class is therefore described as a confounder in epidemiological studies of etiopathogenesis.

In this chapter, we approach etiology in terms of risk factors. In order of importance, the risk is dominated by tobacco use, alcohol abuse and viral infections, frequently in a background of nutritional insufficiencies, all of which have heavy confounding with socioeconomic, cultural, religious, racial and geographic variables. We discuss the issues in a logical sequence, starting with genetic factors before going on to environmental factors. Most of what follows relates to squamous cell carcinoma (SCC) and its precursor lesions and disorders, which are the main focus of this book, and where the risk factors are relatively well understood. We cover other virus-induced malignancies, notably Kaposi's sarcoma (KS). We know relatively little about the etiology of neoplasms of salivary glands, of other soft tissues, of bone and of the odontogenic apparatus.

FAMILIAL AND GENETIC PREDISPOSITION TO ORAL AND OROPHARYNGEAL CANCER

Excluding the major cancer susceptibility syndromes, such as Xeroderma pigmentosum for skin cancers, and Fanconi anemia for a wide range of neoplasms including susceptibility to SCC of the oropharynx and esophagus, there is a real, but not strong, familial and genetic predisposition to oral and oropharyngeal cancer. There is nothing yet to suggest a strong genetic predisposition, even in a minor subset of cases, such as is seen with the carriage of *BRCA1* and/or *BRCA2* in—predominantly familial—but also some cases of sporadic—breast cancer, or of the *APC* gene in familial adenopolyposis coli with high susceptibility to adenocarcinoma of the colon.

While tobacco in all its forms, alcohol drinking and oncogenic viruses are the major risk factors for oral and oropharyngeal cancer, not all individuals exposed to these experience cancer (2). There is epidemiological evidence of the family history of HNC as a marker of increased risk of oral cavity cancer (3). Regarding age, no clear pattern emerges from epidemiological studies, as some have found a stronger association in younger subjects (3) and others the contrary (4). The familial aggregation of oral and pharyngeal cancers, however, may have different genetic and environmental correlates in different populations (3,5). The risk was higher when two or more relatives were affected, and independent from alcohol and tobacco consumption (3), as with earlier reports (6–8). History of oral cancer among first-degree relatives was a strong predictor of increased risk to oral cancer in other family members in several recent studies (9–11).

Lip cancer is among the sites that show the strongest cancer clustering within families in the genealogical records of the Utah database, the others being leukemia, lobular breast cancer, early melanoma and adenocarcinomas of the lung in females (12). Holloway and Sofaer studied surname distributions for 3,658 male cancer cases from the Scottish Cancer Registry for the years 1959–1985, comparing them with distributions for 32,468 male deaths in Scotland for 1976 (13). For cancer of the lip, there is a mild indication of increased isonomy in patients compared with controls, both within and between regions. This might suggest some genetic predisposition, but may also reflect the fact that families tend to have the same occupation—in this case outdoor work such as farming, fishing and forestry, with exposure to ultraviolet light. For cancer of the tongue, there was some evidence of increased isonomy within but not between regions. Although this could result from inherited susceptibility clustering in different regions, a more likely explanation is that environmental risk factors such as tobacco and alcohol are common to families. For cancer of the salivary glands, there was increased isonomy both within and between regions, again suggesting but not proving that genetic factors are involved; this, however, is consistent with reports of the familial occurrence of malignant salivary tumors (14,15).

Chapter 1 described how oral cancer rates are higher in blacks in the U.S.A., and that this is largely explained by social and environmental factors. The same is probably true for the observation that, in Israel, the risk of developing oral cancer is twice as high in Ashkenazic compared with Sephardic and Eastern Jewish ethnic groups. It is interesting that it is the tongue that is the leading site in the Ashkenazi and Sephardi, whereas the lip and alveolar ridges are most affected in the Eastern Jews, perhaps reflecting the type of risk habit.

Perhaps of greater relevance are the studies from Kerala, South India. A familial association was seen in 0.94% of the total oral cancers accrued from January to July 1995, consistent with an autosomal mode of inheritance (11). Further studies of 7 familial cases in comparison with 10 patients with sporadic oral cancer and 14 unaffected first-degree relatives showed no constitutional chromosomal abnormalities. There was a significant difference between patients with oral cancer and unaffected relatives in the sensitivity of chromosomes to bleomycin damage; one unaffected member, who showed enhanced bleomycin sensitivity, later went on to develop an oral cancer, raising the possibility of genetic susceptibility (17). Again, however, a common environmental source of DNA damage is not excluded.

In the Netherlands, Cloos et al. took 617 first-degree relatives of 105 patients with HNC and found among them 31 cases of cancer of the respiratory and upper digestive tract, compared with 10 cases in the control group composed of first-degree relatives of the index patient's spouses (18). This produced a relative risk (RR) of 3.5 ($p = 0.0002$) for first-degree relatives, and RR = 14.6 ($p = 0.0001$) for siblings. Cloos et al. also studied mutagen sensitivity of lymphocytes and found this to be increased in patients with multiple HNC cancers, in comparison to those with single tumors and controls. There was no relation to smoking and drinking histories, and the authors reported that a constitutional factor exists that reflects the way genotoxic compounds are handled (18).

It is important to control for environmental factors in all such studies. This was carefully done in a large case-control study of oral and pharyngeal cancer from the National Cancer Institute in the U.S.A. (6). A similar proportion of patients (46%, $n = 487$) and controls (41%, $n = 485$) reported cancer in a parent or sibling; although trends were apparent, most of these were not statistically significant. The strongest elevated risk was of oral/pharyngeal cancer among those whose sisters developed other cancers (OR = 1.6; 95% confidence interval [CI]: 1.1–2.2). Slightly higher odds ratio (OR) emerged in a study in Puerto Rico, but shared lifestyle risk factors were not excluded (7).

The INHANCE consortium (International Head and Neck Cancer Epidemiology Consortium), http://www.inhance.utah.edu/, an excellent co-operative performing meta-analyses of large databases around the world, reported that the family history of HNC increased the risk of HNC (RR = 1.68; 95% CI: 1.23–2.29; 9,025 cases and 13,739 controls) with adjustment for multiple factors including tobacco and alcohol habits (19). In these pooled data, 5%–10% HNC patients had a family history of cancer in studies largely from Europe, the U.S.A. and South America.

There is rapidly expanding literature describing susceptibility related to inherited capacity to metabolize carcinogens or pro-carcinogens, or impaired ability to repair the consequent DNA damage (20). This especially appears to involve polymorphisms in GST genes (21–24), CYP genes (19,25–27) and the cytochrome P-450 system (28) but not, according to current evidence, in p53 polymorphisms (29,30). The evidence for the involvement of alcohol dehydrogenase genotypes is conflicting (31–33). Therefore, we must conclude that a genetic predisposition to oral cancer is real, but modest. This does not preclude it being of greater importance in a minority of cases, but the effects are swamped by environmental factors on a population basis. Nevertheless, the determination of the reality and nature of these genetic factors would have enormous benefit, not only to at-risk family members, who should take care to avoid other risks, but in unraveling the molecular mechanisms of oral carcinogenesis, opening the way to better prevention and treatment.

OCCUPATION AND RISK OF ORAL AND OROPHARYNGEAL CANCER

Apart from the topic of environmental tobacco smoke (ETS or passive smoking), dealt with below, there is limited literature on occupation and risk of oral cancer. Butchers in Sweden have a small but significantly increased risk (RR 1.6), no doubt partly confounded by lifestyle factors, but possibly involving industrial exposure, for example, to viruses, nitrosamines and polycyclic aromatic hydrocarbons (PAHs). Reported risky occupations include working with vehicles, building, roads, asbestos and the textile industry (34,35). Bricklayers, painters and workers employed in the farming of cattle and dairy farming have been shown to be at increased risk of, particularly, oral and oropharyngeal cancer (36). An association between exposure to cement dust, which is a complex and heterogeneous mixture, and cancer of the pharynx and oral cavity has been shown in some studies (37,38), though interpreted differently by others (39,40). The importance of fossil-fuel combustion in a work setting is confirmed in a large study in 4 areas in the U.S.A. (1,114 cases, 1,268 controls), with OR = ~2.0 for cancers at pharyngeal sites. Male carpet installers emerged as at risk (OR = 7.7; 95% CI = 2.4–24.9; 23 cases, 4 controls) (83).

ASBESTOS AND MAN-MADE VITREOUS FIBERS, WELDING AND CREOSOTE

Asbestos is the commercial name for naturally occurring silicate mineral fibers that were earlier added to many products in the construction industry, including insulation and fire-proofing materials, cement and wallboard (40). Many studies report associations between exposure to asbestos and incidence of oral and oropharyngeal cancer (40–45).

Asbestos fibers, together with smoking and drinking, produce chronic inflammation enhancing the malignant transformation of the pharyngeal mucosa (meta-RR 1.25; 95% CI: 1.10–1.42) (42). On the contrary, a prospective cohort study in the Netherlands reported no such association (46). However, a study of miners in South Africa found a significantly increased risk for cancer of the oral cavity and pharynx in workers exposed to amphibole fibers—the term for a group of asbestos-like fibers (47). Indeed, it is important to note that, while some types of asbestos may be more hazardous than others, all are dangerous. Contact with man-made vitreous fibers, such as glass wool, which have the same physical properties as asbestos, was found significantly associated with increased risk (meta-RR = 1.32; 95% CI: 1.09–1.59) of cancer of the oral cavity and of the pharynx (48).

Workers exposed to creosote were more than two times at risk of lip cancer (49); however, results were not significant in another similar study (50). A case-control study done in Sweden indicates that exposure to welding fumes for more than 8 years increases the risk of pharyngeal cancer by two times (51).

DUSTS

Dusts, defined as small solid particles suspended in air ranging from 1 to 100 μm in diameter (52), are a heterogeneous group of exposures that can be either primarily organic (such as wood or leather dusts) or inorganic (such as metal dusts). Dusts may exert their carcinogenic effect through the induction of chronic inflammation, their intrinsic chemical properties, or by acting as carriers of other carcinogenic compounds (53). Two forms of occupational dust, wood and leather dust, have been classified as type 1 carcinogens by the International Agency for Cancer Research (IARC), and are considered causal for cancers of the nasal cavity and paranasal sinus (53). An increased risk for HNC was found among workers exposed to wood dust in Spain (54) and a dose–response relationship found for those exposed to leather dust in a study from Boston involving 951 incident cases of head and neck squamous cell carcinoma (HNSCC) and 1,193 controls (OR = 1.5, 95% CI: 1.2–1.9) (55); others have questioned such an association (51,56). An association at point estimates was found between leather dust and cancer of the oral cavity, more so with pharyngeal cancer (55).

Most importantly, due to the thoroughness with which the evidence is assessed, the IARC concluded that occupational exposure to wood dust does not seem to have a causal role in cancers of the oropharynx or hypopharynx, whereas the role is clear for nasal, sinus and nasopharyngeal carcinoma (NPC) (53,57).

SOLVENTS

Organic solvents encompass a wide variety of compounds: halogenated hydrocarbons, aliphatic and alicyclic hydrocarbons and aromatic monocyclic hydrocarbons. They are widely used in industry, and their characterization varies in different studies, making clear conclusions difficult. A significant risk was reported between exposure to solvents and incidence of oral and oropharyngeal cancer (44,58), whereas the effects were non-significant in another study (59). Interestingly, in a study of exposure to solvents among construction workers in Arcadia, there appeared to be increased risk for oral cancer, but a decreased risk for pharyngeal cancer (60).

POLYCYCLIC HYDROCARBONS

These are a class of chemicals that include hundreds of compounds. Occupational exposures to these involve many industries and occupations, such as aluminum production, manufacturing of carbon products, paving and roofing (adhesive use), coal tar distillation, coke gasification, iron and steel foundries, chimney sweeps and wood impregnation. A dose–response relationship between cumulative exposure to polycyclic hydrocarbons and incidence for cancer of the oral cavity and the oropharynx was shown in one study from Sweden (51): Others have not shown any significant excess risk (51,61).

EFFECTS OF SOLAR RADIATION

Descriptive studies show that lip cancer is more common in males than females. Incidence rates are higher in light- than dark-skinned populations living in the same geographic area, particularly among those who live or work outdoors, for example, in crop and dairy farming, fishing, forestry, construction, postal delivery and street vendors. Such individuals are exposed to direct sunlight for longer durations (62,63). The lower lip receives considerably more direct sunlight than the upper lip. Also, in the West, the comparatively low incidence of lower lip cancer among females could be attributed to the protective effect of cosmetics and lower outdoor exposures (64,65). Evidence comes from many countries, including those at high latitudes with clean air through which ultraviolet light penetrates easily (albeit for only part of the year), such as Finland (66) or Sweden (67). Furthermore, in countries closer to the equator with regular long hours of sunshine, such as rural Greece, lip cancer can account for 60% of oral cancers (68). In Western Australia, there has been an upward incidence trend with rates of 8.9/100,000 pa and 2.7/100,000 pa for males and females, respectively (69). Similarly, lip cancer has been on the rise among fishermen in India (70) and in Canada and Spain (71,72).

A study from Mexico reported that the proportion of lip cancer cases in women (34.5%) was higher than that reported in the world literature, that is, that 95%–98% of lip cancer occurs in men (71,73). Similarly, a study from California shows that the risk of lip cancer in women is strongly related to a lifetime solar radiation exposure, but that lipstick and other sunscreens are protective (64). The lesions that develop are usually well-differentiated SCC and arise out of long-standing oral potentially malignant disorders (OPMD) usually termed solar keratoses. Histologically, these are characterized by hyperorthokeratosis of the epithelium of the vermilion border, usually of the lower lip, with epithelial atrophy and increased deposition of disorganized elastic fibers in the lamina propria (solar elastosis). With time, the degree of epithelial dysplasia increases and many pass through a demonstrable micro-invasive stage. Lesions at these early stages are readily cured by limited excision.

A decrease in the incidence of lip cancer in the Swiss canton of Vaud is interpreted as mostly due to reduced occupational exposure to sunlight and reduced pipe and cigar smoking (74). Nevertheless, the effects of early life exposure are long standing: for example, New Zealanders have four or more times the relative risk of developing cutaneous melanoma and lip cancer than do residents of England and Wales, and migrants in both directions retain intermediate risks (75).

EFFECTS OF ATMOSPHERIC AIR POLLUTION

Part of the urban/rural difference in the incidence of HNC has been related to atmospheric pollution. For example, in data collected from the West Midland region of England 1950–1990, mean sulfur dioxide and smoke concentrations in the atmosphere were positively correlated with squamous cancer of the larynx and, to a lesser extent, the pharynx (76). There is growing concern globally about air pollution in cities and the impact on public health. Oxides of sulfur and nitrogen, carbon monoxide and carbon dioxide, and hydrocarbon particulates (notably, "PM10s"—particulate material less than 10 μm in diameter, predominantly from diesel engine exhausts) are among the substances causing concern. There is growing evidence that the dramatic rise in the incidence and severity of asthma and of chronic obstructive pulmonary disease around the world is related to poor air quality in built-up areas, arising from industrial and vehicular sources. Malignancies of the lower respiratory tract may also increase as a result. The impact on cancer of the mouth is likely to be less, but merits careful study. Not only those who work, but also those who live in cities and industrial areas will be at increased risk.

In Heidelberg, Germany, Maier et al. reported that blue-collar workers exposed to dust or inhaled organic and inorganic agents are at increased risk for cancers of the mouth, pharynx and larynx (77). Most citizens spend more of their time at home than at their place of work or traveling; the quality of indoor residential air is therefore of prime importance. This, naturally, reflects the quality of outdoor air in the locality, but is added to by-products of the combustion of fossil fuels used for heating and cooking. These factors were addressed in 164 cases of carcinoma of the larynx and 656 controls; 105 cases of pharyngeal cancer and 420 controls and 100 cases of oral cancer and 400 controls (78). In this study, increased risks for air pollution on the job, traffic jams on the way to work, high traffic emissions in residential areas and outdoor air pollution in residential areas were present for all sites but were not statistically significant. However, household heating with fossil-fuel stoves and cooking with fossil fuels produced statistically significant increased risks at all tumor sites. After adjusting for tobacco and alcohol consumption, and excluding socioeconomic differences as confounders the data shown in Table 2.1 are obtained.

Further, evidence also exists for the association between exposure to wood smoke as a risk factor for oral cancer and cancers of the upper aerodigestive tract in China and Southern Brazil (79,80). In high-risk areas of central and eastern Europe, data from a multi-center hospital-based case-control study of 1,065 histologically confirmed upper aerodigestive tract cancer cases and 1,346 controls reported that indoor air pollution from burning of coal for more than 50 years is a risk factor for HNCs (OR = 4.13, 95% CI: 1.99–8.55) (81). From 1989 to 1992, three epidemiologic case-control studies were carried out at the Department of Otorhinolaryngology of the University of Heidelberg, Germany, to determine possible risk factors for the development of HNC (82). From a cohort of 369 cases and 1,476 controls, the maximum risk of pharyngeal cancer was linked to using single stoves (OR = 3.3; 95% CI: 1.43–7.55 after adjusting for potential confounders). Emissions considered to be important were respirable particles to which are bound PAHs, cadmium and nitrosamines, carbon monoxide and volatile organic compounds such as benzenes, styrenes and tetra-chloroethylenes. Hard-coal products were suggested as the most dangerous sources. The importance of fossil-fuel combustion in a work setting was confirmed in a large American study involving 1,114 cases and 1,268 controls where ORs of approximately 2.0 were calculated for cancers at pharyngeal sites. Male carpet installers emerged as at risk (OR = 7.7; 95% CI: 2.4–24.9; 23 cases, 4 controls) (83).

Outdoor air pollution and particulate matter (notably "PM10s"), predominantly from diesel engine exhausts, has been recognized as a Group 1 carcinogen by the IARC (84). Volatile organic compounds, nitrogen-containing and halogenated organic compounds, PAHs, toxic metals and many byproducts of incomplete combustion (e.g., dioxins) are all carcinogens that pollute the air (85). Results from an ARCAGE European case-control study (involving 1,851 cases with incident cancer of the oral cavity, oropharynx, hypopharynx, larynx or esophagus, and 1,949 controls) reported that bricklayers (OR = 1.71; 95% CI: 1.14–2.56) and painters (OR = 2.10; 95% CI: 1.15–3.85) had an increased risk of oral/oropharyngeal cancer (36). There is also evidence of an association between exposure to cement dust,

Table 2.1 Risk of upper aerodigestive cancer from domestic fuels

	Odds ratio	*p*-Value	95% CI
Larynx			
Heating with fossil fuel >40 years	2.0	0.02	1.10–3.46
Cooking with fossil fuel >40 years	1.4	0.3	0.76–2.41
Pharynx			
Heating with fossil fuel >40 years	3.3	0.0005	1.43–7.55
Cooking with fossil fuel >40 years	2.5	0.05	1.03–6.30
Oral cavity			
Heating with fossil fuel >40 years	2.4	0.008	1.26–4.40
Cooking with fossil fuel >40 years	1.6	0.1	0.90–2.97

Source: Raskob G et al. *Otolaryngol Head Neck Surg* 1995;112(2):308–15 (82).

which is a complex and heterogeneous mixture, and cancer of the pharynx and oral cavity (37,38). However, there are some studies that do not support this evidence (39,40).

IMMUNOSUPPRESSION AND RISK OF LIP AND ORAL CANCER

The development of HNSCC is strongly influenced by the host immune system (86,87). The microenvironment of malignant neoplasms arising within the oropharyngeal, nasal or laryngeal mucosa is rich in immune cells and soluble factors these cells produce. The presence of immune cells, primarily dendritic cells, T lymphocytes, B cells and plasma cells, a few natural killer cells (NK), macrophages and eosinophils as well as the proximity of cervical lymph nodes affect the initiation, promotion and progression of neoplasms that arise in this anatomical region (87). Development of cancer can in part be attributed to failure of the immune system to recognize transformed cells as nonself and eliminate them. NK and cytotoxic T cells play critical roles as effector functions in the host defense against neoplasia are often functionally immobilized in HNCs (88). Indeed, reconstitution of these immune responses is the basis for the current explosion in available agents for the immunotherapy of many neoplasms, including HNSCC. The PD-1/PDL-1 pathway is the best known at the time of writing, and the literature is fluid. Very accessible aspects of the current state of the art (and science!) can be found in Warnakulasuriya and Khan (89).

Individuals with HIV/AIDS are at increased risk for a limited number of neoplasms, especially KS, which is commonly present in the mouth, and lymphomas, which are occasionally present in the oral mucosa or as an intrabony lesion in the jaws. In HIV-positive patients, there is an increased incidence of SCC of the mouth and pharynx, which appear, on average, about 10 years earlier, especially in carcinomata driven by high-risk human papillomaviruses (hrHPVs). In HIV-positive patients, the characteristic oral hairy leukoplakia (OHL: driven by Epstein-Barr virus [EBV]) does not appear to undergo malignant transformation (see Chapter 3). Immunosuppressed organ transplant patients are also at increased risk for lip cancer which is principally due to ultraviolet light exposure and smoking (65,78). Aspects of HIV/AIDS are discussed further in the section on viruses below.

TOBACCO USE AND ORAL AND OROPHARYNGEAL CANCER

There is absolutely no doubt that, on a global scale, the use and abuse of tobacco products is the major cause of oral cancer and plays a significant role with keratinizing types of SCC of the oropharynx (90,91). Alcohol use synergizes with tobacco as a risk factor for upper aerodigestive tract SCCs: This synergism is super-multiplicative for the mouth and pharynx, additive for the larynx and between additive and multiplicative for the esophagus (92). Sorting out the independent effects is difficult; however, these habits usually overlap. Many believe that the rising incidence of oral cancer in Europe and elsewhere in the Western world is largely due to increasing alcohol consumption (see below), but HPVs play a role. In many developing countries, particularly in the Islamic world and in Muslim communities everywhere, accurate data on alcohol consumption are impossible to obtain because of religious and cultural inhibitions. The issue of tobacco use in nondrinkers, and of alcohol, and poor diet in nonsmokers (93) is further addressed later in this chapter.

Taken together, the effects of tobacco use in all its myriad culturally distinctive forms, heavy alcohol consumption and poor diet probably explain most cases of oral cancer, with HPV infections contributing a growing proportion of cases in the mouth, more so in the oropharynx. The preventive approach is clear: minimize the use of tobacco and alcohol, try to eat enough fresh fruit and vegetables, and practice sexual hygiene. All health professionals have a responsibility to promote such messages.

Every six seconds another person dies because of tobacco use (94,95). In developed countries as a whole, in the mid-1990s tobacco was estimated to be responsible for 24% of all male deaths and 7% of female deaths, rising to over 40% for men in some of the former socialist countries and 17% for women in the U.S.A. (96). This has been calculated to represent an average loss of life for cigarette smokers of 8 years and, for those whose deaths are directly attributed to tobacco, of 16 years. The proportion of cancer deaths attributed to smoking in developing countries is lower: approximately 21% for men and 4% for women. However, the fall in global tobacco consumption in the West is being matched by growth in developing countries. Of the 1.1 billion smokers in the world, approximately 800 million are in developing countries with at least 300 million in China alone. Today, these numbers are similar to those reported from 2001 (97). In 2010, >6 million deaths per year globally were attributed to tobacco smoking, and this number is expected to rise to 10 million/year by 2040 (96). Of these deaths, approximately 60,000 are due to lip and oral cavity cancer (98). Globally, approximately 350 million people also use smokeless tobacco (99), of which 206 million are in India (100). When the use of oral smokeless tobacco is added to these statistics, tobacco-associated deaths increased to >650,000 globally in 2010, of which 88% were in the South-East Asian Region. Most of these deaths are associated with oral, pharyngeal, laryngeal and esophageal cancer, stomach and cervical cancer, ischemic heart disease and stroke (101). The seriousness of the global epidemic of tobacco-related diseases is even more staggering. We all share a responsibility to help quell this global tobacco epidemic. Doll et al. conducted a long-term study on male British doctors and reported that about half of all regular smokers will be killed

Table 2.2 The major causes of smoking-related deaths

- Cancers of lip, mouth, pharynx, larynx, lung, oesophagus, bladder and pancreas
- Chronic obstructive pulmonary and other respiratory diseases
- Vascular diseases, including coronary artery and peripheral arterial diseases
- Peptic ulceration

by their habit (102). The major causes of such deaths are listed in Table 2.2.

In 1995, among men aged 35–69 years in industrialized countries, smoking was estimated as the cause of 25% of all deaths, 43% of all cancer deaths, 92% of lung cancer deaths, 65% of upper-aero digestive cancer deaths, 75% of chronic obstructive lung disease deaths among men of all ages and 35% of cardiovascular disease deaths (103). While oral and pharyngeal cancers figure prominently, lung cancer, other pulmonary diseases and cardiovascular diseases should be the starting points for counseling patients against tobacco use.

TYPES OF TOBACCO USE: A GLOBAL PERSPECTIVE

The smoking of tobacco in the form of factory-made cigarettes, cigars and cheroots, and loose tobacco in pipes or rolled into hand-made cigarettes, is familiar to all. There is a great variation in the tar, nicotine and nitrosamine contents, depending on tobacco species, curing, additives and method of combustion. Such smoking habits are the predominant form of tobacco use in the West, and in growing millions in developing countries. With government regulation of tobacco advertising, restrictions on smoking in public transport and other public places, and the awarding of damages to individuals and health authorities (particularly in the U.S.A.), manufacturers have been increasingly targeting developing countries for sales, especially of their higher-tar varieties. The morality of this is, of course, appalling.

Despite the WHO promoting its Framework Convention on Tobacco Control since 2003, encouraging countries to adopt a policy package to counter tobacco use, increases in smoking prevalence are occurring in countries that are lagging in policy adoption (104).

SMOKELESS TOBACCO

Much of the tobacco in the world is consumed without combustion, by being placed into contact with mucous membranes, through which nicotine is absorbed to provide the pharmacological "lift." Whereas WHO and the Framework Convention on Tobacco Control, and the Global Adult Tobacco Surveys, periodically updated, have much data on smoking around the world, details on smokeless tobacco are not always present. Fortunately, the Indian Factsheet includes smokeless tobacco: In India alone, it is estimated that 270 million people use tobacco of whom only 70 million smoke, whilst 160 million chew tobacco, and a further 40 million both chew and smoke.

The practice of nasal snuff, popular in the West in the 1700s and 1800s, faded in the 1900s. However, the use of various forms of snuff, either loose or packaged in small portions, placed in the oral vestibule, is common in Scandinavia and the U.S.A. and continues to gain popularity, one reason being public smoking bans. Loose snuff is placed in the mouth in several parts of Africa. Tobacco is also prepared in blocks or flakes for chewing. North Americans use the term "oral smokeless tobacco" for these products. In developing countries, however, tobacco is mostly consumed mixed with other ingredients (Table 2.3). There is extensive evidence for the carcinogenicity of these mixtures (105–108), and there is a wide range of products containing a very wide range of tobacco-specific nitrosamines (TSNAs) between 601 ng/g in many types of Swedish snus and a huge 992,000 ng/g in Sudanese toombak! (109)

Toombak, the form used in Sudan and southern Saudi Arabia, was extensively studied in the 1990s. Indeed, toombak contains unusually high levels of TSNAs, which find their way into the saliva of users (110). A case-control study of 375 patients with SCC of the lip, buccal cavity and floor

Table 2.3 Some common forms of oral smokeless tobacco

Habit	Ingredients	Population
Pan/paan/betel quid	Areca nut, betel leaf/inflorescence, slaked lime, catechu, condiments, with or without tobacco	Indian subcontinent, South-east Asia, Papua New Guinea, part of South America
Khaini	Tobacco and lime	Bihar India
Mishri	Burned tobacco	Maharashtra India
Zarda	Boiled tobacco	India and Arab countries
Gadakhu	Tobacco and molasses	Central India
Mawa	Tobacco, lime and areca	Bhavnagar India
Nass	Tobacco, ash, cotton or sesame oil	Central Asia, Iran, Afghanistan, Pakistan
Naswar/niswar	Tobacco, lime, indigo, cardamom, oil, menthol, etc.	Central Asia, Iran, Afghanistan, Pakistan
Shammah	Tobacco and ash and lime	Saudi Arabia
Toombak	Tobacco and sodium bicarbonate	Sudan

Source: Courtesy of Saman Warnakulasuriya.

of the mouth, and 271 patients with similar cancers of the tongue, palate and maxillary sinus, compared with 204 patients with non-squamous oral and non-oral malignant neoplasms, and with 2,820 disease-free individuals, shows overall adjusted ORs associated with toombak dipping of 7.3 and 3.9, respectively, for the first oral cancer group, compared with hospital and population controls (111). These effects rise to ORs of 11.0 and 4.3, respectively, in the long-term users. No significant ORs were found for the second cancer group where the agent is not in direct contact with the cancer site. These toombak-associated carcinomas show a high prevalence of p53 protein aberration/stabilization but a very low prevalence of HPV carriage (112). Distinctive forms of leukoplakia are common in habitués (Figure 2.1) but, interestingly, these show a low prevalence of epithelial dysplasia and longitudinal studies are still necessary to establish the rate of malignant transformation (113). It is an important question as to the proportion of toombak-related cancers which are preceded by leukoplakias which are sufficiently obvious clinically to provide opportunities for prevention based on habit cessation. Excision of such lesions—as an OPMD with a real risk of malignant transformation—would be, in the present state of our ignorance, ethical and appropriate. However, a cancer may still arise at the same or a different site in the "field"—the whole of the aerodigestive tract—altered by these TSNAs.

Smokeless tobacco is consumed in many forms across the Indian subcontinent, and the local variations are important to understand risks and how best to intervene. We have just concluded a case-control study with a life-course perspective at two hospitals in Pune, India. The sample size ($n = 480$) included 240 histopathologically confirmed cases of upper aerodigestive tract cancers and an equal number of controls, frequency matched with cases by gender and age distribution. Chewing tobacco emerged as the strongest predictor for this group of cancers (OR = 7.61; 95% CI: 4.65–12.45) in comparison to smoking and drinking alcohol. Exposure to second-hand smoke during childhood (<16 years) increased

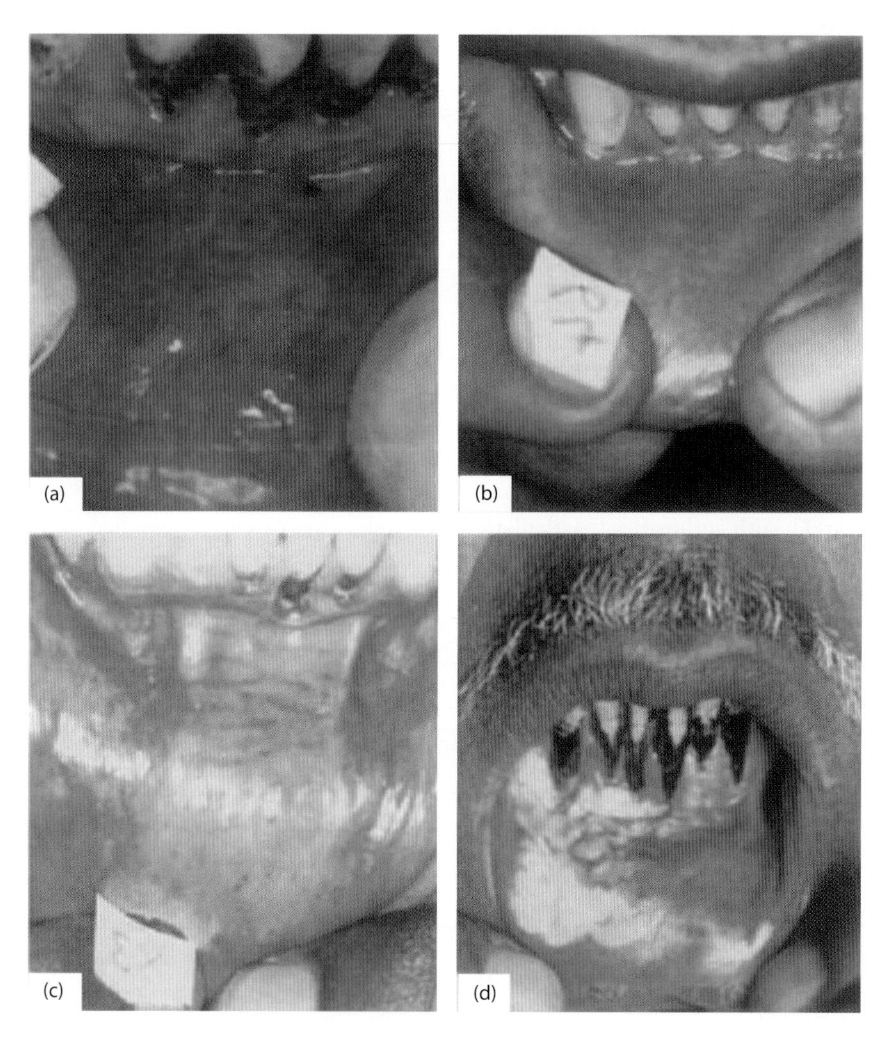

Figure 2.1 Clinical appearance of toombak-associated oral mucosal lesions. **(a)** A superficial lesion with a mild color change and some wrinkling. **(b)** A superficial white lesion with wrinkling. No obvious thickening or roughness. **(c)** A thickened white or yellowish lesion with furrows and wrinkling. **(d)** A marked, elevated white or yellow/brown lesion with heavy thickening and grooving. Note some reddened furrows are also present. (From Idris et al. *J Oral Pathol Med* 1996;25(5):239–44 (113).)

the risk (OR = 4.05; 95% CI: 2.06–7.95). Combined effects of tobacco and alcohol consumption habits elevated the risk by 12-fold (OR = 12.05; 95% CI: 4.61–31.49) in comparison to never users of these habits (114). Such information can readily be used to construct risk profiles for residents (115), but needs to be adjusted to account for the habit mix in the population being considered because these vary considerably across South and South-East Asia and the Western Pacific Islands. In the population dwelling in and around the city of Pune, Maharashtra State, India, the major type of smokeless tobacco used was mawa—but note: this mixture contains areca nut and lime along with tobacco (Table 2.3).

SNUFF IN SCANDINAVIA AND NORTH AMERICA

Relevant observations go back decades in the U.S.A. Brown et al. described "snuff-dipper's cancer" in the South Eastern states of the U.S.A. where the habit of placing snuff in the lower labial sulcus was common (116). This habit was also the basis of the classical description of verrucous carcinoma reported by Ackermann in 1948 (117), and confirmed by McCoy and Waldron in 1981 (118). Women in the textile industry in this area of the U.S.A. had a high prevalence of snuff-dipping and elevated death rates from oral cancer in the late 1970s and early 1980s (119,120). There is clear evidence that this form of oral smokeless tobacco can be topically carcinogenic.

Concern was expressed in the late 1980s at growing use of factory-produced portion-packed snuff in the U.S.A., available since the early 1980s in pouches resembling a then-new low-nitrosamine Swedish product (Figure 2.2), and the oral cancers it might cause, particularly among adolescents (121). Exposure to its advertising has been correlated with curiosity (122) and receptivity (123), leading to a fashion for usage among adolescents in the U.S.A. Chewing tobacco and packaged snuff habits have long been practiced by a proportion of prominent sportsmen, particularly baseball players (124), many of whom are regarded as role models by the young, so the habit is emulated by many youths (125,126).

In 1986, the Surgeon-General of the U.S.A. produced a report which categorically stated that smokeless tobacco carried significant risks to health from oral cancer and other oral lesions and that it could lead to nicotine addiction and dependence (127). In 1986, the American Congress passed an Act that banned the advertising of smokeless tobacco on radio and television, and required health warnings on packages and printed advertisements. After some interesting machinations with the law and its interpretation in several European countries, in 1992 the European Union (EU) banned the sale of portion snuff and loose moist snuff (some of which were imported into Europe from the U.S.A.) in all of its member states: when Sweden joined the EU in 1985, it was exempted from the ban on sales of snus (Swedish moist snuff), but exports were banned (128). In 1985, the same year the IARC stated that there was sufficient evidence that snuff in Europe and the U.S.A. causes cancer (129), the Swedish

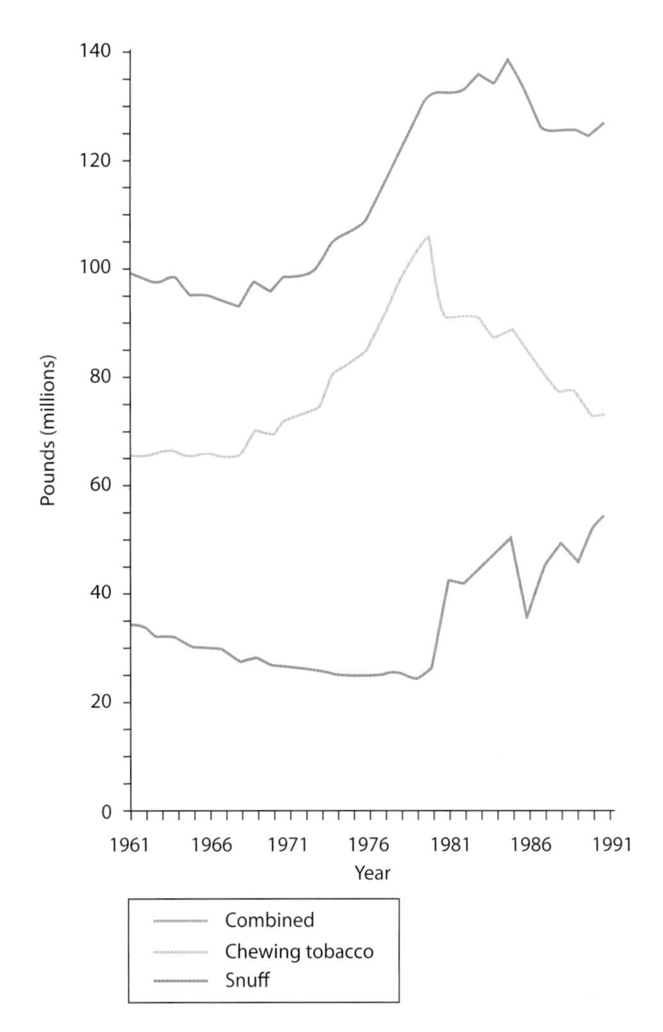

Figure 2.2 Annual consumption of "spitting" tobacco in the USA, 1961–91. (From Sterling et al. *J Clin Epidemiol* 1992;45(3):223–31 (133).)

Government required warning labels to be placed on such products. However, in studies reviewed in 2007 in the subsequent IARC monograph on smokeless tobacco (130), even though Swedish snuff was not found to be associated with oral cancer, the overall evaluation on smokeless tobaccos was that there was sufficient evidence for its carcinogenicity in humans and that smokeless tobacco causes cancer of the oral cavity and pancreas. Remember, however, that all tobacco is not the same!

The association between snuff and HNC remains controversial. American- and Scandinavian-style snuff/snus produces hyperkeratotic lesions in those areas of the oral mucosa in habitual contact with the product (131), and there is a notable prevalence even in teenagers in the U.S.A. where, from a survey of 17,027 children aged 12–17, 2.9% of males and 0.1% of females had lesions associated in a dose-dependent fashion with snuff (particularly) and chewing tobacco (132), although there is usually a long latent period (120). Evidence that emerged during the initial period of rising smokeless tobacco use in the U.S.A. did not support the contention that smokeless tobacco use was a high-risk activity. A study based on combined data of the U.S. National

Mortality Followback Survey (1986, U.S.A., $n = 16{,}598$) and the coincident National Health Interview Survey (1987, U.S.A.), with correction for possible confounders, concluded that the use of smokeless tobacco, either as snuff or chewing tobacco, does not significantly increase the risk of oral cancer or cancer of the digestive organs (133). However, the number of users was small and it is essential to remember that these data relate to Scandinavian- and U.S.-style products. South Asian smokeless tobaccos are definitely highly carcinogenic. Alcohol emerged as a major risk factor for oral cancer in the studies from the U.S.A., with a strong dose–response relationship, as it did to a lesser extent with other digestive cancers. Smoking was associated with risk of oral but not other digestive cancers (Table 2.4). This view of the relatively low cancer risk of smokeless tobacco in the U.S.A. and Sweden led to a movement to advocate this practice as a less dangerous alternative to smoking and as an aid to nicotine withdrawal in those addicted to smoking—a suggestion that is highly controversial because there are undoubtedly safer forms of nicotine replacement.

Table 2.4 Relative risk (RR) and confidence interval (CI) for oral cancer; ICD 9; 140–149; multiplicative model

	RR	CI
Sex		
Male	1.00	
Female	0.52	0.27–1.00
Race		
White	1.00	
Non-white	2.63	1.31–5.27
Age (years)		
25–44	1.00	
45–64	47.22	6.07–367.19
65–84	84.88	10.71–666.38
85+	206.03	20.00–2,122.83
Lifetime smoking (packs)		
0–19 (never)	1.00	
20–11,999	1.07	0.48–2.38
12,000+	2.85	1.41–5.77
Annual drinking		
0–52 (1 drink/week)	1.00	
53–365 (1 drink/day)	2.75	1.26–5.99
366+	7.20	3.74–13.88
Occupation		
Professional/managerial/clerical	1.00	
Blue collar/service/technical	1.06	0.62–1.83
Smokeless tobacco		
0–99 (nonuser)	1.00	
100–9999 times	0.92	0.25–3.42
10,000+	1.21	0.32–4.63

Source: Form Sterling et al. *J Clin Epidemiol* 1992;45(3):223–31 (133).

Newer forms of smokeless tobacco manufactured in Sweden and in the U.S.A. contain even lower levels of harmful substances than traditional American products. For example, total TSNAs found in four new American pouch products ranged from 1.5 to 6.2 μg/g (dry weight), whereas in four American traditional products the range was from 6.3 to 12.0 μg/g. One brand of Swedish snus for comparison averaged 3.1 μg/g. Average nitrite levels were 0.003 mg/g in the new pouch products, 0.037 mg/g in four traditional products and 0.004 mg/g in the Swedish snus (134). A 2002 Swedish study found that the mean amount of TSNAs in 27 brands of Swedish moist snuff was 1.0 μg/g (135). Fortunately, in the U.S.A., newer forms such as pouches, sticks, dissolvable lozenges and pellets have not so far achieved much following (136). Thus, while on a global scale these levels of carcinogens are low, it is worth remembering that nitrosamine levels of newer smokeless tobacco products are still 100–1,000 times higher than any found in food and in beer (134,137). Furthermore, the cardiovascular effects of the newer forms of smokeless tobacco have been demonstrated only to a limited extent (138–140). A small increase in cardiovascular risk appears possible with the available limited evidence (130).

To obtain clearer results on the cancer dangers associated with smokeless tobacco, researchers pooled data from 11 case-control studies from the U.S.A. (1981–2006) and examined the risk of HNC in ever smokeless tobacco users (snuff and chewing tobacco separately) who had never been cigarette smokers (141). They found that ever use of snuff was strongly associated with oral cavity cancers (OR = 3.01; 95% CI: 1.63–5.55) and weakly associated with other HNC (OR = 1.71; 95% CI: 1.08–2.70). Chewing tobacco was also significantly associated with oral cavity cancer (OR = 1.81; 95% CI: 1.04–3.17) but not with the other HNC sites (141). Analyses for the two types of smokeless tobacco among ever cigarette smokers in this study showed that ratios for cancer of the oral cavity and the other head and neck sites were not elevated.

The nature of these products varies considerably. Chewing tobaccos differ distinctly from (moist) snuff, and snuffs as manufactured and used in Europe and North America differ greatly from snuff-like products used in the Middle East, which are made locally in a variety of small-scale industries, by individual vendors, or directly by the users. Products such as toombak, used in Sudan (142), and the shammah of Arabia have, as explained above, exceptionally high TSNAs and are largely responsible for the high incidence of oral cancer (143). There is, however, a paradox in that the characteristic hyperkeratotic lesions of toombak users show a low prevalence of epithelial dysplasia (113), as do those described in the U.S.A. and Scandinavia. We have opined that, in the case of Sudan, this might be because those users most susceptible to cancer have already succumbed to their malignancies by the time epidemiologists begin studying them and so they do not appear in population studies such as those reviewed here.

It is becoming clear that locally manufactured Swedish snuff is no longer a major risk factor for oral cancer. Two

Table 2.5 Oral cancer in Swedish snuff users

References	No. of pairs	Relative risk	95% Confidence interval
Schildt et al. (144)			
Current users	410	0.6	0.3–1.1
Previous users		1.4	0.7–2.8
Lewin et al. (145)			
Current users	128	1.0	0.7–1.6
Previous users		1.2	0.6–1.9

case-control studies of oral cancer in Sweden failed to show an association (Table 2.5) (144,145). In a longitudinal cohort study, Roosaar et al. followed 9,976 men from 1974 to 2002 and showed an excess risk of 3.1 (95% CI: 1.5–6.6) for combined oral cancer and pharyngeal cancer for ever-daily Swedish snuff use based on 11 exposed cases (146). However, these included ever-smokers. The hazard ratio (HR) for never-smokers who ever-used snuff daily (5 cases) was 2.3 (95% CI: 0.7–8.3), which was not significant. Hirsch et al. described 10 Swedish men with oral cancer who never smoked but used snuff (median age 75 years, mean duration of use 43 years), and the cancers were found in the place where the snuff was placed (147). Men in these studies had started using snuff prior to the mid-1980s, before Swedish manufacturers began slowly reducing TSNAs in their products to very low levels by pasteurization to prevent fermentation, requiring that the products be kept under refrigeration in shops and providing "sell by" dates (135).

It has become a valid argument as to whether at least some newer forms of snuff might be used to help smokers quit. This approach has been roundly condemned by the anti-tobacco movement in the U.S.A.; because snuff can lead to nicotine addiction, promote "dual use" (both smoking and smokeless use), or prolong use in ex-smokers who have switched to smokeless tobacco; because it ignores the potential role of snuff in other cancers and in cardiovascular diseases; and that other ethically accepted forms of nicotine replacement therapy (such as chewing gums, skin patches and nasal sprays) are widely available. These are real concerns, which require clarification in well-designed studies. It is, therefore, of interest to note two comparatively recent Swedish studies on heart disease. A case-control study set in Sweden of 585 cases with 10% snuff users and 589 controls with 15% snuff users showed a low relative risk for myocardial infarction (RR = 0.89; 95% CI: 0.62–1.29) in snuff users, compared to smokers (RR = 1.87; 95% CI: 1.40–2.48) (148). Another Swedish study from health screening of 135,036 construction workers identified 6,297 snuff users. The relative risk for death due to cardiovascular disease was minimal (RR = 1.4; 95% CI: 1.2–1.6) and slightly higher (RR = 1.9; 95% CI: 1.7–2.2) for smokers (149). The cohort study by Roosaar et al. (146), mentioned above, showed a non-significant HR for death due to cardiovascular disease (HR = 1.15), and a non-significant HR for death due to any cancer (HR = 1.28), but a significant adjusted all-cause mortality HR among never-smoking Swedish snuff users (HR = 1.23; 95% CI: 1.09–1.40). In a case-control study by Persson et al., no increased risk among snuff users who had never smoked was found among men for the inflammatory bowel diseases, Crohn's disease and ulcerative colitis (150). The possibility of increased risk of cancer at other sites has not yet been fully addressed. A cohort study (1971–2004) by Zendehdel et al. showed an association of Swedish snuff with esophageal and stomach cancers, including among never-smokers (151). In summary, on present evidence, it appears that snuff habits as they exist in Scandinavia today and, probably, to a slightly lesser extent in the U.S.A., carry low risks of serious health hazards, including oral cancer. However, as Axell points out, this does not mean that oral snuff use should be encouraged (152). The absence of evidence of risk does not mean evidence of the absence of risk: snuff almost always produces mucosal lesions, and often affects salivary flow and causes gingival recessions (153). There remains a great need to continue to work towards a tobacco-free society.

Betel quid and areca nut

The recommended terminology (betel quid) is that of the Expert Symposium published in 1997 (154). Betel quids are prepared from areca nut, cured or sun-dried, and chopped (Figure 2.3). These pieces are placed on a leaf of the *Piper betel* vine (in most parts of the world where the habit is indigenous: importantly, this includes emigrant communities), although the inflorescence is used by some, for example in Papua New Guinea (PNG). Slaked lime is an essential ingredient; it raises the pH dramatically and accelerates the release of alkaloids from both tobacco and nut, with enhanced pharmacological "lift." The lime is prepared by baking limestone where available: near coasts this is more often from sea shells or snail shells (such as in Kerala and Sri Lanka) or from coral (as in the Pacific Islands). Customs vary widely. For example, in PNG areca nut is chewed directly, the lime being smeared on the oral mucosa itself; tobacco is rarely added or chewed, although cigars made from rough local tobacco are commonly smoked (155) and the prevalence of cigarette smoking has been increasing (156). The spread of oral cancer from the coasts to the highlands in PNG has followed the trade in coast-grown areca nuts. The effects of long-term, heavy chewing on the mouth are characteristic and are shown in Figure 2.4.

The chewing of areca nut in various forms and mixtures is deeply embedded in the social and cultural history of India, Sri Lanka, Pakistan, Bangladesh, Myanmar, Thailand, Cambodia, Malaysia, Singapore, Indonesia, Philippines, New Guinea, Taiwan and parts of China (Figure 2.5) and in emigrant communities therefrom. Its use appears in ancient Sanskrit literature. Areca nuts contain potent cholinergic muscarinic alkaloids, notably arecoline and guavacoline, with a wide range of parasympatheticomimetic effects: they promote salivation and the passage of wind through the gut; they raise blood pressure and pulse

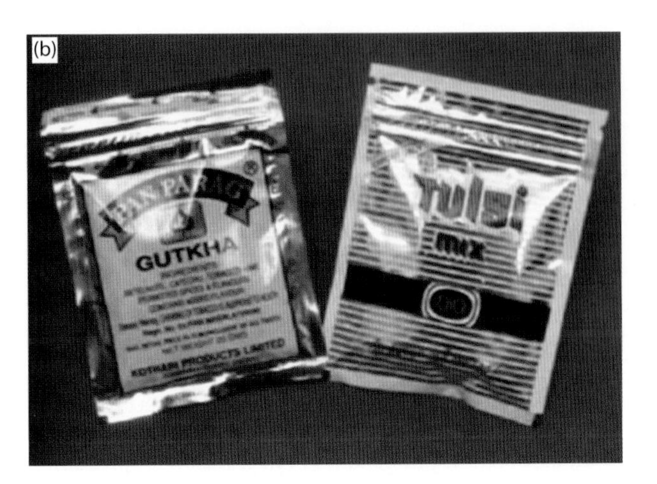

Figure 2.3 **(a)** Ingredients of a traditional betel quid or pan. Chopped areca nut and lime paste are placed on a betel leaf; tobacco and various condiments and sweeteners may be added. (Courtesy of Dr Fali Mehta.) **(b)** These days cheap packets of chopped areca nut are widely available. They usually contain other flavorings and frequently include tobacco, in which case they are likely to carry a government health warning. Use of these products may be even more damaging than traditional betel quids, because the leaf of the latter has antioxidant properties.

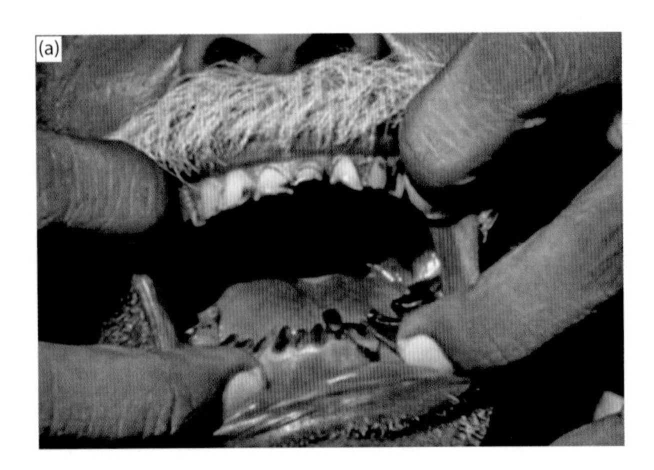

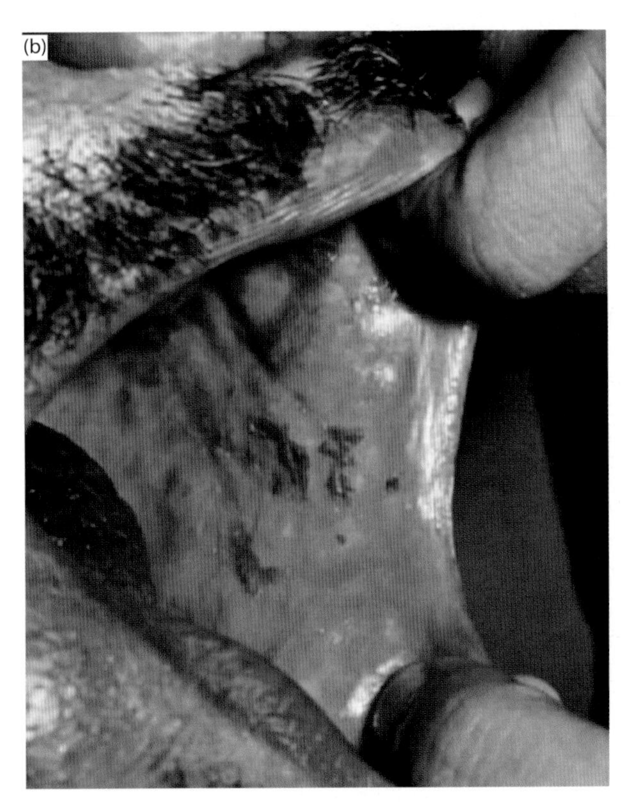

Figure 2.4 **(a)** Severe attrition and tooth staining in a heavy betel quid chewer. **(b)** Atrophic mucosa with superficial plaques of keratin stained by areca extracts.

rate and they elicit a degree of euphoria by virtue of their GABA receptor-inhibitory properties which contribute to dependence and habituation (157). There are also bronchoconstrictor effects, and evidence for a role in precipitating and exacerbating asthma and diabetes, as reviewed by Boucher (158). In addition to aspects of oral cancer and OPMD, the historical, social and general health aspects of betel quid use are well discussed in the excellent monographs of Bedi and Jones (159), Warnakulasuriya (160) and the comprehensive review by Garg et al. (161). Evidence for the carcinogenicity of betel quid has been set out by Daftary et al. (106) in categories of varying epidemiological weight.

Ecological evidence

It has been known, perhaps for over a century, that there is a high frequency of oral cancer in those parts of the world where areca/tobacco-chewing habits are widespread. The association has a strong ethnic basis and remains in emigrant communities from South Asia who continue the

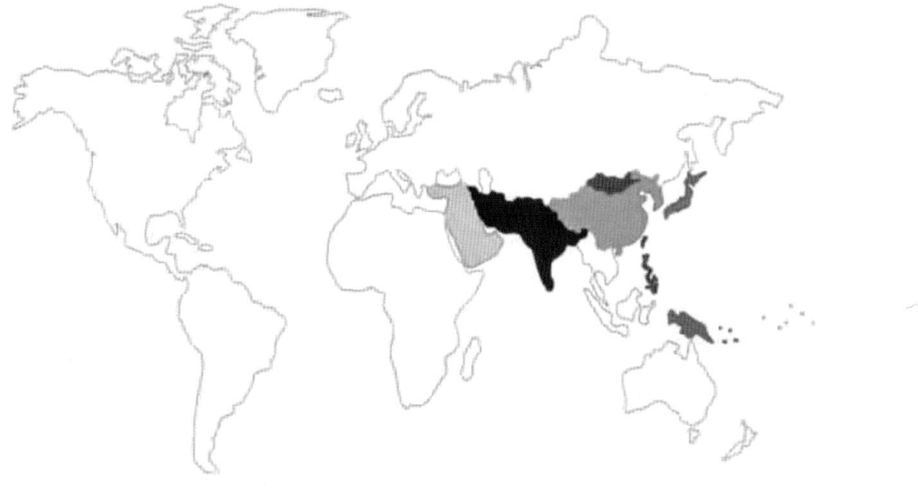

Figure 2.5 Those parts of the globe in which betel quid and other areca nut habits are endemic. These habits are continued among emigrants from those parts of the world and are thus found in immigrant communities worldwide.

habit. Oral submucous fibrosis, for which areca nut itself is the main etiological agent, is almost exclusively found in those ethnic groups who use betel quid or areca in other forms, wherever in the world such people reside.

Chewing habits among patients with oral cancer

Descriptive studies in India going back to the 1960s reported a high prevalence of oral cancer among habitués. For example, in 1962, Paymaster reported that 81% (3412/4212) oral cancer patients used tobacco: 36% were chewers, 23% were smokers and 22% had both habits (162). Many similar observations subsequently have been published. There is a strong association between the site of cancer and the site where the quid is habitually placed—again, quite an old observation (163).

Evidence from cross-sectional studies

Extensive cross-sectional population studies from India, involving over 100,000 individuals, detected 14 oral cancers in chewers of betel quid with tobacco, 24 among other tobacco users and none among nonusers of tobacco (164). In several hospital series in different parts of Thailand, oral cancer ranked second among cancer sites in males in the late 1970s/early 1980s, but by 1990 had dropped to fifth. This has been associated with decreasing use of betel quid, particularly in the cities, as reviewed by Reichart (165); betel quids in Thailand have commonly included tobacco.

Evidence from case-control studies

The carcinogenicity of pan/betel quid mixtures has been clearly established in a meta-analysis of 17 published studies by Thomas and Wilson (166). These show a range of relative risks averaging approximately 10 (Figure 2.6). However, as pointed out by Warnakulasuriya (167), only four studies differentially examine the role of betel quid with and without tobacco, and with and without smoking, in cases of oral cancer in South Asian populations (Table 2.6). While areca nut appears to be increasing the cancer risk, it is clear that tobacco is the major carcinogen, possibly partly because its presence in a mixture adds to the compulsion to chew it more frequently. Our recent analysis (168) of 15 case-control studies (4,553 cases; 8,632 controls) and 4 cohort studies (15,342) showed that chewing tobacco is significantly

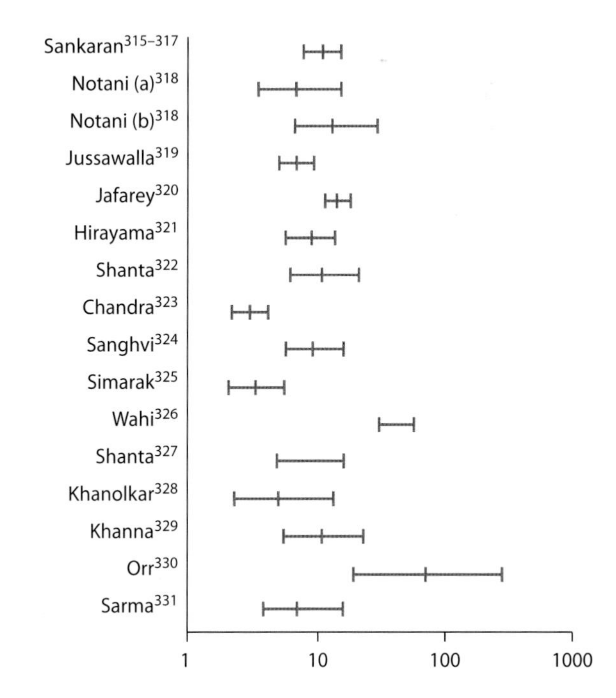

Figure 2.6 Summary of crude odds ratios for the development of oral cancer in populations chewing betel quid in any form, irrespective of smoking habits. (Analysis derived from Thomas S, Wilson A. *Eur J Cancer B Oral Oncol* 1993;29B(4):265–71 (166).)

Table 2.6 Relative risk (RR) of oral cancer from betel quid with or without tobacco

References	Cases/controls	Betel quid with tobacco	Betel quid without tobacco	No chewing habit
Shanta and Krishnamurthi (1959)	Oral cancer	219	33	25
	Controls	35	144	99
	RR	24.8	0.9	1
Chandra (1963)	Oral cancer	138	46	135
	Controls	61	70	256
	RR	4.34*	1.24	1
Hirayama (1966)	Oral cancer	190	35	9
	Controls	215	16	102
	RR	9.1*	1.2	1
Jafarey and Zaidi (1976)	Oral cancer	339	40	88
	Controls	474	216	1690
	RR	13.7*	3.6*	1

Source: Data and cited references from Warnakulasuriya S. In: Bedi R, Jones P (eds). *Betel quid and tobacco chewing among the Bangladeshi Community in the United Kingdom*. London: Centre for Transcultural Oral Health, 1995:61–9 (728).
*$p < 0.01$.

and independently associated with an increased risk of oral SCC (case-control studies OR = 7.46; 95% CI = 5.86–9.50, $p < 0.001$; for cohort studies RR = 5.48; 95% CI: 2.56–11.71, $p < 0.001$). Meta-analysis of fifteen case-control studies (4,648 cases; 7,847 controls) showed betel quid without tobacco to have an independent, but weaker, positive association with oral cancer (OR = 2.82; 95% CI: 2.35–3.40; $p < 0.001$). A meta-analysis focussed on areca products demonstrated that betel quid chewing, with or without added tobacco, increases the risk of oral plus oropharyngeal cancer in an exposure-dependent manner, independently of tobacco and alcohol use: Roughly half of oral cancers in China and Taiwan could be prevented if betel quid (which generally does not contain tobacco in these countries) was no longer chewed (169).

Evidence from prospective studies

Gupta et al. followed 30,000 individuals for approximately 10 years up to 1977 in three areas of India (170). In Ernakulum, Kerala, the annual age-adjusted incidence of oral cancer was 23/100,000 among betel quid/tobacco chewers compared with zero in smokers and non-habitués. A more recent cohort study on oral cavity cancer incidence was conducted in Karunagappally, Kerala, among 66,277 men and 78,140 women aged 30–84 years. The cohort was established during the 1990s and ended in 2005, with an average of about 10 years follow-up. Here also, tobacco chewing was almost always associated with betel quid. Among men, there were 75 cases of oral cancer among 18,692 current chewers (218,673 person-years; RR = 2.4; 95% CI: 1.7–3.3), of which 37 had never smoked beedis (171). Among women, there were 53 cases of oral cancer among 18,612 current chewers (183,749 person-years; RR = 5.5; 95% CI: 3.3–9.0) (172). Since mawa contains areca nut it is most strongly associated with oral submucous fibrosis in users in Chennai, Tamil Nadu State, South India (173).

Evidence from intervention studies

Intensive health education programs among 36,000 betel quid/tobacco chewers and smokers in India showed a significant regression in what were then termed precancerous lesions (174). More significantly, a 10-year follow-up of 12,212 users, producing 77,681 person-years of observation in men and 32,544 among women, successfully achieved habit cessation in 6.5% of the men and 14.4% of the women. There was a substantial drop in the incidence of leukoplakia after cessation (incidence ratio: 0.31), but not for lichen planus or for several other lesions. As leukoplakia is a common well-established potentially malignant disorder in this population, this implies a reduced risk of oral cancer (Table 2.7) (175).

Dose–response relationship

Although this type of evidence is usually regarded as powerful, unfortunately, few studies exist. However, a dose–response relationship was shown in the classical pioneering studies by Orr (176) and by Hirayama (163): the latter showed a relative risk for oral cancer of 8.4 when the number of quids chewed per day was less than 2, rising to 17.6 when the frequency was six times or more per day; individuals who slept with the quid in the mouth had a relative risk of 63. A more recent study (177) provides perhaps the strongest analysis of a dose–response relationship from Indian data (Chennai and Trivandrum), where ORs for oral cancer increased from 2.1 for chewers of 1–3 quids daily on average, to 6.0 for chewers of 4–5 quids, and to as high as 12.0 for chewers of over 5 quids per day.

Areca nut alone as an oral carcinogen

In 1985, the IARC concluded that "there was insufficient evidence that the chewing of betel quid without tobacco was carcinogenic to man" (129). In 2004, this was completely

Table 2.7 Effect of cessation of tobacco habits on incidence of lesions in a 10-year follow-up of 12,212 users

	Stopped		All others		
	Incident cases	Incidence/100000[a]	Incident cases	Incidence/100,000[a]	Incidence ratio
Leukoplakia					
Men	7	92	183	219	0.42
Women	5	63	54	201	0.31
Lichen planus					
Men	7	107	111	143	0.75
Women	19	396	93	294	1.35

Source: From Gupta et al. *Oral Dis* 1995;1(1):54–8 (175).
[a] Age adjusted.

overturned by the IARC when, on the basis of new data, the evidence for the carcinogenicity of betel quid without tobacco and of areca nut by itself, was regarded as "sufficient" (178). Areca nut is certainly the main etiological agent in oral submucous fibrosis (179,180). Also, as seen above from studies in the Indian subcontinent, adding tobacco to betel quids increases their risk considerably.

In Guam, where areca nut is chewed either alone or with betel leaf only, no dramatic increase in oral cancer has been demonstrated (181). Conversely, in Taiwan, most heavy chewers of betel quids do not include tobacco, and yet oral cancer is clearly associated with the habit (182). The risk of malignant transformation of leukoplakia was very high for betel nut chewing in Taiwan (OR = 17; range: 1.94–156.27) (183). In PNG, as already referred to, the predominant chewing habit involves betel vine inflorescence and areca nut, with large quantities of lime applied to the mucosa, but without the addition of tobacco: nevertheless, concurrent cigar smoking is common (184). Furthermore, the synergistic role of alcohol has not been evaluated in the PNG situation (185).

A case-control study from India showed an interaction with alcohol for nonsmokers who chew betel quid with and without tobacco, where oral cancer risk increased from 9.3 for nondrinkers to 24.3 for drinkers among chewers of betel quid with tobacco and from an OR of 3.4 for nondrinkers to 4.4 for drinkers among chewers of betel quid without tobacco (177).

Strong evidence that the chewing of areca alone produces oral cancer comes from South Africa: in a study of 143 cases of oral cancer among the (historic) Indian immigrant community of the Eastern Cape, 39 of 57 with cheek cancer and 21 of 25 with tongue cancer were nut chewers who did not use tobacco in any form (186). Additionally, a small but well-designed case-control ($n = 40 : 160$) study in Taiwan clearly showed a strong carcinogenic effect of the local quids with an OR of 58.4 after adjusting for cigarette smoking and alcohol drinking. Importantly, this showed a strong dose–response relationship, adjusted ORs rising to 275.6 when more than 20 quids were consumed per day, and to 397.5 with more than 40 years of chewing; nevertheless, 18/40 patients drank alcohol and the majority, 32/40, also smoked, so that multiple risk factors are clearly operating in this community (187). The independent role of areca is confirmed in Pakistan (188) and reviewed by Trivedy et al. (189).

A review published in 2015 identified studies published post-2001 that analyzed for betel quid without tobacco and adjusted or stratified for alcohol (190). Three studies were identified that showed significantly elevated ORs for the consumption of betel quid without tobacco, and adjusted for smoking and alcohol drinking: 3 studies for men only (RR = 3.39; 95% CI: 2.04–5.66) (177), another men only (RR = 4.16; 95% CI: 1.46–11.83) and RR for women = 16.42 (4.77–56.48) (191) and the third with RR for men = 3.3 (0.9–12.0) and RR for women = 5.4 (2.1–14.1) (192). Consumption of areca nut (supari) by itself was shown in a fourth study to have an adjusted OR of 11.4 (3.4, 38.2) for both men and women together (193).

The presence of increased numbers of micronucleated epithelial cells, as a putative intermediate marker of oral cancer risk, has been reported in users of areca nut without tobacco in the Philippines (194), and in India (195), in which study chromosomal aberrations and sister chromatid exchanges in phytohemagglutinin-stimulated peripheral blood lymphocytes were found to be progressively increased in areca nut chewers without disease, through chewers with oral submucous fibrosis, to chewers with oral carcinoma.

Animal experiments also support a role for areca nut in the causation of oral cancer. While some early studies produced cancers, such as those by Ranadive and by Shirname (196,197), most of them failed to produce frank neoplasms in the absence of a known artificial/experimental initiator or complete chemical carcinogen and thus evidence for the carcinogenicity of areca nut was limited. With improved methodologies, many later experiments in animals provided clear evidence for the carcinogenicity of areca nut. For example, areca nut fiber and cold aqueous extracts of Taiwan betel quids promoted dimethylbenzanthracene (DMBA)-initiated hamster cheek pouch carcinogenesis, in the absence of tobacco products (198): betel quid alone produced only hyperkeratosis and acanthosis (199). A number of earlier studies in baboons, monkeys, rats and hamsters are reviewed by Warnakulasuriya (167). Eventually, IARC evaluated the accumulated evidence as sufficient for both betel quid and areca nut, as causing cancer in experimental animals (178).

Direct DNA damage has been shown to occur when areca nut extracts are added to human buccal epithelial cells *in vitro* (200), and the tannins have been shown to enhance mucosal permeability (201). The major nitroso compounds formed from areca nut alkaloids are 3-(methylnitrosamino)propionitrile, 3-(methylnitrosamino)propionaldehyde (MNPA), *N*-nitrosoguvacoline (NG) and *N*-nitrosoguvacine (NGV): of these MNPA appears to be the most powerful carcinogen (200). Jeng et al. reviewed the subject comprehensively (202).

In evaluating the dangers of these complex mixtures, it is important to remember that betel leaf itself, like most green leafy vegetables, has been shown to have a protective effect (203). At least two protective compounds have been identified—β-carotene and hydroxychavicol (an astringent antiseptic). In Taiwan, apparently, over 90% of chewers do not consume rolled betel leaf (187).

SMOKING AND ORAL CANCER

There is overwhelming evidence that active smoking, and growing evidence that passive smoking, are both important in bronchogenic carcinoma. The evidence for active smoking is strong for oral cancer, but other factors are clearly involved, and sorting out their relative contributions remains difficult despite continuing research. Discussion in this section relates mostly to studies in the West, avoiding the complications of mixed smoking—often with unusual forms of local tobacco (Figure 2.7)—and chewing habits (discussed above), predominantly in developing countries. These scenarios are helpfully treated separately by Daftary et al. (105) and Binnie (204). The most comprehensive sources of evidence remain the IARC publications of 1986, 2004 and 2012 (178,205,206). This evidence on smoking and cancer is also summarized by the U.S. Surgeon-General's Report of 1989 (207) which lists attributable risk (AR) for cancer at various sites (Table 2.8): the upper aerodigestive sites with which we are here concerned have the highest ARs, in males, of all the many sites for which smoking has been identified as playing a role. Subsequent Surgeon-General's Reports from the U.S.A. have had new messages to communicate. For example, the Report of 2010 informed readers that quitting smoking entirely cuts the risk of cancer of the mouth, throat, esophagus and bladder in half after 5 years (208). This good news needs to be communicated to smokers.

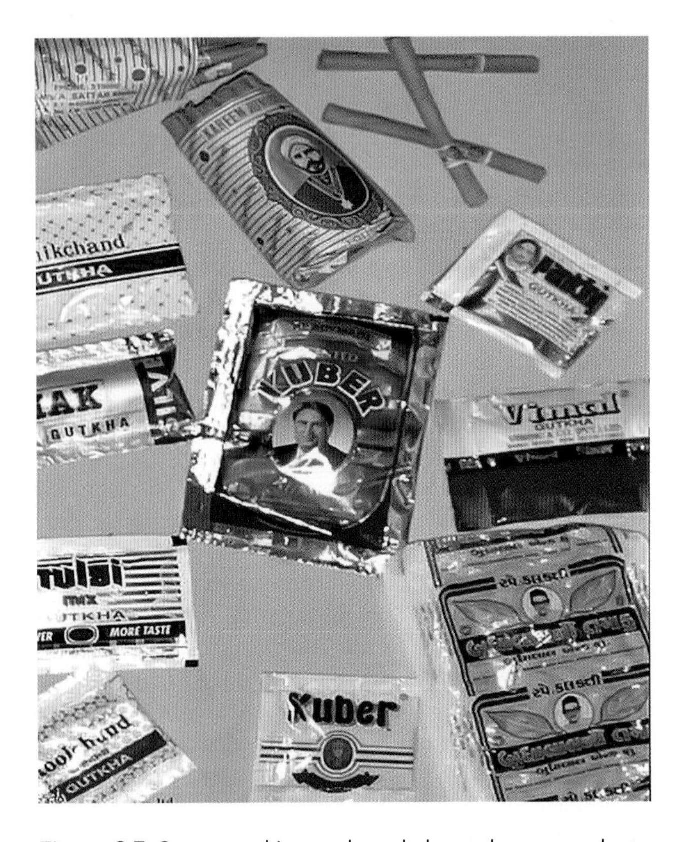

Figure 2.7 Some smoking and smokeless tobacco products common in the Indian subcontinent: packeted snuff, cigars, cut tobacco rolling or pipe, and beedis—cheap tobacco wrapped in a temburni leaf and tied with a cotton thread.

Table 2.8 Cancer deaths due to smoking in the U.S.A., 1985 (U.S. Surgeon-General's report)

Site	% Attributable deaths		Number of deaths pa
	Men	Women	
Lung	90	79	106,000
Lip, oral cavity, pharynx	92	61	7000
Esophagus	78	75	7000
Bladder	47	37	4000
Kidney	48	12	3000
Larynx	81	87	3000

There is confusion in the literature as to the relative importance of different types of smoking. This partly arises because the lip has not always been separated from intra-oral sites. Ultraviolet light is clearly important for the lip, but not for the mouth. Pipe smoking has long been associated with lip cancer, where consideration must be given to the nature of the pipe stem and its permeability, and to heat as cofactors. Most of the literature goes back several decades, perhaps because of the decreased popularity of pipe smoking in recent times in the West (209–212). Some literature suggests that pipes and cigars are less risky for oral cancer than cigarettes (213), but the very extensive study from North Italy shows higher risks associated with these practices for cancer of the mouth and esophagus than with cigarettes. Beedi (beedi) smoking, as practiced in the Indian subcontinent, is more hazardous than cigarette smoking (214,215).

In fact, the large number of beedi smokers, the considerable data on the risks associated with beedi smoking, and its potential for export to other countries, justifies more attention to be given to the beedi (216). The current most comprehensive sources of evidence are the IARC monographs 83 of 2004 (178) and 100E of 2012 (206) and the IARC Handbook on Cancer Prevention of 2007 (217). The IARC Monograph 100 E of 2012 found numerous studies providing evidence for the role of beedi smoking in oral cancer, with increased risks found for higher numbers of beedis smoked per day and longer durations of smoking (206). The cohort study by Jayalekshmy et al. in Kerala, India (171), showed that beedi

Table 2.9 Alcohol and tobacco habits of 690 consecutive cases of oral cancer in Amsterdam, 1971–1991

Tobacco and alcohol	56%
Tobacco only	14%
Alcohol only	5%
Neither	25%

Source: Jovanovic A et al. *Oral Pathol Med* 1993;22(10):459–62 (218).

smoking in men who did not chew tobacco significantly increased oral cancer risk (RR = 2.6; 95% CI = 1.4–4.9). Higher daily consumption ($p < 0.001$), longer duration ($p = 0.001$), and younger age at start of beedi smoking ($p = 0.007$) were associated with higher risks.

A major difficulty in accurately quantifying smoking risks for oral cancer is the strong synergism of tobacco with alcohol. The importance of tobacco can be inferred from the habits associated with patients with oral cancer in a series of cases from Amsterdam (218). This series is valuable because it contains a high proportion of cases without either of these major risk factors (Table 2.9). The relative risk for heavy smoking (more than 20 cigarettes per day), adjusted for the effects of alcohol, is highest for the retromolar area, followed by floor of the mouth, lower lip, lower alveolus, tongue and lowest for the cheek. For heavy alcohol drinking (more than 4 units per day), adjusted for smoking, the risk is highest for floor of the mouth followed by retromolar area, lower alveolus, tongue, lower lip and again lowest for cheek. The differential by the anatomical site is larger for smoking. These locations make intuitive sense.

A large case-control study from the U.S.A. provides good evidence of a dose–response relationship for both tobacco and alcohol (219) (Table 2.10). This is well depicted by the histogram shown in Figure 2.8 (220). The relationship between anatomical site of oral cancer and smoking is less clear-cut than with smokeless tobacco. It has long been stated that the pooling of carcinogens in saliva gives rise to cancers in the "gutter" area and thus affects the floor of the mouth and the ventral and lateral tongue. Mashberg and Meyers (221) reported that in an American cohort, 201/207 (97%) asymptomatic, primarily erythroplastic carcinomas were in three locations: floor of the mouth, ventral or lateral tongue and soft palate complex. In the Amsterdam series (218), the floor of the mouth and retromolar area were significantly more related to tobacco smoking than were cancers of the tongue and cheek. However, in another series of 359 cases among male American Veterans, smoking was more strongly associated with soft palate cancers than anterior sites, and alcohol was associated with floor of the mouth and tongue lesions (222). This is interesting because the long-recognized lesions of stomatitis nicotina (syn. smoker's palate) have a low malignant potential (except in reverse smokers; see below). These lesions predominantly affect the hard palate, producing hyperkeratosis without significant epithelial dysplasia, with plugging of the orifices of minor salivary glands and associated congestion and inflammation. Stomatitis nicotina, in the West, is most commonly associated with pipe smoking and cancers of the hard palate, and sometimes soft palate can arise. A distinction must be made from cancer arising in the palatine tonsil, which is a distinctly different disease, predominantly related to HPV.

Reverse smoking, with the lighted end inside the mouth, particularly among females, has been reported for many years from various parts of the world, and a variety of associated hyperkeratotic and inflammatory changes have been described. A high frequency of dysplastic, potentially malignant, lesions and of SCC has been reported among reverse chutta smokers in India along the coastal districts of Visakhapatnam, Srikakulam (170), East Godavari (223) and in rural Andhra Pradesh (105,224). Elsewhere in India, such as in the state of Goa (225), and in the Caribbean Islands (226), South America (227) and the Philippines (228), cancer is not so commonly reported among reverse smokers.

An analysis by the IARC of four cohort studies and 25 case-control studies of oral cancer shows that the risk of oral cancer decreases after smokers quit, and is lower in former smokers than current smokers. Risk declines with increasing duration of abstinence, in some studies reaching the level of never-smokers after 10 years. In this, smokers can find a good motivation for quitting (217).

Table 2.10 Odds ratios for oral and pharyngeal cancer in U.S. males, adjusted for race, age, study location, and respondent status

	Number of alcoholic drinks per week					
Smoking rate	**<1**	**1–4**	**5–14**	**15–29**	**30+**	**Total**
Nonsmoker	1.0	1.3	1.6	1.4	5.8	1.0
Short duration/former smoker	0.7	2.2	1.4	3.2	6.4	1.1 (0.7–1.7)
1–19/day for 20+ years	1.7	1.5	2.7	5.4	7.9	1.6 (0.9–2.7)
20–39/day for 20+ years	1.9	2.4	4.4	7.2	23.8	2.8 (1.8–4.3)
40+/day for 20+ years	7.4	0.7	4.4	20.2	37.7	4.4 (2.7–7.2)
Pipe and cigar only	0.6	1.0	3.7	4.7	23.0	1.9 (1.1–3.4)
Total	1.0	1.2 (0.7–2.0)	1.7 (1.0–2.7)	3.3 (2.0–5.4)	8.8 (5.4–14.1)	

Source: Blot et al. *Cancer Res* 1988;48(11):3282–7 (219).
Note: Ranges are 95% confidence intervals

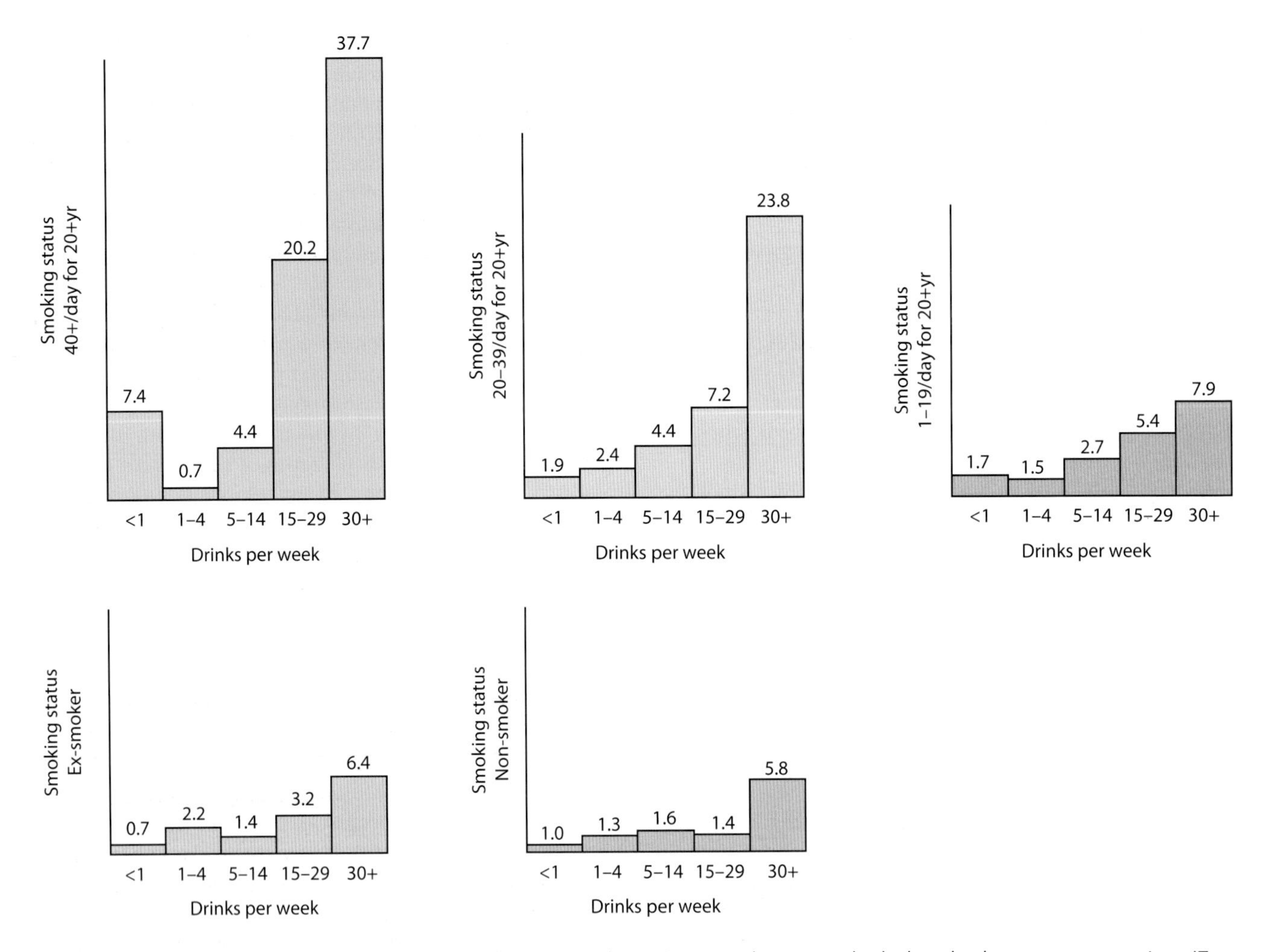

Figure 2.8 Relative risks of oral and pharyngeal cancer in the U.S.A. in relation to alcohol and tobacco consumption. (From the Cancer Research Campaign Factsheet 14.14, 1993; after Blot WJ. *Cancer Res* 1992;52(7 Suppl):2119s–23s (220).)

THE MECHANISMS OF TOBACCO CARCINOGENESIS

There is a vast literature, full coverage of which is outside the scope of this chapter. Over 300 potential carcinogens have been identified in tobacco smoke or in its water-soluble components, which can be expected to leach into saliva (205). A list of the confirmed carcinogens in tobacco smoke is given in Table 2.11 (229). The major and most studied of these are the aromatic hydrocarbon benzo(*a*) pyrene and the TSNAs, *N*′-nitrosonornicotine (NNN), *N*′-nitrosopyrrolidine (NPYR), *N*′-nitrosodimethylamine (NDMA) and 4-(methylnitrosamino)-l-(3-pyridyl)-l-butanone (NNK).

Since the 1920s, it has been known that PAHs were the carcinogenic agents present in tars, and this lies behind the tobacco industry's promotion of "low tar" smoking materials, while continuing to promote "full strength" brands. Benzo(a)pyrene is a powerful carcinogen and is found in amounts of 20–40 ng per cigarette (230). The role of *N*-nitrosamines is reviewed by Hoffman and Hecht (231). The mainstream smoke of a cigarette can contain 310 ng of NNN and 150 ng of NNK (232). In smoking materials these are generated primarily during pyrolysis, but are also produced endogenously from some forms of smokeless tobacco, quite high levels (a range of 20–890 mg/kg being reported by the IARC) being reached in saliva from, as we have seen, Sudanese toombak, for example (142). These agents act locally, on keratinocyte stem cells, and are absorbed and act in many other tissues in the body. They produce DNA adducts, principally *O*-6-methylguanine, and these interfere with the accuracy of DNA replication, leading to mutations, which thus contribute to the molecular chain of events leading to malignant transformation of a cell and its clonal derivatives. There is damage to all replicating cells, including those of the immune response (indeed, DNA adducts, or chromosomal instability, resulting from tobacco are most often studied in lymphocytes from peripheral blood).

The metabolism of these carcinogens usually involves oxygenation by p450 enzymes in cytochromes, and then conjugation, in which the enzyme glutathione-*S*-transferase (GST) is involved. Polymorphisms of the p450 and GST genes are currently under active study in the search for genetic markers of susceptibility to HNC, and indeed to

Table 2.11 A list of confirmed carcinogens in tobacco smoke

Class	Compound
Aromatic hydrocarbons	
Monocyclic	Benzene
Dicyclic and polycyclic	Benzo(*a*)anthracene
	Benzo(*b*)fluoranthene
	Benzo(*p*)fluoranthene
	Benzo(*k*)fluoranthene
	Benzo(*a*)pyrene
	Dibenzo(*a,h*)anthracene
	Dibenzo(*a,e*)pyrene
	Dibenzo(*a,l*)pyrene
	Dibenzo(*a,l*)pyrene
	Idenoil 1,2,3-*c*, dipyrene
	5-Methylchrysene
Aldehydes	Acetaldehyde
	Formaldehyde
Nitrogen compounds	
N-nitroso compounds	4-(Methylnitrosamino)-1-13-pyridyh-1-butanone (NNK)
	N-nitrosodimethylamine (NDMA)
	N-nitrodiethylamine
	N-nitroso-*N*-methylethylamine (NEMA)
	N-nitrosonornicotine (NNN)
	N-nitrosopyrrolidine (NPYR)
	N-nitrosopiperidine
	N-nitroso-*n*-propylamine
Polycyclic aza-arenes	Dibenzo(*a,h*)acridine
	Dibenzo(*a,j*)acridine
Miscellaneous nitrogen compounds	4-Aminobiphenyl ortho-anisidine
	1,1-Dimethylhydrazine
	2-Naphthylamine
	2-Nitropropane
	Urethane
Toxic heavy metals	Particularly Cu, Cd, Cr, Ni and Pb

Source: Davidson et al. *Arch Otolaryngol Head Neck Surg* 1993;119(11):1198–205 (229); Ren et al. *Anal Methods* 2017;9:4033–43 (727).

tobacco-related cancers at many other body sites (233,234). Not all results are consistent, however (235,236).

MARIJUANA USE AND HNC

Although still illegal in most countries, recreational use of various extracts of the plant *Cannabis sativa* is widespread. Cannabis may be smoked in three ways: as marijuana, which is derived from macerated flowers of the plant mixed with tobacco in a cigarette (under which circumstances the concentration of the active intoxicant, Δ9-tetrahydrocannabinol (THC), is of the order of 1%–6% w/v); as hashish, which is dried resin, placed in a pipe (THC 6%–10% w/v); or as hash oil (THC 30%–60%), which is derived from flowers of the female plant. When burned, the cannabinoids are aromatized and absorbed and a wide range of potential carcinogens is released, including PAHs, benzo(*a*)pyrene, phenols, phytosterols, acids and terpenes, including nitrosamines at similar levels to those found in tobacco smoke (237). There are, of course, the products of the tobacco itself.

There are a number of published case reports on aerodigestive tract cancer developing in marijuana users reviewed by Firth (238). There is also a series of 34 patients aged 20–40 treated in California and reported in the German literature (239). Firth himself describes oral cancer in 10/70 patients under the age of 45 years in Melbourne, Australia. Six of these 10 had smoked marijuana at some time, but this is comparable to the proportion of users reported in the young Australian population at that time. Although the majority of these cases have been in young patients, adequate details of tobacco and alcohol use are often missing, although some patients, such as the two with tongue cancers described by Caplan and Brigham in 1990, denied use of the latter two risk factors (240). A study of 173 cases and 176 cancer-free controls at Memorial Sloan-Kettering Cancer Centre in the early 1990s (241) showed ORs for marijuana use, controlling for age, sex, race, education, alcohol and cigarette consumption of 2.6 (1.1–6.6) compared with never users. This rose to OR 3.1 (1.0–9.7) in those aged 55 and under. There was a significant dose–response relationship. Recreational users of marijuana often also enjoy alcohol and tobacco, and tobacco usually forms part of the marijuana smoking mix. It is thus impossible at present to discern an independent risk for the smoking of cannabis products themselves; however, because of their composition, a theoretical risk certainly exists.

A later population-based case-control study on marijuana use and upper aerodigestive cancers and lung cancer conducted in Los Angeles, U.S.A., with 1,212 incident cancer cases and 1,040 cancer-free controls found no association with marijuana after adjusting for confounding variables, including cigarette smoking and alcohol drinking, even among daily users of more than 30 years (242). A later pooled analysis of 4,029 HNC cases and 5,015 controls in five case-control studies conducted in the U.S.A. and Latin America (INHANCE Consortium) found no elevation of risk and no increase in risk for increasing frequency, duration or cumulative consumption of marijuana smoking. Subanalyses focusing first on never tobacco users (493 cases and 1,813 controls) and then on nonsmokers who did not consume alcohol (237 cases and 887 controls) also found no association (243).

A more recent pooled analysis from the INHANCE Consortium, of 9 case-control studies with 1921 oropharyngeal cases, 356 oral tongue cases and 7,639 controls, found a slightly elevated risk for oropharyngeal cancer (OR = 1.24;

95% CI: 1.06–1.47) adjusted for demographic variables, smoking and alcohol use, which remained elevated among never users of tobacco or alcohol. However, when adjusted for HPV exposure, there was no elevated risk of cancer. The risk for tongue cancer was reduced when marijuana was used (OR = 0.47; 95% CI: 0.29–0.75) and remained so when only those who were never users of tobacco or alcohol were analyzed and even after adjusting for HPV exposure (244).

In summary, existing evidence indicates a low cancer risk from marijuana smoking alone. Little evidence exists on the risk of marijuana smoking for the development of OPMD, although (as with more conventional tobacco smokers) leukoedema, nicotinic stomatitis, denture-related stomatitis, angular cheilitis and median rhomboid glossitis are more common (245).

ALCOHOL AND ORAL AND OROPHARYNGEAL CANCER

In the early years of research on the co-carcinogenicity of alcohol, while sufficient evidence was found for the carcinogenicity of alcoholic beverages in humans, which did not depend on the type of alcoholic beverage, pure ethanol was not conclusively shown to be carcinogenic in animal studies (246). It was presumed to act in concert with other, more direct, carcinogens which may be present in the beverage as products of fermentation—so-called congeners—such as other alcohols and acetaldehyde—and with other environmental carcinogens, most notably those derived from tobacco. However, as the designs and conduct of animal studies improved, pure ethanol was found to be a carcinogen in its own right (247,248). As already discussed, most heavy alcohol consumers also use tobacco so that, from epidemiological data, it is difficult to separate the effects. Nevertheless, some cohort and case-control studies have found an increased risk of upper aerodigestive tract cancer associated with alcohol drinking in nonsmokers (249).

The interaction of alcohol use with smokeless tobacco has been difficult to study. This is because in some countries where smokeless tobacco or betel quid are used by alcohol drinkers there is social acceptance of the chewing practice, but not for the use of alcohol: indeed, it is even banned by law in many of these countries. This does not mean that alcohol is not consumed, however. Where it is used, it is likely to be produced illicitly, and may, as a result, contain impurities which add to the risk. In many parts of the Indian subcontinent, for example, local brews distilled from palm juice, "toddy," are widely available, particularly in rural areas where tobacco habitués may be unable to afford factory-made (and therefore quality-controlled) beverages, whether they be of national origin or imported. More recent studies in India demonstrate a clear role for alcohol (177,191,250,251).

The rise in oral cancer incidence in much of the Western world, discussed in Chapter 1, was found to be related to high alcohol consumption, indeed the consumption per capita in Europe was the highest in the world until the turn of the millennium, since when it has steadily declined and been overtaken by the countries of the former Soviet Republics (247,252,253) (Figure 2.9). In England and Wales, alcohol consumption per capita fell from the beginning of the twentieth century to the 1930s, but then more than doubled up to 1973, a phenomenon largely linked to economics. Using mortality from liver cirrhosis as a surrogate measure of damage to health from alcohol, Hindle (254) plotted trends in the U.K. over the twentieth century up until the early 1980s and showed how they match closely the trends in oral cancer mortality (Figure 2.10a).

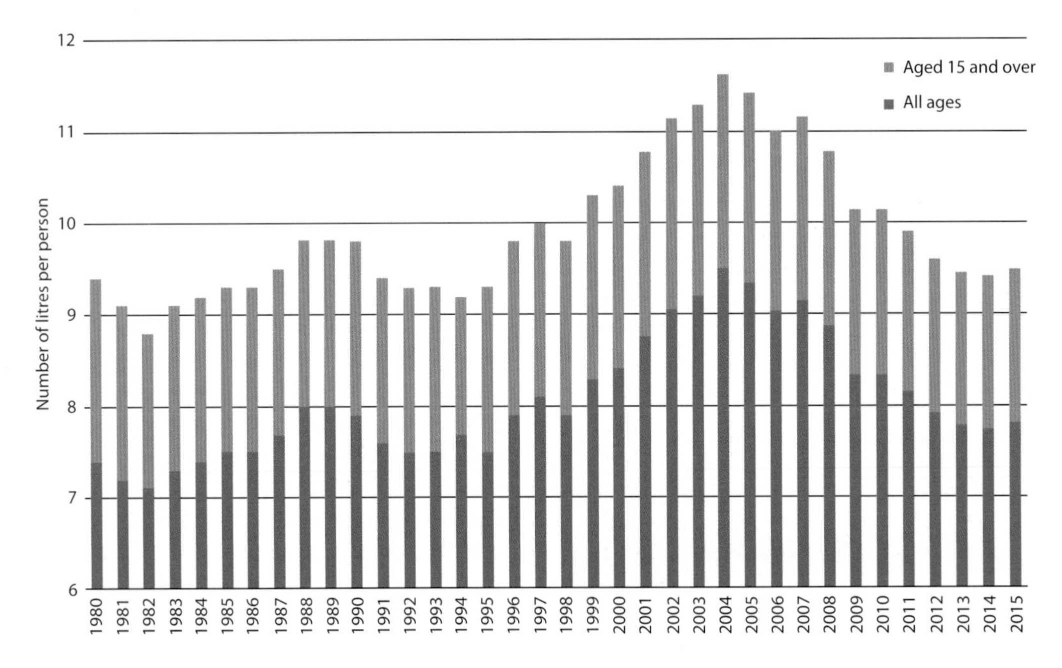

Figure 2.9 Consumption of alcohol, United Kingdom, 1980 to present. (Adapted from The British Beer & Pub Association, *Statistical Handbook*.)

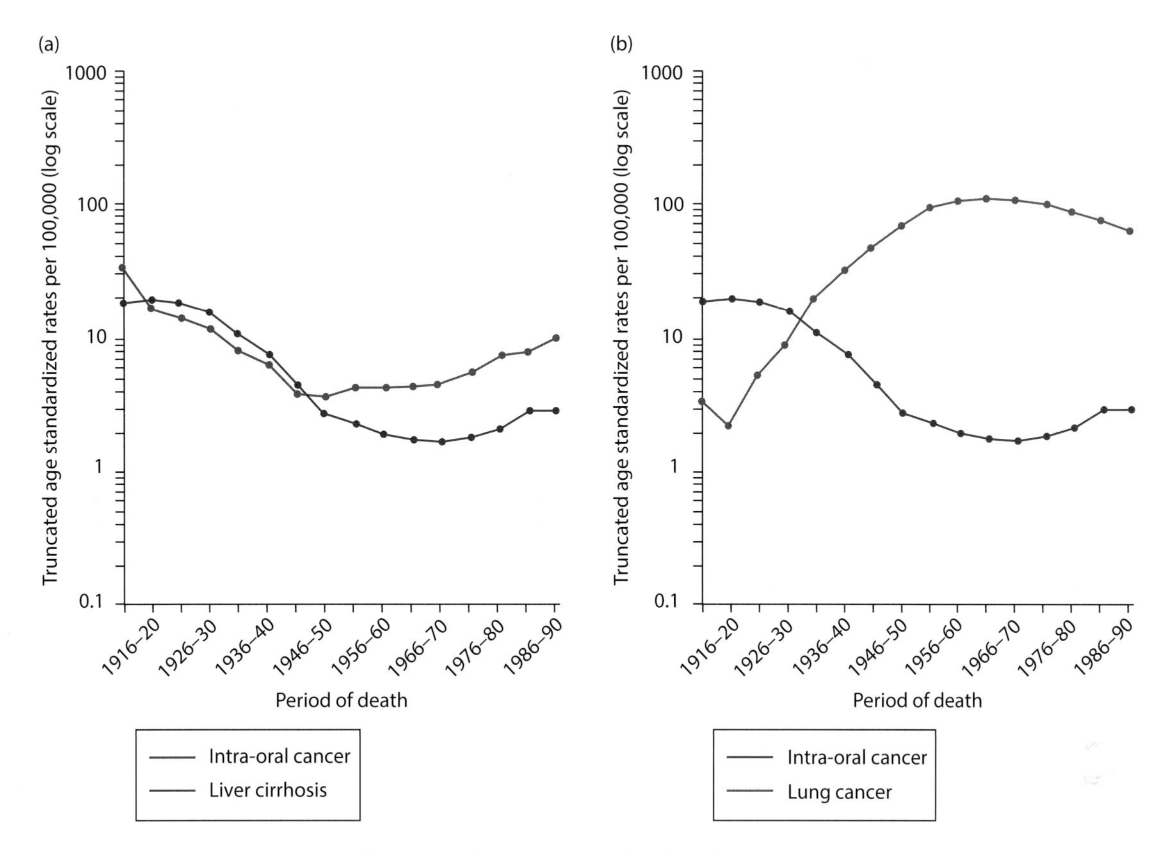

Figure 2.10 **(a)** Trends in the mortality of intra-oral cancer in England and Wales, compared to trends in mortality from liver cirrhosis, 1911–1990, for males aged 35–64. **(b)** Trends in the mortality of intra-oral cancer in England and Wales, compared to lung cancer mortality, 1911–1990, for males aged 35–64. (From Hindle I, Downer MC, Speight PM. *Community Dent Health* 2000;17(2):107–13 (254).)

One has to keep in mind that there is always a time lag between chronic use of a substance and the disease consequences. Taking deaths from lung cancer as a measure of damage due to tobacco smoking, it is striking how the trends for oral cancer move, both down and up in the twentieth century, in opposite directions (Figure 2.10b): this is strong circumstantial evidence that alcohol rather than tobacco was the major factor in the observed trends in oral cancer mortality and, by inference, incidence. Oral cancer mortality has been declining in parts of western Europe, such as France, Italy and Switzerland, since the early 1980s up to at least 2005 (255). This followed a decline in alcohol consumption that began in the early 1970s and continues downward in western Europe (253).

Also since the mid-1970s, per capita alcohol consumption has been increasing rapidly in Belarus, Moldova, Ukraine and Russia (former Soviet areas), and somewhat more slowly in the Western Pacific Region (253), including in Australia (256). According to the analysis by Praud et al., the alcohol attributable fractions for incidence and mortality of oral and pharyngeal cancers are among the highest globally for men in the Western Pacific and the South-East Asian Regions and for women in the Western Pacific and European Regions, as well as the former Soviet areas (257), all of which appears to be a consequence of increasing alcohol consumption in those areas and probably also increasing use of areca nut products in South-East Asia (258).

Some of the effect of alcohol is due to the presence of other carcinogens in the local environment. Apart from those derived from tobacco, beverage congeners include nitrosamines and impurities, the latter particularly in illicit local brews. Brown- or dark-colored drinks may be more dangerous in this respect and it might be useful, if suitable groups could be adequately matched, to compare the risks in consumers of, say, vodka (which is almost pure ethanol) with those who take predominantly whiskeys, which have many congeners (259). The epidemiological evidence shows that all forms of alcoholic drink are dangerous if heavily consumed (260), the most dangerous reflecting the predominant habit in the population under study. Thus, there is evidence for the role of beer (34,219,261–265), wine (264–268) and spirits (211,262,264,265,269,270), which some (270) took as evidence to implicate ethanol itself. Based on many past and current studies, IARC now declares ethanol in alcoholic beverages as a human carcinogen. This is because the carcinogenic effect does not appear to depend on the type of alcoholic beverage, the sufficient evidence that ethanol causes cancer in experimental animals and that acetaldehyde associated with the consumption of alcoholic beverages is also carcinogenic to humans, causing cancers of the upper aerodigestive tract and esophagus (247,248). Among alcoholic beverages, those with higher ethanol concentrations carry a higher risk for consuming the same volume,

Table 2.12 Odds ratios oral and pharyngeal cancer in males, according to alcohol habits: Northern Italy, 1984–89

	Oral cavity ($n = 157$)	Pharynx ($n = 134$)
Wine (drinks/week)		
<20	1	1
21–34	1.1 (0.5–2.3)	0.7 (0.3–1.6)
35–55	1.9 (0.9–3.7)	1.9 (0.9–3.7)
56–83	4.9 (2.6–9.5)	3.1 (1.6–6.1)
84+	8.5 (3.6–20.2)	10.9 (4.7–25.3)
Beer (drinks/week)		
0	1	1
1–13	1.0 (0.6–1.8)	0.5 (0.3–1.0)
14+	0.8 (0.5–1.4)	0.9 (0.5–1.5)
Spirits (drinks/week)		
0	1	1
1–6	0.7 (0.4–1.3)	0.4 (0.2–0.9)
7+	0.9 (0.6–1.3)	1.2 (0.8–1.8)
Total (drinks/week)		
<19	1	1
20–34	1.1 (0.5–2.5)	0.9 (0.4–2.0)
35–59	3.2 (1.6–6.2)	1.5 (0.8–3.1)
60+	3.4 (1.7–7.1)	3.6 (1.8–7.2)

Ranges are 95% confidence intervals.

Source: La Vecchia C et al. *Oral Oncol* 1997;33(5):302–12 (274).

spirits ranking highest, followed by wine and beer (271). The volume of a single drink of any of these types tends to contain the same amount of ethanol, with beer being consumed in larger amounts, wine intermediate amounts and spirits the smallest in a single drink. In an age where natural phytochemicals in grape wine are being praised for their cardiovascular benefits, it is important to note that there is some risk for oral cancer even with light wine drinking, which increases substantially when combined with smoking, suggesting that these phytochemicals in wine are below concentrations required for anti-cancer activity (272). A report from Uruguay, comparing 471 cases of oral and pharyngeal cancer with 471 controls, showed slightly higher ORs for "pure hard liquor" drinking (OR = 3.6; 95% CI: 2.1–6.2) than for "pure wine" drinking (OR = 2.1; 95% CI: 1.3–3.3) (273).

Some of the best evidence for the very significant role of alcohol again comes from the studies in Northern Italy, all reviewed by La Vecchia (92,268,274,275). Table 2.12 extracts data from La Vecchia et al. (274) deriving OR estimates from logistic regression adjusted for age, area of residence, years of education, occupation and smoking habits. It is notable from these data that the 95% CIs for ORs for all beverages for oral and pharyngeal cancer do not exceed unity until the total alcohol consumption per week is quite high—above 55 drinks per week. This is consistent with the earlier data from Paris (276) (Table 2.13). The recent review by Goldstein et al. (277), covering case-control and cohort studies from around the world, reported a clear and consistent relationship across studies with alcohol consumption and HNC. For example, a study pooling data from Europe and North and South America (278) shows similar results to previous studies. Note that, in these studies, even when the tobacco effect is controlled for, heavy alcohol consumption, such as 4 or more drinks per day, itself produces considerable risks. It is the super-multiplicative synergism already described that is really dangerous. It is also worth observing that self-reported alcohol consumption tends to be underestimated (279), implying that alcohol may be an even more important factor than the published data indicate. Table 2.14, again from the Italian studies (92), compares upper aerodigestive sites: the tobacco/alcohol synergism appears to be super-multiplicative for the oral cavity and pharynx, between additive and multiplicative for the esophagus, and close to additive for the larynx which, simplistically, relates to both agents being present in the mouth, alcohol being present in the esophagus with smaller amounts of tobacco products, and tobacco products contacting the larynx with fewer constituents of the beverage.

A cohort study by Boeing et al. (280) [as reviewed in Goldstein et al. (277)] showed a clear dose–response relationship for cancer of the oral cavity, pharynx and esophagus with the amount of alcohol consumed daily (g/day) over the follow-up period: amounts over 30 g per day caused a significant increase in cases (see Table 2.15).

In several western European countries, where a standard drink contains 10 g ethanol, interpreting the table with data

Table 2.13 Relative risk of developing upper aerodigestive tract cancer by alcohol and tobacco habits: Paris registry 1975–82[a]

	Tobacco (g/day; adjusted for alcohol)[b]			Alcohol (g/day[c] adjusted for tobacco)[b]		
	10–19	20–29	≥30	40–99	100–159	≥160
Oropharynx	4.0	7.6	15.2	2.6	15.2	70.3
Hypopharynx	7.1	12.6	35.1	3.3	28.6	143.1
Supraglottis	6.1	19.6	48.8	2.6	11.0	42.1
Glottis	3.0	9.5	28.4	0.8§	1.5§	6.1
Epilarynx	1.7§	6.7	14.8	1.9§	18.7	101.4
Lips	4.5	9.7	21.5	1.8§	4.9	10.5
Mouth	3.9	8.6	15.4	2.7	13.1	70.3

Source: Brugere J et al. *Cancer* 1986;57(2):391–5 (276).

[a] Confidence limits excluded for clarity, but all except § do not cross unity and are thus significant at the 5% level.

[b] 9 g tobacco/day and <40 g alcohol/day taken as RR of 1 respectively.

[c] 15 g alcohol = 1 unit.

from Boeing et al., people who regularly consumed 3 or more drinks per day could be said to be at a significantly higher risk of developing cancer of the oral cavity, pharynx or esophagus.

The IARC Monograph 100E of 2012 summarized evidence from six recent cohort studies from different parts of the world published between 2007 and 2009 that showed alcohol was a risk factor for HNC at higher levels of consumption (248). (See table at http://monographs.iarc.fr/ENG/Monographs/vol100E/100E-06-Table2.3.pdf.) For example, a study in Singapore found a significantly elevated relative risk of cancer of the oropharynx for >7 drinks per week, adjusted for smoking and other confounders (281). Another study in the U.S.A. found a significantly elevated relative risk for cancer of the oral cavity and for cancer of oropharynx and hypopharynx for >3 drinks per day for women and for men, adjusted for smoking and other variables (282). A recent estimate of AR found that 44.7% of oral cavity and pharyngeal cancers in men and 17.2% in women could be attributed to alcohol drinking, using WHO data on alcohol consumption, relative risks from cohort studies and cancer deaths from GLOBOCAN (257,283).

Table 2.14 Odds ratios for upper aerodigestive cancer in males according to smoking and drinking habits: Northern Italy, 1986–1989

	Alcohol intake (drinks/week)			
Smoking practice	**<35**	**35–69**	**60+**	**Total**
Oral cavity/pharynx				
Nonsmokers	1	1.6	2.3	1
Light	3.1	5.4	10.9	3.7
Intermediate	10.9	26.6	36.4	14.1
Heavy	17.6	40.2	79.6	25.0
Total	1	2.3	3.4	
Larynx				
Nonsmokers	1	1.6	–	1
Light	0.9	5.0	5.4	1.0
Intermediate	4.5	7.1	9.5	5.4
Heavy	6.1	10.4	11.7	6.7
Total	1	1.4	2.8	
Esophagus				
Nonsmokers	1	0.8	7.9	1
Light	1.1	7.9	9.4	2.5
Intermediate	2.7	8.8	16.7	4.0
Heavy	6.4	11.0	17.5	6.6
Total	1	3.1	5.7	

Source: Franceschi S et al. *Cancer Res* 1990;50(20):6502–7 (92).

Table 2.15 Results of a cohort study on lifelong consumption of alcohol and cancer of the oral cavity, pharynx and esophagus in western Europe by Boeing et al. (280)

Lifelong alcohol (g/day)	Cases	Hazard RR	95% CI
No alcohol	4	1.0	–
>0–30	83	1.21	0.43–3.40
>30–60	20	3.17	1.00–10.05
>60	17	9.22	2.75–30.93

Source: From Boeing H, Patterns EWGoD. *IARC Sci Publ* 2002;156:151–4 (280).
Note: Adjusted for follow-up time, sex, education, BMI, vegetable and fruit consumption, tobacco smoking, energy intake.

MECHANISMS BY WHICH ALCOHOL CONTRIBUTES TO CARCINOGENESIS

There are several ways in which alcohol is thought to contribute to HNC, by both local and systemic mechanisms. The IARC Monograph No. 44 (1988) deals comprehensively with the evidence up to the late 1980s (246). The mechanisms described there are as follows:

- There is now clear evidence that ethanol increases the permeability of the oral mucosa to water itself (284,285) and to many water-soluble molecules, probably including important carcinogens: indeed, increased passage of nitrosonornicotine has been demonstrated in *in vitro* experiments (286,287). The effect is greater at 15% than at 5%, but is not further enhanced at 40% ethanol, suggesting that the mechanism is related to rearrangement of the epithelial permeability barrier rather than to lipid extraction (288). This means that there will be increased uptake of alcohol itself, and of other carcinogens (such as acetaldehyde in alcoholic drinks and tobacco smoke, TSNAs and other carcinogens from tobacco), with enhanced systemic effects. It also implies a solvent action of ethanol on keratinocyte membranes with likely enhanced penetration of carcinogens into proliferating cells where they may exert a direct mutagenic action (289). A dehydrating effect may contribute (290). Recent animal experiments in which rats were fed ethanol by a stomach tube showed an indirect effect on the permeability of the oral mucosa, because there was a decreased synthesis of lipids contributing to the intercellular permeability barrier, perhaps because of liver damage (291).
- The immediate metabolite of ethanol is acetaldehyde. Some of this is formed locally and damages cells (292). Indeed, considerable amounts of acetaldehyde can be found in saliva after moderate alcohol consumption, owing to the action of bacterial alcohol dehydrogenases (293). Production is significantly reduced after three days' use of an antiseptic mouthwash (chlorhexidine), perhaps helping to explain why poor oral hygiene appears to be an independent risk factor for oral cancer in some studies (294–296). Those genetically predisposed to be more rapid acetylators have been demonstrated to be at increased risk of cancer in one recent U.S. study (297).
- Alcoholic liver disease is common in heavy drinkers and this reduces the detoxification of active carcinogens (249).
- Alcohol is high in calories, which suppresses appetite in heavy drinkers. Those with a serious drinking problem become socially fractured, and many choose to spend available cash on drink rather than food. All of this contributes to inadequate diet. Metabolism is further damaged by liver disease. As a result, nutritional deficiencies are common (298), and, as discussed below, these contribute significantly to lowered resistance to cancer (249).

Further information on mechanisms is provided in the later IARC monographs, vols. 96 (2010) and 100E (2012) (247,248) (see: vol 96, pp 1166–67; 1205, 1277–78)

- The presence of alcohol can induce enzymes that activate tobacco carcinogens in tissues (299).
- Ethanol in the tissues can cause oxidative stress and inflammation resulting in DNA damage and eventually promote malignancy (300).
- Acetaldehyde produced from ethanol can cause DNA adducts, interstrand crosslinks and mutations.

IARC Monograph 96 includes evidence up to 2007 (247, p 1278) and provides an overall evaluation: "There is sufficient evidence in experimental animals for the carcinogenicity of ethanol. There is sufficient evidence in experimental animals for the carcinogenicity of acetaldehyde." The overall evaluation was that "Alcoholic beverages are carcinogenic to humans (Group 1). Ethanol in alcoholic beverages is carcinogenic to humans (Group 1)." While acetaldehyde levels are appreciable in some foods and beverages, such as yoghurt and fruit juices (301), it is clearly the presence of alcohol that is responsible for it entering into oral tissues. Unsurprisingly, alcoholic patients are at special risk for HNC, particularly at sites in direct contact with alcohol (302). If alcohol users quit, however, they reduce their risk, reaching the level of never-drinkers after 20 or more years (303). As with tobacco use, screening and brief interventions for reducing alcohol consumption can effectively be introduced into dental practice and can be linked to screening and counseling for tobacco (304).

MOUTHWASH USE AND RISK OF ORAL CANCER

Since 1979, concern has been expressed about the possibility of high alcohol-containing mouthwashes contributing to oral cancer, when 10 of 11 nonsmoking, nondrinking patients with oral cancer (2 males and 9 females) in the U.S.A. were found to be long-term mouthwash users (305). This was quickly followed up in two case-control studies. The first, among women in North Carolina (206 cases of oral or pharyngeal cancer and 352 controls), found no increased risk when adjusted for snuff-dipping and smoking, but risk increased among women who did not use tobacco (RR = 1.94; 95% CI: 0.8–4.7): no consistent dose–response relationship was observed (306). The second study took 571 cases from the six-city study in the U.S.A. and matched them with 6,047 controls without tobacco-related disease. This showed that daily use of mouthwash was associated with increased risk among females only, regardless of alcohol consumption and/or tobacco use, but the risks were small and showed no dose–response relationship. The study confirmed the strong risks associated with alcohol drinking and tobacco use and, because of confounding by these much more potent factors, these authors concluded that no causal association could be inferred for mouthwash use (307).

Drawing 866 cases from registries in California, Georgia and New Jersey, U.S.A., and matching with 1,249 controls, Winn et al. re-examined the issue some years later (308). They found increased risks associated with the regular use of mouthwash, of 40% for men and 60% for women, after adjusting for alcohol and tobacco use. Risks generally increased in proportion to frequency and duration of mouthwash use and were only apparent when the alcohol content of the mouthwash exceeded 25%: the effects were again stronger in women, revealing a maximum OR of 2.4 (1.5–3.9) in those who began regular use before the age of 20 years. This publication raised considerable discussion in several countries, for example, the U.K. (309), many clinicians expressing concern because, in the West at least, smokers may be inclined to use these products heavily to disguise the smell of tobacco. However, in most of the published studies, rarely do ORs exceed 2 with, in most cases, 95% CIs spanning unity.

A later study, again by Winn et al., with 342 cases and 521 controls in Puerto Rico, showed no increased risk of oral cancer associated with the use of mouthwashes containing >25% ethanol (310). Overall, the risk has to be regarded as small and pales into insignificance compared with those due to tobacco use, heavy alcohol drinking and poor diet. Indeed, critical analysis of all the published literature, including several reviews (311–313), has led the British, Canadian and American Dental Associations (to name just three) to regard the risks, if any, as insignificant and to endorse certain products of this type for control of dental plaque and gingivitis. A meta-analysis conducted in 2012 (314) on mouthwash use and oral cancer, using 18 studies (including 5 published since 2001), found no statistically significant associations between mouthwash use and risk of oral cancer and no trend with daily use. A comment on this paper opined that confounding by smoking and alcohol consumption may be too high for even large-scale studies and sophisticated statistics to detect a small risk posed by mouthwashes containing alcohol (315).

A newer pooled analysis of 8981 cases of HNC and 10,090 controls from 12 case-control studies with comparable information on mouthwash use in the INHANCE consortium (316) found no elevated risk for mouthwash use compared to never use for HNC in general, but slightly elevated risk was found for two subsites: oral cavity (OR = 1.11; 95% CI: 1.00–1.23) and oropharynx (OR = 1.28; 95% CI: 1.06–1.56). For long-term mouthwash use (i.e., >35 years), there was a slight measured association with HNC (OR = 1.15; 95% CI: 1.01–1.30; $p = 0.01$), and comparable to those who used mouthwash more than once a day for >35 years (OR = 1.31; 95% CI: 1.09–1.58; $p < 0.001$), and the mouthwash more than twice a day for >35 years (OR = 1.75; 95% CI: 1.25–2.48). These ORs were adjusted for age, sex, education, tobacco smoking and alcohol drinking. The authors admitted that decoupling mouthwash use from smoking and heavy alcohol use was difficult.

Currie and Farah (317) performed a review of 15 case-control studies in 2014, of which 9 contained evidence supporting an association between mouthwash use and the development of SCC and 6 containing evidence against such an association. They also encapsulated 11 reviews examining the evidence for such associations. Towards the end of their paper, the authors pointed out that the use of mouthwash containing alcohol reduces the contribution of oral flora to the formation of salivary acetaldehyde; nevertheless, those who use such a product briefly show higher levels of salivary acetaldehyde than those who use a nonalcoholic mouthwash. Alcohol-containing mouthwash also increases the permeability of the oral mucosa to carcinogens from tobacco smoke and may induce cytochrome P450 2E1, a (potential) step in carcinogenesis. Smokers are more likely than nonsmokers to use mouthwash to remove the odor of tobacco smoke from the mouth. Mouthwash users who smoke are at greater risk of oral cancer than nonsmoker mouthwash users due to their tobacco use. Currie and Farah pointed out that discovery of an oral lesion might motivate someone to use mouthwash, which in turn might further damage the lesion and make it more dangerous. They concluded that there is a lack of consensus among researchers on a possible relationship between mouthwash containing alcohol and the development of oral squamous cell carcinoma (OSCC). They proposed that this was largely due to poor design and a lack of comparability in the design of the epidemiological studies and limited studies on mechanistic aspects *in vivo* and *in vitro*. They suggested that before any definite conclusion can be reached, it would be wise for clinicians to promote the use of nonalcoholic mouthwashes and discourage the long-term use of those containing high concentrations of alcohol.

Hashim et al. (318) cautioned that mouthwash use is not an essential part of good oral hygiene, while daily tooth brushing (with a fluoridated toothpaste) is. In fact, if mouthwash is used to replace brushing teeth it constitutes bad oral hygiene. Skillful brushing should be adequate for keeping volumes of dental plaque below dangerous levels, but some remain of the opinion that the use of mouthwash once or twice a day can safely contribute to that effort (319). We take the opposite view. Regular use of broad-spectrum antiseptics damages the health-associated oral flora, as well as any potential pathogens present: It disturbs the oral ecology and is not good medicine. In any case, it seems prudent to keep the alcohol content as low as possible in formulating the product (alcohol is necessary to dissolve some of the active antimicrobial agents) and certainly to state the composition on the label.

Incidentally, the levels of alcohol in proprietary mouthwashes are unlikely to influence legal proceedings based on exhaled air analyses (320).

ORAL CANCER IN NONUSERS OF TOBACCO AND ALCOHOL

Because of the overwhelming evidence for the role of tobacco and alcohol, there is great interest in that minority of patients who develop oral cancer in the apparent absence of one or both of these risk factors. Clearly, other factors are operating, as they presumably are in the case of young people who develop these cancers with no exposure, or certainly without the decades of exposure usually associated with high-risk individuals. Lifelong abstainers from both of these prevalent social customs are, in numerical terms, unusual people, and little is known about their wider lifestyle: for example, do they have unusual dietary practices? In addition, we may suspect hereditary, and other environmental factors (including viruses see below). Thus, we have no understanding of the etiology, but differences have been described in the natural history of the disease in these cohorts. Rich and Radden (321) found that Australian patients who had never used tobacco or alcohol developed their carcinomas particularly on the buccal mucosa and upper alveolar ridge, and the Amsterdam data (218) were consistent with this. Hodge et al., in a Kentucky population, described 33/945 cases (3.4%) of HNC in nonusers of tobacco (322). Amongst nonusers of both tobacco and alcohol, there was a definite majority of women, especially older women: this cohort had comparatively few cancers of the floor of the mouth. Other findings in nonuser American cohorts are as follows (323):

- A low incidence of second primaries;
- A higher level of differentiation of the primary lesions;
- A lower frequency of associated oral candidiasis;
- Importantly—*no better overall survival.*

Tan et al. have presented a retrospective study of 59 tobacco nonusers with SCCs of the head and neck and found that, as with the above studies, significantly more women were involved (324). Interestingly, this group comprised significantly more patients with tongue cancers and a relatively *high* rate of second primaries in the head and neck. Most importantly, this group had a high exposure to ETS (passive smoking). None of these studies on the rare cases that occur in nonusers of tobacco and/or alcohol dilute the evidence that these substances are far and away the major risk factors. Viral infections and nutritional inadequacies, which are addressed next, are the main hypothetical factors in this group of patients. Much more research is needed in this intriguing area.

DIET AND NUTRITION IN THE ETIOLOGY OF HNC

Interest here relates to the roles of iron, of the antioxidant or free-radical scavenging vitamins A, C and E, and to trace elements such as zinc and selenium, for which there is evidence of a protective effect. The interest in iron goes back to the beginning of the twentieth century, since the recognition (simultaneously in Scandinavia and in England) of a high incidence of upper gastrointestinal tract cancer in middle-aged women suffering from chronic anemia, with dysphagia and glossitis and atrophy of associated mucosae—the Plummer–Vinson or Patterson–Brown–Kelly syndrome. Both of the original papers were published in 1919. In animals rendered experimentally iron deficient by venesection and a low-iron diet, there is contradictory evidence of the effect on epithelial cell kinetics, with some studies showing increased turnover, theoretically increasing the risk of mutational error (325) and others a decrease (326). There is agreement, however, that this results in epithelial atrophy (327) and increased cancer risk, clearly shown in such animals when challenged with chemical carcinogens (328). On the other hand, there is surprisingly little information on the risks of oral cancer associated with anemia and sideropaenia in human studies: certainly, anemia of chronic blood loss following hookworm infections and other chronic diseases is common in those parts of south Asia where oral cancer prevails, as is mucosal atrophy—which presumably makes tissues more susceptible to tobacco carcinogens (326).

There is a large literature on other possible dietary correlates with upper aerodigestive tract cancer, summary reviews of which have been published by La Vecchia et al. (329). Studies have looked at broad food groups, specific food items, vitamins and other specific micronutrients and, of course, alcohol, which is not discussed further here.

FOOD GROUPS

Of 13 case-control studies that have examined the association between fruit and vegetable consumption and oral/pharyngeal cancer, 11 report a meaningful inverse association (330–332). The reduction in risk with fruits, from the highest to the lowest intake, varies from 20% to 80% (333) and is evident for tongue, mouth and pharynx (334).

Table 2.16 Odds ratios for oral and pharyngeal cancer according to certain food groups: Pordone, Italy, 1984–1989

	Odds ratios for frequency of consumption by tercile[a]	
	Intermediate	High
Pasta or rice	1.1	1.4
Polenta	1.2	1.8
Cheese	1.0	1.7
Eggs	1.4	1.6
Pulses	1.4	1.9
Carrots	0.8	0.7
Fresh tomatoes	0.7	0.5
Green peppers	0.6	0.5

Source: From La Vecchia C et al. *Oral Oncol* 1997;33(5):302–12 (274).
Note: This table includes corrections for age, sex, occupation, smoking and drinking.
[a] Low consumption is reference category with OR set at 1.

With vegetables, the results are less consistent. There is a relationship between total consumption and reduced risk (335,336), and this is most strongly associated with vegetables rich in carotenes (79,267). Again, some of the best results come from the northern Italian studies. Table 2.16 summarizes the data from the high-risk area in Northern Italy, based on 302 cases and 699 controls. In this group, high intake of maize revealed two to three times the risk for low intake of maize, possibly because it is less nutritious than other grains and may cause deficiencies of B-group vitamins. In Milan, an area of intermediate risk, high intakes of milk, meat and cheese were associated with reduced risk, somewhat surprisingly in view of the well-established increased risk of these foods for bowel, breast and other cancers; however, these factors probably indicate the better-nourished individuals. Again, in Milan, carrots (OR 0.4 for highest versus lowest tercile), green vegetables (OR 0.6) and fresh fruit (OR 0.2) were strongly protective, and the effect is clear when expressed in terms of β-carotene intake. A strong protective effect is evident for carotenoids and vitamin C from vegetables and fruit, and of fiber intake in oral cancer risk in an important study from Beijing, China (337).

La Vecchia et al. (274) estimate that approximately 15% of cases of oral and pharyngeal cancers in Europe can be attributed to dietary deficiencies or imbalances, perhaps accounting for 5000 avoidable deaths per year. Artificial supplementation with micronutrients is discussed in Chapter 23. However, it should be noted that obtaining these nutrients from natural foods is more effective than taking dietary supplements. The beneficial effect of high intakes of vegetable and fruits is confirmed, particularly in heavy smokers and alcohol drinkers, in another North-East Italian study (338). On the contrary, a multinational study (339) by International Agency of Research on Cancer showed that this protective effect is restricted only to ever-drinkers and ever-smokers; other studies point to nondrinkers, nonsmokers as well as former smokers and moderate drinkers also benefitting (274,338,340).

DENTAL FACTORS IN THE ETIOLOGY OF ORAL CANCER

Some of the other emerging risk factors, which have been proposed, are chronic irritation from dental factors (poor dentition, trauma due to ill-fitted partial/complete dentures or from a sharp/broken tooth), chronic ulcers, chronic oral infection like periodontitis and low frequency of oral hygiene (79,210,269,341–346). However, the causative role of chronic trauma of the oral mucosa (CTOM) on oral carcinogenesis remains controversial. Some authors proposed it as a cause; on the other hand, some suggest that it is a result of an increase in the volume of tumor (342). In contrast to Lockhart, several case-control studies exhibit a positive relationship between poor oral health status and cancer of the oral cavity (261,341,347–349). However, the nature of association with dental variation is difficult to pinpoint, because of the confounding effect of lifestyle determinants in addition to the socioeconomic and cultural characteristics.

CHRONIC TRAUMA OF THE ORAL MUCOSA

CTOM is the result of a repeated mechanical irritative action of an intra-oral injurious agent. Defective teeth (malpositioned or with sharp or rough surfaces because of decay or fractures), ill-fitting dentures (sharp or rough surfaces, lack of retention, stability or overextended flanges) and/or parafunctional habits (e.g., oral mucosa biting or sucking, tongue interposition or thrusting), acting individually or together, could all be responsible of this mechanical irritation (350).

CTOM could generate lesions on a healthy mucosa or intensify previous oral diseases in addition to its role as promoter or progressor factor of oral neoplasms. Epidemiological (341,347,351,352) and laboratory studies (353,354) described a possible causal relationship between CTOM and cancer of lip plus oral cavity. The mechanism by which CTOM is thought to contribute to carcinogenesis is yet not clearly identified.

A meta-analysis conducted by Manoharan et al. on ill-fitting dentures and oral cancer showed an increased risk by nearly four times (pooled OR = 3.90; 95% CI: 2.48–6.13) (355). The authors also found that the studies that investigated the association between denture use and cancer did not clearly mention if they were investigating removable partial dentures or full dentures. However, the authors reported a slightly increased likelihood of oral cancer with any denture use (OR = 1.42; 95% CI: 1.01–1.99). A major study from Brazil, based on 717 cases of cancer of the mouth, pharynx and larynx, and 1434 controls, reports an OR of 2.3 (95% CI: .2–4.6) for cancer of the mouth and, interestingly, of 2.7 (95% CI: 1.1–6.2) for cancer of the pharynx with a history of oral sores from ill-fitting dentures (341). This latter study also showed that less than daily toothbrushing was associated with an increased risk of tongue neoplasms of 2.1 (95% CI: 1.0–4.3), or of other parts of the mouth of 2.4 (95% CI: 1.0–5.4)—in all cases the logistic regression analyses being carefully controlled for factors such as age, sex, tobacco and alcohol use, ethnicity, income and education. Microorganisms from dental plaque may contribute to chemical carcinogenesis by elaboration of toxins, for example, nitrosating enzymes: it is also likely that infrequent or inadequate oral hygiene fails to dilute tobacco-derived and other carcinogens present. Data from the study in northern Sweden (144) and the U.S.A. (351) also show no increased risk associated with fillings, dentures or fixed prostheses—nor, importantly, in the Swedish study, with experience of dental radiographic procedures.

CHRONIC PERIODONTITIS

Chronic periodontitis is a multifactorial, opportunistic inflammation of the periodontium mostly caused by gram-negative, anaerobic bacteria. Microbial toxins, proteases and endotoxins are secreted, inducing an inflammation through stimulation of monocytes with further excretion of mediators such as prostaglandin E2, thromboxane B2, interleukin-1, 6, 8 and 17, tumor necrosis factor and collagenases (356,357). An induction of OSCC by such chronic bacterial inflammation appears possible since the involved inflammatory mediators, cytokines and bacterial toxins have been shown to have a potential for promoting malignant transformation of keratinocytes *in vitro* (356,358,359).

MICROBES IN THE ETIOLOGY AND PATHOGENESIS OF ORAL AND OROPHARYNGEAL CANCER

There has been an explosion of interest in, and knowledge of, the microorganisms that live on every surface of human beings—both external and internal. This has been fed by the ability to use next-generation sequencing (NGS) to detect, identify and quantitate microbial DNA, as well as an increase in speed and dramatic decrease in costs. There are multiple international collaborations using metagenomics to explore the microbiome, such as those co-ordinated by the U.S. National Institutes of Health: The Human Microbiome Project (https://commonfund.nih.gov/hmp), with a newer international consortium (http://www.human-microbiome.org/). The oral microbiome is one of the prioritized areas, the others being the nasal, skin, gut and urinogenital tract microbiomes.

Estimates of the ratio of prokaryotic organisms (bacteria and fungi) to the number of eukaryotic cells which make up a human body range from 10^9:1 to 10^{14}:1. This ratio likely reflects the much greater number of genes in the human microbiome than in the human genome, not necessarily the number of actual cells. Symbiosis between these microorganisms and the host is essential to health. Damage to the health-associated microflora (e.g., by the overuse of disinfectants and antibiotics) is damaging to human and animal health, hence, the earlier comment on the dangers of disinfectant mouthwashes to oral health. Many of these organisms have never been cultured. So, the adage, "one does not know what one does not know" is apt. It is naïve to believe that we know all about the bacteria that cause dental caries because only about 300 of the 1,000 or so bacterial species that inhabit the human mouth have been cultured, and their physiology and potential pathogenicity studied.

The microorganisms of the mouth comprise, in increasing size, viruses, bacteria, fungi and occasionally multicellular parasites. The latter can cause specific diseases (360), but discussion of them is outside our present purposes as there is no evidence that they play a role in HNC. As contributors to the etiology of human cancers, viruses have been studied for decades. Certain fungi, notably *Candida* spp., have long been associated with oral cancer. NGS and related technologies have rapidly exploded our information base. *Metagenomics* is the field that identifies the organisms present in an environmental sample, using their genomes: for example, soil, water, mouths with or without cancer (or any other disease). *Transcriptomics* quantifies the mRNA levels of genes of interest so one knows what microbes are actually doing in the sample; *proteomics* measures the entire set of proteins, produced as gene products of course, that are produced or modified by an organism or system, which allows interpretation of function; *metabolomics* puts the evidence together to try to understand how a multicellular system, in this case the microbiome, is really functioning and interacting with its host.

VIRUSES AND HNC

It is well established that viruses are etiological agents of human cancers. To date, there are seven known human

Table 2.17 Characteristics and manifestations of the *Herpesviridae* family

Subfamily	Characteristics	Viruses	Diseases
α-Herpesvirinae	Variable host range, short reproductive cycle, destruction of infected cells, latent infection primarily in ganglia	Herpes simplex virus 1 (HSV-1)	Orofacial herpetic blistering, oral cancer
		Herpes simplex virus 2 (HSV-2)	Orofacial herpetic blistering Genital herpes, cervical cancer
		Varicella-zoster virus (VZV) (HSV-3)	Chicken pox, shingles Postherpetic neuralgia
β-Herpesvirinae	Restricted host range, long reproductive cycle, latent infection in secretory cells, lymphoreticular cells, kidneys and other tissues	Cytomegalovirus (CMV) (HHV-5)	Oral ulcers, retinitis/uveítis
		Human herpesvirus 6 (HSV-6)	Exanthem subitum (roseola) Encephalomyelitis
		Human herpesvirus 7 (HHV-7)	Exanthem subitum (roseola)
γ-Herpesvirinae	Infects specifically B or T cells, latent and lytic reproductive cycles	Epstein-Barr virus (EBV) (HHV-4) [Lymphocryptovirus or γ-1 herpesvirus]	Infectious mononucleosis Many B-cell lymphomata Oral cancer
		Human herpesvirus 8 (HHV-8, KSHV) [Rhadinovirus or γ-2 herpesvirus]	Kaposi's sarcoma (KS) Castleman's disease Primary effusion lymphoma (PEL)

Table 2.18 Cancers caused by viruses with sufficient and limited evidence according to the IARC criteria

Virus	Cancers with sufficient evidence	Cancers with limited evidence
EBV	Nasopharyngeal carcinoma Burkitt's lymphoma Immunesuppression-related non-Hodgkin lymphoma Extranodal NK/T-cell lymphoma (nasal type) Hodgkin lymphoma	Gastric carcinoma Lympho-epithelioma-like carcinoma Plasmablastic lymphoma Diffuse large B-cell/immunoblastic lymphoma
HHV-8 (KSHV)	Kaposi's sarcoma Primary effusion lymphoma (classic and solid variants) Plasmablastic lymphomas	Extracavitary KSHV-positive solid lymphoma Early PEL Germinotrophic lymphoproliferation
"High-Risk HPV" HPV-16, 18, 31, 33,35, 39, 45, 51, 52, 56, 58 and 59	Cancers of the cervix, vulva, vagina, penis, anus, oral cavity, oropharynx and tonsil	Cancer of the larynx
HBV	Hepatocellular carcinoma	
HCV	Hepatocellular carcinoma	Oral verrucous carcinoma Oral squamous cell carcinoma
HTLV-1	Adult T-cell leukemia, lymphoma	
MCPyV	Merkel cell carcinoma	

Source: Adapted and modified from Speicher DJ et al. *Oral Dis* 2016;22(Suppl 1):181–92 (368).

"oncoviruses" (aka cancer-causing viruses). In the head and neck, most viral infections manifesting as oral diseases or neoplasms are caused by human herpesviruses (HHVs) and/or HPV (Tables 2.17 and 2.18). Hepatitis virus, particularly hepatitis B virus (HBV) and hepatitis C virus (HCV), are etiological agents of hepatocarcinoma, but their role in oral cancers is speculative at best. Low viral loads of Merkel cell polyomavirus (MCPyV) have been detected in oral and maxillofacial tumors, and a solitary case of Merkel cell carcinoma (MCC) in the oral cavity has been reported, but the role of this novel polyomavirus in oral cancer is also speculative (361,362). Viral diseases of the head and neck include herpes labialis (HSV-1 and 2), herpes zoster or shingles (VZV; HHV-3) infections, oral ulcers and retinitis/uveitis (HCMV; HHV-5), OHL (EBV) and several types of malignant neoplasm caused by the oncoviruses: EBV (HHV-4), human herpesvirus 8 (HHV-8) and "high-risk" HPV's (especially HPV-16, 18, 31 and 33). These malignancies include Burkitt's lymphoma (BL), KS, and a subset of upper aerodigestive tract SCCs, respectively (Table 2.18) (363). "Low-risk" HPVs cause warts and papillomas. While HHVs and HPV are common in the general population and, in some regions, the population prevalence can exceed 50%, in immunocompetent people these viruses are mostly carried asymptomatically due to healthy immunoregulation. However, once an individual becomes immunocompromised by age, illness or HIV infection, these dormant viruses can manifest and produce disease.

Many of these oncoviruses are transmitted through oral–oral contact and are readily detected in saliva. The exceptions are HPV and HHV-8, where detection is primarily in samples reflective of tonsillar and other oropharyngeal lymphoid tissue (tonsillar samples or gargles) (364). Both HSV-1 and HSV-2, as well as HPV, are transmitted through oral–genital contact (365). These oncoviruses work directly through several mechanisms, which include induction of cell proliferation, genomic instability, cell migration and inhibition of apoptosis (Table 2.19). On the other hand, HBV and HCV work indirectly through chronic inflammation.

While this area has been well covered by many extensive reviews and ongoing research, such as that conducted by the IARC (366), and was reviewed at the Sixth and Seventh World Workshop on Oral Health and Disease in AIDS (367,368), much remains unsolved. This section describes the etiological role of viruses in cancers of the whole head and neck region regardless of anatomical location to inform clinicians how to detect opportunistic viral infections associated with oral cancers.

THE ROLE OF HIV AND IMMUNOSUPPRESSION IN HEAD AND NECK CANCERS

The weakening of the host immune system by age, illness, or HIV infection are driving forces in the pathogenesis of HNC (86,87). The ability of the immune system to prevent and control oncogenesis depends upon the presence of immune cells (primarily dendritic cells, T lymphocytes, B-cells and plasma cells, a few natural killer cells (NK), macrophages and eosinophils) within the microenvironment (87). While HIV itself does not cause mortality, infected individuals are at increased risk of acquisition of virus or the emergence of disease due to reactivation from a preexisting latent infection. In fact, prior to the initial detection of HIV in North America and Europe, many viral-associated cancers of the head and neck were rare. Today, many HNCs caused by HHVs and HPV are used

Table 2.19 Established carcinogenic mechanisms of oncogenic viruses

Mechanism	Oncovirus	Carcinogenic properties
Direct	EBV	Cell proliferation, inhibition of apoptosis, genomic instability, cell migration
	HHV-8	Cell proliferation, inhibition of apoptosis, genomic instability, cell migration
	HPV	Immortalization, genomic instability, inhibition of DNA damage response, anti-apoptotic activity
	HBV	Viral replication in nucleus of hepatocytes infects surrounding cells
	HCV	Immortalization via interference with p53 (tumor suppressor gene)
	HTLV-1	Immortalization and transformation of T cells
	HIV	Induce B-cell activation
Indirect through chronic inflammation	HBV	Inflammation, liver cirrhosis, chronic hepatitis
	HCV	Inflammation, liver cirrhosis, liver fibrosis
Indirect through immunosuppression	HIV-1	Immunosuppression
Unknown	MCPyV	Direct integration and transformation of cells is not yet understood

Source: From Speicher DJ et al. *Oral Dis* 2016;22(Suppl 1):181–92 (368).

as AIDS-defining lesions as they are known biomarkers of late-stage HIV infection/AIDS.

While some consider HIV to be an "oncovirus," its role is mainly indirect through increasing immunosuppression. HIV is also associated with immune activation, which can result in chronic inflammation and subsequent carcinogenic effects. Subsequently, this may result in an altered oral microbiome and loss of local immune surveillance and/or chronic inflammation. HIV may also directly induce B-cell activation by up-regulating activation-induced cytidine deaminase (369). Complicating the association with HIV are other cofactors long-associated with HNC. These include tobacco (both smoking and smokeless tobacco), chewing betel quid, the use of alcohol and illicit drugs as well as other viral co-infections (168). Through increased immunosuppression, HIV increases the risk and progression of KS, non-Hodgkin lymphomas, Hodgkin lymphoma, anal and cervical SCC, oral cavity/pharyngeal SCC and liver cancer (366). In the HIV patient, oral disease progression can be defined as a transition from asymptomatic to symptomatic chronic infection or a symptomatic disease that worsens over an accelerated time course (e.g., HPV-associated epithelial dysplasia to invasive carcinoma). Understanding these distinctions remains a challenge as the natural history of these viral infections in the oral cavity is not well understood.

Treatment regimens for HIV/AIDS play a significant role in the natural history of HNC, particularly KS. The use of antiretroviral therapy (ART) causes remission of many, but not all KS lesions. Following the introduction of ART, the incidence of KS was reduced in the U.S.A. from 333 cases/million in 1987 to 28 cases/million by 1998 (370). Since 2000, no further decline in KS has been observed and the number of new cases has plateaued. ART was so effective that 90% of AIDS-KS cases displayed complete remission of cutaneous lesions within 6 months as well as an 81% reduction in mortality (370). However, in a small subset of patients, the initiation of ART can cause an intense rebound of inflammatory responses including those to non-HIV viral infections, a situation now widely recognized as Immune Reconstitution Inflammatory Syndrome (IRIS). IRIS occurs in two forms. If an opportunistic infection worsens despite successful treatment of HIV this is called *paradoxical IRIS*, whereas the emergence of a previously absent infection is called *unmasking IRIS* (371). When KS is associated with IRIS, this is called KS-IRIS. KS-IRIS can occur in up to 11% of newly diagnosed HIV-positive patients initiating ART (372,373). The appearance of KS-IRIS should be treated by maintaining ART and treating the KS with liposomal doxorubicin.

A similar increase in the pathogenesis of HPV-associated HNC has been reported in patients infected with HIV. Recent studies have shown that HIV-infected patients display a 2-fold increase in the incidence of oral HPV infection (374–376) and of HNC (377,378). In 2014, Beachler et al. reported a 15% increase in the prevalence of HPV detected in saliva from HIV-infected individuals and that immunosuppression due to HIV infection may influence HPV-related carcinogenesis at an early stage (379). This increase in incidence was confirmed by a large comprehensive study in the U.S.A. (380). While similar increases in risk and pathogenesis have been reported in diseases caused by the full range of HHVs, this chapter focusses on the etiology of viral-associated HNC irrespective of HIV status.

THE HHVs AND ORAL CANCER

Herpes simplex viruses

The epidemiology of cancer of the uterine cervix has long suggested an infective component; for example, this disease is extremely rare in celibates (such as nuns) and shows a relationship to number of sexual partners (not to simple frequency of intercourse). For some time, this focused attention on a possible role for HSV-2, as this is a common genital tract viral infection in women, and it is known from studies *in vitro* that transfection of epithelial cultures with HSV can immortalize such cells. By implication, a role for HSV-1 and HSV-2 (which can be carried in the mouth) was sought in oral carcinogenesis. Evidence in support of this is the clear demonstration from animal studies that HSV can act as a cocarcinogen with tobacco (321) or other chemical carcinogens such as 4-nitroquinoline *N*-oxide (381) and that immunization against HSV can inhibit the cocarcinogenic effect with DMBA (382).

Several studies in humans have shown that patients with oral cancer have higher antibodies to HSV, but this does not prove a causal relationship (383). Serum IgA antibodies to HSV-1 are higher in smokers, and higher again in smokers with oral or other HNCs, suggesting that prolonged exposure to HSV may sensitize the mucosa to tobacco carcinogens. A more likely explanation, however, is that the generalized immunosuppression, particularly of natural killer-cell (NK) activity, which is induced by smoking favors the acquisition or chronicity of HSV infections/carriage, with consequently raised antibody titers.

Stronger, but still circumstantial, evidence comes from a case-control study of 410 pairs drawn from northern Sweden (144). Univariate analysis showed a slight association for groups with a clearly stated ("certain") history of HSV-1 infection (OR = 1.9; 95% CI: 0.7–4.5) and a strong association for groups with a highly suspected ("certain plus probable") HSV-1 infection (OR = 3.3; 95% CI: 1.6–6.5). Most reports were of recurrent herpes labialis, lip cancer was analyzed separately, and revealed a strong association for the highly suspected group (OR = 4.6; 95% CI: 1.7–13). These associations remained in multivariate analysis, which showed HSV infection (OR = 3.8; 95% CI: 2.0–7.0), alcohol use (OR = 1.5; 95% CI: 1.0–2.3) and current smoking (OR = 1.5; 95% CI: 0.9–2.5) to be the major influences.

Although some studies have claimed to detect HSV antigens, there is little convincing evidence that HSV gene sequences are present in oral cancer cells (384). RNA complementary to HSV DNA has been detected by *in situ* hybridization (ISH), but there is no evidence for integration (385). A hit-and-run hypothesis has long been proposed but is clearly difficult to prove. Currently, there is little emphasis placed on HSV in relation to human oral cancer, but the above observations imply a potential role which is worthy of continued investigation.

Epstein-Barr virus (EBV)

Epstein-Barr virus (EBV) is a Lymphocryptovirus or gamma-1 herpesvirus, and the first human virus to be identified with oncogenic potential (386). EBV usually manifests in the oral cavity and/or head and neck region as infectious mononucleosis, in a high proportion of otherwise healthy children or adolescents, this being the primary infection from which most subsequently become immune. BL often manifests in malnourished children, and OHL is seen with prevalence and disease severity increased in individuals co-infected with HIV (387–389). Genetically, two types of EBV exist: EBV-1 (type A) and EBV-2 (type B). EBV-1 is commonly found in Western populations while both types are common in sub-Saharan Africa and in PNG (390). The EBV genome encodes immediate early (IE), early (E) and

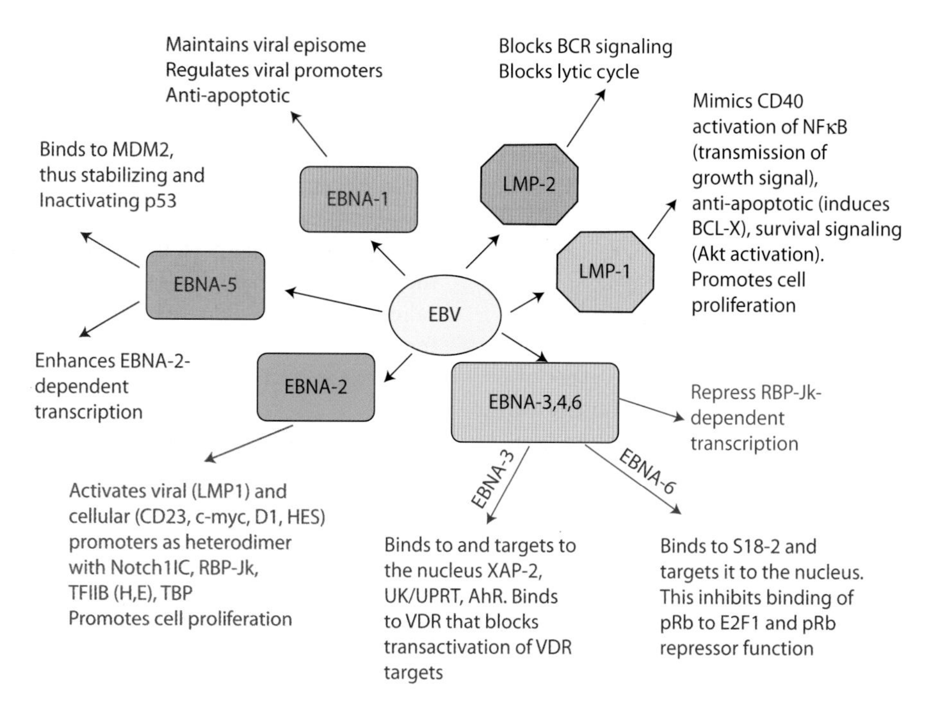

Figure 2.11 Some of the functions of the EBV-encoded proteins expressed in latent infection of B-lymphocytes. (Reproduced from Klein G, Klein E, Kashuba E. *Biochem Biophys Res Commun* 2010;396(1):67–73 (391).)

late (L) proteins, along with nine latent phases including six Epstein-Barr nuclear antigens (EBNA-1 to EBNA-6) and three latent membrane proteins (LMP-1 to LMP-3) (Figure 2.11) (391). Among these, LMP-1, an active transmembrane receptor, mediates EBV-related malignant transformation of cells by activating various signaling pathways, including NF-κB, c-Jun N-terminal kinase and phosphatidylinositol 3-kinase (PI3K)/Akt, *in vitro* and *in vivo* (392).

MECHANISM OF EBV-MEDIATED CARCINOGENESIS

EBV infects both B-lymphocytes circulating in peripheral blood and epithelial cells, particularly those of the nasopharynx, and can be transmitted orally as infectious whole virion because of shedding from periodontal and tonsillar tissues into saliva (393,394). Infectious EBV is then transmitted through intimate oral contact and/or salivary residue left on cups, food, toys or other objects (395). EBV can also be transmitted from donor to recipient during organ transplantation.

Viral entry into oral and oropharyngeal epithelial cells can occur by (i) direct cell-to-cell contact of EBV-infected lymphocytes with apical membranes of oropharyngeal epithelium, (ii) entry of cell-free virions through the basolateral membrane of oral epithelium (mediated by an interaction between β1 and α5β1 integrins and the EBV BMRF-2 proteins) and (iii) by spread of virus across lateral membranes through adjacent epithelial cells (396). Viral entry is facilitated by an envelope glycoprotein binding to the C3d receptor on the cell membrane of B cells and a closely related epitope of the surface of epithelial cells. EBV-infected cells are then immortalized and propagate as tumors in the lymphoid tissue, and lymphoid regions of nasopharyngeal and oropharyngeal mucosae (397). While the exact role of EBV in malignant transformation remains unclear, there is a correlation with over-expression of EBNAs and LMP2 genes as well as with the expression frequency of other genes located on EBV genome (DNA) [spots 61 (BBRF1, BBRF2 and BBRF3) and 68 (BDLF4 and BDLF1)] (398).

EBV and the pathogenesis of OSCC

The relationship between EBV and oral- and oropharyngeal squamous cell carcinoma (OPSCC) is speculative, especially considering reports of EBV DNA detected in some tonsillar carcinomas, supraglottic laryngeal carcinomas and salivary gland carcinomas (399). While early studies failed to detect EBV DNA in OSCC by EBER-ISH (400), possibly due to the low sensitivity of this technique, several studies utilizing PCR have detected EBV DNA in OSCC and OPSCC tissue biopsies (401). Recent studies using nested PCR have shown a higher EBV prevalence in OSCC patients (ranging from 29% to 73%) compared to healthy individuals (19%) (402,403). In 2012, Jalouli et al. reported a high prevalence of EBV in OSCC tissue biopsies from European and African countries (70%–80%), but a low prevalence in OSCC tissue biopsies from South Asia (35%–45%) (404). This lower EBV-association with OSCC in South Asian populations confirmed previous studies. One study from India reported the presence of EBV DNA in 25/103 (24%) oral cancer samples and 13/100 (13%) nonmalignant oral lesions (predominantly leukoplakia), but only 3/76 (4%) normal mucosal specimens from the contralateral side of patients with oral lesions and in 10/141 (7%) of peripheral blood cells (405). An association of EBV with OSCC has also been reported from Japan and Taiwan (406,407). Caution is necessary, however, in interpreting the presence of EBV in tissues because a high proportion of individuals naturally secrete EBV in saliva and, with the high sensitivity of PCR, it is difficult to rule out salivary contamination. Also, we must always remember that association does not prove cause and effect.

BL and nasopharyngeal carcinoma

BL is a disease that characteristically affects the jaws and lymphatic system of malnourished African children, especially in the tropical belt across the whole of the continent. The relationship between EBV and both BL and NPC is well established. The prevalence of both diseases is also exacerbated in the HIV-positive population. Mutalima et al. (2008) found that HIV status increased the risk of BL by 12-fold (408). Among HIV-negative individuals, elevated levels of antibodies for EBV and for malaria were associated with increased risk of BL by 12- and 2.5-fold, respectively. These EBV-positive Hodgkin's and non-Hodgkin lymphomas often manifest in the head and neck. NPCs are also HNCs associated with an EBV infection. NPC, however, is not usually regarded as an EBV-associated AIDS-defining cancer. Hazard ratios for developing NPC have been calculated by association with anti-EBV viral capsid antigen immunoglobulin A: low antibody levels have elevated odds ratios (OR = 9.5; 95% CI: 2.2–40.1) but are much higher when antibody levels are high (OR = 21.4; 95% CI: 2.8–161.7) (409). Transmission of HIV during pregnancy or birth adds complexity to the etiology of EBV-associated cancers and virus-associated oral transmission. In many developing countries, HIV is acquired prior to the first infection with a human oncovirus and this increases the risk of malignancy. Whether HIV has direct biochemical effects on EBV-associated disease beyond modulation of transmission and "seeding" of the latent reservoir of EBV remains a subject of debate.

Oral hairy leukoplakia

OHL is a manifestation of EBV reactivation in association with immunosuppression. It is often asymptomatic and is a pathologic manifestation of permissive EBV infection. OHL is characterized by painless, corrugated, white plaque-like hyperproliferative lesions that are almost always present along the lateral or dorsolateral part of the tongue (410,411) (Figures 2.12 and 2.13). OHL is not confined to HIV-infected people, but can be found in solid-organ transplants and bone marrow transplant recipients (388,412,413).

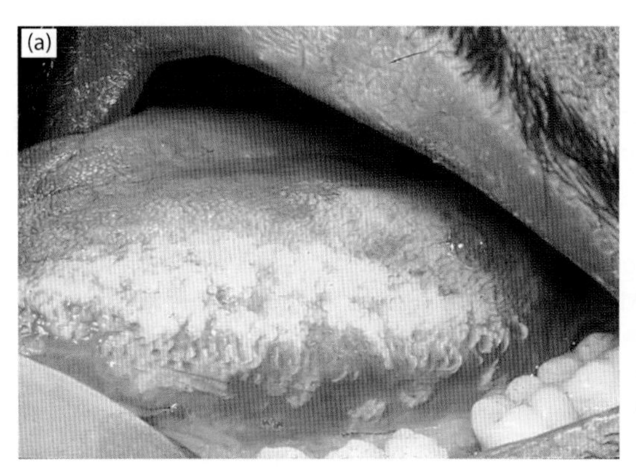
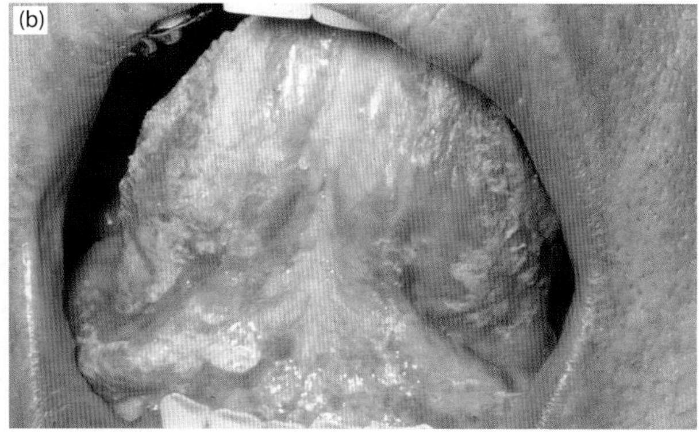

Figure 2.12 **(a)** Oral hairy leukoplakia (Greenspan lesion) on the lateral border of the tongue, mixed with pseudomembranous candidiasis on the dorsum, in an HIV-positive patient. **(b)** A more extensive hairy leukoplakia, affecting lateral and ventral tongue, and floor of the mouth, in an AIDS patient. (Courtesy Dr. Charles Barr, New York.)

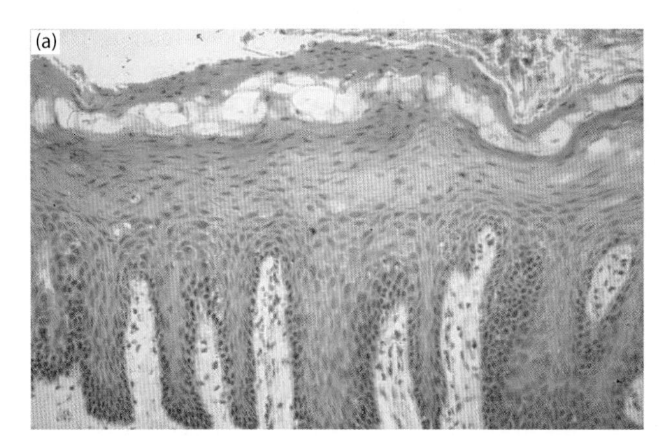
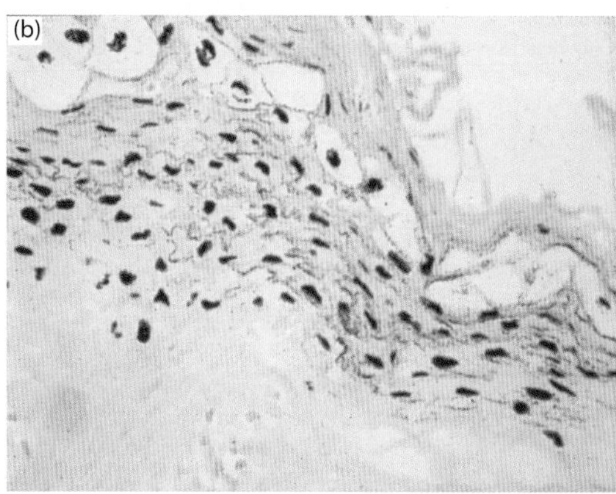

Figure 2.13 **(a)** Histology of oral hairy leukoplakia. Note the modest acanthosis, ballooning of cells in the upper prickle cell layers, a limited hyperparakeratosis, limited rete ridge hyperplasia and absence of an inflammatory infiltrate in the lamina propria. Stained by hematoxylin and eosin. **(b)** An adjacent section to the above, showing EBV in the upper keratinocytes, demonstrated by in situ hybridization.

OHL serves as a clinical biomarker for HIV infection and progression to AIDS. Even in the HAART era, the prevalence of OHL is 12% of the HIV population (414). This is of importance because OHL may serve as an oral indicator, not only of new HIV infections, but of ineffective ART. OHL demonstrates an interesting pattern of gene expression with a combination of lytic and transforming genes (415). OHL lesions have shown the overexpression of EBV-encoded LMP-1 and EBNA-2 genes, thus regulating growth factors and cytokines released from tongue epithelial cells (416). This combined effect may interfere with cell cycle regulation of tongue keratinocytes, induce immunosuppression and inhibit apoptosis (415,416). Nevertheless, malignant transformation has not yet been described.

HUMAN HERPESVIRUS 8 (HHV-8)

Human herpesvirus 8 (HHV-8) is a *Rhadinovirus* or *gamma-2-herpesvirus*. Like other members of the family *Herpesviridae*, HHV-8 displays the typical bulls-eye morphology when viewed by electron microscopy as the virion consists of an electron dense envelope and icosahedral capsid separated by an electron transparent tegument (417,418) (Figure 2.14). HHV-8 was originally named KS-associated herpesvirus (KSHV) as it is the etiological agent of KS (419–421). However, as it is also the etiological agent of multicentric Castleman's disease (MCD) and primary effusion lymphoma (PEL) the term "Human Herpesvirus 8" is more appropriate. Although HHV-8 manifests as KS, MCD and PEL, the latter two rarely present in the head and neck region and are beyond the focus of this chapter.

Kaposi's sarcoma

KS is an angioproliferative disorder manifesting in the oral mucosa (422), skin, lymph nodes (423), the musculoskeletal system (424,425), fibrous and connective tissue and visceral organs (417,426–429). KS is characterized by neoangiogenesis of multifocal origin, edema, erythrocyte extravasation, growth of spindle-shaped cells (endothelial tumor cells), and also with the proliferation of nonmalignant endothelial cells, and inflammatory cell infiltration (430) (Figure 2.15).

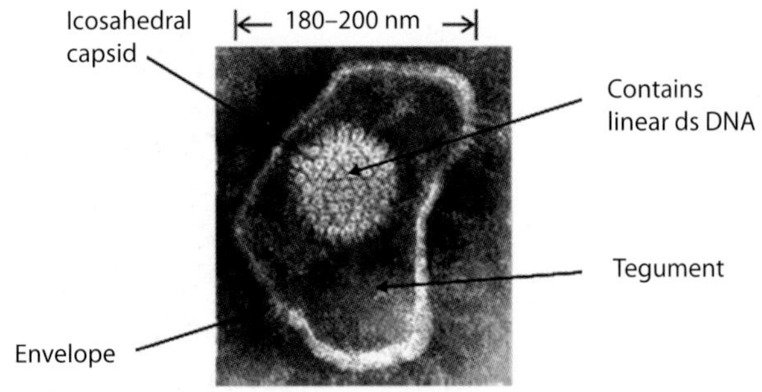

Icosahedral capsid
180–200 nm
Contains linear ds DNA
Tegument
Envelope

Figure 2.14 A typical human herpesvirus virion as viewed under an electron microscope. Micrograph image modified from the Virus Ultra Structure website (Stannard. *Virus Ultra Structure: Electron Micrograph Images*, 1995.)

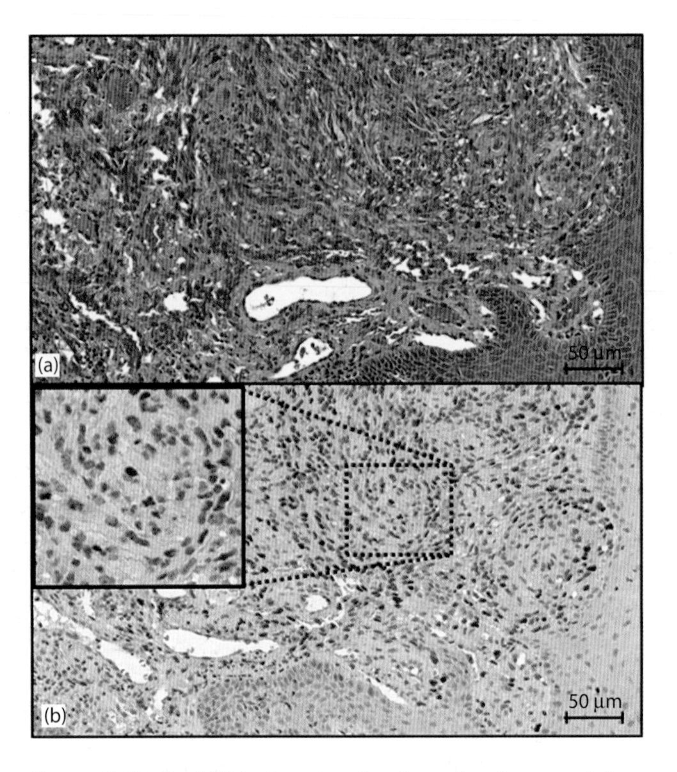

Figure 2.15 Oral KS lesion. A polyp from the dorsum of the tongue of a 37-year-old male (a, H&E; b, HHV-8 IHC). Many of the lining cells of wide, thin-walled vascular channels show strong nuclear staining for LANA-1 antigen, as do most nuclei in hypercellular whorls beneath the epithelium. There is moderate pleomorphism and occasional mitotic figures. Red cell extravasation is limited. Bar = 50 µm. Inset, demonstrates the punctate pattern of nuclear staining, presumably representing clusters of HHV-8 episomes. (Reproduced from Speicher DJ et al. *Journal of Oral Pathology & Medicine: Official Publication of the International Association of Oral Pathologists and the American Academy of Oral Pathology*. 2015;44(10):842–9 (460).)

There are four clinical–epidemiological variants of KS: classic, endemic (African), iatrogenic (transplant-associated) and HIV/AIDS-associated (epidemic). These can be distinguished by the nature and severity of clinical signs and symptoms, manifestations that vary by (i) the extent of anatomical involvement, (ii) the aggressiveness of lesion formation and progression, (iii) patient risk factors (i.e., ethno-geographic origin, age of onset and gender) and (iv) the association with patient morbidity and mortality (Table 2.20). However, all forms of KS have more or less identical, pathognomonic, histological features (431). Classic KS was first described by Dr Moritz Kaposi in 1872 as an "idiopathic multiple pigmented sarcoma of the skin" in five elderly men of Italian, Jewish and Mediterranean origin, long before the onset of the HIV/AIDS epidemic (432). Endemic KS is typically an indolent lesion found across parts of Equatorial Africa known as the "KS belt," encompassing Cameroon, Zaire, Uganda, eastern Zambia, Zimbabwe and Northern South Africa (433,434) (Figure 2.16). Before the HIV epidemic, KS was the most common neoplasm, comprising 3%–9% of all cancers in Ugandan males (370,435,436), and 9%–13% of all cancers in Zaire (434,437–439). Iatrogenic KS follows months to years after the use of immunosuppressant drugs to prevent rejection of renal or other solid-organ allografts (440–442). It has also been described following blood transfusion from an HHV-8-positive donor to an HHV-8-negative recipient (443, 444). Interestingly, the risk of developing iatrogenic KS has genetic and geographical cofactors. It displays an ethno-geographic predominance: a low prevalence of approximately 0.4% of transplant patients is described in the U.S.A. and western Europe (442,445,446), higher, at 1.9%, described in Greece (441) and a surprising 5.3% in Saudi Arabia (447). Compared to the general population, the risks of iatrogenic KS developing in HHV-8 seropositive allograft recipients are increased 28–75-fold in France (446) and 54-fold in Sub-Saharan Africa, whereas in the Middle East is increased 500–1,000-fold (447). AIDS-KS is the most aggressive variant involving skin, bone and widespread dissemination in single or multiple viscera (448–451). Lesions become progressively enlarged due to severe immunosuppression through the reduction of CD4+ cells, and host–virus interactions between HIV-1 *tat*, IL-6, β-FGF and HHV-8, resulting in enhanced HHV-8 replication in KS-derived spindle cells (450–453). KS is AIDS defining and the most frequent AIDS-associated neoplasm worldwide due to the underlying HHV-8 prevalence, limited access to ART and the health delivery infrastructure in many developing nations (454).

Cutaneous KS is defined as lesions on any part of the skin, such as the lower extremities, torso and genitalia (Figure 2.17). Oral KS lesions occur mainly on the palate but also the gingivae and dorsum of the tongue (455–458) (Figure 2.17). While cutaneous KS is more common, oral KS is present in up to 60% of KS cases with up to 45% of cases involving both oral and cutaneous lesions. Oral KS is associated with a higher death rate with mortality occurring 24 months after diagnosis, compared to 72 months as seen in cutaneous lesions (459). While KS does manifest in the mouth one must be cautious to not make a diagnosis based upon clinical appearance and histological staining of lesions, especially in communities with a high prevalence of HIV and of HHV-8-associated diseases. In a study from Kenya, Speicher et al. identified 12/28

Table 2.20 Epidemiological forms of Kaposi's sarcoma

Epidemiological variant	Clinical form	Clinical behavior	Anatomical involvement	Age of onset	Primary geographical location	Patient risk factors
Classical	Cutaneous-nodular	Indolent	Cutaneous	50–70 years	Mediterranean, Jewish, Eastern European	Ethnicity and geographical cofactors
Endemic (African)	Generalized and/or locally aggressive Cutaneous-nodular or plaques	Indolent and/ or aggressive	Cutaneous, but lymphadenopathic form: also includes viscera	35 years Infants approximately 3 years for lymphadenopathic form	Sub-Saharan Africa	Ethnicity and geographical cofactors
Iatrogenic	Generalized aggressive	Aggressive	Cutaneous and multiple organ involvement	Any	Worldwide	Immunosuppression Ethno-geographic predominance
AIDS (epidemic)	Generalized aggressive	Aggressive	Cutaneous and multiple organ involvement	Most descriptions average age is 30–40 years, but can be as low as 18 years	Worldwide	HIV immunosuppression

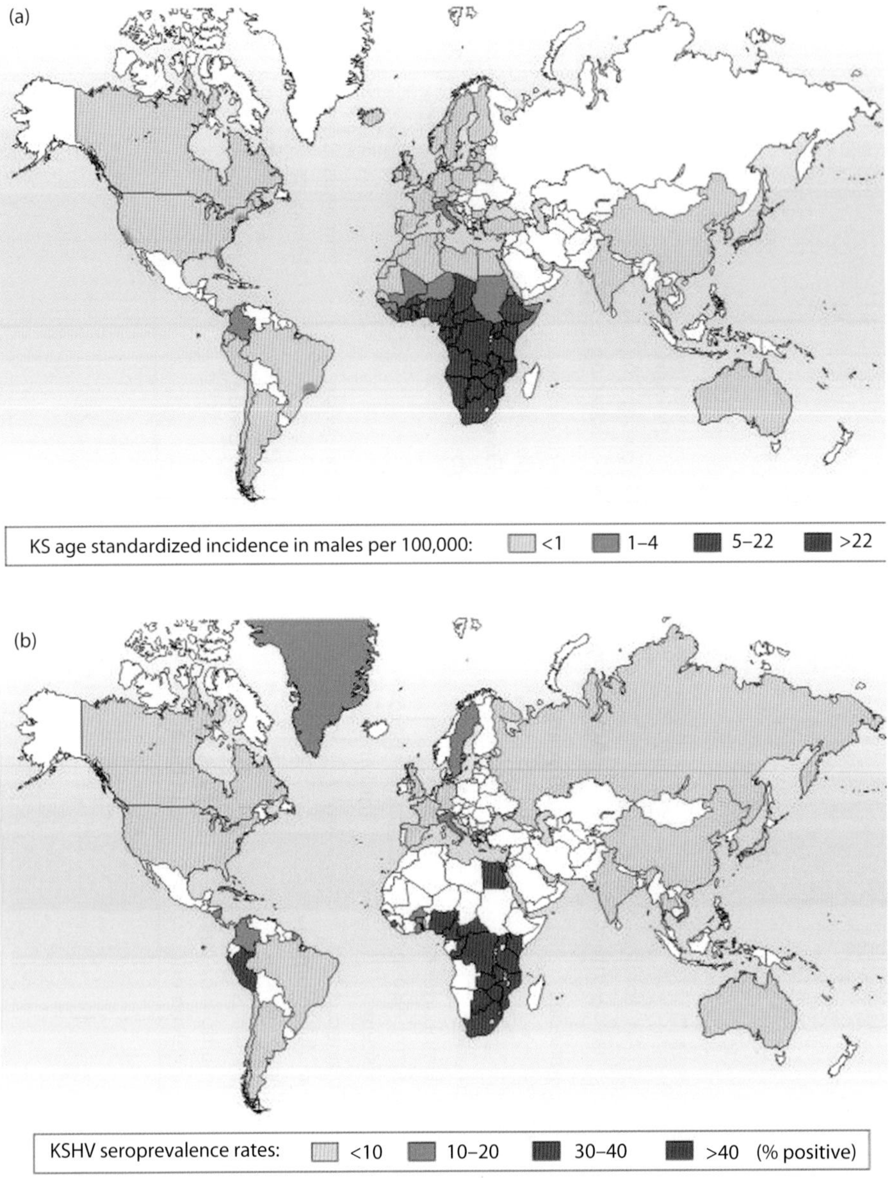

Figure 2.16 Geographical **(a)** incidence of Kaposi's sarcoma and **(b)** seroprevalence of HHV-8. (From Mesri EA, Cesarman E, Boshoff C. Kaposi's sarcoma and its associated herpesvirus. *Nat Rev Cancer* 2010;10(10):707–19 (729).)

oral and 4/21 cutaneous lesions that displayed clinical and histological features of KS but were negative to HHV-8 IHC (460). Of the oral lesions that were misdiagnosed, 6/12 were actually pyogenic granulomata. This emphasizes that HHV-8 IHC is essential for the correct diagnosis of KS and allows discrimination against similar clinical manifestations like pyogenic granulomata (Table 2.21).

Epidemiology and risk factors

Globally, the prevalence of KS usually mirrors the seroprevalence of HHV-8 and HIV, except for in Amazon Amerindian populations of South America, and in India (Figure 2.16). In the HIV-negative Amazon Amerindian populations of Brazil, Ecuador and French Guiana, HHV-8 is endemic (i.e., 75.4% seroprevalence) but clinical KS is rare (461). In 2012, the Government of India estimated that 2.4 million Indians are living with HIV with an adult prevalence of 0.31% (462), but KS has only been documented in the literature a total of eight times in this vast nation (463–468), the first suspected case being seen at YRG CARE in Chennai (469), and only recently has a case of KS been confirmed by immunehistochemical detection of HHV-8 itself (468). In 1999, Ablashi et al. reported a 4% HHV-8 seropositivity rate in blood collected from 108 healthy individuals at blood bank facilities in Bombay, Chennai and New Delhi (470). This is comparable to rates of seropositivity found in blood donors in the U.S.A. (5.2%; 7/135) as reported in the same study. Later studies have shown that the seroprevalence of HHV-8 in the HIV-positive ART-naïve population in India ranges

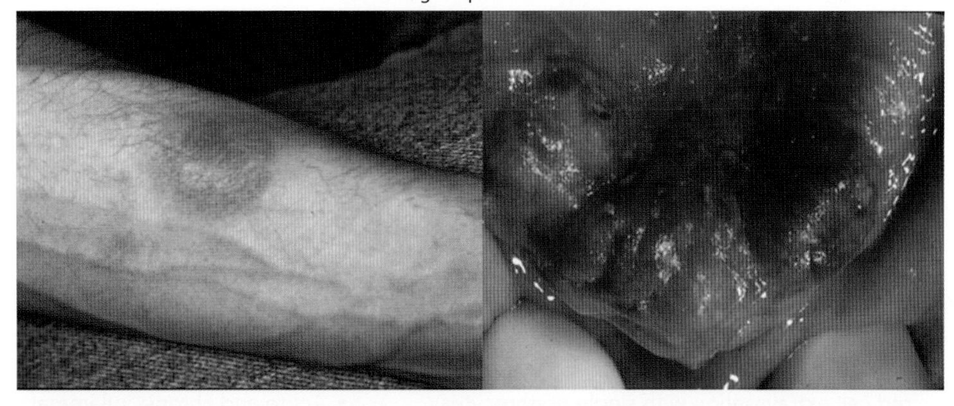

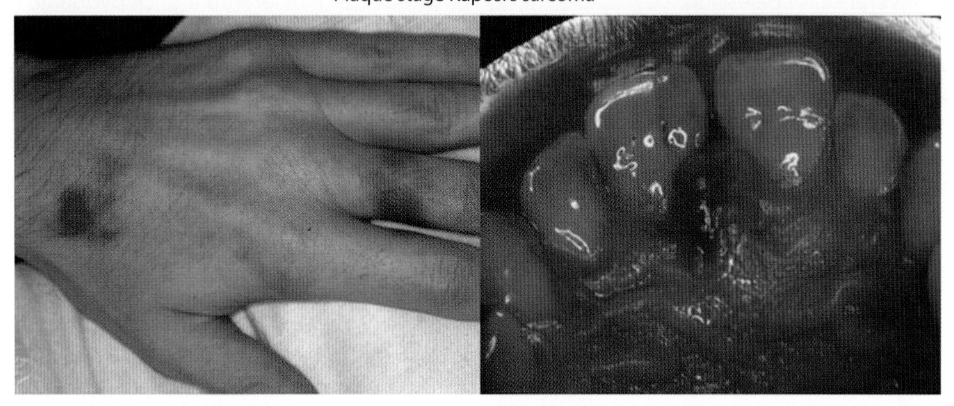

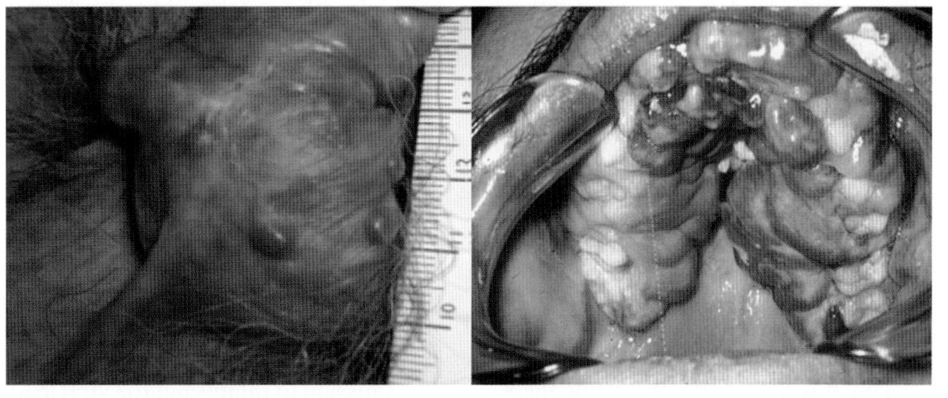

Figure 2.17 Cutaneous and oral clinical manifestations of KS at the early patch and plaque and late nodular stages. All photos courtesy of Professor Newell Johnson except the scrotal KS. (From Curatolo P et al. *Dermatol Surg* 2008;34:839–42; discussion 42–3 (730).)

between 11% (471) and 26% (472). Thus, HHV-8 is circulating in India, but rarely expresses itself as KS.

In developed nations, such as the U.S.A. and Australia, the prevalence of HHV-8 is low, and one-third of KS cases develop in patients (mostly older homosexual males) on suppressive ART (473). It is the high-risk sexual practices of these homosexual males and their multiple sexual partners that encourage HHV-8 transmission (474–477). In developing nations, such as Kenya, KS is endemic and HHV-8 is transmitted *via* non-sexual routes, vertically from mother to child, horizontally between siblings and childhood playmates, or perinatally between mother and newborn (479).

Transmission

During the 1980s, KS was thought to be sexually transmitted among men having sex with men (MSM) as they were 300 times more likely to develop KS than other immunosuppressed groups and 20,000 times more likely than the general population (482). KS was higher in MSM because they were more sexually active and involved in high-risk sexual activities such as oral–anal sex resulting in a higher risk for developing KS and other sexually transmitted diseases than other men with AIDS (477,483–486). Some MSM also had up to 60 sexual partners over a 5-year period, severely

Table 2.21 Differential diagnosis of oral Kaposi's sarcoma and oral pyogenic granuloma

Oral Kaposi's sarcoma	Oral pyogenic granuloma
1. Clinical appearance • Range from dusky purple patches, to macular plaques, to exophytic polyps • Occur on any mucosal area, commonly flat surfaces such as the hard palate or edentulous ridges • Highly vascularized so larger lesions appear red and granular • Large lesions commonly ulcerate 2. Histological features • Fascicular arrangements of spindle-shaped cells and slit-like vessels • Characteristic red cell extravasation with single erythrocytes or clumps of several cells coalescing • If ulcerated a thick pyogenic membrane 3. Immunohistochemistry • Positive markers for endothelial cells • Modest inflammatory cell numbers • HHV-8 antigen positive	1. Clinical appearance • Polypoid, sometimes pedunculated • Frequently arise from gingival margins of teeth • Variable size mm to cm • Highly vascularized so appear red and granular • Most lesions ulcerate 2. Histological features • Immature fibroblastic stroma • Florid capillary proliferation • Areas of hemorrhage • Acute and chronic inflammatory cell infiltrates • If ulcerated a thick pyogenic membrane 3. Immunohistochemistry • Positive markers for endothelial cells • Large numbers of inflammatory cells • HHV-8 antigen negative

Source: Table reproduced from Speicher DJ et al. *J Oral Pathol Med* 2015;44(10):842–9 (460).

increasing the risk of transmission (477,487). While these high-risk activities are well documented, the route of transmission is still uncertain as it is still unclear which body fluid contains infectious HHV-8: this could include saliva. Unlike other sexually transmitted diseases, including HIV, which is transmitted primarily *via* genital fluids during sexual activities, this may not be the case with HHV-8. Examinations into the viral load of HHV-8 in various bodily fluids have found that HHV-8 virion in semen is infectious when present, but difficult to detect, even under ideal conditions, especially when the viral load is low. This perhaps indicates that genital secretions may not be the primary route of HHV-8 transmission (488). HHV-8 has been found in cervicovaginal secretions from female prostitutes at a lower detection rate but at a much higher viral load compared to semen from homosexual males, casting further doubt on the initial thought that HHV-8 was passed *via* genital fluids during sexual activities (475,489). It is noteworthy that while these female prostitutes were HHV-8 positive, none were known to have developed KS, raising the question of genetic or herd immunity. Increased prevalence among MSM is potentially due to a combination of immunosuppression with HIV and the increased HHV-8 lytic cycle of replication due to interactions with the HIV-1 tat glycoprotein providing a more suitable host for HHV-8 (490,491).

In developing nations where HHV-8 is endemic, such as Sub-Sahara Africa and South America, familial and vertical transmission appears to be the dominant route of HHV-8 transmission in the general population. In these countries, many children appear to be HHV-8 seropositive due to close personal contact with an HHV-8 infected mother. It has been shown that a child of an HHV-8 infected mother is three times more likely to be HHV-8 seropositive than a child of an HHV-8 seronegative mother (492,493), and one wonders if the virus is being transmitted *via* saliva. The transmission rate of HHV-8 *via* saliva from mother to child may be as high as 30% (494). There is also a correlation between a child's age and HHV-8 seropositivity. During pregnancy, the increased HHV-8 viral load in mothers is thought to be due to pregnancy lowering the immune system (480,481,495). High seroprevalence to HHV-8 in neonates is due to passive immunity derived from the mother, which declines until around 9 months of age before seroprevalence again increases as the infant matures, due to close contact with their infected mother, siblings and playmates (478). Examination of various body fluids using both serological and molecular assays revealed high viral loads in saliva from both mothers and their children, suggesting that the oral route plays a dominant role in HHV-8 transmission, like the transmission of another HHV, EBV (496). Breast milk may contribute to HHV-8 transmission to infants but the viral loads are substantially lower than in saliva: nevertheless, infants are exposed to high volumes of breast milk (497). The viral load is also higher in saliva than breast milk, further supporting this route of transmission. Like in MSM in developed countries, HHV-8 has been rarely detected in peripheral blood mononuclear cells or genital secretions and when present, is in low viral loads. Investigations into the role of the oral mucosa as a route for HHV-8 transmission showed that, like EBV, HHV-8 replication occurs predominately in the mucosa of the oropharynx with the tonsils and adenoids being a reservoir for infection (493,498–500). Unlike EBV, the difficulty in detecting HHV-8 in the oral cavity is the intermittent viral shedding and the lack of "gold standard" assay (497). While the primary reservoir of HHV-8 is the oropharynx, and thus transmission is primarily *via* oral fluids—usually simplistically described as saliva—it is still unclear why HHV-8 is not transmitted between normal, otherwise healthy, heterosexual adults (498,501,502).

HUMAN PAPILLOMAVIRUS (HPV)

The *Papillomaviridae* are a large family of small circular, non-enveloped double-stranded DNA viruses that are species specific and preferentially infect epithelial cells of the skin and mucous membranes of higher vertebrates, including humans (503). HPV is a member of this *Papillomaviridae* family, with a genome of 7200–8000 base pairs in length and 55 nm in diameter (504). In the HPV genome, all putative viral protein-coding sequences, termed as open-reading frames (ORFs), are located on one strand that serves as a template for transcription. This transcriptional strand consists of three regions: (1) an upstream regulatory region or long control region or non-coding region, which has no ORFs but incorporates sequences that regulate viral transcription and replication; (2) an early region with ORFs (E1, E2, E4, E5, E6 and E7) that are engaged in various functions including transactivation of transcription, transformation, replication and viral adaptation; and (3) a late region coding for L1 and L2 capsid proteins that are involved in the formation of virion structure and facilitate selective encapsidation and maturation of viral DNA (505,506) (Figure 2.18).

The association of HPV with benign squamous epithelial lesions was first identified in humans in 1956 (507). However, Zur Hausen was the first to describe the oncogenic potential of these viruses (506). HPVs are common pathogens that are associated with several cutaneous and mucosal infections in both adults and children. Based on their tissue tropism, they are classified into cutaneous and mucosal HPVs (508). However, according to their nucleotide sequence homology of the L1 gene, which is the most conserved gene, HPVs are classified into more than 160 different genotypes (509). Approximately, 60 of these are mucosal HPVs that are preferentially found in cancerous and precancerous lesions (509, 510). Current convention is that, when <90% homology of the E6, E7 and L1 ORFs exist, a new type is designated and numbered in the order of discovery. Homology >90% defines a subtype and >98% a variant. Depending on their oncogenic potential or association with malignancy, HPV genotypes are further segregated into two groups: "high-risk" types (hrHPV) and "low-risk" types (lrHPV). The hrHPVs are types 16, 18, 31, 33, 34, 35, 39, 45, 51, 52, 53, 56, 58, 59, 66, 68, 73 and 82, whereas lrHPVs are types 6, 11, 40, 42, 43, 44, 61, 81 and 89 (510). The hrHPVs are commonly associated with malignant squamous epithelial lesions of the cervix, genital, anogenital and head and neck regions, whereas the lrHPVs are seen in benign lesions of skin and mucous membranes, such as verruca vulgaris, common infectious warts and genital warts.

HPV and HNC

In 1983, the association of HPV with a subset of HNCs was first documented (511). It is widely accepted that HPV-16

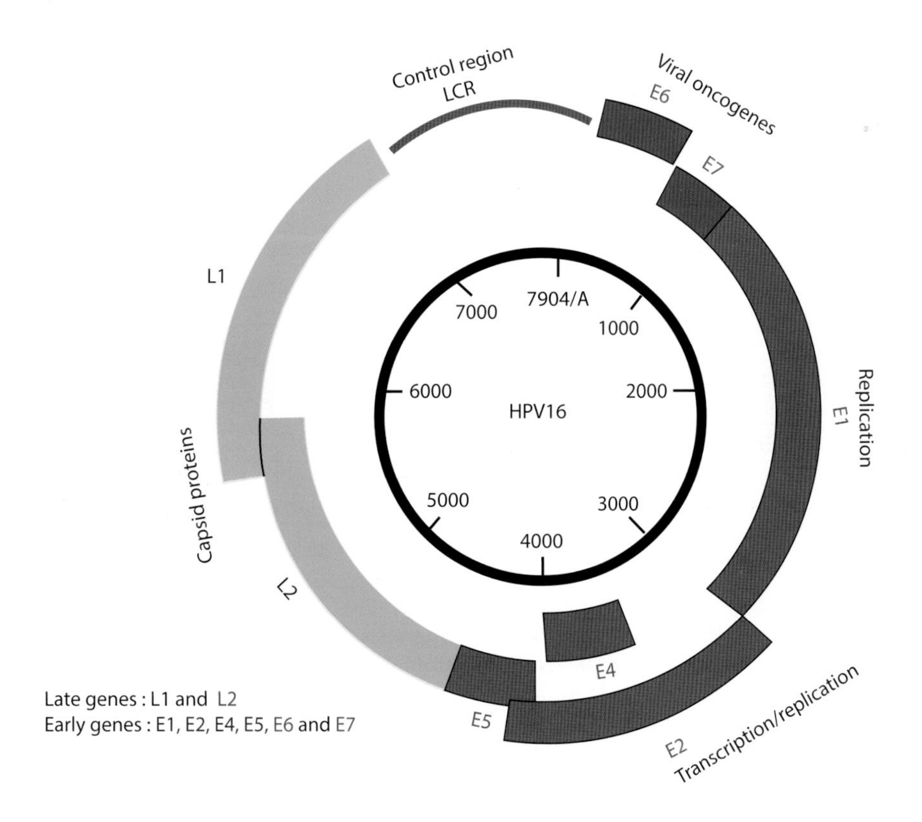

Figure 2.18 The structure and organization of an HPV genome. A schematic picture of a representative α-HPV genome is shown. The reference HPV-16 genome is a circular, double-stranded 7908 bp molecule. (Reproduced from Shaikh MH, McMillan NA, Johnson NW. *Cancer Epidemiol* 2015;39(6):923–38 (544).)

and HPV-18 are responsible for 70%–90% of cancers of the uterine cervix (512) and are strongly associated with anal, vulvar and penile cancers (513,514). Recently, a growing body of evidence suggests that approximately 20% of oral cancers and 60%–80% of oropharyngeal cancers are associated with HPVs (515–517). The IARC has declared HPV as a proven etiological factor for the development of OPSCC (518). Approximately 25 HPV types are associated with oral lesions and >90% of cases of HPV-related HNSCC are associated with HPV-16 (519–521).

HPV-positive and HPV-negative HNSCC are now regarded as two distinctly separate entities. There is better prognosis with HPV-positive HNSCC, but the specific mechanism behind this remains unknown (522,523). One possible explanation might be the reliance of HPV-associated HNSCC on *E6* and *E7* oncogenes, which inactivate or down-regulate *p53* gene and pRB protein, respectively (Figure 2.19). Whereas, in HPV-negative HNSCC, *p53* and pRb genes are frequently mutated, resulting in wider genomic instability and resistance to treatment (524). The mutation of the pRb protein in HPV-negative HNSCC occurs through the inactivation of *CDKN2A*, the gene that encodes two other cell cycle regulatory genes *p16* (INK4A) and *p14* (Arf/INK4B) (525). The functional loss of *CDKN2A* eventually leads to the down-regulation of the *p16* gene, which is related to the poor prognosis of non-HPV-associated HNSCC (526,527). However, recent studies have shown a poor outcome even with HPV-associated HNC patients who have a smoking history (528,529). This indicates that tobacco might potentiate the transformation effect of HPV, and that viral copy numbers in the infected cells could play an important role in disease progression. Usually, much lower viral loads are seen in HPV-associated HNSCC compared to cervical cancer. The highest viral loads and better survival rates have been reported in those with tonsillar cancer (530). Studies suggest that HPV infection is an early event in the pathogenesis of HPV-associated cancers. An *in vitro* model of an HPV-positive cancer cell line (UT-DEC1) has shown that HPV remains episomal much of the time, but becomes fully integrated only after 20 passages (531). Therefore, it is thought that in early HPV infections, both the episomal and integrated forms exist in the same cell. It is the integration of HPV that acts as the key factor in HPV-mediated carcinogenesis (532).

Epidemiology of HPV-associated NPC

HNC has long been a serious problem in many parts of the world, with increases in recent time. According to GLOBOCAN 2012 data, the estimated burden of HNC is

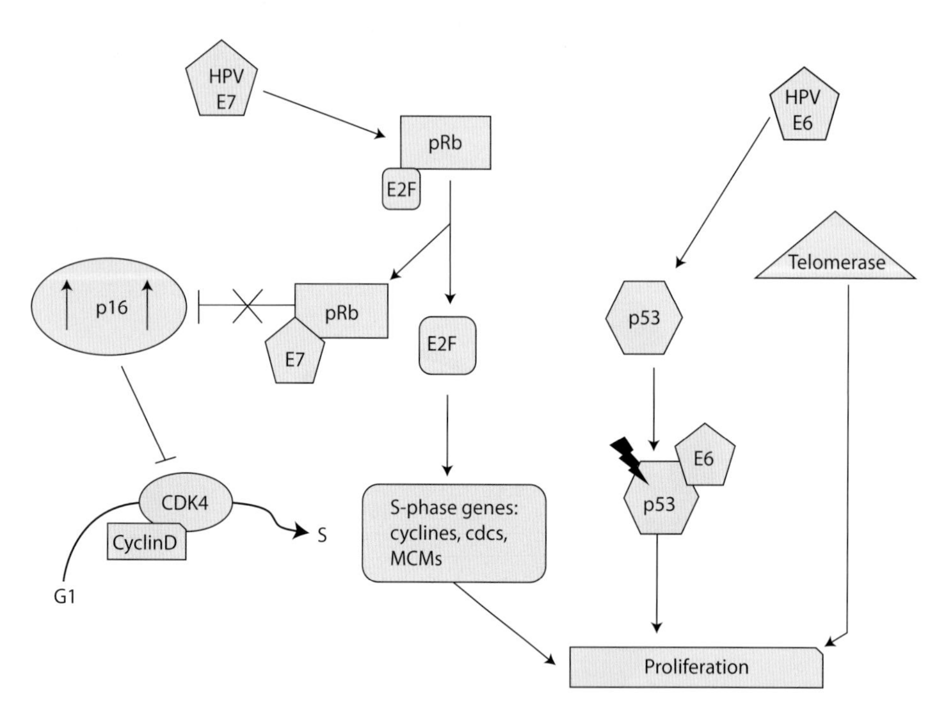

Figure 2.19 A schematic diagram of the process of HPV carcinogenesis. The diagram presents two HPV oncoproteins E6 and E7 targeting cell cycle regulatory protein (pRb—retinoblastoma protein) and tumor suppressor gene (*p53*) respectively. E7 binds with pRb, which inactivates pRb leading to the release of E2F transcription factor that drives the expression of S-phase genes and ultimately progresses to uncontrolled cell proliferation. In addition, a reciprocal relationship has been observed between pRb and p16 protein where inactivation of pRb leads to over expression of the *p16* gene [p16(INK4)]. P16 protein binds to CDK4 & CDK6 (cyclin-dependent kinases) and inhibits their ability to interact with cyclin D and stimulates passage through the G1 phase to S phase. E7 also degrades p21 protein function, which is thought to play a major role in cellular response to DNA damage. On the other hand, oncoprotein E6 binds to p53 protein and leads to its degradation, allowing the cancer cell to escape apoptosis. The *E6* gene also increases telomerase activity. These changes ultimately promote cancer progression.

approximately 634,766 new cases per annum worldwide, including approximately 263,020 for oral cavity, 150,677 for larynx, 136,622 for oropharynx, excluding the nasopharynx because of its distinctive biological characteristics (283). While the majority of these are observed in developing countries, there is considerable geographical variation in incidence. South Asia falls into the high-incidence category for HNC. The annual incidence is 143,152 new cases p.a. (70,283). The age-standardized incidence rate of HNC in South Asian countries (approximately 17.27 per 100,000 persons p.a.) is higher than other parts of the world, because of the extensive use of tobacco, areca nut and poor oral health (283).

Although HPV-related cancers are mostly seen in the uterine cervix, as more than 99% of these harbor HPV (533), a significant association of HPV with HNSCC is now well recognized, with an overall prevalence of approximately 25%–35% with a substantial variability (534–536). The HPV association with HNSCC was first reported in 1983 (511) with the association validated by Loning et al. and de Villers et al. on oral cavity (OSCC) and OPSCC in 1985 (537,538). However, recent rising rates of OPSCC, especially of the tonsil and base of the tongue, have been reported in Europe and in the U.S.A., many of which showed a clear association with HPV (539–542). Similar trends have been described in Australia where the prevalence of HPV-related oropharyngeal cancer increased from approximately 19% in 1982 to approximately 29% in 2005 (543). Although a high incidence of oral cavity cancer in South Asia has been recognized for decades due to the pervasive use of tobacco (smoking and smokeless forms) and areca nut, some recent data show significant association of HPV with HNSCC in the South Asian region. Studies from South Asia present a striking variability of the prevalence of HPV-associated HNSCC ranging from 3% to 74% (544). Studies from India also reported variability in the prevalence of HPV in OPSCC, ranging from 23% to 74% (545–547). A study from the western part of India showed approximately 28.6% prevalence of HPV in OSCC (548). The prevalence of HPV in laryngeal SCC (LSCC) also varies widely across the world. The reported prevalence of HPV in LSCC has ranged from 9.4% to 27% in the U.S.A., 4.4%–52% in Europe and slightly higher in South America, ranging from 32% to 37.3% (549–560). There are a few studies from South Asia reporting the prevalence of HPV in LSCC ranging from 34% to 47% (561, 562).

Risk factors for HPV-associated HNSCC

Current evidence across the world indicates that patients with HPV-related HNSCC are generally younger, male, of comparatively high socioeconomic status, are nonsmokers, non- or light-drinkers and are of Caucasian ethnicity (563–569). Several studies indicate that sexual behavior is the most important risk factor for HPV-positive HNSCC. The prevalence of HPV in HNSCC is 5–10-fold lower than that of cervical cancers and the transmission of hrHPVs in both these cancers is highly correlated with sexual behavior (570,571). These include sexual debut at early age, high number of lifetime vaginal or oral sex partners, open-mouth kissing, oral sex in both oral–oral and oral–genital forms (571–573). Case-control studies indicate a 2-fold increase in those individuals who have had more than one lifetime oral sexual partner and a 5-fold increase in individuals who had more than six (574–576). Further, homosexuals are more commonly infected than heterosexuals, as they tend to have a greater number of sexual partners (577). Another study shows a significant association of HPV with head and neck cancers in MSM who have regular oral–genital contact (578).

HPV prevalence in HNSCC tends to be higher in Caucasians, 34%, compared to the black population (4%) in a recent comprehensive study in the USA (579). Although it seems that HPV-positive HNSCC is more likely to develop in Caucasians, a significant prevalence has also been noted in South Asian populations, probably due to the changing of traditional sexual behaviors and the rapid infiltration of Western culture (575). The actual mechanism of HPV transmission remains unknown. However, unprotected sexual intercourse could be a leading cause, especially with oro-genital sex where the genital mucosa could be infected by HPVs and during the intercourse it would transmit from the genital region to the oral cavity (580,581). Other possibilities could be direct skin–skin contact, considering that anogenital warts (caused by lrHPVs), are often spread by self-inoculation from other skin sites by contaminated objects (fomites) and/or by hands to the genital region (577,582,583). HPVs can also be transmitted by other non-sexual routes, most commonly mother-to-child transmission during birth. Vertical transmission of HPV DNA may occur while the fetus passes through the infected cervix and birth canal of the mother, which can lead to the development of laryngeal papillomatosis in the newborn (583,584).

Current understanding suggests that tobacco use, marijuana use and alcohol abuse could be regarded as further risk factors as they might contribute to the transmission of HPV virus and cancer progression (365,583). Recent studies have demonstrated a decrease in the progress-free survival rate of HPV-associated HNC patients who have used tobacco for more than 10 pack-years (585,586). This indicates a potential interplay between chemical carcinogens and the HPV. Several studies have reported that men are at a 2–3-fold greater risk of developing HPV-associated HNC compared to women (365,571,573). HPVs have a high predilection for the mucosal epithelium of the oropharynx compared to the other parts of head and neck region (540,587). The oropharynx, especially the tonsils and base of the tongue, provide a particularly suitable microenvironment for HPV infection. These sites contain lymphoid tissues and are part of Waldeyer's ring (550,588). Lymphoid aggregations are lined by non-keratinized epithelium containing crypts (588). The crypts, lined by basal keratinocytes, function as traps for antigens but may also be a target for nuclear integration of HPV DNA (520,588). Another possibility could be that this region of the oropharynx acts as an embryonic transformation zone for which HPVs may have a predilection (520). Consistent with such origins, HPV-positive HNSCCs exhibit poorly differentiated, non-keratinized morphology with many basaloid tumor cells (589–591).

HPV entry and replication in basal epithelial cells

HPVs are commonly present in the normal genital mucosa as well as in the oral cavity and oropharynx, especially in tonsillar crypts (588, 592). It has been suggested that crypt epithelium of human palatine tonsils is part of a specialized mucosa, which contains stratified squamous non-keratinized epithelium, patches of reticulated and sponge-like epithelium (resembling intraepithelial passages, filled by non-epithelial cells) (593,594). These discontinuities apparently make the tonsils susceptible to viral and bacterial infections. Contrarily, reticulated epithelium lining the tonsillar crypt functions as a first-line immune defense by providing a favorable environment for the effector cells of immune response. The crypts also facilitate direct transport of antigens and contain a pool of immunoglobulins (594).

HPVs critically depend on the cellular machinery of the host for replication of their genome (595). The initiation of replication of HPV DNA follows the similar mechanism of eukaryotic chromosomes. The HPV E2 gene acts as the initiating factor for replication, which facilitates the recruitment of E1 gene by binding to LCR in HPV. The E1 gene then exploits host cell replication machinery proteins: replication protein A, topoisomerase 1 and polymerase α-primers, and interacts with cellular genes to coordinate viral replication at S phase of cell cycle (595,596) (Figure 2.20).

HPV can only initiate infection once it successfully binds and integrates into host epithelial cells. Typically, non-enveloped DNA viruses are internalized by the clathrin-mediated endocytosis pathway (597), sometimes also *via* caveola-mediated endocytosis (598). In squamous epithelium, HPVs infect undifferentiated basal cells after trauma or erosion and exist as a long-term latent infection. During an active viral DNA replication phase (productive phase), HPVs can generate more than 1000 DNA copies/cell (599). This leads to the expression of L1 and the production of mature viral particles in the cells of the uppermost layers of differentiated epithelia. The L2 gene is important for viral infectivity and the endosomal escape of the viral genome, which ultimately allows the virus to enter into the host nucleus (600,601). A recent concept on cellular receptor binding suggests the presence of HPV receptors for α6β4 integrins and sulfate proteoglycans (HSPGs; syndecan-1) (602). Overexpression of α6β4 integrins and syndecan-1 has been noticed in migrating cells and basal cells, respectively,

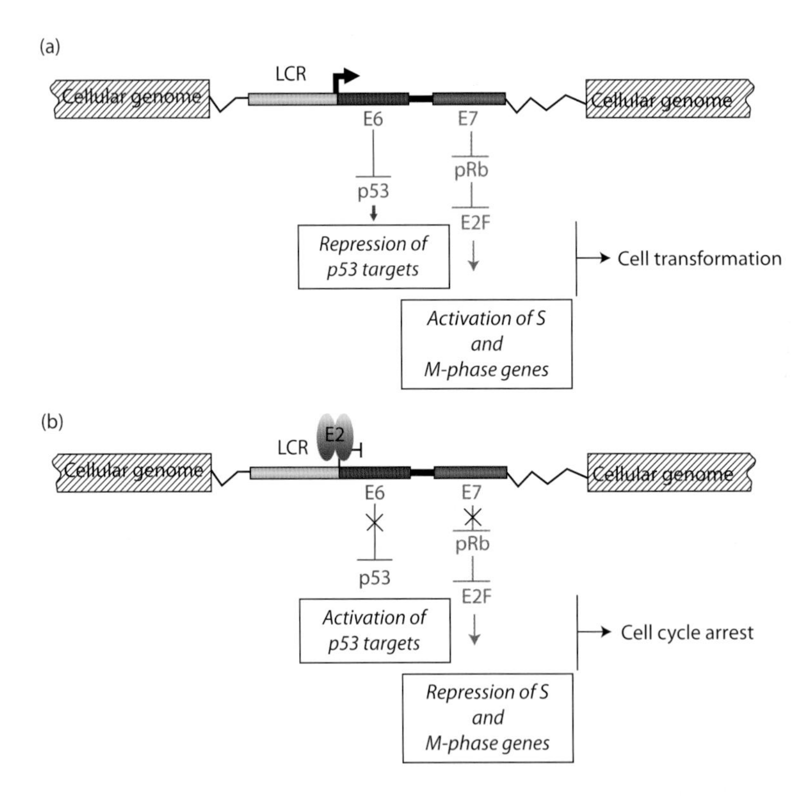

Figure 2.20 Schematic representation of the fragment of HPV18 genome integrated in the cellular genome as in the HeLa cervical carcinoma cells. **(a)** The E6 and E7 genes are transcribed from the P105 promoter and the products of these genes negatively interfere with p53 and pRb respectively, thus inducing cell cycle deregulation and cell transformation. **(b)** When expressed in HeLa cells, the viral E2 transcription factor represses the E6 and E7 transcription thereby inhibiting their effects on p53 and pRb and inducing cell cycle arrest and senescence. (Reproduced from Thierry F. *Virology* 2009;384(2):375–9 (595).)

following trauma (602,603). It is thought that HPVs might bind to α6β4 integrins and syndecan-1 during their cellular entry process. Once the cell entry has been achieved, HPV undergoes endosomal acidification for viral uncoating followed by effective infection (603,604).

Mechanism of HPV-mediated carcinogenesis

The exact pathogenesis of HPV-associated cancers is not completely understood, but is thought to commence with the integration of HPV DNA into the host keratinocyte genome. Two of the early genes, *E6* and *E7*, are responsible for malignant transformation (Figures 2.19 and 2.20). Suppression of the transcriptional repressor HPV *E2* gene allows continuous expression of *E6* and *E7*, which then function as oncogenes throughout the life of malignant keratinocytes (605). It has been suggested that the HPV *E6* and *E7* oncogenes of hrHPVs bind to the *p53* gene and Rb protein, respectively, with approximately 10-fold higher affinity than those of lrHPVs (606,607). This alone has been shown to be sufficient to immortalize primary human genital and oral keratinocytes *in vitro* (608,609). However, additional alterations, including activated *ras* gene mutations or deletions of the *DCC* gene, are also required *in vivo* (610,611). The HPV *E6* oncogene, localized in the nuclear matrix, targets and degrades the *p53* tumor suppressor gene, thus inhibiting *p53*-dependent cell cycle arrest and induction of apoptosis (612,613). The HPV *E6* oncogene also enhances telomerase activity, favoring immortalization of affected keratinocytes. The other viral oncogene *E7* promotes cellular proliferation by down-regulating the cyclin-dependent kinase (CDK) inhibitors p21 and p27, and by inactivating the Rb (retinoblastoma) protein by binding with the hypophosphorylated forms of Rb: pRb, p130 and p107 (614–616). Thus, the loss of both p53 and Rb function ultimately lead to malignancy (Figure 2.19). The *E7* oncogene also downregulates another CDK inhibitor (inhibits *p16* gene transcription) that upregulates CDKN2A, which ultimately mediates the overexpression of $p16^{INK4A}$ gene in HPV-positive cancers (617,618). The *p16* activity is used as a surrogate marker for diagnosing HPV-positive HNSCC (619,726).

Since the mucosae of the head and neck are more exposed to environmental, chemical carcinogens than the genital region, it is possible that additional, different carcinogenic mechanisms are involved in HPV-associated HNC than in cervical and other genital cancers. Recent studies have suggested that apart from p53 and pRb pathways, HPV oncoproteins E5, E6 and E7, coordinately target multiple pathways in the development of HPV-induced HNSCC. These include the EGFR pathway, TGFβ pathway, PI3-PTEN-AKT pathway (evading apoptosis, this providing survival for HPV-positive cancer cells) and angiogenesis including hypoxia-inducible factor (605,620,621) (Figure 2.21). Activation of WNT pathways by E6 and E7 in HNC has also been reported (622). HPV interference in these pathways leads to mutations of cellular genes, which cause genomic instability and ultimately full transformation (623). Understanding the molecular mechanisms is essential for effective bio-prevention and individualized biotherapies.

HPV AND BENIGN AND POTENTIALLY MALIGNANT DISORDERS OF THE ORAL MUCOSA

These benign proliferative lesions are slow-growing enlargements of the oral mucosa that are typically well defined, asymptomatic and may hamper the normal function of the oral cavity. Condylomas, warts (verrucae), focal epithelial hyperplasia (FEH), koilocytic dysplasia and oral papillomas are caused by lrHPVs.

Oral squamous cell papilloma

Oral squamous cell papillomas (OSCP) are small, benign growths that originate from squamous epithelium. They affect both genders, at any age, but particularly in the third to fifth decades (624). OSCP can present as a single lesion (usually <1–2 mm in diameter) or as multiple cohesive lesions, with exophytic growth and either a wide base or, usually, are pedunculated (Figure 2.22). OSCPs occur on the soft palate, dorsal or lateral borders of tongue and lower lip in adults, while in children the laryngotracheobronchial complex is the more common site (625). Histopathology shows papillary proliferations of squamous epithelium with prominent acanthosis, parakeratin lining deep crypts and classical koilocytosis. They have a central fibrovascular core (625).

The cytological hallmark of HPV infection is the presence of koilocytic atypia of the prickle cell (intermediate) layers of stratified squamous epithelia. This is manifested as ballooning of keratinocytes with densely staining irregular nuclei, often pressed to the side of the cell, surrounded by a perinuclear halo with condensed, amphophilic cytoplasm at its margins. A distinction should be made between true koilocytosis and vacuolization of cells, such as that seen in white sponge naevus of the oral mucosa, which is not HPV related. In HPV infection, there may also be parakeratinized (dyskeratotic) cells singly or in clusters below the surface layers. Both koilocytotic and dyskeratotic cells may be bi- or multinucleate and show enlarged nuclei. The association of koilocytosis with the presence of HPV DNA can be confirmed by ISH. HPV particles (by electron microscopy), HPV antigens (by immunocytochemistry) and HPV DNA (by nucleic acid testing) have been found in approximately 80% of lesions (626). HPV-6 and 11 are the most common types in OSCP.

Condyloma acuminatum

Condyloma acuminata (CA) are in effect venereal warts identical to those on the genital mucosa. They present as multiple, small, pink nodules, sometimes with a verrucous surface, which may proliferate and coalesce to form soft sessile growths up to 1 cm in diameter (627). CA have predilection for tongue, lips, palate and floor of the mouth (628). HPV particles, HPV structural antigens and HPV DNA

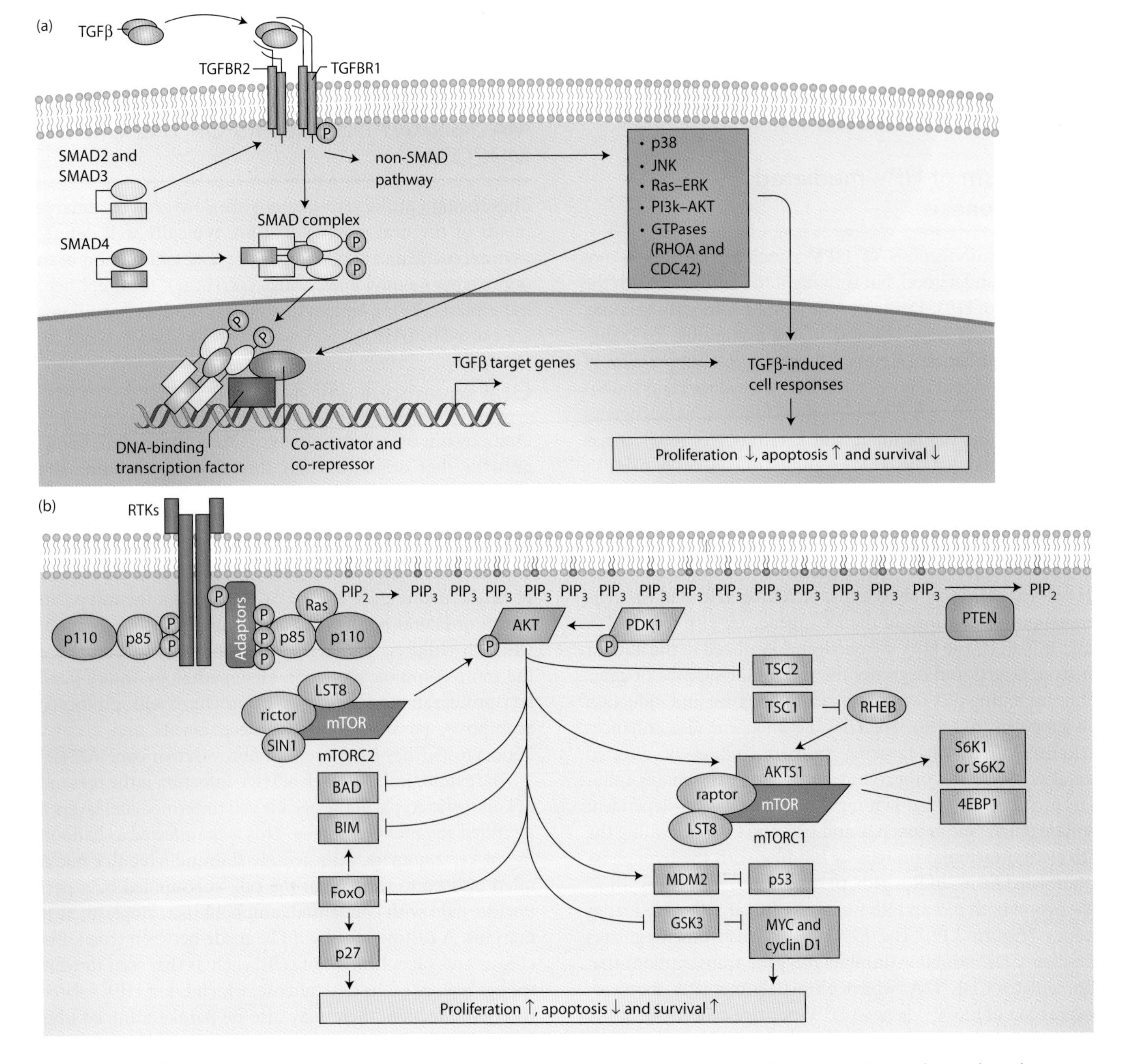

Figure 2.21 Schematic representation of the transforming growth factor-β (TGFβ) pathway. TGFβ signaling relayed through the SMAD pathway seems to be most important for head and neck squamous cell carcinoma (HNSCC). (Reproduced from Leemans CR et al. *Nat Rev Cancer* 2011;11(1):9–22 (623).)

6 and 11 have been found in up to 85% of these lesions (627). People who practice regular oral sex have up to 50% chance of developing oral condylomata (628). Histologically, they are similar to oral papillomata, with acanthosis, parakeratosis and koilocytosis (629). Treatment is not always necessary as 60% are self-limiting and regress spontaneously within 6 months to 1 year (628).

Verruca vulgaris

The common wart of skin, verruca vulgaris (VV), is relatively rare in the upper aerodigestive tract but can be found on the lips, hard palate, tongue, oral mucosa and larynx in adults (624,630) and on the lips in children (624). VV may be difficult to distinguish from papillomata, verrucous hyperplasia and verrucous carcinoma. A true verruca shows, histologically, a prominent granular layer, containing numerous keratohyaline granules, just beneath a layer of koilocytes, and layers of orthokeratin. They have thin rete ridges, which often curl inwards at the margins of the lesion. In the connective tissue, slight infiltration of lymphocytes and some dilated capillaries may be seen (631). VV of the skin has a clear association with HPV-2 and HPV-4 types and the designation of oral warts should be limited to lesions with these types (632). Oral and labial VV are usually associated with HPV-2, rarely with HPV-4. Most oral warts are

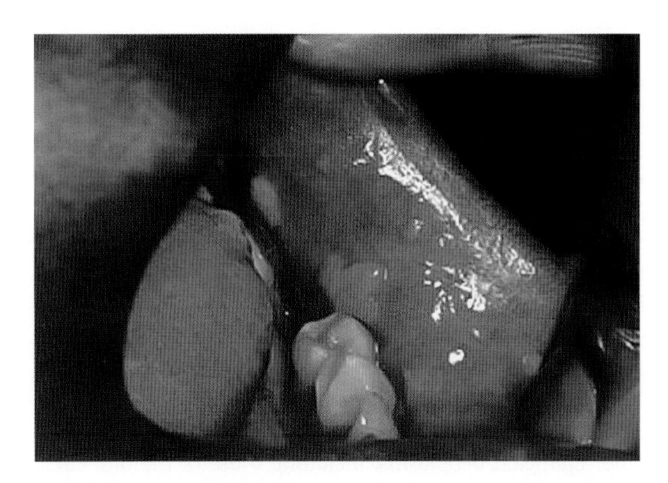

Figure 2.22 Flat papillomas of the buccal mucosa in a patient who had multiple lesions on the lips and elsewhere in the mouth.

self-limiting and may disappear within 2 years. Esthetic discomfort or bite injuries may cause patients to seek treatment.

Focal (or multifocal) epithelial hyperplasia

FEH (aka Heck's disease) is a virus-induced benign hyperplasia of the oral mucosa with an ethnic predilection, preponderantly described in Eskimos in Greenland, Northern Canada and Alaska (where the prevalence may be as high as 10%), among Native Americans (prevalence more than 3%), and descendants of Khoi-San in South Africa (7%–13%); only occasional cases have been described in Caucasians (633,634). FEH can affect all age groups, but is more common in children, adolescents and, inexplicably, in females (635).

Clinically, there are two types of FEH: circumscribed, sessile, soft, nodular elevations; well-demarcated, soft, slightly elevated papules with a flat surface. Lesional size ranges between 0.1 and 1.0 cm and both types show an irregular periphery. FEH commonly affects oral mucosa, tongue and lips (particularly the lower lip). In the Eskimos, approximately 50% of the lesions may be on the tongue, whereas in American Indians, the lip is described as the most common site (636). Most patients have had lesions for many years that are not painful.

Histologically, the lesions demonstrate acanthosis, slight parakeratosis and elongation of rete ridges with horizontal anastomoses. Distinctive ballooning of keratinocytes at various levels in the epithelium is described, with mitosis-like aberrations (so-called FEH cells, a form of koilocytosis). Inclusion bodies may be seen in these nuclei and electron microscopy demonstrates HPV-like particles with a diameter of 40–60 nm (626,637,624,638); lrHPV types 13 and 32 are found in approximately 90% of cases (635). HPV-1 and 11 are rare and may indicate malignant potential.

Recurrent respiratory papillomatosis

Recurrent respiratory papillomatosis (RRP) affects the mucosa of large areas of the upper aerodigestive tract, with multiple benign, wart-like growths (639). It is mainly associated with lrHPV types HPV-6 and HPV-11 (640). Sometimes RRP associated with HPV-type 11 presents with an aggressive clinical course and may result in hoarseness and airway obstruction (641). Frequent recurrence and rapid papilloma growth are common. RRP affects both children and adults. In 75% of child cases, RRP is diagnosed before the fifth birthday and the virus is thought to be vertically transmitted during childbirth (642–644). However, in adults, RRP may be observed in the fourth decade of life and may arise because of the practice of oral sex (645).

Koilocytic dysplasia

Koilocytic dysplasia (KD) is believed to be a subtype of oral dysplasia with unique histological features predictive of the presence of HPV DNA (646). Microscopy shows the simultaneous presence of acanthosis, koilocytosis, keratinocyte multinucleation, nuclear pleomorphism and basal cell hyperplasia. There is a striking male predominance (80%) and relatively adult aged presentation (39 years) (646). Lesions occur mostly on the tongue, lips and buccal mucosa (647).

These lesions may be misdiagnosed as flat condylomata, Bowen's disease or bowenoid papulosis. HIV seropositivity or risk activities for HIV infection have been found in a quarter of the patients. HPV DNA is detected more often in KD than in conventional oral epithelial dysplasia with the presence of hrHPV types HPV-16, HPV-18, HPV-31, HPV-33 and HPV-51, whether or not they may contain lrHPV types HPV-6 and HPV-11 (646).

ORAL POTENTIALLY MALIGNANT DISORDERS

The term OPMDs was recommended for any oral mucosal situation that carries the risk of malignant transformation, in a WHO workshop, held in 2005. The term OPMDs includes lesions/conditions previously called oral precancerous conditions (lichen planus and submucous fibrosis) or oral premalignant lesions (oral leukoplakia [OL], oral erythroplakia and oral verrucous hyperplasia [OVH]) (648,649). It is well documented that HPV is one of the major risk factors for HNSCC. However, recent studies have revealed significant detection rates of HPV DNA in some OPMDs and the prevalence of HPV association with OPMDs is thought to be approximately 25.4% worldwide, with significant regional variation (650). A recent comprehensive meta-analysis suggests a significant association of HPV with these OPMDs with an OR of 3.69 compared to healthy control subjects (516). Here we briefly discuss some OPMDs and their potential relation with the HPVs.

Oral leukoplakia

OL is the most common OPMD found in the oral cavity. The word "leukoplakia" simply means white patch (from the Greek: leuko-white and plakia-patch). Approximately

3.5% of white patches that histologically exhibit a degree of epithelial dysplasia undergo malignant transformation, as a global average (651). OL is characterized by a distinct white/greyish keratotic patch that is granular or nodular in appearance. The prevalence of OL may be higher in females and the common risk factors include the long-term use of tobacco or alcohol, chronic friction, including by restorative materials and ultraviolet radiation (for the lip vermillion) (652–654). Some 22%–25% cases of OL worldwide have been shown to be associated with HPV-16 and/or HPV-18 (655,656).

Proliferative verrucous leukoplakia

Proliferative verrucous leukoplakia is a distinct form of oral leukoplakia, characterized by slow-growing hyperkeratotic, multifocal, wart-like lesions. Gingiva and alveolar ridges are the most common sites and females are mostly affected (657,658). The exact aetiopathogenesis is unknown but an association with HPV has been described from various studies ranging from 24% to 89% of cases (658,659).

Oral verrucous carcinoma

OVC, also known as Akerman's tumor, is a variant of HNSCC, a slow-growing white plaque characterized by painless, soft, fungating, exophytic growths with a cauliflower appearance (660). It is well demarcated, but expansive (661). The most common sites are buccal mucosa, gingivae, lips and mandibular alveolar crest. OVC predominantly affects males 50–80 years of age (662). Histologically, there is considerable surface keratinization with keratin plugging and acanthosis. Cellular atypia is minimal and there is a subepithelial nonspecific inflammatory infiltrate (662). The exact etiology is unknown but the association with HPV has been widely described and HPV types 6, 11, 16 and/or 18 are commonly identified (662,663).

Oral Lichen planus

Oral lichen planus (OLP) is an immunologically mediated chronic mucocutaneous disorder, characterized by hyperkeratotic oral mucosa with striated or annular appearance. Malignant transformation rates of OLP (especially, with the erosive variant) are controversial, studies having reported 0.8%–2.9% over a variable number of years (664–666). OLP commonly affects females between 30 and 60 years of age (667,668). Histologically, acanthosis may be present, while hydropic degeneration of the basal layer and strong subepithelial lymphocytic infiltrate are distinguishing features observed (669). The exact aetiopathogenesis is unknown, but association with HPV has been reported, ranging between 9.2% and 42.6% (mean 25.3%). HPV types HPV-11 and HPV-16 have been found (670,671). As these are lr and hr, respectively, it will be important for newer studies to assess the virology in longitudinal samples for a better understanding of etiology and risk of malignant transformation. This applies to other OPMD, in particular to oral submucous fibrosis for which, although areca nut and genetic predisposition are clearly the main etiological factors, a viral contribution has not yet been researched.

HEPATITIS VIRUSES AND ORAL MALIGNANCIES

HBV, a double-stranded DNA virus of the family *Hepadnaviridae*, and HCV, a small, enveloped, single-stranded, positive-sense RNA virus of the family *Flaviviridae*, are etiological agents of liver cirrhosis and hepatocellular carcinoma, and possibly pancreatic cancer. There is also speculation that these oncoviruses contribute to increased risk of other epithelial neoplasms, including those of the oral cavity (672,673). In 1994, Gandolfo et al. reported a high prevalence of HCV in OLP patients (674). Lodi et al. also published a comprehensive meta-analysis showing 16.8% of HCV prevalence in 5,516 lichen planus patients (675). Two other meta-analyses also suggest a strong association of HCV with lichen planus; pooled OR of lichen planus patient versus control 2.8 (95% CI: 2.4–3.2) and 5.4 (95% CI: 3.5–8.3), respectively (676,677). Further studies suggest that HCV infection may precede the development of OLP (678). Several studies have also suggested a link between HCV infection and OVC and OSCC (679–681). Although the exact mechanism is not well understood, it is thought that the HCV NS3 protein accumulates in the nuclei of infected cells and binds to wild-type, but not mutant p53, thus dysregulating the cell cycle (682). Other theoretical molecular interactions can be speculated upon, but there is yet no evidence that suggests a direct role of HCV on oral carcinogenesis.

MERKEL CELL POLYOMAVIRUS

MCPyV, a member of the family *Polyomaviridae*, is the most recent human oncovirus discovered, and the etiological agent of MCC; a rare but aggressive neuroendocrine neoplasm (683,684). While only a single case of MCC manifesting in the mandibular gingiva in an HIV-positive patient has been reported (361), MCPyV has been detected in saliva and tissue biopsies from oral lesions of both transplant and non-transplant patients (362,685). Evidence shows an association with the presence of both CMV and HHV-6 in the saliva and tissue biopsies of transplant patients (685). There is evidence that MCPyV replicates in oral lymphoid tissue and in salivary glands, indicating the need to elucidate the role of MCPyV in HNCs.

THE EMERGING ROLE OF BACTERIA AND FUNGI IN ORAL AND OROPHARYNGEAL CARCINOGENESIS

EMERGING ROLE OF ORAL BACTERIA

A significant proportion of cases of oral cancer (around 15%) has no history of exposure to any of the major risk factors delineated above (686), suggesting that there are other factors as yet undiscovered. The possible role of oral bacteria is one such factor that has gained increasing attention recently, inspired by convincing evidence in the literature of association between certain bacteria and cancer. A typical example is the etiological role of *Helicobacter pylori* in gastric cancer and mucosa-associated lymphoid tissue lymphomas (687). The associations between *Chlamydia trachomatis* and cervical cancer (688), *Salmonella typhi* and gallbladder cancer (689) and *Bacteroides fragilis* and Fusobacteria with colon cancer (690,691) are further examples.

Possible mechanisms by which bacteria are believed to contribute to oral carcinogenesis include induction of chronic inflammation, inhibition of apoptosis, activation of cell proliferation, promotion of cellular invasion and production of carcinogens (Figure 2.23). For example, oral bacteria are capable of producing carcinogenic levels of acetaldehyde from ethanol. In primary epithelial culture, *Porphyromonas gingivalis* has been found to suppress apoptosis by activation of JAK/STAT and PI3K/Akt signaling and upregulation of miR-203 (692–694), and to induce cell cycle progression by modification of cyclin/CDK activity and inhibition of tumor suppressor P53 (695). In OSCC lines, *P. gingivalis* has also been shown to promote cellular invasion by upregulation and activation of matrix metalloproteinase 9 (MMP-9) (696). In OSCC cell lines, *P. gingivalis*, upregulates B7-H1 and B7-DC receptors, both of which are known to contribute to chronic inflammation (697). There is also evidence to suggest that infection of OSCC by *P. gingivalis* can result in increased metastatic potential and resistance to treatment with Taxol, a chemotherapeutic agent (698). *Fusobacterium nucleatum* also has attributes consistent with a potential carcinogenic role. *In vitro*, *F. nucleatum* has been demonstrated to increase proliferation of colorectal cancer *in vitro* by activation of β-catenin signaling (699) and to promote tumor invasiveness by stimulating secretion of MMP-9 and MMP-13 (700). *F. nucleatum* has been found to be associated with high cytokine levels in CRC and to create an inflammatory microenvironment supportive of tumor progression (691,701). The potentially oncogenic effects of *P. gingivalis* and *F. nucleatum* on epithelial cells are illustrated in Figure 2.24.

Epidemiological studies exploring bacteria associated with OSCC are summarized in Table 2.22. The first attempt to characterize bacteria associated with OSCC was by Nagy et al. (704) in which OSCC lesion surface was shown, using culture techniques, to be colonized by *Porphyromonas* spp. and *Fusobacterium* spp. at significantly higher frequency compared to the adjacent healthy mucosa. In line with this, Katz et al. (705) found that sections of gingival squamous cell carcinoma, immunohistochemically stained for *P. gingivalis*, displayed higher intensity than those of healthy gingival tissue samples, suggesting denser invasion of cancerous epithelium by this bacterium. Interestingly, *P. gingivalis* as well as *F. nucleatum* have been linked to other types of cancer, namely pancreatic and colorectal cancers, respectively (691,706–708). *Streptococcus anginosus* has also been implicated in OSCC. Tateda et al. (709) identified this species by

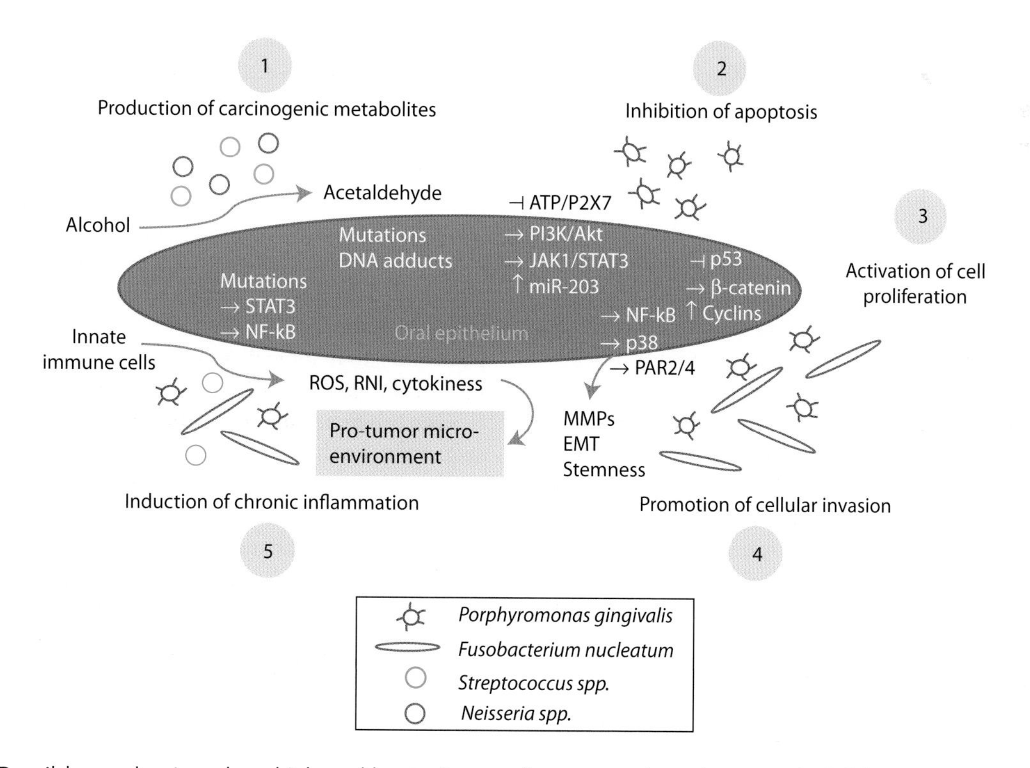

Figure 2.23 Possible mechanisms by which oral bacteria contribute to oral carcinogenesis. ROS, reactive oxygen species; RNI, reactive nitrogen intermediates, MMPs, matrix metalloproteinases; PAR, protease-associated receptor; EMT, epithelial to mesenchymal transition. (Adapted with permission from Perera M et al. *J Oral Microbiol* 2016;8:32762 (702).)

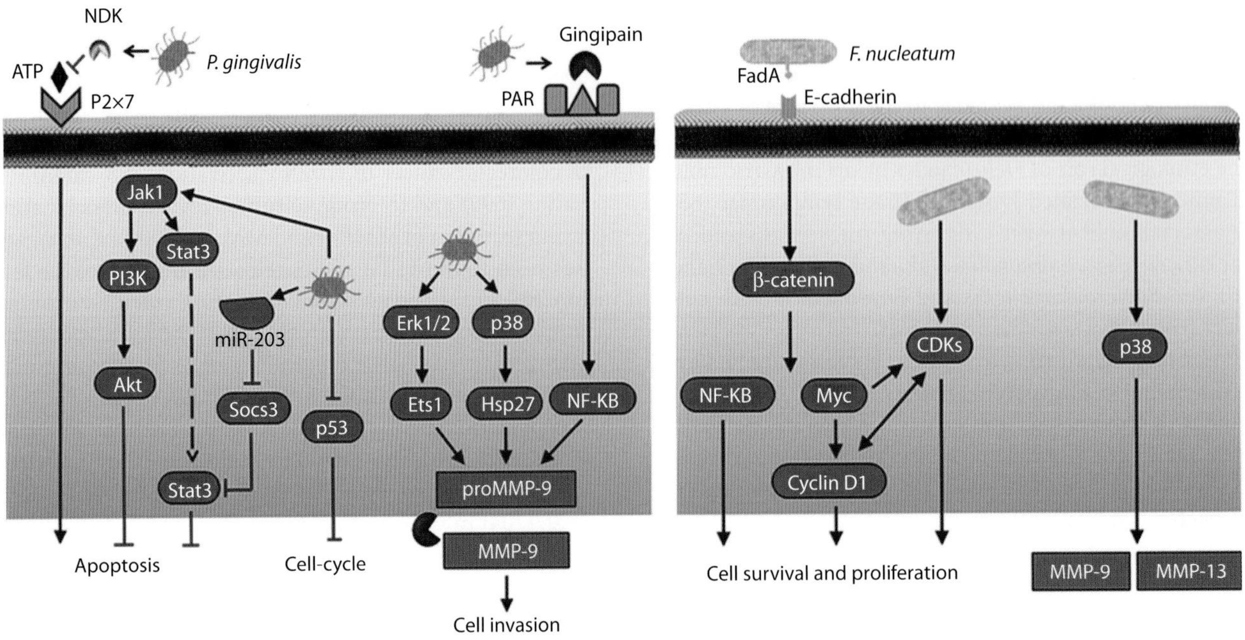

Figure 2.24 Potentially oncogenic effects of *P. gingivalis* and *F. nucleatum* on epithelial cells. (Adapted with permission from Whitmore SE, Lamont RJ. *PloS Pathog* 2014;10(3):e1003933 (703).)

PCR in 100% of 217 HNSCC DNA samples included in their study. Consistently, Sasaki et al. (710), using the same technology, detected *S. anginosus* in 19 out of 42 OSCC samples, but not in leukoplakia or other cancer types. In contrast, however, Morita et al. (711) identified the species less frequently in oral cancer (13%) compared to esophageal cancer (44%). Furthermore, more recent studies detected *S. anginosus* at equal and even higher frequencies in non-tumorous control samples than in tumorous controls (712,713), suggesting that *S. anginosus* may be a normal colonizer of oral epithelium.

Using checkerboard DNA–DNA hybridization, Mager et al. (714) profiled 40 species in saliva samples from individuals with and without OSCC. Three species, *Capnocytophaga gingivalis*, *Prevotella melaninogenica* and *Streptococcus mitis*, were found to be significantly elevated in the OSCC individuals and able to predict cancer cases with 80% sensitivity and 83% specificity. These were thus described as diagnostic markers rather than putative etiological agents of OSCC; however, the results have not been replicated in any other study. In 2006, Hooper et al. (715), using cultivation methods, demonstrated for the first time the presence of 80 viable species within OSCC tissues. Two years later, the same group, using Sanger sequencing of 16S rRNA gene clone libraries (i.e., a metagenomics analysis), identified an additional 28 species in the same samples (712), bringing the bacterial diversity within OSCC tissues to 108 species. Of these, *Ralstonia insidiosa*, *Micrococcus luteus*, *P. melaninogenica*, *Exiguobacterium oxidotolerans*, *Fusobacterium naviforme*, *Staphylococcus aureus*, *Veillonella parvula*, *Peptostreptococcus micros*, *Clavibacter michiganensis* subsp. *Tessellarius*, *Capnocytophaga sp. oral strain S3* and *Prevotella sp. oral clone BE073* were detected in either or both studies at >10% higher prevalence in tumorous than in non-tumorous tissues. The majority of species identified in the tumors, however, were saccharolytic and aciduric, probably reflecting a selection process by the tumor microenvironment, rather than a causal association with OSCC. To add to this complexity, another group, again using metagenomics, detected a further 35 species within OSCC tissues (713), increasing the number of species detected in OSCC to over 140. A different group of species were found to be associated with tumor samples in this study including *Parvimonas* sp. oral taxon 110, *Eubacterium infirmum*, *Eubacterium brachy*, *Gemella haemolysans*, *Gemella morbillorum*, *Gemella sanguinis*, *Johnsonella ignava*, *Peptostreptococcus stomatis*, *Streptococcus gordonii*, *Streptococcus parasanguinis I* and *Streptococcus salivarius*. Although all of these species are oral taxa that are probably adapting to the tumor tissue microenvironment, the possibility that some may contribute to the development of OSCC or modify its clinical course cannot be excluded.

One inherent limitation to culture techniques and Sanger sequencing is the limited number of strains/clones that can be feasibly analyzed, which hinders reproducible detection of potentially relevant species, particularly those with low abundance. Fortunately, the advent of next-generation sequencing (NGS) technologies has recently revolutionized the study of microbial communities by allowing analysis of samples at unprecedented depth (no. of sequences per sample) and breadth (number of samples analyzed) (716). Four studies have so far employed NGS to characterize the oral bacteriome—the collective community of oral bacteria—in association with OSCC. In one study that involved salivary samples from three cases and two healthy controls, the genera *Streptococcus*, *Rothia*, *Gemella* and *Porphyromonas* were

Table 2.22 Summary of epidemiological studies that assessed the association between bacteria and oral cancer

Study	*N*	Technology used	Case sample	Control sample	Taxa associated with oral cancer
Nagy et al. (704)	21	Cultivation; biochemical identification	Tumor surface swabs	Contiguous mucosa surface swabs	*Fusobacterium*, *Porphyromonas*, *Actinomyces*, *Propionibacterium* spp. and *Candida albicans*
Katz et al. (705)	15	Immunohistochemical staining	FFPE gingival carcinoma tissue	FFPE normal tissue	*Porphyromonas gingivalis*
Tateda et al. (709)	270	Cultivation, PCR and Southern-blot	Tumor tissue; gingival smears; oropharyngeal swabs	None	*Streptococcus anginosus*
Sasaki et al. (710)	49	PCR	Fresh tumor tissue; dental plaque; saliva	Fresh tissue: leukoplakia; lymphoma; rhabdomyosarcoma	*S. anginosus*
Morita et al. (711)	63	Real-time PCR	Fresh tumor tissue	Fresh non-cancerous tissue	Association with *S. anginosus* ruled out
Mager et al. (687)	274	Checkerboard DNA–DNA hybridization	Unstimulated saliva	Unstimulated saliva	*Capnocytophaga gingivalis*, *Prevotella melaninogenica* and *Streptococcus mitis*
Hooper et al. (715)	51	Cultivation; 16S rRNA gene sequencing	Fresh tumor tissue	Fresh contagious tissue	*Micrococcus luteus*, *Prevotella melaninogenica*, *Exiguobacterium oxidotolerans*, *Fusobacterium naviforme*, *Staphylococcus aureus* and *Veillonella parvula*
Hooper et al. (712)	20	16S rRNA metagenomics: Sanger sequencing	Fresh tumor tissue	Fresh contiguous tissue	*Ralstonia insidiosa*, *Fusobacterium naviforme*, *Peptostreptococcus micros*, *Clavibacter michiganensis subsp. tessellarius*, *Capnocytophaga sp. oral strain S3* and *Prevotella sp. oral clone BE073*
Pushalkar et al. (713)	20	16S rRNA metagenomics: Sanger sequencing; DGGE	Fresh tumor tissue	Fresh contiguous tissue	*Parvimonas sp. oral taxon 110*, *Eubacterium infirmum*, *Eubacterium brachy*, *Gemella haemolysans*, *Gemella morbillorum*, *Gemella sanguinis*, *Johnsonella ignava*, *Peptostreptococcus stomatis*, *Streptococcus gordonii*, *Streptococcus parasanguinis I* and *Streptococcus salivarius*

(*Continued*)

Table 2.22 (*Continued*) Summary of epidemiological studies that assessed the association between bacteria and oral cancer

Study	*N*	Technology used	Case sample	Control sample	Taxa associated with oral cancer
Pushalkar et al. (717)	05	16S rRNA metagenomics: NGS (454); DGGE	Stimulated saliva	Stimulated saliva	Genera *Streptococcus*, *Rothia*, *Gemella*, *Peptostreptococcus*, *Lactobacillus*, *Micromonas* and *Porphyromonas*
Schmidt et al. (718)	94	16S rRNA metagenomics: NGS (Illumina)	Tumor surface swabs	Surface swabs: contralateral normal; healthy and precancer subjects	Genus *Fusobacterium*; phylum Bacteriodetes; (*Streptococcus* and *Rothia* showed inverse association)
Al-hebshi et al. (719)	03	16S rRNA metagenomics: NGS (454)	Fresh tumor tissue	None	*Bacteroides fragilis*
Al-hebshi et al.	40	16S rRNA metagenomics: NGS (Illumina)	Fresh tumor tissue	Deep epithelial swabs	*Fusobacterium nucleatum*, *Pseudomonas aeruginosa*, *Campylobacter* spp., *Leptotrichia trevisanii*, *Aggregatibacteria* spp., *Parvimonas micra*, *Haemophilus influenzae*, *Staphylococcus aureus*, *Bacteroides fragilis* and *Escherichia coli*. *Functionally*: an inflammatory bacteriome was identified

Source: Adapted with modification from Perera M et al. *J Oral Microbiol* 2016;8:32762 (702).
Abbreviations: PCR: polymerase chain reaction; FFPE: formalin-fixed, paraffin-embedded; DGGE: denaturing gradient gel electrophoresis; NGS: next-generation sequencing.

found to be more abundant in the OSCC cases, whereas *Prevotella*, *Neisseria* and *Leptotrichia* outnumbered in the controls (717). A more comprehensive study, involving analysis of surface swabs of lesion and contralateral normal mucosae from 18 OSCC and 8 precancer cases as well as of mucosae from nine healthy controls, was carried out by Schmidt et al. (718). In this study, the abundance of the genera *Streptococcus* and *Rothia* was significantly lower in the tumor samples compared to the contralateral normal as well as the precancer samples, while that of *Fusobacterium* was significantly higher. However, none of these differences were observed when compared with samples from healthy normal subjects. On the other hand, the phylum Bacteriodetes was characteristically more abundant in both cancerous and normal tissues of OSCC patients compared to precancer and healthy controls, suggesting certain species within this phylum may predispose oral mucosa to malignancy.

One problem with the two studies described above was the low taxonomic resolution: i.e., inability to classify sequences to the species level, which is more pertinent to exploring the link between bacteria and oral cancer. This has, in fact, been a limitation to most oral microbiome studies employing NGS, inherent in the classical bioinformatics approach used for taxonomic assignment of the sequences. Recently, Al-hebshi et al. (719) introduced a bioinformatic algorithm that exploits well-curated 16S rRNA reference sequence datasets, including the Human Oral Microbiome Database for classification of individual NGS reads to the species level. Applying the algorithm in a pilot study involving three samples of OSCC DNA revealed the presence of 228 species, of which 35 were present in all samples. *B. fragilis*, a species seldom isolated from the oral cavity, was identified in two of the samples. Six proteins from this species have been previously detected in the saliva of OSCC patients (720): in addition, it has been recently linked to colon cancer (690). Therefore, *B. fragilis* could be of potential relevance to oral carcinogenesis, a possibility being currently explored.

The same algorithm was employed in a subsequent, larger-scale study involving 20 OSCC biopsies and 20 control oral epithelium swabs. This study provided the first epidemiological evidence for the association of *F. nucleatum* with OSCC. Many other species were also found to be significantly more abundant in the tumor tissues including *Pseudomonas aeruginosa*, *Campylobacter* oral taxon 44, *Leptotrichia trevisanii* and *Campylobacter showae*. In addition, many human pathogens such as *Haemophilus influenzae*, *S. aureus*, *B. fragilis* and *Escherichia coli* were exclusively found in the tumors. The control samples, on the other hand, were associated with higher abundance of, among others, *S. mitis*, *Rothia mucilaginosa* and *Haemophilus parainfluenzae*. More important, functional analysis of the bacterial community profiles revealed enrichment of metabolic pathways involved in bacterial mobility, flagellar assembly, bacterial chemotaxis and LPS synthesis in the tumor tissue, indicating that the bacteriome associated with OSCC is inflammatory in nature, which has significant implication for oral carcinogenesis given the established role of inflammation in cancer.

In conclusion, there is as yet no consensus among studies on particular species to link unequivocally with oral cancer. Putting evidence from *in vitro* and epidemiological studies together, *P. gingivalis* and *F. nucleatum* are the strongest candidates, but other species, such as *Campylobacter ssp.*, *P. aeruginosa and B. fragilis,* may soon find their way to the list. It may well be that microbial community dysbiosis at the function, rather than at the composition level is what matters. In other words, it may be that particular bacterial functions are associated with OSCC regardless of what species are contributing them. Employing high-resolution, NGS technologies coupled with reliable functional analysis will probably help improve our understanding of the association between the oral bacteriome and oral cancer in the near future.

Fungal infections

Several species of *Candida*, especially *C. albicans*, are common commensals of the oral cavity. They become opportunistic pathogens when there is immunosuppression, either local (e.g., by the use of steroid inhalers) or systemic (e.g., by drugs in transplant patients, or in HIV disease), reduction of competing oral flora (such as in the long-term use of antibiotics), or local changes favoring their proliferation and adherence to the oral mucosa: such changes include poor denture hygiene, and the presence of surface roughening or hyperkeratosis, or both.

In a proportion of cases of leukoplakia, there is superficial invasion by fungal hyphae (Figure 2.25), particularly those of nodular leukoplakia, and it has been demonstrated that these have a higher risk of malignant transformation. Of 4,724 mucosal biopsies accessed by one service in London between 1991 and 1995, periodic acid–Schiff (PAS)-positive fungal hyphae were found in 223 (4.7%), with a significant positive association with moderate or severe dysplasia (722). A number of subsequent studies found a similar association not only with dysplasia but with OSCC itself (721–723). Furthermore, some of these studies showed the salivary levels of *C. albicans* to correlate with the severity of dysplasia and of having OSCC (721,722). A more recent study involving analysis of DNA from OSCC tissues and control fibroepithelial polyps using next-generation sequencing of the 16S rRNA gene revealed the presence of a dysbiotic (imbalanced) fungal community (mycobiome) dominated by *C. albicans* in association with OSCC; another two species, were also significantly more abundant in the tumor tissues: *Candida etchellsii* and *Hannaella luteola*-like species (724).

There is also a clear association between smoking and the risk of acquiring a candidal infection in the mouth: this also applies to HIV-positive individuals, compounding the risk. Patients with iron deficiency, clearly at increased risk for oral cancer (see below), are also more prone to oral candidiasis, indicating an interactive, multifactorial process in oral carcinogenesis, as pointed out by Binnie (204). Whether

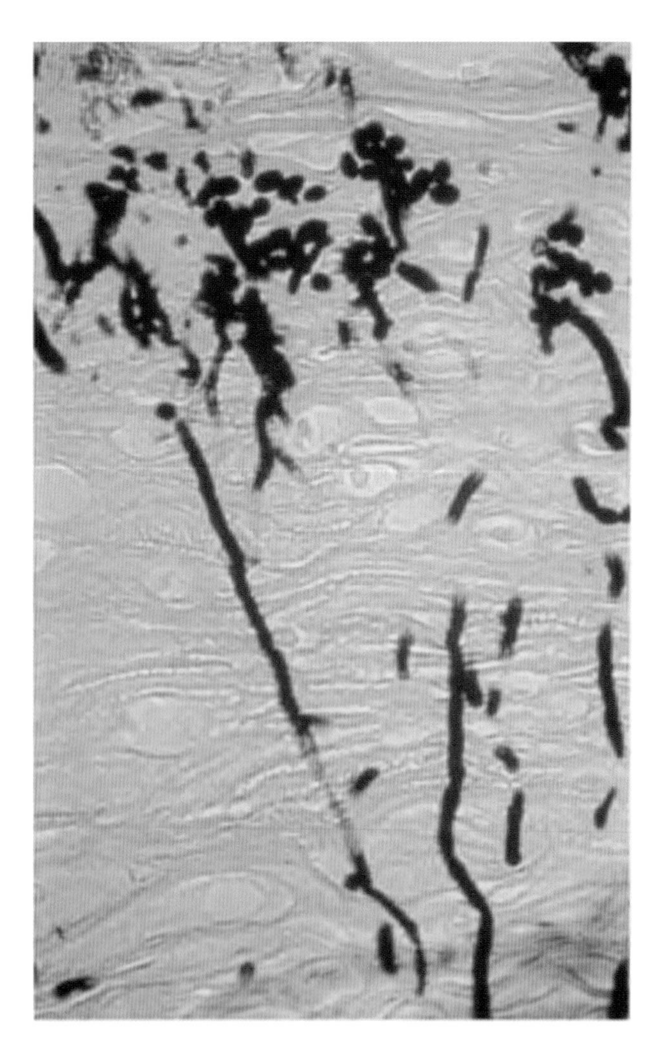

Figure 2.25 Yeasts and hyphae of *Candida albicans*, penetrating the upper layers of the epithelium in a clinical leukoplakia, demonstrated in this section by Grocot's reaction, in which the walls of the organisms are stained black with silver.

Candida spp. invade oral potentially malignant lesions as a secondary event, or are causal in the lesion or the subsequent cancer (or both), remains uncertain. However, a mechanism clearly exists, as these organisms have the enzymes necessary to promote the nitrosation of dietary substrates. Recently, oral isolates of both *C. albicans* and non-albicans candida spp. have been found to be capable of producing carcinogenic amounts of acetaldehyde (16,725).

REFERENCES

1. Burt BA. Definitions of risk. *J Dent Educ* 2001;65(10):1007–8.
2. Lacko M, Braakhuis BJ, Sturgis EM et al. Genetic susceptibility to head and neck squamous cell carcinoma. *Int J Radiat Oncol Biol Phys* 2014;89(1):38–48.
3. Garavello W, Foschi R, Talamini R et al. Family history and the risk of oral and pharyngeal cancer. *Int J Cancer* 2008;122(8):1827–31.
4. Negri E, Boffetta P, Berthiller J et al. Family history of cancer: pooled analysis in the International Head and Neck Cancer Epidemiology Consortium. *Int J Cancer* 2009;124(2):394–401.
5. Copper MP, Jovanovic A, Nauta JJ et al. Role of genetic factors in the etiology of squamous cell carcinoma of the head and neck. *Arch Otolaryngol Head Neck Surg* 1995;121(2):157–60.
6. Goldstein AM, Blot WJ, Greenberg RS et al. Familial risk in oral and pharyngeal cancer. *Eur J Cancer B Oral Oncol* 1994;30B(5):319–22.
7. Brown LM, Gridley G, Diehl SR et al. Family cancer history and susceptibility to oral carcinoma in Puerto Rico. *Cancer* 2001;92(8):2102–8.
8. Goldgar DE, Easton DF, Cannon-Albright LA, Skolnick MH. Systematic population-based assessment of cancer risk in first-degree relatives of cancer probands. *J Natl Cancer Inst* 1994;86(21):1600–8.
9. Radoi L, Paget-Bailly S, Guida F et al. Family history of cancer, personal history of medical conditions and risk of oral cavity cancer in France: the ICARE study. *BMC Cancer* 2013;13:560.
10. Krishna Rao S, Mejia GC, Logan RM et al. A screening model for oral cancer using risk scores: development and validation. *Community Dent Oral Epidemiol* 2016;44(1):76–84.
11. Ankathil R, Mathew A, Joseph F, Nair M. Is oral cancer susceptibility inherited? report of five oral cancer families. *Eur J Cancer B Oral Oncol* 1996;32(1):63–7.
12. Cannon-Albright LA, Thomas A, Goldgar DE et al. Familiality of cancer in Utah. *Cancer Res* 1994;54(9):2378–85.
13. Holloway SM, Sofaer JA. Coefficients of relationship by isonymy among oral cancer registrations in Scottish males. *Community Dent Oral Epidemiol* 1992;20(5):284–7.
14. Merrick Y, Albeck H, Nielsen NH, Hansen HS. Familial clustering of salivary gland carcinoma in Greenland. *Cancer* 1986;57(10):2097–102.
15. Newman AN, Calcaterra TC, Bhuta S. Familial carcinoma of the submandibular gland. A case report and an epidemiologic review. *Arch Otolaryngol* 1981;107(3):169–71.
16. Nieminen MT, Uittamo J, Salaspuro M, Rautemaa R. Acetaldehyde production from ethanol and glucose by non-*Candida albicans* yeasts in vitro. *Oral Oncol* 2009;45(12):e245–8.
17. Ankathil R, Bhattathiri NV, Francis JV et al. Mutagen sensitivity as a predisposing factor in familial oral cancer. *Int J Cancer* 1996;69(4):265–7.
18. Cloos J, Braakhuis BJ, Steen I et al. Increased mutagen sensitivity in head-and-neck squamous-cell carcinoma patients, particularly those with multiple primary tumors. *Int J Cancer* 1994;56(6):816–9.
19. Sato M, Sato T, Izumo T, Amagasa T. Genetically high susceptibility to oral squamous cell carcinoma

in terms of combined genotyping of CYP1A1 and GSTM1 genes. *Oral Oncol* 2000;36(3):267–71.
20. Scully C, Bedi R. Ethnicity and oral cancer. *Lancet Oncol* 2000;1(1):37–42.
21. Buch SC, Notani PN, Bhisey RA. Polymorphism at GSTM1, GSTM3 and GSTT1 gene loci and susceptibility to oral cancer in an Indian population. *Carcinogenesis* 2002;23(5):803–7.
22. Gronau S, Konig-Greger D, Rettinger G, Riechelmann H. GSTM1 gene polymorphism in patients with head and neck tumors. *Laryngorhinootologie* 2000;79(6):341–4.
23. Kietthubthew S, Sriplung H, Au WW. Genetic and environmental interactions on oral cancer in Southern Thailand. *Environ Mol Mutagen* 2001;37(2):111–6.
24. Park LY, Muscat JE, Kaur T et al. Comparison of GSTM polymorphisms and risk for oral cancer between African-Americans and Caucasians. *Pharmacogenetics* 2000;10(2):123–31.
25. Liu S, Park JY, Schantz SP, Stern JC, Lazarus P. Elucidation of CYP2E1 5′ regulatory RsaI/PstI allelic variants and their role in risk for oral cancer. *Oral Oncol* 2001;37(5):437–45.
26. Sreelekha TT, Ramadas K, Pandey M, Thomas G, Nalinakumari KR, Pillai MR. Genetic polymorphism of CYP1A1, GSTM1 and GSTT1 genes in Indian oral cancer. *Oral Oncol* 2001;37(7):593–8.
27. Topcu Z, Chiba I, Fujieda M et al. CYP2A6 gene deletion reduces oral cancer risk in betel quid chewers in Sri Lanka. *Carcinogenesis* 2002;23(4):595–8.
28. Bouchardy C, Hirvonen A, Coutelle C, Ward PJ, Dayer P, Benhamou S. Role of alcohol dehydrogenase 3 and cytochrome P-4502E1 genotypes in susceptibility to cancers of the upper aerodigestive tract. *Int J Cancer* 2000;87(5):734–40.
29. Summersgill KF, Smith EM, Kirchner HL, Haugen TH, Turek LP. P53 polymorphism, human papillomavirus infection in the oral cavity, and oral cancer. *Oral Surg Oral Med Oral Pathol Oral Radiol Endod* 2000;90(3):334–9.
30. Tandle AT, Sanghvi V, Saranath D. Determination of p53 genotypes in oral cancer patients from India. *Br J Cancer* 2001;84(6):739–42.
31. Nomura T, Noma H, Shibahara T, Yokoyama A, Muramatusu T, Ohmori T. Aldehyde dehydrogenase 2 and glutathione S-transferase M 1 polymorphisms in relation to the risk for oral cancer in Japanese drinkers. *Oral Oncol* 2000;36(1):42–6.
32. Schwartz SM, Doody DR, Fitzgibbons ED, Ricks S, Porter PL, Chen C. Oral squamous cell cancer risk in relation to alcohol consumption and alcohol dehydrogenase-3 genotypes. *Cancer Epidemiol Biomarkers Prev* 2001;10(11):1137–44.
33. Sturgis EM, Dahlstrom KR, Guan Y et al. Alcohol dehydrogenase 3 genotype is not associated with risk of squamous cell carcinoma of the oral cavity and pharynx. *Cancer Epidemiol Biomarkers Prev* 2001;10(3):273–5.
34. Merletti F, Boffetta P, Ciccone G, Mashberg A, Terracini B. Role of tobacco and alcoholic beverages in the etiology of cancer of the oral cavity/oropharynx in Torino, Italy. *Cancer Res* 1989;49(17):4919–24.
35. Andreotti M, Rodrigues AN, Cardoso LM, Figueiredo RA, Eluf-Neto J, Wunsch-Filho V. Occupational status and cancer of the oral cavity and oropharynx. *Cad Saude Publica* 2006;22(3):543–52.
36. Richiardi L, Corbin M, Marron M et al. Occupation and risk of upper aerodigestive tract cancer: the ARCAGE study. *Int J Cancer* 2012;130(10):2397–406.
37. Meo SA. Health hazards of cement dust. *Saudi Med J* 2004;25(9):1153–9.
38. World Health Organization. *Chrysotile Asbestos.* Environmental Health Criteria 203, Geneva, 1998.
39. Krewski D, Burnett RT, Goldberg MS et al. Overview of the reanalysis of the Harvard Six Cities Study and American Cancer Society study of particulate air pollution and mortality. *J Toxicol Environ Health Part A* 2003;66(16–19):1507–51.
40. Purdue MP, Järvholm B, Bergdahl IA, Hayes RB, Baris D. Occupational exposures and head and neck cancers among Swedish construction workers. *Scand J Work Environ Health* 2006;32(4):270–5.
41. Maier H, Tisch M, Kyrberg H, Conradt C, Weidauer H. Occupational hazardous substance exposure and nutrition. Risk factors for mouth, pharyngeal and laryngeal carcinomas? *Hno* 2002;50(8):743–52.
42. Paget-Bailly S, Cyr D, Luce D. Occupational exposures to asbestos, polycyclic aromatic hydrocarbons and solvents, and cancers of the oral cavity and pharynx: a quantitative literature review. *Int Arch Occup Environ Health* 2012;85(4):341–51.
43. Ulvestad B, Kjaerheim K, Martinsen JI et al. Cancer incidence among workers in the asbestos-cement producing industry in Norway. *Scand J Work Environ Health* 2002;28(6):411–7.
44. Tarvainen L, Kyyronen P, Kauppinen T, Pukkala E. Cancer of the mouth and pharynx, occupation and exposure to chemical agents in Finland [in 1971–95]. *Int J Cancer* 2008;123(3):653–9.
45. Reid A, Ambrosini G, de Klerk N, Fritschi L, Musk B. Aerodigestive and gastrointestinal tract cancers and exposure to crocidolite (blue asbestos): incidence and mortality among former crocidolite workers. *Int J Cancer* 2004;111(5):757–61.
46. Offermans NS, Vermeulen R, Burdorf A et al. Occupational asbestos exposure and risk of oral cavity and pharyngeal cancer in the prospective Netherlands Cohort Study. *Scand J Work Environ Health* 2014;40(4):420–7.
47. Sluis-Cremer GK, Liddell FD, Logan WP, Bezuidenhout BN. The mortality of amphibole miners in South Africa, 1946–80. *Br J Ind Med* 1992; 49(8):566–75.

48. Lipworth L, La Vecchia C, Bosetti C, McLaughlin JK. Occupational exposure to rock wool and glass wool and risk of cancers of the lung and the head and neck: a systematic review and meta-analysis. *J Occup Environ Med* 2009;51(9):1075–87.
49. Karlehagen S, Andersen A, Ohlson CG. Cancer incidence among creosote-exposed workers. *Scand J Work Environ Health* 1992;18(1):26–9.
50. Wong O, Harris F. Retrospective cohort mortality study and nested case-control study of workers exposed to creosote at 11 wood-treating plants in the United States. *J Occup Environ Med* 2005;47(7):683–97.
51. Gustavsson P, Jakobsson R, Johansson H, Lewin F, Norell S, Rutkvist LE. Occupational exposures and squamous cell carcinoma of the oral cavity, pharynx, larynx, and oesophagus: a case-control study in Sweden. *Occup Environ Med* 1998;55(6):393–400.
52. WHO. *Hazard Prevention and Control in the Work Environment: Airborne Dust*. Geneva, Switzerland: World Health Organization (WHO) Prevention and Control Exchange (PACE), 1999.
53. International Agency for Research on Cancer. Arsenic, metals, fibres and dusts. *A Review of Human Carcinogens* 2012;100 C.
54. Pollan M, Lopez-Abente G. Wood-related occupations and laryngeal cancer. *Cancer Detect Prev* 1995;19(3):250–7.
55. Langevin SM, McClean MD, Michaud DS, Eliot M, Nelson HH, Kelsey KT. Occupational dust exposure and head and neck squamous cell carcinoma risk in a population-based case-control study conducted in the greater Boston area. *Cancer Med* 2013;2(6):978–86.
56. Deitmer T. Laryngeal carcinoma caused by exposure to wood dust? *Laryngo–Rhino–Otologie* 1995;74(6):365–70.
57. International Agency for Research on Cancer. *Wood Dust and Formaldehyde*. IARC Monographs on the Evaluation of Carcino-Genic Risk to Humans, 1995, 62.
58. Coble JB, Brown LM, Hayes RB et al. Sugarcane farming, occupational solvent exposures, and the risk of oral cancer in Puerto Rico. *J Occup Environ Med* 2003;45(8):869–74.
59. Blair A, Hartge P, Stewart PA, McAdams M, Lubin J. Mortality and cancer incidence of aircraft maintenance workers exposed to trichloroethylene and other organic solvents and chemicals: extended follow up. *Occup Environ Med* 1998;55(3):161–71.
60. Purdue MP, Jarvholm B, Bergdahl IA, Hayes RB, Baris D. Occupational exposures and head and neck cancers among Swedish construction workers. *Scand J Work Environ Health* 2006;32(4):270–5.
61. Merletti F, Boffetta P, Ferro G, Pisani P, Terracini B. Occupation and cancer of the oral cavity or oropharynx in Turin, Italy. *Scand J Work Environ Health* 1991;17(4):248–54.
62. International Agency for Research on Cancer. IARC Monographs on the Evaluation of Carcinogenic Risks to Humans: Solar and Ultraviolet Radiation, 1992, 55.
63. Ariyawardana A, Johnson NW. Trends of lip, oral cavity and oropharyngeal cancers in Australia 1982–2008: overall good news but with rising rates in the oropharynx. *BMC Cancer* 2013;13:333.
64. Pogoda JM, Preston-Martin S. Solar radiation, lip protection, and lip cancer risk in Los Angeles County women (California, United States). *Cancer Causes & Control: CCC* 1996;7(4):458–63.
65. de Visscher JG, van der Waal I. Etiology of cancer of the lip. A review. *Int J Oral Maxillofac Surg* 1998;27(3):199–203.
66. Laakkonen A, Pukkala E. Cancer incidence among Finnish farmers, 1995–2005. *Scand J Work Environ Health* 2008;34(1):73–9.
67. Ji J, Hemminki K. Occupation and upper aerodigestive tract cancers: a follow-up study in Sweden. *J Occup Environ Med* 2005;47(8):785–95.
68. Antoniades DZ, Styanidis K, Papanayotou P, Trigonidis G. Squamous cell carcinoma of the lips in a northern Greek population. Evaluation of prognostic factors on 5-year survival rate – I. *Eur J Cancer B Oral Oncol* 1995;31B(5):333–9.
69. Abreu L, Kruger E, Tennant M. Lip cancer in Western Australia, 1982–2006: a 25-year retrospective epidemiological study. *Aust Dent J* 2009;54(2):130–5.
70. Gupta B, Ariyawardana A, Johnson NW. Oral cancer in India continues in epidemic proportions: evidence base and policy initiatives. *Int Dent J* 2013; 63(1):12–25.
71. Moore S, Johnson N, Pierce A, Wilson D. The epidemiology of lip cancer: a review of global incidence and aetiology. *Oral Dis* 1999;5(3):185–95.
72. Perea-Milla Lopez E, Minarro-Del Moral RM, Martinez-Garcia C et al. Lifestyles, environmental and phenotypic factors associated with lip cancer: a case-control study in southern Spain. *Br J Cancer* 2003;88(11):1702–7.
73. Luna-Ortiz K, Guemes-Meza A, Villavicencio-Valencia V, Mosqueda-Taylor A. Lip cancer experience in Mexico. An 11-Year Retrospective Study. *Oral Oncol* 2004;40(10):992–9.
74. Levi F, La Vecchia C, Te VC, Franceschi S. Trends in lip cancer incidence in Vaud, Switzerland. *Br J Cancer* 1993;68(5):1012–3.
75. Swerdlow AJ, Cooke KR, Skegg DC, Wilkinson J. Cancer incidence in England and Wales and New Zealand and in migrants between the two countries. *Br J Cancer* 1995;72(1):236–43.
76. Wake M. The urban/rural divide in head and neck cancer – the effect of atmospheric pollution. *Clin Otolaryngol Allied Sci* 1993;18(4):298–302.
77. Maier H, de Vries N, Weidauer H. Occupation and cancer of the oral cavity, pharynx and larynx. *Hno* 1990;38(8):271–8.

78. King GN, Healy CM, Glover MT et al. Increased prevalence of dysplastic and malignant lip lesions in renal-transplant recipients. *N Engl J Med* 1995;332(16): 1052–7.
79. Franco EL, Kowalski LP, Oliveira BV et al. Risk factors for oral cancer in Brazil: a case-control study. *Int J Cancer* 1989;43(6):992–1000.
80. Pintos J, Franco EL, Kowalski LP, Oliveira BV, Curado MP. Use of wood stoves and risk of cancers of the upper aero-digestive tract: a case-control study. *Int J Epidemiol* 1998;27(6):936–40.
81. Sapkota A, Zaridze D, Szeszenia-Dabrowska N et al. Indoor air pollution from solid fuels and risk of upper aerodigestive tract cancers in central and eastern Europe. *Environ Res* 2013;120:90–5.
82. Raskob G, Dietz R, Senneweld E, Maier H. Indoor air pollution by emissions of fossil fuel single stoves: possibly a hitherto underrated risk factor in the development of carcinomas in the head and neck. *Otolaryngol Head Neck Surg* 1995;112(2):308–15.
83. Huebner WW, Schoenberg JB, Kelsey JL et al. Oral and pharyngeal cancer and occupation: a case-control study. *Epidemiology* 1992;3(4):300–9.
84. IARC: The International Agency for Research on Cancer. Outdoor air pollution a leading environmental cause of cancer deaths. Available from: http://www.iarc.fr/en/mediacentre/pr/2013/pdfs/pr221_E.pdf.
85. Straif K, Benbrahim-Tallaa L, Baan R et al. A review of human carcinogens – Part C: metals, arsenic, dusts, and fibres. *Lancet Oncol* 2009;10(5):453–4.
86. Hoffmann TK, Bier H, Whiteside TL. Targeting the immune system: novel therapeutic approaches in squamous cell carcinoma of the head and neck. *Cancer Immunol Immunother* 2004;53(12):1055–67.
87. Whiteside TL. Immunobiology of head and neck cancer. *Cancer Metastasis Rev* 2005;24(1):95–105.
88. Jewett A, Cacalano NA, Teruel A et al. Inhibition of nuclear factor kappa B (NFkappaB) activity in oral tumor cells prevents depletion of NK cells and increases their functional activation. *Cancer Immunol Immunother* 2006;55(9):1052–63.
89. Warnakulasuriya S, Khan Z. *Squamous Cell Carcinoma: Molecular Therapeutic Targets*. Springer, 2017.
90. Winn DM. Tobacco use and oral disease. *J Dent Educ* 2001;65(4):306–12.
91. Johnson N. Tobacco use and oral cancer: a global perspective. *J Dent Educ* 2001;65(4):328–39.
92. Franceschi S, Talamini R, Barra S et al. Smoking and drinking in relation to cancers of the oral cavity, pharynx, larynx, and esophagus in northern Italy. *Cancer Res* 1990;50(20):6502–7.
93. Fioretti F, Bosetti C, Tavani A, Franceschi S, La Vecchia C. Risk factors for oral and pharyngeal cancer in never smokers. *Oral Oncol* 1999;35(4):375–8.
94. Mathers CD, Loncar D. Projections of global mortality and burden of disease from 2002 to 2030. *PLoS Med* 2006;3(11):e442.
95. Organization WH. WHO report on the global tobacco epidemic, 2015: raising taxes on tobacco, 2015.
96. Peto R, Lopez AD, Boreham J, Thun M, Heath C Jr, Doll R. Mortality from smoking worldwide. *Br Med Bull* 1996;52(1):12–21.
97. World Health Organization. *WHO Report on the Global Tobacco Epidemic*. Geneva, 2015.
98. Collaborators GBDRF. Global, regional, and national comparative risk assessment of 79 behavioural, environmental and occupational, and metabolic risks or clusters of risks, 1990–2015: a systematic analysis for the Global Burden of Disease Study 2015. *Lancet* 2016;388(10053):1659–724.
99. Sinha DN, Suliankatchi RA, Gupta PC et al. Global burden of all-cause and cause-specific mortality due to smokeless tobacco use: systematic review and meta-analysis. *Tob Control* 2018;27(1):35–42. doi: 10.1136/tobaccocontrol-2016-053302. Epub November 30, 2016.
100. Sinha DN, Palipudi KM, Gupta PC et al. Smokeless tobacco use: a meta-analysis of risk and attributable mortality estimates for India. *Indian J Cancer* 2014;51(Suppl 1):S73–7.
101. Sinha DN, Abdulkader RS, Gupta PC. Smokeless tobacco-associated cancers: a systematic review and meta-analysis of Indian studies. *Int J Cancer* 2016;138(6):1368–79.
102. Doll R, Peto R, Wheatley K, Gray R, Sutherland I. Mortality in relation to smoking: 40 years' observations on male British doctors. *BMJ (Clinical Research Ed)* 1994;309(6959):901–11.
103. Peto R, Lopez A, Boreham J, Thun M, Heath C. *Mortality from Smoking in Developed Countries 1950–2000. Indirect Estimates from National Statistics*. Oxford, New York, Tokyo: Oxford University Press, 1994.
104. Ng M, Freeman MK, Fleming TD et al. Smoking prevalence and cigarette consumption in 187 countries, 1980–2012. *JAMA* 2014;311(2):183–92.
105. Daftary D, Murti P, Bhonsle R, Gupta P, Mehta F, Pindborg J. Risk factors and risk markers for oral cancer in high incidence areas of the world. In: *Risk Markers for Oral Diseases*. Volume 2, Oral Cancer, Edited by NW Johnson, Cambridge University Press, 1991, 29–63.
106. Daftary D, Murti P, Bhonsle R, Gupta P, Mehta F, Pindborg JJ. Oral squamous cell carcinoma. In: *Oral Diseases in the Tropics*. Oxford University Press, New Delhi, 1992. Revised reprint, 2017, from www.jaypeebrothers.com/pgDetails.aspx?book_id=9789386150554.
107. Gupta PC, Hamner JE, Murti P (eds). Control of tobacco-related cancers and other diseases. In: *Proceedings of an International Symposium Mumbai*. Oxford University Press, 1992.

108. Mehta FS, Hamner JE. *Tobacco-related Oral Mucosal Lesions and Conditions in India: A Guide for Dental Students, Dentists, and Physicians: Basic Dental Research Unit*. Tata Institute of Fundamental Research, 1993.
109. Stanfill SB, Connolly GN, Zhang L et al. Global surveillance of oral tobacco products: total nicotine, unionised nicotine and tobacco-specific N-nitrosamines. *Tob Control* 2011;20(3):e2.
110. Idris AM, Nair J, Friesen M et al. Carcinogenic tobacco-specific nitrosamines are present at unusually high levels in the saliva of oral snuff users in Sudan. *Carcinogenesis* 1992;13(6):1001–5.
111. Idris AM, Ahmed HM, Malik MO. Toombak dipping and cancer of the oral cavity in the Sudan: a case-control study. *Int J Cancer* 1995;63(4):477–80.
112. Idris AM, Warnakulasuriya KAAS, Johnson NW et al. 1998; personal communication.
113. Idris AM, Warnakulasuriya KA, Ibrahim YE, Nielsen R, Cooper D, Johnson NW. Toombak-associated oral mucosal lesions in Sudanese show a low prevalence of epithelial dysplasia. *J Oral Pathol Med* 1996;25(5):239–44.
114. Gupta B, Kumar N, Johnson NW. Relationship of lifetime exposure to tobacco, alcohol and second hand tobacco smoke with upper aero-digestive tract cancers in India: a case-control study with a life-course perspective. *Asian Pac J Cancer Prev* 2017; 18(2):347–56.
115. Gupta B, Kumar N, Johnson NW. A risk factor-based model for upper aerodigestive tract cancers in India: Predicting and validating the receiver operating characteristic curve. *J Oral Pathol Med* 2017;46(6):465–71.
116. Brown RL, Suh JM, Scarborough JE, Wilkins SA, Smith RR. Snuff dippers' intraoral cancer: clinical characteristics and response to therapy. *Cancer* 1965; 18(1):2–13.
117. Ackerman LV. Verrucous carcinoma of the oral cavity. *Surgery* 1948;23(4):670–8.
118. McCoy JM, Waldron CA. Verrucous carcinoma of the oral cavity. a review of forty-nine cases. *Oral Surg Oral Med Oral Pathol* 1981;52(6):623–9.
119. Blot WJ, Fraumeni JF Jr. Geographic patterns of oral cancer in the United States: etiologic implications. *J Chronic Dis* 1977;30(11):745–57.
120. Winn DM, Blot WJ, Shy CM, Pickle LW, Toledo A, Fraumeni JF Jr. Snuff dipping and oral cancer among women in the southern United States. *N Engl J Med* 1981;304(13):745–9.
121. Winn DM. Smokeless tobacco and cancer: the epidemiologic evidence. *CA Cancer J Clin* 1988;38(4):236–43.
122. Portnoy DB, Wu CC, Tworek C, Chen J, Borek N. Youth curiosity about cigarettes, smokeless tobacco, and cigars: prevalence and associations with advertising. *Am J Prev Med* 2014;47(2 Suppl 1):S76–86.
123. Timberlake DS. Advertising receptivity and youth initiation of smokeless tobacco. *Subst Use Misuse* 2016;51(9):1077–82.
124. Conrad AK, Hutton SB, Munnelly M, Bay RC. Screening for smokeless tobacco use and presence of oral lesions in major league baseball athletes. *J Calif Dent Assoc* 2015;43(1):14–20.
125. Connolly GN, Orleans CT, Kogan M. Use of smokeless tobacco in major-league baseball. *N Engl J Med* 1988;318(19):1281–5.
126. Agaku IT, Singh T, Jones SE et al. Combustible and smokeless tobacco use among high school athletes – United States, 2001–2013. *MMWR Morb Mortal Wkly Rep* 2015;64(34):935–9.
127. U.S. Department of Health and Human Services, Public Health Service. *The health consequences of using smokeless tobacco: a report of the advisory committee to the Surgeon General*. U.S. Department of Health and Human Services, Public Health Service, National Institutes of Health, National Cancer Institute. DHHS Publication No. (NIH), 1986.
128. McCarten B. Smokeless tobacco: the Irish experience and Eu experience. *Oral Dis* 1998;4:56–7.
129. IARC. Tobacco habits other than smoking; betel-quid and areca-nut chewing and some related nitrosamines (*IARC Monographs on the Evaluation of Carcinogenic Risk to Humans*, Vol. 37). Lyon, France: International Agency for Research on Cancer (IARCPress), 1985.
130. IARC Monographs on the Evaluation of Carcinogenic Risks to Humans Volume 89. *Smokeless Tobacco and Some Tobacco-specific N-nitrosamines*, World Health Organization, 2007.
131. Grady D, Greene J, Daniels TE et al. Oral mucosal lesions found in smokeless tobacco users. *J Am Dent Assoc* 1990;121(1):117–23.
132. Tomar SL, Winn DM, Swango PA, Giovino GA, Kleinman DV. Oral mucosal smokeless tobacco lesions among adolescents in the United States. *J Dent Res* 1997;76(6):1277–86.
133. Sterling TD, Rosenbaum WL, Weinkam JJ. Analysis of the relationship between smokeless tobacco and cancer based on data from the National Mortality Followback Survey. *J Clin Epidemiol* 1992;45(3):223–31.
134. Stepanov I, Jensen J, Hatsukami D, Hecht SS. New and traditional smokeless tobacco: comparison of toxicant and carcinogen levels. *Nicotine Tob Res* 2008;10(12):1773–82.
135. Osterdahl BG, Jansson C, Paccou A. Decreased levels of tobacco-specific N-nitrosamines in moist snuff on the Swedish market. *J Agric Food Chem* 2004;52(16):5085–8.
136. Biener L, Roman AM, Mc Inerney SA et al. Snus use and rejection in the USA. *Tob Control* 2016;25(4):386–92.
137. Bartsch H, Spiegelhalder B. Environmental exposure to N-nitroso compounds (NNOC) and precursors: an overview. *Eur J Cancer Prev* 1996;5 Suppl 1:11–7.

138. Rodu B. *For Smokers Only: How Smokeless Tobacco can Save Your Life.* Sulzburger & Graham Publishing Company, New York, USA, 1995.
139. Timberlake DS, Zell JA. Review of epidemiologic data on the debate over smokeless tobacco's role in harm reduction. *BMC Med* 2009;7:61.
140. Lee PN, Hamling J. Systematic review of the relation between smokeless tobacco and cancer in Europe and North America. *BMC Med* 2009;7:36.
141. Wyss AB, Hashibe M, Lee YA et al. Smokeless tobacco use and the risk of head and neck cancer: pooled analysis of US studies in the INHANCE consortium. *Am J Epidemiol* 2016, October 15. [Epub ahead of print].
142. Idris AM, Nair J, Ohshima H et al. Unusually high levels of carcinogenic tobacco-specific nitrosamines in Sudan snuff (toombak). *Carcinogenesis* 1991;12(6):1115–8.
143. Idris AM, Prokopczyk B, Hoffmann D. Toombak: a major risk factor for cancer of the oral cavity in Sudan. *Prev Med* 1994;23(6):832–9.
144. Schildt EB, Eriksson M, Hardell L, Magnuson A. Oral infections and dental factors in relation to oral cancer: a Swedish case-control study. *Eur J Cancer Prev* 1998;7(3):201–6.
145. Lewin F, Norell SE, Johansson H et al. Smoking tobacco, oral snuff, and alcohol in the etiology of squamous cell carcinoma of the head and neck: a population-based case-referent study in Sweden. *Cancer* 1998;82(7):1367–75.
146. Roosaar A, Johansson AL, Sandborgh-Englund G, Axell T, Nyren O. Cancer and mortality among users and nonusers of snus. *Int J Cancer* 2008;123(1):168–73.
147. Hirsch JM, Wallstrom M, Carlsson AP, Sand L. Oral cancer in Swedish snuff dippers. *Anticancer Res* 2012; 32(8):3327–30.
148. Huhtasaari F, Asplund K, Lundberg V, Stegmayr B, Wester PO. Tobacco and myocardial infarction: is snuff less dangerous than cigarettes? *BMJ (Clinical Research Ed)* 1992;305(6864):1252–6.
149. Bolinder G, Alfredsson L, Englund A, de Faire U. Smokeless tobacco use and increased cardiovascular mortality among Swedish construction workers. *Am J Public Health* 1994;84(3):399–404.
150. Persson PG, Hellers G, Ahlbom A. Use of oral moist snuff and inflammatory bowel disease. *Int J Epidemiol* 1993;22(6):1101–3.
151. Zendehdel K, Nyren O, Luo J et al. Risk of gastroesophageal cancer among smokers and users of Scandinavian moist snuff. *Int J Cancer* 2008;122(5):1095–9.
152. Axell TE. Smokeless tobacco and oral health: The Swedish experience. *Oral Dis* 1998;4:55–6.
153. Axell TE. Oral mucosal changes related to smokeless tobacco usage: research findings in Scandinavia. *Eur J Cancer B Oral Oncol* 1993;29B(4):299–302.
154. Zain RB, Ikeda N, Gupta PC et al. Oral mucosal lesions associated with betel quid, areca nut and tobacco chewing habits: consensus from a workshop held in Kuala Lumpur, Malaysia, November 25–27, 1996. *J Oral Pathol Med* 1999;28(1):1–4.
155. Thomas SJ, Bain CJ, Battistutta D, Ness AR, Paissat D, Maclennan R. Betel quid not containing tobacco and oral cancer: a report on a case-control study in Papua New Guinea and a meta-analysis of current evidence. *Int J Cancer* 2007;120(6):1318–23.
156. Hou X, Xu X, Anderson I. Determinants of tobacco consumption in Papua New Guinea: challenges in changing behaviours. *Asia Pac Policy Stud* 2015;2(2):255–65.
157. Warnakulasuriya S, Chaturvedi P, Gupta PC. Addictive behaviours need to include areca nut use. *Addiction (Abingdon, England)* 2015;110(9):1533.
158. Boucher BJ. Betel quid, smokeless tobacco and general health. In: Bedi R, Jones P. (eds). *Betel Quid and Tobacco Chewing Among the Bangladeshi Community in the United Kingdom; Usage and Health Issues.* London: Centre for Transcultural Oral Health, 1995, 53–8.
159. R. Bedi. Betel-quid and tobacco chewing among the United Kingdom's Bangladeshi community. *Br J Cancer.* 1996;29:S73–S77. PMCID: PMC2149859.
160. Warnakulasuriya S, Peters T. Introduction: biology, medical and socio-economic aspects of areca nut use. *Addict Biol* 2002;7(1):75–6.
161. Garg A, Chaturvedi P, Gupta PC. A review of the systemic adverse effects of areca nut or betel nut. *Indian J Med Paediatr Oncol* 2014;35(1):3–9.
162. Paymaster JC. Some observations on oral and pharyngeal carcinomas in the State of Bombay. *Cancer* 1962;15:578–83.
163. Hirayama T. An epidemiological study of oral and pharyngeal cancer in Central and South-East Asia. *Bull World Health Organ* 1966;34(1):41–69.
164. Mehta FS, Gupta PC, Daftary DK, Pindborg JJ, Choksi SK. An epidemiologic study of oral cancer and precancerous conditions among 101,761 villagers in Maharashtra, India. *Int J Cancer* 1972;10(1):134–41.
165. Reichart PA. Oral cancer and precancer related to betel and Miang Chewing in Thailand: a review. *J Oral Pathol Med* 1995;24(6):241–3.
166. Thomas S, Wilson A. A quantitative evaluation of the aetiological role of betel quid in oral carcinogenesis. *Eur J Cancer B Oral Oncol* 1993;29B(4):265–71.
167. Warnakulasuriya S. *The Role of Betel-quid in Oral Carcinogenesis.* Usage and Health Issues Center for Transcultural Oral Health, London, UK, 1995.
168. Gupta B, Johnson NW. Systematic review and meta-analysis of association of smokeless tobacco and of betel quid without tobacco with incidence of oral cancer in South Asia and the Pacific. *PloS One* 2014;9(11):e113385.
169. Guha N, Warnakulasuriya S, Vlaanderen J, Straif K. Betel quid chewing and the risk of oral and oropharyngeal cancers: a meta-analysis with implications for cancer control. *Int J Cancer* 2014;135(6):1433–43.

170. Gupta PC, Mehta FS, Daftary DK et al. Incidence rates of oral cancer and natural history of oral precancerous lesions in a 10-year follow-up study of Indian villagers. *Community Dent Oral Epidemiol* 1980;8(6):283–333.
171. Jayalekshmi PA, Gangadharan P, Akiba S, Koriyama C, Nair RR. Oral cavity cancer risk in relation to tobacco chewing and bidi smoking among men in Karunagappally, Kerala, India: Karunagappally cohort study. *Cancer Sci* 2011;102(2):460–7.
172. Jayalekshmi PA, Gangadharan P, Akiba S, Nair RR, Tsuji M, Rajan B. Tobacco chewing and female oral cavity cancer risk in Karunagappally cohort, India. *Br J Cancer* 2009;100(5):848–52.
173. Junaid M, Periyanan K, Raj A, Madan Kumar PD. Patterns of tobacco usage among subjects with potentially malignant oral lesions or conditions in Chennai city: a comparative study. *J Cancer Res Ther* 2017;13(2):230–4.
174. Mehta FS, Gupta MB, Pindborg JJ, Bhonsle RB, Jalnawalla PN, Sinor PN. An intervention study of oral cancer and precancer in rural Indian populations: a preliminary report. *Bull World Health Organ* 1982;60(3):441–6.
175. Gupta PC, Murti PR, Bhonsle RB, Mehta FS, Pindborg JJ. Effect of cessation of tobacco use on the incidence of oral mucosal lesions in a 10-yr follow-up study of 12,212 users. *Oral Dis* 1995;1(1):54–8.
176. Orr I. Oral cancer in betel nut chewers in Travancore: its aetiology, pathology, and treatment. *The Lancet* 1933;222(5741):575–80.
177. Znaor A, Brennan P, Gajalakshmi V et al. Independent and combined effects of tobacco smoking, chewing and alcohol drinking on the risk of oral, pharyngeal and esophageal cancers in Indian men. *Int J Cancer* 2003;105(5):681–6.
178. Humans IWGotEoCRt. Betel-quid and areca-nut chewing and some areca-nut derived nitrosamines. *IARC Monogr Eval Carcinog Risks Hum* 2004;85:1.
179. Maher R, Lee AJ, Warnakulasuriya KA, Lewis JA, Johnson NW. Role of areca nut in the causation of oral submucous fibrosis: a case-control study in Pakistan. *J Oral Pathol Med* 1994;23(2):65–9.
180. Murti PR, Bhonsle RB, Gupta PC, Daftary DK, Pindborg JJ, Mehta FS. Etiology of oral submucous fibrosis with special reference to the role of areca nut chewing. *J Oral Pathol Med* 1995;24(4):145–52.
181. Stich HF, Rosin MP, Brunnemann KD. Oral lesions, genotoxicity and nitrosamines in betel quid chewers with no obvious increase in oral cancer risk. *Cancer Lett* 1986;31(1):15–25.
182. Ko YC, Chiang TA, Chang SJ, Hsieh SF. Prevalence of betel quid chewing habit in Taiwan and related sociodemographic factors. *J Oral Pathol Med* 1992;21(6):261–4.
183. Shiu MN, Chen TH, Chang SH, Hahn LJ. Risk factors for leukoplakia and malignant transformation to oral carcinoma: a leukoplakia cohort in Taiwan. *Br J Cancer* 2000;82(11):1871–4.
184. Atkinson L, Purohit R, Reay-Young P, Scott GC. Cancer reporting in Papua New Guinea: 1958–70 and 1971–78. *Natl Cancer Inst Monogr* 1982;62:65–71.
185. Thomas S, Kearsley J. Betel quid and oral cancer: a review. *Oral Oncol, Eur J Cancer* 1993;29B(4):251–5.
186. van Wyk CW, Stander I, Padayachee A, Grobler-Rabie AF. The areca nut chewing habit and oral squamous cell carcinoma in South African Indians. a retrospective study. *S Afr Medl J* 1993;83(6):425–9.
187. Lu CT, Yen YY, Ho CS et al. A case-control study of oral cancer in Changhua County, Taiwan. *J Oral Pathol Med* 1996;25(5):245–8.
188. Merchant A, Husain SS, Hosain M et al. Paan without tobacco: an independent risk factor for oral cancer. *Int J Cancer* 2000;86(1):128–31.
189. Trivedy CR, Craig G, Warnakulasuriya S. The oral health consequences of chewing areca nut. *Addict Biol* 2002;7(1):115–25.
190. Gupta PC, Ray CS. Areca nut use and cancer in India. *Biomed Res J* 2015;2(2):140–65.
191. Balaram P, Sridhar H, Rajkumar T et al. Oral cancer in southern India: the influence of smoking, drinking, paan-chewing and oral hygiene. *Int J Cancer* 2002;98(3):440–5.
192. Muwonge R, Ramadas K, Sankila R et al. Role of tobacco smoking, chewing and alcohol drinking in the risk of oral cancer in Trivandrum, India: a nested case-control design using incident cancer cases. *Oral Oncol* 2008;44(5):446–54.
193. Mahapatra S, Kamath R, Shetty BK, Binu VS. Risk of oral cancer associated with gutka and other tobacco products: a hospital-based case-control study. *J Cancer Res Ther* 2015;11(1):199–203.
194. Stich HF, Stich W, Parida BB. Elevated frequency of micronucleated cells in the buccal mucosa of individuals at high risk for oral cancer: betel quid chewers. *Cancer Lett* 1982;17(2):125–34.
195. Dave BJ, Trivedi AH, Adhvaryu SG. Role of areca nut consumption in the cause of oral cancers. a Cytogenetic Assessment. *Cancer* 1992;70(5):1017–23.
196. Ranadive KJ, Ranadive SN, Shivapurkar NM, Gothoskar SV. Betel quid chewing and oral cancer: experimental studies on hamsters. *Int J Cancer* 1979;24(6):835–43.
197. Shirname LP, Menon MM, Nair J, Bhide SV. Correlation of mutagenicity and tumorigenicity of betel quid and its ingredients. *Nutr Cancer* 1983;5(2):87–91.
198. Jin YT, Tsai ST, Wong TY, Chen FF, Chen RM. Studies on promoting activity of Taiwan betel quid ingredients in hamster buccal pouch carcinogenesis. *Eur J Cancer B Oral Oncol* 1996;32B(5):343–6.
199. Lin LM, Chen YK, Lai DR, Huang YL, Chen HR. Cancer-promoting effect of Taiwan betel quid in hamster buccal pouch carcinogenesis. *Oral Dis* 1997;3(4):232–5.

200. Sundqvist K, Liu Y, Nair J, Bartsch H, Arvidson K, Grafström RC. Cytotoxic and genotoxic effects of areca nut-related compounds in cultured human buccal epithelial cells. *Cancer Research* 1989;49(19):5294–8.
201. van der Bijl P, van Eyk AD. Areca nut extract lowers the permeability of vaginal mucosa to reduced arecoline and arecaidine. *J Oral Pathol Med* 2001;30(9):537–41.
202. Jeng JH, Chang MC, Hahn LJ. Role of areca nut in betel quid-associated chemical carcinogenesis: current awareness and future perspectives. *Oral Oncol* 2001;37(6):477–92.
203. Nagabhushan M, Amonkar AJ, D'Souza AV, Bhide SV. Nonmutagenicity of betel leaf and its antimutagenic action against environmental mutagens. *Neoplasma* 1987;34(2):159–67.
204. Binnie W. Risk factors and risk markers for oral cancer in low incidence areas of the world. *Oral Cancer* 1991;2:64–87.
205. IARC. *Tobacco Smoking (IARC Monographs on the Evaluation of the Carcinogenic Risk of Chemicals to Humans, Vol. 38)*. Lyon, France: International Agency for Research on Cancer (IARCPress), 1986.
206. IARC. Personal habits and indoor combustions. *IARC Monogr Eval Carcinog Risks Hum* 2012;100:319–31.
207. USDHHS. *Reducing the Health Consequences of Smoking, 25 years of progress*. A report of the Surgeon General of the United States, 1989.
208. USDHHS. *How tobacco smoke causes disease: the biology and behavioral basis for smoking-attributable disease*. A report of the Surgeon General, 2010.
209. Levin ML, Goldstein H, Gerhardt PR. Cancer and tobacco smoking; a preliminary report. *J Am Med Assoc* 1950;143(4):336–8.
210. Wynder EL, Bross IJ, Feldman RM. A study of the etiological factors in cancer of the mouth. *Cancer* 1957;10(6):1300–23.
211. Clemmesen J. Statistical studies in the aetiology of malignant neoplasms. I. Review and results. Supplement 174. I. *Acta Pathologica et Microbiologica Scandinavica Supplementum* 1965;174:1–543.
212. Spitzer WO, Hill GB, Chambers LW, Helliwell BE, Murphy HB. The occupation of fishing as a risk factor in cancer of the lip. *N Engl J Med* 1975;293(9):419–24.
213. Wynder EL, Mushinski MH, Spivak JC. Tobacco and alcohol consumption in relation to the development of multiple primary cancers. *Cancer* 1977;40(4 Suppl):1872–8.
214. Dikshit RP, Kanhere S. Tobacco habits and risk of lung, oropharyngeal and oral cavity cancer: a population-based case-control study in Bhopal, India. *Int J Epidemiol* 2000;29(4):609–14.
215. Duong M, Rangarajan S, Zhang X et al. Effects of bidi smoking on all-cause mortality and cardiorespiratory outcomes in men from south Asia: an observational community-based substudy of the Prospective Urban Rural Epidemiology Study (PURE). *Lancet Glob Health* 2017;5(2):e168–76.
216. Gupta PC, Asma S. *Bidi Smoking and Public Health*. New Delhi: Ministry of Health and Family Welfare, Government of India, 2008, 1–238.
217. IARC. *Tobacco Control: Reversal of Risk After Quitting Smoking*. IARC Handbooks of Cancer Prevention No. 11. World Health Organization, 2007.
218. Jovanovic A, Schulten EA, Kostense PJ, Snow GB, van der Waal I. Tobacco and alcohol related to the anatomical site of oral squamous cell carcinoma. *J Oral Pathol Med* 1993;22(10):459–62.
219. Blot WJ, McLaughlin JK, Winn DM et al. Smoking and drinking in relation to oral and pharyngeal cancer. *Cancer Res* 1988;48(11):3282–7.
220. Blot WJ. Alcohol and cancer. *Cancer Res* 1992; 52(7 Suppl):2119s–23s.
221. Mashberg A, Meyers H. Anatomical site and size of 222 early asymptomatic oral squamous cell carcinomas: A continuing prospective study of oral cancer. II. *Cancer* 1976;37(5):2149–57.
222. Boffetta P, Mashberg A, Winkelmann R, Garfinkel L. Carcinogenic effect of tobacco smoking and alcohol drinking on anatomic sites of the oral cavity and oropharynx. *Int J Cancer* 1992;52(4):530–3.
223. Bharath TS, Kumar NG, Nagaraja A, Saraswathi TR, Babu GS, Raju PR. Palatal changes of reverse smokers in a rural coastal Andhra population with review of literature. *J Oral Maxillofac Pathol* 2015;19(2):182–7.
224. van der Eb MM, Leyten EM, Gavarasana S, Vandenbroucke JP, Kahn PM, Cleton FJ. Reverse smoking as a risk factor for palatal cancer: a cross-sectional study in rural Andhra Pradesh, India. *Int J Cancer* 1993;54(5):754–8.
225. Bhonsle RB, Murti PR, Gupta PC, Mehta FS. Reverse dhumti smoking in Goa: an epidemiologic study of 5,449 villagers for oral precancerous lesions. *Indian J Cancer* 1976;13(4):301–5.
226. Quigley LF Jr, Shklar G, Cobb CM. Reverse cigarette smoking in Caribbeans: clinical, histologic, and cytologic observations. *J Am Dent Assoc* 1966;72(4):867–73.
227. Morrow RC, Suarez G. Mucosal changes and cancer in intra-oral smoking. *Laryngoscope* 1971;81(7):1020–8.
228. Ortiz GM, Pierce AM, Wilson DF. Palatal changes associated with reverse smoking in Filipino women. *Oral Dis* 1996;2(3):232–7.
229. Davidson BJ, Hsu TC, Schantz SP. The genetics of tobacco-induced malignancy. *Arch Otolaryngol Head Neck Surg* 1993;119(11):1198–205.
230. Hecht SS, Carmella SG, Murphy SE, Foiles PG, Chung FL. Carcinogen biomarkers related to smoking and upper aerodigestive tract cancer. *J Cell Biochem Suppl* 1993;17F:27–35.
231. Hoffmann D, Hecht SS. Nicotine-derived N-nitrosamines and tobacco-related cancer: current status and future directions. *Cancer Res* 1985;45(3):935–44.
232. Hoffmann D, Adams JD, Brunnemann KD, Hecht SS. Assessment of tobacco-specific N-nitrosamines

in tobacco products. *Cancer Res* 1979;39(7 Pt 1): 2505–9.
233. Lafuente A, Maristany M, Arias C et al. Glutathione and glutathione S-transferases in human squamous cell carcinomas of the larynx and GSTM1 dependent risk. *Anticancer Res* 1998;18(1A):107–11.
234. Hung HC, Chuang J, Chien YC et al. Genetic polymorphisms of CYP2E1, GSTM1, and GSTT1; environmental factors and risk of oral cancer. *Cancer Epidemiol Biomarkers Prev* 1997;6(11):901–5.
235. Oude Ophuis MB, van Lieshout EM, Roelofs HM, Peters WH, Manni JJ. Glutathione S-transferase M1 and T1 and cytochrome P4501A1 polymorphisms in relation to the risk for benign and malignant head and neck lesions. *Cancer* 1998;82(5):936–43.
236. Veneroni S, Silvestrini R, Costa A, Salvatori P, Faranda A, Molinari R. Biological indicators of survival in patients treated by surgery for squamous cell carcinoma of the oral cavity and oropharynx. *Oral Oncol* 1997;33(6):408–13.
237. Nahas G, Latour C. The human toxicity of marijuana. *Med J Aust* 1992;156(7):495–7.
238. Firth NA. Marijuana use and oral cancer: a review. *Oral Oncol* 1997;33(6):398–401.
239. aWengen DF. Marijuana and malignant tumors of the upper aerodigestive tract in young patients. On the risk assessment of marijuana. *Laryngorhinootologie* 1993;72(5):264–7.
240. Caplan GA, Brigham BA. Marijuana smoking and carcinoma of the tongue. Is there an association? *Cancer* 1990;66(5):1005–6.
241. Zhang ZF, Morgenstern H, Spitz MR et al. Marijuana use and increased risk of squamous cell carcinoma of the head and neck. *Cancer Epidemiol Biomarkers Prev* 1999;8(12):1071–8.
242. Hashibe M, Morgenstern H, Cui Y et al. Marijuana use and the risk of lung and upper aerodigestive tract cancers: results of a population-based case-control study. *Cancer Epidemiol Biomarkers Prev* 2006;15(10):1829–34.
243. Berthiller J, Lee YC, Boffetta P et al. Marijuana smoking and the risk of head and neck cancer: pooled analysis in the INHANCE consortium. *Cancer Epidemiol Biomarkers Prev* 2009;18(5):1544–51.
244. Marks MA, Chaturvedi AK, Kelsey K et al. Association of marijuana smoking with oropharyngeal and oral tongue cancers: pooled analysis from the INHANCE consortium. *Cancer Epidemiol Biomarkers Prev* 2014;23(1):160–71.
245. Darling MR, Arendorf TM. Effects of cannabis smoking on oral soft tissues. *Community Dent Oral Epidemiol* 1993;21(2):78–81.
246. Alcohol drinking. IARC working Group, Lyon, 13–20 October 1987. *IARC Monogr Eval Carcinog Risks Hum* 1988;44:1–378.
247. Humans IWGotEoCRt. Alcohol consumption and ethyl carbamate. *IARC Monogr Eval Carcinog Risks Hum* 2010;96:3–1383.
248. Humans IWGotEoCRt. Personal habits and indoor combustions. Volume 100 E. A Review of Human Carcinogens. *IARC Monogr Eval Carcinog Risks Hum* 2012;100(Pt E):1–538.
249. Kato I, Nomura AM. Alcohol in the aetiology of upper aerodigestive tract cancer. *Eur J Cancer B Oral Oncol* 1994;30B(2):75–81.
250. Iype EM, Pandey M, Mathew A, Thomas G, Sebastian P, Nair MK. Oral cancer among patients under the age of 35 years. *J Postgrad Med* 2001;47(3):171–6.
251. Pednekar MS, Sansone G, Gupta PC. Association of alcohol, alcohol and tobacco with mortality: findings from a prospective cohort study in Mumbai (Bombay), India. *Alcohol (Fayetteville, NY)* 2012;46(2):139–46.
252. Hindle I, Downer MC, Moles DR, Speight PM. Is alcohol responsible for more intra-oral cancer? *Oral Oncol* 2000;36(4):328–33.
253. Monteiro MG, Rehm J, Shield KD, Stockwell T. Alcohol consumption: an overview of international trends. In: Stella RQ, William CC. (eds). *International Encyclopedia of Public Health*. Oxford: Academic Press, 2017, 45–57. ISBN: 978-0-12-803708-9.
254. Hindle I, Downer MC, Speight PM. The association between intra-oral cancer and surrogate markers of smoking and alcohol consumption. *Community Dent Health* 2000;17(2):107–13.
255. Garavello W, Bertuccio P, Levi F et al. The oral cancer epidemic in central and eastern Europe. *Int J Cancer* 2010;127(1):160–71.
256. Chikritzhs TN, Allsop SJ, Moodie AR, Hall WD. Per capita alcohol consumption in Australia: will the real trend please step forward? *Med J Aust* 2010;193(10):594–7.
257. Praud D, Rota M, Rehm J et al. Cancer incidence and mortality attributable to alcohol consumption. *Int J Cancer* 2016;138(6):1380–7.
258. Gupta PC, Ray CS, Murti PR, Sinha DN. Rising incidence of oral cancer in Ahmedabad city. *Indian J Cancer* 2014;51(Suppl 1):S67–72.
259. Rothman KJ. The effect of alcohol consumption on risk of cancer of the head and neck. *Laryngoscope* 1978;88(1 Pt 2 Suppl 8):51–5.
260. Schlecht NF, Pintos J, Kowalski LP, Franco EL. Effect of type of alcoholic beverage on the risks of upper aerodigestive tract cancers in Brazil. *Cancer Causes Control* 2001;12(7):579–87.
261. Bundgaard T, Wildt J, Frydenberg M, Elbrond O, Nielsen JE. Case-control study of squamous cell cancer of the oral cavity in Denmark. *Cancer Causes Control* 1995;6(1):57–67.
262. Mashberg A, Boffetta P, Winkelman R, Garfinkel L. Tobacco smoking, alcohol drinking, and cancer of the oral cavity and oropharynx among U.S. Veterans. *Cancer* 1993;72(4):1369–75.

263. Kabat GC, Wynder EL. Type of alcoholic beverage and oral cancer. *Int J Cancer* 1989;43(2):190–4.
264. Altieri A, Bosetti C, Gallus S et al. Wine, beer and spirits and risk of oral and pharyngeal cancer: a case-control study from Italy and Switzerland. *Oral Oncol* 2004;40(9):904–9.
265. Purdue MP, Hashibe M, Berthiller J et al. Type of alcoholic beverage and risk of head and neck cancer – a pooled analysis within the INHANCE Consortium. *Am J Epidemiol* 2009;169(2):132–42.
266. Andre K, Schraub S, Mercier M, Bontemps P. Role of alcohol and tobacco in the aetiology of head and neck cancer: a case-control study in the Doubs region of France. *Eur J Cancer B Oral Oncol* 1995;31B(5):301–9.
267. Franceschi S, Barra S, La Vecchia C, Bidoli E, Negri E, Talamini R. Risk factors for cancer of the tongue and the mouth. A case-control study from northern Italy. *Cancer* 1992;70(9):2227–33.
268. Barra S, Franceschi S, Negri E, Talamini R, La Vecchia C. Type of alcoholic beverage and cancer of the oral cavity, pharynx and oesophagus in an Italian area with high wine consumption. *Int J Cancer* 1990;46(6):1017–20.
269. Zheng TZ, Boyle P, Hu HF et al. Tobacco smoking, alcohol consumption, and risk of oral cancer: a case-control study in Beijing, People's Republic of China. *Cancer Causes Control* 1990;1(2):173–9.
270. Boyle P, Macfarlane GJ, Blot WJ et al. European School of Oncology Advisory report to the European Commission for the Europe Against Cancer Programme: oral carcinogenesis in Europe. *Eur J Cancer B Oral Oncol* 1995;31B(2):75–85.
271. Castellsague X, Quintana MJ, Martinez MC et al. The role of type of tobacco and type of alcoholic beverage in oral carcinogenesis. *Int J Cancer* 2004;108(5):741–9.
272. Varoni EM, Lodi G, Iriti M. Ethanol versus phytochemicals in wine: oral cancer risk in a light drinking perspective. *Int J Mol Sci* 2015;16(8):17029–47.
273. De Stefani E, Boffetta P, Oreggia F, Fierro L, Mendilaharsu M. Hard liquor drinking is associated with higher risk of cancer of the oral cavity and pharynx than wine drinking. A case-control study in Uruguay. *Oral Oncol* 1998;34(2):99–104.
274. La Vecchia C, Tavani A, Franceschi S, Levi F, Corrao G, Negri E. Epidemiology and prevention of oral cancer. *Oral Oncol* 1997;33(5):302–12.
275. Talamini R, La Vecchia C, Levi F, Conti E, Favero A, Franceschi S. Cancer of the oral cavity and pharynx in nonsmokers who drink alcohol and in nondrinkers who smoke tobacco. *J Natl Cancer Inst* 1998;90(24):1901–3.
276. Brugere J, Guenel P, Leclerc A, Rodriguez J. Differential effects of tobacco and alcohol in cancer of the larynx, pharynx, and mouth. *Cancer* 1986;57(2):391–5.
277. Goldstein BY, Chang SC, Hashibe M, La Vecchia C, Zhang ZF. Alcohol consumption and cancers of the oral cavity and pharynx from 1988 to 2009: an update. *Eur J Cancer Prev* 2010;19(6):431–65.
278. Hashibe M, Brennan P, Chuang SC et al. Interaction between tobacco and alcohol use and the risk of head and neck cancer: pooled analysis in the International Head and Neck Cancer Epidemiology Consortium. *Cancer Epidemiol Biomarkers Prev* 2009;18(2):541–50.
279. Tuyns AJ. Alcohol and cancer. *Proc Nutr Soc* 1990;49(2):145–51.
280. Boeing H, Patterns EWGoD. Alcohol and risk of cancer of the upper gastrointestinal tract: first analysis of the EPIC data. *IARC Sci Publ* 2002;156:151–4.
281. Friborg JT, Yuan JM, Wang R, Koh WP, Lee HP, Yu MC. A prospective study of tobacco and alcohol use as risk factors for pharyngeal carcinomas in Singapore Chinese. *Cancer* 2007;109(6):1183–91.
282. Freedman ND, Abnet CC, Leitzmann MF, Hollenbeck AR, Schatzkin A. Prospective investigation of the cigarette smoking-head and neck cancer association by sex. *Cancer* 2007;110(7):1593–601.
283. Ferlay J, Soerjomataram I, Ervik M et al. GLOBOCAN 2012 v1.0: Cancer Incidence and Mortality Worldwide: IARC Cancer Base No. 11 (International Agency for Research on Cancer, Lyon, France, 2013). http://globocaniarcfr. 2012.
284. Lesch CA, Squier CA, Cruchley A, Williams DM, Speight P. The permeability of human oral mucosa and skin to water. *J Dent Res* 1989;68(9):1345–9.
285. Hsu TC, Furlong C, Spitz MR. Ethyl alcohol as a cocarcinogen with special reference to the aerodigestive tract: a cytogenetic study. *Anticancer Res* 1991;11(3):1097–101.
286. Squier CA, Cox P, Hall BK. Enhanced penetration of nitrosonornicotine across oral mucosa in the presence of ethanol. *J Oral Pathol* 1986;15(5):276–9.
287. Du X, Squier CA, Kremer MJ, Wertz PW. Penetration of N-nitrosonornicotine (NNN) across oral mucosa in the presence of ethanol and nicotine. *J Oral Pathol Med* 2000;29(2):80–5.
288. Howie NM, Trigkas TK, Cruchley AT, Wertz PW, Squier CA, Williams DM. Short-term exposure to alcohol increases the permeability of human oral mucosa. *Oral Dis* 2001;7(6):349–54.
289. McCoy GD, Wynder EL. Etiological and preventive implications in alcohol carcinogenesis. *Cancer Res* 1979;39(7 Pt 2):2844–50.
290. Siilverman S Jr, Shillitoe EH. Aetiology and predisposing factors. In: Silverman S Jr (ed.). *Oral Cancer.* Atlanta: The American Cancer Society, 1990, 7–39.
291. Squier CA, Kremer MJ, Wertz PW. Effect of ethanol on lipid metabolism and epithelial permeability barrier of skin and oral mucosa in the rat. *J Oral Pathol Med* 2003;32(10):595–9.
292. Enwonwu CO, Meeks VI. Bionutrition and oral cancer in humans. *Crit Rev Oral Biol Med* 1995;6(1):5–17.

293. Homann N, Tillonen J, Meurman JH et al. Increased salivary acetaldehyde levels in heavy drinkers and smokers: a microbiological approach to oral cavity cancer. *Carcinogenesis* 2000;21(4):663–8.
294. Homann N, Tillonen J, Rintamaki H, Salaspuro M, Lindqvist C, Meurman JH. Poor dental status increases acetaldehyde production from ethanol in saliva: a possible link to increased oral cancer risk among heavy drinkers. *Oral Oncol* 2001;37(2):153–8.
295. Moreno-Lopez LA, Esparza-Gomez GC, Gonzalez-Navarro A, Cerero-Lapiedra R, Gonzalez-Hernandez MJ, Dominguez-Rojas V. Risk of oral cancer associated with tobacco smoking, alcohol consumption and oral hygiene: a case-control study in Madrid, Spain. *Oral Oncol* 2000;36(2):170–4.
296. Homann N, Jousimies-Somer H, Jokelainen K, Heine R, Salaspuro M. High acetaldehyde levels in saliva after ethanol consumption: methodological aspects and pathogenetic implications. *Carcinogenesis* 1997;18(9):1739–43.
297. Chen C, Ricks S, Doody DR, Fitzgibbons ED, Porter PL, Schwartz SM. N-Acetyltransferase 2 polymorphisms, cigarette smoking and alcohol consumption, and oral squamous cell cancer risk. *Carcinogenesis* 2001;22(12):1993–9.
298. Harris C, Warnakulasuriya KA, Gelbier S, Johnson NW, Peters TJ. Oral and dental health in alcohol misusing patients. *Alcohol Clin Exp Res* 1997;21(9):1707–9.
299. Farinati F, Lieber CS, Garro AJ. Effects of chronic ethanol consumption on carcinogen activating and detoxifying systems in rat upper alimentary tract tissue. *Alcohol Clin Exp Res* 1989;13(3):357–60.
300. Seitz HK, Stickel F. Risk factors and mechanisms of hepatocarcinogenesis with special emphasis on alcohol and oxidative stress. *Biol Chem* 2006;387(4):349–60.
301. Miyake T, Shibamoto T. Quantitative analysis of acetaldehyde in foods and beverages. *J Agric Food Chem* 1993;41(11):1968–70.
302. Boffetta P, Ye W, Adami HO, Mucci LA, Nyren O. Risk of cancers of the lung, head and neck in patients hospitalized for alcoholism in Sweden. *Br J Cancer* 2001;85(5):678–82.
303. Marron M, Boffetta P, Zhang ZF et al. Cessation of alcohol drinking, tobacco smoking and the reversal of head and neck cancer risk. *Int J Epidemiol* 2010;39(1):182–96.
304. McAuley A, Goodall CA, Ogden GR, Shepherd S, Cruikshank K. Delivering alcohol screening and alcohol brief interventions within general dental practice: rationale and overview of the evidence. *Br Dent J* 2011;210(9):E15.
305. Weaver A, Fleming SM, Smith DB. Mouthwash and oral cancer: carcinogen or coincidence? *J Oral Surg* 1979;37(4):250–3.
306. Blot WJ, Winn DM, Fraumeni JF Jr. Oral cancer and mouthwash. *J Natl Cancer Inst* 1983;70(2):251–3.
307. Wynder EL, Kabat G, Rosenberg S, Levenstein M. Oral cancer and mouthwash use. *J Natl Cancer Inst* 1983;70(2):255–60.
308. Winn DM, Blot WJ, McLaughlin JK et al. Mouthwash use and oral conditions in the risk of oral and pharyngeal cancer. *Cancer Res* 1991;51(11):3044–7.
309. Johnson NW. Alcohol in mouthwashes: a health hazard. *Br Dent J* 1994;177(4):124.
310. Winn DM, Diehl SR, Brown LM et al. Mouthwash in the etiology of oral cancer in Puerto Rico. *Cancer Causes Control* 2001;12(5):419–29.
311. Gagari E, Kabani S. Adverse effects of mouthwash use. a review. *Oral Surg Oral Med Oral Pathol Oral Radiol Endod* 1995;80(4):432–9.
312. Elmore JG, Horwitz RI. Oral cancer and mouthwash use: Evaluation of the epidemiologic evidence. *Otolaryngol Head Neck Surg* 1995;113(3):253–61.
313. Shapiro S, Castellana JV, Sprafka JM. Alcohol-containing mouthwashes and oropharyngeal cancer: a spurious association due to underascertainment of confounders? *Am J Epidemiol* 1996;144(12):1091–5.
314. Gandini S, Negri E, Boffetta P, La Vecchia C, Boyle P. Mouthwash and oral cancer risk quantitative meta-analysis of epidemiologic studies. *Ann Agric Environ Med* 2012;19(2):173–80.
315. Lachenmeier DW. Alcohol-containing mouthwash and oral cancer – can epidemiology prove the absence of risk? *Ann Agric Environ Med* 2012;19(3):609–10.
316. Boffetta P, Hayes RB, Sartori S et al. Mouthwash use and cancer of the head and neck: a pooled analysis from the International Head and Neck Cancer Epidemiology Consortium. *Eur J Cancer Prev* 2016;25(4):344–8.
317. Currie S, Farah C. Alcohol-containing mouthwash and oral cancer risk: a review of current evidence. *Oa Alcohol* 2014;2(1):4.1–9.
318. Hashim D, Sartori S, Brennan P et al. The role of oral hygiene in head and neck cancer: results from International Head and Neck Cancer Epidemiology (INHANCE) consortium. *Ann Oncol* 2016;27(8):1619–25.
319. Boyle P, Koechlin A, Autier P. Mouthwash use and the prevention of plaque, gingivitis and caries. *Oral Dis* 2014;20(Suppl 1):1–68.
320. Bhatti SA, Walsh TF, Douglas CW. Ethanol and pH levels of proprietary mouthrinses. *Community Dent Health* 1994;11(2):71–4.
321. Rich AM, Radden BG. Squamous cell carcinoma of the oral mucosa: a review of 244 cases in Australia. *J Oral Pathol* 1984;13(5):459–71.
322. Hodge KM, Flynn MB, Drury T. Squamous cell carcinoma of the upper aerodigestive tract in nonusers of tobacco. *Cancer* 1985;55(6):1232–5.
323. Ng SK, Kabat GC, Wynder EL. Oral cavity cancer in non-users of tobacco. *J Natl Cancer Inst* 1993;85(9):743–5.

324. Tan EH, Adelstein DJ, Droughton ML, Van Kirk MA, Lavertu P. Squamous cell head and neck cancer in nonsmokers. *Am J Clin Oncol* 1997;20(2):146–50.
325. Rennie JS, MacDonald DG. Cell kinetics of hamster ventral tongue epithelium in iron deficiency. *Arch Oral Biol* 1984;29(3):195–9.
326. Ranasinghe AW, Warnakulasuriya KA, Tennekoon GE, Seneviratna B. Oral mucosal changes in iron deficiency anemia in a Sri Lankan female population. *Oral Surg Oral Med Oral Pathol* 1983;55(1):29–32.
327. Ranasinghe AW, Johnson NW, Scragg MA, Williams RA. Iron deficiency reduces cytochrome concentrations of mitochondria isolated from hamster cheek pouch epithelium. *J Oral Pathol Med* 1989;18(10):582–5.
328. Prime SS, MacDonald DG, Rennie JS. The effect of iron deficiency on experimental oral carcinogenesis in the rat. *Br J Cancer* 1983;47(3):413–8.
329. Bravi F, Edefonti V, Randi G, Ferraroni M, La Vecchia C, Decarli A. Dietary patterns and upper aerodigestive tract cancers: an overview and review. *Ann Oncol* 2012;23(12):3024–39.
330. Block G, Patterson B, Subar A. Fruit, vegetables, and cancer prevention: a review of the epidemiological evidence. *Nutr Cancer* 1992;18(1):1–29.
331. La Vecchia C, Tavani A. Fruit and vegetables, and human cancer. *Eur J Cancer Prev* 1998;7(1):3–8.
332. Potter JD, Steinmetz K. Vegetables, fruit and phytoestrogens as preventive agents. *IARC Sci Publ* 1996;(139):61–90.
333. Winn DM. Diet and nutrition in the etiology of oral cancer. *Am J Clin Nutr* 1995;61(2):437S–45S.
334. McLaughlin JK, Gridley G, Block G et al. Dietary factors in oral and pharyngeal cancer. *J Natl Cancer Inst* 1988;80(15):1237–43.
335. Oreggia F, De Stefani E, Correa P, Fierro L. Risk factors for cancer of the tongue in Uruguay. *Cancer* 1991;67(1):180–3.
336. Takezaki T, Hirose K, Inoue M et al. Tobacco, alcohol and dietary factors associated with the risk of oral cancer among Japanese. *Jpn J Cancer Res* 1996;87(6):555–62.
337. Zheng T, Boyle P, Willett WC et al. A case-control study of oral cancer in Beijing, People's Republic of China. Associations with nutrient intakes, foods and food groups. *Eur J Cancer B Oral Oncol* 1993;29B(1):45–55.
338. Tavani A, Gallus S, La Vecchia C et al. Diet and risk of oral and pharyngeal cancer. An Italian case-control study. *Eur J Cancer Prev* 2001;10(2):191–5.
339. Guha N, Boffetta P, Wunsch Filho V et al. Oral health and risk of squamous cell carcinoma of the head and neck and esophagus: results of two multicentric case-control studies. *Am J Epidemiol* 2007;166(10):1159–73.
340. Kreimer AR, Randi G, Herrero R et al. Diet and body mass, and oral and oropharyngeal squamous cell carcinomas: analysis from the IARC multinational case-control study. *Int J Cancer* 2006;118(9):2293–7.
341. Velly AM, Franco EL, Schlecht N et al. Relationship between dental factors and risk of upper aerodigestive tract cancer. *Oral Oncol* 1998;34(4):284–91.
342. Thumfart W, Weidenbecher M, Waller G, Pesch HG. Chronic mechanical trauma in the aetiology of oro-pharyngeal carcinoma. *J Maxillofac Surg* 1978;6(3):217–21.
343. Warnakulasuriya S. Causes of oral cancer – an appraisal of controversies. *Br Dent J* 2009;207(10):471–5.
344. Marshall JR, Graham S, Haughey BP et al. Smoking, alcohol, dentition and diet in the epidemiology of oral cancer. *Eur J Cancer B Oral Oncol* 1992;28B(1):9–15.
345. Graham S, Dayal H, Rohrer T et al. Dentition, diet, tobacco, and alcohol in the epidemiology of oral cancer. *J Natl Cancer Inst* 1977;59(6):1611–8.
346. Maier H, Zoller J, Herrmann A, Kreiss M, Heller WD. Dental status and oral hygiene in patients with head and neck cancer. *Otolaryngol Head Neck Surg* 1993;108(6):655–61.
347. Rosenquist K, Wennerberg J, Schildt EB, Bladstrom A, Goran Hansson B, Andersson G. Oral status, oral infections and some lifestyle factors as risk factors for oral and oropharyngeal squamous cell carcinoma. A population-based case-control study in southern Sweden. *Acta Otolaryngol* 2005;125(12):1327–36.
348. Zheng TZ, Boyle P, Hu HF et al. Dentition, oral hygiene, and risk of oral cancer: a case-control study in Beijing, People's Republic of China. *Cancer Causes Control* 1990;1(3):235–41.
349. Talamini R, Vaccarella S, Barbone F et al. Oral hygiene, dentition, sexual habits and risk of oral cancer. *Br J Cancer* 2000;83(9):1238–42.
350. Piemonte ED, Lazos JP, Brunotto M. Relationship between chronic trauma of the oral mucosa, oral potentially malignant disorders and oral cancer. *J Oral Pathol Med* 2010;39(7):513–7.
351. Lockhart PB, Norris CM Jr, Pulliam C. Dental factors in the genesis of squamous cell carcinoma of the oral cavity. *Oral Oncol* 1998;34(2):133–9.
352. Dayal, Reddy R, Anuradha Bhat K. Malignant potential of oral submucous fibrosis due to intraoral trauma. *Indian J Med Sci* 2000;54(5):182–7.
353. Konstantinidis A, Smulow JB, Sonnenschein C. Tumorigenesis at a predetermined oral site after one intraperitoneal injection of N-nitroso-N-methylurea. *Science* 1982;216(4551):1235–7.
354. Jones RB, Pomrehn PR, Mecklenburg RE, Lindsay EA, Manley M, Ockene JK. The COMMIT dental model: tobacco control practices and attitudes. *J Am Dent Assoc* 1993;124(9):92–104; discussion 6–8.
355. Manoharan S, Nagaraja V, Eslick GD. Ill-fitting dentures and oral cancer: a meta-analysis. *Oral Oncol* 2014;50(11):1058–61.

356. Sharma M, Bairy I, Pai K et al. Salivary IL-6 levels in oral leukoplakia with dysplasia and its clinical relevance to tobacco habits and periodontitis. *Clin Oral Investig* 2011;15(5):705–14.
357. Champagne CM, Buchanan W, Reddy MS, Preisser JS, Beck JD, Offenbacher S. Potential for gingival crevice fluid measures as predictors of risk for periodontal diseases. *Periodontol 2000* 2003;31:167–80.
358. Coussens LM, Werb Z. Inflammation and cancer. *Nature* 2002;420(6917):860–7.
359. Guerra L, Guidi R, Frisan T. Do bacterial genotoxins contribute to chronic inflammation, genomic instability and tumor progression? *FEBS J* 2011;278(23):4577–88.
360. Prabhu S, Wilson D, Daftary D, Johnson N. *Oral Diseases in the Tropics*. Jaypee Brothers Medical Publishers, 2017.
361. Li M, Saghafi N, Freymiller E, Basile JR, Lin YL. Metastatic Merkel cell carcinoma of the oral cavity in a human immunodeficiency virus-positive patient and the detection of Merkel cell polyomavirus. *Oral Surg Oral Med Oral Pathol Oral Radiol* 2013;115(5):e66–71.
362. Tanio S, Matsushita M, Kuwamoto S et al. Low prevalence of Merkel cell polyomavirus with low viral loads in oral and maxillofacial tumours or tumour-like lesions from immunocompetent patients: absence of Merkel cell polyomavirus-associated neoplasms. *Mol Clin Oncol* 2015;3(6):1301–6.
363. Johnson NW. The mouth in HIV/AIDS: markers of disease status and management challenges for the dental profession. *Aust Dent J* 2010;55(Suppl 1):85–102.
364. Duray A, Descamps G, Bettonville M et al. High prevalence of high-risk human papillomavirus in palatine tonsils from healthy children and adults. *Otolaryngol Head Neck Surg* 2011;145(2):230–5.
365. Pickard RK, Xiao W, Broutian TR, He X, Gillison ML. The prevalence and incidence of oral human papillomavirus infection among young men and women, aged 18–30 years. *Sex Transm Dis* 2012;39(7):559–66.
366. IARC Working Group on the Evaluation of Carcinogenic Risks to Humans. *A Review of Human Carcinogens. Part B: Biological Agents*. Lyon France: International Agency for Research on Cancer, 2009.
367. Patton LL, Ranganathan K, Naidoo S et al. Oral lesions, HIV phenotypes, and management of HIV-related disease: Workshop 4A. *Adv Dent Res* 2011;23(1):112–6.
368. Speicher DJ, Ramirez-Amador V, Dittmer DP, Webster-Cyriaque J, Goodman MT, Moscicki AB. Viral infections associated with oral cancers and diseases in the context of HIV: a workshop report. *Oral Dis* 2016;22(Suppl 1):181–92.
369. He B, Qiao X, Klasse PJ et al. HIV-1 envelope triggers polyclonal Ig class switch recombination through a CD40-independent mechanism involving BAFF and C-type lectin receptors. *J Immunol* 2006;176(7):3931–41.
370. Ziegler JL, Newton R, Katongole-Mbidde E et al. Risk factors for Kaposi's sarcoma in HIV-positive subjects in Uganda. *AIDS* 1997;11(13):1619–26.
371. Tappuni AR. Immune reconstitution inflammatory syndrome. *Adv Dent Res* 2011;23(1):90–6.
372. Speicher DJ, Sehu MM, Johnson NW, Shaw DR. Successful treatment of an HIV-positive patient with unmasking Kaposi's sarcoma immune reconstitution inflammatory syndrome. *J Clin Virol* 2013;57(3):282–5.
373. Achenbach CJ, Harrington RD, Dhanireddy S, Crane HM, Casper C, Kitahata MM. Paradoxical immune reconstitution inflammatory syndrome in HIV-infected patients treated with combination antiretroviral therapy after AIDS-defining opportunistic infection. *Clin Infect Dis* 2012;54(3):424–33.
374. Kreimer AR, Alberg AJ, Daniel R et al. Oral human papillomavirus infection in adults is associated with sexual behavior and HIV serostatus. *J Infect Dis* 2004;189(4):686–98.
375. Beachler DC, Weber KM, Margolick JB et al. Risk factors for oral HPV infection among a high prevalence population of HIV-positive and at-risk HIV-negative adults. *Cancer Epidemiol Biomarkers Prev* 2012;21(1):122–33.
376. Read TR, Hocking JS, Vodstrcil LA et al. Oral human papillomavirus in men having sex with men: risk-factors and sampling. *PloS One* 2012;7(11):e49324.
377. Grulich AE, van Leeuwen MT, Falster MO, Vajdic CM. Incidence of cancers in people with HIV/AIDS compared with immunosuppressed transplant recipients: a meta-analysis. *Lancet* 2007;370(9581):59–67.
378. Frisch M, Biggar RJ, Goedert JJ. Human papillomavirus-associated cancers in patients with human immunodeficiency virus infection and acquired immunodeficiency syndrome. *J Natl Cancer Inst* 2000;92(18):1500–10.
379. Beachler DC, Abraham AG, Silverberg MJ et al. Incidence and risk factors of HPV-related and HPV-unrelated head and neck squamous cell carcinoma in HIV-infected individuals. *Oral Oncol* 2014;50(12):1169–76.
380. Beachler DC, Sugar EA, Margolick JB et al. Risk factors for acquisition and clearance of oral human papillomavirus infection among HIV-infected and HIV-uninfected adults. *Am J Epidemiol* 2015;181(1):40–53.
381. Larsson PA, Johansson SL, Vahlne A, Hirsch JM. Snuff tumorigenesis: effects of long-term snuff administration after initiation with 4-nitroquinoline-N-oxide and herpes simplex virus type 1. *J Oral Pathol Med* 1989;18(4):187–92.
382. Park K, Cherrick HM, Min BM, Park NH. Active HSV-1 immunization prevents the cocarcinogenic activity of HSV-1 in the oral cavity of hamsters. *Oral Surg Oral Med Oral Pathol* 1990;70(2):186–91.
383. Larsson PA, Edstrom S, Westin T, Nordkvist A, Hirsch JM, Vahlne A. Reactivity against herpes simplex virus

in patients with head and neck cancer. *Int J Cancer* 1991;49(1):14–8.
384. Eskinazi DP, Cantin EM. Monoclonal antibodies to HSV-infection-related antigens cross-react with tumor cell lines and tumor tissue sections. *Oral Surg Oral Med Oral Pathol* 1988;65(3):308–15.
385. Eglin RP, Scully C, Lehner T, Ward-Booth P, McGregor IA. Detection of RNA complementary to herpes simplex virus in human oral squamous cell carcinoma. *Lancet* 1983;2(8353):766–8.
386. Epstein MA, Barr YM, Achong BG. A second virus-carrying tissue culture strain (EB2) of lymphoblasts from Burkitt's lymphoma. *Pathol Biol* 1964;12:1233–4.
387. Andersson J. An overview of Epstein-Barr virus: from discovery to future directions for treatment and prevention. *Herpes* 2000;7(3):76–82.
388. King GN, Healy CM, Glover MT et al. Prevalence and risk factors associated with leukoplakia, hairy leukoplakia, erythematous candidiasis, and gingival hyperplasia in renal transplant recipients. *Oral Surg Oral Med Oral Pathol* 1994;78(6):718–26.
389. Henle G, Henle W, Diehl V. Relation of Burkitt's tumor-associated herpes-type virus to infectious mononucleosis. *Proc Natl Acad Sci USA* 1968;59(1):94–101.
390. Zimber-Strobl U, Kempkes B, Marschall G et al. Epstein-Barr virus latent membrane protein (LMP1) is not sufficient to maintain proliferation of B cells but both it and activated CD40 can prolong their survival. *EMBO J* 1996;15(24):7070–8.
391. Klein G, Klein E, Kashuba E. Interaction of Epstein-Barr virus (EBV) with human B-lymphocytes. *Biochem Biophys Res Commun* 2010;396(1):67–73.
392. Thornburg NJ, Kulwichit W, Edwards RH, Shair KH, Bendt KM, Raab-Traub N. LMP1 signaling and activation of NF-kappaB in LMP1 transgenic mice. *Oncogene* 2006;25(2):288–97.
393. Contreras A, Zadeh HH, Nowzari H, Slots J. Herpesvirus infection of inflammatory cells in human periodontitis. *Oral Microbiol Immunol* 1999; 14(4):206–12.
394. Frangou P, Buettner M, Niedobitek G. Epstein-Barr virus (EBV) infection in epithelial cells in vivo: rare detection of EBV replication in tongue mucosa but not in salivary glands. *J Infect Dis* 2005;191(2):238–42.
395. Balfour HH Jr, Holman CJ, Hokanson KM et al. A prospective clinical study of Epstein-Barr virus and host interactions during acute infectious mononucleosis. *J Infect Dis* 2005;192(9):1505–12.
396. Tugizov SM, Berline JW, Palefsky JM. Epstein-Barr virus infection of polarized tongue and nasopharyngeal epithelial cells. *Nat Med* 2003;9(3):307–14.
397. Thompson MP, Kurzrock R. Epstein-Barr virus and cancer. *Clin Cancer Res* 2004;10(3):803–21.
398. Li C, Shi Z, Zhang L et al. Dynamic changes of territories 17 and 18 during EBV-infection of human lymphocytes. *Mol Biol Rep* 2010;37(5):2347–54.
399. Boulter A, Johnson NW, Birnbaum W, Teo CG. Epstein-Barr virus (EBV) associated lesions of the head and neck. *Oral Dis* 1996;2(2):117–24.
400. Talacko AA, Teo CG, Griffin BE, Johnson NW. Epstein-Barr virus receptors but not viral DNA are present in normal and malignant oral epithelium. *J Oral Pathol Med* 1991;20(1):20–5.
401. Al-Hebshi NN, Nasher AT, Speicher DJ, Shaikh MH, Johnson NW. Possible interaction between tobacco use and EBV in oral squamous cell carcinoma. *Oral Oncol* 2016;59:e4–5.
402. Kis A, Feher E, Gall T et al. Epstein-Barr virus prevalence in oral squamous cell cancer and in potentially malignant oral disorders in an eastern Hungarian population. *Eur J Oral Sci* 2009;117(5):536–40.
403. Polz-Gruszka D, Morshed K, Stec A, Polz-Dacewicz M. Prevalence of Human papillomavirus (HPV) and Epstein-Barr virus (EBV) in oral and oropharyngeal squamous cell carcinoma in south-eastern Poland. *Infect Agents Cancer* 2015;10:37.
404. Jalouli J, Jalouli MM, Sapkota D, Ibrahim SO, Larsson PA, Sand L. Human papilloma virus, herpes simplex virus and Epstein-Barr virus in oral squamous cell carcinoma from eight different countries. *Anticancer Res* 2012;32(2):571–80.
405. D'Costa J, Saranath D, Sanghvi V, Mehta AR. Epstein-Barr virus in tobacco-induced oral cancers and oral lesions in patients from India. *J Oral Pathol Med* 1998;27(2):78–82.
406. Higa M, Kinjo T, Kamiyama K, Iwamasa T, Hamada T, Iyama K. Epstein-Barr virus (EBV) subtype in EBV related oral squamous cell carcinoma in Okinawa, a subtropical island in southern Japan, compared with Kitakyushu and Kumamoto in mainland Japan. *J Clin Pathol* 2002;55(6):414–23.
407. Yen CY, Lu MC, Tzeng CC et al. Detection of EBV infection and gene expression in oral cancer from patients in Taiwan by microarray analysis. *J Biomed Biotechnol* 2009;2009:904589.
408. Mutalima N, Molyneux E, Jaffe H et al. Associations between Burkitt lymphoma among children in Malawi and infection with HIV, EBV and malaria: results from a case-control study. *PloS One* 2008;3(6):e2505.
409. Hsu WL, Chen JY, Chien YC et al. Independent effect of EBV and cigarette smoking on nasopharyngeal carcinoma: a 20-year follow-up study on 9,622 males without family history in Taiwan. *Cancer Epidemiol Biomarkers Prev* 2009;18(4):1218–26.
410. Greenspan JS, Greenspan D, Lennette ET et al. Replication of Epstein-Barr virus within the epithelial cells of oral "hairy" leukoplakia, an AIDS-associated lesion. *N Engl J Med* 1985;313(25):1564–71.
411. Boulter AW, Soltanpoor N, Swan AV, Birnbaum W, Johnson NW, Teo CG. Risk factors associated with Epstein-Barr virus replication in oral epithelial cells of HIV-infected individuals. *AIDS* 1996;10(9):935–40.

412. Itin P, Rufli T, Rudlinger R et al. Oral hairy leukoplakia in a HIV-negative renal transplant patient: a marker for immunosuppression? *Dermatologica* 1988;177(2):126–8.
413. Epstein JB, Sherlock CH, Greenspan JS. Hairy leukoplakia-like lesions following bone-marrow transplantation. *AIDS* 1991;5(1):101–2.
414. Shiboski CH, Chen H, Secours R et al. High accuracy of common HIV-related oral disease diagnoses by non-oral health specialists in the AIDS clinical trial group. *PloS One* 2015;10(7):e0131001.
415. Webster-Cyriaque J, Middeldorp J, Raab-Traub N. Hairy leukoplakia: an unusual combination of transforming and permissive Epstein-Barr virus infections. *J Virol* 2000;74(16):7610–8.
416. Walling DM, Ling PD, Gordadze AV, Montes-Walters M, Flaitz CM, Nichols CM. Expression of Epstein-Barr virus latent genes in oral epithelium: determinants of the pathogenesis of oral hairy leukoplakia. *J Infect Dis* 2004;190(2):396–9.
417. Monini P, de Lellis L, Fabris M, Rigolin F, Cassai E. Kaposi's sarcoma-associated herpesvirus DNA sequences in prostate tissue and human semen. *N Engl J Med* 1996;334(18):1168–72.
418. Wu L, Lo P, Yu X, Stoops JK, Forghani B, Zhou ZH. Three-dimensional structure of the human herpesvirus 8 capsid. *J Virol* 2000;74(20):9646–54.
419. Levy JA. A new human herpesvirus: KSHV or HHV8? *Lancet* 1995;346(8978):786.
420. Moore PS, Chang Y. Detection of herpesvirus-like DNA sequences in Kaposi's sarcoma in patients with and those without HIV infection. *N Engl J Med* 1995;332(18):1181–5.
421. Moore PS, Gao SJ, Dominguez G et al. Primary characterization of a herpesvirus agent associated with Kaposi's sarcoma. *J Virol* 1996;70(1):549–58.
422. Bottler T, Kuttenberger J, Hardt N, Oehen HP, Baltensperger M. Non-HIV-associated Kaposi's sarcoma of the tongue. Case report and review of the literature. *Int J Oral Maxillofac Surg* 2007;36(12):1218–20.
423. Pantanowitz L, Duke WH. Lymphoedematous variants of Kaposi's sarcoma. *J Eur Acad Dermatol Venereol* 2008;22(1):118–20.
424. Caponetti G, Dezube BJ, Restrepo CS, Pantanowitz L. Kaposi sarcoma of the musculoskeletal system: a review of 66 patients. *Cancer* 2007;109(6):1040–52.
425. Pantanowitz L, Dezube BJ. Editorial comment: bone lesions in Kaposi sarcoma. *AIDS Read* 2007;17(4):204.
426. Blackbourn DJ, Levy JA. Human herpesvirus 8 in semen and prostate. *AIDS* 1997;11(2):249–50.
427. Charfi S, Krichen-Makni S, Yaich S et al. Successful treatment of post-renal transplant gastric and pulmonary Kaposi's sarcoma with conversion to rapamycin treatment. *Saudi J Kidney Dis Transpl* 2007;18(4):617–20.
428. Garay SM, Belenko M, Fazzini E, Schinella R. Pulmonary manifestations of Kaposi's sarcoma. *Chest* 1987;91(1):39–43.
429. Gunawardena KA, al-Hasani MK, Haleem A, al-Suleiman M, al-Khader AA. Pulmonary Kaposi's sarcoma in two recipients of renal transplants. *Thorax* 1988;43(8):653–6.
430. Lebbe C, de Cremoux P, Rybojad M, Costa da Cunha C, Morel P, Calvo F. Kaposi's sarcoma and new herpesvirus. *Lancet* 1995;345(8958):1180.
431. Ablashi DV, Chatlynne LG, Whitman JE Jr, Cesarman E. Spectrum of Kaposi's sarcoma-associated herpesvirus, or human herpesvirus 8, diseases. *Clin Microbiol Rev* 2002;15(3):439–64.
432. Kaposi M. Idiopatiches multiple pigment sarcom der Haut. *Arch Derm Syphilol* 1872;4:265–72.
433. Biryahwaho B, Dollard SC, Pfeiffer RM et al. Sex and geographic patterns of human herpesvirus 8 infection in a nationally representative population-based sample in Uganda. *J Infect Dis* 2010;202(9):1347–53.
434. Cook-Mozaffari P, Newton R, Beral V, Burkitt DP. The geographical distribution of Kaposi's sarcoma and of lymphomas in Africa before the AIDS epidemic. *Br J Cancer* 1998;78(11):1521–8.
435. Lothe F. Kaposi's sarcoma in Uganda Africans. *Acta Pathol Microbiol Scand Suppl* 1963;(Suppl 161):1.
436. Taylor JF, Templeton AC, Vogel CL, Ziegler JL, Kyalwazi SK. Kaposi's sarcoma in Uganda: a clinico-pathological study. *Int J Cancer* 1971;8(1):122–35.
437. Kestens L, Melbye M, Biggar RJ et al. Endemic African Kaposi's sarcoma is not associated with immunodeficiency. *Int J Cancer* 1985;36(1):49–54.
438. Oettle AG. Geographical and racial differences in the frequency of Kaposi's sarcoma as evidence of environmental or genetic causes. *Acta Unio Int Contra Cancrum* 1962;18:330–63.
439. Olweny CL. Etiology of endemic Kaposi's sarcoma. *IARC Sci Publ* 1984;(63):543–8.
440. Montagnino G, Bencini PL, Tarantino A, Caputo R, Ponticelli C. Clinical features and course of Kaposi's sarcoma in kidney transplant patients: report of 13 cases. *Am J Nephrol* 1994;14(2):121–6.
441. Panayiotakopoulos GD, Papaconstantinou I, Mavroyianni D, Kostakis A, Kordossis T. Pretransplantation prevalence of human herpesvirus 8 antibodies in kidney donors and recipients in Athens, Greece. *Transplant Proc* 2005;37(10):4180–2.
442. Penn I. Kaposi's sarcoma in organ transplant recipients: report of 20 cases. *Transplantation* 1979;27(1):8–11.
443. Caterino-de-Araujo A, Magri MC, Santos-Fortuna E, Souza JF, Sens YA, Jabur P. Human herpesvirus-8 infection in hemodialysis patients from Sao Paulo, Brazil: preliminary results. *Transplant Proc* 2007;39(10):3044–6.
444. Friedman-Kien AE, Saltzman BR. Clinical manifestations of classical, endemic African, and epidemic AIDS-associated Kaposi's sarcoma. *J Am Acad Dermatol* 1990;22(6 Pt 2):1237–50.
445. Ahmadpoor P, Ilkhanizadeh B, Sharifzadeh P et al. Seroprevalence of human herpesvirus-8 in renal

transplant recipients: a single center study from Iran. *Transplant Proc* 2007;39(4):1000–2.
446. Farge D. Kaposi's sarcoma in organ transplant recipients. The Collaborative Transplantation Research Group of Ile de France. *Eur J Med* 1993;2(6):339–43.
447. Qunibi W, Akhtar M, Sheth K et al. Kaposi's sarcoma: the most common tumor after renal transplantation in Saudi Arabia. *Am J Med* 1988;84(2):225–32.
448. Aoki Y, Tosato G. HIV-1 Tat enhances Kaposi sarcoma-associated herpesvirus (KSHV) infectivity. *Blood* 2004;104(3):810–4.
449. Attia S, Dezube BJ, Torrealba JR et al. AIDS-related Kaposi's sarcoma of the gastrointestinal tract. *J Clin Oncol* 2010;28(16):e250–1.
450. Ensoli B, Barillari G, Salahuddin SZ, Gallo RC, Wong-Staal F. Tat protein of HIV-1 stimulates growth of cells derived from Kaposi's sarcoma lesions of AIDS patients. *Nature* 1990;345(6270):84–6.
451. Ensoli B, Gendelman R, Markham P et al. Synergy between basic fibroblast growth factor and HIV-1 Tat protein in induction of Kaposi's sarcoma. *Nature* 1994;371(6499):674–80.
452. Ensoli B, Salahuddin SZ, Gallo RC. AIDS-associated Kaposi's sarcoma: a molecular model for its pathogenesis. *Cancer Cells* 1989;1(3):93–6.
453. Boivin G, Cote S, Cloutier N, Abed Y, Maguigad M, Routy JP. Quantification of human herpesvirus 8 by real-time PCR in blood fractions of AIDS patients with Kaposi's sarcoma and multicentric Castleman's disease. *J Med Virol* 2002;68(3):399–403.
454. Dittmer DP, Damania B. Kaposi sarcoma associated herpesvirus pathogenesis (KSHV) – an update. *Curr Opin Virol* 2013;3(3):238–44.
455. Aldenhoven M, Barlo NP, Sanders CJ. Therapeutic strategies for epidemic Kaposi's sarcoma. *Int J STD AIDS* 2006;17(9):571–8.
456. Lager I, Altini M, Coleman H, Ali H. Oral Kaposi's sarcoma: a clinicopathologic study from South Africa. *Oral Surg Oral Med Oral Pathol Oral Radiol Endod* 2003;96(6):701–10.
457. Reznik DA. Oral manifestations of HIV disease. *Top HIV Med* 2005;13(5):143–8.
458. Rohrmus B, Thoma-Greber EM, Bogner JR, Rocken M. Outlook in oral and cutaneous Kaposi's sarcoma. *Lancet* 2000;356(9248):2160.
459. Jindal JR, Campbell BH, Ward TO, Almagro US. Kaposi's sarcoma of the oral cavity in a non-AIDS patient: case report and review of the literature. *Head Neck* 1995;17(1):64–8.
460. Speicher DJ, Wanzala P, D'Lima M et al. Diagnostic challenges of oral and cutaneous Kaposi's sarcoma in resource-constrained settings. *J Oral Pathol Med* 2015;44(10):842–9.
461. Borges JD, Souza VA, Giambartolomei C et al. Transmission of human herpesvirus type 8 infection within families in American indigenous populations from the Brazilian Amazon. *J Infect Dis* 2012;205(12):1869–76.
462. Joint United Nations Programme on HIV/AIDS (UNAIDS). *The Gap Report*. Geneva, 2014.
463. Vaishnani JB, Bosamiya SS, Momin AM. Kaposi's sarcoma: a presenting sign of HIV. *Indian J Dermatol Venereol Leprol* 2010;76(2):215.
464. Dongre A, Montaldo C. Kaposi's sarcoma in an HIV-positive person successfully treated with paclitaxel. *Indian J Dermatol Venereol Leprol* 2009;75(3):290–2.
465. Kharkar V, Gutte RM, Khopkar U, Mahajan S, Chikhalkar S. Kaposi's sarcoma: a presenting manifestation of HIV infection in an Indian. *Indian J Dermatol Venereol Leprol* 2009;75(4):391–3.
466. Kura MM, Khemani UN, Lanjewar DN, Raghuwanshi SR, Chitale AR, Joshi SR. Kaposi's sarcoma in a patient with AIDS. *J Assoc Physicians India* 2008;56:262–4.
467. Soufiane M, Fadl TM, Nawfel M et al. Kaposi's sarcoma: HIV-negative man with isolated penile localization. *Indian J Pathol Microbiol* 2010;53(3):535–6.
468. Bhatia R, Shubhdarshini S, Yadav S, Ramam M, Agarwal S. Disseminated Kaposi's sarcoma in a human immunodeficiency virus-infected homosexual Indian man. *Indian J Dermatol Venereol Leprol* 2017;83(1):78–83.
469. Kumarasamy N, Solomon S, Yesudian PK, Sugumar P. First report of Kaposi's sarcoma in an AIDS patient from Madras, India. *Indian J Dermatol* 1996;41(1):23–5.
470. Ablashi D, Chatlynne L, Cooper H et al. Seroprevalence of human herpesvirus-8 (HHV-8) in countries of Southeast Asia compared to the USA, the Caribbean and Africa. *Br J Cancer* 1999;81(5):893–7.
471. Speicher DJ, Nandagopal P, Saravanan S, Kumarasamy N, Ranganathan K, Johnson NW (eds). Detection of Human Herpesviruses in HIV-positive patients from Southeast India. *Seventh World Workshop on Oral Health & Disease in AIDS*, 2014 November 6–9, 2014; Hyderabad, India.
472. Munawwar A, Sharma SK, Gupta S, Singh S. Seroprevalence and determinants of Kaposi sarcoma-associated human herpesvirus 8 in Indian HIV-infected males. *AIDS Res Hum Retroviruses* 2014;30(12):1192–6.
473. Krown SE, Lee JY, Dittmer DP, Consortium AM. More on HIV-associated Kaposi's sarcoma. *N Engl J Med* 2008;358(5):535–6; author reply 6.
474. Cannon MJ, Dollard SC, Black JB et al. Risk factors for Kaposi's sarcoma in men seropositive for both human herpesvirus 8 and human immunodeficiency virus. *AIDS* 2003;17(2):215–22.
475. Grulich AE, Cunningham P, Munier ML et al. Sexual behaviour and human herpesvirus 8 infection in homosexual men in Australia. *Sex Health* 2005;2(1):13–8.

476. Grulich AE, Kaldor JM, Hendry O, Luo K, Bodsworth NJ, Cooper DA. Risk of Kaposi's sarcoma and oroanal sexual contact. *Am J Epidemiol* 1997;145(8):673–9.
477. Grulich AE, Olsen SJ, Luo K et al. Kaposi's sarcoma-associated herpesvirus: A sexually transmissible infection? *J Acquir Immune Defic Syndr Hum Retrovirol* 1999;20(4):387–93.
478. Bourboulia D, Whitby D, Boshoff C et al. Serologic evidence for mother-to-child transmission of Kaposi sarcoma-associated herpesvirus infection. *JAMA* 1998;280(1):31–2.
479. Mbulaiteye SM, Goedert JJ. Transmission of Kaposi sarcoma-associated herpesvirus in sub-Saharan Africa. *AIDS* 2008;22(4):535–7.
480. Mbulaiteye SM, Pfeiffer RM, Whitby D, Brubaker GR, Shao J, Biggar RJ. Human herpesvirus 8 infection within families in rural Tanzania. *J Infect Dis* 2003;187(11):1780–5.
481. Plancoulaine S, Abel L, van Beveren M et al. Human herpesvirus 8 transmission from mother to child and between siblings in an endemic population. *Lancet* 2000;356(9235):1062–5.
482. Beral V, Peterman TA, Berkelman RL, Jaffe HW. Kaposi's sarcoma among persons with AIDS: a sexually transmitted infection? *Lancet* 1990;335(8682):123–8.
483. Beral V, Bull D, Jaffe H et al. Is risk of Kaposi's sarcoma in AIDS patients in Britain increased if sexual partners came from United States or Africa? *BMJ (Clinical Research Ed)* 1991;302(6777):624–5.
484. Kasolo FC, Monze M, Obel N, Anderson RA, French C, Gompels UA. Sequence analyses of human herpesvirus-8 strains from both African human immunodeficiency virus-negative and -positive childhood endemic Kaposi's sarcoma show a close relationship with strains identified in febrile children and high variation in the K1 glycoprotein. *J Gen Virol* 1998;79(Pt 12):3055–65.
485. Meng YX, Spira TJ, Bhat GJ et al. Individuals from North America, Australasia, and Africa are infected with four different genotypes of human herpesvirus 8. *Virology* 1999;261(1):106–19.
486. Goedert JJ, Vitale F, Lauria C et al. Risk factors for classical Kaposi's sarcoma. *J Natl Cancer Inst* 2002;94(22):1712–8.
487. Grulich AE, Vajdic CM. The epidemiology of non-Hodgkin lymphoma. *Pathology* 2005;37(6):409–19.
488. Hayward GS. KSHV strains: the origins and global spread of the virus. *Semin Cancer Biol* 1999;9(3): 187–99.
489. Drago F, Rebora A. Human herpesvirus as a sexually transmitted agent. *Lancet* 2001;357(9252): 307.
490. Koelle DM, Huang ML, Chandran B, Vieira J, Piepkorn M, Corey L. Frequent detection of Kaposi's sarcoma-associated herpesvirus (human herpesvirus 8) DNA in saliva of human immunodeficiency virus-infected men: Clinical and immunologic correlates. *J Infect Dis* 1997;176(1):94–102.
491. Bagasra O, Patel D, Bobroski L et al. Localization of human herpesvirus type 8 in human sperms by in situ PCR. *J Mol Histol* 2005;36(6–7):401–12.
492. Calabro ML, Fiore JR, Favero A et al. Detection of human herpesvirus 8 in cervicovaginal secretions and seroprevalence in human immunodeficiency virus type 1-seropositive and -seronegative women. *J Infect Dis* 1999;179(6):1534–7.
493. Taylor MM, Chohan B, Lavreys L et al. Shedding of human herpesvirus 8 in oral and genital secretions from HIV-1-seropositive and -seronegative Kenyan women. *J Infect Dis* 2004;190(3):484–8.
494. Casper C, Meier AS, Wald A, Morrow RA, Corey L, Moscicki AB. Human herpesvirus 8 infection among adolescents in the REACH cohort. *Arch Pediatr Adolesc Med* 2006;160(9):937–42.
495. Mbulaiteye S, Marshall V, Bagni RK et al. Molecular evidence for mother-to-child transmission of Kaposi sarcoma-associated herpesvirus in Uganda and K1 gene evolution within the host. *J Infect Dis* 2006;193(9):1250–7.
496. Lisco A, Barbierato M, Fiore JR et al. Pregnancy and human herpesvirus 8 reactivation in human immunodeficiency virus type 1-infected women. *J Clin Microbiol* 2006;44(11):3863–71.
497. Dedicoat M, Newton R, Alkharsah KR et al. Mother-to-child transmission of human herpesvirus-8 in South Africa. *J Infect Dis* 2004;190(6):1068–75.
498. Chagas CA, Endo LH, Sakano E, Pinto GA, Brousset P, Vassallo J. Detection of herpesvirus type 8 (HHV8) in children's tonsils and adenoids by immunohistochemistry and *in situ* hybridization. *Int J Pediatr Otorhinolaryngol* 2006;70(1):65–72.
499. Mbulaiteye SM, Pfeiffer RM, Engels EA et al. Detection of Kaposi sarcoma-associated herpesvirus DNA in saliva and buffy-coat samples from children with sickle cell disease in Uganda. *J Infect Dis* 2004;190(8):1382–6.
500. Pak F, Mwakigonja AR, Kokhaei P et al. Kaposi's sarcoma herpesvirus load in biopsies of cutaneous and oral Kaposi's sarcoma lesions. *Eur J Cancer* 2007;43(12):1877–82.
501. Martin JN. Kaposi sarcoma-associated herpesvirus/human herpesvirus 8 and Kaposi sarcoma. *Adv Dent Res* 2011;23(1):76–8.
502. Triantos D, Horefti E, Paximadi E et al. Presence of human herpesvirus-8 in saliva and non-lesional oral mucosa in HIV-infected and oncologic immunocompromised patients. *Oral Microbiol Immunol* 2004;19(3):201–4.
503. Bernard HU, Burk RD, Chen Z, van Doorslaer K, zur Hausen H, de Villiers EM. Classification of papillomaviruses (PVs) based on 189 PV types and proposal of taxonomic amendments. *Virology* 2010;401(1):70–9.

504. McCance DJ. Human papillomaviruses and cancer. *Biochim Biophys Acta* 1986;823(3):195–205.
505. zur Hausen H. Human papillomaviruses and their possible role in squamous cell carcinomas. *Curr Top Microbiol Immunol* 1977;78:1–30.
506. Burk RD. Human papillomavirus and the risk of cervical cancer. *Hosp Pract (Minneap)* 1999;34(12):103–11; quiz 12.
507. Koss LG, Durfee GR. Unusual patterns of squamous epithelium of the uterine cervix: cytologic and pathologic study of koilocytotic atypia. *Ann N Y Acad Sci* 1956;63(6):1245–61.
508. Suzich JA, Ghim SJ, Palmer-Hill FJ et al. Systemic immunization with papillomavirus L1 protein completely prevents the development of viral mucosal papillomas. *Proc Natl Acad Sci USA* 1995;92(25):11553–7.
509. Burk RD, Harari A, Chen Z. Human papillomavirus genome variants. *Virology* 2013;445(1–2):232–43.
510. de Villiers EM, Fauquet C, Broker TR, Bernard HU, zur Hausen H. Classification of papillomaviruses. *Virology* 2004;324(1):17–27.
511. Syrjanen K, Syrjanen S, Lamberg M, Pyrhonen S, Nuutinen J. Morphological and immunohistochemical evidence suggesting human papillomavirus (HPV) involvement in oral squamous cell carcinogenesis. *Int J Oral Surg* 1983;12(6):418–24.
512. zur Hausen H. Papillomaviruses and cancer: from basic studies to clinical application. *Nat Rev Cancer* 2002;2(5):342–50.
513. Kayes O, Ahmed HU, Arya M, Minhas S. Molecular and genetic pathways in penile cancer. *Lancet Oncol* 2007;8(5):420–9.
514. Crum CP, McLachlin CM, Tate JE, Mutter GL. Pathobiology of vulvar squamous neoplasia. *Curr Opin Obstet Gynecol* 1997;9(1):63–9.
515. Ang KK, Harris J, Wheeler R et al. Human papillomavirus and survival of patients with oropharyngeal cancer. *N Engl J Med* 2010;363(1):24–35.
516. Syrjanen S, Lodi G, von Bultzingslowen I et al. Human papillomaviruses in oral carcinoma and oral potentially malignant disorders: a systematic review. *Oral Dis* 2011;17(Suppl 1):58–72.
517. Mehanna H, Beech T, Nicholson T et al. Prevalence of human papillomavirus in oropharyngeal and nonoropharyngeal head and neck cancer – systematic review and meta-analysis of trends by time and region. *Head Neck* 2013;35(5):747–55.
518. Dalianis T. Human papillomavirus (HPV) and oropharyngeal squamous cell carcinoma. *Presse Med* 2014;43(12 Pt 2):e429–34.
519. Syrjanen S. Human papillomavirus infections and oral tumors. *Med Microbiol Immunol* 2003;192(3):123–8.
520. Gillison ML, Koch WM, Capone RB et al. Evidence for a causal association between human papillomavirus and a subset of head and neck cancers. *J Natl Cancer Inst* 2000;92(9):709–20.
521. Marur S, D'Souza G, Westra WH, Forastiere AA. HPV-associated head and neck cancer: a virus-related cancer epidemic. *Lancet Oncol* 2010;11(8):781–9.
522. Lewis JS Jr, Thorstad WL, Chernock RD et al. P16 positive oropharyngeal squamous cell carcinoma: an entity with a favorable prognosis regardless of tumor HPV status. *Am J Surg Pathol* 2010;34(8):1088–96.
523. Harris SL, Thorne LB, Seaman WT, Hayes DN, Couch ME, Kimple RJ. Association of p16(INK4a) overexpression with improved outcomes in young patients with squamous cell cancers of the oral tongue. *Head Neck* 2011;33(11):1622–7.
524. Bolt J, Vo QN, Kim WJ et al. The ATM/p53 pathway is commonly targeted for inactivation in squamous cell carcinoma of the head and neck (SCCHN) by multiple molecular mechanisms. *Oral Oncol* 2005;41(10):1013–20.
525. Rocco JW, Sidransky D. P16(MTS-1/CDKN2/INK4a) in cancer progression. *Exp Cell Res* 2001;264(1):42–55.
526. Agrawal N, Frederick MJ, Pickering CR et al. Exome sequencing of head and neck squamous cell carcinoma reveals inactivating mutations in NOTCH1. *Science* 2011;333(6046):1154–7.
527. Stransky N, Egloff AM, Tward AD et al. The mutational landscape of head and neck squamous cell carcinoma. *Science* 2011;333(6046):1157–60.
528. Fakhry C, Westra WH, Li S et al. Improved survival of patients with human papillomavirus-positive head and neck squamous cell carcinoma in a prospective clinical trial. *J Natl Cancer Inst* 2008;100(4):261–9.
529. Sinha P, Logan HL, Mendenhall WM. Human papillomavirus, smoking, and head and neck cancer. *Am J Otolaryngol* 2012;33(1):130–6.
530. Mellin H, Dahlgren L, Munck-Wikland E et al. Human papillomavirus type 16 is episomal and a high viral load may be correlated to better prognosis in tonsillar cancer. *Int J Cancer* 2002;102(2):152–8.
531. Ruutu M, Peitsaro P, Johansson B, Syrjanen S. Transcriptional profiling of a human papillomavirus 33-positive squamous epithelial cell line which acquired a selective growth advantage after viral integration. *Int J Cancer* 2002;100(3):318–26.
532. Kadaja M, Isok-Paas H, Laos T, Ustav E, Ustav M. Mechanism of genomic instability in cells infected with the high-risk human papillomaviruses. *PLoS Pathog* 2009;5(4):e1000397.
533. Walboomers JM, Jacobs MV, Manos MM et al. Human papillomavirus is a necessary cause of invasive cervical cancer worldwide. *J Pathol* 1999;189(1):12–9.
534. McKaig RG, Baric RS, Olshan AF. Human papillomavirus and head and neck cancer: epidemiology and molecular biology. *Head Neck* 1998;20(3):250–65.
535. Gillison ML, Shah KV. Human papillomavirus-associated head and neck squamous cell carcinoma: mounting evidence for an etiologic role for human

papillomavirus in a subset of head and neck cancers. *Curr Opin Oncol* 2001;13(3):183–8.
536. Kreimer AR, Johansson M, Waterboer T et al. Evaluation of human papillomavirus antibodies and risk of subsequent head and neck cancer. *J Clin Oncol* 2013;31(21):2708–15.
537. Loning T, Ikenberg H, Becker J, Gissmann L, Hoepfer I, zur Hausen H. Analysis of oral papillomas, leukoplakias, and invasive carcinomas for human papillomavirus type related DNA. *J Invest Dermatol* 1985;84(5):417–20.
538. de Villiers EM, Weidauer H, Otto H, zur Hausen H. Papillomavirus DNA in human tongue carcinomas. *Int J Cancer* 1985;36(5):575–8.
539. Hammarstedt L, Lindquist D, Dahlstrand H et al. Human papillomavirus as a risk factor for the increase in incidence of tonsillar cancer. *Int J Cancer* 2006;119(11):2620–3.
540. Chaturvedi AK, Engels EA, Pfeiffer RM et al. Human papillomavirus and rising oropharyngeal cancer incidence in the United States. *J Clin Oncol* 2011;29(32):4294–301.
541. Shiboski CH, Schmidt BL, Jordan RC. Tongue and tonsil carcinoma: increasing trends in the U.S. population ages 20–44 years. *Cancer* 2005;103(9):1843–9.
542. Braakhuis BJ, Visser O, Leemans CR. Oral and oropharyngeal cancer in The Netherlands between 1989 and 2006: Increasing incidence, but not in young adults. *Oral Oncol* 2009;45(9):e85–9.
543. Hocking JS, Stein A, Conway EL et al. Head and neck cancer in Australia between 1982 and 2005 show increasing incidence of potentially HPV-associated oropharyngeal cancers. *Br J Cancer* 2011;104(5):886–91.
544. Shaikh MH, McMillan NA, Johnson NW. HPV-associated head and neck cancers in the Asia Pacific: a critical literature review & meta-analysis. *Cancer Epidemiol* 2015;39(6):923–38.
545. Balaram P, Nalinakumari KR, Abraham E et al. Human papillomaviruses in 91 oral cancers from Indian betel quid chewers – high prevalence and multiplicity of infections. *Int J Cancer* 1995;61(4):450–4.
546. Bahl A, Kumar P, Dar L et al. Prevalence and trends of human papillomavirus in oropharyngeal cancer in a predominantly north Indian population. *Head Neck* 2014;36(4):505–10.
547. Nagpal JK, Patnaik S, Das BR. Prevalence of high-risk human papilloma virus types and its association with p53 codon 72 polymorphism in tobacco addicted oral squamous cell carcinoma (OSCC) patients of Eastern India. *Int J Cancer* 2002;97(5):649–53.
548. Koppikar P, deVilliers EM, Mulherkar R. Identification of human papillomaviruses in tumors of the oral cavity in an Indian community. *Int J Cancer* 2005;113(6):946–50.
549. Shen J, Tate JE, Crum CP, Goodman ML. Prevalence of human papillomaviruses (HPV) in benign and malignant tumors of the upper respiratory tract. *Mod Pathol* 1996;9(1):15–20.
550. Paz IB, Cook N, Odom-Maryon T, Xie Y, Wilczynski SP. Human papillomavirus (HPV) in head and neck cancer. An association of HPV 16 with squamous cell carcinoma of Waldeyer's tonsillar ring. *Cancer* 1997;79(3):595–604.
551. Baumann JL, Cohen S, Evjen AN et al. Human papillomavirus in early laryngeal carcinoma. *Laryngoscope* 2009;119(8):1531–7.
552. Stephen JK, Chen KM, Shah V et al. Human papillomavirus outcomes in an access-to-care laryngeal cancer cohort. *Otolaryngol Head Neck Surg* 2012;146(5):730–8.
553. de Oliveira DE, Bacchi MM, Macarenco RS, Tagliarini JV, Cordeiro RC, Bacchi CE. Human papillomavirus and Epstein-Barr virus infection, p53 expression, and cellular proliferation in laryngeal carcinoma. *Am J Clin Pathol* 2006;126(2):284–93.
554. Torrente MC, Ampuero S, Abud M, Ojeda JM. Molecular detection and typing of human papillomavirus in laryngeal carcinoma specimens. *Acta Otolaryngol* 2005;125(8):888–93.
555. Salam MA, Rockett J, Morris A. General primer-mediated polymerase chain reaction for simultaneous detection and typing of human papillomavirus DNA in laryngeal squamous cell carcinomas. *Clin Otolaryngol Allied Sci* 1995;20(1):84–8.
556. Venuti A, Manni V, Morello R, De Marco F, Marzetti F, Marcante ML. Physical state and expression of human papillomavirus in laryngeal carcinoma and surrounding normal mucosa. *J Med Virol* 2000;60(4):396–402.
557. Snijders PJ, Scholes AG, Hart CA et al. Prevalence of mucosotropic human papillomaviruses in squamous-cell carcinoma of the head and neck. *Int J Cancer* 1996;66(4):464–9.
558. Koskinen WJ, Brondbo K, Mellin Dahlstrand H et al. Alcohol, smoking and human papillomavirus in laryngeal carcinoma: a Nordic prospective multicenter study. *J Cancer Res Clin Oncol* 2007; 133(9):673–8.
559. Hoffmann M, Scheunemann D, Fazel A, Gorogh T, Kahn T, Gottschlich S. Human papillomavirus and p53 polymorphism in codon 72 in head and neck squamous cell carcinoma. *Oncol Rep* 2009;21(3):809–14.
560. Morshed K, Polz-Dacewicz M, Szymanski M, Smolen A. Usefulness and efficiency of formalin-fixed paraffin-embedded specimens from laryngeal squamous cell carcinoma in HPV detection by IHC and PCR/DEIA. *Folia Histochem Cytobiol* 2010;48(3):398–402.
561. Jacob SE, Sreevidya S, Chacko E, Pillai MR. Cellular manifestations of human papillomavirus infection in laryngeal tissues. *J Surg Oncol* 2002;79(3):142–50.
562. Talukdar FR, Ghosh SK, Laskar RS, Kannan R, Choudhury B, Bhowmik A. Epigenetic pathogenesis

of human papillomavirus in upper aerodigestive tract cancers. *Mol Carcinog* 2015;54(11):1387–96.
563. Benard VB, Johnson CJ, Thompson TD et al. Examining the association between socioeconomic status and potential human papillomavirus-associated cancers. *Cancer* 2008;113(10 Suppl):2910–8.
564. Gillison ML, D'Souza G, Westra W et al. Distinct risk factor profiles for human papillomavirus type 16-positive and human papillomavirus type 16-negative head and neck cancers. *J Natl Cancer Inst* 2008;100(6):407–20.
565. Llewellyn CD, Johnson NW, Warnakulasuriya KA. Risk factors for squamous cell carcinoma of the oral cavity in young people – a comprehensive literature review. *Oral Oncol* 2001;37(5):401–18.
566. Ryerson AB, Peters ES, Coughlin SS et al. Burden of potentially human papillomavirus-associated cancers of the oropharynx and oral cavity in the US, 1998–2003. *Cancer* 2008;113(10 Suppl):2901–9.
567. Gillison ML. Human papillomavirus and prognosis of oropharyngeal squamous cell carcinoma: Implications for clinical research in head and neck cancers. *J Clin Oncol* 2006;24(36):5623–5.
568. Klozar J, Kratochvil V, Salakova M et al. HPV status and regional metastasis in the prognosis of oral and oropharyngeal cancer. *Eur Arch Oto-Rhino-Laryngol* 2008;265(Suppl 1):S75–82.
569. Lindel K, Beer KT, Laissue J, Greiner RH, Aebersold DM. Human papillomavirus positive squamous cell carcinoma of the oropharynx: a radiosensitive subgroup of head and neck carcinoma. *Cancer* 2001;92(4):805–13.
570. Satterwhite CL, Torrone E, Meites E et al. Sexually transmitted infections among U.S. women and men: prevalence and incidence estimates, 2008. *Sex Transm Dis* 2013;40(3):187–93.
571. D'Souza G, Agrawal Y, Halpern J, Bodison S, Gillison ML. Oral sexual behaviors associated with prevalent oral human papillomavirus infection. *J Infect Dis* 2009;199(9):1263–9.
572. Rosenquist K, Wennerberg J, Annertz K et al. Recurrence in patients with oral and oropharyngeal squamous cell carcinoma: human papillomavirus and other risk factors. *Acta Otolaryngol* 2007;127(9):980–7.
573. Sanders AE, Slade GD, Patton LL. National prevalence of oral HPV infection and related risk factors in the U.S. adult population. *Oral Dis* 2012;18(5):430–41.
574. D'Souza G, Kreimer AR, Viscidi R et al. Case-control study of human papillomavirus and oropharyngeal cancer. *N Engl J Med* 2007;356(19):1944–56.
575. Rajkumar T, Sridhar H, Balaram P et al. Oral cancer in Southern India: the influence of body size, diet, infections and sexual practices. *Eur J Cancer Prev* 2003;12(2):135–43.
576. Smith EM, Ritchie JM, Summersgill KF et al. Age, sexual behavior and human papillomavirus infection in oral cavity and oropharyngeal cancers. *Int J Cancer* 2004;108(5):766–72.
577. Esquenazi D, Bussoloti Filho I, Carvalho Mda G, Barros FS. The frequency of human papillomavirus findings in normal oral mucosa of healthy people by PCR. *Braz J Otorhinolaryngol* 2010;76(1):78–84.
578. Zou H, Tabrizi SN, Grulich AE et al. Site-specific human papillomavirus infection in adolescent men who have sex with men (HYPER): an observational cohort study. *Lancet Infect Dis* 2015;15(1):65–73.
579. Settle K, Posner MR, Schumaker LM et al. Racial survival disparity in head and neck cancer results from low prevalence of human papillomavirus infection in black oropharyngeal cancer patients. *Cancer Prev Res* 2009;2(9):776–81.
580. Feller L, Khammissa RA, Wood NH, Lemmer J. Epithelial maturation and molecular biology of oral HPV. *Infect Agents Cancer* 2009;4:16.
581. Sanchez-Vargas LO, Diaz-Hernandez C, Martinez-Martinez A. Detection of Human Papilloma Virus (HPV) in oral mucosa of women with cervical lesions and their relation to oral sex practices. *Infect Agents Cancer* 2010;5(1):25.
582. Durzynska J, Pacholska-Bogalska J, Kaczmarek M et al. HPV genotypes in the oral cavity/oropharynx of children and adolescents: cross-sectional survey in Poland. *Eur J Pediatr* 2011;170(6):757–61.
583. Sinclair KA, Woods CR, Kirse DJ, Sinal SH. Anogenital and respiratory tract human papillomavirus infections among children: age, gender, and potential transmission through sexual abuse. *Pediatrics* 2005;116(4):815–25.
584. Rombaldi RL, Serafini EP, Mandelli J, Zimmermann E, Losquiavo KP. Perinatal transmission of human papilomavirus DNA. *Virol J* 2009;6:83.
585. Gillison ML, Alemany L, Snijders PJ et al. Human papillomavirus and diseases of the upper airway: head and neck cancer and respiratory papillomatosis. *Vaccine* 2012;30(Suppl 5):F34–54.
586. Maxwell JH, Kumar B, Feng FY et al. Tobacco use in human papillomavirus-positive advanced oropharynx cancer patients related to increased risk of distant metastases and tumor recurrence. *Clin Cancer Res* 2010;16(4):1226–35.
587. Chaturvedi AK, Engels EA, Anderson WF, Gillison ML. Incidence trends for human papillomavirus-related and -unrelated oral squamous cell carcinomas in the United States. *J Clin Oncol* 2008;26(4):612–9.
588. Syrjanen S. HPV infections and tonsillar carcinoma. *J Clin Pathol* 2004;57(5):449–55.
589. Wilczynski SP, Lin BT, Xie Y, Paz IB. Detection of human papillomavirus DNA and oncoprotein overexpression are associated with distinct morphological patterns of tonsillar squamous cell carcinoma. *Am J Pathol* 1998;152(1):145–56.
590. Barnes L, Ferlito A, Altavilla G, MacMillan C, Rinaldo A, Doglioni C. Basaloid squamous cell carcinoma

of the head and neck: clinicopathological features and differential diagnosis. *Ann Otol Rhinol Laryngol* 1996;105(1):75–82.
591. Andl T, Kahn T, Pfuhl A et al. Etiological involvement of oncogenic human papillomavirus in tonsillar squamous cell carcinomas lacking retinoblastoma cell cycle control. *Cancer Res* 1998;58(1):5–13.
592. Begum S, Cao D, Gillison M, Zahurak M, Westra WH. Tissue distribution of human papillomavirus 16 DNA integration in patients with tonsillar carcinoma. *Clin Cancer Res* 2005;11(16):5694–9.
593. Kim SH, Koo BS, Kang S et al. HPV integration begins in the tonsillar crypt and leads to the alteration of p16, EGFR and c-myc during tumor formation. *Int J Cancer* 2007;120(7):1418–25.
594. Surjan L Jr. Immunohistochemical markers of tonsillar crypt epithelium. *Acta Otolaryngol Suppl* 1988;454:60–3.
595. Thierry F. Transcriptional regulation of the papillomavirus oncogenes by cellular and viral transcription factors in cervical carcinoma. *Virology* 2009;384(2):375–9.
596. Doorbar J. The papillomavirus life cycle. *J Clin Virol* 2005;32(Suppl 1):S7–15.
597. Day PM, Lowy DR, Schiller JT. Papillomaviruses infect cells via a clathrin-dependent pathway. *Virology* 2003;307(1):1–11.
598. Bousarghin L, Touze A, Sizaret PY, Coursaget P. Human papillomavirus types 16, 31, and 58 use different endocytosis pathways to enter cells. *J Virol* 2003;77(6):3846–50.
599. Wang HK, Duffy AA, Broker TR, Chow LT. Robust production and passaging of infectious HPV in squamous epithelium of primary human keratinocytes. *Genes Dev* 2009;23(2):181–94.
600. Kamper N, Day PM, Nowak T et al. A membrane-destabilizing peptide in capsid protein L2 is required for egress of papillomavirus genomes from endosomes. *J Virol* 2006;80(2):759–68.
601. Sapp M, Bienkowska-Haba M. Viral entry mechanisms: human papillomavirus and a long journey from extracellular matrix to the nucleus. *FEBS J* 2009;276(24):7206–16.
602. Shafti-Keramat S, Handisurya A, Kriehuber E, Meneguzzi G, Slupetzky K, Kirnbauer R. Different heparan sulfate proteoglycans serve as cellular receptors for human papillomaviruses. *J Virol* 2003;77(24):13125–35.
603. Letian T, Tianyu Z. Cellular receptor binding and entry of human papillomavirus. *Virol J* 2010;7:2.
604. Yang R, Day PM, Yutzy WHt, Lin KY, Hung CF, Roden RB. Cell surface-binding motifs of L2 that facilitate papillomavirus infection. *J Virol* 2003;77(6):3531–41.
605. Munger K, Baldwin A, Edwards KM et al. Mechanisms of human papillomavirus-induced oncogenesis. *J Virol* 2004;78(21):11451–60.
606. Farthing AJ, Vousden KH. Functions of human papillomavirus E6 and E7 oncoproteins. *Trends Microbiol* 1994;2(5):170–4.
607. Brachman DG, Graves D, Vokes E et al. Occurrence of p53 gene deletions and human papilloma virus infection in human head and neck cancer. *Cancer Res* 1992;52(17):4832–6.
608. Munger K, Phelps WC, Bubb V, Howley PM, Schlegel R. The E6 and E7 genes of the human papillomavirus type 16 together are necessary and sufficient for transformation of primary human keratinocytes. *J Virol* 1989;63(10):4417–21.
609. Barbosa MS, Schlegel R. The E6 and E7 genes of HPV-18 are sufficient for inducing two-stage *in vitro* transformation of human keratinocytes. *Oncogene* 1989;4(12):1529–32.
610. Crook T, Storey A, Almond N, Osborn K, Crawford L. Human papillomavirus type 16 cooperates with activated ras and fos oncogenes in the hormone-dependent transformation of primary mouse cells. *Proc Natl Acad Sci USA* 1988;85(23):8820–4.
611. Klingelhutz AJ, Hedrick L, Cho KR, McDougall JK. The DCC gene suppresses the malignant phenotype of transformed human epithelial cells. *Oncogene* 1995;10(8):1581–6.
612. Werness BA, Levine AJ, Howley PM. Association of human papillomavirus types 16 and 18 E6 proteins with p53. *Science* 1990;248(4951):76–9.
613. Klingelhutz AJ, Foster SA, McDougall JK. Telomerase activation by the E6 gene product of human papillomavirus type 16. *Nature* 1996;380(6569):79–82.
614. Dyson N, Howley PM, Munger K, Harlow E. The human papilloma virus-16 E7 oncoprotein is able to bind to the retinoblastoma gene product. *Science* 1989;243(4893):934–7.
615. Davies R, Hicks R, Crook T, Morris J, Vousden K. Human papillomavirus type 16 E7 associates with a histone H1 kinase and with p107 through sequences necessary for transformation. *J Virol* 1993;67(5):2521–8.
616. Claudio PP, Howard CM, Baldi A et al. P130/pRb2 has growth suppressive properties similar to yet distinctive from those of retinoblastoma family members pRb and p107. *Cancer Res* 1994;54(21):5556–60.
617. Wiest T, Schwarz E, Enders C, Flechtenmacher C, Bosch FX. Involvement of intact HPV16 E6/E7 gene expression in head and neck cancers with unaltered p53 status and perturbed pRb cell cycle control. *Oncogene* 2002;21(10):1510–7.
618. Benevolo M, Mottolese M, Marandino F et al. Immunohistochemical expression of p16(INK4a) is predictive of HR-HPV infection in cervical low-grade lesions. *Mod Pathol* 2006;19(3):384–91.
619. Kuo KT, Hsiao CH, Lin CH, Kuo LT, Huang SH, Lin MC. The biomarkers of human papillomavirus infection in tonsillar squamous cell carcinoma-molecular

basis and predicting favorable outcome. *Mod Pathol* 2008;21(4):376–86.

620. Moody CA, Laimins LA. Human papillomavirus oncoproteins: pathways to transformation. *Nat Rev Cancer* 2010;10(8):550–60.
621. Maufort JP, Shai A, Pitot HC, Lambert PF. A role for HPV16 E5 in cervical carcinogenesis. *Cancer Res* 2010;70(7):2924–31.
622. Rampias T, Boutati E, Pectasides E et al. Activation of Wnt signaling pathway by human papillomavirus E6 and E7 oncogenes in HPV16-positive oropharyngeal squamous carcinoma cells. *Mol Cancer Res* 2010;8(3):433–43.
623. Leemans CR, Braakhuis BJ, Brakenhoff RH. The molecular biology of head and neck cancer. *Nat Rev Cancer* 2011;11(1):9–22.
624. Castro TP, Bussoloti Filho I. Prevalence of human papillomavirus (HPV) in oral cavity and oropharynx. *Braz J Otorhinolaryngol* 2006;72(2):272–82.
625. Jaju PP, Suvarna PV, Desai RS. Squamous papilloma: case report and review of literature. *Int J Oral Sci* 2010;2(4):222–5.
626. Chang F, Syrjanen S, Kellokoski J, Syrjanen K. Human papillomavirus (HPV) infections and their associations with oral disease. *J Oral Pathol Med* 1991;20(7):305–17.
627. Swan RH, McDaniel RK, Dreiman BB, Rome WC. Condyloma acuminatum involving the oral mucosa. *Oral Surg Oral Med Oral Pathol* 1981;51(5):503–8.
628. Scheurer ME, Tortolero-Luna G, Adler-Storthz K. Human papillomavirus infection: biology, epidemiology, and prevention. *Int J Gynecol Cancer* 2005;15(5):727–46.
629. Anderson KM, Perez-Montiel D, Miles L, Allen CM, Nuovo GJ. The histologic differentiation of oral condyloma acuminatum from its mimics. *Oral Surg Oral Med Oral Pathol Oral Radiol Endod* 2003;96(4):420–8.
630. Syrjanen S. The role of human papillomavirus infection in head and neck cancers. *Ann Oncol* 2010;21(Suppl 7):vii243–5.
631. Praetorius F. HPV-associated diseases of oral mucosa. *Clin Dermatol* 1997;15(3):399–413.
632. Adler-Storthz K, Newland JR, Tessin BA, Yeudall WA, Shillitoe EJ. Identification of human papillomavirus types in oral verruca vulgaris. *J Oral Pathol* 1986;15(4):230–3.
633. Harris AM, van Wyk CW. Heck's disease (focal epithelial hyperplasia): a longitudinal study. *Community Dent Oral Epidemiol* 1993;21(2):82–5.
634. Michael EJ, Husain S, Zalar G, Nuovo G. Focal epithelial hyperplasia in an Ecuadorian girl. *Cutis* 1999;64(6):395–6.
635. Vera-Iglesias E, Garcia-Arpa M, Sanchez-Caminero P, Romero-Aguilera G, Cortina de la Calle P. Focal epithelial hyperplasia. *Actas Dermosifiliogr* 2007;98(9):621–3.
636. Clausen FP, Mogeltoft M, Roed-Petersen B, Pindborg JJ. Focal epithelial hyperplasia of the oral mucosa in a south-west Greenlandic population. *Scand J Dent Res* 1970;78(3):287–94.
637. Lamey PJ, Lewis MA, Rennie JS, Beattie AD. Heck's disease. *Br Dent J* 1990;168(6):251–2.
638. Bassioukas K, Danielides V, Georgiou I, Photos E, Zagorianakou P, Skevas A. Oral focal epithelial hyperplasia. *Eur J Dermatol* 2000;10(5):395–7.
639. Silverberg MJ, Thorsen P, Lindeberg H, Ahdieh-Grant L, Shah KV. Clinical course of recurrent respiratory papillomatosis in Danish children. *Arch Otolaryngol Head Neck Surg* 2004;130(6):711–6.
640. Hartley C, Hamilton J, Birzgalis AR, Farrington WT. Recurrent respiratory papillomatosis – the Manchester experience, 1974–1992. *J Laryngol Otol* 1994;108(3):226–9.
641. Wiatrak BJ, Wiatrak DW, Broker TR, Lewis L. Recurrent respiratory papillomatosis: a longitudinal study comparing severity associated with human papilloma viral types 6 and 11 and other risk factors in a large pediatric population. *Laryngoscope* 2004;114(11 Pt 2 Suppl 104):1–23.
642. Cohn AM, Kos JT, 2nd, Taber LH, Adam E. Recurring laryngeal papillopa. *Am J Otolaryngol* 1981;2(2):129–32.
643. Silverberg MJ, Thorsen P, Lindeberg H, Grant LA, Shah KV. Condyloma in pregnancy is strongly predictive of juvenile-onset recurrent respiratory papillomatosis. *Obstet Gynecol* 2003;101(4):645–52.
644. Winckworth LC, Nichol R. Question 2: do caesarean sections reduce the maternal-fetal transmission rate of human papillomavirus infection? *Arch Dis Child* 2010;95(1):70–3.
645. Ruiz R, Achlatis S, Verma A et al. Risk factors for adult-onset recurrent respiratory papillomatosis. *Laryngoscope* 2014;124(10):2338–44.
646. Fornatora M, Jones AC, Kerpel S, Freedman P. Human papillomavirus-associated oral epithelial dysplasia (koilocytic dysplasia): an entity of unknown biologic potential. *Oral Surg Oral Med Oral Pathol Oral Radiol Endod* 1996;82(1):47–56.
647. Klingbeil MF, De Lima MD, Gallottini MH, Dos Santos Pinto D Jr, Lemos CA Jr. Oral koilocytic dysplasia: long-term clinical control. A case report. *Minerva Stomatol* 2012;61(6):289–94.
648. Warnakulasuriya S, Johnson NW, van der Waal I. Nomenclature and classification of potentially malignant disorders of the oral mucosa. *J Oral Pathol Med* 2007;36(10):575–80.
649. van der Waal I. Potentially malignant disorders of the oral and oropharyngeal mucosa; terminology, classification and present concepts of management. *Oral Oncol* 2009;45(4–5):317–23.
650. Syrjanen S, Puranen M. Human papillomavirus infections in children: the potential role of maternal transmission. *Crit Rev Oral Biol Med* 2000;11(2):259–74.
651. Warnakulasuriya S, Ariyawardana A. Malignant transformation of oral leukoplakia: a systematic

review of observational studies. *J Oral Pathol Med* 2016;45(3):155–66.
652. Maserejian NN, Joshipura KJ, Rosner BA, Giovannucci E, Zavras AI. Prospective study of alcohol consumption and risk of oral premalignant lesions in men. *Cancer Epidemiol Biomarkers Prev* 2006;15(4):774–81.
653. Napier SS, Speight PM. Natural history of potentially malignant oral lesions and conditions: an overview of the literature. *J Oral Pathol Med* 2008;37(1):1–10.
654. Holmstrup P, Vedtofte P, Reibel J, Stoltze K. Long-term treatment outcome of oral premalignant lesions. *Oral Oncol* 2006;42(5):461–74.
655. Kashima HK, Kutcher M, Kessis T, Levin LS, de Villiers EM, Shah K. Human papillomavirus in squamous cell carcinoma, leukoplakia, lichen planus, and clinically normal epithelium of the oral cavity. *Ann Otol Rhinol Laryngol* 1990;99(1):55–61.
656. Acay R, Rezende N, Fontes A, Aburad A, Nunes F, Sousa S. Human papillomavirus as a risk factor in oral carcinogenesis: a study using in situ hybridization with signal amplification. *Oral Microbiol Immunol* 2008;23(4):271–4.
657. Bagan J, Scully C, Jimenez Y, Martorell M. Proliferative verrucous leukoplakia: a concise update. *Oral Dis* 2010;16(4):328–32.
658. Campisi G, Giovannelli L, Ammatuna P et al. Proliferative verrucous vs conventional leukoplakia: no significantly increased risk of HPV infection. *Oral Oncol* 2004;40(8):835–40.
659. Palefsky JM, Silverman S Jr, Abdel-Salaam M, Daniels TE, Greenspan JS. Association between proliferative verrucous leukoplakia and infection with human papillomavirus type 16. *J Oral Pathol Med* 1995;24(5):193–7.
660. Lubbe J, Kormann A, Adams V et al. HPV-11- and HPV-16-associated oral verrucous carcinoma. *Dermatology* 1996;192(3):217–21.
661. Alkan A, Bulut E, Gunhan O, Ozden B. Oral verrucous carcinoma: a study of 12 cases. *Eur J Dent* 2010;4(2):202–7.
662. Santoro A, Pannone G, Contaldo M et al. A troubling diagnosis of verrucous squamous cell carcinoma ("the bad kind" of keratosis) and the need of clinical and pathological correlations: a review of the literature with a case report. *J Skin Cancer* 2011;2011:370605.
663. Shroyer KR, Greer RO, Fankhouser CA, McGuirt WF, Marshall R. Detection of human papillomavirus DNA in oral verrucous carcinoma by polymerase chain reaction. *Mod Pathol* 1993;6(6):669–72.
664. Eisen D. The clinical features, malignant potential, and systemic associations of oral lichen planus: a study of 723 patients. *J Am Acad Dermatol* 2002;46(2):207–14.
665. Bornstein MM, Kalas L, Lemp S, Altermatt HJ, Rees TD, Buser D. Oral lichen planus and malignant transformation: a retrospective follow-up study of clinical and histopathologic data. *Quintessence Int* 2006;37(4):261–71.
666. Ingafou M, Leao JC, Porter SR, Scully C. Oral lichen planus: a retrospective study of 690 British patients. *Oral Dis* 2006;12(5):463–8.
667. Nico MM, Fernandes JD, Lourenco SV. Oral lichen planus. *An Bras Dermatol* 2011;86(4):633–41; quiz 42–3.
668. Farhi D, Dupin N. Pathophysiology, etiologic factors, and clinical management of oral lichen planus, part I: facts and controversies. *Clin Dermatol* 2010;28(1):100–8.
669. van der Waal I. Oral lichen planus and oral lichenoid lesions; a critical appraisal with emphasis on the diagnostic aspects. *Med Oral Patol Oral Cir Bucal* 2009;14(7):E310–4.
670. Ostwald C, Rutsatz K, Schweder J, Schmidt W, Gundlach K, Barten M. Human papillomavirus 6/11, 16 and 18 in oral carcinomas and benign oral lesions. *Med Microbiol Immunol* 2003;192(3):145–8.
671. Gorsky M, Epstein JB. Oral lichen planus: malignant transformation and human papilloma virus: a review of potential clinical implications. *Oral Surg Oral Med Oral Pathol Oral Radiol Endod* 2011;111(4):461–4.
672. Johnson NW, Ranasinghe AW, Warnakulasuriya KA. Potentially malignant lesions and conditions of the mouth and oropharynx: natural history – cellular and molecular markers of risk. *Eur J Cancer Prev* 1993;2(Suppl 2):31–51.
673. Alavian SM, Mahboobi N, Mahboobi N, Karayiannis P. Oral conditions associated with hepatitis C virus infection. *Saudi J Gastroenterol* 2013;19(6):245–51.
674. Gandolfo S, Carbone M, Carrozzo M, Gallo V. Oral lichen planus and hepatitis C virus (HCV) infection: is there a relationship? A report of 10 cases. *J Oral Pathol Med* 1994;23(3):119–22.
675. Lodi G, Pellicano R, Carrozzo M. Hepatitis C virus infection and lichen planus: a systematic review with meta-analysis. *Oral Dis* 2010;16(7):601–12.
676. Petti S, Rabiei M, De Luca M, Scully C. The magnitude of the association between hepatitis C virus infection and oral lichen planus: meta-analysis and case control study. *Odontology* 2011;99(2):168–78.
677. Shengyuan L, Songpo Y, Wen W, Wenjing T, Haitao Z, Binyou W. Hepatitis C virus and lichen planus: a reciprocal association determined by a meta-analysis. *Arch Dermatol* 2009;145(9):1040–7.
678. Nagao Y, Myoken Y, Katayama K, Tanaka J, Yoshizawa H, Sata M. Epidemiological survey of oral lichen planus among HCV-infected inhabitants in a town in Hiroshima Prefecture in Japan from 2000 to 2003. *Oncol Rep* 2007;18(5):1177–81.
679. Nagao Y, Sata M, Noguchi S et al. Various extrahepatic manifestations caused by hepatitis C virus infection. *Int J Mol Med* 1999;4(6):621–5.
680. Porter SR, Lodi G, Chandler K, Kumar N. Development of squamous cell carcinoma in

hepatitis C virus-associated lichen planus. *Oral Oncol* 1997;33(1):58–9.

681. Carrozzo M, Carbone M, Gandolfo S, Valente G, Colombatto P, Ghisetti V. An atypical verrucous carcinoma of the tongue arising in a patient with oral lichen planus associated with hepatitis C virus infection. *Oral Oncol* 1997;33(3):220–5.
682. Ishido S, Muramatsu S, Fujita T et al. Wild-type, but not mutant-type, p53 enhances nuclear accumulation of the NS3 protein of hepatitis C virus. *Biochem Biophys Res Commun* 1997;230(2):431–6.
683. Chang Y, Moore PS. Merkel cell carcinoma: a virus-induced human cancer. *Annu Rev Pathol* 2012;7:123–44.
684. Feng H, Shuda M, Chang Y, Moore PS. Clonal integration of a polyomavirus in human Merkel cell carcinoma. *Science* 2008;319(5866):1096–100.
685. Baez CF, Guimaraes MA, Martins RA et al. Detection of Merkel cell polyomavirus in oral samples of renal transplant recipients without Merkel cell carcinoma. *J Med Virol* 2013;85(11):2016–9.
686. Chocolatewala N, Chaturvedi P, Desale R. The role of bacteria in oral cancer. *Indian J Med Paediatr Oncol* 2010;31(4):126–31.
687. Mager DL. Bacteria and cancer: cause, coincidence or cure? A review. *J Transl Med* 2006;4:14.
688. Markowska J, Fischer N, Markowski M, Nalewaj J. The role of *Chlamydia trachomatis* infection in the development of cervical neoplasia and carcinoma. *Medycyny Wieku Rozwojowego* 2005;9(1):83–6.
689. Nagaraja V, Eslick GD. Systematic review with meta-analysis: the relationship between chronic *Salmonella typhi* carrier status and gall-bladder cancer. *Aliment Pharmacol Ther* 2014;39(8):745–50.
690. Toprak NU, Yagci A, Gulluoglu BM et al. A possible role of Bacteroides fragilis enterotoxin in the aetiology of colorectal cancer. *Clin Microbiol Infect* 2006;12(8):782–6.
691. Kostic AD, Gevers D, Pedamallu CS et al. Genomic analysis identifies association of *Fusobacterium* with colorectal carcinoma. *Genome Res* 2012;22(2):292–8.
692. Mao S, Park Y, Hasegawa Y et al. Intrinsic apoptotic pathways of gingival epithelial cells modulated by *Porphyromonas gingivalis*. *Cell Microbiol* 2007;9(8):1997–2007.
693. Moffatt CE, Lamont RJ. *Porphyromonas gingivalis* induction of microRNA-203 expression controls suppressor of cytokine signaling 3 in gingival epithelial cells. *Infect Immun* 2011;79(7):2632–7.
694. Yilmaz O, Jungas T, Verbeke P, Ojcius DM. Activation of the phosphatidylinositol 3-kinase/Akt pathway contributes to survival of primary epithelial cells infected with the periodontal pathogen *Porphyromonas gingivalis*. *Infect Immun* 2004;72(7):3743–51.
695. Kuboniwa M, Hasegawa Y, Mao S et al. *P. gingivalis* accelerates gingival epithelial cell progression through the cell cycle. *Microbes Infect* 2008;10(2):122–8.
696. Inaba H, Sugita H, Kuboniwa M et al. *Porphyromonas gingivalis* promotes invasion of oral squamous cell carcinoma through induction of proMMP9 and its activation. *Cell Microbiol* 2014;16(1):131–45.
697. Groeger S, Domann E, Gonzales JR, Chakraborty T, Meyle J. B7-H1 and B7-DC receptors of oral squamous carcinoma cells are upregulated by *Porphyromonas gingivalis*. *Immunobiology* 2011;216(12):1302–10.
698. Woo BH, Kim DJ, Choi JI et al. Oral cancer cells sustainedly infected with *Porphyromonas gingivalis* exhibit resistance to Taxol and have higher metastatic potential. *Oncotarget* 2017;8(29):46981–92.
699. Rubinstein MR, Wang X, Liu W, Hao Y, Cai G, Han YW. *Fusobacterium nucleatum* promotes colorectal carcinogenesis by modulating E-cadherin/beta-catenin signaling via its FadA adhesin. *Cell Host Microbe* 2013;14(2):195–206.
700. Uitto VJ, Baillie D, Wu Q et al. *Fusobacterium nucleatum* increases collagenase 3 production and migration of epithelial cells. *Infect Immun* 2005;73(2):1171–9.
701. McCoy AN, Araujo-Perez F, Azcarate-Peril A, Yeh JJ, Sandler RS, Keku TO. Fusobacterium is associated with colorectal adenomas. *PloS One* 2013;8(1):e53653.
702. Perera M, Al-Hebshi NN, Speicher DJ, Perera I, Johnson NW. Emerging role of bacteria in oral carcinogenesis: a review with special reference to perio-pathogenic bacteria. *J Oral Microbiol* 2016;8:32762.
703. Whitmore SE, Lamont RJ. Oral bacteria and cancer. *PLoS Pathog* 2014;10(3):e1003933.
704. Nagy KN, Sonkodi I, Szoke I, Nagy E, Newman HN. The microflora associated with human oral carcinomas. *Oral Oncol* 1998;34(4):304–8.
705. Katz J, Onate MD, Pauley KM, Bhattacharyya I, Cha S. Presence of *Porphyromonas gingivalis* in gingival squamous cell carcinoma. *Int J Oral Sci* 2011;3(4):209–15.
706. Ahn J, Segers S, Hayes RB. Periodontal disease, *Porphyromonas gingivalis* serum antibody levels and orodigestive cancer mortality. *Carcinogenesis* 2012;33(5):1055–8.
707. Castellarin M, Warren RL, Freeman JD et al. *Fusobacterium nucleatum* infection is prevalent in human colorectal carcinoma. *Genome Res* 2012;22(2):299–306.
708. Michaud DS, Izard J, Wilhelm-Benartzi CS et al. Plasma antibodies to oral bacteria and risk of pancreatic cancer in a large European prospective cohort study. *Gut* 2013;62(12):1764–70.
709. Tateda M, Shiga K, Saijo S et al. *Streptococcus anginosus* in head and neck squamous cell carcinoma: implication in carcinogenesis. *Int J Mol Med* 2000;6(6):699–703.
710. Sasaki M, Yamaura C, Ohara-Nemoto Y et al. Streptococcus anginosus infection in oral cancer and its infection route. *Oral Dis* 2005;11(3):151–6.
711. Morita E, Narikiyo M, Yano A et al. Different frequencies of *Streptococcus anginosus* infection in

oral cancer and esophageal cancer. *Cancer Sci* 2003;94(6):492–6.
712. Hooper SJ, Crean SJ, Fardy MJ et al. A molecular analysis of the bacteria present within oral squamous cell carcinoma. *J Med Microbiol* 2007;56(Pt 12):1651–9.
713. Pushalkar S, Ji X, Li Y et al. Comparison of oral microbiota in tumor and non-tumor tissues of patients with oral squamous cell carcinoma. *BMC Microbiol* 2012;12:144.
714. Mager DL, Haffajee AD, Devlin PM, Norris CM, Posner MR, Goodson JM. The salivary microbiota as a diagnostic indicator of oral cancer: a descriptive, non-randomized study of cancer-free and oral squamous cell carcinoma subjects. *J Transl Med* 2005;3:27.
715. Hooper SJ, Crean SJ, Lewis MA, Spratt DA, Wade WG, Wilson MJ. Viable bacteria present within oral squamous cell carcinoma tissue. *J Clin Microbiol* 2006;44(5):1719–25.
716. Siqueira JF Jr, Fouad AF, Rocas IN. Pyrosequencing as a tool for better understanding of human microbiomes. *J Oral Microbiol* 2012;4(1).
717. Pushalkar S, Mane SP, Ji X et al. Microbial diversity in saliva of oral squamous cell carcinoma. *FEMS Immunol Med Microbiol* 2011;61(3):269–77.
718. Schmidt BL, Kuczynski J, Bhattacharya A et al. Changes in abundance of oral microbiota associated with oral cancer. *PloS One* 2014;9(6):e98741.
719. Al-Hebshi NN, Nasher AT, Idris AM, Chen T. Robust species taxonomy assignment algorithm for 16S rRNA NGS reads: application to oral carcinoma samples. *J Oral Microbiol* 2015;7:28934.
720. Xie H, Onsongo G, Popko J et al. Proteomics analysis of cells in whole saliva from oral cancer patients via value-added three-dimensional peptide fractionation and tandem mass spectrometry. *Mol Cell Proteomics* 2008;7(3): 486–98.
721. Hebbar PB, Pai A, Sujatha D, Mycological and histological associations of candida in oral mucosal lesions. *J Oral Sci* 2013;55(2):157–60.
722. McCullough M, Jaber M, Barrett AW, Bain L, Speight PM, Porter SR. Oral yeast carriage correlates with presence of oral epithelial dysplasia. *Oral Oncol* 2002;38(4):391–3.
723. Spolidorio LC, Martins VR, Nogueira RD, Spolidorio DM. The frequency of Candida sp. in biopsies of oral mucosal lesions. *Pesqui OdontolBras* 2003;17(1):89–93.
724. Perera M, Al-hebshi NN, Perera I et al. A dysbiotic mycobiome dominated by *Candida albicans* is identified within oral squamous cell carcinomas. *J Oral Microbiol.* 2017 Oct 27;9(1):1385369. doi: 10.1080/20002297.2017.1385369. eCollection 2017. PMID: 29152157.
725. Gainza-Cirauqui ML, Nieminen MT, Novak Frazer L, Aguirre-Urizar JM, Moragues MD, Rautemaa R. Production of carcinogenic acetaldehyde by *Candida albicans* from patients with potentially malignant oral mucosal disorders. *J Oral Pathol Med* 2013;42(3):243–9.
726. Shaikh MH, Khan AI, Sadat A et al. Prevalence and types of high-risk human papillomaviruses in head and neck cancers from Bangladesh. *BMC Cancer* 2017;17(1):792. doi:10.1186/s12885-017-3789-0. PMID: 29178862.
727. Ren et al. *Anal Methods* 2017;9: 4033–43.
728. Warnakulasuriya S. In: Bedi R, Jones P (eds). *Betel quid and tobacco chewing among the Bangladeshi Community in the United Kingdom.* London: Centre for Transcultural Oral Health, 1995,61–9.
729. Mesri EA, Cesarman E, Boshoff C. Kaposi's sarcoma and its associated herpesvirus. *Nat Rev Cancer* 2010;10(10):707–19. doi: 10.1038/nrc2888.
730. Curatolo P, Mancini M, Ruggiero A, Clerico R, Di Marco P, Calvieri S. Successful treatment of penile Kaposi's sarcoma with electrochemotherapy. *Dermatol Surg* 2008;34:839–42; discussion 42–3.

3

Clinical features and diagnosis

CAMILE S. FARAH, MARYAM JESSRI, KEZIAH JOHN, YASTIRA LALLA, AN VU, AND OMAR KUJAN

INTRODUCTION

Oral cancer is a major global health burden, with more than 275,000 new cases estimated to be diagnosed annually (1). Oral cancer has been associated with a group of lesions and conditions that may develop into malignancy and are called oral potentially malignant disorders (OPMDs) (2). These disorders have previously been described by different names and terminologies such as precancer, precancerous, premalignant lesions and conditions, intra-epithelial neoplasia and precursor lesions in addition to oral potentially malignant lesions (OPMLs). This has attracted confusion in the international published literature and, as of yet, there is no consensus relating to the use of these terms in describing oral lesions that carry likelihood of malignant transformation (MT). What does make these oral lesions unique from other premalignant lesions in the body is that only a small proportion of OPMDs genuinely transform into cancer (2,3). In fact, the synonyms of precancer such as "premalignant" and "precancerous" literally mean that these lesions will transform into cancer at some stage. However, this is not an absolute in the context of oral carcinogenesis (2,4). Added to this ambiguity are the current gaps in our full understanding of the natural history of oral carcinogenesis (3,5).

International leading researchers have previously gathered in conjunction with the World Health Organization (WHO) Collaborating Centre for Oral Cancer and Precancer in the U.K. with the aim of incorporating the knowledge of advanced biology into the understanding of oral precancerous lesions to achieve a consensus in terms of diagnosis in clinical practice. As a result, consensus definitions and a classification emerged. The term "potentially malignant disorders" was adopted and has since been applied broadly in the world of oral carcinogenesis (4). Historically, several attempts have been made to agree on terminology of lesions that might lead to oral cancer. An early attempt dates back to 1978 when the WHO Collaborating Centre for Oral Precancerous Lesions subdivided OPMDs into two broad groups: precancerous lesion defined as "a morphologically altered tissue in which oral cancer is likely to occur than in its apparently normal counterpart" and precancerous condition defined as "a generalised state associated with a significantly increased risk of cancer" (6). Even earlier, the first edition of the WHO Histological Typing of Oral and Oropharyngeal Tumours published a histological classification of oral cancer and precancer using the terminology "precancerous" (7). At the time, the International Histological Classification of Tumours' publication contained morphological code numbers of the International Classification of Diseases for Oncology (ICD-O) and the Systematized Nomenclature of Medicine (SNOMED) to promote the use of unified terms that may facilitate communication between cancer researchers and clinicians (8). The second edition of the WHO Histological Typing of Oral Cancer and Precancer in 1997 described precancerous lesions and conditions (8). The precancerous lesions were termed clinically as leukoplakia, erythroplakia and palatal keratosis associated with reverse smoking, and histologically as squamous epithelial dysplasia, squamous cell carcinoma (SCC) *in situ* and solar keratosis. On the other hand, precancerous conditions were listed as sideropenic dysphagia, lichen planus, oral submucous fibrosis (OSF), syphilis, discoid lupus erythematosus (DLE), xeroderma pigmentosum and epidermolysis bullosa (8). Interestingly, the most recent edition of the WHO monograph on Head and Neck Tumours (2005) has adopted the term "epithelial precursor lesion" (9). To the best of our knowledge at the time of writing this chapter, the WHO monograph on Head and Neck Tumours is being revised and the term "potentially malignant disorders" will be used.

This chapter aims to provide an in-depth assessment of the clinical presentations and diagnostic approaches for oral cancer and OPMDs and to discuss the emerging role of optical and molecular imaging approaches in the visualization, identification and early detection of these lesions.

ORAL POTENTIALLY MALIGNANT LESIONS

LEUKOPLAKIA

The WHO defines oral leukoplakia (OL) as "a white plaque of questionable risk having excluded other known diseases or disorders that carry no risk" (4). It is merely a clinical term and histopathologically may be used distinctly with atrophy, hyperplasia or dysplasia and excludes all frictional disorders (10). It is the most common OPML; however, a recent study found an incidence of OL of under 0.1% (three patients) in a sample of 3,142 dental patients (0.9% had a final diagnosis of OPMDs) (11). The risk of MT of OL is around 5% or more (12); the most recent study of a 10-year follow-up showed 12.19% of cases undergoing MT in untreated patients, while only 1.41% of lesions in treated patients underwent MT (13). Ho et al. reported an MT rate of 22% at 5 years among 91 patients diagnosed with oral epithelial dysplasia (OED), with the median time to MT being 48 months (14,15). The frequency of OED, carcinoma *in situ* or invasive SCC in leukoplakias has been reported to be between 8.6% and 60% (16–19). This wide range of variation in the presence/absence of OED is perhaps population/risk factor dependent. For example, Lee and colleagues (2006) from Taiwan (17) defined subjects who had one or more alcoholic drinks three times or more per week, chewed one betel quid or more or smoked one cigarette or more per day for at least 1 year as habitual drinkers, chewers or smokers, respectively. The male to female ratio was 10.6 to 1. The study reported 75.9% of all 1,046 OL patients had chewed betel quid. The rate of epithelial dysplasia was 45.6%. In contrast, Schepman et al. (1998) undertook a study (1973–1993) of 166 Dutch patients over a median follow-up period of 29 months (18) and showed a small female preponderance. The rates of smokers and alcohol drinkers of more than two units/day were 61.5% and 33%, respectively. OED of several grades was diagnosed in 56.6% of all biopsied lesions (18).

There are two main recognized clinical variants of leukoplakia—homogeneous and non-homogeneous. Homogeneous leukoplakia presents as a predominantly white lesion of uniform, flat, thin appearance that may manifest shallow cracks and has a smooth, wrinkled or corrugated surface with a consistent texture throughout (Figure 3.1). Non-homogeneous leukoplakia (Figure 3.2) may be speckled leukoplakia (Figure 3.3), erythroleukoplakia (Figure 3.4), nodular leukoplakia, verrucous leukoplakia (Figure 3.5) and proliferative verrucous leukoplakia (PVL) (Figure 3.6) (4). Non-homogeneous leukoplakia is predominantly white or red and white and may be irregularly flat, nodular or exophytic. Nodular lesions have slightly raised, rounded, red and/or white excrescences. Exophytic lesions have irregular blunt or sharp projections. Erythroleukoplakia, a red and white lesion, seems to contain a higher risk of MT (10). PVL (20), which presents with multiple verruciform white plaques, is a distinct entity displaying a tendency to expand and recur and has a predilection

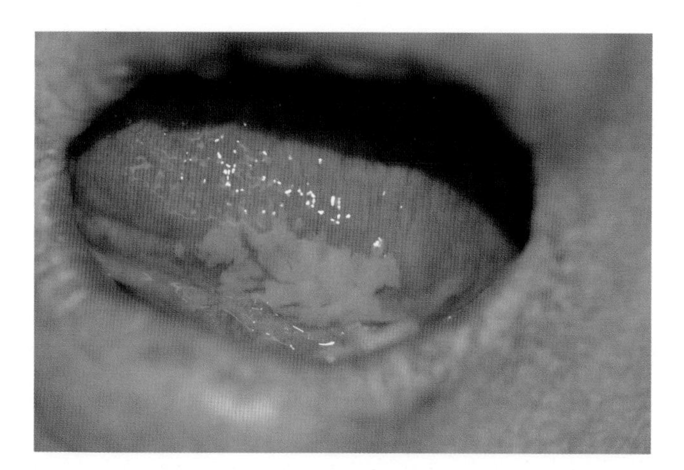

Figure 3.1 Homogenous leukoplakia involving left lateral tongue in a 53-year-old male smoker; biopsy-proven no epithelial dysplasia.

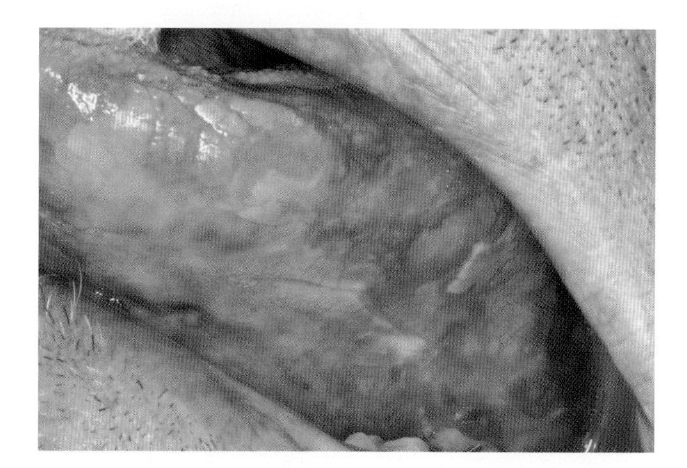

Figure 3.2 Non-homogenous leukoplakia involving left lateral tongue in a 66-year-old male smoker; biopsy-proven oral lichen planus.

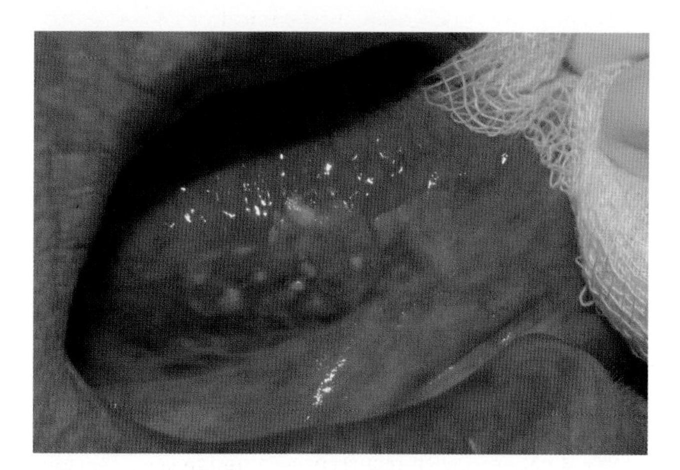

Figure 3.3 Speckled erythroleukoplakia on right lateral tongue in a 74-year-old female ex-smoker; biopsy-proven oral squamous cell carcinoma.

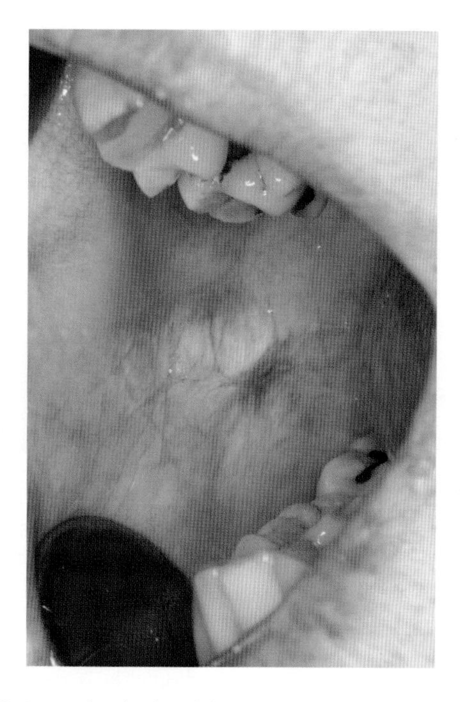

Figure 3.4 Erythroleukoplakia involving right buccal mucosa in a 46-year-old female smoker; biopsy-proven oral lichen planus.

for non-smokers and women around 50–60 years (10,12,21). These lesions have been linked to approximately 100% rates of MT in short periods (12,22).

The rarer of the two, non-homogeneous leukoplakia, is associated with a higher risk of MT (four- to seven-fold) and presence of OED compared to homogeneous leukoplakia

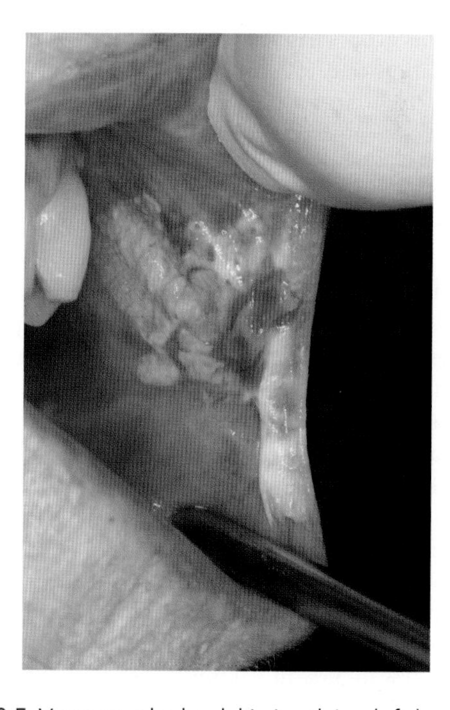

Figure 3.5 Verrucous leukoplakia involving left buccal mucosa and commissure with an area of ulceration in a 93-year-old female non-smoker; biopsy-proven moderate epithelial dysplasia.

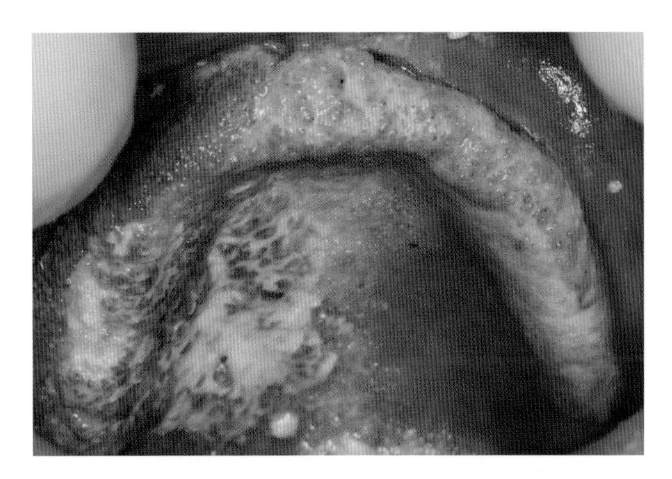

Figure 3.6 Proliferative verrucous leukoplakia involving the palate and maxillary alveolar ridge in an 81-year-old female non-smoker; biopsy-proven moderate epithelial dysplasia.

(2,3,14,23–25). Homogeneous leukoplakia is deemed to be less sinister, but is to be treated with greater degree of caution if occurring in high-risk areas such as the floor of the mouth (Figure 3.7a) and the ventral (Figure 3.7b) and lateral borders of the tongue (Figure 3.7c) in high-risk patients (high tobacco and alcohol exposure) (2,3,14,23–25). A change in the clinical diagnosis from homogeneous to non-homogeneous leukoplakia is associated with a 4.2-times increase in the risk of diagnosing dysplasia on histopathological analysis (24). The most frequent forms of non-homogeneous leukoplakia are nodular leukoplakia and erythroleukoplakia.

The malignant potential of OL is undisputed but the rate at which this occurs has been reported variably. The annual transformation rate was reported to be 2.9% in a Dutch study and 3.38% in a Chinese study (18,26). In Australia, the annual MT rate is about 1% (16). While the incidence of leukoplakia is higher in smokers, the rate of MT in established lesions is higher in non-smokers, especially among women (18,19,27). In general, the risk of MT of leukoplakia is higher in women (18). Significant predictors of MT were reported by a recent longitudinal observational study to be non-smoking status, site, non-homogeneous appearance, size of lesion >200 mm^2 and (of borderline significance) high grade of dysplasia (14). Age, gender, number of lesions and alcohol history were not found to be predictors of MT (14). The authors suggested that non-smoking patients with OED have an inherited or acquired predisposition for MT and should undergo more aggressive treatment, forming the focus for further investigation (14).

Surgical excision is the preferred treatment in the presence of moderate or severe dysplasia (28). Several studies have reported variable recurrence rates after surgery ranging from 10% to 35% in variable follow-up periods up to 10 years (19,29–31). In widespread lesions, photodynamic therapy may be considered, which does not damage collagenous tissue, yielding more esthetic results after treatment (3,32,33). Cryotherapy is also a suggested destructive method (34). One study observed complete responses in 72.9% of patients, with recurrence occurring in 27.1% cases when treated with cryotherapy, while 89.2% of lesions treated with photodynamic treatment displayed complete response, with recurrence occurring in 24.3% of cases in a

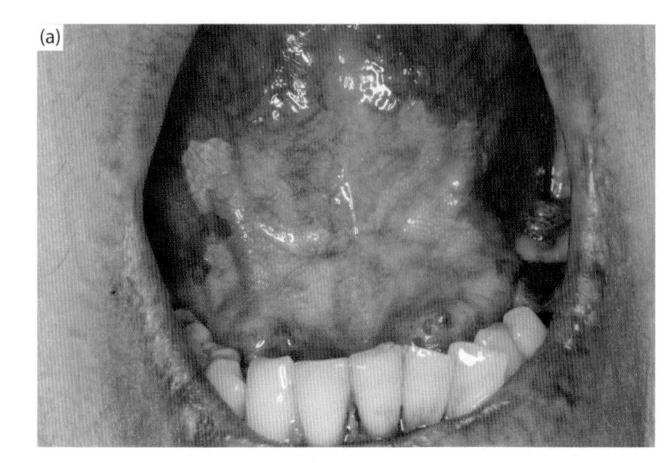

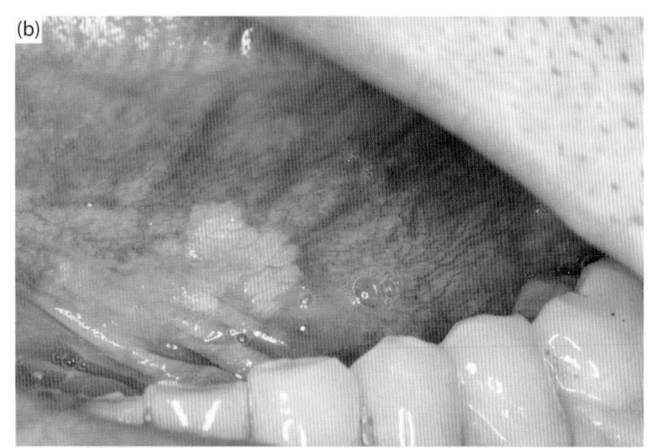

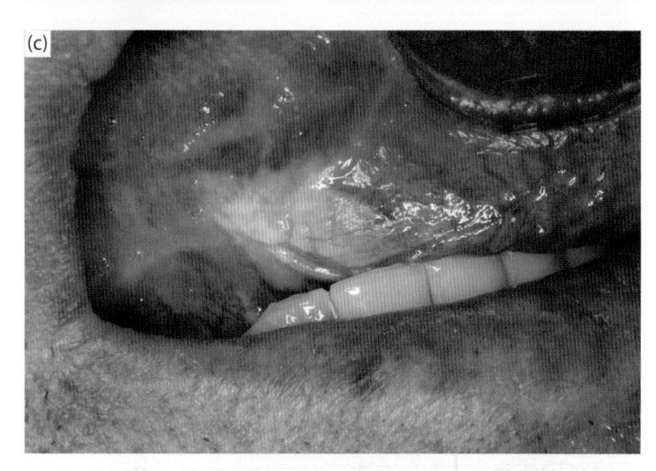

Figure 3.7 **(a)** Homogenous leukoplakia involving the floor of mouth in 46-year-old female smoker; biopsy-proven orthokeratosis with no epithelial dysplasia. **(b)** Homogenous leukoplakia involving left ventral tongue in a 60-year-old male smoker; biopsy-proven moderate epithelial dysplasia. **(c)** Non-homogenous leukoplakia involving the anterior right lateral border of tongue in a 45-year-old male non-smoker; biopsy-proven mild epithelial dysplasia.

median follow-up period of 52 months (32). Non-invasive treatment modalities include carotenoids (β-carotene and lycopene), vitamins (vitamins C, E and A and fenretinide) and bleomycin (35). Topical retinoic acid has been shown to have some success, but recurrence has been reported in about 50% of cases after ceasing its use (28,36).

ERYTHROPLAKIA

Erythroplakia, analogous to leukoplakia, has been defined as a "fiery red patch which cannot be characterised clinically or pathologically as any other definable disease" (Figure 3.8) (4,27,37). It mainly occurs in the middle aged and the elderly, with males affected more than females (28). The lesion may be flat or depressed and is mostly found on the floor of mouth, soft palate, ventral tongue and tonsillar fauces (38). Lesions are usually asymptomatic, but patients may complain of a burning sensation and/or soreness (38). A solitary lesion distinguishes erythroplakia from systemic conditions (27). They may present as mixed red and white lesions, termed erythroleukoplakia (4). The epithelium may be atrophic and non-keratinized (38). Hyperplasia may be noted occasionally (38). The redness is due to epithelial thinning, which allows for the underlying microvasculature to show through (38).

Studies from various countries including the USA, Denmark, India and Thailand have indicated erythroplakia, a purely red lesion, to have a high malignant potential, though low in prevalence (0.01%–0.20%), with up to 55%–65% reported to have undergone MT over a follow-up period of 12 years (38,39). At first biopsy, greater than 90% of erythroplakia contain OED, carcinoma *in situ* or invasive SCC (38). A large proportion of those cases that display dysplasia undergo MT (27). Owing to the high transformation rate, expeditious biopsy or surgical excision is recommended.

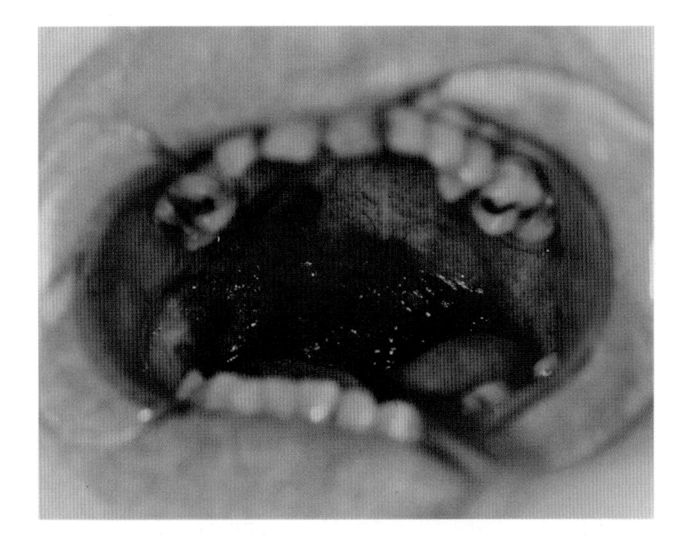

Figure 3.8 Erythroplakia involving the right soft and hard palate in a 79-year-old male smoker; biopsy-proven severe epithelial dysplasia. (Courtesy of Dr Anastasia Georgiou, Sydney Skin Clinic, Sydney, Australia.)

CHRONIC HYPERPLASTIC CANDIDOSIS

The *Candida* spp. of yeasts are commensal organisms found in about 40% of individuals, with *Candida albicans* being the most frequently isolated species (40). Chronic hyperplastic candidosis, one of the oral mucosal lesions associated with *Candida* and also known as candidal leukoplakia (40), presents as "an adherent chronic white patch on the commissures of the oral mucosa" (41). *Candida*-associated leukoplakia is often erosive or ulcerated (Figure 3.9a) or of

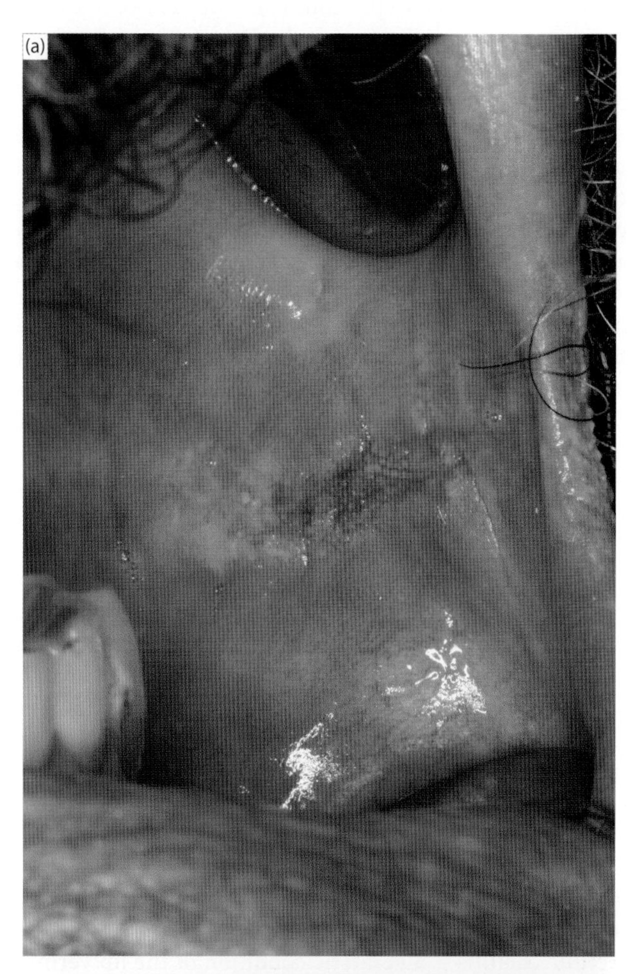

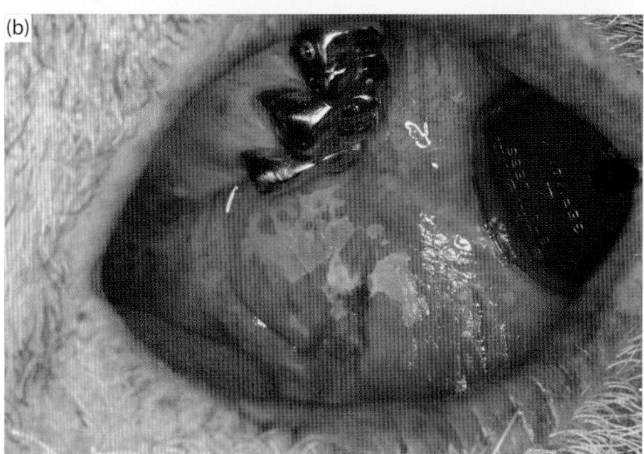

Figure 3.9 **(a)** Erosive form and **(b)** non-homogenous type of chronic hyperplastic candidosis on the left buccal mucosa.

the non-homogeneous type (Figure 3.9b). Associations have been found between oral yeast load and OED (40,42,43). It has been shown that in patients with OED, the degree of dysplasia correlates positively with the amount of yeast in the oral cavity (40). One study found that in 21.9% of patients with concurrent fungal infection, OED progressed in severity compared with patients without fungal elements (7.6%) (42). It has also been shown that the lesion site itself may harbor candidal infection (44), suggesting that the fungus itself does not initiate or exacerbate the malignant process, but that the dysplastic epithelium provides a favorable environment for the species to grow in. Despite this, it has been estimated that up to 10% of candidal leukoplakia progress to malignancy over a period of 10 years (43,45,46).

The link between *Candida* infection and MT remains unclear. *C. albicans* may influence carcinogenesis by producing carcinogens (such as nitrosamines), promoting carcinogenesis in initiated epithelium, metabolizing precarcinogens (e.g. conversion of ethanol to acetaldehyde, a known carcinogen) (47) or modifying the microenvironment and inducing chronic inflammation (41). It has also been recently found that *C. albicans* genotype A strains were significantly more prevalent in oral cancer patients, while *C. albicans* genotype B strains occurred more frequently in non-oral cancer patients, implying that the former strain may possess characteristics conducive to neoplastic changes (48). Localized increases in concentration of acetylaldehyde, particularly in the event of the highly significant joint additive effect of *Candida* presence and current/daily alcohol exposure (48), may initiate malignant changes in the oral epithelium, as acetaldehyde is known to produce mutagenic effects such as DNA adducts, DNA cross-linking, aneuploidy or chromosomal aberrations (49,50). While the details of the linkage remain unclear, there is a plausible association between oral *Candida* colonization and the pathogenesis of alcohol-related carcinogenesis, resulting in chronic hyperplastic candidosis being considered an OPML.

ACTINIC CHEILITIS

Actinic cheilitis is a keratotic condition of the lip vermilion that is considered to be potentially malignant. Patients may present with a variety of clinical signs and symptoms, the most commonly reported being dryness of the lip, atrophy and ulceration, erythema, edema and blurring of the vermilion border (Figure 3.10a), in addition to leukoplakia of the lower lip (Figure 3.10b) (51–53). This condition mostly occurs in fair-skinned, middle-aged men with a high lifetime exposure to UV radiation (51,52). Due to the etiology of this condition, actinic cheilitis occurs most often on the lower lip and is rarely seen on the upper lip. While rates of MT have not been reported, it is noted that most cancers of the lip (Figure 3.10c) are associated with pre-existing actinic cheilitis (52). It is to be noted that the demographic and clinical appearance of this condition has been found to be unrelated to histopathological grading for dysplasia (54,55).

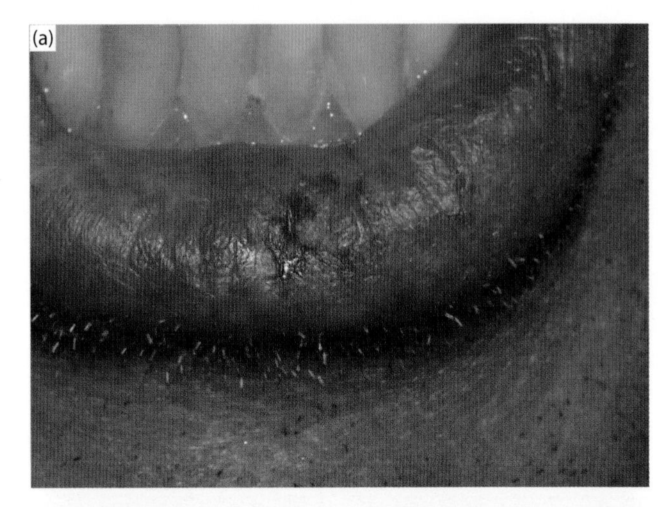

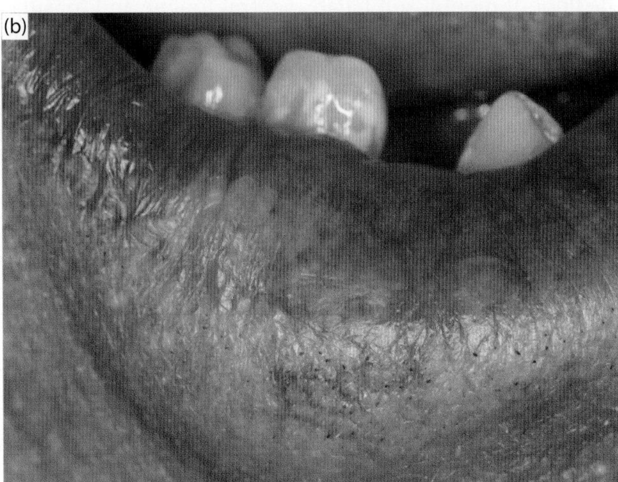

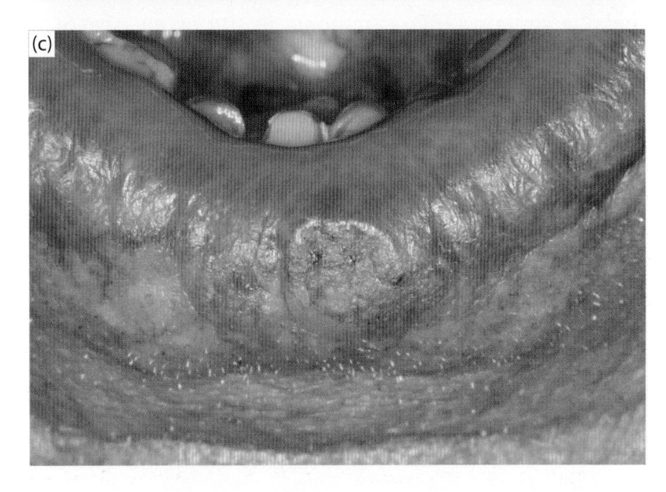

Figure 3.10 Actinic cheilitis on lower lip presenting as areas of ulceration and crusting **(a)** or leukoplakia involving the vermilion border **(b)**. Lower lip squamous cell carcinoma developing on a background of actinic cheilitis **(c)**; note the area of central ulceration and blurring of the vermilion.

ORAL LICHEN PLANUS

Oral lichen planus (OLP) is a chronic inflammatory condition with an established immune-mediated pathogenesis (56,57). It commonly affects oral mucosa, usually

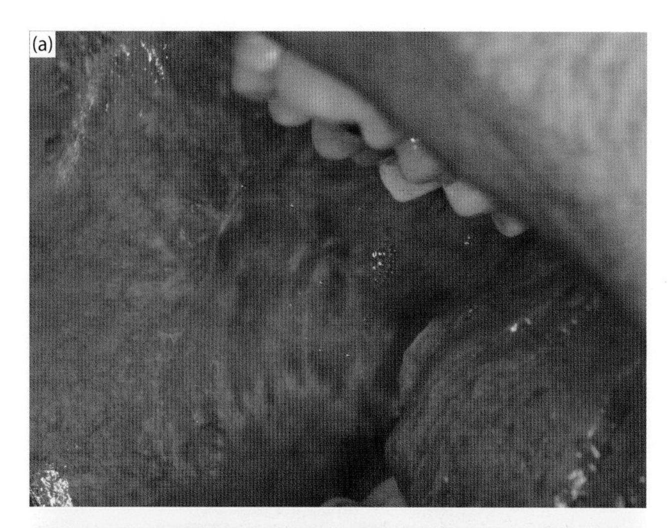

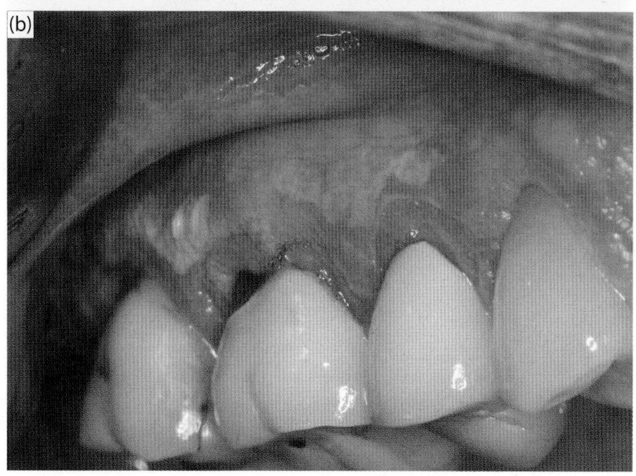

Figure 3.11 Reticular oral lichen planus on the buccal mucosa **(a)** and plaque-type oral lichen planus on the labial gingiva and attached mucosa **(b)**.

buccal mucosa, tongue, gingiva, palate and lips, but can also involve the skin, genital mucosa and nails (56,58). It affects middle-aged people and predominates in women, with reported prevalence rates varying from 0.1%–4% of individuals, depending on the population sampled (59). Clinically, OLP is typically bilateral and symmetric (60,61). OLP is divided into six different forms. The reticular (Figure 3.11a), papular and plaque-like (Figure 3.11b) types are typically asymptomatic and go unnoticed by patients, while the atrophic (Figure 3.12a), ulcerative (Figure 3.12b) and bullous types (which are commonly grouped together as erosive lichen planus) are associated with burning, pain and complaints in taste alteration (56,62).

Oral lichenoid lesions (OLLs) (Figure 3.13a and b) are similar to OLP but do not demonstrate the entire typical clincopathological requirements of OLP (61,63). OLL can be reactive where there is a known cause, such as reaction to an amalgam restoration, drugs or graft-versus-host disease, or can be idiopathic (57,63–65). OLP and OLLs have been termed in the literature collectively as "oral lichenoid mucositis" or "oral lichenoid disease" (60,63,66). Likewise, all these lichenoid conditions (including lichenoid dysplasia

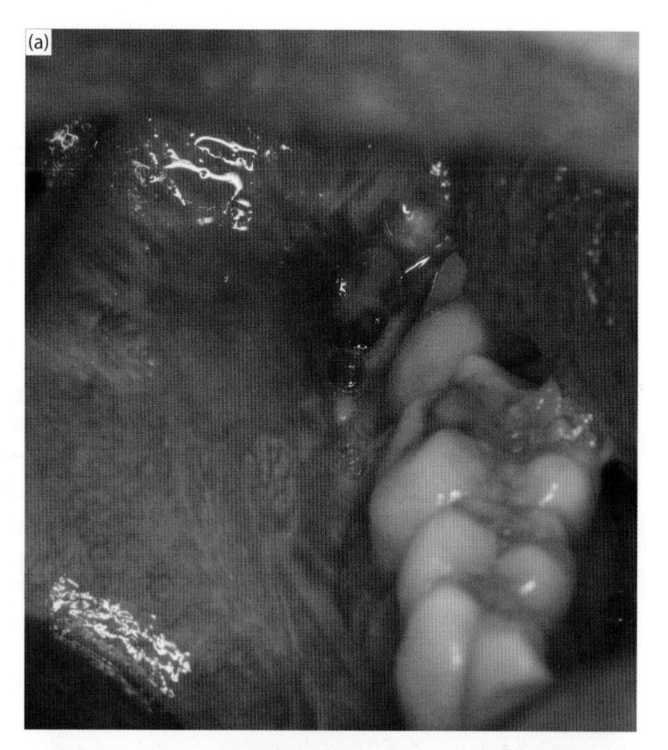

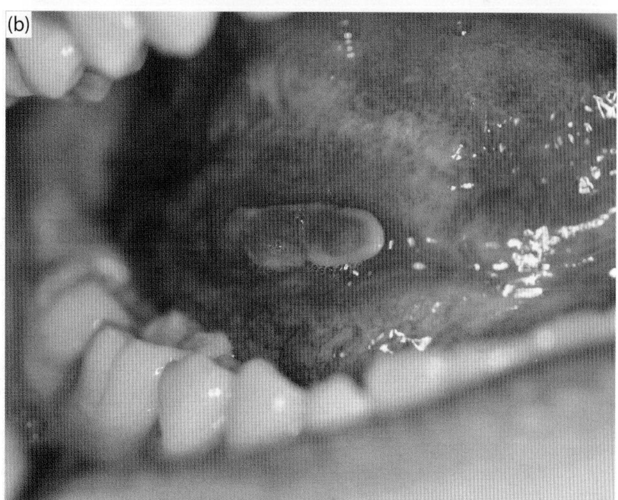

Figure 3.12 Erosive oral lichen planus involving the lower sulcus and buccal mucosa **(a)** and ulcerative oral lichen planus on the ventrolateral border of the tongue **(b)**.

[LD]) have been referred to as OLLs, generating confusion in terminology and understanding, comparison and translation of results.

A key issue relating to OLP is its potential for MT. Transformation rates have been reported to vary between 0% and 9% in a period of up to 10 years of follow-up (56,67–71). It is necessary to verify initial diagnosis with a biopsy and compare developed oral SCC (OSCC) to the original anatomical location of the OLP (56,72). The presence of dysplasia at the initial diagnosis must also be noted (56). Interestingly, there have been reports that OLLs have a greater risk of MT than OLP (65,73–76), making it imperative that these lesions be diagnosed accurately. As such,

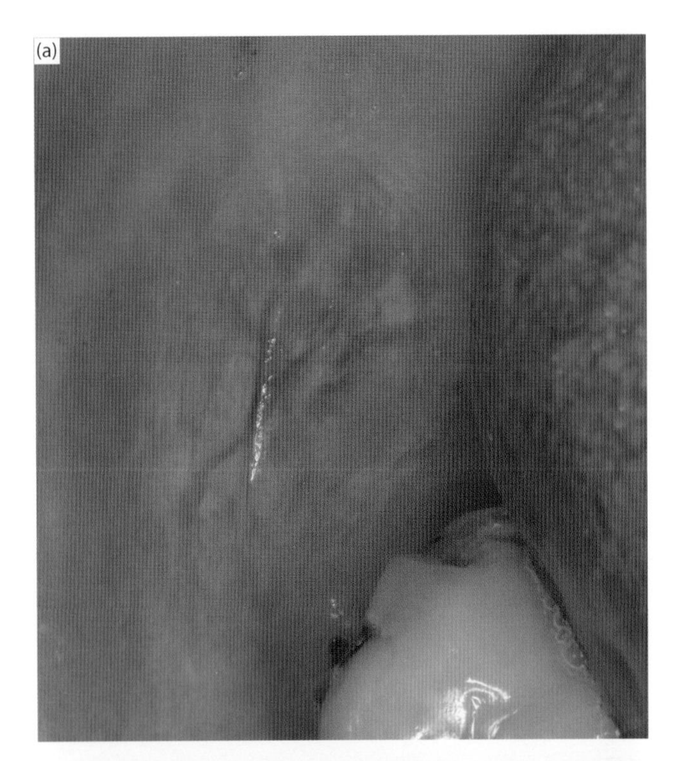

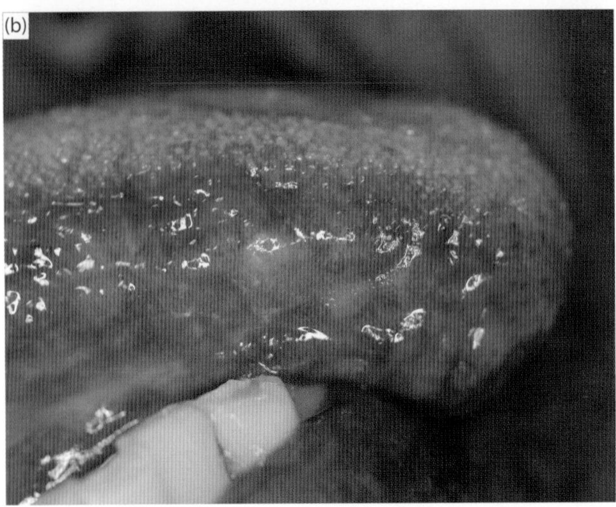

Figure 3.13 Oral lichenoid lesion on the right buccal mucosa adjacent to a heavily restored tooth **(a)** and the right lateral border of tongue **(b)**, both demonstrating reticular striations with minor background erythema.

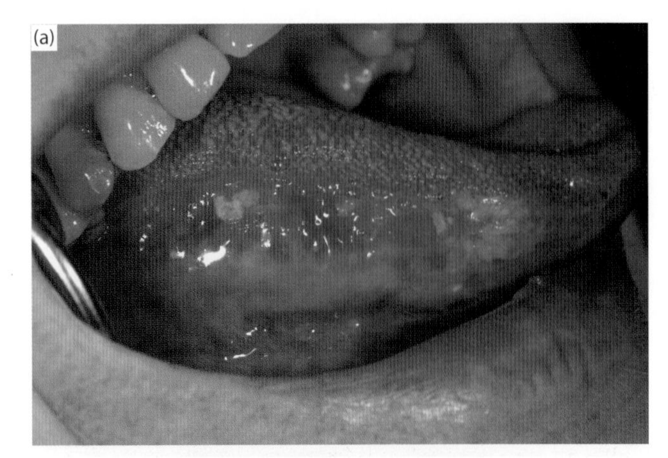

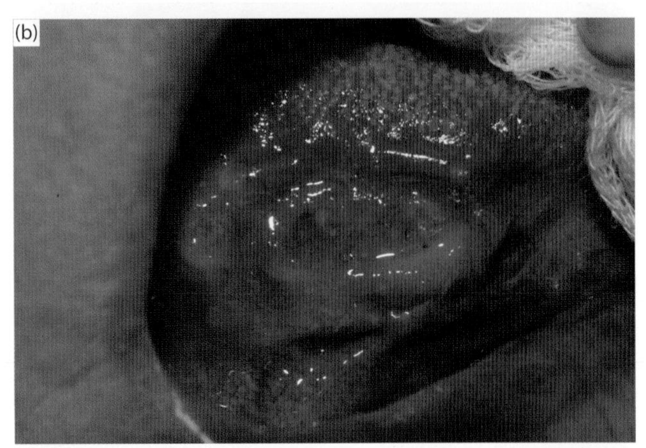

Figure 3.14 Non-homogenous leukoplakia on the right lateral border of the tongue in a non-smoking female patient **(a)** diagnosed clinically with oral lichen planus in 1996 aged 50, histopathologically with mild epithelial dysplasia in 2002 and subsequently developed an oral squamous cell carcinoma in 2009 at age 63 **(b)**.

these lesions, which are contact lesions, must be managed differently to OLP (57). Nevertheless, it is generally accepted that both OLP and OLLs are associated with increased risk of cancer development (57,66).

Krutchkoff and Eisenberg (77) reported that lesions showing lichenoid features with epithelial dysplasia in a cohort of U.S. patients are a distinct histopathological entity termed LD, postulating that OLP cases evolving to malignancy are linked to this lesion and LD was neither a variant nor a transitional form of OLP. In other words, OLP lesions that are thought to undergo MT are likely to represent red and white lesions that clinically and histologically mimic OLP, but are dysplastic from their inception (Figure 3.14a and b) (78). LD may correspond to either OLP showing dysplasia or a leukoplakia on biopsy showing both epithelial dysplasia and lichenoid features (79).

Histologically, OLP is classically represented by hyperkeratosis, liquefactive degeneration of the basal epithelial cells, colloid bodies and the presence of a well-defined band-like zone of cellular infiltration (56,80). This infiltrate is confined to the superficial part of the connective tissue and consists mainly of lymphocytes, with activated CD8+ T lymphocytes found in the epithelium or near damaged basal keratinocytes and CD4+ T cells occurring in small clusters deeper in the subepithelial, lymphocyte-rich band (56,80,81).

The MT of OLP and, consequently, its inclusion as an OPML in the WHO classification (4) have been of some debate, with some arguing that pathologists have not been strict in the use of the term "lichen planus" (82). While it is considered that the presence of dysplasia in OLP-like lesions increases the risk of MT (83), excluding the OLP label from cases that exhibit both dysplasia and lichenoid features warrants deliberation, as this might lead to underestimation of the rate of MT of OLP. A recent systematic review by Fitzpatrick et al. (66) excluded all patients who had dysplasia on initial biopsy of OLP or OLLs. They reported MT of OLP to be 1.09% (85 out of 7,806 patients with OLP developed SCC), which was reported from 0% to 3.5% in individual studies in an average period of 51.4 months from the time of diagnosis. In the one study evaluated involving OLLs, the transformation rate was 3.2% in a mean follow-up period of 53.8 months and the annual transformation rate was calculated at 0.71% (76).

Assessing the MT of OLP in reported cases is difficult due to the lack of application of universally accepted criteria for the diagnosis of OLP (61,84–86), which would reveal whether malignancies arise from this particular small cohort (57).

In a recent retrospective analysis by Patil et al. (57) aiming to quantify the presence of OED in a large series of OLP and OLLs, a pro forma document was used to achieve consistency in arriving at each diagnosis based on previously described histological features of each lesion (37,75,87). OLP was diagnosed if there was no dysplasia present, with histological evidence of a well-defined band-like zone of cellular infiltration confined to the superficial part of the connective tissue, consisting mainly of lymphocytes, and signs of liquefaction degeneration in the basal cell layer. OLLs would feature the presence of a diffuse cellular infiltration, consisting of either lymphocytes or a combination of lymphocytes and plasma cells, extending to the deeper part of the connective tissue, showing signs of liquefaction degeneration in the basal cell layer. The presence of epithelial dysplasia, even though other features typify OLP, would make it an OLL. Epithelial dysplasia is defined as per the WHO Collaborating Centre criteria for the assessment of dysplastic features (87). Lichenoid features in OED would contain dysplastic features, as well as either a well-defined band-like zone of cellular infiltration confined to the superficial part of the connective tissue or the presence of a diffuse cellular infiltration that extends to the deeper part of the connective tissue, containing lymphocytes or a mixture of lymphocytes and plasma cells. LD was diagnosed after using the above criteria and confirming the evidence of an oral lichenoid response and then applying the WHO Collaborating Centre criteria for the assessment of dysplastic features. Cases exhibiting any lichenoid features were reclassified as LD. Patil et al. (57) supported the proposal of dysplasia being deemed a disqualifying feature of OLP and called for the specific and deliberate use of terminology to aid in future analysis of the malignant potential of OLP and/or LD.

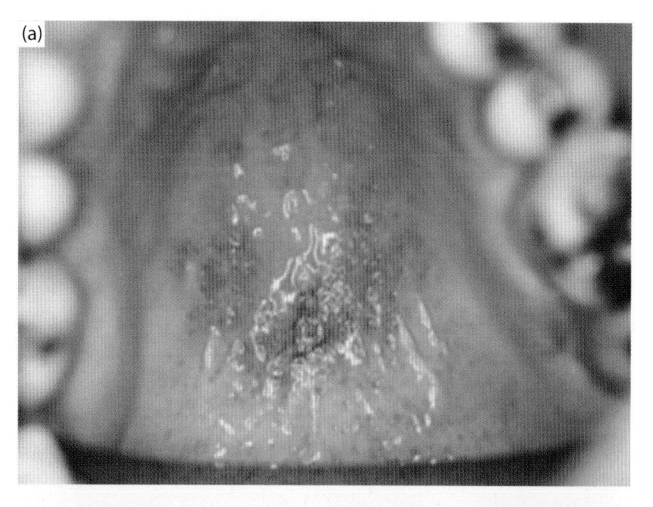

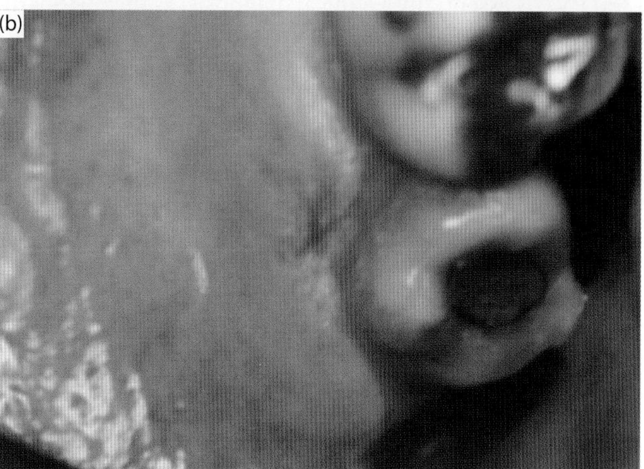

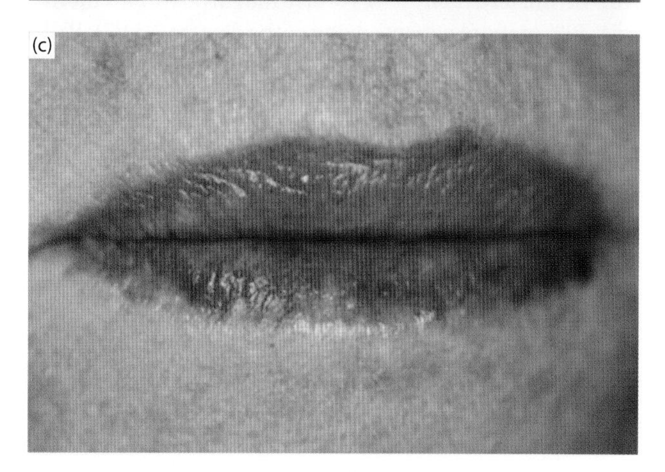

Figure 3.15 Female patient displaying erosive and ulcerative features of discoid lupus erythematosus involving the mid hard palate **(a)**, palatal gingiva **(b)** and lips **(c)**.

DISCOID LUPUS ERYTHEMATOSUS

DLE is a chronic autoimmune, scarring, mucocutaneous disease of unknown etiology characterized by white keratinized plaques with raised rims, radiating white striae and telangiectasia. The clinical features of DLE sometimes make it difficult to distinguish DLE from either lichen planus or erythroplakia (Figure 3.15a–c) (88). The majority of oral DLE lesions are found on the buccal mucosa, followed by the gingival mucosa, labial mucosa and vermilion border of the lip (89). The prevalence of DLE is less than 24 cases per 100,000 population and it is more common in females than males, with a ratio of 1.8:1 (90). DLE has been considered an OPMD for many years; however, data from the published literature are based on individual cases of DLE-related OSCC, with MT taking up to 20 years. Epidemiological studies estimate that DLE-related OSCCs range from 2.3% to 3.3% (88).

Males are more frequently affected than females, with an estimated ratio of 2.2 to 1. The lower lip is reported to be the most frequent site for MT (91), with a third of transformed DLE cases occurring at multiple sites (88). The mechanism of DLE progression to OSCC is poorly understood; however, sun exposure, scarring, epithelial atrophy, depigmentation, chronic inflammation and aberrant healing processes have been considered to be factors that increase the risk of SCC development (92).

PROLIFERATIVE VERRUCOUS LEUKOPLAKIA

Because of the considerable oncologic danger associated with oral PVL, it is singled out for special consideration. Oral PVL is essentially a clinical diagnosis, as the histopathologic features of any lesion along the spectrum of the disease are indistinguishable from non-PVL-associated lesions of the same type.

PVL is considered to be a progressive type of OL that is impossible to recognize in its nascent stages (20). The condition typically begins as non-dysplastic keratosis and develops over time (sometimes 20 or more years) into a confluent, multifocal and widespread oral keratosis with stubborn recurrence and persistence and a high frequency of malignant change (93–95). The progressive oral mucosal involvement is accompanied by an exophytic and verrucous character of the lesional tissues. There has been some recent consideration that PVL may mimic OLP or OLLs initially (96). Ultimately, many PVLs evolve into invasive carcinoma, with 30% or more patients dying of the disease (93,97). PVLs warrant a high degree of clinical suspicion (98).

Although irreversibility is probably intrinsic even in the early, flat, non-verrucous form of PVL, it cannot be predicted with reasonable certainty until the leukoplakia has evolved to the exophytic, verrucous form from which it derives its name. The clinical continuum from hyperkeratosis to carcinoma is also reflected in the spectrum of histologic appearances manifested by PVL. Verrucous carcinoma (VC), conventional well-differentiated SCC and histologic verrucous hyperplasia can all exist concurrently within oral PVL. There may also be a progressive dysplasia, but a clinical leukoplakia that shows severe dysplasia at its initial appearance does not qualify (20).

Studies from the U.K. and USA have found that PVL is most commonly seen in elderly women (age range, 36–90 years; mean, 70.2 years). Patients often indicate a longtime awareness of leukoplakia, sometimes for more than 20 years. Tobacco use history is variable, but abstinence is often claimed (20,93,95).

The buccal mucosa is most often the site of initial involvement (Figure 3.16a), followed by the hard and soft (Figure 3.16b) palate, alveolar mucosa, tongue, floor of mouth, gingiva (Figure 3.16c) and lip. In its early form, especially with isolated lesions, the clinical findings of PVL cannot be distinguished from any of the more common types of clinical leukoplakia (99). These early forms are flat, thickened

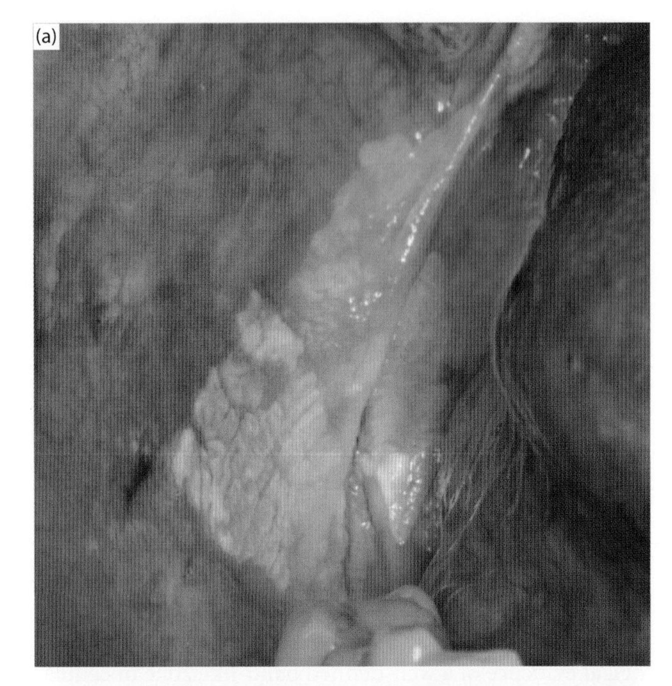

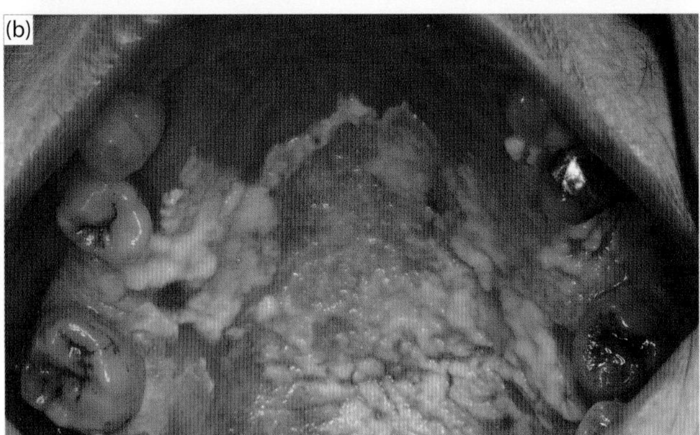

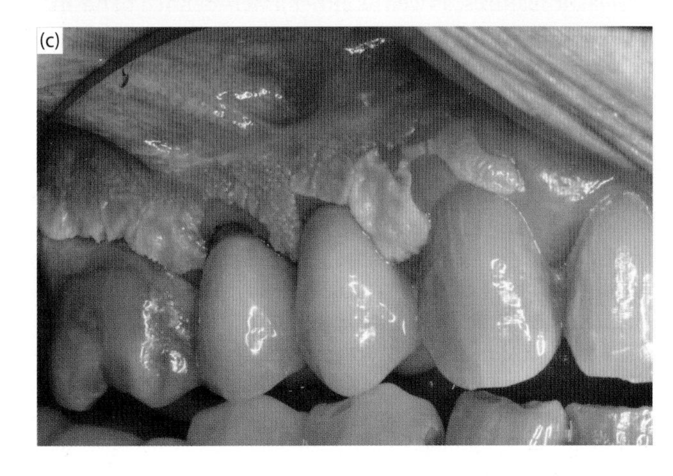

Figure 3.16 Proliferative verrucous leukoplakia involving the buccal mucosa and retromolar trigone **(a)** and palate and alveolar mucosa **(b)** in a 68-year-old female; both sites were biopsy-proven orthokeratosis with mild epithelial dysplasia. Proliferative verrucous leukoplakia involving the buccal gingiva and attached mucosa in an 80-year-old female **(c)**.

keratoses. Progression of the disorder is manifested by confluence of lesions, wider mucosal involvement and an exophytic topography.

The often-noted absence of risk factors ordinarily associated with oral SCC, the preponderance of women among the patients and the occurrence at an older age have suggested that the pathogenesis of carcinomas arising in patients with PVL may differ from that of non-PVL-associated carcinomas (100–102). Using polymerase chain reaction for human papillomavirus (HPV) DNA, Palefsky et al. (101) studied nine lesions from seven patients with PVL, histologically diagnosed with focal keratosis, papilloma, epithelial dysplasia and SCC, and found that eight lesions (89%) were HPV positive, seven for HPV-16. This frequency was higher than the HPV detection rates in non-PVL lesions.

The surgical management of PVL is bedeviled by high recurrence rates and a widespread mucosal involvement that makes total excision often impossible (103). Only three of the 30 patients studied by Hansen et al. (20) remained disease free after treatment. Irradiation has not been effective.

VERRUCOUS HYPERPLASIA

Here, we restrict the term "verrucous hyperplasia" to a histopathologic context only, but include it as one of the evolutionary stages in oral PVL (93). It need not, however, be part of that peculiar leukoplakia. Outside of the oral cavity, in the sinonasal tract and larynx, verrucous hyperplasia occurs either as an apparently *de novo* lesion or in association with papillomas. In our opinion, verrucous hyperplasia is an irreversible lesion, often histologically indistinguishable from VC (i.e. an early form of that neoplasm), although the characteristic feature of a blunted epithelial front pushing into the underlying lamina propria seen in VC is absent in verrucous hyperplasia.

At any of the mucosal sites, verrucous hyperplasia is a lesion of mature adults. In the oral cavity, it is diagnosed most often in patients who are in the sixth through eighth decades. There is a male preponderance. Studies from The Netherlands, China and India highlight the gingiva and alveolar mucosa as sites of predilection (Figure 3.17), followed by the buccal mucosa, tongue, floor of mouth, lips and palate (97,104,105). The true and false vocal cords are the laryngeal areas of preference (93).

Shear and Pindborg (106) have indicated two clinicopathologic patterns in the oral cavity. The patterns are also applicable to sinonasal and laryngeal lesions. The growth patterns are primarily distinguished by the height and degree of keratinization of the verrucous processes. Either a sharp or blunt form may dominate. In the oral cavity and paranasal sinuses, the sharp verrucous hyperplasia is most often seen; there is seemingly no particular preference in laryngeal lesions. Combinations of the two forms are also seen (105).

Prior to the sharp or blunt architecture, verrucous hyperplasia undergoes a sequence of histologic changes that starts with a keratotic, non-dysplastic mucosal thickening and then progresses through hyperplasia, mucosal clefting, downgrowth and a verrucous pattern. Areas of a homogeneous leukoplakia are usually adjacent to (or found elsewhere in) oral verrucous hyperplasia. These are usually absent in the sinonasal lesions, but are found with verrucous hyperplasias of the larynx.

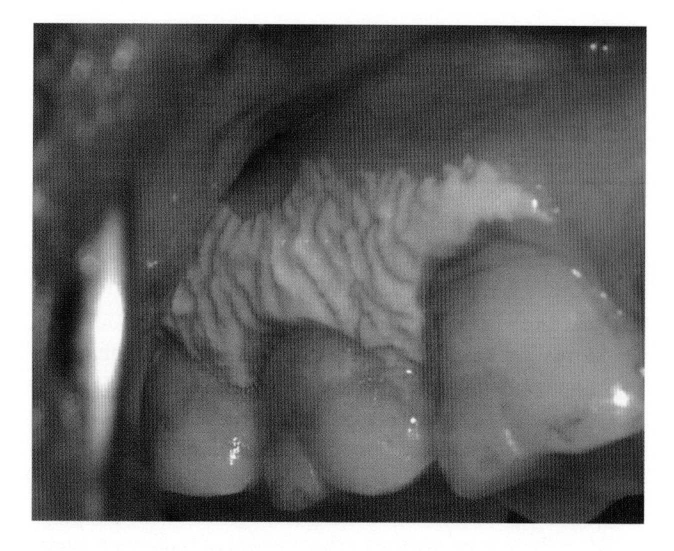

Figure 3.17 Verrucous hyperplasia involving the buccal gingiva with evidence of mild epithelial dysplasia on biopsy.

Besides the apparent irreversibility of verrucous hyperplasia, the progression to, or the association with, carcinoma is notable (107). Of 68 patients studied by Shear and Pindborg (106), seven had coexistent VC, and in seven others there was a conventional SCC. Slootweg and Müller (97) record similar findings: 37% of their patients had a coexisting or separately occurring SCC and in 26% epithelial dysplasia was also present. On the basis of these considerations, together with histologic and clinical data, Slootweg and Müller (97) opine that both verrucous hyperplasia and VC are variants of the same disease—VC.

It is likely that the same principle applies to the lesions of the larynx and Schneiderian mucosa. Schneiderian papillomas are nearly always devoid of a surface keratosis or even of other areas of cellular keratinization. Keratinization of these papillomas, therefore, has to be regarded as an atypical histologic finding with an ominous portent (93). Keratotic Schneiderian papillomas are associated with quick recurrences and an eventual verrucous hyperplasia, with coexistent or subsequent VC or invasive, conventional SCC of various degrees of differentiation. Verrucous hyperplasia in the larynx either is a persistently recurrent lesion or contains a VC arising from its matrix.

It is accepted that the lesions of verrucous hyperplasia and VC may, at times, be indistinguishable (97,106,107). With verrucous hyperplasia, the exophytic processes and the majority of the hyperplastic epithelium are entirely superficial to the adjacent normal epithelium. VC shows the same superficial exophytic processes, but the retia are broader and extend deeper than the adjacent uninvolved epithelium. As an additional feature, the verrucous processes in VC often retract a margin of normal epithelium down with them into the underlying stroma. A recent study found keratin plugging, epithelial dysplasia and subepithelial lymphocytic infiltration to be significantly different in verrucous hyperplasia compared to VC. The study also reported dysplasia in verrucous hyperplasia specimens (108).

HPVs have been implicated in the genesis of verrucous hyperplasia. Greer et al. (100) reported that six of 30 verrucous hyperplasias and four of 20 VCs expressed HPV DNA. Shroyer and Greer (102) also found four of an additional 14 verrucous hyperplasias to be HPV DNA positive. The surgical management of verrucous hyperplasia should be at least similar to that used for VC.

ORAL SUBMUCOUS FIBROSIS

OSF is a chronic condition of the mucosa of the upper digestive tract (27,109). It is characterized by fibrosis of the lamina propria and submucosal layers of the mucosal lining of the oral cavity (Figure 3.18a and b), oropharynx and, at times, the esophagus, resulting in loss of tissue mobility and trismus (110,111). A burning sensation is a common symptom, while clinical signs include loss of pigmentation of the vermilion border of the lips and the oral mucosa, leathery texture and blanching of the oral mucosa (112). OSF presents with features of autoimmune disease and is therefore thought to be immune mediated; however, onset is often in the presence of environmental risk factors, such as exposure to areca nut (113,114). It is estimated that OSF affects 2.5 million individuals, primarily in India and other south Asian countries, where exposure to etiological factors is common (109,115). OSF is seen increasingly in Melanesia and other Pacific islands and, given the rapid rates of migration, it is now more frequently seen in other countries with a significant diaspora from the Indian subcontinent (111,116). Between 7% and 25% of cases present with OED on histopathological examination and approximately 7.6% of OSF cases develop an oral malignancy (109). Oral mucosal depigmentation has been considered as a possible early manifestation of OSF in a report involving 2–3-year-olds from Sri Lanka (112).

ORAL HAIRY LEUKOPLAKIA

Oral hairy leukoplakia (OHL) is the most recently defined form of leukoplakia. The histopathologic features are distinctive and unlike those of any previously defined oral white lesion (117–120). They do, however, resemble skin warts and uterine condylomata, both of which are associated with papilloma viruses. Although these lesions were initially thought to be limited to homosexual men, subsequent reports have acknowledged their existence in other populations at risk for AIDS, including those with hemophilia and other transfusion recipients. Some may dispute the adjective "hairy," but the disorder has become (in nearly all instances) a marker of host immunosuppression, either natural or iatrogenically induced. Nevertheless, examples in immunocompetent subjects have been reported (117).

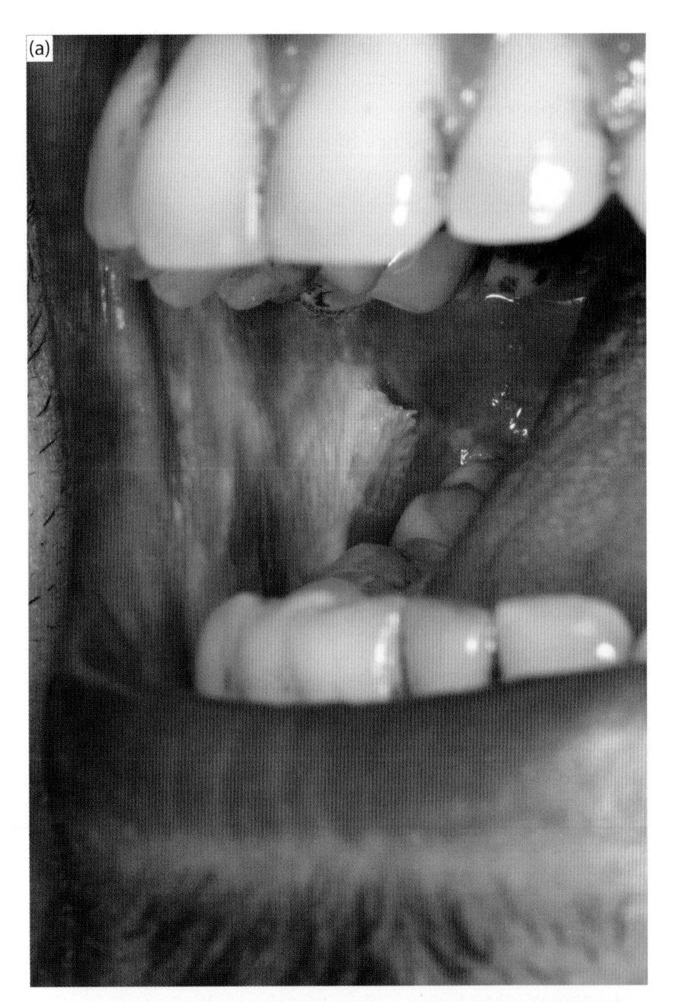

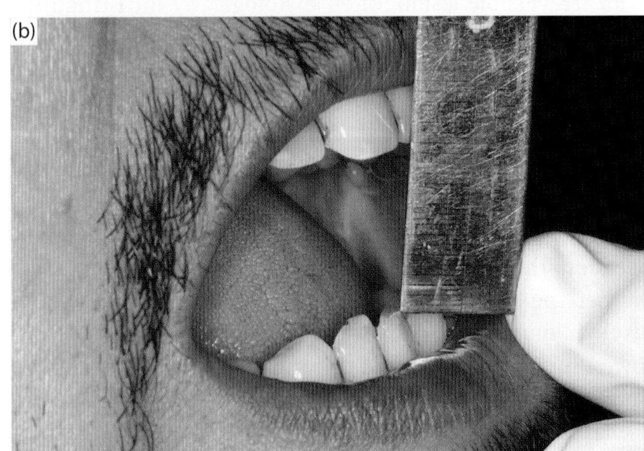

Figure 3.18 Oral submucous fibrosis in a 34-year-old Indian male involving the buccal mucosa with evidence of hyperkeratosis on a background of marbled like pallor **(a)**, presenting with scarring and limited opening of 16 mm **(b)**.

The lesions are located mainly on the lateral surface of the tongue and appear as white, slightly raised plaques with a corrugated "hairy" surface (Figure 3.19). The plaques range in size from a few millimeters to 3 cm, do not rub off and are usually not symptomatic. The lesions may also be noted on the buccal or labial mucosa.

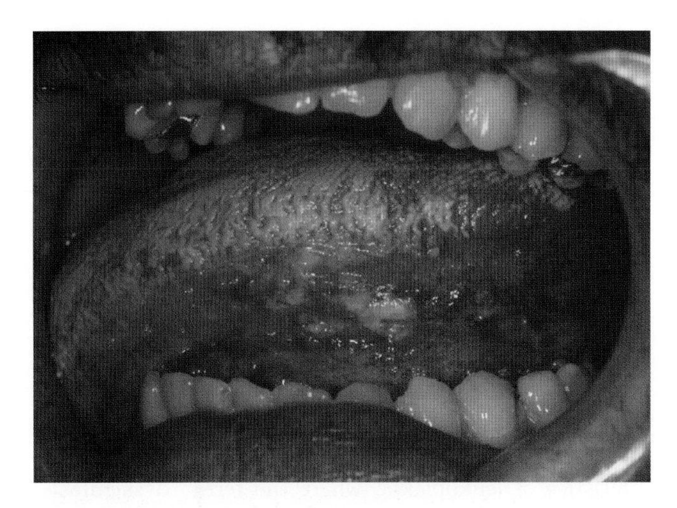

Figure 3.19 Oral hairy leukoplakia on the lateral border of the tongue in a HIV-positive male.

Histologically, the free surface is heavily parakeratotic with slender surface projections and corrugations and acanthosis. Beneath the parakeratotic layer is a band of large, pale-staining (balloon) cells that form the superior portion of the spinous layer, which is generally thickened. There is a characteristic nuclear chromatin change exemplified by a peripheral condensation of chromatin along the nuclear membrane. Central to this altered chromatin pattern is an amphophilic homogeneous deposit that consists of viral aggregates consistent with Epstein–Barr virus (EBV). Electron microscopy of the balloon cells reveals numerous virions typical of EBV, but HPVs are also found (121). There is no evidence of dysplasia, nor is there any reported association with MT of this form of leukoplakia over time. Candidal organisms are frequently found on the surface and, in fact, hairy leukoplakia was initially thought to be a severe form of oral thrush.

The differential diagnoses include leukoplakias with atypia, candidosis, white sponge nevus, OLP and geographic tongue. The parakeratosis and koilocytosis of hairy leukoplakia and the presence of EBV and HPV help to confirm the diagnosis.

The importance of a correct diagnosis is not so much related to confusion with malignancy, but more because OHL seems to be a precursor of AIDS and can serve as a reasonably reliable marker for the presence of HIV.

Management of OHL is generally unsatisfactory, but is usually not necessary beyond routine observation unless esthetics dictate otherwise. Some lesions recede with antifungal therapy, presumably owing to the eradication of candidal organisms. There is, however, never a complete resolution and a return occurs following cessation of treatment.

The significance of a mixed viral (EBV and HPV) infection is unresolved. It may be that a papilloma virus facilitates entry and subsequent replication of EBV in infected cells.

OHL should not be confused with hairy tongue, which commonly presents in patients with a history of smoking, topical antibiotic use, astringent mouthwash use, or with a local pH of 6 or less. It is said to develop also in subjects who have had radiotherapy to the head and neck (122). In contrast to a low incidence generally found in healthy subjects, hairy tongue appears to be much more common in patients with advanced cancer. Farman (122) has recorded a 22% incidence in such patients. General ill health is also a factor. Although infection with *Candida* species has been implicated as a factor, hairy tongue is not associated with vegetative *Candida* species. Hairy tongue in contrast to OHL, has no cancerous potential.

TYLOSIS

A relationship between tylosis (palmoplantar keratoderma) and carcinoma of the esophagus has been known since 1954 (123). Subsequently, abnormal oral lesions were described in tylotic patients (age range 4–59 years) (123). The oral lesions that presented in childhood were called "preleukoplakia" and had clinical as well as histologic characteristics similar to those seen in other epithelial disorders such as white sponge nevus and pachyonychia congenita. The adult oral lesions were called leukoplakia, but they also had associated areas of abnormal mucosa, resembling those seen in affected children.

The lesions designated preleukoplakia are clinically reminiscent of those seen in leukoedema with a gray–white, opalescent appearance, particularly affecting the buccal mucosa. Histologically, there are similarities to leukoedema, morsicatio mucosae oris (cheek biting) and white sponge nevus. There is no inflammatory cell reaction in the lamina propria. The adult form, originally described as "leukoplakia," is clinically non-specific; in other words, it is a benign keratosis without special features.

Although it is now recognized that the association of palmoplantar keratoderma with oral mucosal changes is an important clinical sign in the diagnosis of different patterns of focal palmoplantar keratoderma, the relationship with oral cancer is unknown, since risk factors such as smoking and alcohol drinking are nearly always present.

Because of the problems with the confusing earlier nomenclature, Field et al. (123) recommend use of the term "leukokeratosis" for the spectrum of diffuse oral lesions seen in the group of tylotic patients and also for the other clinical patterns of focal palmoplantar keratoderma.

EPITHELIAL HYPERPLASIA

The nomenclature applied to histologic epithelial abnormalities of the oral cavity, other than invasive carcinoma, encompasses the terms "hyperplasia," "dysplasia" and "carcinoma *in situ*." For each, there is the inevitable problem of subjectivity on the part of the surgical pathologist. In addition, for too long there has been the assumption that one can transfer criteria for the lesions from those used to define uterine cervical lesions to lesions of the head and neck mucosa.

It should be also appreciated that there are always varying degrees of histologic overlap. Indeed, pseudoepitheliomatous hyperplasia, an exaggerated response to injury, can be one of the most difficult differential diagnoses in oral pathology.

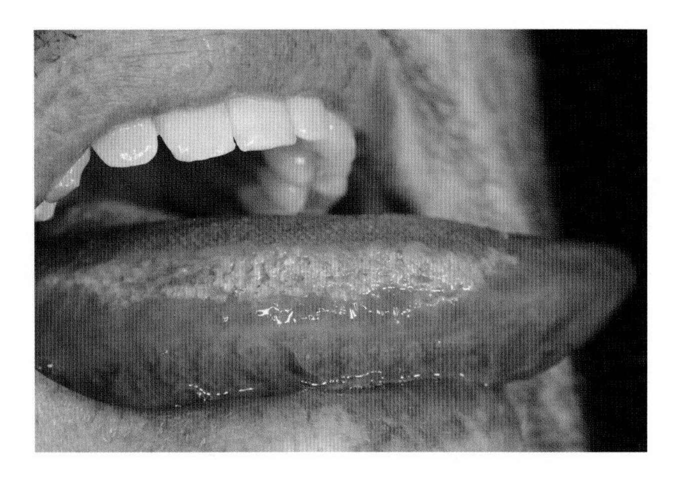

Figure 3.20 Reactive epithelial hyperplasia and keratosis on the lateral border of the tongue in a male non-smoker.

A reactive hyperplasia of the squamous mucosa of the oral cavity is its most common response to injury (Figure 3.20). A keratotic surface is a usual, but not inevitable, accompaniment. The reactive hyperplasia is characterized by epithelial thickening with a resulting readily identified and intact basal layer. Cellular maturation with a manifest orderly progression is typical. Cytologic atypia is minimal or absent. Division figures are normally found only adjacent to the basal layer of the epithelium. This form of hyperplasia is reversible and should be readily distinguishable from forms of dysplasia (mild, moderate and severe).

ORAL EPITHELIAL DYSPLASIA AND CARCINOMA *IN SITU*

Given the recent advances in molecular and biological studies on cancer, it is well accepted that MT from normal epithelium to invasive carcinoma is a "multiyear, multistep and multipath" process associated with progressive genetic and associated tissue damage (124–126). In addition, despite the fact that cancerous and premalignant lesions share similar biological characteristics, the ability to differentiate between these two entities is extremely important (126). Previous work by Vogelstein and others shows that cancer develops in a progressive fashion, evolving from hyperplasia to gradual degrees of dysplasia to carcinoma *in situ* and, ultimately, to invasive cancer (125). Although molecular and biological analyses have revealed additional complex genetic and epigenetic aberrations, the full molecular picture of premalignant lesions remains to be determined. Nonetheless, current knowledge allows us to understand the potential mechanisms of normal tissue's progression to malignancy (126).

Several types of cancer have benefited from our understanding of the molecular events of carcinogenesis, which has allowed the implementation of interventions designed to detect early cancer or premalignant lesions. Such interventions have resulted in improved outcomes, as in the case of HPV screening for cervical cancer (126).

Interestingly, many oral mucosal changes, such as leukoplakia, erythroplakia or erythroleukoplakia, may appear clinically benign, but histological examination may reveal cellular atypia and altered maturation that is histologically diagnosed as epithelial dysplasia (127). Despite the large volume of existing knowledge on molecular markers and their usefulness in providing information on the prediction and prognosis of potentially malignant oral lesions, these markers have not found their way into routine diagnostics (128). Biopsy and histological grading of epithelial dysplasia is still considered the gold standard, although there are current limitations in the management of OPMDs (128,129).

The history of OED dates back to the work of Shafer and Waldron (1961) on the clinical and histopathological characteristics of leukoplakia, where the term "dyskeratosis" was used to describe lesions with cellular atypia (130). Years later, dyskeratosis was replaced with the term "epithelial dysplasia." It was Smith and Pindborg (1969) who first defined OED (8). The collective work of the first WHO monograph on oral and oropharyngeal tumors specified the primary particulars of precancerous oral lesions (7). However, continued efforts by the WHO Collaborating Centre produced a more advanced monograph on the histological typing of oral cancer and precancer with illustrations explaining the different grades of OED and how this system could be adopted into routine diagnostic practice. Several attempts were made at methods for classifying OED to minimize disputes surrounding its significance (131).

The WHO definition of epithelial dysplasia as "a precancerous lesion of stratified squamous epithelium characterized by cellular atypia and loss of normal maturation and stratification short of carcinoma *in situ*" is still in use (8). Currently, for their diagnostic decisions, pathologists apply the defined architecture and cellular criteria described in the most recent monograph of the WHO's *Pathology and Genetics of Head and Neck Tumours* (9). It is always a challenge for pathologists to accurately assess the degree of dysplasia in OPMDs for reliable prediction and management. The histopathological diagnosis of OED is divided into four different categories: mild, moderate, severe and carcinoma *in situ*. This classification is based on the pathologist's interpretation of the presence and severity of the observed cellular atypia and chaotic architecture. For example, mild dysplasia refers to a lesion where the changes are limited only to the lower third of the epithelium, whereas moderate dysplasia refers to changes appearing in the lower two-thirds of the epithelium (Figure 3.21a–d) (9).

OED grading is still an issue that is debated between various researchers, pathologists and clinicians and among scientific peers (132). The current histopathological grading of OED notoriously lacks reliability. Grading is hampered by the arbitrary division into distinct categories of a continually progressing process without naturally and sharply defined borders. Several reports have demonstrated variable interobserver agreement on the grading of OED lesions. These variations might be due to a lack of objectivity in the evaluation of established criteria, arbitrary division of

Figure 3.21 Homogenous leukoplakia on the right soft palate in a 59-year-old male smoker diagnosed histopathologically as mild epithelial dysplasia **(a)**. Non-homogenous leukoplakia on the left ventral tongue in a 79-year-old female ex-smoker diagnosed histopathologically as moderate epithelial dysplasia **(b)**. Erythroleukoplakia on the right lateral tongue in a 62-year-old male smoker diagnosed histopathologically as severe epithelial dysplasia **(c)**. Erythroleukoplakia involving the labial gingiva between 34 and 35 in a 74-year-old male non-smoker diagnosed histopathologically as carcinoma *in situ* **(d)**.

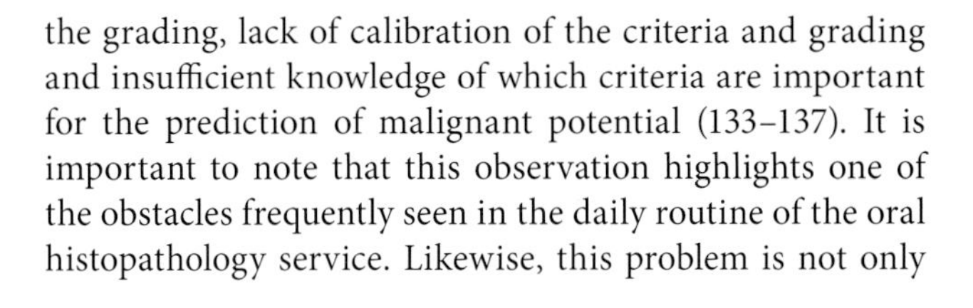

the grading, lack of calibration of the criteria and grading and insufficient knowledge of which criteria are important for the prediction of malignant potential (133–137). It is important to note that this observation highlights one of the obstacles frequently seen in the daily routine of the oral histopathology service. Likewise, this problem is not only present in the oral field, but it is also observed in the grading of epithelial dysplasia in other parts of the body, such as cervical intraepithelial neoplasia, vulvar intraepithelial neoplasia and Barrett's esophagus dysplasia (138,139).

Recently, many criticisms have been raised against the conventional role of histopathological evaluation in the grading of OED. It is widely accepted that the microscopic assessment of OED indicates only that a lesion has an increased risk of MT, but cannot confidently predict malignant changes in individual cases (133,140). There is, therefore, a critical need for the use of adjunctive markers to augment the determination of the MT of OPMDs (133,140).

There is, as yet, no consensus when it comes to the management of OPMDs. Decisions are ultimately dependent upon the individual experience of the clinicians at a single healthcare center employing patient characteristics, lesion features and histopathological findings (3,132,141). Several protocols compiling the personal clinical experience of these well-developed centers in managing patients with OPMDs were recently published (129,133,142–146). The dilemma of the management of OEDs persists as two crucial questions have not yet been reasonably answered: What is the likelihood of an oral lesion with OED undergoing MT to SCC? What intervention(s) can be used to mitigate this risk (142)? Traditionally, OPMDs with moderate to severe OED are treated surgically, if possible, while the mild ones are mostly left to "watch and wait"; this is due to the notion that lesions harboring higher grades of dysplasia have a greater potential for MT and therefore require immediate intervention. However, this is not true in all cases. There are many cases of either no apparent epithelial dysplasia or mild cases progressing into carcinoma. The threshold of MT varies from study to study. Yet, the pooled evidence from a meta-analysis on 14 non-randomized studies showed that the MT rate of OPMDs ranges from 0% to 36% with a mean of 12.1% in a mean follow-up of 4.3 years (147). Another interesting finding from this study highlights the importance of treatment of all OED cases, as it was observed that non-excised lesions demonstrated considerably higher MT than those that were excised (147).

OED has a long history of having predictive value, but this is now questionable given the well-known shortcomings with regard to sampling errors, the lack of interobserver agreement on grading and an incomplete understanding of the natural history of oral carcinogenesis (87,132,133). Therefore, a reliable method to guide clinicians when deciding to treat or not to treat is needed. There still is no reliable method for determining whether a particular OPMD may develop into OSCC, persist unchanged for the lifetime of the patient, enlarge to cover more of the oral mucosa or reduce in size or even disappear altogether. Improvement to the standard of the histopathological reporting of OED lesions is needed to provide insightful information to guide OPMD management decisions (134,148,149). This can be achieved by considering several points. There is a need for a universal definition of the architectural and cytological features that are the basis of any OED grading process. In addition, a consensus on the scoring process between two or more observers should be encouraged as this would not only improve interobserver agreement, but also help to eliminate errors (134,149).

Loss of heterozygosity (LOH) has shown a validated role in discriminating OPMDs into high-risk and low-risk groups after a median follow-up time of 44.6 months (144). However, more evidence is needed before this test can be recommended in routine diagnostic practice (144). DNA ploidy has shown good correlation with epithelial grading, but has shown better predictive value for the progression of OED lesions into carcinoma (149,150). Like LOH, evidence must still be accumulated in favor of DNA ploidy testing before it can find its way into routine practice.

It is often said that prevention is better than cure. Primary prevention attempts to eliminate disease risk factors, while secondary prevention aims for early detection of OPMD to cure or to significantly reduce morbidity and mortality. Additionally, appropriate surveillance to monitor "at-risk" patients is regarded as tertiary prevention, as it is aimed at reducing recurrence risks (143).

The philosophy beyond treating OPMDs is to eliminate the lesions either surgically or non-surgically in an attempt to prevent MT (27). The most commonly used treatment modalities consist of cold knife surgical excision or laser therapy. Additionally, along with the watch-and-wait protocol, chemoprevention—either topically or systemically—with retinoid vitamins A, C and E, carotenes or lycopene, mouthwash therapy containing an attenuated adenovirus and photodynamic therapy offer alternative treatment modalities (152). Unfortunately, no substantial evidence based on randomized controlled studies exists to support any of the previously mentioned modalities (152). Furthermore, there are no scientific data about the value of follow-up visits and the optimal intervals after leukoplakia treatment (27).

What makes management of OPMDs difficult for the clinician is the current limited knowledge of the natural history of OPMD, grading OED, risk profiling and unpredictable clinical outcomes (143).

Establishment of an accurate diagnosis allows the clinician to develop a treatment plan that is based on the best available evidence and is most appropriate for the patient's needs and desires. Dependence of the patient's treatment plan on the histological assessment of OED is questionable. Molecular tests should accompany the pathological diagnosis of OPMDs to help in their future management in terms of prevention, treatment, surveillance and discriminating between progressive versus non-progressive lesions.

Until either evidence-based guidelines or a universal consensus on the management of OPMDs emerges, clinicians have to update their management philosophy by leveraging all of the recent advances concerning adjunctive diagnostic aids, molecular techniques, biomarkers, treatment modalities and chemoprevention. Though optimal OPMD management should be individually tailored based on the assessment of the patient's history of risk factors and compliance, clinical presentation, histopathological and molecular parameters, some may regard surgical intervention for mild OED as necessary, while others may regard this as overtreatment. What is certain is that management of OED generally, and mild OED specifically, is still debatable.

ORAL CANCER

Oral cancer is the 11th most prevalent malignancy in the world (153). As in most malignancies, the risk of oral cancer increases with age advancement; the peak occurrence is around the age of 60 and its incidence is higher in males compared with females (154,155). Melanesia has the world's highest incidence of oral cancer with 31.5 cases per 100,000 men and 20.2 cases per 100,000 women. In many parts of India, Pakistan, Bangladesh and Sri Lanka, oral cancer is the most common form of cancer among men (156). In addition, a high rate of oral cancer is registered in Hong Kong, Singapore and the Philippines (157). Although the majority of cases are observed in developing countries, in several regions of Europe, Japan and Australia, the incidence and mortality of oral cancer are rising (153). According to the WHO, tumors of the oral cavity may originate from epithelium, connective or hematolymphoid tissues (9). This section covers oral epithelial malignancies, which include tumors of the oral epithelial lining, with special emphasis on OSCC and its subtypes and oropharyngeal carcinoma.

ORAL SQUAMOUS CELL CARCINOMA (ICD-O CODE: 8070/3)

OSCC is an invasive neoplasm of the epithelial lining of the oral cavity and may show varying grades of squamous differentiation. These tumors account for more than 90% of all malignant tumors of the oral cavity and have a tendency for extensive and early lymph node metastases. Although it has not been possible to prove conclusively a causative agent or factor (carcinogen) for OSCC, intrinsic and extrinsic carcinogens considered as significant or speculative risk factors include tobacco, alcohol, betel quid, OPMD, infections, diet and deficiency states and genetic disorders.

Similar to other upper aerodigestive tract malignancies, the majority of the disease burden of oral and oropharyngeal malignancies is attributed to tobacco consumption (153). A widely used substance, tobacco can be consumed as smokeless (e.g. chewing and snuff) or smoked (e.g. cigarettes, cigars and pipes). There are considerable variations in the adverse consequences of tobacco consumption depending on the amount and form in which tobacco is used. Cigarette smokers are at an increased risk (sixfold) for developing oral cancer (158). Unlike cigarette smoking in which there is no specific site for oral lesions, pipe smoking, smokeless tobacco and reverse smoking cause oral lesions (both OPMLs and OSCCs) in specific locations. Since many alcohol users are smokers as well, exploring the independent influence of alcohol consumption in OSCC is challenging. By adjusting odds ratios for confounding factors, however, the existence of alcohol consumption as an independent risk factor for OSCC has been "statistically" shown (159–176). The combination of heavy smoking (2+ packs/day for 20+ years) and heavy drinking (4+ alcoholic beverages/day) has been shown to have a synergistic and strong association with OSCC (an increase of 35-fold) (159). In the same population, the separately adjusted risks of developing OSCC for heavy smoking and drinking were significantly lower than the combined risk (159).

Although no viral infection has been shown to directly cause oral cancer, the oncogenic potential of some viruses has been identified (177). Once, adenoviruses, retroviruses, herpes simplex viruses and HPVs were thought to have a role in the development of oral cancer. Currently, considerable evidence exists for an increase in risk associated with infection with oncogenic subtypes of HPV (HPV-16). HPV-positive cases now form a small but nevertheless distinct group of OSCCs (178–185). Although infection with OSCC implies incorporation of one or more of the functional genes of the virus into the host DNA, of interest is the lower rate of genetic changes (including TP53 mutations) in HPV-positive OSCCs compared to HPV-negative cases (186–189).

Tertiary syphilis infection has also been associated with an increased risk of developing syphilitic leukoplakia which, in turn, has a 30%–100% chance of MT (177,190). Due to the significant decline in the prevalence of tertiary syphilis, this association and its details, however, cannot be further explored (177).

Similarly, chronic candidosis has been proposed as a potential risk factor for developing chronic hyperplastic candidosis (also known as candidal leukoplakia), which has a propensity for MT (40). *C. albicans* has also been directly associated with a higher risk for the development of oral neoplasia (191,192). Nevertheless, many variants of *Candida* are commensal fungi and the mere presence of the microorganism does not imply MT.

Malnutrition, especially iron and vitamin A deficiency, may be associated with a risk of developing OSCC (193). Last but not least, in preparing the inventory of cancer risk factors and studying what one might call a cancer epidemic, the effect of longer life expectancy and an aging population should not be overlooked. More than 90% of oral cancers are diagnosed in persons over the age of 40; this and the mean diagnosis age of 60 once more emphasize the role of accumulative environmental carcinogens in development of oral cancer (194).

OPMDs and the lesions associated with them may precede OSCC. Not all OPMLs undergo MT and the exact nature of progression of OPMLs to OSCC is yet to be fully clarified. Prediction of cancer risk is often based on population estimates rather than on an individual basis (5). To date, the best indication of MT of OPMLs remains the presence and not the grade of dysplasia (133–135,195).

The traditional clinical impression of a Caucasian patient with OSCC has been depicted as an elderly male with a history of long-term tobacco and excessive alcohol consumption. Early or small OSCC lesions are often asymptomatic and this may partly explain the delay in seeking care and the consequent late diagnosis of these lesions. Hence, a high clinical suspicion and informed use of diagnostic adjunctive tools is required to ensure the timely diagnosis and management of early OSCC.

The majority (70%) of OSCCs are found in the lower part of the mouth (i.e. lateral borders of the tongue, floor of the mouth and the lingual alveolar mucosa), which forms only 20% of the oral cavity. This distribution pattern, which represents the most likely locations in the oral cavity for pooling of carcinogens, has been linked with the current hypotheses that propose OSCC carcinogenesis to be the result of the accumulation of mutations in response to environmental mutagens (196).

Diagnosis of OSCC, particularly in the early stages, presents a real challenge to clinicians. Early lesions are often painless and, in most cases, an early OSCC appears as a red, speckled or white patch. The clinical appearance of erythroplakic, erythroleukoplakic and leukoplakic OSCCs is identical to that of their OPML namesakes; however, the clinical similarities between these early OSCC lesions and OPMLs could be due to the common keratinization process and should not be merely attributed to pre-existing OPMLs (177). As malignancy progresses, mucosal changes may result in a raised nodule (exophytic OSCC) or ulcerated surface (ulcerated, invasive or burrowing OSCC). An exophytic OSCC is the result of inflammation, infiltration and fibrosis and may be of irregular, fungating, papillary or verruciform appearance (Figure 3.22). The color varies from normal to white or red and depends on the amount of fibrosis, keratinization or vascularity. Ulcerated lesions are usually irregular in shape and present with a depressed, necrotic center and rolled (indurated) borders, which indicate invasion of the tumor downward and laterally under the epithelium (Figure 3.23). Extremely advanced lesions may extend and resorb surrounding structures (including underlying bone) (Figure 3.24) and patients may present with pain or referred pain to the ear, dysphasia, dysphagia, bleeding, swelling of the neck and weight loss (9).

Based on the affected site and degree of invasion, patients with OSCC may present with varying signs and symptoms. Lingual squamous carcinoma constitutes 50% of all intraoral cancers and, in descending order, it presents on the posterior lateral (Figure 3.25), anterior lateral, ventral (Figure 3.26) and dorsal surfaces. The tongue is the most affected site in younger patients (under 40 years of age) (197) and is the only location in which congenital OSCC has been reported (198). Squamous carcinomas of the floor of the mouth (Figure 3.27) are most likely to be preceded by an OPML; they usually start in the midline near the frenum and are most often associated with development of a secondary tumor. Patients with carcinomas of the tongue and floor of the mouth usually seek professional care in advanced stages when the lesion has spread beyond the tongue and turned into a necrotic ulcer with a diameter of 2 cm or more with poor prognosis (177). In advanced stages, the tumor becomes increasingly fixed to the surrounding tissues, infiltrates the tongue and makes it stiffer; at this stage, pain generally becomes the patient's chief complaint with a high chance for lymph node involvement. In such circumstances, the 5-year survival rate is as low as 16% (177).

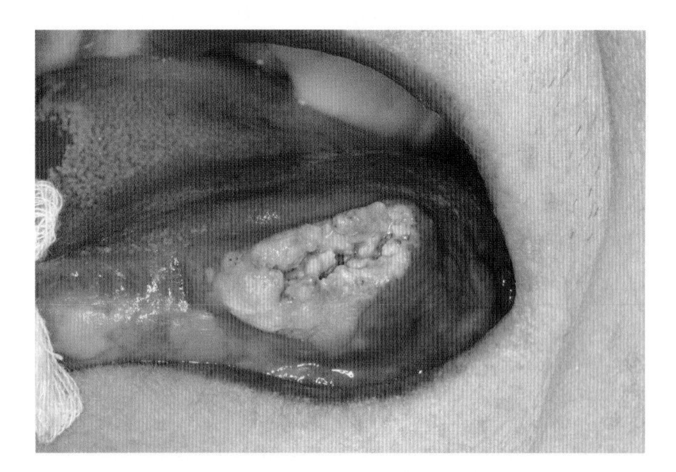

Figure 3.22 Exophytic lesion with a central crater, rolled margins and extensive keratosis on the left lateral border of the tongue in a 68-year-old female non-smoker; biopsy-proven well-differentiated oral squamous cell carcinoma.

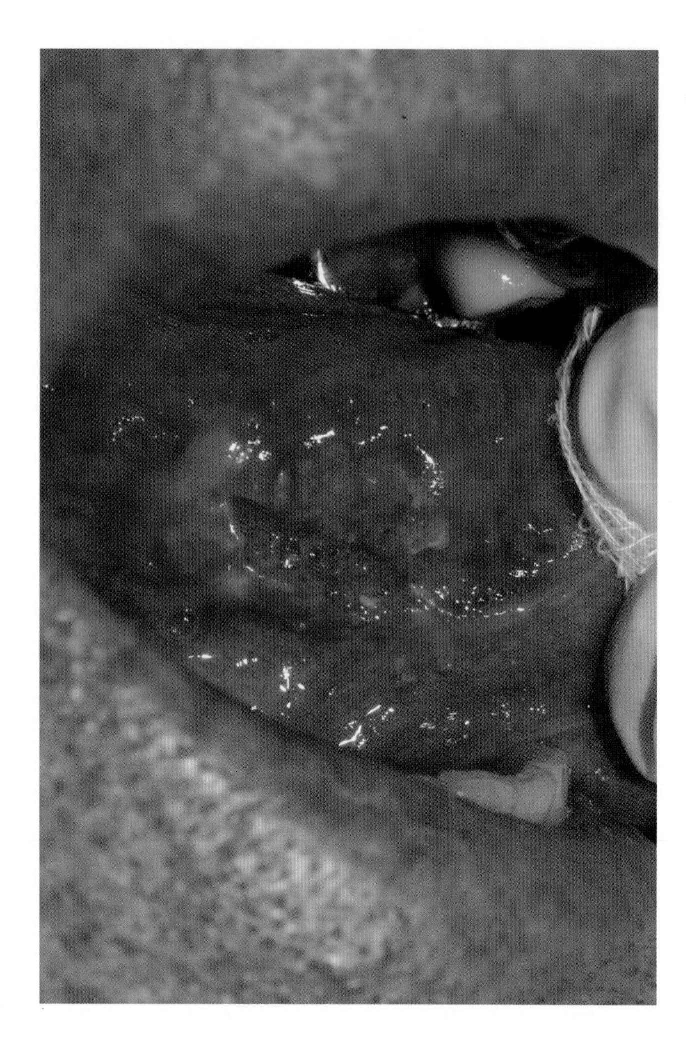

Figure 3.23 Ulcerated lesion with raised margins and induration on the posterior right lateral border of the tongue in a 59-year-old male non-smoker; biopsy-proven poorly differentiated oral squamous cell carcinoma.

SCC of buccal mucosa (Figure 3.28) is the most common cancer of central to East Asia and is generally found upon the preferential side of chewing and placement of betel quid (199). Most buccal cancers are preceded by previous mucosal lesions; leukoplakic/erythroplakic lesions are

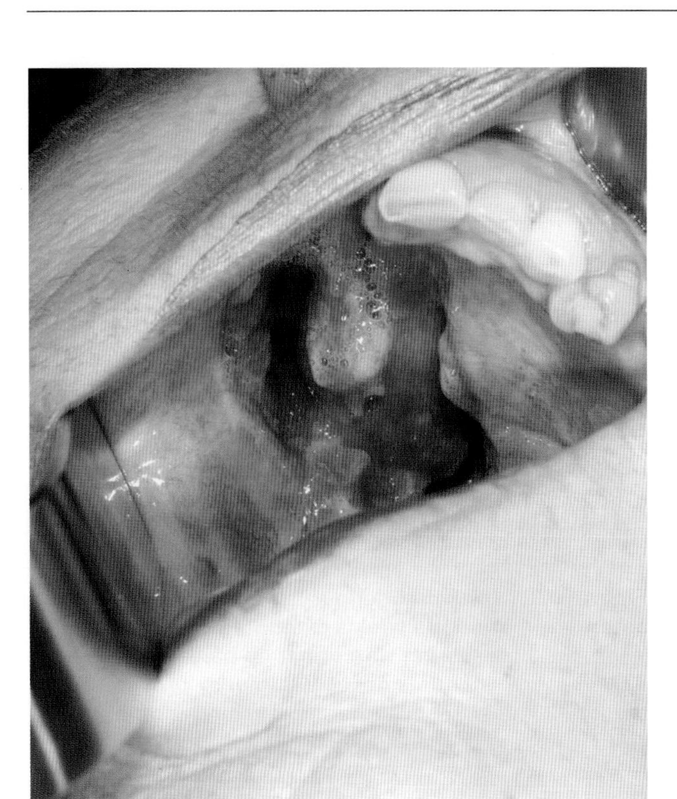

Figure 3.24 Oral squamous cell carcinoma of the right maxillary alveolus treated with inferior structure hemi-maxillectomy. The patient uses an obturator satisfactorily and is 4 years post-treatment. (Courtesy of Dr Chady Sader, Department of Otolaryngology, Head and Neck Surgery, Sir Charles Gairdner Hospital, Perth, Australia.)

more commonly found in the anterior regions of the buccal mucosa, while posterior buccal SCC generally follow lichen planus or traumatic ulcers (194). These cancers clinically appear as ulcerated lesions with indurated raised borders and exophytic or verrucous growths (9). In advanced stages,

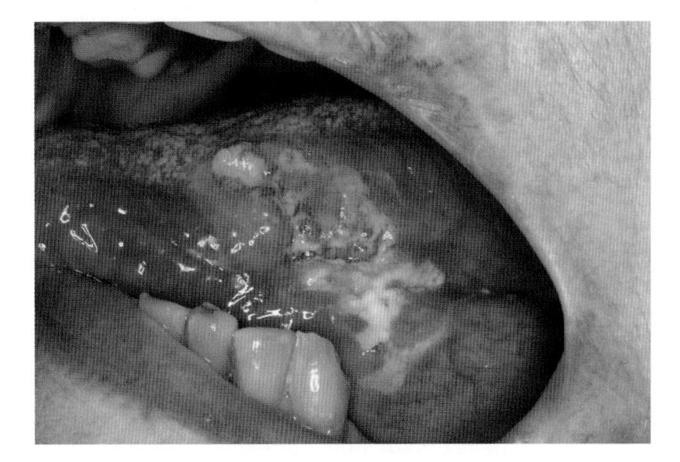

Figure 3.25 Erythroleukoplakia displaying rolled margins, necrotic center and induration, involving the posterior left lateral border of the tongue extending onto the floor of mouth in an 82-year-old female ex-smoker; biopsy-proven moderately differentiated squamous cell carcinoma.

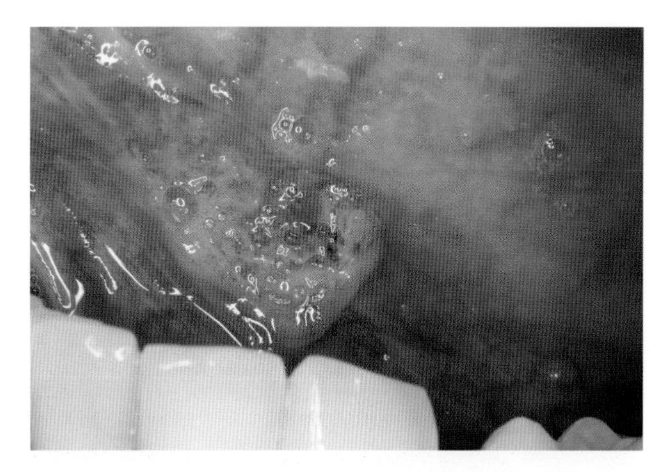

Figure 3.26 Chronic ulcer on the left anterior ventral tongue in a 24-year-old male non-smoker; biopsy-proven moderately differentiated squamous cell carcinoma.

the lesions progress into the adjacent bone or overlying skin and advanced cases often progress to oro-cutaneous fistulas.

Primary gingival (Figure 3.29) or alveolar SCC (Figure 3.30) present as painless lesions that highly resemble inflammatory lesions such as angiogranuloma or white reactive lesions. Carcinomas of the alveolar mucosa and hard palate have a higher propensity for bone invasion at earlier stages, which complicates management of these lesions. As a result of bone invasion, these lesions may cause tooth mobility and some are only diagnosed after tooth extraction, when they proliferate out of the socket and resemble hyperplastic granulation tissue of epulis granulomatosa.

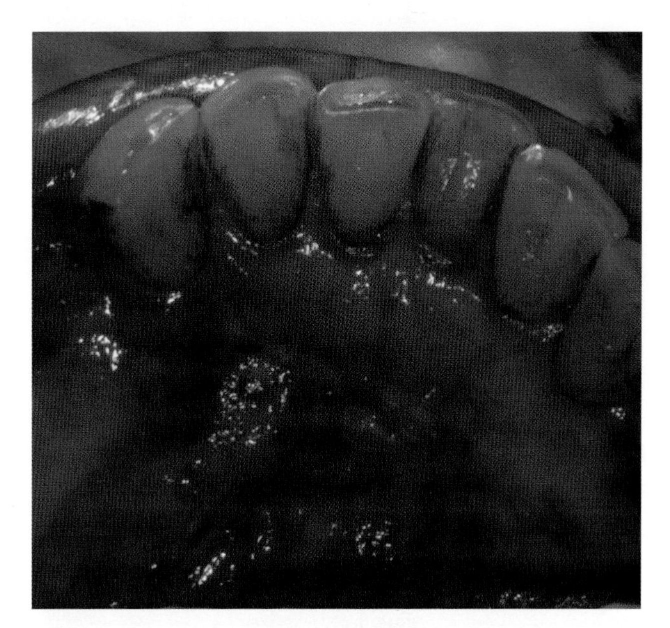

Figure 3.27 Friable erythroleukoplakic lesion involving the anterior floor of mouth extending onto the alveolar mucosa in an 80-year-old female smoker; T1 biopsy-proven moderately differentiated squamous cell carcinoma.

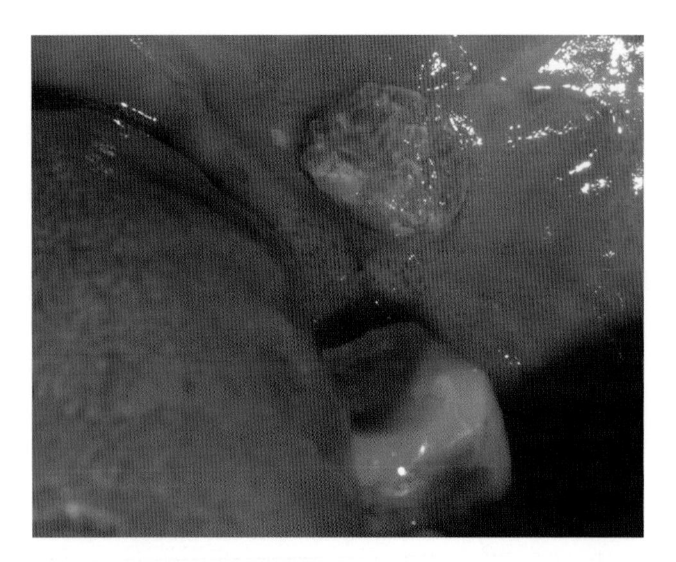

Figure 3.28 Soft tissue lump on the buccal mucosa in an 83-year-old female smoker; biopsy-proven papillary squamous cell carcinoma.

OSCC invades by direct infiltration and extension and although bone forms an initial barrier in the early stages of invasion, superficial erosion eventually will result in invasion along the medullary cavity (200–202). Perineural invasion and vascular infiltration are not commonly seen; nonetheless, they have been associated with regional metastasis (203). In tissues that have not previously been irradiated, due to the high influence of anatomical features, local spread of early OSCC is relatively predictable (9).

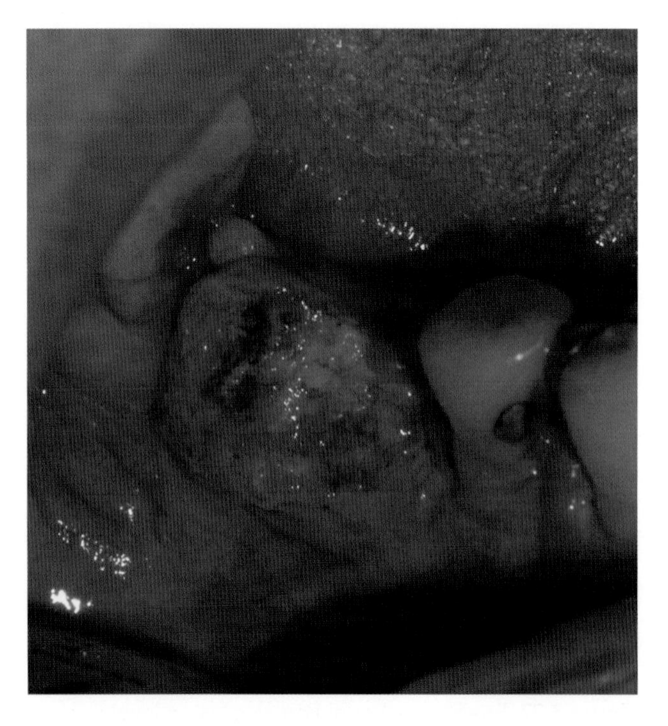

Figure 3.29 Ulcerated gingival lump in an 83-year-old female smoker (same patient demonstrated in Figure 3.28); T4 biopsy-proven moderately differentiated keratinizing squamous cell carcinoma.

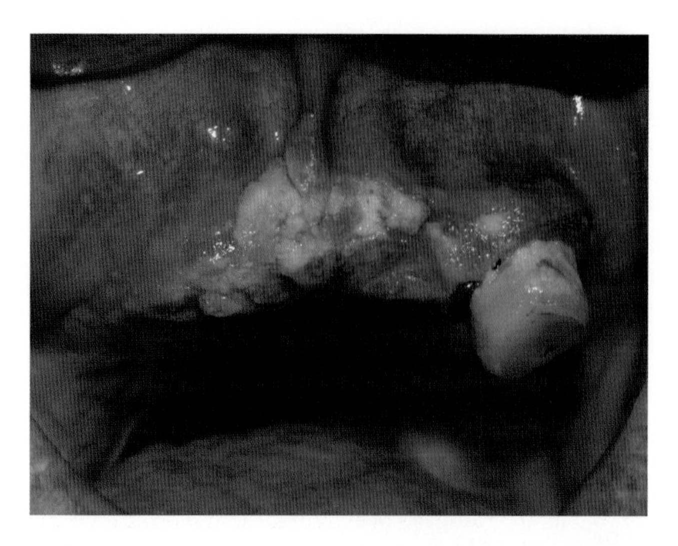

Figure 3.30 Non-homogenous leukoplakic lesion on the anterior edentulous alveolus extending to involve the left maxilla presenting with upper lip paresthesia in a 77-year-old male non-smoker; T4a biopsy-proven squamous cell carcinoma with perineural infiltration of the VII cranial nerve.

The clinical appearance and superficial involvement of most OSCC lesions except those of the tongue are reliable indications of tumor spread. Early SCC of the floor of the mouth and palate are unlikely to invade the underlying mylohyoid muscle or the sublingual glands. In contrast, tumors of the lateral border of the tongue, whether primary or as a result of local spread from the floor of the mouth, spread in depth (9).

Pierre Denoix first classified malignant tumors based on the extent of the primary tumor (T), involvement of regional lymph nodes (N) and distant metastasis (M) in the 1940s (204). Individual TNM classifications are used for most human cancers. Recent changes have been made to accommodate micrometastasis, the presence of isolated tumor cells, findings in sentinel nodes and tumor detection by molecular methods (9,205). Once each of the three parameters of TNM has been determined, the collective effect is used to determine management and prognosis.

Clinical staging and tumor location are both important factors in guiding the treatment of OSCC, which consists of wide-margin surgical removal, radiation therapy or a combination of the two. Positive indications for radiation therapy include regional metastasis, poorly differentiated lesions and perineural or angiolymphatic invasion (198). Chemotherapeutic agents such as platinum-containing compounds (e.g. cisplatin and carboplatin), 5-fluorouracil and taxanes (e.g. paclitaxel and docetaxel) are only administered as adjuncts to radiation. The overall 5-year survival rate for oral cancer continues to be about 50%, with survivors experiencing poor quality of life (206–208). Generally, patients with advanced disease and higher TNM grading have a poor prognosis and high locoregional and distant recurrences (209,210).

VERRUCOUS CARCINOMA (ICD-O CODE: 8051/3)

VC is a low-grade variant of SCC with a deceptively benign appearance. It was first described in detail by Ackerman in 1948 as a carcinoma predominantly seen in the buccal mucosa and lower gingivae of older males (211). VC is uncommon and accounts for 1%–10% of all OSCCs. This carcinoma is not limited to the oral cavity and other anatomic sites such as the larynx, urinary bladder, anogenital region, vulvovaginal region and skin of the breasts can also be affected.

VC is a disease of the elderly and most patients with VC report a history of chewing tobacco, ill-fitting dentures and poor oral hygiene (212). Tobacco is not a contributing factor to the carcinogenesis of extraoral VC and other etiological factors should be considered for these lesions. Infection with HPV subtypes 16 and 18, although in a minority (up to 40%) of the cases, has been reported (213,214).

The average age of patients presenting with VC is 67 years (215). The most common sites of involvement in the oral cavity include the mandibular vestibule and gingivae (Figure 3.31a) followed by the buccal mucosa, tongue (Figure 3.31b) and hard palate (Figure 3.31c) (107). The lesion may exist in the mouth for 2–3 years prior to diagnosis and, unless the surface is infected or ulcerated, appears as a painless, diffuse, keratotic plaque with well-defined borders and papillary (blunted tips) or verruciform (pointed tips) surface projections (Figure 3.32). Lesions are typically white but, based on the amount of keratin and inflammation, may appear erythematous or pink.

Surgical removal without neck dissection is the treatment of choice for VC (215,216). Although the extent of surgical margins for removal of VC is still a controversial subject (217), most authors agree that surgery for VC does not generally need to be as extensive as that for OSCC. Metastasis is a rare occurrence in VC and this malignancy has a good prognosis with a 5-year survival rate of 90%, during which only 8% of the patients required additional surgery (218,219). Although no molecular biomarker is currently known to help with the prognosis of VC, clinicians should be aware that in 20% of the cases, VC contains a co-existing OSCC that may complicate the course of treatment and prognosis (219). If left untreated, VC may develop an invasive focus that may lead to metastasis (177).

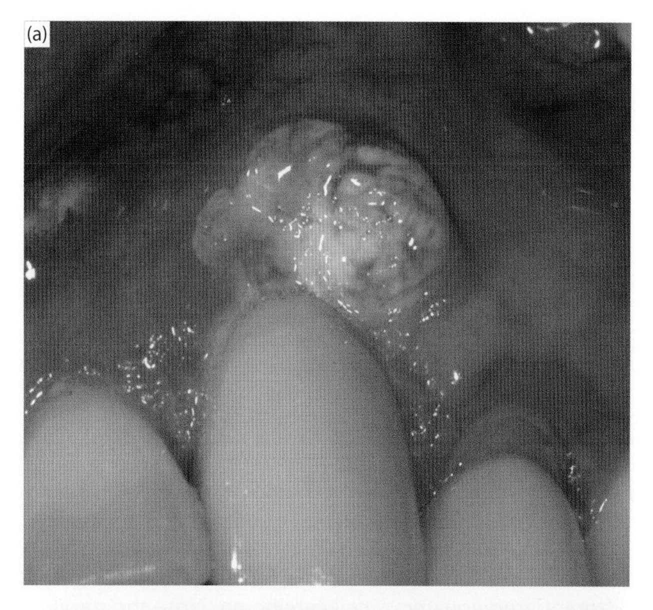

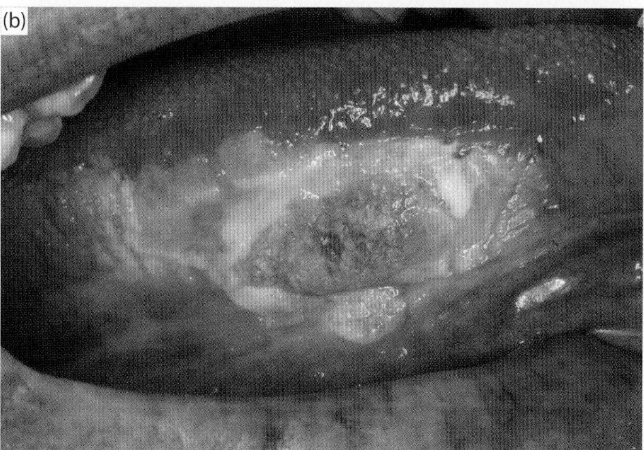

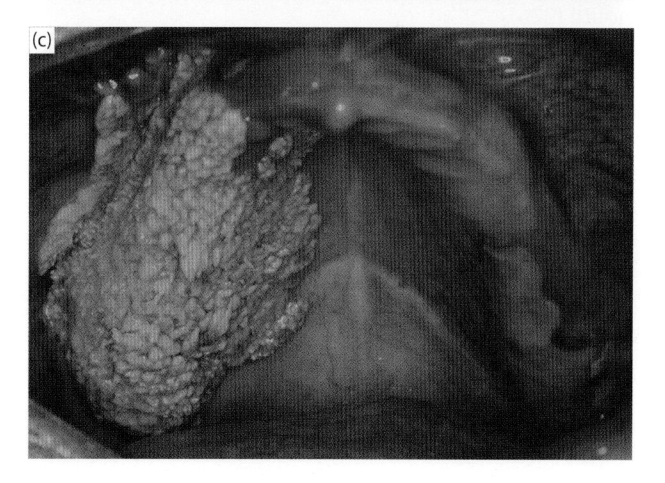

Figure 3.31 Verrucous carcinoma of the gingiva **(a)**, tongue **(b)** and hard palate **(c)**. Note the papillary (blunted tips) in (a) and the verruciform (pointed tips) surface projections in (b) and (c).

BASALOID SQUAMOUS CELL CARCINOMA (ICD-O CODE: 8083/3)

The most recently defined variant of SCC, basaloid SCC (BSCC) was first described by Wain et al. in 1986 (220). BSCC is an aggressive tumor and most frequently presents in the upper aerodigestive tract, particularly in the larynx and hypopharynx and the base of the tongue (221). Oral BSCCs are uncommon in the oral cavity and more so in the gingivae. According to the WHO, BSCC contains basaloid and squamous components (222) and histologically mimics other malignancies such as adenoid cystic carcinoma, basal cell adenocarcinoma and small-cell neuroendocrine carcinoma (221).

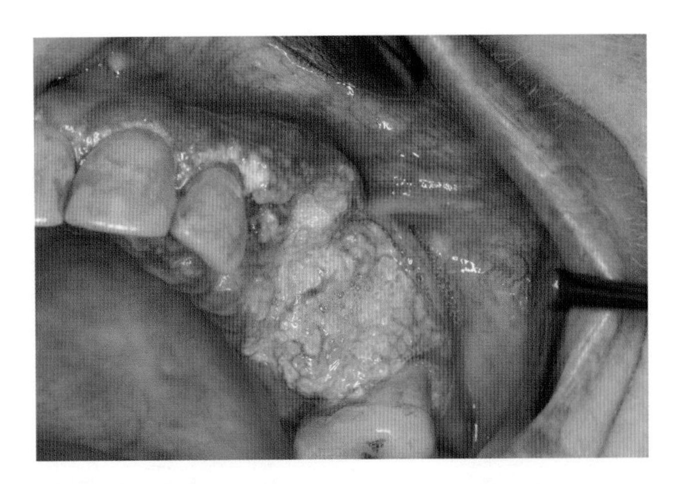

Figure 3.32 Biopsy-proven verrucous carcinoma involving the alveolar ridge and gingiva of quadrant 2 in a 57-year-old female non-smoker. The lesion had been present for at least 14 months before a second biopsy confirmed well-differentiated squamous cell carcinoma. Note the papillary (blunted tips) surface projections.

Most patients with BSSC give a history of tobacco use and alcohol consumption (223). Although infection with HPV has been suggested to predispose individuals to developing BSCC (224), this is inconclusive (223).

Oral BSCC is a distinct and highly aggressive subtype of OSCC that tends to affect individuals older than 40 years of age. Clinical features of BSCC are very similar to those of OSCC; hence, in most cases, final diagnosis is made through histological and immunohistochemical evaluations (225). BSCC is uncommon in the oral cavity and intraoral cases are mostly found at the base of the tongue and floor of the mouth (226).

Due to its aggressive nature, surgery followed by radiotherapy is the treatment of choice for oral BSCC and chemotherapy is advised for distant metastases. While some estimate the mean survival time of patients with oral BSCC to be significantly shorter than those with conventional OSCC, others have found similar survival rates between the two (227). Since Fritsch and Lentsch (227) matched lesions by stage and anatomical site, one might attribute the worse outcome reported by Neville et al. (198) to the poorer stage at which oral BSCC is diagnosed.

PAPILLARY SQUAMOUS CELL CARCINOMA (ICD-O CODE: 8052/3)

Papillary SCC (PSCC) is a rare variant of SCC that generally presents as a solitary exophytic lesion (Figure 3.28) (228). Because of its rarity, the bulk of our current knowledge about oral PSCC is obtained from published case reports that have discussed less than 100 cases in small and isolated groups. Unlike conventional SCC, a positive association between smoking and alcohol consumption has not been observed in oral PSCC (228,229). This could be partly due to the small number of samples, which challenges the power of any statistical analysis performed.

The mean age of patients with oral PSCC is between 63.3 (229) and 72.9 years (228) and, in most reports, most affected individuals are male (228,229). PSCC is extremely rare in the oral cavity and most frequently presents in the larynx and hypopharynx. In the oral cavity, the gingiva is the most commonly affected site (228,229). This tumor has an exophytic appearance with finger-like projections that consist of tumor epithelium surrounding a fibrovascular core (9).

Most reported cases of oral PSCC have been treated by surgery with or without neck dissection (228). Although there is no statistically reliable data in regard to prognosis and survival of oral PSCC, it is believed that in location- and stage-matched cases, patients with PSCC generally have a better prognosis (228).

SPINDLE CELL CARCINOMA (ICD-O CODE: 8074/3)

Spindle cell carcinoma (SpCC) or polypoid SCC is a rare variant of SCC that generally affects the larynx (9). Similar to PSCC and due to the low number of reported cases, the etiologic factors involved in the carcinogenesis of SpCC have not been elucidated. The large number of spindle cells present in the lesion makes it indistinguishable from connective tissue sarcomas; however, to date, this neoplasm is clearly categorized as a variant of conventional SCC (198).

SpCC has no sex predilection and is generally diagnosed during the sixth decade of life (230). The most common intraoral site of involvement is the lower lip and the lesion may appear as a polypoid pedunculated mass, as well as a sessile nodule or even an ulcer (198). SpCC is extremely aggressive—it frequently recurs and metastasizes and has a poorer prognosis compared to conventional SCC (231). Therefore, surgical removal with wider margins is advisable. In a study of 18 SpCCs, survival was highly dependent upon the stage at the time of diagnosis and while stage I and II lesions had a 100% 3-year survival rate, this rate was 0% for stages III and IV (231).

ADENOSQUAMOUS CARCINOMA (ICD-O CODE: 8560/3)

A rare variant of SCC, oral adenosquamous carcinoma shows clear areas of adenocarcinoma in addition to regions characterizing classic SCC. While the SCC features normally dominate, the adenoid pattern has also been clearly demonstrated in metastatic lesions (9). Although the role of HPV in the carcinogenesis of cervical adenosquamous carcinoma is clearly demonstrated, its contribution to oral adenosquamous carcinoma is still unclear (232).

Adenosquamous carcinoma has a slight propensity to affect older males (233). It has been reported in most sites of the oral cavity and presents as a nodular mass that may or may not be painful or ulcerated (233).

The first study to describe adenosquamous carcinoma reported that 80% of cases developed distant metastases (234). In most cases of adenosquamous carcinoma, nodes are involved at the time of diagnosis and, as a result, prognosis is generally poor. Patients are treated with radical surgical removal of the tumor, which may be combined with radiotherapy.

OROPHARYNGEAL SQUAMOUS CELL CARCINOMA

Oropharyngeal SCC (OPSCC) includes carcinomas arising in the soft palate (Figure 3.33), base of the tongue (Figure 3.34), tonsillar region (tonsil, tonsillar fossa and pillars) (Figure 3.35) and posterior pharyngeal wall (235). The tonsillar region subsite currently accounts for the majority of cases (approximately 70%–80%) (235), while traditionally

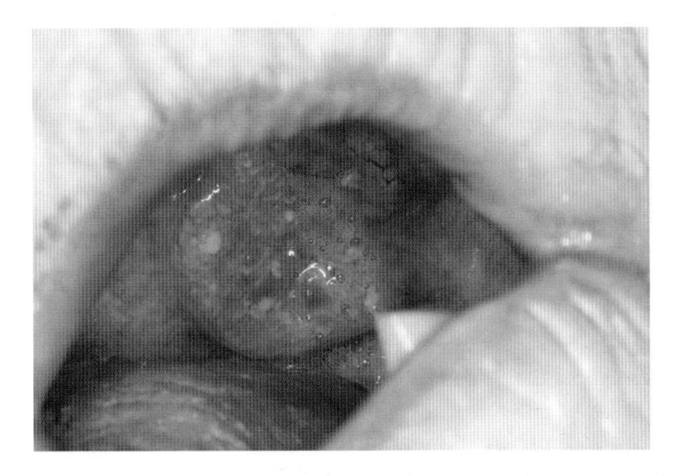

Figure 3.33 Chronic fungating non-healing ulcer displaying rolled raised margins and a necrotic center occurring on the posterior left soft palate extending beyond the posterior surface of a full upper denture in a 68-year-old female smoker; biopsy-proven well differentiated squamous cell carcinoma.

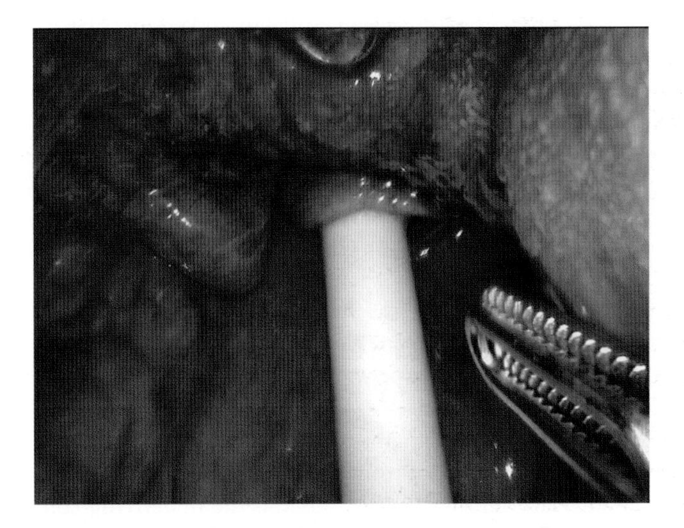

Figure 3.34 T1 left tonsillolingual sulcus squamous cell carcinoma amenable to trans-oral robotic resection (intra-operative endoscopic photo). (Courtesy of Dr Chady Sader, Department of Otolaryngology, Head and Neck Surgery, Sir Charles Gairdner Hospital, Perth, Australia.)

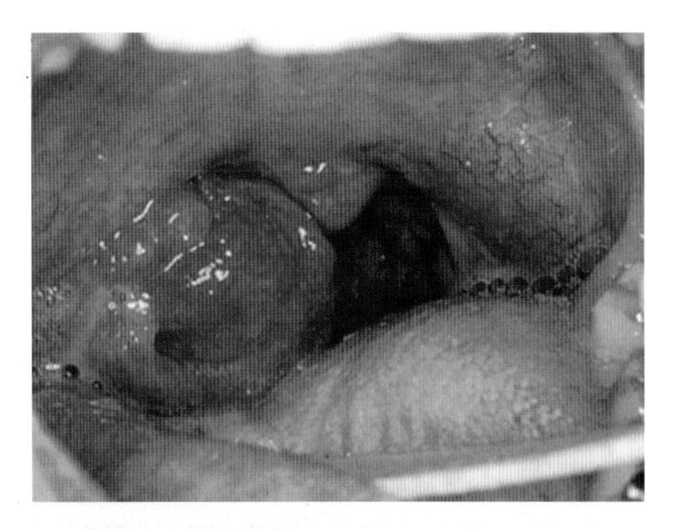

Figure 3.35 T2 right palatine tonsil squamous cell carcinoma. This patient presented with a unilateral enlarged tonsil. (Courtesy Dr of Chady Sader, Department of Otolaryngology, Head and Neck Surgery, Sir Charles Gairdner Hospital, Perth, Australia).

primary tumors of the oropharynx have arisen in the "high-risk" base of the tongue subsite (236).

Epidemiological studies indicate tonsillar and oropharyngeal tumors related to HPV to be on the rise (237–241). The etiological role of HPV in the carcinogenesis of the oral cavity and similarities in molecular mechanisms to those found in cervical cancer are bases for ongoing investigations (242,243). A history of cervical cancer increases the risk of oral cavity and oropharyngeal cancer development to over six-times that of the general female population (relative risk of head and neck cancer [HNC] development subsequent to cervical cancer was 6.7), further increasing the suspicion that the two cancers share similar etiological factors (244).

The predilection for high-risk HPV subtypes to infect and affect changes specifically in the oropharynx and tonsils and the high propensity for these carcinomas to result in early metastases are thought to be related to the nature of the tonsillar microanatomy (243). The surface of the tonsil is covered with epithelium-lined pits—tonsillar crypts—that pass into the underlying lymphoid tissue (245). Tonsillar epithelium originates from the mesoderm and ectoderm with crypts that are populated by lymphocytes (246). The palatine and lingual tonsils are lined with stratified squamous epithelium also in the crypts (246). The pharyngeal tonsils, however, are lined by ciliated, pseudostratified columnar epithelium, similar to that of the respiratory passages, have shallow infoldings called pleats instead of crypts and tend to atrophy after childhood (246,247). The stratified squamous epithelium extends into the crypt for some distance, but as it merges with the underlying lymphoid tissue, the epithelial cells assume a more basaloid appearance (i.e. high nuclear-to-cytoplasmic ratio and absence of cytoplasmic keratinization) with vesicular nuclei and loss of distinct cytoplasmic borders and intercellular bridges, which would facilitate metastasis (245,248). It is considered that HPV-related OPSCCs arise from this crypt epithelium, particularly of the lingual and palatine tonsils, both of which lie within the oropharynx (245). The preferential targeting possibly reflects the complex biological interactions between HPV and the specialized lympho-epithelium lining of the tonsillar crypts, known as reticulated epithelium (248).

Clinically, OPSCC appears as an ulcerated mass, fullness or irregular erythematous mucosal change (249,250) and is preceded by mucosal changes and the presence of an OPML (207). OPSCC is notoriously difficult to detect, is often present at more advanced stages compared to OSCC and is likely to metastasize (249). It is not uncommon for patients to present with significant metastatic neck disease and a small, as-yet undetected primary tumor (249). This tendency to remain hidden is related to the anatomy of the region, with many tumors arising in the tonsillar crypt epithelium, which is difficult to examine clinically by the dental or medical physician (243). The use of flexible nasoendoscopy to visualize the base of the tongue and nasopharynx is useful in this regard. The chief symptoms are the presence of a neck mass (from metastatic disease) (Figure 3.36), sore throat, difficulty in swallowing (dysphagia) and pain on swallowing (odynophagia) (235,236,249). The pain may be dull or sharp with frequent referred pain to the ear (235). However, the most featured symptom differs between HPV-positive and -negative OPSCCs (251). Patients with HPV-positive OPSCC most frequently complain about the development of a neck mass (51%), followed by a sore throat (28%) and dysphagia (10%), while patients with HPV-negative OPSCC tend to present with a sore throat (53%), followed by dysphagia (41%) and a neck mass (18%) (251).

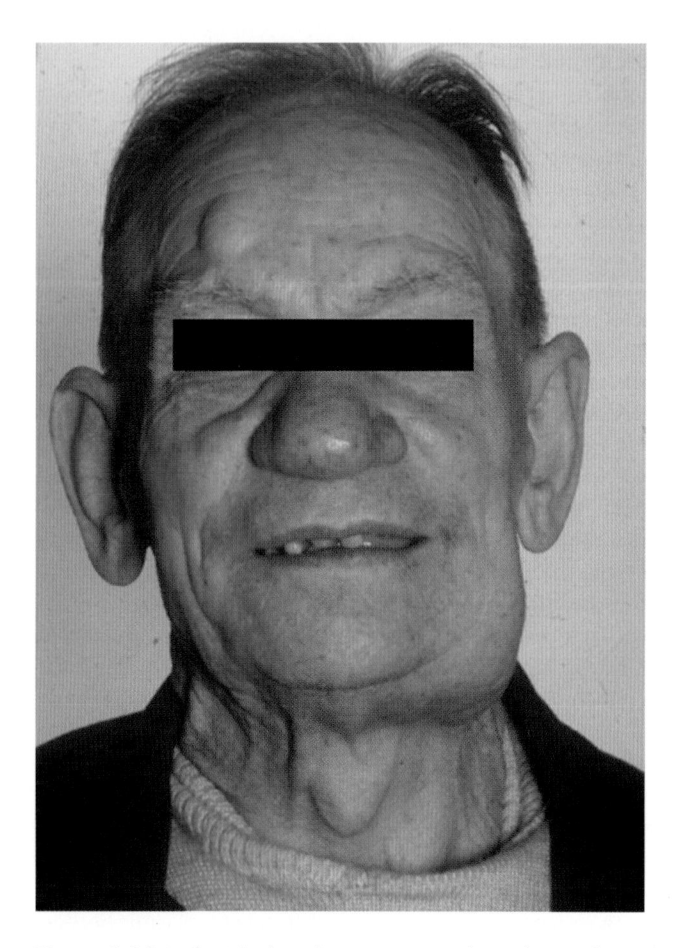

Figure 3.36 Left-sided neck mass in a male with oropharyngeal squamous cell carcinoma.

HPV-related head and neck squamous cell carcinoma (HNSCC) has not been well characterized microscopically. Islands of squamous epithelial cells without keratinization, compared to conventional severe dysplasia, and invasive growth are features of this tumor (252,253). Cells typically lack maturation and display moderate to significant atypia with "koilocytic" features (252–254). HPV-related tumors have characteristic Bowenoid histologic features (resembling Bowen's disease of the skin) described as "basaloid" with diffuse, full-thickness loss of squamous differentiation and a high proliferation index throughout the basal and suprabasal epithelial layers (253,255). Mitotic figures and mitotic-like structures, multinucleated cells, dyskeratotic cells and apoptosis can be seen throughout the thickness of the epithelium (253,255,256). Secondary morphologic features have been described by Westra (248) to include the presence of central necrosis with cystic change, tumor-infiltrating lymphocytes and basaloid features. He adds that surface dysplasia and prominent stromal desmoplasia may also be absent. El-Mofty (257) describes some of the variants in the histological presentation of HPV-related SCC. Quantitative reverse transcriptase polymerase chain reaction for high-risk HPV E6 and E7 mRNA, immunohistochemical staining for p16 (a surrogate marker for transcriptionally active, high-risk HPV infection in OPSCC) and *in situ* hybridization demonstrating the presence of intranuclear HPV-16 DNA are current methods for diagnosing HPV-related OPSCC (249,258).

The T-stage in OPSCC correlates with prognosis and the best opportunity for cure is when the tumors are asymptomatic and small (<2 cm), but visible or palpable, allowing recognition by the examining clinician (251). Most OSCCs and OPSCCs present with tumors <2 cm in size (stage T1) and the presence of symptoms suggests more advanced disease (259,260). These symptoms included pain, referred otalgia, dysphagia, odynophagia and a sore throat. Base of the tongue OPSCC symptoms include a neck mass (25.7%), dysphagia (25%), ear pain (17.6%), a sore tongue (15.4%), a lump on the tongue (11.8%), voice changes (3.7%) and bleeding (0.7%) (261).

MUCOSAL MALIGNANT MELANOMA (ICD-O CODE: 8720/3)

Melanoma is the malignant proliferation of melanocytic or melanocyte precursors from the epithelial–connective tissue interface into the epithelium and the underlying connective tissues (9). Melanoma is the third most common skin cancer and may occur at any site where melanocytes are present. Only 1% of all melanomas involve the mucous membranes of the head and neck, from which 50% arise in the oral cavity (9).

Damage from UV radiation, a fair complexion and sun sensitivity are considered major contributing factors in the pathogenesis of cutaneous melanoma (9). Etiology of oral malignant melanoma, however, is independent of UV radiation and some authors have associated it with other causes such as ill-fitting dentures, betel nut, tobacco, formaldehyde, nevi at traumatic regions and racial pigmentation (262).

Mucosal melanomas usually present approximately a decade later than cutaneous melanomas at the average age of 67 years and, unlike cutaneous melanomas, they have an equal distribution amongst light- and dark-skinned individuals (263). Differences between cutaneous and mucosal melanomas are not limited to epidemiology and the role of UV radiation; an increasing number of reports suggest molecular and biological differences between the two (264). The palate and upper alveolar ridge are the most commonly affected sites, while the tongue is rarely affected. Oral melanomas are usually pigmented (black, brown, gray or purple) (Figure 3.37) and rarely (15%–20% of cases) amelanotic. Typical melanomas progress in a predictable pattern: they start as asymmetric, flat, pigmented lesions with irregular borders that spread laterally within the epithelium to form multiple or widespread areas of macular pigmentation. The macules eventually become nodular as a result of vertical growth (9). Unless the surface is ulcerated, pain is not a common feature of melanoma and, as a result of bone invasion, the underlying bone may present a moth-eaten destruction pattern on radiographic imaging (198). Surgical removal is the treatment of choice for oral malignant melanomas. Due to their long asymptomatic period and the fact that they may be hard to distinguish from the oral mucosa, in 75% of cases, cervical lymph node metastasis has already occurred upon diagnosis (9). A late diagnosis in addition to the aggressive nature of the tumor results in an extremely poor 5-year survival rate as low as 13% (198).

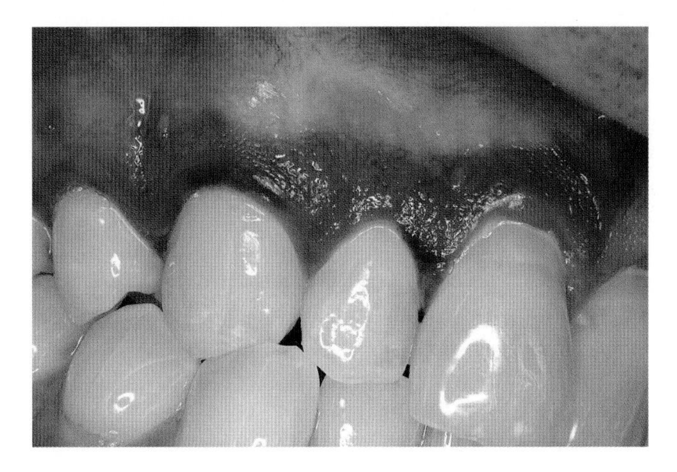

Figure 3.37 Brown and black pigmentation of the labial gingiva in anterior quadrant 1 in a 67-year-old male with biopsy-proven oral malignant melanoma and a past history of melanoma *in situ* excised from the lower back 15 years prior.

KAPOSI SARCOMA (ICD-O CODE: 9140/3)

Kaposi sarcoma was first described in 1872 by Moritz Kaposi as a multiple-pigmented sarcoma of the skin in people of Mediterranean or Jewish origin. It is an unusual and locally aggressive connective tissue neoplasm that most frequently presents as multiple cutaneous patches and nodules, but can also involve the mucous membrane and is commonly noted in the palate (Figure 3.38), lymph nodes and visceral organs. Kaposi sarcoma is uniformly believed to be caused by human herpesvirus 8 and, prior to the advent of AIDS, Kaposi sarcoma was a rare tumor.

Based on clinical presentations, Kaposi sarcomas are classified into four distinct groups: classic, endemic (or African), iatrogenic and AIDS-related. A rare tumor, classic Kaposi sarcoma is predominantly seen in males (10–15 males to 1 female) with an onset age of 50–70 years (265). It involves the lower extremities and has a relatively benign pattern, although almost a third of patients with classic Kaposi sarcoma develop a second malignancy such as non-Hodgkin lymphoma (266,267). African Kaposi sarcoma accounts for 9% of all cancers of Ugandan males (265). It can be as indolent as classic Kaposi sarcoma or present as an aggressive tumor that may invade underlying bone (265). Iatrogenic Kaposi sarcoma is seen in organ recipients (up to 5% of renal transplant patients) and, similar to classic Kaposi sarcoma, it most frequently affects individuals with Jewish and Mediterranean descent (268). AIDS-related Kaposi sarcoma may involve the skin, oral mucosa, lymph nodes and visceral organs.

Kaposi sarcoma is usually the first manifestation of HIV infection; the disease generally progresses in a predictable fashion, starting from a few localized lesions that grow to more numerous lesions that involve the skin, lymph nodes and gastrointestinal tract. The most frequent intraoral site is the palate and the tumor may present as dark purple nodules that bleed easily and resemble oral purpura, pyogenic granuloma or bacillary angiomatosis (177).

Clinical subtype and stage of disease are the most important factors in determining the suitable treatment for Kaposi

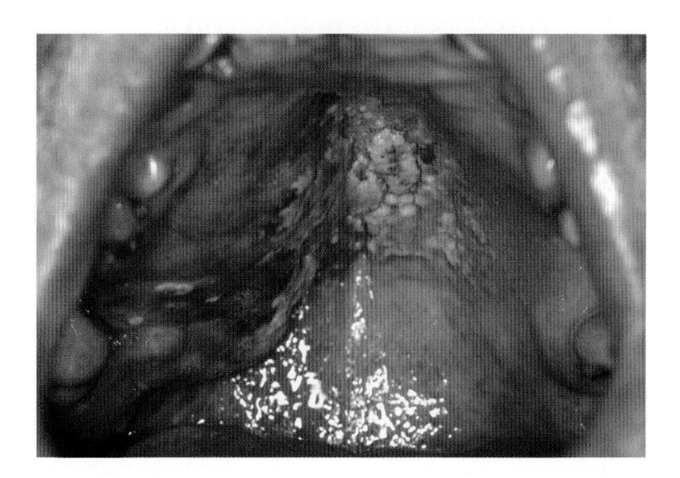

Figure 3.38 Kaposi sarcoma involving the right palate.

sarcoma. While radiation therapy is the treatment of choice for skin lesions, the same treatment for oral lesions may cause severe mucositis (198). Alternative treatments include surgical excision for solitary lesions of the skin or mucosa and systemic chemotherapy.

Prognosis is also highly dependent upon the subtype and the patient's immune status. While patients with the classic form have a mean survival time of 10–15 years, iatrogenic, AIDS-related and most African Kaposi sarcomas are more aggressive and have a poorer prognosis (265).

DIAGNOSTIC APPROACHES

Current clinical practices for the detection and surveillance of oral cancer and potentially malignant disorders are mainly dependent on the clinician's individual experience with conventional oral examination (COE), which involves visual examination and digital palpation of oral tissues under chairside light. If a suspicious lesion is identified, the patient is then referred to a specialist, who may take a biopsy to confirm the diagnosis. Delay in diagnosis has been associated with a poor prognosis, as more advanced cases are often due to poor routine oral examinations (269–271). COE has a low specificity and often fails to detect lesions that lack visible changes. COE also requires special training (272). Opportunistic screening for oral cancer and OPMDs is advocated as part of the patient's routine dental visit. Early detection has shown efficacy in improving the clinical outcomes of OSCC (273). The major challenge for early detection is distinguishing those lesions that have a high risk of developing into malignancy from those with low risk. Extensive research has been undertaken to evaluate some adjunctive tools, devices and techniques for improving the efficacy of early detection of oral cancer, while others remain untested.

IMAGING TECHNIQUES

It has now been established that molecular profiling of tissue changes enable clinicians to "visualize" more of the disease and indeed diagnose altered tissue early. While macroscopic changes may be detected under white light examination and tissue/cell-level changes through histopathology, molecular dysregulation may be identified using special imaging techniques. While most current methods assess tissue in the plane parallel to the lesion, methods aiding assessment in the vertical cross-section (plane perpendicular to the mucosal surface) are required to detect lesions below the mucosal surface and evaluate submucosal tumor invasion (274).

All optical imaging techniques detect and analyze backscattered photons from mucosa (274). Visible light (400–700 nm) is used for conventional white light inspection; however, shorter wavelengths in UV and longer wavelengths in the near-infrared (NIR) regions of the light spectrum can also be used for imaging. UV and blue light are absorbed by biomolecules to produce fluorescence (274). In order to detect targeted tumor cells, the tumor-specific signal must be significantly discriminated from the non-specific background signals, thus optimizing the signal-to-background ratio (SBR) (275). The visible light spectrum has relatively short penetration depths useful for imaging (<100 μm) as it is mostly absorbed by hemoglobin and is significantly associated with a high level of non-specific surrounding signals, resulting in a low SBR (274,275). NIR light is less susceptible to tissue scattering and hemoglobin absorption, yielding penetration depths >1000 μm through the mucosa and a high SBR, with an optical imaging window of about 650–900 nm in which the absorption coefficient is at a minimum (274,275).

Optical imaging techniques using optical fluorescence imaging (OFI) and narrow band imaging (NBI) reflect tissue changes at the microscopic and molecular levels. Optical coherence tomography (OCT) and angle-resolved low-coherence interferometry (a/LCI) non-invasively provide information in the vertical and axial planes. Raman spectroscopy is a point detection technique based on the inelastic scattering of light also enabling molecular histopathological examination. Computed tomography (CT) and magnetic resonance imaging (MRI) are methods traditionally used to detect carcinoma and metastasis (hence staging) and to assess treatment response, providing anatomical and physiological information. Positron emission tomography (PET) is a true form of molecular imaging, opening the door for drug delivery and molecular surgical guidance. Hybrid imaging methods—PET/CT and PET/MRI—offer the best of both these imaging approaches. All these methods, collectively termed "optical biopsy," are non-destructive, *in situ* assays of mucosal histopathologic states using the spectral and spatial properties of scattered light to measure cellular and/or tissue morphology, providing an instantaneous diagnosis (274,276).

REFLECTANCE VISUALIZATION

Reflectance visualization in its simplest and purest form is encountered by use of traditional incandescent or halogen light commonly found in the dental operatory. More recently, there has been increased understanding and acceptance that white light-emitting diode (LED) light is more useful for examination of oral mucosal tissues. This has been adopted either with or without magnification (Figure 3.39) (277,278).

There are two commercially available devices that utilize reflectance visualization in conjunction with an acetic acid mouthwash to improve detection of OPMDs. ViziLite™ (Zila Pharmaceuticals, Phoenix, AZ, USA.) and Microlux/DL™ (AdDent, Danbury, CT, USA.) systems incorporate initial use of an acetic acid mouthwash prior to inspection of the oral cavity using the devices (279,280). The 1% acetic acid mouthwash desiccates cells within the oral mucosa, increasing the nuclear-to-cytoplasmic ratio and altering the refractile properties of OPMDs. Lesions become more

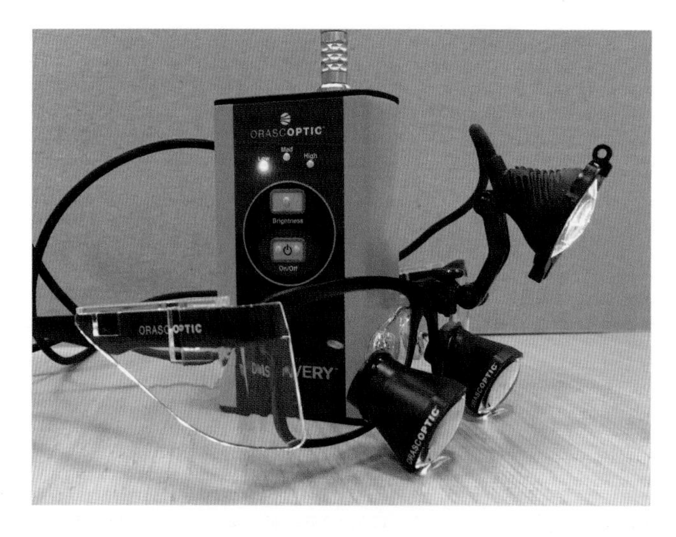

Figure 3.39 White light-emitting diode headlight with 2.5× magnification loupes (Orascoptic™ Discovery™, which can emit either 3,000, 5,000 or 7,000 foot candle of light output at 460 and 555 nm).

visible as they appear "aceto-white" against the normal oral mucosa (277,279,281,282).

VIZILITE™ AND VIZILITE PLUS™

ViziLite™ utilizes a chemiluminescent light stick containing an inner glass vial of hydrogen peroxide and an outer plastic capsule of acetyl salicylic acid to assess the oral cavity (281,283). The updated version, ViziLite Plus™, includes Toluidine blue (TB), which the manufacturers claim enhances the delineation effect of the ViziLite™ system by marking abnormal areas of suspicious lesions (280). TB is a metachromatic, acidophilic dye that selectively stains acidic tissue components such as nucleic acids (284). It has been used for decades as an adjunctive technique for the diagnosis of OSCCs, as well as to delineate the margins and extension of lesions more effectively (285).

Farah and McCullough used ViziLite™ to examine patients referred for assessment of leukoplakic oral mucosal lesions in a specialist oral medicine setting (281). Details such as lesion size, location, ease of visibility and the presence of satellite lesions were recorded during an initial COE and after use of the complete ViziLite™ system. All lesions were biopsied and the presence of OED was considered a positive finding. ViziLite™ did not affect visualization of lesion size or the distinctiveness of margins, and thus did not influence decisions about biopsy site. However, there was one instance where the device aided in the identification of a satellite lesion that was not detected by COE. Conversely, Chainani-Wu et al. conducted a similar protocol on a similar patient cohort and found an 88% reduction in clear margin delineation and a 78% decrease in lesion brightness (286).

Both studies reported that ViziLite™ could not distinguish between malignant and benign lesions, making all appear "aceto-white." Farah et al. interpreted this result as all lesions displaying a ViziLite™-positive result and

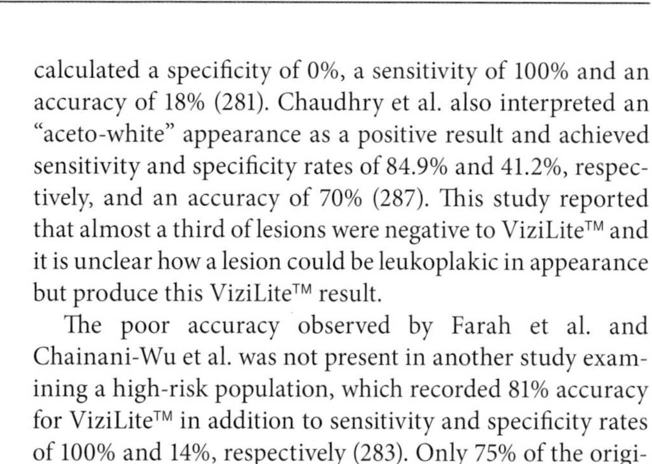

calculated a specificity of 0%, a sensitivity of 100% and an accuracy of 18% (281). Chaudhry et al. also interpreted an "aceto-white" appearance as a positive result and achieved sensitivity and specificity rates of 84.9% and 41.2%, respectively, and an accuracy of 70% (287). This study reported that almost a third of lesions were negative to ViziLite™ and it is unclear how a lesion could be leukoplakic in appearance but produce this ViziLite™ result.

The poor accuracy observed by Farah et al. and Chainani-Wu et al. was not present in another study examining a high-risk population, which recorded 81% accuracy for ViziLite™ in addition to sensitivity and specificity rates of 100% and 14%, respectively (283). Only 75% of the original lesions were biopsied; therefore, the accuracy of these results cannot be determined and this study was given a low quality rating by a subsequent review (288).

Epstein and colleagues assessed 84 patients using ViziLite™ in 2008 (289) and this study methodology was adopted by Mojsa et al. in 2012 (290). Both studies reported increased brightness or sharpness of lesions in 58%–62% of cases. ViziLite™ was only used on lesions visible during COE and both studies noted that sensitivity and specificity were not significant as negative results on initial COE were excluded on ethical grounds.

ViziLite™ has also been utilized to assess erythroplakic and erythroleukoplakic lesions in a study by Awan and colleagues (291). The device demonstrated reduced efficacy for the detection of lesions of this type compared to leukoplakic lesions (281,283), with sensitivity and specificity findings of 77% and 27%, respectively. Only 75% of lesions assessed in this study were detected, enhanced or appeared aceto-white during examination using the ViziLite™ system. This study was the first to acknowledge that use of the acetic acid mouthwash increased salivary flow, which enhanced mucosal reflectance and hindered delineation of lesion margins. As expected, Awan et al. concluded that ViziLite™ could not discriminate between low- and high-risk lesions and, as such, vigilant interpretation of the results of ViziLite™ examination is required (291).

ViziLite™ has also been assessed in two opportunistic screening studies that utilized OralCDx® brush biopsy for evaluation of lesions that could not be diagnosed clinically (292,293). Following initial COE, Oh and Laskin re-examined patients using incandescent light and the acetic acid solution followed by examination using both the solution and the light component of the ViziLite™ system (292). The lesions detected at each stage were noted, as well as whether the lesions could be diagnosed clinically. Use of the acetic acid rinse in conjunction with incandescent light alone detected 12 new lesions and the addition of the ViziLite™ light did not detect any further lesions. Thirty-two lesions could not be diagnosed clinically and were submitted to OralCDx® and of these only two returned atypical results, but proved to be benign following scalpel biopsy.

Huber et al. conducted COE followed by examination using the complete ViziLite™ system (293). The majority of lesions were clinically diagnosed as linea alba and leukoedema and were accentuated by ViziLite™. Two out of 14 lesions clinically diagnosed as frictional irritation were amplified by ViziLite™ and the provisional diagnoses of all lesions were confirmed *via* OralCDx®. The authors noted one instance of an amplified lesion in a high-risk patient that displayed cellular atypia following scalpel biopsy, as well as another lesion only detected by ViziLite™ that returned a result of mild atypia following evaluation with OralCDx®.

Finally, subjective comparisons of lesion size, discreteness and sharpness have been used to assess the efficacy of ViziLite™ for visualizing oral mucosal lesions (294,295). Epstein and colleagues conducted COE and examinations using ViziLite™ on patients with a history of mucosal lesions or newly detected lesions (294). ViziLite™ failed to detect three lesions and of these two were erythroplakic but not suspicious of malignancy, while histology confirmed the third as OLP. Two lesions were only visible following ViziLite™ examination, but only one was biopsied and confirmed to be recurrent OSCC. The second was clinically determined to be benign. The device improved the brightness of 54% of lesions, 40% had more distinct borders and 36% had a more defined texture when using the device. An increase in size was noted in 15% of lesions, although the difference in lesion size was not statistically significant.

Kerr and colleagues conducted COE followed by ViziLite™ examination in high-risk patients (295). Examination with ViziLite™ resulted in visual enhancement of 61% of lesions clinically determined to be suspicious compared to 6% of non-suspicious lesions. The study established that the appearance, size, location and type of lesion determined if it would be detected by ViziLite™, with red lesions the least likely to be detected. As expected, the study concluded that ViziLite™ resulted in a significant increase in the sharpness of lesions, but differences in lesion brightness and texture were not statistically significant.

The literature indicates that ViziLite™ cannot differentiate between malignant, premalignant or benign lesions (281,291), but is capable of improving the visibility of lesions (289,290,294,295). Studies involving larger cohorts of participants and with uniform histopathological correlation are required before the device can be recommended as an adjunctive method for early detection.

MICROLUX™/DL

Microlux™/DL (Figure 3.40) consists of a battery-powered LED transilluminator that produces diffuse light (279). Thus far, two studies have been undertaken to assess Microlux™/DL using similar protocols.

Farah and colleagues assessed the efficacy of Microlux™/DL in the visualization of oral mucosal lesions using a previously published methodology (281) with the addition of examination under a LED head light prior to the use of the acetic mouth rinse (277). Microlux™/DL produced an 81% increase in the percentage of lesions with distinct borders and a 64% improvement in the visibility of lesions. Use of the acetic acid component provided further enhancement

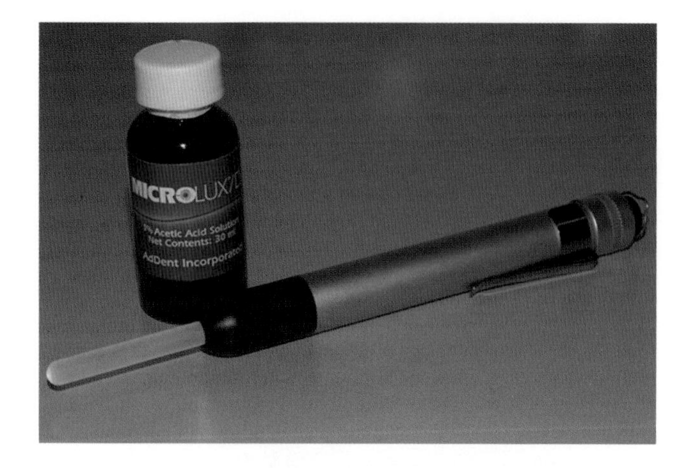

Figure 3.40 Battery-operated intraoral light-emitting diode Microlux™/DL (AdDent, Danbury, CT, USA.) with trans-illuminator attachment emits diffused light at 460 and 555 nm.

in 12% of cases, but had no effect on lesion size, choice of biopsy site or detection of satellite lesions. The authors found that an LED head light provided further enhanced visibility and border distinctness and a more intense white light than the Microlux™/DL, with and without the use of the acetic acid mouthwash (277). The device had a sensitivity of 78% and a specificity of 71% for the detection of dysplasia.

These results are different from the findings of a parallel cohort study involving screening of participants with a history of smoking by oral medicine specialists and general dentists (296). Using the protocol set by Farah and colleagues in 2007 (281), Microlux™/DL provided statistically significant improvement in lesion visibility and border distinctness when compared to COE and displayed sensitivity and specificity rates for the detection of dysplasia of 100% and 39.4%, respectively. Ibrahim et al. also reported that Microlux™/DL subjectively enhanced lesion visibility and uncovered new lesions, but did not alter the chosen biopsy site or provisional diagnosis (296).

The results of both studies indicate that Microlux™/DL provides a poor indication of the underlying pathology of lesions and does not provide any additional benefit to oral examinations beyond improved lesion visibility and border distinctness.

Farah et al.'s study (281) was also the first to demonstrate that white light provides superior visibility of oral mucosal lesions compared to incandescent lighting and supports the use of a white light source during oral mucosal examination (Figure 3.41a and b).

It should be noted that despite strict manufacturer instructions regarding the use of the acetic acid mouthwashes with both ViziLite™ and Microlux™/DL, Farah and colleagues found no evidence that rinsing with acetic acid enhanced visualization of oral lesions on inspection with Microlux™/DL (281). This is reportedly the same with the ViziLite™ system (Farah, unpublished observation). This then begs the question as to the usefulness and cost-effectiveness of incorporation of the acetic acid rinses with these systems.

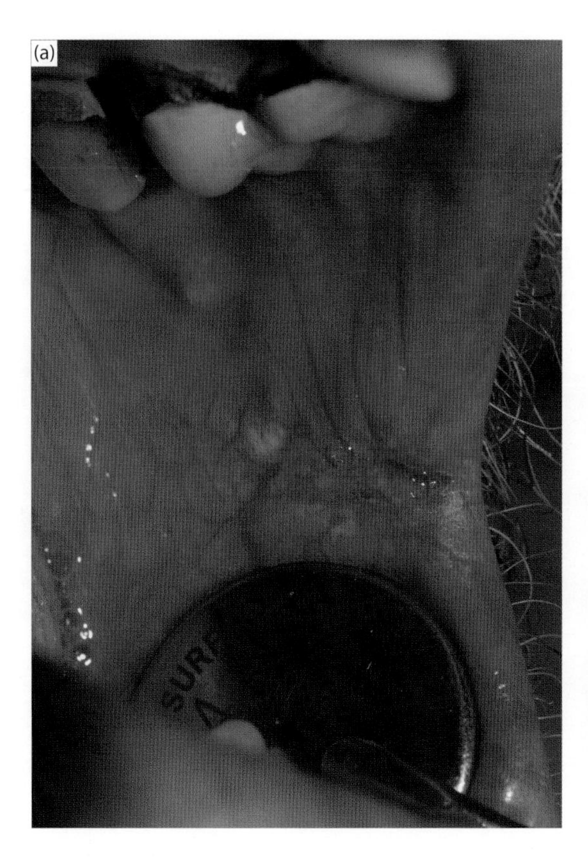

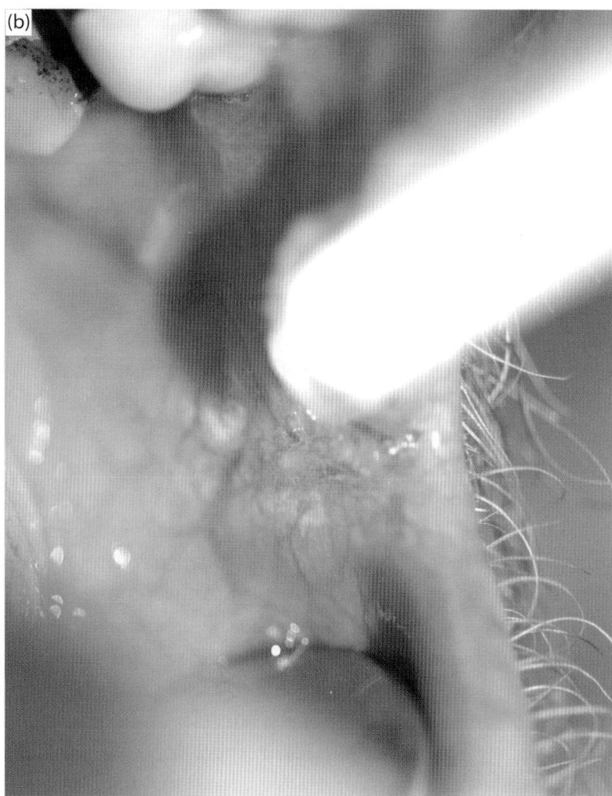

Figure 3.41 Chronic hyperplastic candidosis on left buccal commissure visualized without **(a)** and with **(b)** Microlux™/DL (AdDent, Danbury, CT, USA.) diffused light source.

OPTICAL FLUORESCENCE IMAGING

The basis of optical imaging techniques is the ability of photons to travel through tissue and interact with tissue components (297). Fluorescence is the property of certain molecules to absorb light at a particular wavelength and to emit light of a longer wavelength after a brief interval called the fluorescence lifetime (297). Fluorescence spectroscopy, a major form of optical imaging, is a non-invasive diagnostic tool that evaluates the biochemical composition and structure of tissue autofluorescence (AF) (298). It is relatively simple, fast and accurate and can aid in real-time cancer detection (298). While microscopic imaging systems for intraoperative surgical margin assessment based on endogenous contrast or AF are useful, high resolution of the diseased tissue is limited to a small field of view, making it difficult to survey the entire surgical excision margin intraoperatively (299). Extrinsic approaches are more effective, which use fluorescent dyes detected by probes (299). The signals can also be integrated into the white light image, which enables real-time intraoperative visualization (299).

OFI is advantageous and convenient as it can be used intraoperatively for surgical guidance in resecting malignant tissue and for pathological sampling (300). Various devices implementing OFI, both commercially available as well as those developed by researchers, using visible light or NIR light and with or without excitable dyes, have been investigated, mostly in breast cancer (300,301), but are now being tested in HNSCC as well (302–310).

Assessment of mucosal AF properties involves illumination of the tissue using the visible light spectrum. This causes absorption of a portion of the photons by molecules within the tissue called fluorophores (311) located in the epithelial layer, such as nicotinamide adenine dinucleotide (NADH) and flavin adenine dinucleotide (FAD), or the stroma, such as elastin and collagen cross-links (312). The fluorophores then emit lower-energy photons that can be detected from the mucosal surface as fluorescence (311).

The presence of disease can alter the absorption properties of tissue due to changes in blood concentration or nuclear size distribution. Changes in epithelial thickness, such as epithelial hyperplasia, can limit the fluorescence signal produced by the strongly fluorescent collagen layer and these lesions will display loss of AF (LAF) (313).

Malignant lesions display reduced fluorescence due a reduction in the number of collagen and elastin cross-links present, as well as altered concentrations of FAD or an imbalance between fluorescent NADH and non-fluorescent NAD+. This affects the distribution and concentration of fluorophores within the epithelium and stroma and influences the ability of the epithelium to emit fluorescence after stimulation with an excitation light (311,313–316).

Preliminary research indicated that AF was a suitable adjunct to COE in the early detection of OSCC and OPMDs

(306,311,316–318). This technology has now been incorporated in two adjunctive devices aimed at early detection of OPMDs and OSCCs.

Francisco et al. (298) recently showed that fluorescence spectroscopy could discriminate between oral mucosa, injury, margins and areas of recurrence using a homemade fluorescence spectroscopy system at a wavelength of 406 nm (298) without using injectable dyes, providing macroscopic visualization of affected and unaffected tissue.

The Visually Enhanced Lesion Scope (VELscope™), Identafi® and others are commercially available tools that use the principles of AF and tissue reflectance to discriminate between normal and abnormal tissue. These tools are described below in order to illustrate LAF and diascopic fluorescence as indicators of tissue change, which provide the clinician with additional information aiding diagnosis. Miyamoto et al. investigated intraoperative molecular imaging (multispectral fluorescence images) to identify tumor extensions in a murine HNC model (319). They reported 86% sensitivity and 100% specificity in the diagnostic accuracy analysis compared to histology, the gold standard. They also reported a 60-day improvement in survival rate when using molecular imaging during surgery compared to standard surgery (37% versus 5%, respectively). Thus, fluorescence can be used both for diagnosis and for surgical guidance to improve patient outcomes.

VELSCOPE™ AND VELSCOPE® VX

The VELscope™ (Figure 3.42) and the updated, cordless, handheld VELscope® Vx (LED Medical Diagnostics, Inc., Vancouver, BC, Canada) (Figure 3.43) are intended for use by trained clinicians to enhance oral mucosal abnormalities under direct tissue AF (320). The VELscope™ was developed in partnership between LED Medical Diagnostics, Inc., and the British Columbia Cancer Agency, a system marketed as an extraoral device that utilizes a blue light of 400–460 nm in wavelength to view oral tissues. The blue light causes normal tissues to fluoresce bright green whereas abnormal tissue appears dark (321).

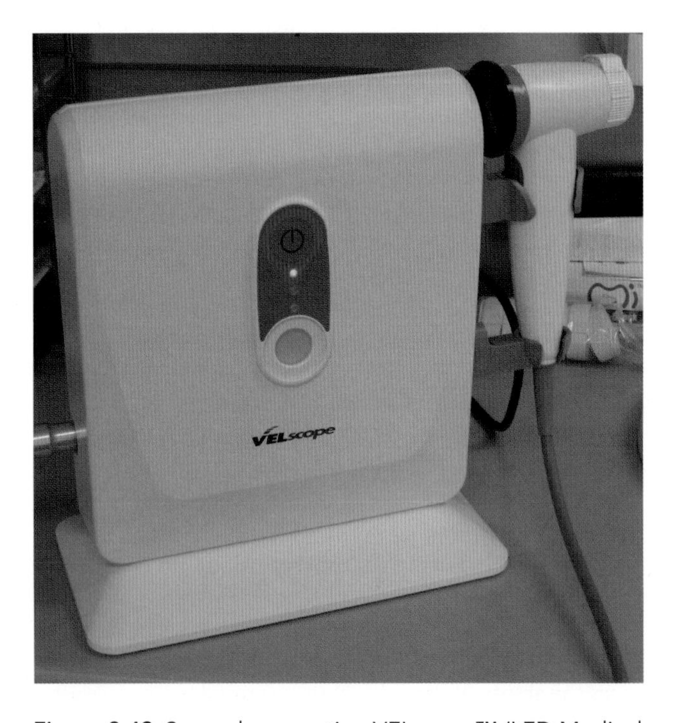

Figure 3.42 Second-generation VELscope™ (LED Medical Diagnostics, Inc., Vancouver, Canada) with fixed cord handset.

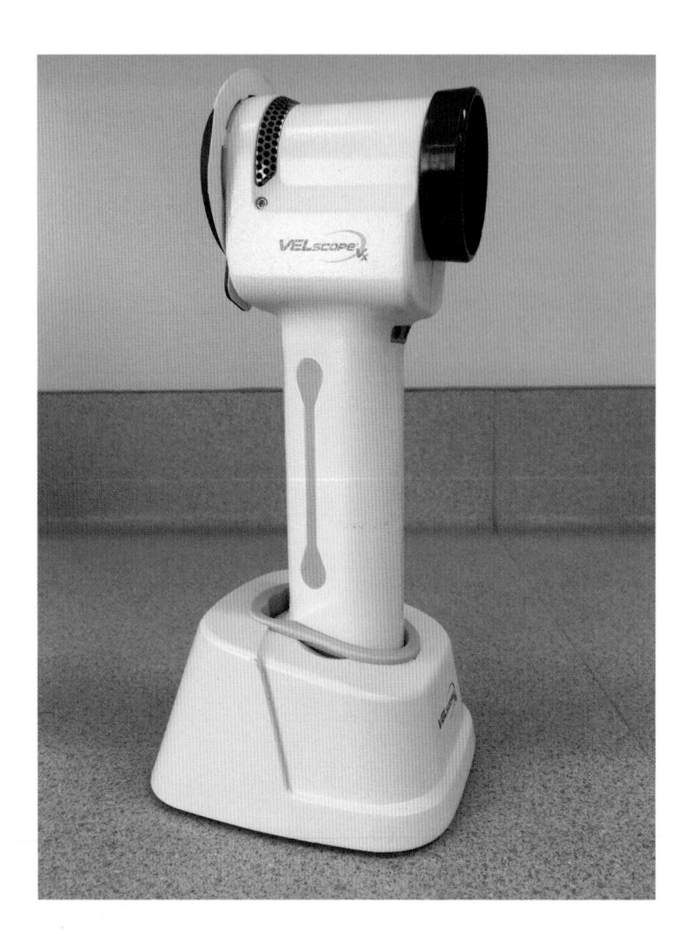

Figure 3.43 Third-generation cordless rechargeable handheld VELscope® Vx (LED Medical Diagnostics, Inc., Vancouver, Canada) which emits blue light at 400–460 nm. The visualization filter is embedded in the handset of the extraoral device.

An external light source, in this case blue light excitation between 400 and 460 nm, is used to excite endogenous fluorophores (typically NADH and FAD) in the oral epithelium and collagen cross-links in the underlying stroma, which absorb the extrinsic photons and emit lower-energy photons that appear clinically as fluorescence (311–314,322,323). Since each fluorophore is associated with specific excitation and emission wavelengths, changes in tissue architecture and concentrations of fluorophores (as in the case of mucosal abnormalities and neoplastic development) result in altered absorption and scattering properties of the tissue (320), with decreased tissue AF being reported in OED and mucosal inflammation (309,314,324). Under the

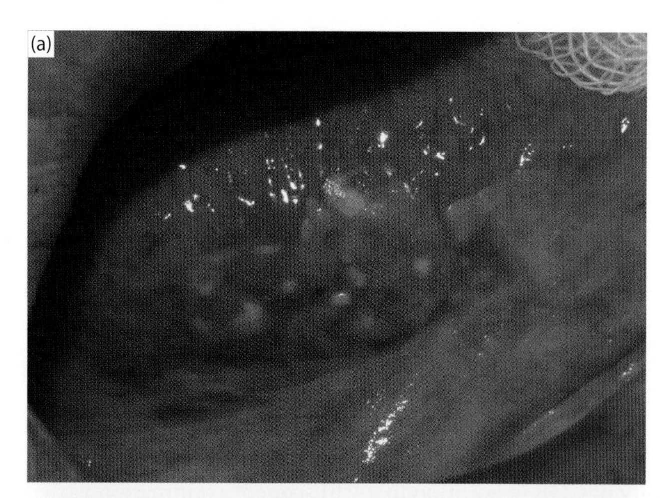

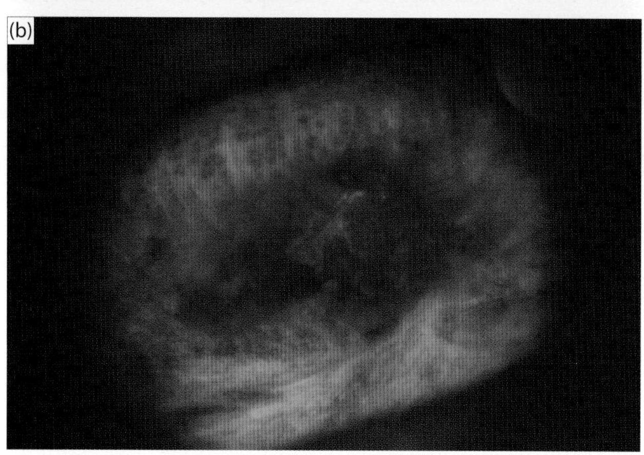

Figure 3.44 Speckled erythroleukoplakia on right lateral tongue as shown in Figure 3.3 visualized under normal incandescent operatory light **(a)** and with VELscope™ **(b)**. Under incandescent light, the lesion displays a diffuse margin. Under VELscope™, normal tissue fluoresces green, while the abnormal tissue displays loss of fluorescence with a well-defined border delineating the true extension of the lesion. Lesion was biopsy-proven oral squamous cell carcinoma.

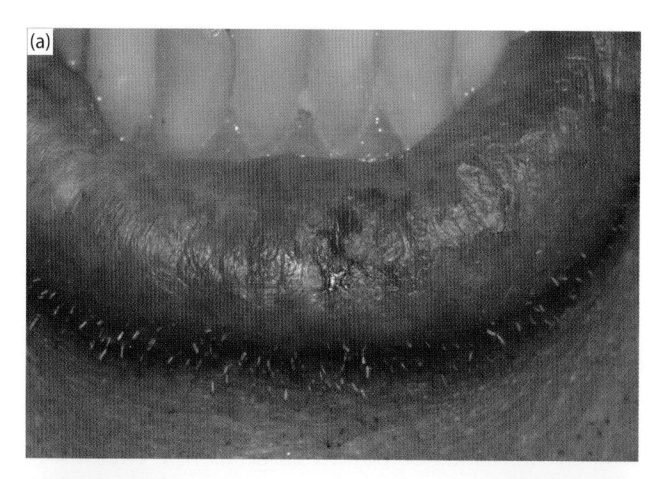

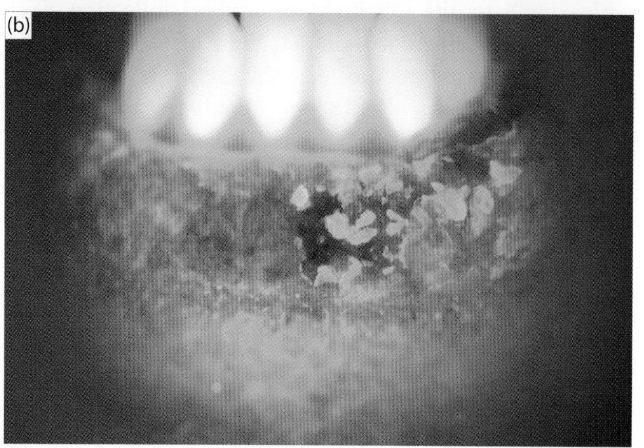

Figure 3.45 Actinic cheilitis on lower lip presenting as areas of ulceration and crusting visualized with normal incandescent operatory light **(a)** and with VELscope™ **(b)**. Note the loss of fluorescence of the ulcerated area and the gain of fluorescence of the keratotic tissue.

VELscope™, normal oral mucosa appears pale green when viewed under a filter, while abnormal tissue exhibits LAF and appears dark (Figure 3.44a and b). Hyperkeratosis, which is commonly seen when involving oral tissues, appears bright green/white and displays gain of fluorescence (Figure 3.45a and b).

While the VELscope™ has assisted in the detection of OED and OSCC not visible by COE, warranting tissue biopsy and aiding in demarcating margins (309,325), clinicians have been advised to use the VELscope™ in conjunction with COE, as LAF may also be displayed in tissues with mucosal inflammation (326). Complete diascopic fluorescence, wherein tissues display normal fluorescence patterns with the application of pressure, can differentiate inflammatory lesions from neoplastic lesions (326). However, the challenge of completely blanching tissues and interoperator variation in the interpretation of partial blanching (i.e. low specificity and variable sensitivity) grades the VELscope™ as a useful clinical tool for clinically visualizing abnormalities, but not an accurate discriminator of the condition of the mucosa under inspection (326). Nevertheless, a recent clinical study suggested that the use of a decision-making protocol incorporating the VELscope™ in routine general dental practice allows for the detection of additional oral mucosal lesions requiring specialist referral (327).

The efficacy of the VELscope™ has been extensively assessed at a specialist level in high-risk patient groups. One of these studies found that 81% of areas displaying LAF histologically displayed benign features, although LAF was significantly associated with OED and OSCC compared to normal tissue (328). The sensitivity and specificity rates of the device in detecting moderate to severe OED or OSCC were 100% and 80%, respectively. The authors acknowledged that differentiating between LAF and diminished fluorescence was related to the experience of the user, who in this study were surgeons experienced in using the device. These results are similar to the findings of another single-blind study also examining a high-risk group using both COE and VELscope™ (329). Biopsies were conducted on the basis of COE alone, VELscope™ examination alone or both techniques. VELscope™ displayed a sensitivity of 92% and a specificity of 77%, whereas COE displayed sensitivity and specificity rates of 62% and 88%, respectively.

Awan and colleagues achieved different results evaluating VELscope™ in a population selected on the basis of having mucosal lesions requiring biopsy (330). VELscope™ displayed sensitivity and specificity rates for detection of OED of 84% and 15%, respectively. The study concluded that the device was unable to discriminate between high- and low-risk lesions, although it could confirm the presence of leukoplakia and erythroplakia, as well as other mucosal lesions.

Hanken et al. conducted a single-blind study and found that, in the hands of trained surgeons, the addition of VELscope™ to the examination process following COE increased the sensitivity for detection of OED/OSCC by 22%, but decreased the specificity by 8.4% (331). There were also 13 cases in which VELscope™ could not discriminate between OED and healthy mucosa. They recommended that the device be restricted to use by experienced clinicians and only be used to exclude suspicious lesions, not for mucosal screening by general dentists.

Mehrotra et al. conducted a cross-sectional study assessing the ViziLite™ and VELscope™ systems on lesions displaying innocuous clinical appearance using Sciubba's classification of Class 1 and Class 2 lesions (332,333). ViziLite™ had sensitivity and specificity rates of 0% and 76%, respectively, whereas VELscope™ had a sensitivity of 50% and a specificity of 39%. The poor results could be attributed to the authors' decision to screen only innocuous lesions as they asserted that screening lesions that displayed high levels of clinical suspicion and required immediate biopsy "would be meaningless" (333).

The manufacturer's instructions for VELscope™ include blanching of lesions as part of the examination process. Blanching of lesions allows for evaluation of diascopic fluorescence, which refers to cases in which lesions display LAF, but regain complete fluorescence of all areas of the lesion under application of pressure (Figure 3.46a–h). This phenomenon highlights the absorptive features of hemoglobin associated with edema and inflammation, which can mimic LAF (334). Despite the importance of this step, only three studies have incorporated blanching of lesions as part of the examination process (326,327,335).

In the first study, Farah and colleagues examined patients selected on the basis of having leukoplakic, erythroplakic or erythroleukoplakic lesions that required evaluation by an oral medicine specialist (326). Patients with known cases of OSCC or OED were excluded. COE was conducted in accordance with previous publications (277,281). The results of COE were used to group lesions into categories such as homogeneous leukoplakia, non-homogeneous leukoplakia, lesions with lichenoid features and other lesions such as chronic hyperplastic candidosis. The second was a cross-sectional study that featured a similar patient cohort to that reported by Farah et al. with the addition of randomization of the participants into COE or VELscope™ examination groups (335). In this study, Rana et al. attempted to reduce the incidence of false-positive findings by incorporating blanching of lesions into the examination process as well as reviewing lesions of suspected acute inflammatory origin after 2 weeks.

Farah and colleagues calculated an accuracy of 69% for COE and 55% for VELscope™ alone. Qualitative data indicated that VELscope™ enhanced the visualization of 35% of lesions and uncovered five clinically undetected lesions, one of which displayed moderate OED. There were no differences noted regarding border distinctness or visibility between benign lesions and OED. VELscope™ examination resulted in a change of biopsy site in four cases and a change in provisional diagnosis in 22 cases. The combined sensitivity of COE in addition to a VELscope™ examination varied significantly, with Farah et al. determining 46% sensitivity, while Rana and colleagues established 100% sensitivity. Both studies criticized the diagnostic value of diascopic fluorescence, with Farah et al. noting that of the 38 lesions that displayed diascopic fluorescence there were 10 cases of OED and one OSSC, indicating that blanching cannot rule out malignancy.

It is apparent that success using VELscope™ requires operator experience, careful interpretation and consideration of the results of COE as even lesions that display retained AF or diascopic fluorescence may be dysplastic (326,335).

The sample populations assessed in the previous studies could have overstated the positive predictive value of the device (336) and, as such, evaluation of VELscope™ at a general practitioner level is vital (337,338). A parallel cohort study assessing COE and VELscope™ in a general practice setting established a 0.83% prevalence of mucosal abnormalities using COE, none of which were OPMDs, and a 1% prevalence of mucosal abnormalities using VELscope™, of which 83% were OPMDs (339). OralCDx® brush biopsy or liquid-based brush cytology were performed on the eight lesions detected by COE and 12 lesions detected using VELscope™ as these lesions could not be diagnosed clinically as benign. Two of the eight lesions detected by COE initially displayed mild atypia but were later confirmed as pigmentation and hyperkeratosis. Conversely, all 12 lesions detected using VELscope™ displayed abnormal cells and subsequent histology confirmed the presence of OED in 10 cases. Another opportunistic screening study focused on lesions detected by VELscope™ that were not visible during COE (340). Areas of LAF reported as normal during COE were noted in 69 patients. Assessment of normal variations in tissue characteristics were used to exclude 41 cases; however, blanching was not utilized as a diagnostic criterion and, as such, false-positive findings due to inflammation-induced LAF were not eliminated. Five patients consented to immediate biopsy and four patients had areas of persistent LAF biopsied at a 2-week review. Five cases of mild to moderate OED were noted as well as two cases of OLP and two inflammatory lesions.

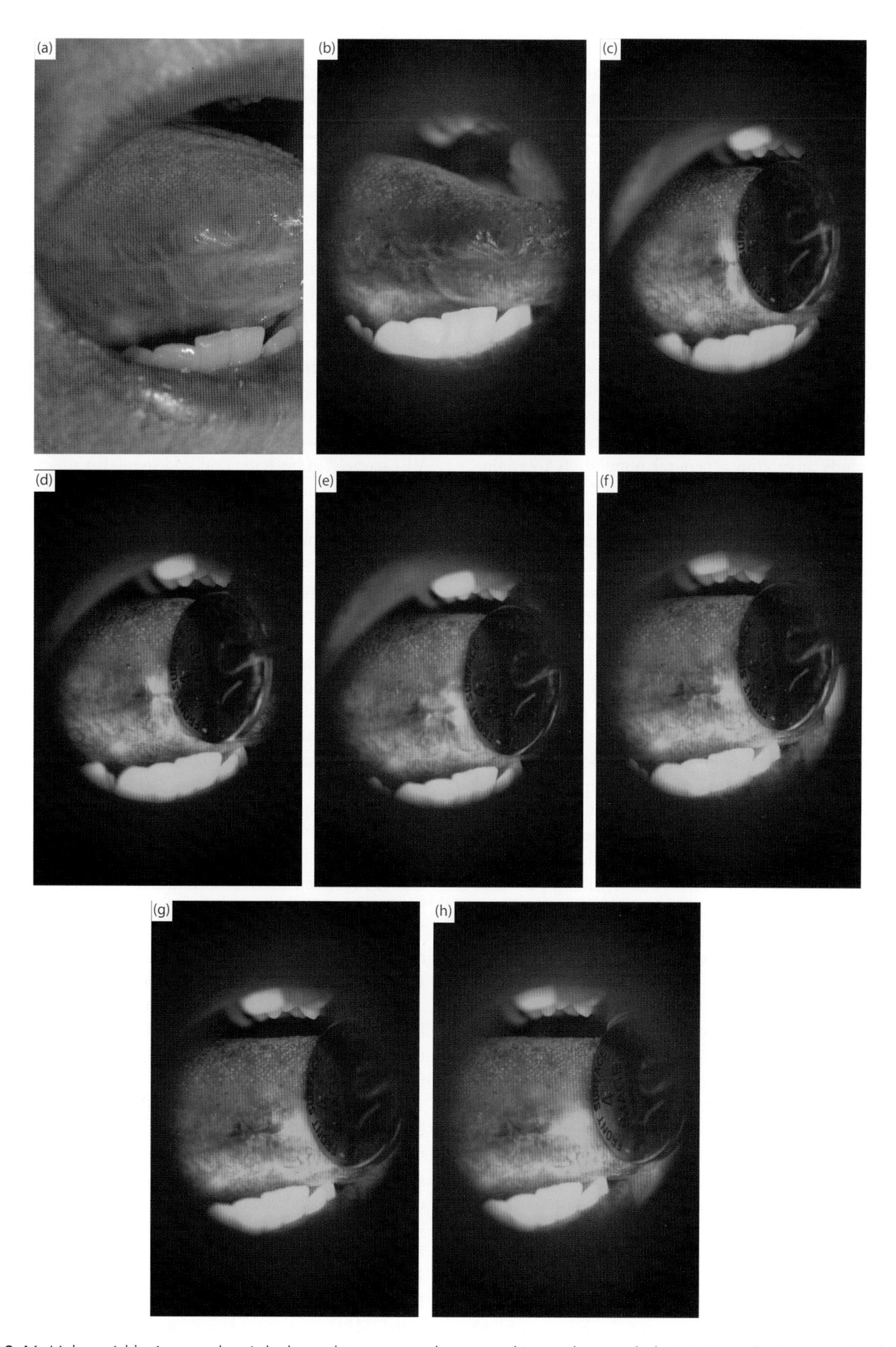

Figure 3.46 Lichenoid lesion on the right lateral tongue under normal incandescent light **(a)**. Same lesion visualized with VELscope™ demonstrating diffuse loss of fluorescence and ill-defined borders **(b)**. Application of blanching with mirror head demonstrates complete regain of green fluorescence under pressure (diascopic fluorescence) over entire length of lesion **(c–h)**. Lesion was biopsy-proven oral lichen planus with no epithelial dysplasia.

Only two general population studies assessing VELscope™ have calculated sensitivity and specificity rates for the device. In one study, all lesions detected by VELscope™ were also visible using COE and all lesions displaying LAF upon 2-week review were biopsied (341). Only two of the 32 samples taken were positive for malignancy or dysplasia and sensitivity and specificity rates were calculated at 67% and 6%, respectively; one of the poorest results for VELscope™ thus far. Clearly, the presence of LAF needs to be evaluated in conjunction with the results of COE to identify and eliminate obvious false-positive findings and prevent patient harm through unnecessary biopsies.

Thus far, the limitations of current studies assessing VELscope™ are the use of high-risk populations that could overestimate the positive predictive value of the device and the lack of inclusion of diascopic fluorescence as an assessment criterion. Bhatia et al. have addressed this in a screening study involving a general population to evaluate an algorithm for the use of VELscope™ to reduce the incidence of false-positive findings (327). Utilizing a similar protocol to Farah et al. (326), the results of diascopic fluorescence were used to determine if lesions required follow-up with an oral medicine specialist based on the VELscope™ findings alone and the combined results of COE and VELscope™. Lesions that displayed LAF were photographed and reviewed at 2 weeks and a decision was made to refer based on the results of COE, VELscope™ and a combined examination result. Lesions that displayed partial blanching were recommended for referral to the oral medicine specialist. Following a protocol of reviewing lesions to exclude trauma and including analyses of the results of diascopic fluorescence and COE removed a large proportion of over-referrals that cause unnecessary patient stress and unnecessary biopsies, which cause patient harm. Combining the results of COE and VELscope™ also increased the positive predictive value and specificity rate from 15% and 54% for VELscope™ alone to 81% and 97.9% for COE and VELscope™, respectively.

VELscope™ is intended for use by suitably qualified, trained clinicians. Ayoub et al. have undertaken the only study involving examination of high-risk patients entirely by hygienists trained in the use of the device (342). Although 30 patients with a history of heavy smoking were examined, no lesion was found using either examination method.

The manufacturers of VELscope™ claim that it can also be used to ascertain biopsy margins for suspicious lesions. Elvers et al. evaluated this claim by using VELscope™ to analyze the margins of 26 oral leukoplakic lesions (343). Three punch biopsies were taken for each lesion: the center of the lesion, 2.5 mm from the clinically visible borders of the lesion and from an adjacent area that was normal clinically using COE and VELscope™. Lesions were divided into two groups on the basis of the presence of AF surrounding the lesion. None of the lesions displayed underlying OED; therefore, the study was only able to establish that LAF can be used to detect mucosal inflammation that extends beyond the clinically visible borders of a lesion, not just OED.

The literature indicates that VELscope™ cannot differentiate between high- and low-risk lesions (326,330,335,340,341) and that interpretation of the results achieved using VELscope™ is dependent on the experience of the clinician (326,328). Furthermore, its usefulness seems to currently be centered on the examination of high-risk patients with suspicious oral mucosal lesions in a specialist setting. Farah even noted in his closing remarks on this device that perhaps it was potentially more suited in a specialist oral cancer clinic instead of a general dental or medical practice, although further studies were indicated in this context (326). Clearly, further studies assessing the efficacy of VELscope™ by general dentists and in a general population are required before the effectiveness and clinical significance of this device can be fully established.

Given the wide range of studies examining the utility of VELscope™ in both general and specialist practice and the variability in sensitivity and specificity of the device compared to either COE or the presence of OED on histopathological assessment, there is a need for a clinically defined protocol that will provide clinicians with more certainty in using the device, given its widespread use despite the variability noted. Farah and colleagues were the first to test such a clinical protocol in the form of a decision-making protocol in general dental practice (327). The study recruited 305 patients to determine the value of VELscope™ as an adjunct to COE in a general dental practice setting. The devised clinical protocol featured five steps: (1) background and risk assessment; (2) COE; (3) VELscope™ examination; (4) combined examination; and (5) review appointment. The study makes major contributions to the understanding of VELscope™ and its use. The results confirm that using VELscope™ alone for screening patients in routine general dental practice has overestimated the burden of significant oral mucosal abnormalities and has resulted in over-referral. The devised clinical protocol, with particular emphasis on careful clinical interpretation and reviewing lesions where appropriate helped in reducing the number of unnecessary referrals that may occur if relying on LAF alone. This study has also shown that VELscope™ may aid in the detection of underlying tissue dysplasia, which may not be identified by COE alone (327).

Farah and colleagues have extended their work on fluorescence visualization and conducted an interesting study that examined molecular profiling using RNA next-generation sequencing for three different histopathological groups of oral lesions visualized under direct tissue AF (344). It was the first report on the identification of candidate genes involved in LAF and diascopic fluorescence (DF) patterns in OPMDs. By excluding OSCC samples and by using supervised differential expression analysis, the authors were able to segregate OMPD specimens based on fluorescence patterns (loss of AF versus retained fluorescence). Their data showed that LAF in oral epithelial hyperplasia is mostly due to changes in inflammation, cell cycle regulation and apoptosis pathways, while in OED, this is due to inflammation, angiogenesis and extracellular matrix (ECM) remodeling. Furthermore, AF has a higher sensitivity for high-grade dysplasia compared to low-grade dysplasia (344).

Although not within the scope of this chapter, it is noteworthy to comment on the utility of VELscope™ in assisting with the determination of surgical margins. One study in oral cancer patients showed that all their tumor samples (confirmed by histopathology) had displayed LOH intraorally when a simple handheld device, similar to a VELscope™ was used (309). Molecular analysis in this study on margins with low-grade or no dysplasia showed a significant association between LAF samples and LOH at 3p and/or 9p, which is strongly associated with tumor recurrence after tumor removal (309). Furthermore, this study found that LAF extended beyond the clinical visible lesion and these areas displayed dysplasia/cancer on histology and/or genetic alterations associated with molecular risk, thus showing that the VELscope™ can distinguish between dysplasia and normal oral mucosa (309). In a more recent report by the same research group, using the VELscope™ handheld device for fluorescence visualization of the resected tumor margins significantly improved the locoregional recurrence and survival rates of T1 or T2 OSCCs (345). However, this study has limitations due to its retrospective nature.

IDENTAFI®

The Identafi® (DentalEZ, PA,USA) (Figure 3.47) is a multispectral screening device that uses direct fluorescence as well as tissue reflectance to visualize intraoral tissues by incorporating three different lights that are to be used sequentially (320,346). In addition to an LED white light, the device also includes violet and green–amber lights to induce tissue fluorescence and reflectance, respectively. The white light enables superior visualization of oral tissues but cannot differentiate between OPMLs and other more

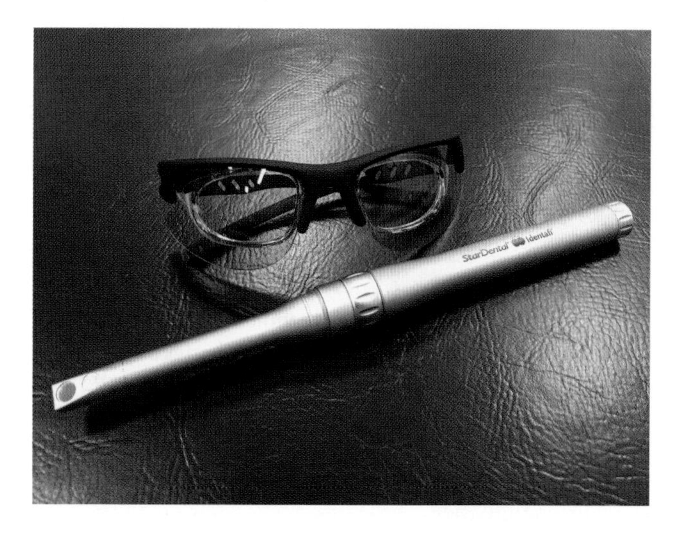

Figure 3.47 Second-generation intraoral Identafi® (DentalEZ, PA, USA.) multispectral device with pink-colored filter glasses worn by the operator for visualization of lesions under violet light emitted at 405 nm.

benign abnormalities of the oral mucosa, in a manner similar to that displayed by Microlux™/DL (320,347,348). The high-intensity white light can be used during initial oral examination and the inclusion of this feature is supported by existing evidence that white light produces superior visualization of mucosal lesions compared to incandescent light (277). Lalla et al. have shown that the Identafi® white light can highlight new lesions not seen during COE and provide improved lesion visibility and border distinctness compared to incandescent light (349). COE and Identafi® were utilized by a general dental practitioner to examine 342 patients presenting for routine dental treatment. The Identafi® white light provided enhanced visualization compared to white light in 14 cases and highlighted 15 lesions previously undetected using incandescent light.

A violet light is used to assess the AF properties of oral tissues. The device is accompanied by photosensitive glasses that filter out the violet light, allowing normal mucosa to exhibit natural fluorescence while abnormal tissue appears darker compared to surrounding tissue due to diminished AF properties, in a similar fashion to VELscope™ (320).

Visualization of oral mucosa under violet light (405-nm wavelength) through the accompanying photosensitive filter glasses assesses the AF properties of tissue, with normal mucosa exhibiting natural fluorescence and abnormal tissues displaying LAF in a similar fashion to VELscope™ (Figure 3.48a–c) (320). Despite the dubious sensitivity and specificity of this wavelength of light (311), areas of LAF visualized were often larger than what was clinically visible, which might be due to the visualization of deeper neovascularization and stromal changes that accompany lesion progression, thus having a potential application in the determination of surgical margins for lesion excision (305). Roblyer and colleagues have demonstrated that light of 405-nm wavelength can display high sensitivity and specificity for differentiation of normal and abnormal mucosa, with 96%–100% calculated for sensitivity and 91%–96% for specificity (311). Sweeny and colleagues reported significantly different results when assessing the device on a population with a history of head and neck cancer using COE as a comparison (350).

Eighty-eight patients were recruited and 17 lesions were identified using the device, although all lesions were also detected by COE. Nine of the 17 lesions underwent biopsy but the histological findings were not explicitly discussed and it was only mentioned that four patients had "positive disease" with no indication whether this was OSCC, OED or the number of lesions these patients had. The study reported that the violet light had a sensitivity of 50% and a specificity of 81%, whereas COE had sensitivity and specificity rates of 50% and 98%, respectively. The white light function of the device was not evaluated and the authors attributed the low sensitivity noted to post-radiation-induced changes, such as fibrosis and pigmentation.

Lane and colleagues have released two papers using samples of a larger database of clinical images from ongoing trials of a prototype of Identafi® (305,351). Clinical images of lesions from a high-risk population were analyzed by

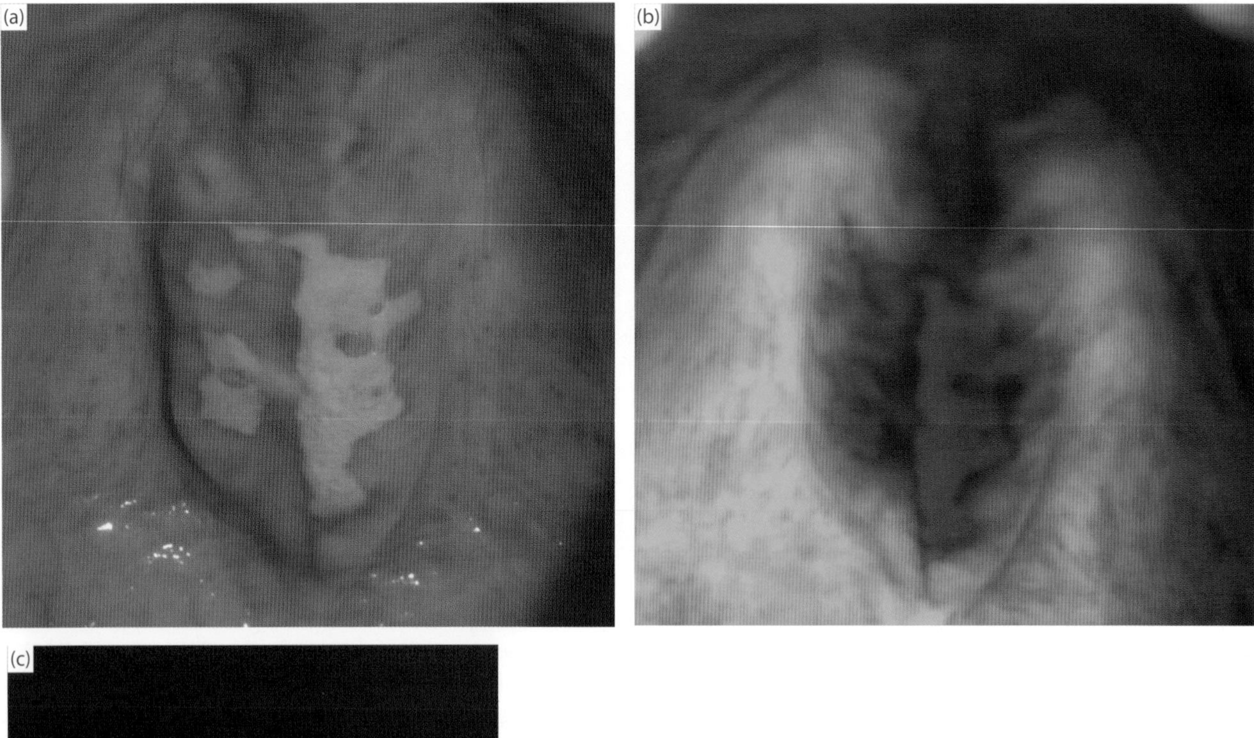

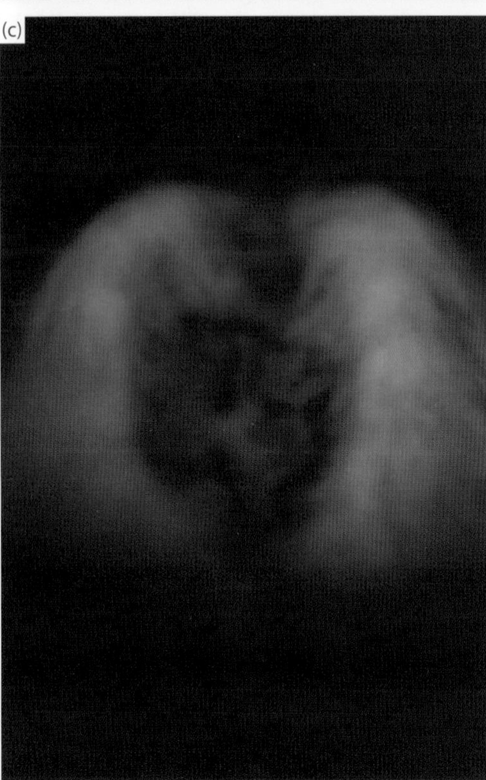

Figure 3.48 Hyperplastic lesion on palatal torus viewed under normal incandescent light **(a)** and VELscope™ demonstrating loss of fluorescence at borders **(b)**. Same lesion viewed with Identafi® violet light and filter **(c)** demonstrates a similar autofluorescence pattern of tissue compared to that of VELscope™, with normal mucosa exhibiting natural blue fluorescence and abnormal tissues displaying maroon loss of fluorescence.

investigators. The larger study aim was to correlate the features noted in the clinical images with histological findings. Early results indicate that the violet 405-nm light aided in identification of characteristics indicative of OSCC and OED and that areas of LAF associated with these lesions were often larger than the clinically visible lesion under COE. This was attributed to visualization of the deeper neovascularization and stromal changes that accompany progression of lesions and it was therefore suggested that the device could assist in delineating the margins of lesions for surgical management.

Lalla et al. (349) noted that the violet light provided only a minimal increase in lesion size and changed the provisional diagnosis in only two cases. This was also the first study to indicate the issues regarding the effect of ambient light on the intensity of the violet light; however, the violet light did detect new lesions, but none of these were suspicious for malignancy.

The green–amber light of 545-nm wavelength utilizes reflectance spectroscopy to delineate the vasculature of the underlying connective tissue (320). The process of carcinogenesis involves angiogenesis, resulting in altered vascular morphology, and it has been suggested that these tissue changes can be used to determine the prognosis of oral lesions, enabling the differentiation between benign lesions and OPMLs (320,352–354). Reflectance spectroscopy uses light within the absorption spectrum of hemoglobin (400–600 nm), which would reflect the degree of angiogenesis in the tissue (334). Significantly reduced reflectance spectra are observed in OSCC and OPMLs due to greater light absorption from the increased microvasculature density and oxygenated hemoglobin content in neoplastic tissue (320). Existing evidence indicates that tumor-induced angiogenesis results in altered vascular morphology and is therefore pertinent in determining the status of oral lesions (353,354). This supports assessment of angiogenesis in OPMDs to increase the efficacy of early detection and to improve the prognosis of these lesions. A significant increase in microvessel count has been associated with the development of OPMDs (353) and the increased microvessel count noted in mild/moderate OED indicates that angiogenesis may be an early step in tumor progression (352–354).

There are significant reductions in the reflectance spectra of OSCCs and OPMDs at 577 and 542 nm, which can be attributed to increased light absorption due to increased microvasculature and oxygenated hemoglobin in these lesions. While other imaging modalities evaluating tissue angiogenesis are available, such as NBI (320), Identafi® is the only commercially available device utilizing tissue reflectance to visualize mucosal vasculature.

Lane et al. found that the green–amber light enhanced the visibility of the surface vasculature and the keratotic features of lesions, making them larger and more visible (305). High-resolution images of lesions illuminated using green–amber light allowed the examiners to visualize vasculature specific to neoplasia. Another study reported 0% sensitivity and 86% specificity compared to COE, although this study had low power and further research is required (350). In addition, taking detailed clinical images using the Identafi® violet and green–amber lights is technique sensitive and retrospective analyses of such detailed clinical images may not be practical in general practice.

Messadi and colleagues have shown that the visibility of increased tissue vasculature using the green–amber light was significantly associated with increased histological vascularity (355). Tissue sections of 25 lesions were treated with endothelial cell marker CD34, which is mainly used to identify positive endothelial cells and to quantify vascularity in tissue sections. These findings were compared to the clinical appearance of tissue vasculature using the green–amber light. This study reported similar clinical findings regarding the enhanced clinical appearance of keratinization using the green–amber light as noted by Lane et al. (351). The authors did comment that increased vascularity was not restricted to OSCC, as hyperkeratotic lesions and OLP also presented with increased clinical vascularity. Despite the association between clinical visibility of lesions using the green–amber light and an underlying increase in microscopic vasculature, the green–amber light appears to provide limited clinical information about oral lesions in a general practice setting. Lalla et al. (349) commented that, following examination of 342 patients using the green–amber light, only 15 lesions were detected, all of which were visible during COE or violet light examination. Identafi® is the most recent development in commercially available oral cancer screening devices, incorporating assessment of tissue AF and tissue reflectance spectroscopy. The manufacturer of Identafi® specifies that the device is intended for use in mucosal screening but further studies are needed.

The underlying principles have enormous potential for application. A clinical study by our group showed excellent lesion visibility compared to COE under incandescent light (349). Violet light examination provided improved lesion visibility compared to COE, improved visualization of lesion borders and a slight increase in lesion size compared to incandescent and white light (Figure 3.49a and b). It also demonstrated a high level of clinical utility for evaluating inflammatory pathology. However, a high level of clinical experience is required to interpret the results of LAF examination, as the violet light displays low sensitivity for detection of OED. The green light helps uncover subtle vascular and inflammatory patterns, providing additional clinical information (Figure 3.50a and b). In the only clinical study designed to assess Identafi® for examining and monitoring patients with oral mucosal lesions in a specialist setting, Lalla et al. demonstrated the value of blanching (diascopy) in differentiating between lesions (348). They found a high correlation between lesion size and measures of lesion visibility ($p = .0001$) and border distinctness ($p = .0001$) using Identafi's white light and the overhead white light source compared to Identafi's violet and green–amber lights. Their findings also showed that non-homogeneous lesions were more likely to display incomplete blanching, whereas lesions with lichenoid features more commonly displayed diascopic fluorescence. Lalla et al. suggested Identafi® has the potential for use as an adjunctive screening device, as it provided intraoral white light visibility of oral mucosal lesions equivalent to the high standard of LED white light and 2.5× magnification used in the study (348).

Other OFI devices are available on the market such as Forward Science's OralID™, AdDent's Bio/Screen® and DenMat's ViziLite® PRO, which operate by emitting blue excitation light at 450 nm and require visualization through a filter incorporated into the device or worn by the operator.

NARROW BAND IMAGING

NBI (Olympus Medical Systems Corporation, Tokyo, Japan) (Figure 3.51) utilizes the concept that the depth of light penetration is dependent on its wavelength to enhance mucosal surface texture and underlying vasculature (356–358). The spectral bandwidth of the filtered light is narrowed (357). The system has two modes: white light and NBI (358). In NBI mode, only blue light (400–430 nm) and green light (525–555 nm) are emitted in parallel, which make blood

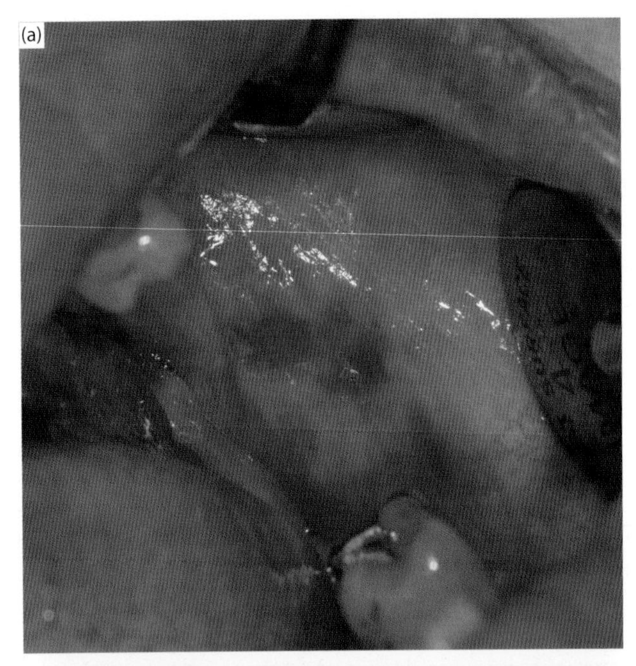

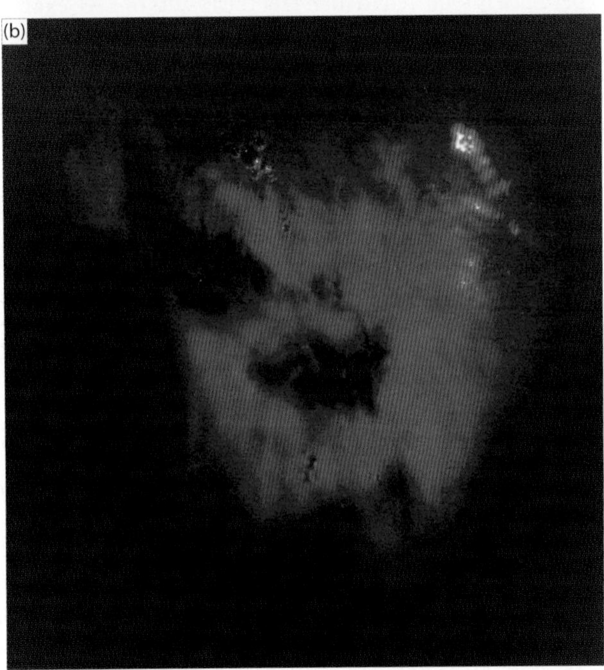

Figure 3.49 Atrophic lichenoid lesion on the left buccal mucosa under normal incandescent light **(a)** and same lesion viewed with Identafi® violet light and filter **(b)** demonstrating maroon loss of fluorescence compared to normal-appearing tissue in blue. Violet light examination provides improved lesion visibility compared to conventional oral examination, improved visualization of lesion borders and a slight increase in lesion size compared to incandescent light.

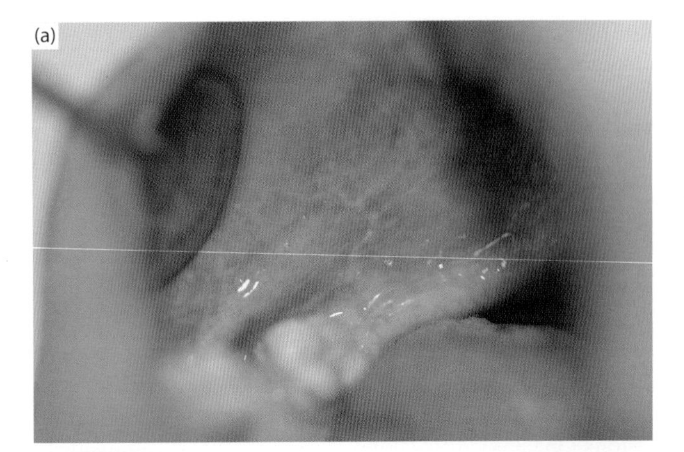

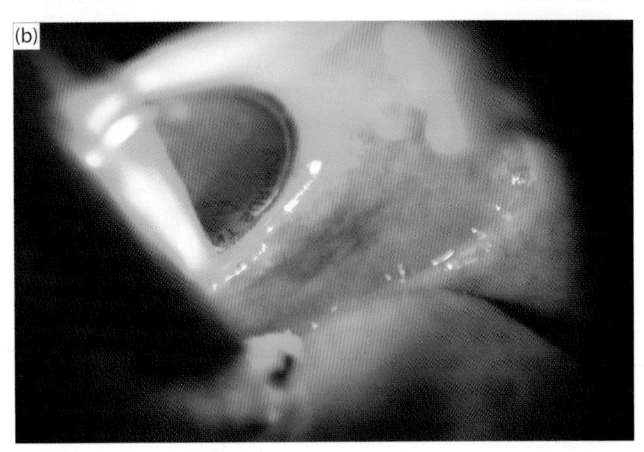

Figure 3.50 Subtle lichenoid lesion on the right buccal mucosa visualized with white light **(a)** and using Identafi® green–amber light **(b)**. The green light helps uncover subtle submucosal inflammatory changes evident as an area of diffuse redness.

vessels in the superficial mucosa appear brown and the deeper, larger vessels in the submucosa appear cyan (357). Blue light (centered at 415 nm) penetrates shallowly and corresponds to the peak absorption spectrum of hemoglobin, while green light (centered at 540 nm) penetrates deeper (357). In NBI mode, inflammatory lesions have an ill-demarcated border and can be differentiated from neoplastic lesions that appear as areas with scattered dark spots and a well-demarcated border (359,360). These scattered dark brown spots represent superficial blood vessels: interpapillary capillary loops (IPCLs) (Figure 3.52a and b) (358). Visualization of the vasculature as well as the degree of dilation, meandering, tortuosity and caliber of IPCLs all indicate the true extent of lesions and severity of pathology, thus guiding the position of biopsy and resection margins (359,361–363). It has been recommended that lesions with Type III and IV IPCL patterns must always be biopsied (364). The presence of keratinized tissue can hinder optimal visualization of the lesion itself (358).

Gono et al. (357) used NBI in colonoscopy and upper gastrointestinal endoscopy and concluded that magnified NBI enhanced the capillary pattern and the crypt pattern on the mucosa, which are useful features for diagnosing early cancer (365). Later, Muto et al. reported that carcinoma *in situ* at oropharyngeal and hypopharyngeal mucosal sites can be clinically recognized using magnified NBI endoscopy, confirming the usefulness of evaluating *in situ*

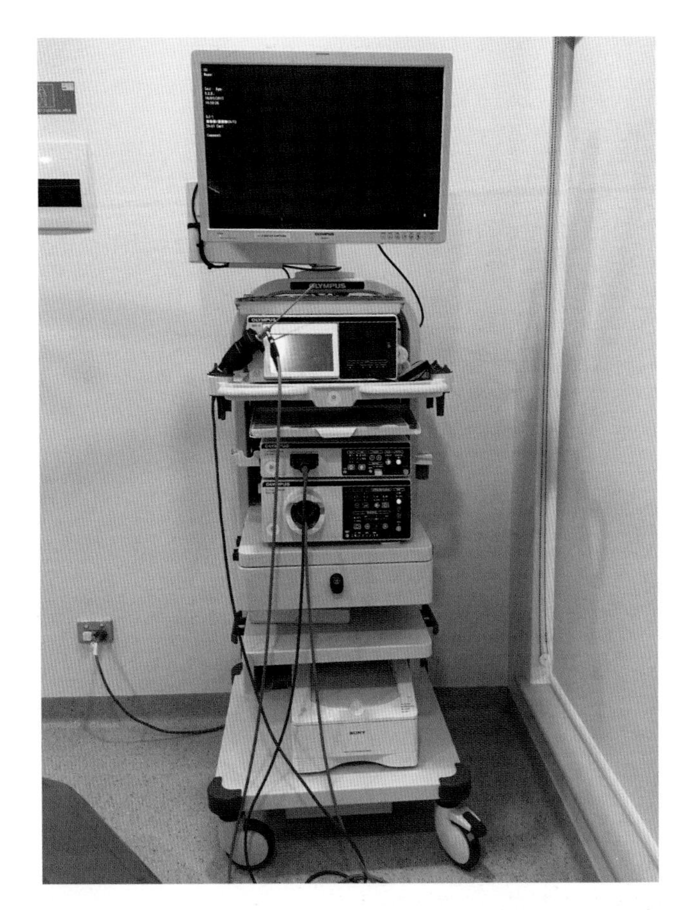

Figure 3.51 Narrow band imaging (NBI; Olympus Medical Systems Corporation, Tokyo, Japan) endoscopic system allows examination of oral and oropharyngeal lesions under white light and in NBI mode. Blue light (400–430 nm) and green light (525–555 nm) are emitted in parallel, which make blood vessels in the superficial mucosa appear brown and the deeper, larger vessels in the submucosa appear cyan. The device allows video and still digital recording of endoscopic examination with either a rigid or flexible endoscope.

angiogenesis in solid tumors in the head and neck region (366,367). Yoshida et al. validated the use of NBI with magnifying endoscopy in esophageal lesions (368). A case report by Katada et al. showed the usefulness of NBI combined with gastrointestinal endoscopy in detecting OSCC in the floor of the mouth (362). Further case reports and investigations also supported the use of NBI in the oropharynx (369), nasopharynx (370,371), hypopharynx (308), larynx (372) and esophagus (373). Its use in determining tumor sizes and margins in gastrointestinal cancers of the bile duct (374,375), duodenal papilla (376) and stomach (377,378) was also investigated, all with encouraging results boasting higher sensitivities and specificities than the current detection method used at the time. All these studies hailed NBI as a method with improved detection and diagnostic accuracy of cancers in areas that are difficult to examine and, critically, allowing for early diagnosis and having an impact on treatment options, quality of life and patient survival (379).

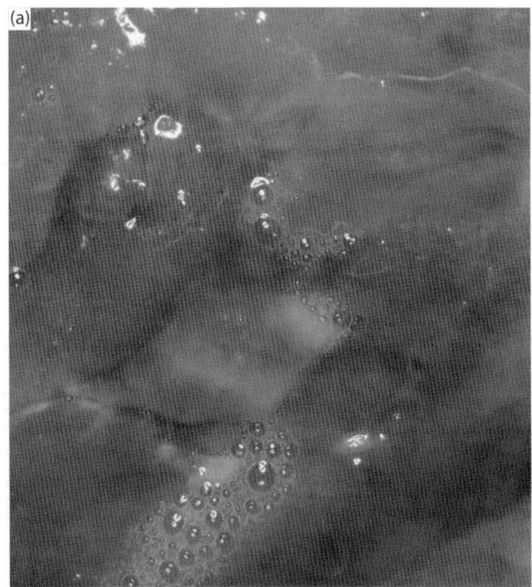

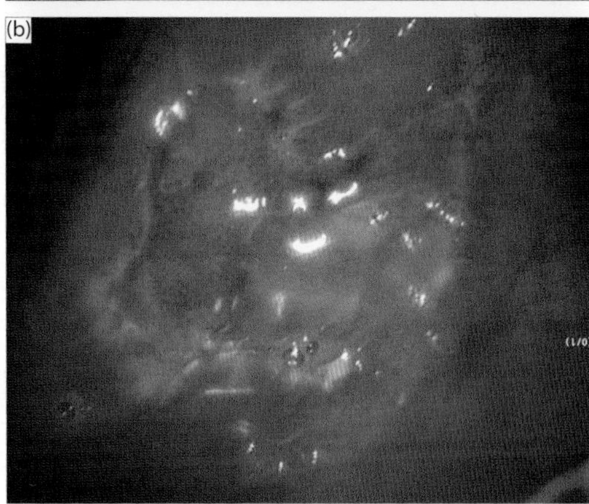

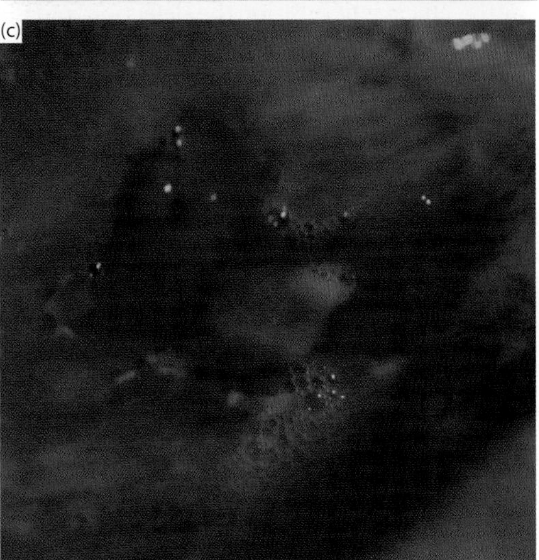

Figure 3.52 Ulcerated lesion on the lateral border of tongue viewed with endoscopic white light **(a)** and in narrow band imaging mode **(b)**. Note the scattered dark brown spots in (b) representing superficial blood vessels and interpapillary capillary loops (type III) consistent with the presence of dysplasia. Same lesion visualized with VELscope® Vx **(c)** demonstrating loss of fluorescence of area with interpapillary capillary loop type III pattern under narrow band imaging. Biopsy-proven severe epithelial dysplasia.

It was considered that NBI would develop into a useful tool in the future pre-, intra- and post-operative endoscopic assessment of neoplastic lesions in the upper aerodigestive tract (380).

In a multicenter, prospective, randomized controlled trial (n = 320), Muto et al. (381) found that NBI detected superficial cancer more frequently than white light imaging in both the head and neck region (100% versus 8%) and the esophagus (97% versus 55%). They reported a sensitivity rate and accuracy of 100% and 86.7% in the detection of superficial cancer in the head and neck region using NBI and of 97.2% and 88.9% in the esophagus, respectively (381). Piazza et al. (382) showed that 27% (26 of 96) of patients with OSCC and OPSCC had a diagnostic advantage by applying NBI and high-definition television (HDTV) compared to white light and HDTV. In a later study (383), they concluded that NBI and HDTV were of value in defining superficial tumor extension, in the detection of synchronous lesions in the pre-/intra-operative settings and in post-treatment surveillance for early detection of persistence, recurrence and metachronous tumors.

Fielding et al. combined white light and AF to the bronchoscopic and laryngoscopic assessments of head and neck cancer patients and reported improved sensitivity but low specificity, increasing the number of unnecessary biopsies (384). A later study combined AF and NBI for the detection of mucosal lesions during panendoscopy in head and neck cancer patients and reported higher specificity than when using AF or white light alone, thus directly impacting patient management (385).

A recently published systematic review by Vu and Farah (386) on the efficacy of NBI for the detection and surveillance of OPMLs analyzed data from a prospective cohort study by Piazza et al. (383) and a retrospective cohort study by Yang et al. (387), both of which aimed to evaluate the efficacy of NBI endoscopy compared to white light in oral mucosal examination. Vu and Farah concluded that, based on available evidence, there is a demonstrable improvement in the ability of NBI visualization to stage tumors, assess margins and detect synchronous, metachronous and recurrent lesions compared to visualization using broadband white light (386).

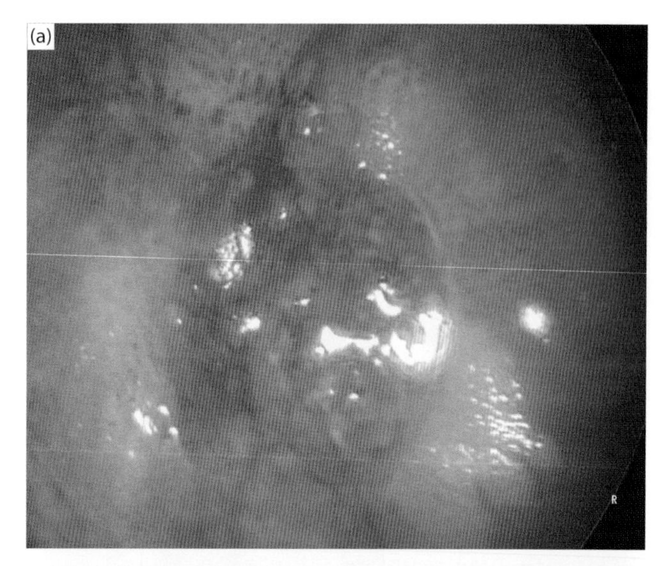

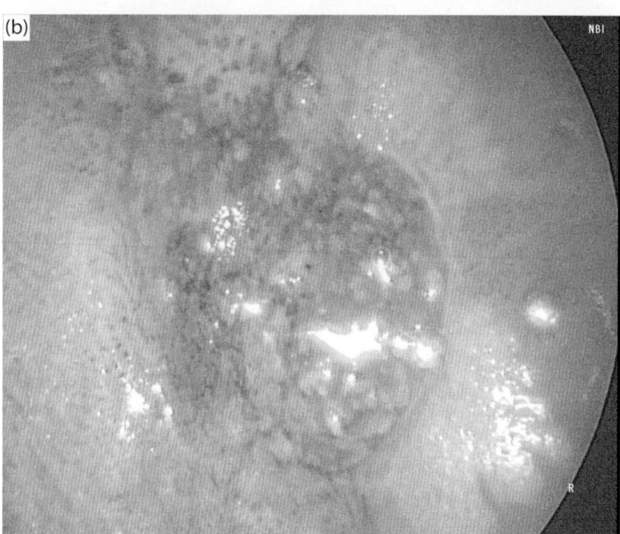

Figure 3.53 Lesion on the lateral border of the tongue viewed with endoscopic white light **(a)** and in narrow band imaging mode **(b)**. Note the scattered dark brown spots representing superficial blood vessels and interpapillary capillary loops (type IV) consistent with presence of malignancy. Biopsy-proven well-differentiated squamous cell carcinoma.

In the only prospective study examining the utility of NBI in the detection of OPMLs (278), Farah and colleagues found NBI to be excellent at detecting and monitoring OPMLs (Figure 3.53a,b), particularly those that were undetected by COE or white light endoscopy. In this prospective study, 96 patients were recruited to a single-site oral medicine specialist referral practice and examined by COE, white light and NBI consecutively. The sensitivity, specificity and accuracy rates of NBI for detecting OPMDs were 100%, 87.50% and 97.43%, respectively, when compared to white light as a gold standard. A similar finding reported high values for NBI compared to COE as a gold standard. However, NBI has a lower correlation with the histological evaluation of OPMDs. The study presented evidence that NBI enhances the visualization of lesions detected by COE and white light and assists in the detection of lesions that were undetected by COE and white light (388).

A prospective study by Nguyen et al. utilized white light, NBI and AF to inspect the oral cavity, larynx/hypopharynx and bronchus of 73 patients with known HNSCC, patients with SCC of unknown primary origin and surgically treated HNSCC patients requiring panendoscopy for suspected recurrent disease (385). The authors found a significant improvement in the detection of moderate dysplasia or worse by NBI compared to white light and that the combined use of AF and NBI had significant implications upon mapping and guiding the surgical resection borders of three assessed oral cases (385). This study demonstrated increased specificity with NBI for the detection of mucosal lesions (385).

Moreover, NBI has great potential in accurately assisting in the real-time assessment of new and existing OPMLs, OSCCs and OPSCCs and, ultimately, influencing their treatment (358,389). Farah and colleagues performed a prospective bioinformatic study of mRNA expression data for tissue biopsies of tumor core and white light-determined surgical margin and NBI-determined surgical margin samples obtained from 18 patients during primary resection of intraoral SCC (390). The results of this study provide evidence that the surgical margins determined by NBI possess fewer molecular abnormalities than the more conservative surgical margins determined by white light examination. In other words, surgical margins that are determined by NBI rather than by white light examination leave less potentially malignant residual tissue and thereby increase the likelihood of surgical success (390).

OPTICAL COHERENCE TOMOGRAPHY

OCT is a non-invasive optical imaging technology that utilizes NIR light and the principle of low-coherence interferometry to provide real-time, high-resolution, cross-sectional images of tissue microstructure—a direct analogue of ultrasound (391,392).

OCT is based on the principle of low-coherence interferometry (274). It provides high-resolution (~1–20-μm) cross-sectional images of tissue *in situ*, higher than conventional ultrasound, MRI or CT and comparable to conventional histology but, being non-destructive, it aids real-time surgical diagnostics and "optical biopsy" of the tissue (393). Initial success with this modality was with retinal pathology (394) and bronchopulmonary diseases (395). More recently, it has been deemed useful in diagnosing diseases of the oropharynx/larynx and other oral tissues (393,396,397).

OCT is similar to ultrasound B-mode imaging except that OCT uses light instead of acoustic waves, measuring the echo time delay and intensity of backscattered light (398). The system uses NIR light, split into reference and sample beams, and plots the back-reflected light from structures within the tissue against depth (up to 2–3 mm) (394,398,399). Since the velocity of light is extremely high, optical echoes cannot be measured directly by electronic detection, but instead OCT uses low-coherence interferometry—the backscattered light waves interfere with the reference beam and this interference pattern is used to measure the light echoes versus the depth profile of the tissue *in vivo* (399). OCT also uses fiber-optic technology, allowing for low-profile imaging to be performed through small optical fibers attached directly to a scalpel, tissue probe, endoscope or microscope (399). The device is compact and portable (399).

The low-power NIR light (between 750 and 1,300 nm) incorporated in the technology has reference and sample beams (320,391). Depending on the tissue, the light typically penetrates to a depth of 1–3 mm and scatters as it interacts with the tissue (320,391). The backscattered light combines with reflected light from the reference, is measured using a Michelson-type interferometer and an image is generated based on its echo time delay and intensity (320). The fact that this portable device can provide subsurface tomographic visualization of tissue *in vivo* without the need for tissue preparation has enabled it to not only provide an "optical biopsy" of tissues, but also to aid the detection of neoplasias and guide surgical intervention (391,393). Early applications of this technology in ophthalmology led to significant clinical impact (394). More recently, OCT has been used for evaluating bronchopulmonary diseases, inflammatory diseases and cancers in the breast, skin, vulva, prostate and head and neck (320,391,400–405).

The use of OCT in the oral cavity and oropharyngeal region has only been a fairly recent development (393,396,397). Healthy oral mucosa has an easily distinguished basement membrane at the junction of the lamina propria, which appears bright, and epithelium, which appears dark (303). In contrast, changes in the thickness of epithelial and keratin cell layers and in the integrity of the basement membrane and architectural changes in the rete pegs and lamina propria are visible with OCT, hence it is possible for clinicians to assess the mucosa for neoplastic lesions (406,407).

In healthy mucosa, the basement membrane can be easily identified at the junction of the bright lamina propria and the darker epithelium, which is lost in the presence of invasive cancer (303). However, one study had inconsistent results, showing a deceptive change in the histological layers when compared to conventional biopsy of oral lesions (various anatomical sites) (393). The authors also noted that OCT image analysis is unique, requiring special training and associated with a wide range of variability when interpreting its parameters (mainly epithelium thickness and status of basement membrane) (393). The authors previously aimed to generate a bank of normative and pathological OCT data from oral tissues to identify cellular structures of normal and pathological processes, thus creating a diagnostic algorithm (406).

While OCT is useful for clinical detection of OSCCs and OPMLs (407), it also has potential in evaluating surgical margins for Minimal Residual Disease (MRD) in HNSCC, just as it has been proven useful in cancers of other tissues, such as breast (402,404), skin (400,401), vulva (408) and prostate (403).

Although one early study (409) reported 93% sensitivity and 97% specificity for OCT in aiding the diagnosis of OSCC when compared to histology, a later study (393) reported only 85% sensitivity and 78% specificity for detecting OPMDs in *ex vivo* biopsies. This suggests that unlike OSCC, the more subtle cellular and histological changes in OPMDs cannot be easily detected with OCT, and thus it is more difficult to grade and differentiate between OPMDs (406,407). However, OCT has been found to be capable of differentiating between benign lesions and OPMDs of epithelial origin in some tissue types (405). A more recent study (410) optically scanned OSCC resection margins in 28 patients in the immediate *ex vivo* phase and compared the four margins in each section to the gold standard—histopathology. The authors reported the overall sensitivity, specificity, positive predictive value and negative predictive value to be 81.5%, 87%, 61.5% and 95%, respectively. When using OCT, the mean epithelial thickness in tumor-free resection margins was 360 μm, while it was 567 μm in tumor-involved margins (410).

Learning how to use and interpret OCT images requires special training as many variations and parameters need to be considered regarding epithelium thickness and the status of the basement membrane (393,411). Lee et al. (412) have developed a handheld, side-looking, fiber-optic rotary pull-back catheter enabling wide-field view of features such as epithelial thickness and continuity of the basement membrane, which could prove useful for chairside management of oral lesions. Pande et al. (413) formulated automated algorithms for quantifying structural features associated with MT of oral epithelium based on image processing of OCT data, reporting a sensitivity of 90.2% and a specificity of 76.3% when distinguishing malignant lesions from benign lesions. Further research is required to produce a set of reference OCT profiles for normal and pathological oral and oropharyngeal tissues, which can be used for diagnosis in the future. Moreover, analysis of OCT profiles for OSCC has found that the technology can be used to delineate OSCC margins. In addition to investigating the use of OCT for the detection and diagnosis of OPMDs, OSCC and OPSCC, research into the other clinical applications of OCT in the oral cavity and oropharynx is warranted.

ANGLE-RESOLVED LOW-COHERENCE INTERFEROMETRY

a/LCI is a light-scattering technique that isolates the angle-scattering distribution from cellular nuclei at various tissue depths (276). In doing so, it is able to provide biomarkers based on morphology that are highly correlated with the presence of dysplasia (276). It measures the angular intensity distribution of light scattered by a tissue sample, quantifying subcellular morphology as a function of depth in the tissue (276). For each depth layer, signatures from cell nuclei are extracted by collecting and processing the angular scattering signal using a Mie theory-based light-scattering model to produce measurements of average nuclear diameter with submicron-level accuracy (276). Studies that have investigated the use of a/LCI have confirmed that neoplastic tissue transformation is accompanied by an increase in the average cell nucleus size (276,414–416), thus detecting potentially malignant lesions as well as malignant lesions. The diameter of a non-dysplastic epithelial cell nucleus is typically 5–10 μm, while dysplastic nuclei can be as large as 20 μm across (417). When this is optimized to 11.84 μm for the classification of tissue health, a/LCI yields a sensitivity of 100%, a specificity of 84%, overall accuracy of 86%, a positive predictive value of 34% and a negative predictive value of 100% in esophageal epithelium *in vivo* (276,415). This technique has been studied in animal models, *ex vivo* human studies and, more recently, in *in vivo* studies, predominantly associated with cases of Barrett's esophagus (which is associated with an increased risk of esophageal adenocarcinoma) and esophageal epithelium (276). The system is portable and the probe can be used through the accessory channel of a standard endoscope, thus providing surgical guidance (276).

a/LCI could have a role in assessing surgical margins in HNSCC by assessing the size of nuclei in the margins, although currently there are no studies that have investigated this, nor have there been studies assessing this technology for the detection and visualization of OPMDs.

CONFOCAL MICROSCOPY

Confocal reflectance microscopy (CM) is an enhanced optical imaging, non-invasive technique for superficial soft tissues in near real-time. What makes this method different from other conventional microscope techniques is that CM has light penetration to approximate depths of 200–400 μm (418,419). CM allows for detailed images of cell morphology and tissue architecture by using the backscattering of various tissue components to provide contrast (420). The CM components are a light source, a condenser, an objective lens and a detector (418). This technology is based on a tightly focused beam of light focused into a small spot at a chosen depth within a sample. Only the light from the chosen spot at the chosen depth is in focus at the pinhole, enabling it to pass through unimpeded (420). In theory, CM can visualize the tissue in a similar fashion to conventional histological evaluation, but in a non-invasive, non-stained, three-dimensional, subcellular resolution (421). CM has been shown to be a promising tool for diagnosing and for helping to manage oral mucosal lesions (420,422–424). A systematic review by Maher et al. identified 25 papers that met the inclusion criteria, with the papers being mostly case reports or case series. They concluded that the current scope and evidence for *in vivo* applications of CM in diagnosing and managing patients with oral mucosal lesions is limited, as the main focus was on the appearance of normal oral epithelium (425). However, potential areas of *in vivo* clinical applications of CM, such as OED, OSCC and oral vesiculobullous disorders, have been postulated (425).

CYTOLOGY TECHNIQUES

The survival rate of patients with OSCC is highly dependent upon the clinical stage at the time of diagnosis. Patients diagnosed at an early stage have a significantly better 5-year survival rate (80%) compared to those diagnosed when distant metastasis is present (20%) (426). Despite dramatic improvements in our understanding of the early changes of the surface epithelium in the process of carcinogenesis, early detection rates and, as a consequence, prognosis of OSCC have remained unchanged for the past three decades (427). A thorough clinical examination of the oral cavity is a non-invasive technique that can be performed by a multitude of healthcare professionals after appropriate training and bears no additional expense to patients; hence, it remains the preferred approach for the detection of oral abnormalities. Despite this preference, the efficacy of unaided visual examination in the timely detection of oral lesions is controversial (428).

Final diagnosis of OSCC and OPMLs is almost exclusively established through scalpel biopsy, which, due to its invasive nature, is only indicated in cases with highly suspicious clinical appearance (e.g. erythroplakia, non-homogeneous leukoplakia and erythroleukoplakia). It also confines the sampling to a limited area, which is particularly problematic in case of multiple lesions. Lastly, a false-negative rate of up to 23% poses a serious challenge to the current complete reliance on scalpel biopsy (429,430); this and the above-mentioned limitations may partly be responsible for the late detection and consequent poor prognosis of OSCC. An important adjunctive diagnostic technique is oral cytology, which has been defined as microscopic examination of surface epithelium that has been harvested *via* non-invasive methods such as brush, spatula and curette (431). The first record of cancer cytology dates to 1860 when L.S. Beale published an illustration of cells harvested from oral cancer (432). Since that time, cytodiagnosis has slowly become an integral component of oral cancer diagnosis and its application has been extended to aiding the diagnosis of not only oral lesions, but also lesions of several other organs. Due to its ease of use and its inexpensive and non-invasive nature, exfoliative cytology can be routinely used for the screening and early diagnosis of oral lesions, in addition to the identification of potential biomarkers. Cytology is advantageous as it can be repeated for follow-up and research purposes and, although a definitive diagnosis is generally reached by conventional scalpel biopsy, Exfoliative Cytology (EC) has a supportive role in the management of OSCC.

SUPRAVITAL STAINING

TB (also known as tolonium chloride) is an acidophilic dye that specifically binds to and stains the acidic components of the cell such as nucleic acids. During the 1960s, it was suggested that since dysplastic and, in particular, neoplastic cells have a higher nuclear content, TB could stain these cells more strongly than their normal counterparts (433). Since this method can be used on live tissues without obtaining a biopsy, it is referred to as a vital or supravital technique. To perform the staining *in vivo*, TB can be used as either a 1% or 2% oral rinse after application of a mucolytic agent (1% citric acid wipe). The oral mucosa is then blotted dry and the clinician assesses the oral cavity. A 1% TB solution may be prepared from laboratory-grade TB or purchased as pharmaceutical-grade TB in single-use swab kits. Various commercial preparations of TB include AdDent's OralBlu™ and Zila's ViziLite™ TB (Figure 3.54). The difference in the appearance between normal and malignant cells should be considered as a relative rather than an absolute measure (433). Clinical applications of TB staining include

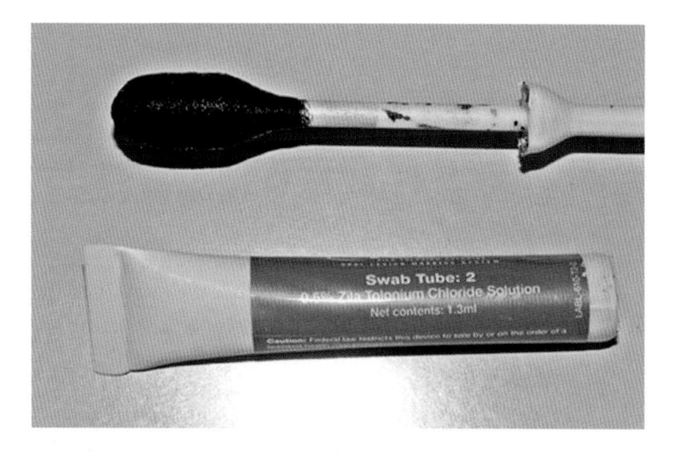

Figure 3.54 Tolonium chloride swab (Zila TBlue[630]). (Courtesy of Clinical Professor A. Ross Kerr, Department of Oral and Maxillofacial Pathology, Radiology & Medicine, New York University College of Dentistry, NY, USA.)

surveillance in high-risk patients (434), identifying and highlighting early OPMLs and defining the extent of oral lesions prior to excision (273).

In comparison with unaided clinical examination in a large cohort (4080 TB versus 3895 clinical examination participants), 5% more OPMLs and 79% more OSF cases were detected in the TB group; nevertheless, after a 5-year follow-up period, the difference in cancer incidence between the two groups was non-significant (435). Although a recent large review of the literature also suggested TB to be an unreliable technique due to its subjectivity and large dependence on examiners' experience (436), others have found it to be a useful adjunct to incisional biopsy in diagnosing oral lesions (437). TB staining, although unreliable on its own, seems to be a valuable tool when used and interpreted in combination with a precise clinical history and conventional biopsy.

CONVENTIONAL EXFOLIATIVE CYTOLOGY

Compared to incisional biopsy, exfoliative cytology provides the diagnostician with a rich collection of cells harvested from a wider area. Although the concept is the same, based on different collecting devices, the sensitivity and specificity of exfoliative cytology differs.

The most commonly used exfoliative cytology instruments include wooden tongue depressors, metal spatulas and cotton-tipped applicators. Both the wooden tongue depressors and metal/plastic spatulas are readily available in a dental practice and can be used with relative ease; however, when scraped over sensitive areas such as gingival margins or the muco-gingival junction they can cause discomfort. In addition, due to their inflexibility, size and shape, the wooden tongue depressors and metal spatulas cannot be adapted to all parts of the oral cavity. Cytoplasmic and nuclear distortion have been reported in smears collected using wooden tongue depressors and metal spatulas due to collection of epithelial cells in a thick aggregate (438). Cotton-tipped applicators are more convenient for the patient; however, fewer cells are harvested with their use and many remain trapped in the cotton, resulting in a smaller number of cells for diagnostic purposes, and these are mostly collected from superficial layers, thus limiting accurate interpretation of the presence of epithelial dysplasia.

Different types of staining techniques are used in exfoliative cytology. The most widely used stain is the Papanicolaou (PAP), which is a particularly useful tool in monitoring cervical cancer (439). The PAP stain was first developed in 1942 by George Papanicolaou to stain vaginal smears (440). While the main uses of this technique remain diagnosing and monitoring cervical cancer (439), PAP staining has also been used in the diagnosis and screening of oral lesions and, in particular, OSCC (441).

Silver-binding nuclear organizing region (AgNOR staining) is another staining method used in exfoliative cytology. AgNORs are exclusively seen in the nucleus and their number in each cell is correlated with nucleolar and cell proliferative activity of tumors (442). The number and scatter of AgNORs have also been associated with severity of oral lesions (443). Despite a whole myriad of tests and biomarkers that can be used for assessing the harvested cells, the most important aspect of EC remains the quality and quantity of the collected cells. Hence, ensuring the sample is taken from the full thickness of the epithelium is of prime importance; this is especially crucial in dysplastic lesions in which changes start at the basal layer.

BRUSH BIOPSY CYTOLOGY

To overcome the innate limitations of conventional exfoliative cytology, pathologists have striven to improve cytology-associated techniques and instrumentation. The oral Cytobrush was modified from the cytobrush used in obstetrics (Figure 3.55) and, in most comparisons, has proven advantageous over the wooden/metallic spatula (438,444,445) and even comparable with incisional biopsy (444). Efficacy of brush biopsy is particularly confirmed in small OSCC lesions with a diameter of less than 20 mm (446). In general, oral brush biopsy has been used with different degrees of success and its sensitivity is reported to range from 71% (447) to 97.2% (448). Although brush biopsy has the advantage of collecting cells from a wide area and all three layers of epithelium by accessing the basement membrane (449), potential disadvantages of this technique include difficulty detaching cells in ulcerated and necrotic surfaces and visualizing cells out of context (449). Similar to other techniques, the efficacy of brush biopsy is highly dependent upon adequate training of the operator.

OralCDx® (OralCDx Laboratories, Suffern, NY, USA.) (Figure 3.56) is a patented modification of the brush biopsy that uses a computerized program to interpret the morphologic and cytologic changes of collected cells (332). OralCDx® comes with the promise of overcoming the inherent limitations of conventional brush biopsy, particularly the tedious visual search for potentially rare abnormalities through using an image analysis system (332). In the first and still largest study assessing the sensitivity and specificity of OralCDx® in the detection of cancerous and precancerous oral mucosal lesions, Sciubba and colleagues from across the United States conducted a multicenter, double-blind study comparing the results of OralCDx® analysis with those of scalpel biopsy of suspicious oral lesions, as well as using OralCDx® on oral lesions that appeared benign clinically (332). In 945 patients, OralCDx® independently detected every case of histologically confirmed oral dysplasia and carcinoma with a sensitivity of 100%. Every OralCDx® "positive" result was subsequently confirmed by histology as dysplasia or carcinoma. The specificity for the OralCDx® "positive" results was 100%, while the specificity for the OralCDx® "atypical" results was 92.9%. In 4.5% of clinically benign-appearing lesions that would not have received additional testing or attention other than clinical follow-up, OralCDx® uncovered dysplasia or carcinoma

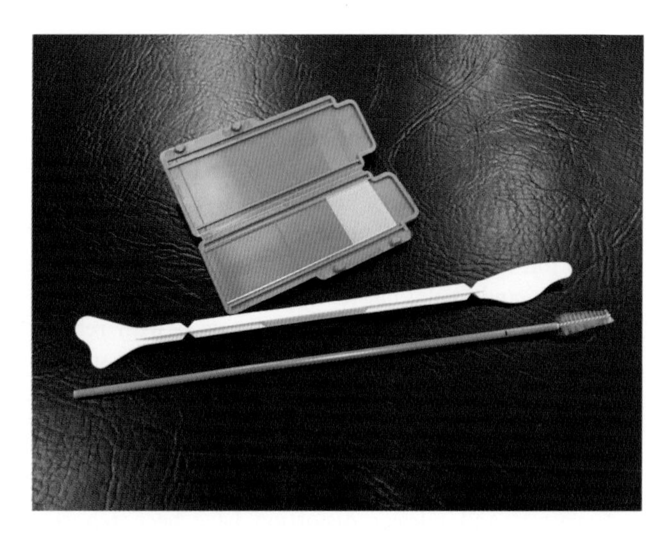

Figure 3.55 Cervical cytology kit including a plastic spatula and Cytobrush.

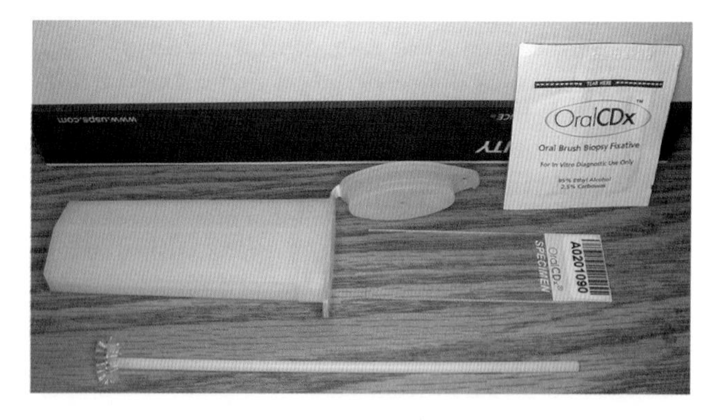

Figure 3.56 OralCDx™ (OralCDx Laboratories®, Suffern, NY, USA.) kit comprising brush, fixative and glass slide. (Courtesy of Clinical Professor A. Ross Kerr, Department of Oral and Maxillofacial Pathology, Radiology & Medicine, New York University College of Dentistry, NY, USA.)

(sensitivity >96%; specificity for the OralCDx® "positive" results >97% and for the "atypical" results >90%) (332). The study concluded that OralCDx® was a highly accurate method for detecting oral cancerous and precancerous lesions and could aid in confirming the nature of apparently benign oral mucosal lesions and, more significantly, reveal those that are precancerous and cancerous when they are not clinically suspected of being so.

Four subsequent studies have assessed the utility of OralCDx® in clinical settings for the assessment of oral mucosal lesions. Scheifele et al. compared 103 OralCDx® results with the histological findings of 96 clinical sites in 80 patients demonstrating histological findings compatible with OL, OLP, OED and OSCC (450). After excluding 6.8% of specimens that were inadequate for cell assessment, the sensitivity and specificity rates of OralCDx® for detecting dysplasia and OSCC were 92.3% and 94.3%, respectively. The positive and negative likelihood ratios were 16.2 (95% confidence interval [CI]: 6.2–42.1) and 0.08 (95% CI: 0.02–0.31), supporting the findings of the Sciubba study and the use of OralCDx® as a screening tool for oral mucosal lesions (450). Mehrotra et al. (451) assessed 85 consecutive patients presenting with an oral lesion deemed to be minimally suspicious by clinical examination and undertook OralCDx® brush biopsy followed immediately by a matched scalpel biopsy at the same location. The sensitivity of the brush biopsy was 96.3%, while the specificity of a "positive" brush result was 100% and that of an "atypical" result 90.4%. The positive predictive value and negative predictive value were 84% and 98%, respectively (451).

These two studies are contrasted by a retrospective audit undertaken by Poate et al. (447) in a group of 112 patients attending a specialist oral medicine unit for assessment of OPMD and a smaller study by Seijas-Naya and colleagues on 24 patients attending a specialist university clinic (452). Poate et al. found that the sensitivity and specificity rates of OralCDx® for the detection of OED or OSCC were 71.4% and 32%, respectively, while the positive predictive value of an abnormal brush biopsy result (positive or atypical) was 44.1% and the negative predictive value was 60%. Unlike others, these authors concluded that not all OPMDs are detected with the OralCDx® oral brush biopsy system (447). These latter findings are supported in part by Seijas-Naya and colleagues, who reported a sensitivity, specificity, positive predictive value and negative predictive value of 72.7%, 92.3%, 88.8% and 80%, respectively, for OralCDx®, with a biopsy diagnostic κ coefficient of 0.66 compared to histopathological assessment of scalpel biopsy specimens, concluding that although OralCDx® was a good tool for monitoring OL, the most reliable method for confirmation of the exact diagnosis of lesions and their anatomical and pathological characteristics was still conventional scalpel biopsy (452).

Although significant discussion still rages as to the applicability of OralCDx® in routine clinical practice for the assessment of oral mucosal lesions, it must be emphasized that the proprietary OralCDx® collection brush must be used with the computer-assisted neural network software analysis system for maximum potential and accurate results. Attempting to use the brush without the computer-assisted software, with other software packages or using a different brush with the neural network software or with liquid-based cytology (LBC) will compromise sensitivity and specificity findings and therefore the overall utility of the OralCDx® oral brush biopsy system. Despite this, many authors have used the OralCDx® brush to obtain cellular material for various applications, including LBC, DNA image cytometry and molecular biomarker analysis.

Other specifically designed brush systems include Orcellex® Brush Oral Cell Sampler (Rovers Medical Devices, The Netherlands) (Figure 3.57). The Rovers® brush manufacturer designed the Orcellex® Brush to specifically collect representative cells from all epithelial layers. Kujan et al. have investigated the capability of Orcellex® to obtain an adequate number of cells from the oral mucosa for subsequent LBC and DNA studies in a cohort of normal subjects (453). Their findings revealed that the Orcellex® brush was tolerable and well-accepted by patients and was capable of obtaining a mean of 55,500 cells per sample (range 35,000–90,000 cells). Furthermore, all specimens were constituted from populations of cells representative of all layers of normal epithelium: basal/parabasal, spinosal (intermediate) and superficial cells. Keratin products such as parakeratin, single keratosis and keratin pearls were documented, in addition to anucleate cells suggestive of ortho-keratinization. The Orcellex® brush yielded genomic DNA of higher molecular weight with minimal protein contamination. Another study investigated the yield and quality of RNA extracted from oral samples obtained using the Orcellex® brush and the results showed satisfactory quantitative Polymerase Chain Reaction (qPCR) results (454). The use of the Orcellex® brush produced an adequate sample for a chip-based approach to quantitatively assess malignancy risk in a cohort of 714 patients with OPMLs (455). Further studies are currently underway to assess the

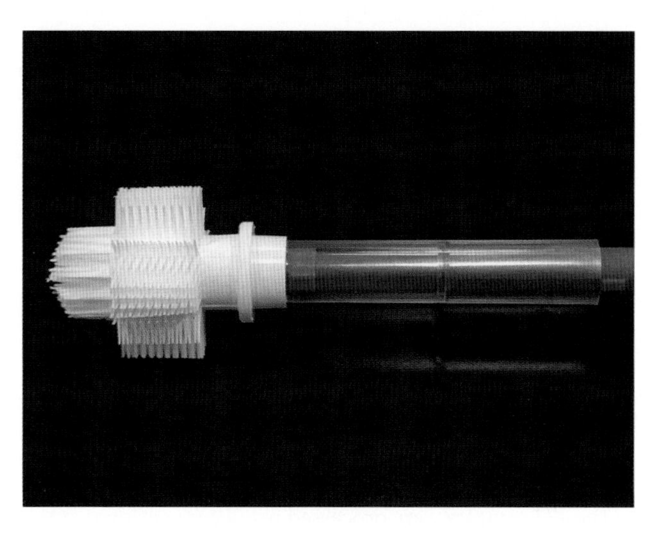

Figure 3.57 Orcellex® Brush Oral Cell Sampler (Rovers Medical Devices, The Netherlands)

clinical utility of the Orcellex® brush in assessing, monitoring and mapping OPMDs.

LIQUID-BASED CYTOLOGY

To improve the characteristics of conventional exfoliative cytology through reducing cell necrosis, blood contamination and inflammation, LBC was developed. In this technique, after collection, cells are transferred into a vial containing preservative liquids to ensure immediate fixation, an even distribution and a significantly higher number of collected cells. Despite its extensive use in detecting cervical cancer, LBC is not commonly used in the oral health setting. Hayama et al., in one of the few articles discussing the differences between LBC and conventional cytology, suggested LBC smears have better preserved cell morphology and less cellular overlap and blood contamination (456). Kujan et al. found similar results; in addition, they reported lower bacterial count and mucous contamination in association with LBC (453). In a more recent comparative study assessing Cytobrush®, OralCDx® and dermatological curette for LBC, Reboiras-López and colleagues did not find any correlation between the average number of cells and the type of instrument used when assessing cytological samples from normal oral mucosa of healthy volunteers. Furthermore, all preparations showed appropriate preparation quality, with cells being distributed uniformly and showing no mucus, bleeding, inflammatory exudate or artefacts. The samples generally consisted of superficial and intermediate cells, but surprisingly no basal cells in any of the analyzed samples. Furthermore, no differences were found among the cytological preparations of these three instruments (458). They then furthered their work by comparing the three systems in their ability to harvest enough cellular material to undertake downstream molecular analysis using quantitative real-time polymerase chain reaction analysis of a housekeeping gene. Adequate samples were more likely to be obtained with a curette (90.6%) or OralCDx® (80.0%) than a Cytobrush® (48.6%; $p < .001$). Similarly, the RNA quantification was higher with a curette or OralCDx® compared with the Cytobrush®. There were statistically significant differences between the Cytobrush® and curette ($p = .008$) and between the Cytobrush® and OralCDx® ($p = .034$). Although material was obtained with all three instruments, adequate samples were more likely to be obtained with the curette or OralCDx® than with the Cytobrush®. Furthermore, they reported that the OralCDx® brush was a less aggressive instrument than the curette, so could be a useful tool in a clinical setting, particularly as molecular biomarkers found their way into clinical practice (459).

Navone et al. (460) used LBC and conventional cytology to study 473 patients referred for presence of OSCC or OPMLs. All patients, after sampling for cytology, received surgical biopsy and histological examination. Eighty-nine of the 473 samples were processed using conventional cytology and 384 by LBC (ThinPrep®, Figure 3.58). In total, 12.4% of cases were inadequate in conventional oral cytology compared with 8.8% in LBC. The sensitivity, specificity and positive and negative predictive values were 85.7%, 95.9%, 95.4% and 87.0%, respectively, for conventional samples, versus 95.1%, 99.0%, 96.3% and 98.7% for LBC. This has been supported by Delavarian et al. (461) who assessed 25 patients and obtained values of 88.8%, 100%, 100% and 80.0%, respectively.

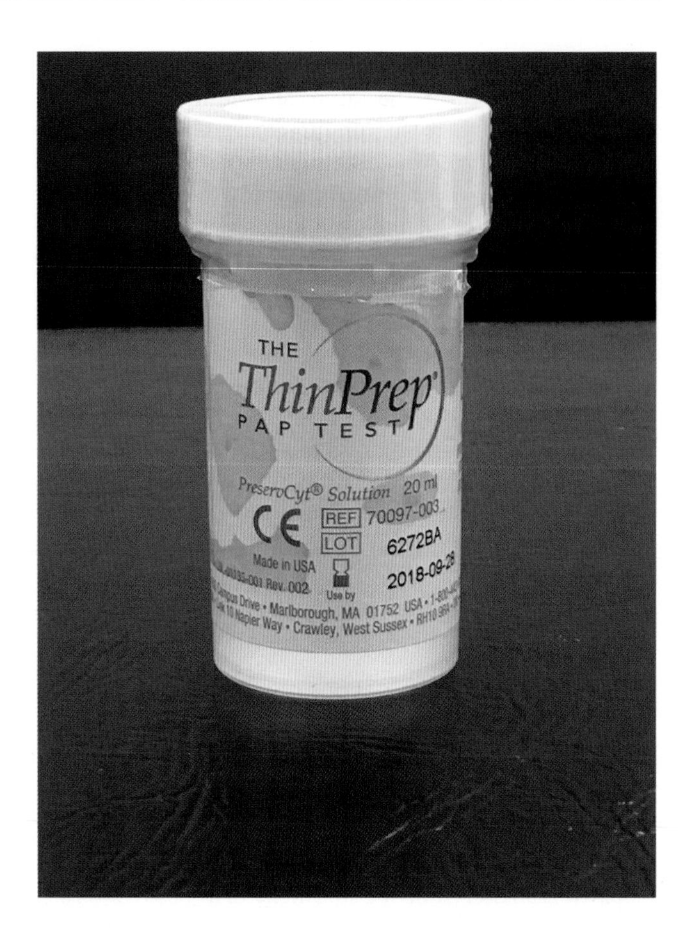

Figure 3.58 ThinPrep® PreservCyt® Solution (Hologic, Inc., MA, USA.) solution used for cell preservation liquid-based cytology preparations.

DNA ANALYSIS AND IMAGE CYTOMETRY

DNA cellular content (ploidy) has been reported to be a reliable marker for both malignant and premalignant lesions. DNA ploidy has been studied by both flow and image cytometry. Marsico et al. (462) combined LBC and flow cytometry to examine 211 OPMLs compared to a conventional histopathological diagnosis on scalpel biopsy. Flow cytometry demonstrated aneuploidy in 54.8% of OSCCs, 15.1% of OPMLs without dysplasia and in 50% of OPMLs with dysplasia.

McCullough and Farah took advantage of the positive characteristics of LBC and assessed DNA content using a Cytobrush® and virtual microscopy for the early detection of OED and neoplasia in oral mucosal lesions (463). They compared the usefulness of ploidy analysis of Feulgen-stained cytological ThinPrep® specimens with incisional biopsy and histopathological examination of 17 OPMDs/OSCCs and were unable to observe variation between abnormal samples compared to a database of 100 normal controls. They concluded that DNA content assessment of oral cytology utilizing Cytobrush®, LBC and virtual microscopy was not useful as an adjunctive prognostic tool in the analysis of the malignant potential of oral mucosal lesions.

More recently, Kämmerer and colleagues assessed the ability of DNA image cytometry (DNA-ICM) to enhance the morphological interpretation of pure oral brush biopsies (464). They found that DNA-ICM has the potential to substantially improve the sensitivity of a pure morphological interpretation of oral brush biopsies (from 55% to 76%), while the combination of DNA-ICM and brush biopsy had a specificity of 100%, similar to that of brush biopsy or DNA-ICM alone for the detection of dysplasia. In an effort to increase cell numbers, Navone et al. (465) used a dermatological curette approach (scraping/micro-biopsy) and LBC in a prospective study of 164 patients with OPMLs to detect the presence of dysplasia/carcinoma. Micro-biopsy diagnosis was in agreement with scalpel biopsy in 91.14% of cases and showed a better sensitivity than scalpel biopsy (97.65% versus 85.88%), corresponding to two of 158 false-negative cases by micro-biopsy versus 12 of 158 by scalpel biopsy (465).

Given the disparate results surrounding the use of the OralCDx® oral brush biopsy system with computer-assisted neural network analysis and DNA-ICM in diagnosing oral cancer and precancerous conditions, a recent meta-analysis was conducted to compare the accuracy of the two systems in diagnosing both conditions. Bibliographic databases were systematically searched for original relevant studies on the early diagnosis of oral cancer and precancer. Thirteen studies (eight of OralCDx® brush biopsy and five of DNA-ICM) were identified as having reported on 1981 oral mucosal lesions. The meta-analysis found that the areas under the summary receiver operating characteristic curves of the OralCDx® brush biopsy and DNA-ICM were 0.8879 and 0.9885, respectively. The pooled sensitivity and specificity rates and diagnostic odds ratio of the OralCDx® brush biopsy were 86%, 81% and 20.36, respectively, while these were 89%, 99% and 446.08 for DNA-ICM, respectively. Results of a pairwise comparison between each modality demonstrated that specificity, area under the curve and Q^* index of DNA-ICM were significantly higher than those of the OralCDx® brush biopsy, but no significant difference in sensitivity was found. The authors concluded that based on available published studies, DNA-ICM was more accurate than OralCDx® brush biopsy in diagnosing oral cancer and precancerous mucosal lesions (466).

FINE NEEDLE ASPIRATION BIOPSY

Exfoliative cytology is best reserved for epithelial abnormalities, but for palpable nodules, especially those with difficult access, fine needle aspiration biopsy (FNAB) is indicated (Figure 3.59). Although in theory FNAB is indicated in deep oral mucosal abnormalities, its application in the head and neck region is mostly limited to thyroid, major salivary glands and lymph nodes and is very rarely used in the oral cavity (467). The most common oral cavity lesions approached using FNAB are odontogenic tumors, salivary gland tumors and intra-osseous lesions (468).

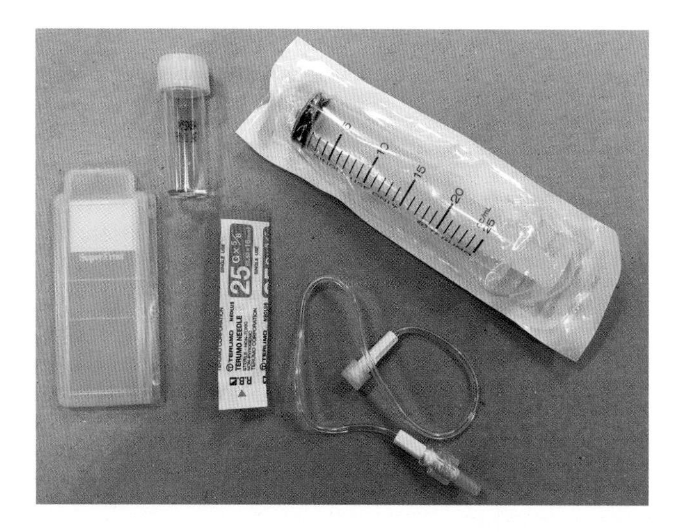

Figure 3.59 A fine needle aspiration biopsy kit.

Amongst the advantages of FNAB, the most commonly discussed are preoperative diagnosis, patient comfort, follow-up, preserving the integrity of the oral cavity and the lower risk of infection and tissue damage (469,470). In contrast, the lack of adequate space to perform the FNAB properly and the difficulty fixing the lesion have been counted as disadvantages of this technique (469,470). However, the most important challenge facing diagnosticians using FNAB is that the technique may yield insufficient material for analysis (469). The sensitivity of FNAB in the oral cavity varies between 80% and 100% and its specificity varies between 60% and 100% (469,470).

CYTOLOGIC EVALUATION

Historically, cytology has been utilized mostly in cervical pathology. To avoid the inevitable confusion caused by multiple classification systems, the Bethesda system (TBS) was developed in 1988 to provide a uniform terminology for the diagnosis and reporting of cervical/vaginal cytologic changes (471). TBS received much input from cytologists and cytotechnologists and was updated in 1991 and again in 2001 (472). Despite the great success of TBS, there has been little drive to adapt or develop a universal system for reporting and grading of oral cytology findings. This lack of enthusiasm could be explained by the great variation in quality and cellularity of oral cytology, which in turn results in relatively unreliable results and consequently a lack of interest in oral cytology as a field.

A tiered classification system (positive, suspicious and negative with or without unsatisfactory class) has been used successfully in the past (332,473). As an example, all suspicious FNA samples from Scher et al.'s investigation were proven to be malignant with incisional biopsy (473). Although OralCDx® is a specifically designed algorithm for analysis of exfoliative biopsy, TBS seems to be more informative in comparison. TBS requires the specimen to be of adequate quantity and quality and categorizes the smears as: (a) normal; (b) reactive; (c) atypical—probably reactive/low-grade squamous intraepithelial lesion; (d) atypical—probably high grade; (e) high-grade squamous intraepithelial lesion; (f) invasive SCC; and (g) other neoplasms (474). While these definitions can be extended and applied to the oral cavity, TBS is tailored for cervical lesions. The need for a universal grading system for oral cytology with the emergence of new technologies is now greater than ever.

LIMITATIONS

An ideal diagnostic technique is user-friendly, inexpensive, time effective and causes minimal discomfort for the patient. When used correctly by a trained healthcare provider and supplemented with appropriate interpretation and analysis tools, cytology can potentially meet all the above criteria. However, in real-world scenarios and in less-than-optimal conditions, cytology—similar to most other diagnostic techniques—is subject to shortcomings and limitations. In a recent Cochrane review assessing the diagnostic tests for oral cancer and OPMLs in patients presenting with clinically evident lesions, 1,622 samples from 1,554 patients discussed in 13 studies revealed an overall sensitivity of 91% (81%–96%) and a specificity of 91% (81%–95%) (475). Although none of the adjunctive methods reviewed in the Cochrane meta-analysis were alternatives to scalpel biopsy, the overall high sensitivity and specificity of cytology presented it as a valuable asset in oral diagnostics (475). However, despite all the improvements made to the technique and the interpretation of cytologic results, there are still major hindrances and limitations that need to be addressed.

Lesion-related limitations include site selection, inaccessible sites and lesion characteristics. Most early oral lesions have a deceptively innocuous appearance and some are larger than they appear clinically (449). Failure in site selection due to overlooking lesions or inaccessible sites may result in false-negative findings and under-diagnosis of oral lesions. Lesion characteristics such as keratosis, ulcerated surface, presence of blood clots and infection may also result in inadequate sampling. Operator-related limitations include procedural (e.g. superficial sampling, obscuring the smear due to inappropriate thickness or debris, artefacts and poor staining) and interpretation errors (476).

Although most of these limitations could be overcome by careful patient selection and appropriate handling of tissues and samples, some are inevitable and inherent to the technique. Oral diagnosticians may choose to overcome their evidence-founded aversion for cytology by learning from the cervical cancer experience. At this point in time, cytology does not routinely serve as a replacement for scalpel biopsy; nevertheless, it is a useful tool that could provide beneficial information in the diagnosis and management of oral lesions.

BIOMARKERS

While macroscopic and microscopic changes in neoplastic and transforming tissues have captured our attention for decades, the imprint of molecular signatures in diseased tissue has more recently come to the limelight. Research into transcriptomics, proteomics and methylomics using assays and, more recently, high-throughput sequencing has uncovered a medley of putative biomarkers and discriminatory genes for HNSCC and OPMDs. Clarity for distinct biomarker pattern(s) is as yet evasive, albeit imminent, and considerable ongoing work is contributing to this wide and varied knowledge base.

It is currently accepted that the accumulation of genetic and epigenetic changes within a clonal population of cells drives carcinogenesis by altering oncogene and tumor suppressor gene (TSG) function (477–480). These genotypic alterations can affect hundreds of genes, causing genomic instability through chromosomal rearrangement, amplification, deletion, methylation or mutation and leading to phenotypic changes in critical cellular functions such as resistance to cell death, increased proliferation, induction of angiogenesis and the ability to invade and metastasize (481,482).

Potential molecular markers for OSCC or OED include protein markers (e.g. TP53 (483–489), MMP9 (490), CDKN2A [p16] (484,491–493) and EIF4E (494)) and epigenetic markers (promoter hypermethylation (492,495–497)), microRNA expression [e.g. miR-16, miR-125a and miR-184] (498), DNA copy number changes (486,499–502) and LOH [e.g. 3p, 9p, 13q, 11q, 17p] (309,500,503,504).

PROTEINS

Several proteins, encoding genes and subsequent mRNA transcripts have been found to be dysregulated in OED and HNSCC. p53, one such protein and a TSG located on chromosome 17p13, plays a major role in cell cycle progression, cellular differentiation and DNA repair and apoptosis (505,506). Loss of p53 function impairs cell cycle regulation and apoptosis and, as a result, alters the ability of cells to respond to stress or cell damage (such as DNA damage, hypoxia and oncogene activation) (505,506). This can lead to genomic instability and the accumulation of additional genetic alterations (507). Loss of p53 has long been implicated in early carcinogenesis, including HNSCC (508).

The proto-oncogene eIF4E is a eukaryotic translation initiation factor (509). eIF4E regulates the translation of cap-dependent mRNAs. An aberrant increase in eIF4E shifts the balance in favor of translation of transcripts that promote cell proliferation and malignancy (300,509). eIF4E protein is often elevated in HNSCCs (510) and its overexpression in surgical margins has been found in a number of studies associated with increased risk of local recurrence (300).

EPIGENETIC EVENTS

Unlike genetic alterations, epigenetic changes are heritable but potentially reversible (511). Any heritable modifications in gene expression without alterations of the DNA sequence are referred to as epigenetic changes—they occur more frequently than gene mutations, often persisting for the duration of cell life and even through several generations (479). In the chromatin context, transcription of genes may change from high-level expression to total silencing depending on the influence of the "epimutations" that interfere with the action of activators and suppressors on specific promoters (477). Epigenetic inheritance includes DNA methylation, histone modifications, changes in chromatin conformation and RNA-mediated silencing (481).

Promoter hypermethylation is well documented as a mechanism for tumor-specific alteration of TSG activity in head and neck cancer (512). In normal tissues, unmethylated cytosine is found in high densities in CpG islands—areas with high concentrations of cytosine and guanine that map close to a promoter region in 40% of mammalian genes (477). This unmethylated state is associated with a high rate of transcriptional activity, which is vital for maintaining TSG levels. Hypermethylation of TSG (*via* the enzyme DNA methyltransferase) is associated with stable transcriptional silencing of tumor suppressor activity (478,511).

As an example, studies have shown that methylation of the *p16INK4a* gene is a frequent event in primary HNC, with hypermethylation occurring in 50%–73% of cases (513,514). Surgical margin studies have shown p16 methylation to occur in clear margins (497,515); however, its prognostic significance has been debated (492,497). A recent systematic review and meta-analysis of the literature concluded that, based on six studies analyzed, significantly better overall survival rates were seen in p16-positive OPSCC tumors (516). Differences in methodologies and cut-off points for analysis between the studies remain a limitation for analysis and there remains inadequate evidence at this time to determine whether or not hypermethylation of p16 can be used as a biomarker in the determination of clear surgical resection margins, the ability to predict the risk of local relapse or indeed even in the accurate diagnosis and prognostication of OPMLs or OSCCs.

microRNA

There has been increasing evidence of the role of non-coding microRNAs (miRs) in the regulation of fundamental cellular processes and the impact of their dysregulation on carcinogenesis, with there also being current interest in the interaction between miRs and the HPV in HPV-associated HNSCC (517–524). miRs are single-stranded, endogenous, non-coding RNA (ncRNA) sequences transcribed from DNA and range between 18 and 24 nucleotides in length. They have the ability to regulate the expression of other genes on a post-transcriptional level through various processes, by degradation or repression of target mRNA, thereby influencing organ development, cell differentiation, proliferation, apoptosis and stress responses (188,525). Recent studies have suggested that miRs may also regulate mRNA targets through less stringent mechanisms, such as binding to non-complementary regions and to sites located within the coding regions of transcripts (514). Given their pivotal function as post-transcriptional regulators of gene expression, miRs affect almost every cellular process and have been implicated in numerous disease types, including cancer (188,519,526).

The role of miRs in cancer development was first established in a study that reported that a specific miR cluster (miR-15/16) was deleted and/or downregulated in the majority of chronic lymphocytic leukemia cases (499). The link to cancer was further strengthened by the discovery that miR genomic positioning appeared to be non-random (499,526) and that a significant number of miR genes were located at fragile sites or genomic regions that have been linked to cancers (527). One miR can have multiple targets; for example, *RAS*, *HMGA2* and *MYC* oncogenes have been identified as let-7 targets, indicating significant tumor-suppressive importance for this family of miRs (525,527).

There have been many molecular studies investigating the expression and dysregulation of miRs in HNSCC (518–520,528–530). Using a candidate gene approach, most have attempted to examine the role of the expression and the proposed targets of specific miRs in HNSCC cell lines compared to normal samples (520,529–532). The underlying process by which miR deregulation affects the process of transition from dysplasia to HNSCC has not yet been fully elucidated, with a main impediment being the multifactorial etiology of HNSCC and the wide heterogeneity of lesions. However, one theory is that upregulation of the enzymes involved in processing miRNA, such as Dicer and Drosha, may be implicated in carcinogenesis (173). It is pertinent to note that most studies to date investigating miR expression profiles in HNSCC have used cancer cell lines and only a few have been in solid tumor samples (520,533). Cell lines may not reflect the miR profiles of solid tumors, as particular culture conditions and clonal selection may radically change miR expression (532).

Despite the increasing number of studies into miR expression in HNSCC, there are only a few that investigate the role of miRs in tissue transformation from dysplasia to malignancy. Upregulation of both miR-31 and its complementary strand miR-31* has been found to occur in OL (534). This was consistent with miR expression profile findings in another prospective translational study that examined global miR expression in a series of consecutive tumors and biopsies obtained from patients with OSCC and OPSCC, concluding that the upregulation of miR-31 and the downregulation of miR-375 were the most significant aberrations (532). Thus, there is evidence to suggest that the upregulation of miR-31 may be an early event in the transition process from dysplasia to OSCC.

LOSS OF HETEROZYGOSITY

When one copy of a polymorphic marker with two slightly different alleles is lost or amplified (allelic gain), LOH may occur (535). LOH in key chromosomal loci represents one of the more promising markers, consistently being identified as a potentially independent risk predictor, supported by data from several laboratories, including studies by Sidransky, Califano, Mao, Hong, Lippman and Lee (393,536–540).

Califano and Sidransky (537,541) reported LOH at 9p21, 3p and 17p13 in squamous hyperplasia and at 13q11, 13q21 and 14q31 in dysplasia, with loss of chromosomal region 9p21 being the most common genetic alteration in HNSCC (occurring in 70%–80% of dysplastic lesions of the oral mucosa) (537,541). There is a general consensus that LOH at 3p and 9p provides evidence of the accumulation of genetic damage in potentially malignant lesions (542–544). Lesions with greater disturbance in cellular architecture and organization seem to harbor more genetic alterations at 3p and 9p; however, this is not noted in all studies (536–538,542).

The predictive and prognostic capacity of LOH at 3p and 9p for risk of transition from OED to malignancy has also been explored (485,545,546). High-risk (3p and/or 9p LOH) lesions have been found to have a 22.6-fold increased risk of progression when compared with the low-risk (3p and 9p retention) lesions. These findings are consistent with a previous study (88,545). It has also been demonstrated that low-grade lesions showing retention of 9p had an approximately 5% risk of progression over 5 years to severe dysplasia or more advanced disease (88). This finding has important implications, as it could suggest that individuals falling into this category might not require aggressive treatment or monitoring, despite having a histologic diagnosis of dysplasia. Conversely, a high progression rate (approximately 65%) for high-risk lesions was found and would suggest that this group should be aggressively monitored for clinical progression (88).

Ultimately, comparison amongst existing studies is hindered by methodological differences, adjustment for confounders, and controls. While early evidence appears promising, the clinical utility of LOH in 3p and 9p as a predictive tool to screen for progression of OED still requires further long-term prospective validation and/or investigation (535,545).

SALIVARY MARKERS

In addition to its known constituents, saliva has recently been shown to accommodate unique molecular markers capable of discriminating oral and systemic diseases, similar to blood, augmenting recent research in salivaomics (547–555). At the basic mechanistic level in a rodent pancreatic cancer model, it is considered that exosome-like vesicles carry, drive and deliver tumor-specific biomarkers into saliva (547,556). One of the key motivations for research into saliva diagnostics is that it is a non-invasive, simple and low-cost method for disease screening and detection (547,557–560). Due to low RNA abundance, small sample volumes, highly fragmented mRNA and the profusion of bacterial contents challenging downstream RNA sequencing assays, ncRNAs have proven to be the ideal group of salivary biomarkers, being short in size, located mainly within exosomes and possessing good body fluid stability (547,561–565). miRs in particular (small ncRNAs 18–23 nucleotides long with a critical role in mRNA regulation, thus influencing biological processes) have been widely investigated in saliva (521,566).

A study by Weber et al. investigating the miR profile in 12 body fluids discovered that saliva had a high number of detectable miR species and the miR spectrum in plasma was different to most other body fluids (567). There is a differentiation of saliva in studies, with some using whole saliva (WS), which includes cell content and cell debris, including all bacterial material, while others investigate cell-free saliva (CFS). Patel et al. reported miR-223, miR-191, miR-16, miR-203 and miR-24 to be the most highly expressed miRs in WS, which was corroborated in other studies (563,568–570). Spielmann et al. used massively parallel sequencing to compare WS to CFS miR contents and found measurable differences between them, with the greatest difference being in percentage of reads aligning to microbial genomes (higher in WS than in CFS), which noticeably decreases the sensitivity of human RNA in WS analysis (561).

Park et al. found miR-125a and miR-200a to be differentially expressed in both CFS and WS when comparing patients with and without oral cancer (569). Wiklund et al. reported aberrant expression of miR-375 and miR-200a and miR-200c-141 methylation when comparing oral rinse and saliva from patients with OSCC and healthy controls, suggesting a potential miR signature in oral fluids (571). Liu et al. investigated miR-31 as a biomarker for OSCC in oral lesions, plasma and saliva and found that miR-31 was significantly increased in saliva from patients with oral carcinoma at all clinical stages, including small tumors (572). However, this did not hold true in patients with verrucous leukoplakia compared with controls. Furthermore, miR-31 was found more abundantly in saliva than in plasma, suggesting miR-31 to be a more sensitive marker for oral malignancy. They also reported that salivary miR-31 was reduced after excision of oral carcinoma, suggesting that most of the upregulated salivary miR-31 was transcripted from tumor tissue. Yang et al. identified 25 differentially expressed miRs between progressive and non-progressive low grade dysplasia in OPMLs, progressing to high-grade dysplasia or OSCC: miR-10b-5p, miR-99a-5p, miR-99b-5p, miR-145-5p, miR-100-5p, miR-125b-5p, miR-181b, miR-181c, miR-197-3p, miR-331-3p, miR-15a-5p, miR-708, miR-150-5p, miR-30e-3p, miR-30a-3p, miR-21, let-7a-5p, miR-335-5p, miR-144*, miR-25-3p, miR-19a-3p, miR-660-5p, miR-140-5p, miR-590-5p and miR-9 (573). Momen-Heravi et al. identified 11 downregulated miRs (miR-136, miR-147, miR-1250, miR-148a, miR-632, miR-646, miR668, miR-877, miR-503, miR-220a and miR-323-5p) and two overexpressed miRs (miR-24 and miR-27b) in the saliva of patients with OSCC compared with healthy controls (574). Salazar et al. reported miR-9, miR-134 and miR-191 to be differentially expressed in saliva of HNSCC patients compared to healthy controls, with good discriminative capacity (575).

Xiao et al. reported 17 and 15 proteins to be consistently upregulated and downregulated in malignant and epithelial dysplasia, respectively, when compared to adjacent normal oral epithelium, of which cornulin, myoglobin and S100A8 have been validated (576). Notably, this study found cornulin to be downregulated in the saliva of oral cancer patients, providing the ability to differentiate between oral cancer patients and non-oral cancer patients ($p < .005$), while myoglobin and S100A8 could also significantly differentiate between epithelial dysplasia and oral cancer (576). Increased abundances of myosin and actin in saliva have previously been found, enabling differentiation between premalignant and malignant oral lesions (577).

Salivary levels of IL-6 have been found to be higher in 20 patients with OSCC than in 20 patients with PVL compared to 20 normal controls (578). Another study found significantly higher levels of IL-8 in the saliva of patients with OSCCs compared to patients with OPMLs and healthy controls (579). The detection of IL-6 and IL-8 in saliva and their potential as biomarkers for HNSCC have previously been reported (580,581).

A recent study by Wang et al. (582) investigated the potential value of tumor-specific DNA (defined as somatic mutations or HPV genes) in saliva or plasma as a biomarker for HNSCC. One hundred percent of patients with early-stage disease ($n = 10$) had detectable tumor DNA, while this statistic was 95% in patients with late-stage disease ($n = 37$). In patients with tumors of the oral cavity ($n = 15$), oropharynx ($n = 22$), larynx ($n = 7$) and hypopharynx ($n = 3$), tumor DNA was detected in 100%, 91%, 100% and 100%, respectively. Tumor DNA was found in WS in 100% of patients with oral cavity cancers and in 47%–70% of patients with cancers from other sites, while in plasma, these figures were 80% and 86%–100%, respectively. This suggests that saliva is preferentially enriched for tumor DNA from the oral cavity, while plasma is preferentially enriched for tumor DNA from the other sites. Furthermore, tumor DNA was found post-surgically in the saliva of three patients before clinical diagnosis of recurrence, but in none of the five patients without recurrence. Thus, tumor DNA in plasma and saliva appears to be a potentially valuable biomarker for the detection of HNSCC. The authors claim that a biomarker panel including HPV-16 DNA sequences, *TP53*, *PIK2CA*, *NOTCH1* and *CDKN2A* would be able to detect >95% of invasive HNSCCs (582).

Epigenetic changes are also thought to be reflected in the saliva of patients with HNSCC (481). Rettori et al. (583) compared the DNA hypermethylation status of 24 genes in salivary rinses collected from HNSCC patients at diagnosis, immediately after the last curative treatment and in the patient follow-up visit at 6 months after treatment. The analysis of the salivary rinses taken at the time of diagnosis showed five genes with sensitivity and specificity: *CCNA1*, *DAPK*, *DCC*, *MGMT* and *TIMP3*. The authors reported that *TIMP3* methylation in samples collected 6 months after treatment was significantly associated with lower recurrence-free survival, with multivariate analysis confirmed *TIMP3* hypermethylation to be an independent prognostic factor for local recurrence (583). This was corroborated in another study (457) investigating DNA hypermethylation in salivary rinses from 197 patients with HNSCC, which reported that the detection of hypermethylation of *CCNA1*, *MGMT* and *MINT31* was significantly associated with poor overall survival, *TIMP3* was significantly associated with local recurrence-free survival and *MINT31* was significantly associated with poor disease-free survival, all in univariate analyses. In multivariate analyses, detection of hypermethylation of *TIMP3* in the salivary rinse was found to have an independent, significant association with local recurrence-free survival (457).

When investigating differences in salivary miR profiles between benign and malignant parotid gland tumors, Matse et al. found 57 of 750 investigated miRs were differentially expressed, 54 of which were overexpressed in the saliva of patients with malignant parotid gland tumors, while only three were underexpressed in this group (miR-519b-3p, miR-520C-3p and miR-520D-3p), compared to the saliva of patients with benign parotid gland tumors (151).

In the absence of a validated biomarker for predicting the MT of OPMDs, an excellent COE along with the patient's history risk stratification associated with an objective histopathological evaluation of a biopsy taken from a suspicious lesion is still the gold standard for the early detection of oral cancer. Extensive research has been carried out to identify promising adjunctive aids and biomarkers for the early detection of oral cancer. However, longitudinal, multicenter, well-designed studies to assess the utility of these adjunctive methods and biomarkers are required before they can become part of routine daily practice.

REFERENCES

1. GLOBOCAN 2012 v1.0, Cancer Incidence and Mortality Worldwide: IARC CancerBase No. 11 [Internet]. Lyon, France: International Agency for Research on Cancer, 2013. Available from: http://globocan.iarc.fr, accessed on 05/05/2016. 2013.
2. Napier SS, Speight PM. Natural history of potentially malignant oral lesions and conditions: an overview of the literature. *J Oral Pathol Med* 2008;37(1):1–10.
3. van der Waal I. Potentially malignant disorders of the oral and oropharyngeal mucosa; present concepts of management. *Oral Oncol* 2010;46(6):423–5.
4. Warnakulasuriya S, Johnson NW, van der Waal I. Nomenclature and classification of potentially malignant disorders of the oral mucosa. *J Oral Pathol Med* 2007;36(10):575–80.
5. Warnakulasuriya S. Lack of molecular markers to predict malignant potential of oral precancer. *J Pathol* 2000;190(4):407–9.

6. Kramer IR, Lucas RB, Pindborg JJ, Sobin LH. Definition of leukoplakia and related lesions: an aid to studies on oral precancer. *Oral Surg Oral Med Oral Pathol* 1978;46(4):518–39.
7. Wahi PN, World Health Organization. *Histological Typing of Oral and Oropharyngeal Tumours*: World Health Organization, Geneva, Switzerland, 1971.
8. Pindborg JJ, Sobin LH, Reichart PA, Smith CJ, van der Waal I. *Histological Typing of Cancer and Precancer of the Oral Mucosa: In Collaboration with L.H. Sobin and Pathologists in 9 Countries*. Berlin Heidelberg: Springer, 1997.
9. Barnes L, Eveson JW, Reichart P. (eds) SD. World health organization classification of tumours. *Pathology and Genetics of Head and Neck Tumours* (9th Edition). Lyon: IARC Press, 2005.
10. Farah CS, Woo SB, Zain RB, Sklavounou A, McCullough MJ, Lingen M. Oral cancer and oral potentially malignant disorders. *Int J Dent* 2014;2014:853479.
11. Villa A, Gohel A. Oral potentially malignant disorders in a large dental population. *J Appl Oral Sci* 2014;22(6):473–6.
12. Parlatescu I, Gheorghe C, Coculescu E, Tovaru S. Oral leukoplakia—an update. *Maedica (Buchar)* 2014;9(1):88–93.
13. Starzynska A, Pawlowska A, Renkielska D, Michajlowski I, Sobjanek M, Blazewicz I. Oral premalignant lesions: epidemiological and clinical analysis in the northern Polish population. *Postepy Dermatol Alergol* 2014;31(6):341–50.
14. Ho MW, Field EA, Field JK et al. Outcomes of oral squamous cell carcinoma arising from oral epithelial dysplasia: rationale for monitoring premalignant oral lesions in a multidisciplinary clinic. *Br J Oral Maxillofac Surg* 2013;51(7):594–9.
15. Ho MW, Risk JM, Woolgar JA et al. The clinical determinants of malignant transformation in oral epithelial dysplasia. *Oral Oncol* 2012;48(10):969–76.
16. Dost F, Le Cao K, Ford PJ, Ades C, Farah CS. Malignant transformation of oral epithelial dysplasia: a real-world evaluation of histopathologic grading. *Oral Surg Oral Med Oral Pathol Oral Radiol* 2014;117(3):342–52.
17. Lee JJ, Hung HC, Cheng SJ et al. Carcinoma and dysplasia in oral leukoplakias in Taiwan: prevalence and risk factors. *Oral Surg Oral Med Oral Pathol Oral Radiol Endod* 2006;101(4):472–80.
18. Schepman KP, Van Der Meij EH, Smeele LE, Van Der Waal I. Malignant transformation of oral leukoplakia: a follow-up study of a hospital-based population of 166 patients with oral leukoplakia from The Netherlands. *Oral Oncol* 1998;34(4):270–5.
19. Silverman S Jr, Gorsky M, Lozada F. Oral leukoplakia and malignant transformation. A follow-up study of 257 patients. *Cancer* 1984;53(3):563–8.
20. Hansen LS, Olson JA, Silverman S Jr. Proliferative verrucous leukoplakia. A long-term study of thirty patients. *Oral Surg Oral Med Oral Pathol* 1985;60(3):285–98.
21. Akrish S, Ben-Izhak O, Sabo E, Rachmiel A. Oral squamous cell carcinoma associated with proliferative verrucous leukoplakia compared with conventional squamous cell carcinoma—a clinical, histologic and immunohistochemical study. *Oral Surg Oral Med Oral Pathol Oral Radiol* 2014;119(3):318–25.
22. Bagan J, Scully C, Jimenez Y, Martorell M. Proliferative verrucous leukoplakia: a concise update. *Oral Dis* 2010;16(4):328–32.
23. Amagasa T, Yamashiro M, Uzawa N. Oral premalignant lesions: from a clinical perspective. *Int J Clin Oncol* 2011;16(1):5–14.
24. Dost F, Le Cao KA, Ford PJ, Farah CS. A retrospective analysis of clinical features of oral malignant and potentially malignant disorders with and without oral epithelial dysplasia. *Oral Surg Oral Med Oral Pathol Oral Radiol* 2013;116(6):725–33.
25. Reibel J. Prognosis of oral pre-malignant lesions: Significance of clinical, histopathological, and molecular biological characteristics. *Crit Rev Oral Biol Med* 2003;14(1):47–62.
26. Liu W, Wang YF, Zhou HW, Shi P, Zhou ZT, Tang GY. Malignant transformation of oral leukoplakia: a retrospective cohort study of 218 Chinese patients. *BMC Cancer* 2010;10:685.
27. van der Waal I. Potentially malignant disorders of the oral and oropharyngeal mucosa; terminology, classification and present concepts of management. *Oral Oncol* 2009;45(4–5):317–23.
28. Yardimci G, Kutlubay Z, Engin B, Tuzun Y. Precancerous lesions of oral mucosa. *World J Clin Cases* 2014;2(12):866–72.
29. Pindborg JJ, Jolst O, Renstrup G, Roed-Petersen B. Studies in oral leukoplakia: a preliminary report on the period pervalence of malignant transformation in leukoplakia based on a follow-up study of 248 patients. *J Am Dent Assoc* 1968;76(4):767–71.
30. Wang YY, Tail YH, Wang WC et al. Malignant transformation in 5071 southern Taiwanese patients with potentially malignant oral mucosal disorders. *BMC Oral Health* 2014;14:99.
31. Vedtofte P, Holmstrup P, Hjorting-Hansen E, Pindborg JJ. Surgical treatment of premalignant lesions of the oral mucosa. *Int J Oral Maxillofac Surg* 1987;16(6):656–64.
32. Kawczyk-Krupka A, Waskowska J, Raczkowska-Siostrzonek A et al. Comparison of cryotherapy and photodynamic therapy in treatment of oral leukoplakia. *Photodiagnosis Photodyn Ther* 2012;9(2):148–55.
33. Pietruska M, Sobaniec S, Bernaczyk P et al. Clinical evaluation of photodynamic therapy efficacy in the treatment of oral leukoplakia. *Photodiagnosis Photodyn Ther* 2014;11(1):34–40.

34. Krahl D, Altenburg A, Zouboulis CC. Reactive hyperplasias, precancerous and malignant lesions of the oral mucosa. *J Dtsch Dermatol Ges* 2008;6(3):217–32.
35. Ribeiro AS, Salles PR, da Silva TA, Mesquita RA. A review of the nonsurgical treatment of oral leukoplakia. *Int J Dent* 2010;2010:186018.
36. Gorsky M, Epstein JB. The effect of retinoids on premalignant oral lesions: focus on topical therapy. *Cancer* 2002;95(6):1258–64.
37. Buerki N, Gautier L, Kovac M et al. Evidence for breast cancer as an integral part of lynch syndrome. *Genes Chromosomes Cancer* 2012;51(1):83–91.
38. Villa A, Villa C, Abati S. Oral cancer and oral erythroplakia: an update and implication for clinicians. *Aust Dent J* 2011;56(3):253–6.
39. Reichart PA, Philipsen HP. Oral erythroplakia—a review. *Oral Oncol* 2005;41(6):551–61.
40. McCullough M, Jaber M, Barrett AW, Bain L, Speight PM, Porter SR. Oral yeast carriage correlates with presence of oral epithelial dysplasia. *Oral Oncol* 2002;38(4):391–3.
41. Mohd Bakri M, Mohd Hussaini H, Rachel Holmes A, David Cannon R, Mary Rich A. Revisiting the association between candidal infection and carcinoma, particularly oral squamous cell carcinoma. *J Oral Microbiol* 2010;2.
42. Barrett AW, Kingsmill VJ, Speight PM. The frequency of fungal infection in biopsies of oral mucosal lesions. *Oral Dis* 1998;4(1):26–31.
43. Sitheeque MA, Samaranayake LP. Chronic hyperplastic candidosis/candidiasis (candidal leukoplakia). *Crit Rev Oral Biol Med* 2003;14(4):253–67.
44. Nagy K, Szoke I, Sonkodi I et al. Inhibition of microflora associated with oral malignancy. *Oral Oncol* 2000;36(1):32–6.
45. Hooper SJ, Wilson MJ, Crean SJ. Exploring the link between microorganisms and oral cancer: a systematic review of the literature. *Head Neck* 2009;31(9):1228–39.
46. Cawson RA, Lehner T. Chronic hyperplastic candidiasis—candidal leukoplakia. *Br J Dermatol* 1968;80(1):9–16.
47. Gainza-Cirauqui ML, Nieminen MT, Novak Frazer L, Aguirre-Urizar JM, Moragues MD, Rautemaa R. Production of carcinogenic acetaldehyde by *Candida albicans* from patients with potentially malignant oral mucosal disorders. *J Oral Pathol Med* 2013;42(3):243–9.
48. Alnuaimi AD, Wiesenfeld D, O'Brien-Simpson NM, Reynolds EC, McCullough MJ. Oral *Candida* colonization in oral cancer patients and its relationship with traditional risk factors of oral cancer: a matched case–control study. *Oral Oncol* 2015;51(2):139–45.
49. Homann N, Tillonen J, Meurman JH et al. Increased salivary acetaldehyde levels in heavy drinkers and smokers: a microbiological approach to oral cavity cancer. *Carcinogenesis* 2000;21(4):663–8.
50. Tillonen J, Homann N, Rautio M, Jousimies-Somer H, Salaspuro M. Role of yeasts in the salivary acetaldehyde production from ethanol among risk groups for ethanol-associated oral cavity cancer. *Alcohol Clin Exp Res* 1999;23(8):1409–15.
51. Cavalcante ASR, Anbinder AL, Carvalho YR. Actinic cheilitis: clinical and histological features. *J Oral Maxillofac Surg* 2008;66(3):498–503.
52. Savage NW, McKay C, Faulkner C. Actinic cheilitis in dental practice. *Aust Dent J* 2010;55(Suppl 1):78–84.
53. Markopoulos A, Albanidou-Farmaki E, Kayavis I. Actinic cheilitis: clinical and pathologic characteristics in 65 cases. *Oral Dis* 2004;10(4):212–6.
54. de Santana Sarmento DJ, da Costa Miguel MC, Queiroz LM, Godoy GP, da Silveira EJ. Actinic cheilitis: clinicopathologic profile and association with degree of dysplasia. *Int J Dermatol* 2014;53(4):466–72.
55. Lopes ML, Silva Junior FL, Lima KC, Oliveira PT, Silveira EJ. Clinicopathological profile and management of 161 cases of actinic cheilitis. *An Bras Dermatol* 2015;90(4):505–12.
56. Casparis S, Borm JM, Tektas S et al. Oral lichen planus (OLP), oral lichenoid lesions (OLL), oral dysplasia, and oral cancer: retrospective analysis of clinicopathological data from 2002–2011. *Oral Maxillofac Surg* 2015;19(2):149–56. doi: 10.1007/s10006-014-0469-y. Epub October 14, 2014.
57. Patil S, Rao RS, Sanketh DS, Warnakulasuriya S. Lichenoid dysplasia revisited—evidence from a review of Indian archives. *J Oral Pathol Med* 2015;44(7):507–14. doi: 10.1111/jop.12258. Epub September 15, 2014.
58. Bagan-Sebastian JV, Milian-Masanet MA, Penarrocha-Diago M, Jimenez Y. A clinical study of 205 patients with oral lichen planus. *J Oral Maxillofac Surg* 1992;50(2):116–8.
59. Scully C, Beyli M, Ferreiro MC et al. Update on oral lichen planus: etiopathogenesis and management. *Crit Rev Oral Biol Med* 1998;9(1):86–122.
60. Fitzpatrick SG, Honda KS, Sattar A, Hirsch SA. Histologic lichenoid features in oral dysplasia and squamous cell carcinoma. *Oral Surg Oral Med Oral Pathol Oral Radiol* 2014;117(4):511–20.
61. van der Meij EH, van der Waal I. Lack of clinicopathologic correlation in the diagnosis of oral lichen planus based on the presently available diagnostic criteria and suggestions for modifications. *J Oral Pathol Med* 2003;32(9):507–12.
62. Andreasen JO. Oral lichen planus. 1. A clinical evaluation of 115 cases. *Oral Surg Oral Med Oral Pathol* 1968;25(1):31–42.
63. Cortes-Ramirez DA, Gainza-Cirauqui ML, Echebarria-Goikouria MA, Aguirre-Urizar JM. Oral lichenoid disease as a premalignant condition: the controversies and the unknown. *Med Oral Patol Oral Cir Bucal* 2009;14(3):E118–22.

64. Aguirre Urizar JM. Letter to the editor: oral lichenoid disease. A new classification proposal. *Med Oral Patol Oral Cir Bucal* 2008;13(4):E224.
65. Al-Hashimi I, Schifter M, Lockhart PB et al. Oral lichen planus and oral lichenoid lesions: diagnostic and therapeutic considerations. *Oral Surg Oral Med Oral Pathol Oral Radiol Endod* 2007;103(Suppl):S25.e1–12.
66. Fitzpatrick SG, Hirsch SA, Gordon SC. The malignant transformation of oral lichen planus and oral lichenoid lesions: a systematic review. *J Am Dent Assoc* 2014;145(1):45–56.
67. Barnard NA, Scully C, Eveson JW, Cunningham S, Porter SR. Oral cancer development in patients with oral lichen planus. *J Oral Pathol Med* 1993;22(9):421–4.
68. Holmstrup P, Thorn JJ, Rindum J, Pindborg JJ. Malignant development of lichen planus-affected oral mucosa. *J Oral Pathol* 1988;17(5):219–25.
69. Lo Muzio L, Mignogna MD, Favia G, Procaccini M, Testa NF, Bucci E. The possible association between oral lichen planus and oral squamous cell carcinoma: a clinical evaluation on 14 cases and a review of the literature. *Oral Oncol* 1998;34(4):239–46.
70. Mignogna MD, Lo Muzio L, Lo Russo L, Fedele S, Ruoppo E, Bucci E. Clinical guidelines in early detection of oral squamous cell carcinoma arising in oral lichen planus: a 5-year experience. *Oral Oncol* 2001;37(3):262–7.
71. Silverman S Jr, Gorsky M, Lozada-Nur F, Giannotti K. A prospective study of findings and management in 214 patients with oral lichen planus. *Oral Surg Oral Med Oral Pathol* 1991;72(6):665–70.
72. Bornstein MM, Kalas L, Lemp S, Altermatt HJ, Rees TD, Buser D. Oral lichen planus and malignant transformation: a retrospective follow-up study of clinical and histopathologic data. *Quintessence Int* 2006;37(4):261–71.
73. Acay RR, Felizzola CR, de Araujo N, de Sousa SO. Evaluation of proliferative potential in oral lichen planus and oral lichenoid lesions using immunohistochemical expression of p53 and Ki67. *Oral Oncol* 2006;42(5):475–80.
74. Thornhill MH, Sankar V, Xu XJ et al. The role of histopathological characteristics in distinguishing amalgam-associated oral lichenoid reactions and oral lichen planus. *J Oral Pathol Med* 2006;35(4):233–40.
75. van der Meij EH, Schepman KP, van der Waal I. The possible premalignant character of oral lichen planus and oral lichenoid lesions: a prospective study. *Oral Surg Oral Med Oral Pathol Oral Radiol Endod* 2003;96(2):164–71.
76. van der Meij EH, Mast H, van der Waal I. The possible premalignant character of oral lichen planus and oral lichenoid lesions: a prospective five-year follow-up study of 192 patients. *Oral Oncol* 2007;43(8):742–8.
77. Krutchkoff DJ, Eisenberg E. Lichenoid dysplasia—a distinct histopathologic entity. *Oral Surg Oral Med Oral Pathol Oral Radiol Endod* 1985;60(3):308–15.
78. Lovas JG, Harsanyi BB, ElGeneidy AK. Oral lichenoid dysplasia: a clinicopathologic analysis. *Oral Surg Oral Med Oral Pathol* 1989;68(1):57–63.
79. Lodi G, Scully C, Carrozzo M, Griffiths M, Sugerman PB, Thongprasom K. Current controversies in oral lichen planus: report of an international consensus meeting. Part 2. Clinical management and malignant transformation. *Oral Surg Oral Med Oral Pathol Oral Radiol Endod* 2005;100(2):164–78.
80. Eisenberg E. Oral lichen planus: a benign lesion. *J Oral Maxillofac Surg* 2000;58(11):1278–85.
81. Jungell P, Konttinen YT, Nortamo P, Malmstrom M. Immunoelectron microscopic study of distribution of T cell subsets in oral lichen planus. *Scand J Dent Res* 1989;97(4):361–7.
82. Allen CM. Is lichen planus really premalignant? *Oral Surg Oral Med Oral Pathol Oral Radiol Endod* 1998;85(4):347.
83. Epstein JB, Wan LS, Gorsky M, Zhang L. Oral lichen planus: progress in understanding its malignant potential and the implications for clinical management. *Oral Surg Oral Med Oral Pathol Oral Radiol Endod* 2003;96(1):32–7.
84. Sousa FA, Rosa LE. Oral lichen planus: clinical and histopathological considerations. *Braz J Otorhinolaryngol* 2008;74(2):284–92.
85. van der Waal I. Oral lichen planus and oral lichenoid lesions; a critical appraisal with emphasis on the diagnostic aspects. *Med Oral Patol Oral Cir Bucal* 2009;14(7):E310–4.
86. Gonzalez-Moles MA, Scully C, Gil-Montoya JA. Oral lichen planus: controversies surrounding malignant transformation. *Oral Dis* 2008;14(3):229–43.
87. Warnakulasuriya S, Reibel J, Bouquot J, Dabelsteen E. Oral epithelial dysplasia classification systems: predictive value, utility, weaknesses and scope for improvement. *J Oral Pathol Med* 2008;37(3):127–33.
88. Tao J, Zhang X, Guo N et al. Squamous cell carcinoma complicating discoid lupus erythematosus in Chinese patients: review of the literature, 1964–2010. *J Am Acad Dermatol* 2012; 66(4):695–6.
89. Savage NW, Boras VV, Zaini ZM. Oral squamous cell carcinoma with discoid lupus erythematosus. *Oral Oncol Extra* 2006;42(1):32–5.
90. Kyriakis KP, Michailides C, Palamaras I, Terzoudi S, Evangelou G, Damoulaki E. Lifetime prevalence distribution of chronic discoid lupus erythematosus. *J Eur Acad Dermatol Venereol* 2007;21(8):1108–9.
91. Makita E, Akasaka E, Sakuraba Y et al. Squamous cell carcinoma on the lip arising from discoid lupus erythematosus: a case report and review of Japanese patients. *Eur J Dermatol* 2016;26(4):395–6.

92. Molomo EM, Bouckaert M, Khammissa RA, Motswaledi HM, Lemmer J, Feller L. Discoid lupus erythematosus-related squamous cell carcinoma of the lip in an HIV-seropositive black male. *J Cancer Res Ther* 2015;11(4):1036.
93. Batsakis JG, Suarez P, el-Naggar AK. Proliferative verrucous leukoplakia and its related lesions. *Oral Oncol* 1999;35(4):354–9.
94. Hall JM, Cohen MA, Moreland AA. Multiple and confluent lesions of oral leukoplakia. Proliferative verrucous leukoplakia. *Arch Dermatol* 1991;127(6):887–90.
95. Zakrzewska JM, Lopes V, Speight P, Hopper C. Proliferative verrucous leukoplakia: a report of ten cases. *Oral Surg Oral Med Oral Pathol Oral Radiol Endod* 1996;82(4):396–401.
96. Lopes MA, Feio P, Santos-Silva AR, Vargas PA. Proliferative verrucous leukoplakia may initially mimic lichenoid reactions. *World J Clin Cases* 2015;3(10):861–3.
97. Slootweg PJ, Müller H. Verrucous hyperplasia or verrucous carcinoma. An analysis of 27 patients. *J Maxillofac Surg* 1983;11(1):13–9.
98. Owosho AA, Bilodeau EA, Summersgill KF. 7 cases of proliferative verrucous leukoplakia: the need for a high clinical suspicion among dental practitioners. *Pa Dent J (Harrisb)* 2015;82(1):26–31.
99. Arduino PG, Bagan J, El-Naggar AK, Carrozzo M. Urban legends series: oral leukoplakia. *Oral Dis* 2013;19(7):642–59.
100. Greer RO Jr, Eversole LR, Crosby LK. Detection of human papillomavirus-genomic DNA in oral epithelial dysplasias, oral smokeless tobacco-associated leukoplakias, and epithelial malignancies. *J Oral Maxillofac Surg* 1990;48(11):1201–5.
101. Palefsky JM, Silverman S Jr, Abdel-Salaam M, Daniels TE, Greenspan JS. Association between proliferative verrucous leukoplakia and infection with human papillomavirus type 16. *J Oral Pathol Med* 1995;24(5):193–7.
102. Shroyer KR, Greer RO Jr. Detection of human papillomavirus DNA by *in situ* DNA hybridization and polymerase chain reaction in premalignant and malignant oral lesions. *Oral Surg Oral Med Oral Pathol* 1991;71(6):708–13.
103. Sciubba JJ, Helman JI. Current management strategies for verrucous hyperkeratosis and verrucous carcinoma. *Atlas Oral Maxillofac Surg Clin North Am* 2013;25(1):77–82. vi.
104. Zhu LK, Ding YW, Liu W, Zhou YM, Shi LJ, Zhou ZT. A clinicopathological study on verrucous hyperplasia and verrucous carcinoma of the oral mucosa. *J Oral Pathol Med* 2012;41(2):131–5.
105. Hazarey VK, Ganvir SM, Bodhade AS. Verrucous hyperplasia: a clinico-pathological study. *J Oral Maxillofac Pathol* 2011;15(2):187–91.
106. Shear M, Pindborg JJ. Verrucous hyperplasia of the oral mucosa. *Cancer* 1980;46(8):1855–62.
107. Alkan A, Bulut E, Gunhan O, Ozden B. Oral verrucous carcinoma: a study of 12 cases. *Eur J Dent* 2010;4(2):202–7.
108. Patil S, Warnakulasuriya S, Raj T, Sanketh DS, Rao RS. Exophytic oral verrucous hyperplasia: a new entity. *J Investig Clin Dent* 2016;7(4):417–23. doi: 10.1111/jicd.12166. Epub June 15, 2015.
109. Cox SC, Walker DM. Oral submucous fibrosis. A review. *Aust Dent J* 1996;41(5):294–9.
110. Agrawal A, Airen Sarkar P, Shigli A. Oral submucous fibrosis in a 9-year-old Indian girl. *BMJ Case Rep* 2011;September 28:2011. pii: bcr0820114588. doi: 10.1136/bcr.08.2011.4588.
111. Aziz SR. Coming to America: betel nut and oral submucous fibrosis. *J Am Dent Assoc* 2010;141(4):423–8.
112. Sitheeque M, Ariyawardana A, Jayasinghe R, Tilakaratne W. Depigmentation of oral mucosa as the earliest possible manifestation of oral submucous fibrosis in Sri Lankan preschool children. *J Investig Clin Dent* 2010;1(2):156–9.
113. Maher R, Lee AJ, Warnakulasuriya KA, Lewis JA, Johnson NW. Role of areca nut in the causation of oral submucous fibrosis: a case–control study in Pakistan. *J Oral Pathol Med* 1994; 23(2):65–9.
114. Gupta B, Johnson NW. Systematic review and meta-analysis of association of smokeless tobacco and of betel quid without tobacco with incidence of oral cancer in South Asia and the Pacific. *PLoS One* 2014;9(11):e113385.
115. International Agency on Research for Cancer. *Betel Quid and Areca Nut Chewing and Some Areca-nut-derived Nitrosamines. IARC Monographs on the Evaluation of Carcinogenic Risks to Humans.* Vol. 85. Lyon: world Health Organisation International Agency on Research for Cancer, 2004.
116. Oliver AJ, Radden BG. Oral submucous fibrosis. Case report and review of the literature. *Aust Dent J* 1992;37(1):31–4.
117. Eisenberg E, Krutchkoff D, Yamase H. Incidental oral hairy leukoplakia in immunocompetent persons. A report of two cases. *Oral Surg Oral Med Oral Pathol* 1992;74(3):332–3.
118. Eversole LR, Jacobsen P, Stone CE, Freckleton V. Oral condyloma planus (hairy leukoplakia) among homosexual men: a clinicopathologic study of thirty-six cases. *Oral Surg Oral Med Oral Pathol* 1986;61(3):249–55.
119. Schiodt M, Greenspan D, Daniels TE, Greenspan JS. Clinical and histologic spectrum of oral hairy leukoplakia. *Oral Surg Oral Med Oral Pathol* 1987;64(6):716–20.
120. Sciubba J, Brandsma J, Schwartz M, Barrezueta N. Hairy leukoplakia: an AIDS-associated opportunistic infection. *Oral Surg Oral Med Oral Pathol* 1989;67(4):404–10.

121. Ficarra G, Gaglioti D, Di Pietro M, Adler-Storthz K. Oral hairy leukoplakia: clinical aspects, histologic morphology and differential diagnosis. *Head Neck* 1991;13(6):514–21.
122. Farman AG. Hairy tongue (lingua villosa). *J Oral Med* 1977;32(3):85–91.
123. Field EA, Ellis A, Friedmann PS, Leigh IM, Field JK. Oral tylosis: a re-appraisal. *Oral Oncol* 1997;33(1):55–7.
124. Hanahan D, Weinberg RA. Hallmarks of cancer: the next generation. *Cell* 2011;144(5):646–74.
125. Vogelstein B, Kinzler KW. The multistep nature of cancer. *Trends Genet* 1993;9(4):138–41.
126. Ryan BM, Faupel-Badger JM. The hallmarks of premalignant conditions: a molecular basis for cancer prevention. *Semin Oncol* 2016;43(1):22–35.
127. Noonan VL, Kabani S. Diagnosis and management of suspicious lesions of the oral cavity. *Otolaryngol Clin North Am* 2005;38(1):21–35. vii.
128. van der Waal I. Oral potentially malignant disorders: is malignant transformation predictable and preventable? *Med Oral Patol Oral Cir Bucal* 2014;19(4):e386–90.
129. Lee JJ, Hong WK, Hittelman WN et al. Predicting cancer development in oral leukoplakia: ten years of translational research. *Clin Cancer Res* 2000;6(5):1702–10.
130. Shafer WG, Waldron CA. A clinical and histopathologic study of oral leukoplakia. *Surg Gynecol Obstet* 1961;112:411–20.
131. Rastogi V, Puri N, Mishra S, Arora S, Kaur G, Yadav L. An insight to oral epithelial dysplasia. *Int J Head Neck Surg* 2013;4(2):74–82.
132. Edwards PC. The natural history of oral epithelial dysplasia: perspective on Dost et al. *Oral Surg Oral Med Oral Pathol Oral Radiol* 2014;117(3):263–6.
133. Dost F, Lê Cao K, Ford PJ, Ades C, Farah CS. Malignant transformation of oral epithelial dysplasia: a real-world evaluation of histopathologic grading. *Oral Surg Oral Med Oral Pathol Oral Radiol* 2014;117(3):343–52.
134. Kujan O, Oliver RJ, Khattab A, Roberts SA, Thakker N, Sloan P. Evaluation of a new binary system of grading oral epithelial dysplasia for prediction of malignant transformation. *Oral Oncol* 2006;42(10):987–93.
135. Brothwell DJ, Lewis DW, Bradley G et al. Observer agreement in the grading of oral epithelial dysplasia. *Community Dent Oral Epidemiol* 2003;31(4):300–5.
136. Katz HC, Shear M, Altini M. A critical evaluation of epithelial dysplasia in oral mucosal lesions using the Smith-Pindborg method of standardization. *J Oral Pathol* 1985;14(6):476–82.
137. Pindborg JJ, Reibel J, Holmstrup P. Subjectivity in evaluating oral epithelial dysplasia, carcinoma *in situ* and initial carcinoma. *J Oral Pathol* 1985;14(9):698–708.
138. McCluggage WG, Bharucha H, Caughley LM et al. Interobserver variation in the reporting of cervical colposcopic biopsy specimens: comparison of grading systems. *J Clin Pathol* 1996;49(10):833–5.
139. Montgomery E, Bronner MP, Goldblum JR et al. Reproducibility of the diagnosis of dysplasia in Barrett esophagus: a reaffirmation. *Hum Pathol* 2001;32(4):368–78.
140. Dionne KR, Warnakulasuriya S, Zain RB, Cheong SC. Potentially malignant disorders of the oral cavity: current practice and future directions in the clinic and laboratory. *Int J Cancer* 2015;136(3):503–15.
141. Brennan M, Migliorati CA, Lockhart PB et al. Management of oral epithelial dysplasia: a review. *Oral Surg Oral Med Oral Pathol Oral Radiol Endod* 2007;103(Suppl):S19.e1–2.
142. Field EA, McCarthy CE, Ho MW et al. The management of oral epithelial dysplasia: the Liverpool algorithm. *Oral Oncol* 2015;51(10):883–7.
143. Thomson PJ. Managing oral potentially malignant disorders: a question of risk. *Fac Dent J* 2015;6(4):186–91.
144. Zhang L, Poh CF, Williams M et al. Loss of heterozygosity (LOH) profiles—validated risk predictors for progression to oral cancer. *Cancer Prev Res* 2012;5(9):1081–9.
145. Diajil A, Robinson CM, Sloan P, Thomson PJ. Clinical outcome following oral potentially malignant disorder treatment: a 100 patient cohort study. *Int J Dent* 2013;2013:809248.
146. Goodson ML, Sloan P, Robinson CM, Cocks K, Thomson PJ. Oral precursor lesions and malignant transformation—who, where, what, and when? *Br J Oral Maxillofac Surg* 2015;53(9):831–5.
147. Mehanna HM, Rattay T, Smith J, McConkey CC. Treatment and follow-up of oral dysplasia—a systematic review and meta-analysis. *Head Neck* 2009;31(12):1600–9.
148. Kujan O, Khattab A, Oliver RJ, Roberts SA, Thakker N, Sloan P. Why oral histopathology suffers interobserver variability on grading oral epithelial dysplasia: an attempt to understand the sources of variation. *Oral Oncol* 2007;43(3):224–31.
149. Sperandio M, Brown AL, Lock C et al. Predictive value of dysplasia grading and DNA ploidy in malignant transformation of oral potentially malignant disorders. *Cancer Prev Res* 2013;6(8):822–31.
150. Torres-Rendon A, Stewart R, Craig GT, Wells M, Speight PM. DNA ploidy analysis by image cytometry helps to identify oral epithelial dysplasias with a high risk of malignant progression. *Oral Oncol* 2009;45(6):468–73.
151. Matse JH, Yoshizawa J, Wang X et al. Discovery and prevalidation of salivary extracellular microRNA biomarkers panel for the noninvasive detection of benign and malignant parotid gland tumors. *Clin Cancer Res.* 2013;19(11):3032–8.

152. Lodi G, Sardella A, Bez C, Demarosi F, Carrassi A. Interventions for treating oral leukoplakia. *Cochrane Database Syst Rev* 2001(4):CD001829.
153. World Health Organization (WHO). Global Data on Incidence of Oral Cancer, WHO/NMH/CHP/HPR/ORH2005. http://www.who.int/oral_health/publications/cancer_maps/en/
154. Parkin DM, Pisani P, Ferlay J. Estimates of the worldwide incidence of 25 major cancers in 1990. *Int J Cancer* 1999;80(6):827–41.
155. Parkin DM, Bray F, Ferlay J, Pisani P. Global cancer statistics, 2002. *CA Cancer J Clin* 2005;55(2):74–108.
156. Malaovalla AM, Silverman S, Mani NJ, Bilimoria KF, Smith LW. Oral cancer in 57,518 industrial workers of Gujarat, India: a prevalence and followup study. *Cancer* 1976;37(4):1882–6.
157. La Vecchia C, Tavani A, Franceschi S, Levi F, Corrao G, Negri E. Epidemiology and prevention of oral cancer. *Oral Oncol* 1997;33(5):302–12.
158. Hirayama T. An epidemiological study of oral and pharyngeal cancer in central and South-East Asia. *Bull World Health Organ* 1966;34(1):41–69.
159. Blot WJ, McLaughlin JK, Winn DM et al. Smoking and drinking in relation to oral and pharyngeal cancer. *Cancer Res* 1988;48(11):3282–7.
160. Talamini R, Franceschi S, Barra S, Lavecchia C. The role of alcohol in oral and pharyngeal cancer in non-smokers, and of tobacco in non-drinkers. *Int J Cancer* 1990;46(3):391–3.
161. Franceschi S, Levi F, Dal Maso L et al. Cessation of alcohol drinking and risk of cancer of the oral cavity and pharynx. *Int J Cancer* 2000;85(6):787–90.
162. Fernandez Garrote L, Herrero R, Ortiz Reyes RM et al. Risk factors for cancer of the oral cavity and oropharynx in Cuba. *Br J Cancer* 2001;85(1):46–54.
163. Zavras AI, Douglass CW, Joshipura K et al. Smoking and alcohol in the etiology of oral cancer: gender-specific risk profiles in the south of Greece. *Oral Oncol* 2001;37(1):28–35.
164. Balaram P, Sridhar H, Rajkumar T et al. Oral cancer in southern India: the influence of smoking, drinking, paan-chewing and oral hygiene. *Int J Cancer* 2002;98(3):440–5.
165. Huang WY, Winn DM, Brown LM et al. Alcohol concentration and risk of oral cancer in Puerto Rico. *Am J Epidemiol* 2003;157(10):881–7.
166. Pelucchi C, Talamini R, Negri E et al. Folate intake and risk of oral and pharyngeal cancer. *Ann Oncol* 2003;14(11):1677–81.
167. Lissowska J, Pilarska A, Pilarski P et al. Smoking, alcohol, diet, dentition and sexual practices in the epidemiology of oral cancer in Poland. *Eur J Cancer Prev* 2003;12(1):25–33.
168. Castellsague X, Quintana MJ, Martinez MC et al. The role of type of tobacco and type of alcoholic beverage in oral carcinogenesis. *Int J Cancer* 2004;108(5):741–9.
169. Maserejian NN, Joshipura KJ, Rosner BA, Giovannucci E, Zavras AI. Prospective study of alcohol consumption and risk of oral premalignant lesions in men. *Cancer Epidemiol Biomark Prev* 2006;15(4):774–81.
170. Castellsague X, Munoz N, De Stefani E et al. Independent and joint effects of tobacco smoking and alcohol drinking on the risk of esophageal cancer in men and women. *Int J Cancer* 1999;82(5):657–64.
171. Hashibe M, Brennan P, Benhamou S et al. Alcohol drinking in never users of tobacco, cigarette smoking in never drinkers, and the risk of head and neck cancer: pooled analysis in the international head and neck cancer epidemiology consortium. *J Natl Cancer Inst* 2007;99(10):777–89.
172. Lubin JH, Purdue M, Kelsey K et al. Total exposure and exposure rate effects for alcohol and smoking and risk of head and neck cancer: a pooled analysis of case–control studies. *Am J Epidemiol* 2009;170(8):937–47.
173. Hashibe M, Brennan P, Chuang SC et al. Interaction between tobacco and alcohol use and the risk of head and neck cancer: pooled analysis in the international head and neck cancer epidemiology consortium. *Cancer Epidemiol Biomark Prev* 2009;18(2):541–50.
174. Wight AJ, Ogden GR. Possible mechanisms by which alcohol may influence the development of oral cancer—a review. *Oral Oncol* 1998;34(6):441–7.
175. Boffetta P, Hashibe M. Alcohol and cancer. *Lancet Oncol* 2006;7(2):149–56.
176. Gillison ML. Current topics in the epidemiology of oral cavity and oropharyngeal cancers. *Head Neck J Sci Spec* 2007;29(8):779–92.
177. Cawson RA. *E.W. O. Cawson's Essentials of Oral Pathology and Oral Medicine*. New York: churchill Livingstone, 2008.
178. Lingen MW, Xiao W, Schmitt A et al. Low etiologic fraction for high-risk human papillomavirus in oral cavity squamous cell carcinomas. *Oral Oncol* 2013;49(1):1–8.
179. Siebers TJH, Merkx MAW, Slootweg PJ, Melchers WJG, van Cleef P, Wilde PCM. No high-risk HPV detected in SCC of the oral tongue in the absolute absence of tobacco and alcohol—a case study of seven patients. *Oral Maxillofac Surg* 2008;12(4):185–8.
180. Salem A. Dismissing links between HPV and aggressive tongue cancer in young patients. *Ann Oncol* 2010;21(1):13–7.
181. Kabeya M, Furuta R, Kawabata K, Takahashi S, Ishikawa Y. Prevalence of human papillomavirus in mobile tongue cancer with particular reference to young patients. *Cancer Sci* 2012;103(2):161–8.
182. Gillison ML, Koch WM, Capone RB et al. Evidence for a causal association between human papillomavirus and a subset of head and neck cancers. *J Natl Cancer Inst* 2000;92(9):709–20.

183. Herrero R, Castellsagué X, Pawlita M et al. Human papillomavirus and oral cancer: the international agency for research on cancer multicenter study. *J Natl Cancer Inst* 2003;95(23):1772–83.
184. Neville BW, Day TA. Oral cancer and precancerous lesions. *CA Cancer J Clin* 2002;52(4):195–215.
185. D'Souza G, Kreimer AR, Viscidi R et al. Case–control study of human papillomavirus and oropharyngeal cancer. *N Engl J Med* 2007;356(19):1944–56.
186. Smeets SJ, Brakenhoff RH, Ylstra B et al. Genetic classification of oral and oropharyngeal carcinomas identifies subgroups with a different prognosis. *Cell Oncol* 2009;31(4):291–300.
187. Stransky N, Egloff AM, Tward AD et al. The mutational landscape of head and neck squamous cell carcinoma. *Science* 2011;333(6046):1157–60.
188. Agrawal N, Frederick MJ, Pickering CR et al. Exome sequencing of head and neck squamous cell carcinoma reveals inactivating mutations in NOTCH1. *Science* 2011;333(6046):1154–7.
189. Chaturvedi AK, Anderson WF, Lortet-Tieulent J et al. Worldwide trends in incidence rates for oral cavity and oropharyngeal cancers. *J Clin Oncol* 2013;31(36):4550–9.
190. Leao JC, Gueiros LA, Porter SR. Oral manifestations of syphilis. *Clinics (Sao Paulo, Brazil)* 2006;61(2):161–6.
191. Roed-Petersen B, Renstrup G, Pindborg JJ. Candida in oral leukoplakias. A histologic and exfoliative cytologic study. *Scand J Dent Res* 1970;78(4):323–8.
192. Renstrup G. Occurrence of *Candida* in oral leukoplakias. *Acta Pathol Microbiol Scand B Microbiol Immunol* 1970;78(4):421–4.
193. Chainani-Wu N, Epstein J, Touger-Decker R. Diet and prevention of oral cancer: strategies for clinical practice. *J Am Dent Assoc* 2011;142(2):166–9.
194. Nicolás B, Fabián LF, Silvia A, López de Blanc, Rosana AM, María AO. *Oral Squamous Cell Carcinoma Clinical Aspects*. Oral cancer. Ogbureke KUE (ed.) InTech, Rijeka, Croatia. March 14, 2012. doi: 10.5772/32968.
195. Speight PM, Abram TJ, Floriano PN et al. Interobserver agreement in dysplasia grading: toward an enhanced gold standard for clinical pathology trials. *Oral Surg Oral Med Oral Pathol Oral Radiol* 2015;120(4):474–82 e2.
196. Sugerman PB, Savage NW. Current concepts in oral cancer. *Aust Dent J* 1999;44(3):147–56.
197. Muller S, Pan Y, Li R, Chi AC. Changing trends in oral squamous cell carcinoma with particular reference to young patients: 1971–2006. The Emory University experience. *Head Neck Pathol* 2008;2(2):60–6.
198. Neville BW, Damm DD, Allen CM, Bouquot JE. *Oral and Maxillofacial Pathology*. (3rd Edition). St. Louis: Saunders, 2009.
199. Diaz EM Jr, Holsinger FC, Zuniga ER, Roberts DB, Sorensen DM. Squamous cell carcinoma of the buccal mucosa: one institution's experience with 119 previously untreated patients. *Head Neck* 2003;25(4):267–73.
200. Woolgar JA, Scott J, Vaughan ED, Brown JS, West CR, Rogers S. Survival, metastasis and recurrence of oral cancer in relation to pathological features. *Ann R Coll Surg Engl* 1995;77(5):325–31.
201. Shaw RJ, Brown JS, Woolgar JA, Lowe D, Rogers SN, Vaughan ED. The influence of the pattern of mandibular invasion on recurrence and survival in oral squamous cell carcinoma. *Head Neck* 2004;26(10):861–9.
202. Quan J, Zhou C, Johnson NW, Francis G, Dahlstrom JE, Gao J. Molecular pathways involved in crosstalk between cancer cells, osteoblasts and osteoclasts in the invasion of bone by oral squamous cell carcinoma. *Pathology* 2012;44(3):221–7.
203. Dik EA, Ipenburg NA, Adriaansens SO, Kessler PA, van Es RJ, Willems SM. Poor correlation of histologic parameters between biopsy and resection specimen in early stage oral squamous cell carcinoma. *Am J Clin Pathol* 2015;144(4):659–66.
204. van Meerbeeck JP, Janssens A. The seventh tumour–node–metastasis staging system for lung cancer: sequel or prequel? *Eur J Cancer Suppl* 2013;11(2):150–8.
205. Compton CC, Byrd DR, Garcia-Aguilar J et al. *AJCC Cancer Staging Atlas: a Companion to the Seventh Editions of the AJCC Cancer Staging Manual and Handbook*. New York: Springer New York: Imprint: Springer, 2012.
206. Nagadia R, Pandit P, Coman WB, Cooper-White J, Punyadeera C. miRNAs in head and neck cancer revisited. *Cell Oncol* 2013;36(1):1–7.
207. Mashberg A. Diagnosis of early oral and oropharyngeal squamous carcinoma: obstacles and their amelioration. *Oral Oncol* 2000;36(3):253–5.
208. Farah CS, Simanovic B, Dost F. Oral cancer in Australia 1982–2008: a growing need for opportunistic screening and prevention. *Aust Dent J* 2014;59(3):349–59.
209. de Carvalho AC, Kowalski LP, Campos AH, Soares FA, Carvalho AL, Vettore AL. Clinical significance of molecular alterations in histologically negative surgical margins of head and neck cancer patients. *Oral Oncol* 2012;48(3):240–8.
210. Leemans CR, Tiwari R, Nauta JJP, Vanderwaal I, Snow GB. Recurrence at the primary site in head and neck-cancer and the significance of neck lymph-node metastases as a prognostic factor. *Cancer* 1994;73(1):187–90.
211. Ackerman LV. Verrucous carcinoma of the oral cavity. *Surgery* 1948;23(4):670–78.
212. Addante RR, McKenna SJ. Verrucous carcinoma. *Atlas Oral Maxillofac Surg Clin North Am* 2006;18(4):513–9.
213. Szentirmay Z, Polus K, Tamas L et al. Human papillomavirus in head and neck cancer: molecular

biology and clinicopathological correlations. *Cancer Metastasis Rev* 2005;24(1):19–34.
214. Torrente MC, Rodrigo JP, Haigentz M Jr et al. Human papillomavirus infections in laryngeal cancer. *Head Neck* 2011;33(4):581–6.
215. Tornes K, Bang G, Stromme Koppang H, Pedersen KN. Oral verrucous carcinoma. *Int J Oral Surg* 1985;14(6):485–92.
216. Medina JE, Dichtel W, Luna MA. Verrucous-squamous carcinomas of the oral cavity. A clinicopathologic study of 104 cases. *Arch Otolaryngol* 1984;110(7):437–40.
217. Kang CJ, Chang JT, Chen TM, Chen IH, Liao CT. Surgical treatment of oral verrucous carcinoma. *Chang Gung Med J* 2003;26(11):807–12.
218. Candau-Alvarez A, Dean-Ferrer A, Alamillos-Granados FJ et al. Verrucous carcinoma of the oral mucosa: an epidemiological and follow-up study of patients treated with surgery in 5 last years. *Med Oral Patol Oral Cir Bucal* 2014;19(5):e506–11.
219. Odell EW, Jani P, Sherriff M et al. The prognostic value of individual histologic grading parameters in small lingual squamous cell carcinomas. The importance of the pattern of invasion. *Cancer* 1994;74(3):789–94.
220. Wain SL, Kier R, Vollmer RT, Bossen EH. Basaloid-squamous carcinoma of the tongue, hypopharynx, and larynx: report of 10 cases. *Hum Pathol* 1986;17(11):1158–66.
221. Sundharam BS, Krishnan PA. Basaloid squamous cell carcinoma report of a case and review of literature. *Indian J Dent Res* 2003;14(3):184–6.
222. Shanmugaratnam K, Sobin LH. The World Health Organization histological classification of tumours of the upper respiratory tract and ear. A commentary on the second edition. *Cancer* 1993;71(8):2689–97.
223. Jayasooriya PR, Tilakaratne WM, Mendis BR, Lombardi T. A literature review on oral basaloid squamous cell carcinomas, with special emphasis on etiology. *Ann Diagn Pathol* 2013;17(6):547–51.
224. El-Mofty SK. Histopathologic risk factors in oral and oropharyngeal squamous cell carcinoma variants: an update with special reference to HPV-related carcinomas. *Med Oral Patol Oral Cir Bucal* 2014;19(4):e377–85.
225. Yu GY, Gao Y, Peng X, Chen Y, Zhao FY, Wu MJ. A clinicopathologic study on basaloid squamous cell carcinoma in the oral and maxillofacial region. *Int J Oral Maxillofac Surg* 2008;37(11):1003–8.
226. Shivakumar B, Dash B, Sahu A, Nayak B. Basaloid squamous cell carcimoma: a rare case report with review of literature. *J Oral Maxillofac Pathol* 2014;18(2):291–4.
227. Fritsch VA, Lentsch EJ. Basaloid squamous cell carcinoma of the head and neck: location means everything. *J Surg Oncol* 2014;109(6):616–22.
228. Ding Y, Ma L, Shi L, Feng J, Liu W, Zhou Z. Papillary squamous cell carcinoma of the oral mucosa: a clinicopathologic and immunohistochemical study of 12 cases and literature review. *Ann Diagn Pathol* 2013;17(1):18–21.
229. Bao Z, Yang X, Shi L, Feng J, Liu W, Zhou Z. Clinicopathologic features of oral squamous papilloma and papillary squamous cell carcinoma: a study of 197 patients from eastern China. *Ann Diagn Pathol* 2012;16(6):454–8.
230. Romanach MJ, Azevedo RS, Carlos R, de Almeida OP, Pires FR. Clinicopathological and immunohistochemical features of oral spindle cell carcinoma. *J Oral Pathol Med* 2010;39(4):335–41.
231. Su HH, Chu ST, Hou YY, Chang KP, Chen CJ. Spindle cell carcinoma of the oral cavity and oropharynx: factors affecting outcome. *J Chin Med Assoc* 2006;69(10):478–83.
232. Klussmann JP, Weissenborn S, Fuchs PG. Human papillomavirus infection as a risk factor for squamous-cell carcinoma of the head and neck. *N Engl J Med* 2001;345(5):376; author reply 7.
233. Schick U, Pusztaszeri M, Betz M et al. Adenosquamous carcinoma of the head and neck: report of 20 cases and review of the literature. *Oral Surg Oral Med Oral Pathol Oral Radiol* 2013;116(3):313–20.
234. Gerughty RM, Hennigar GR, Brown FM. Adenosquamous carcinoma of the nasal, oral and laryngeal cavities. A clinicopathologic survey of ten cases. *Cancer* 1968;22(6):1140–55.
235. Mendillo ML, Putnam CD, Mo AO et al. Probing DNA- and ATP-mediated conformational changes in the MutS family of mispair recognition proteins using deuterium exchange mass spectrometry. *J Biol Chem* 2010;285(17):13170–82.
236. Uzcudun AE, Bravo Fernandez P, Sanchez JJ et al. Clinical features of pharyngeal cancer: a retrospective study of 258 consecutive patients. *J Laryngol Otol* 2001;115(2):112–8.
237. Ernster JA, Sciotto CG, O'Brien MM et al. Rising incidence of oropharyngeal cancer and the role of oncogenic human Papilloma virus. *Laryngoscope* 2007;117(12):2115–28.
238. Hammarstedt L, Lindquist D, Dahlstrand H et al. Human papillomavirus as a risk factor for the increase in incidence of tonsillar cancer. *Int J Cancer* 2006;119(11):2620–3.
239. Thomas J, Primeaux T. Is p16 immunohistochemistry a more cost-effective method for identification of human papilloma virus-associated head and neck squamous cell carcinoma? *Ann Diagn Pathol* 2012;16(2):91–9.
240. Westra WH. The changing face of head and neck cancer in the 21st century: the impact of HPV on the epidemiology and pathology of oral cancer. *Head Neck Pathol* 2009;3(1):78–81.
241. Chaturvedi AK. Epidemiology and clinical aspects of HPV in head and neck cancers. *Head Neck Pathol* 2012;6:S16–24.

242. Angiero F, Gatta LB, Seramondi R et al. Frequency and role of HPV in the progression of epithelial dysplasia to oral cancer. *Anticancer Res* 2010;30(9):3435–40.
243. Feng ZH, Hu WW, Marnett LJ, Tang MS. Malondialdehyde, a major endogenous lipid peroxidation product, sensitizes human cells to UV- and BPDE-induced killing and mutagenesis through inhibition of nucleotide excision repair. *Mutat Res* 2006;601(1–2):125–36.
244. Dost F, Ford PJ, Farah CS. Heightened risk of second primary carcinoma of the head and neck following cervical neoplasia. *Head Neck* 2014;36(8):1132–7. doi: 10.1002/hed.23417. Epub October 4, 2013.
245. Konopka JB, Watanabe SM, Singer JW. Cell lines and clinical isolates derived from Ph1-positive chronic myelogenous leukemia patients express c-abl proteins with a common structural alteration. *Proc Natl Acad Sci USA* 1985;82(6):1810–4.
246. Syrjanen S. HPV infections and tonsillar carcinoma. *J Clin Pathol* 2004;57(5):449–55.
247. Köberle B, Ditz C, Kausch I, Wollenberg B, Ferris RL, Albers AE. Metastases of squamous cell carcinoma of the head and neck show increased levels of nucleotide excision repair protein XPF *in vivo* that correlate with increased chemoresistance *ex vivo*. *Int J Oncol* 2010;36(5):1277–84.
248. Westra WH. The morphologic profile of HPV-related head and neck squamous carcinoma: implications for diagnosis, prognosis, and clinical management. *Head Neck Pathol* 2012;6(Suppl 1):S48–54.
249. Chi AC, Day TA, Neville BW. Oral cavity and oropharyngeal squamous cell carcinoma-an update. *CA Cancer J Clin* 2015;65(5):401–21.
250. Sood AJ, McIlwain W, O'Connell B, Nguyen S, Houlton JJ, Day T. The association between T-stage and clinical nodal metastasis in HPV-positive oropharyngeal cancer. *Am J Otolaryngol* 2014;35(4):463–8.
251. McIlwain WR, Sood AJ, Nguyen SA, Day TA. Initial symptoms in patients with HPV-positive and HPV-negative oropharyngeal cancer. *JAMA Otolaryngol* 2014;140(5):441–7.
252. Cardesa A, Nadal A. Carcinoma of the head and neck in the HPV era. *Acta Dermatovenerol Alp Panonica Adriat* 2011;20(3):161–73.
253. Chernock RD, Nussenbaum B, Thorstad WL et al. Extensive HPV-related carcinoma *in situ* of the upper aerodigestive tract with "nonkeratinizing" histologic features. *Head Neck Pathol* 2014;8(3):322–8.
254. Fornatora M, Jones AC, Kerpel S, Freedman P. Human papillomavirus-associated oral epithelial dysplasia (koilocytic dysplasia): an entity of unknown biologic potential. *Oral Surg Oral Med Oral Pathol Oral Radiol Endod* 1996;82(1):47–56.
255. McCord C, Xu J, Xu W et al. Association of high-risk human papillomavirus infection with oral epithelial dysplasia. *Oral Surg Oral Med Oral Pathol Oral Radiol* 2013;115(4):541–9.
256. Woo SB, Cashman EC, Lerman MA. Human papillomavirus-associated oral intraepithelial neoplasia. *Modern Pathol* 2013;26(10):1288–97.
257. El-Mofty SK. HPV-related squamous cell carcinoma variants in the head and neck. *Head Neck Pathol* 2012;6(Suppl 1):S55–62.
258. Bishop JA, Lewis JS Jr, Rocco JW, Faquin WC. HPV-related squamous cell carcinoma of the head and neck: an update on testing in routine pathology practice. *Semin Diagn Pathol* 2015;32(5):344–51.
259. Mashberg A, Meyers H. Anatomical site and size of 222 early asymptomatic oral squamous cell carcinomas: a continuing prospective study of oral cancer. II. *Cancer* 1976;37(5):2149–57.
260. Guggenheimer J, Verbin RS, Johnson JT, Horkowitz CA, Myers EN. Factors delaying the diagnosis of oral and oropharyngeal carcinomas. *Cancer* 1989;64(4):932–5.
261. Gorsky M, Epstein JB, Oakley C, Le ND, Hay J, Stevenson-Moore P. Carcinoma of the tongue: a case series analysis of clinical presentation, risk factors, staging, and outcome. *Oral Surg Oral Med Oral Pathol Oral Radiol Endod* 2004;98(5):546–52.
262. Bentham G, Aase A. Incidence of malignant melanoma of the skin in Norway, 1955–1989: associations with solar ultraviolet radiation, income and holidays abroad. *Int J Epidemiol* 1996;25(6):1132–8.
263. Chang AE, Karnell LH, Menck HR. The national cancer data base report on cutaneous and noncutaneous melanoma: a summary of 84,836 cases from the past decade. The American college of surgeons commission on cancer and the American cancer society. *Cancer* 1998;83(8):1664–78.
264. Grozinger G, Mann S, Mehra T et al. Metastatic patterns and metastatic sites in mucosal melanoma: a retrospective study. *Eur Radiol* 2016;26(6):1826–34. doi: 10.1007/s00330-015-3992-9. Epub September 15, 2015.
265. *Kaposi Sarcoma Treatment (PDQ®): Health Professional Version*. https://www.cancer.gov/types/soft-tissue-sarcoma/hp/kaposi-treatment-pdq.
266. Safai B, Good RA. Kaposi's sarcoma: a review and recent developments. *Clin Bull* 1980;10(2):62–9.
267. Safai B, Mike V, Giraldo G, Beth E, Good RA. Association of Kaposi's sarcoma with second primary malignancies: possible etiopathogenic implications. *Cancer* 1980;45(6):1472–9.
268. Penn I. Kaposi's sarcoma in organ transplant recipients: report of 20 cases. *Transplantation* 1979;27(1):8–11.
269. Panzarella V, Pizzo G, Calvino F, Compilato D, Colella G, Campisi G. Diagnostic delay in oral squamous cell carcinoma: the role of cognitive and psychological variables. *Int J Oral Sci* 2014;6(1):39–45.
270. Pitchers M, Martin C. Delay in referral of oropharyngeal squamous cell carcinoma to secondary care correlates with a more advanced stage at presentation, and is associated with poorer survival. *Br J Cancer* 2006;94(7):955–8.

271. Gomez I, Seoane J, Varela-Centelles P, Diz P, Takkouche B. Is diagnostic delay related to advanced-stage oral cancer? a meta-analysis. *Eur J Oral Sci* 2009;117(5):541–6.
272. Epstein JB, Guneri P, Boyacioglu H, Abt E. The limitations of the clinical oral examination in detecting dysplastic oral lesions and oral squamous cell carcinoma. *J Am Dent Assoc* 2012;143(12):1332–42.
273. Lingen MW, Kalmar JR, Karrison T, Speight PM. Critical evaluation of diagnostic aids for the detection of oral cancer. *Oral Oncol* 2008;44(1):10–22.
274. Wang TD, Van Dam J. Optical biopsy: a new frontier in endoscopic detection and diagnosis. *Clin Gastroenterol Hepatol* 2004;2(9):744–53.
275. Keereweer S, Kerrebijn JD, van Driel PB et al. Optical image-guided surgery—where do we stand? *Mol Imaging Biol* 2011;13(2):199–207.
276. Zhu Y, Terry NG, Wax A. Angle-resolved low-coherence interferometry: an optical biopsy technique for clinical detection of dysplasia in Barretts esophagus. *Expert Rev Gastroenterol Hepatol* 2012;6(1):37–41.
277. McIntosh L, McCullough MJ, Farah CS. The assessment of diffused light illumination and acetic acid rinse (Microlux/DL™) in the visualisation of oral mucosal lesions. *Oral Oncol* 2009;45(12):e227–31.
278. Vu AN, Matias MA, Farah CS. Diagnostic accuracy of narrow band imaging for detection of oral potentially malignant disorders. *Oral Dis* 2015;21(4):519–29.
279. Microlux/DL™. http://www.addent.com/microluxdl/.
280. ViziLite™. https://www.pattersondental.com/Supplies/ProductFamilyDetails/PIF_84128.
281. Farah CS, McCullough MJ. A pilot case control study on the efficacy of acetic acid wash and chemiluminescent illumination (ViziLite™) in the visualisation of oral mucosal white lesions. *Oral Oncol* 2007;43(8):820–4.
282. ViziLite™ TBlue. https://www.denmat.com/Oral%20Hygiene/Lesion%20Detection/ViziLite/Pack.
283. Ram S, Siar CH. Chemiluminescence as a diagnostic aid in the detection of oral cancer and potentially malignant epithelial lesions. *Int J Oral Maxillofac Surg* 2005;34(5):521–7.
284. Herlin P, Marnay J, Jacob JH, Ollivier JM, Mandard AM. A study of the mechanism of the Toluidine blue dye test. *Endoscopy* 1983;15(1):4–7.
285. Mashberg A. Final evaluation of tolonium chloride rinse for screening of high-risk patients with asymptomatic squamous carcinoma. *J Am Dent Assoc* 1983;106(3):319–23.
286. Chainani-Wu N, Madden E, Cox D, Sroussi H, Epstein J, Silverman S Jr. Toluidine blue aids in detection of dysplasia and carcinoma in suspicious oral lesions. *Oral Dis* 2015;21(7):879–85.
287. Chaudhry A, Manjunath M, Ashwatappa D, Krishna S, Krishna AG. Comparison of chemiluminescence and toluidine blue in the diagnosis of dysplasia in leukoplakia: a cross-sectional study. *J Investig Clin Dent* 2014.
288. Patton LL, Epstein JB, Kerr AR. Adjunctive techniques for oral cancer examination and lesion diagnosis: a systematic review of the literature. *J Am Dent Assoc* 2008;139(7):896–905.
289. Epstein JB, Silverman S Jr, Epstein JD, Lonky SA, Bride MA. Analysis of oral lesion biopsies identified and evaluated by visual examination, chemiluminescence and toluidine blue. *Oral Oncol* 2008;44(6):538–44.
290. Mojsa I, Kaczmarzyk T, Zaleska M, Stypulkowska J, Zapala-Pospiech A, Sadecki D. Value of the ViziLite Plus System as a diagnostic aid in the early detection of oral cancer/premalignant epithelial lesions. *J Craniofac Surg* 2012;23(2):e162–4.
291. Awan KH, Morgan PR, Warnakulasuriya S. Utility of chemiluminescence (ViziLite) in the detection of oral potentially malignant disorders and benign keratoses. *J Oral Pathol Med* 2011;40(7):541–4.
292. Oh ES, Laskin DM. Efficacy of the ViziLite system in the identification of oral lesions. *J Oral Maxillofac Surg* 2007;65(3):424–6.
293. Huber MA, Bsoul SA, Terezhalmy GT. Acetic acid wash and chemiluminescent illumination as an adjunct to conventional oral soft tissue examination for the detection of dysplasia: a pilot study. *Quintessence Int* 2004;35(5):378–84.
294. Epstein JB, Gorsky M, Lonky S, Silverman S Jr, Epstein JD, Bride M. The efficacy of oral lumenoscopy (ViziLite) in visualizing oral mucosal lesions. *Spec Care Dentist* 2006;26(4):171–4.
295. Kerr AR, Sirois DA, Epstein JB. Clinical evaluation of chemiluminescent lighting: an adjunct for oral mucosal examinations. *J Clin Dent* 2006;17(3):59–63.
296. Ibrahim SS, Al-Attas SA, Darwish ZE, Amer HA, Hassan MH. Effectiveness of the Microlux/DL™ chemiluminescence device in screening of potentially malignant and malignant oral lesions. *Asian Pac J Cancer Prev* 2014;15(15):6081–6.
297. Weissleder R, Pittet MJ. Imaging in the era of molecular oncology. *Nature* 2008;452(7187):580–9.
298. Francisco AL, Correr WR, Pinto CA et al. Analysis of surgical margins in oral cancer using *in situ* fluorescence spectroscopy. *Oral Oncol* 2014;50:593–9.
299. Hussain T, Nguyen QT. Molecular imaging for cancer diagnosis and surgery. *Adv Drug Deliv Rev* 2014;66:90–100.
300. Bydlon TM, Barry WT, Kennedy SA et al. Advancing optical imaging for breast margin assessment: an analysis of excisional time, cautery, and patent blue dye on underlying sources of contrast. *PLoS One* 2012;7(12):e51418.
301. Pleijhuis R, Timmermans A, De Jong J, De Boer E, Ntziachristos V, Van Dam G. Tissue-simulating phantoms for assessing potential near-infrared fluorescence imaging applications in breast cancer surgery. *J Vis Exp* 2014;(91):51776. doi: 10.3791/51776.

302. Chen HM, Chiang CP, You C, Hsiao TC, Wang CY. Time-resolved autofluorescence spectroscopy for classifying normal and premalignant oral tissues. *Lasers Surg Med* 2005;37(1):37–45.
303. Hughes OR, Stone N, Kraft M, Arens C, Birchall MA. Optical and molecular techniques to identify tumor margins within the larynx. *Head Neck* 2010;32(11):1544–53.
304. Keereweer S, Sterenborg HJ, Kerrebijn JD, Van Driel PB, Baatenburg de Jong RJ, Lowik CW. Image-guided surgery in head and neck cancer: current practice and future directions of optical imaging. *Head Neck* 2012;34(1):120–6.
305. Lane P, Follen M, MacAulay C. Has fluorescence spectroscopy come of age? A case series of oral precancers and cancers using white light, fluorescent light at 405 nm, and reflected light at 545 nm using the Trimira Identafi 3000. *Gend Med* 2012;9(1 Suppl):S25–35.
306. Lane PM, Gilhuly T, Whitehead P et al. Simple device for the direct visualization of oral-cavity tissue fluorescence. *J Biomed Opt* 2006;11(2):024006.
307. Olivo M, Bhuvaneswari R, Keogh I. Advances in bio-optical imaging for the diagnosis of early oral cancer. *Pharmaceutics* 2011;3(3):354–78.
308. Orita Y, Kawabata K, Mitani H et al. Can narrow-band imaging be used to determine the surgical margin of superficial hypopharyngeal cancer? *Acta Med Okayama* 2008;62(3):205–8.
309. Poh CF, Zhang L, Anderson DW et al. Fluorescence visualization detection of field alterations in tumor margins of oral cancer patients. *Clin Cancer Res* 2006;12(22):6716–22.
310. Ragazzi M, Piana S, Longo C et al. Fluorescence confocal microscopy for pathologists. *Mod Pathol* 2014;27(3):460–71.
311. Roblyer D, Kurachi C, Stepanek V et al. Objective detection and delineation of oral neoplasia using autofluorescence imaging. *Cancer Prev Res (Phila)* 2009;2(5):423–31.
312. Richards-Kortum R, Sevick-Muraca E. Quantitative optical spectroscopy for tissue diagnosis. *Annu Rev Phys Chem* 1996;47:555–606.
313. De Veld DC, Witjes MJ, Sterenborg HJ, Roodenburg JL. The status of *in vivo* autofluorescence spectroscopy and imaging for oral oncology. *Oral Oncol* 2005;41(2):117–31.
314. Pavlova I, Williams M, El-Naggar A, Richards-Kortum R, Gillenwater A. Understanding the biological basis of autofluorescence imaging for oral cancer detection: high-resolution fluorescence microscopy in viable tissue. *Clin Cancer Res* 2008;14(8):2396–404.
315. Shin D, Vigneswaran N, Gillenwater A, Richards-Kortum R. Advances in fluorescence imaging techniques to detect oral cancer and its precursors. *Future Oncol* 2010;6(7):1143–54.
316. Schwarz RA, Gao W, Stepanek VM et al. Prospective evaluation of a portable depth-sensitive optical spectroscopy device to identify oral neoplasia. *Biomed Opt Express* 2010;2(1):89–99.
317. Roblyer D, Richards-Kortum R, Sokolov K et al. Multispectral optical imaging device for *in vivo* detection of oral neoplasia. *J Biomed Opt* 2008;13(2):024019.
318. Jayaprakash V, Sullivan M, Merzianu M et al. Autofluorescence-guided surveillance for oral cancer. *Cancer Prev Res (Phila)* 2009;2(11):966–74.
319. Miyamoto S, Sperry S, Yamashita T, Reddy NP, O'Malley BW Jr, Li D. Molecular imaging assisted surgery improves survival in a murine head and neck cancer model. *Int J Cancer* 2012;131(5):1235–42.
320. Bhatia N, Lalla Y, Vu AN, Farah CS. Advances in optical adjunctive aids for visualisation and detection of oral malignant and potentially malignant lesions. *Int J Dent* 2013;2013:194029.
321. LED Inc. VELscope, The Oral Cancer Screening System, http://www.velscope.com/.
322. Rethman MP, Carpenter W, Cohen EEW et al. Evidence-based clinical recommendations regarding screening for oral squamous cell carcinomas. *J Am Dent Assoc* 2010;141(5):509–20.
323. Poh CF, MacAulay CE, Zhang L, Rosin MP. Tracing the "at-risk" oral mucosa field with autofluorescence: steps toward clinical impact. *Cancer Prev Res* 2009;2(5):401–4.
324. Pavlova I, Weber CR, Schwarz RA, Williams MD, Gillenwater AM, Richards-Kortum R. Fluorescence spectroscopy of oral tissue: Monte Carlo modeling with site-specific tissue properties. *J Biomed Opt* 2009;14(1):014009.
325. Kois JC, Truelove E. Detecting oral cancer: a new technique and case reports. *Dent Today* 2006;25(10):94–7.
326. Farah CS, McIntosh L, Georgiou A, McCullough MJ. Efficacy of tissue autofluorescence imaging (VELScope) in the visualization of oral mucosal lesions. *Head Neck* 2012;34(6):856–62.
327. Bhatia N, Matias MA, Farah CS. Assessment of a decision making protocol to improve the efficacy of VELscope in general dental practice: a prospective evaluation. *Oral Oncol* 2014;50(10):1012–9.
328. Scheer M, Neugebauer J, Derman A, Fuss J, Drebber U, Zoeller JE. Autofluorescence imaging of potentially malignant mucosa lesions. *Oral Surg Oral Med Oral Pathol Oral Radiol Endod* 2011;111(5):568–77.
329. Marzouki HZ, Tuong Vi Vu T, Ywakim R, Chauvin P, Hanley J, Kost KM. Use of fluorescent light in detecting malignant and premalignant lesions in the oral cavity: a prospective, single-blind study. *J Otolaryngol Head Neck Surg* 2012;41(3):164–8.

330. Awan KH, Morgan PR, Warnakulasuriya S. Evaluation of an autofluorescence based imaging system (VELscope) in the detection of oral potentially malignant disorders and benign keratoses. *Oral Oncol* 2011;47(4):274–7.
331. Hanken H, Kraatz J, Smeets R et al. The detection of oral pre-malignant lesions with an autofluorescence based imaging system (VELscope)—a single blinded clinical evaluation. *Head Face Med* 2013;9:23.
332. Sciubba JJ. Improving detection of precancerous and cancerous oral lesions. Computer-assisted analysis of the oral brush biopsy. U.S. Collaborative OralCDx study group. *J Am Dent Assoc* 1999;130(10):1445–57.
333. Mehrotra R, Singh M, Thomas S et al. A cross-sectional study evaluating chemiluminescence and autofluorescence in the detection of clinically innocuous precancerous and cancerous oral lesions. *J Am Dent Assoc* 2010;141(2):151–6.
334. Subhash N, Mallia JR, Thomas SS, Mathews A, Sebastian P, Madhavan J. Oral cancer detection using diffuse reflectance spectral ratio R540/R575 of oxygenated hemoglobin bands. *J Biomed Opt* 2006;11(1):014018.
335. Rana M, Zapf A, Kuehle M, Gellrich NC, Eckardt AM. Clinical evaluation of an autofluorescence diagnostic device for oral cancer detection: a prospective randomized diagnostic study. *Eur J Cancer* 2012;21(5):460–6.
336. Balevi B. Assessing the usefulness of three adjunctive diagnostic devices for oral cancer screening: a probabilistic approach. *Community Dent Oral Epidemiol* 2011;39(2):171–6.
337. Seoane Leston J, Diz Dios P. Diagnostic clinical aids in oral cancer. *Oral Oncol* 2010;46(6):418–22.
338. Fedele S. Diagnostic aids in the screening of oral cancer. *Head Face Med* 2009;1:5.
339. Huff K, Stark PC, Solomon LW. Sensitivity of direct tissue fluorescence visualization in screening for oral premalignant lesions in general practice. *Gen Dent* 2009;57(1):34–8.
340. Truelove EL, Dean D, Maltby S et al. Narrow band (light) imaging of oral mucosa in routine dental patients. part I: assessment of value in detection of mucosal changes. *Gen Dent* 2011;59(4):281–9. quiz 90–1, 319–20.
341. McNamara KK, Martin BD, Evans EW, Kalmar JR. The role of direct visual fluorescent examination (VELscope) in routine screening for potentially malignant oral mucosal lesions. *Oral Surg Oral Med Oral Pathol Oral Radiol* 2012;114(5):636–43.
342. Ayoub HM, Newcomb TL, McCombs GB, Bonnie M. The use of fluorescence technology versus visual and tactile examination in the detection of oral lesions: a pilot study. *J Dent Hyg* 2015;89(1):63–71.
343. Elvers D, Braunschweig T, Hilgers RD et al. Margins of oral leukoplakia: autofluorescence and histopathology. *Br J Oral Maxillofac Surg* 2015;53(2):164–9.
344. Kordbacheh F, Bhatia N, Farah CS. Patterns of differentially expressed genes in oral mucosal lesions subjected to autofluorescence (VELscope™). *Oral Dis* 2016;22(4):285–96. doi: 10.1111/odi.12438. Epub February 9, 2016.
345. Poh CF, Anderson DW, Durham JS et al. Fluorescence visualization-guided surgery for early-stage oral cancer. *JAMA Otolaryngol Head Neck Surg* 2016;142(3):209–16.
346. Dental EZ. Identafi—Multispectral, Oral Cancer Screening Device 2013 [cited 2013 20/03]. Available from: http://www.identafi.net/.
347. McIntosh L, McCullough MJ, Farah CS. The assessment of diffused light illumination and acetic acid rinse (Microlux/DL) in the visualisation of oral mucosal lesions. *Oral Oncol* 2009;45(12):e227–31.
348. Lalla Y, Matias MA, Farah CS. Assessment of oral mucosal lesions with autofluorescence imaging and reflectance spectroscopy. *J Am Dent Assoc* 2016;147(8):650–60. doi: 10.1016/j.adaj.2016.03.013. Epub April 23, 2016.
349. Lalla Y, Matias M, Farah CS. Oral mucosal disease in an Australian urban indigenous community using autofluorescence imaging and reflectance spectroscopy. *Aust Dent J* 2015;60(2):216–24.
350. Sweeny L, Dean NR, Magnuson JS, Carroll WR, Clemons L, Rosenthal EL. Assessment of tissue autofluorescence and reflectance for oral cavity cancer screening. *Otolaryngol Head Neck Surg* 2011;145(6):956–60.
351. Lane P, Lam S, Follen M, MacAulay C. Oral fluorescence imaging using 405-nm excitation, aiding the discrimination of cancers and precancers by identifying changes in collagen and elastic breakdown and neovascularization in the underlying stroma. *Gend Med* 2012;9(1 Suppl):S78–82.e1–8.
352. Pazouki S, Chisholm DM, Adi MM et al. The association between tumour progression and vascularity in the oral mucosa. *J Pathol* 1997;183(1):39–43.
353. Raica M, Cimpean AM, Ribatti D. Angiogenesis in pre-malignant conditions. *Eur J Cancer* 2009;45(11):1924–34.
354. Shetty DC, Ahuja P, Taneja DK et al. Relevance of tumor angiogenesis patterns as a diagnostic value and prognostic indicator in oral precancer and cancer. *Vasc Health Risk Manag* 2011;7(1):41–7.
355. Messadi DV, Younai FS, Liu HH, Guo G, Wang CY. The clinical effectiveness of reflectance optical spectroscopy for the *in vivo* diagnosis of oral lesions. *Int J Oral Sci* 2014;6(3):162–7.
356. Wong Kee Song LM, Adler DG, Conway JD et al. Narrow band imaging and multiband imaging. *Gastrointest Endosc* 2008;67(4):581–9.

357. Gono K, Yamazaki K, Doguchi N et al. Endoscopic observation of tissue by narrowband illumination. *Opt Rev* 2003;10(4):211–5.
358. Vu A, Farah CS. Narrow band imaging: clinical applications in oral and oropharyngeal cancer. *Oral Dis* 2016;22(5):383–90. doi: 10.1111/odi.12430. Epub January 25, 2016, Review.
359. Takano JH, Yakushiji T, Kamiyama I et al. Detecting early oral cancer: narrowband imaging system observation of the oral mucosa microvasculature. *Int J Oral Maxillofac Surg* 2010;39(3):208–13.
360. Tan NC, Herd MK, Brennan PA, Puxeddu R. The role of narrow band imaging in early detection of head and neck cancer. *Br J Oral Maxillofac Surg* 2012;50(2):132–6.
361. Fujii S, Yamazaki M, Muto M, Ochiai A. Microvascular irregularities are associated with composition of squamous epithelial lesions and correlate with subepithelial invasion of superficial-type pharyngeal squamous cell carcinoma. *Histopathology* 2010;56(4):510–22.
362. Katada C, Nakayama M, Tanabe S et al. Narrow band imaging for detecting superficial oral squamous cell carcinoma: a report of two cases. *Laryngoscope* 2007;117(9):1596–9.
363. Tan NCW, Mellor T, Brennan PA, Puxeddu R. Use of narrow band imaging guidance in the management of oral erythroplakia. *Br J Oral Maxillofac Surg* 2011;49(6):488–90.
364. Yang SW, Lee YS, Chang LC, Chien HP, Chen TA. Clinical appraisal of endoscopy with narrow-band imaging system in the evaluation and management of homogeneous oral leukoplakia. *ORL J Otorhinolaryngol Relat Spec* 2012;74(2):102–9.
365. Gono K, Obi T, Yamaguchi M et al. Appearance of enhanced tissue features in narrow-band endoscopic imaging. *J Biomed Opt* 2004;9(3):568–77.
366. Muto M, Nakane M, Katada C et al. Squamous cell carcinoma *in situ* at oropharyngeal and hypopharyngeal mucosal sites. *Cancer* 2004;101(6):1375–81.
367. Muto M, Katada C, Sano Y, Yoshida S. Narrow band imaging: a new diagnostic approach to visualize angiogenesis in superficial neoplasia. *Clin Gastroenterol Hepatol* 2005;3(7 Suppl):S16–20.
368. Yoshida T, Inoue H, Usui S, Satodate H, Fukami N, Kudo SE. Narrow-band imaging system with magnifying endoscopy for superficial esophageal lesions. *Gastrointest Endosc* 2004;59(2):288–95.
369. Matsumura M, Uedo N, Ishihara R, Iishi H, Fujii T, Tomita Y. A case of intraepithelial neoplasia in the oropharynx detected by endoscopic screening with narrow-band imaging videoendoscopy. *Gastrointest Endosc* 2008;68(1):146–7.
370. Lin YC, Wang WH. Narrow-band imaging for detecting early recurrent nasopharyngeal carcinoma. *Head Neck* 2011;33(4):591–4.
371. Piazza C. Is narrow band imaging the ideal screening tool for mucosal head and neck cancer? *Oral Oncol* 2011;47(5):313.
372. Watanabe A, Taniguchi M, Tsujie H, Hosokawa M, Fujita M, Sasaki S. The value of narrow band imaging for early detection of laryngeal cancer. *Eur Arch Oto-Rhino-Laryngol* 2009;266(7):1017–23.
373. Watanabe A, Taniguchi M, Tsujie H, Hosokawa M, Fujita M, Sasaki S. The value of narrow band imaging endoscope for early head and neck cancer. *Otolaryngol Head Neck Surg* 2008;138(4):446–51.
374. Igarashi Y, Okano N, Ito K, Suzuki T, Mimura T. Effectiveness of peroral cholangioscopy and narrow band imaging for endoscopically diagnosing the bile duct cancer. *Dig Endosc* 2009;21(Suppl 1):S101–2.
375. Itoi T, Sofuni A, Itokawa F, Tsuchiya T, Kurihara T. Evaluation of peroral videocholangioscopy using narrow-band imaging for diagnosis of intraductal papillary neoplasm of the bile duct. *Dig Endosc* 2009;21(Suppl 1):S103–7.
376. Itoi T, Tsuji S, Sofuni A et al. A novel approach emphasizing preoperative margin enhancement of tumor of the major duodenal papilla with narrow-band imaging in comparison to indigo carmine chromoendoscopy (with videos). *Gastrointest Endosc.* 2009;69(1):136–41.
377. Kiyotoki S, Nishikawa J, Satake M et al. Usefulness of magnifying endoscopy with narrow-band imaging for determining gastric tumor margin. *J Gastroenterol Hepatol* 2010;25(10):1636–41.
378. Nagahama T, Yao K, Maki S et al. Usefulness of magnifying endoscopy with narrow-band imaging for determining the horizontal extent of early gastric cancer when there is an unclear margin by chromoendoscopy (with video). *Gastrointest Endosc* 2011;74(6):1259–67.
379. Muto M, Horimatsu T, Ezoe Y, Morita S, Miyamoto S. Improving visualization techniques by narrow band imaging and magnification endoscopy. *J Gastroenterol Hepatol* 2009;24(8):1333–46.
380. Piazza C, Dessouky O, Peretti G, Cocco D, De Benedetto L, Nicolai P. Narrow-band imaging: a new tool for evaluation of head and neck squamous cell carcinomas. Review of the literature. *Acta Otorhinolaryngol Ital* 2008;28(2):49–54.
381. Muto M, Minashi K, Yano T et al. Early detection of superficial squamous cell carcinoma in the head and neck region and esophagus by narrow band imaging: a multicenter randomized controlled trial. *J Clin Oncol* 2010;28(9):1566–72.
382. Piazza C, Cocco D, Del Bon F et al. Narrow band imaging and high definition television in evaluation of oral and oropharyngeal squamous cell cancer: a prospective study. *Oral Oncol* 2010;46(4):307–10.
383. Piazza C, Cocco D, Del Bon F, Mangili S, Nicolai P, Peretti G. Narrow band imaging and high definition

television in the endoscopic evaluation of upper aero-digestive tract cancer. *Acta Otorhinolaryngol Ital* 2011;31(2):70–5.
384. Fielding D, Agnew J, Wright D, Hodge R. Autofluorescence improves pretreatment mucosal assessment in head and neck cancer patients. *Otolaryngol Head Neck Surg* 2010;142(3):S20–6.
385. Nguyen P, Bashirzadeh F, Hodge R et al. High specificity of combined narrow band imaging and autofluorescence mucosal assessment of patients with head and neck cancer. *Head Neck* 2013;35(5):619–25.
386. Vu AN, Farah CS. Efficacy of narrow band imaging for detection and surveillance of potentially malignant and malignant lesions in the oral cavity and oropharynx: a systematic review. *Oral Oncol* 2014;50(5):413–20. doi: 10.1016/j.oraloncology.2014.02.002. Epub 2014 March 4, 2014, Review.
387. Yang SW, Lee YS, Chang LC, Chien HP, Chen TA. Light sources used in evaluating oral leukoplakia: broadband white light versus narrowband imaging. *Int J Oral Maxillofac Surg* 2013;42(6):693–701.
388. Vu AN, Matias M, Farah CS. Diagnostic accuracy of narrow band imaging for the detection of oral potentially malignant disorders. *Oral Dis* 2015;21(4):519–29.
389. Vu A, Farah CS. Narrow band imaging: clinical applications in oral and oropharyngeal cancer. *Oral Dis* 2016;22(5):383–90.
390. Farah CS, Dalley AJ, Nguyen P et al. Improved surgical margin definition by narrow band imaging for resection of oral squamous cell carcinoma: a prospective gene expression profiling study. *Head Neck* 2016;38(6):832–9.
391. Feng ZH, Hu WW, Tang MS. Trans-4-hydroxy-2-nonenal inhibits nucleotide excision repair in human cells: a possible mechanism for lipid peroxidation-induced carcinogenesis. *Proc Natl Acad Sci USA* 2004;101(23):8598–602.
392. Green B, Cobb AR, Brennan PA, Hopper C. Optical diagnostic techniques for use in lesions of the head and neck: review of the latest developments. *Br J Oral Maxillofac Surg* 2014;52(8):675–80.
393. Hamdoon Z, Jerjes W, Upile T, McKenzie G, Jay A, Hopper C. Optical coherence tomography in the assessment of suspicious oral lesions: an immediate *ex vivo* study. *Photodiagnosis Photodyn Ther* 2013;10(1):17–27.
394. Adhi M, Duker JS. Optical coherence tomography—current and future applications. *Curr Opin Ophthalmol* 2013;24(3):213–21.
395. Whiteman SC, Yang Y, Gey van Pittius D, Stephens M, Parmer J, Spiteri MA. Optical coherence tomography: real-time imaging of bronchial airways microstructure and detection of inflammatory/neoplastic morphologic changes. *Clin Cancer Res.* 2006;12(3 Pt 1): 813–8.
396. Lee CK, Tsai MT, Lee HC et al. Diagnosis of oral submucous fibrosis with optical coherence tomography. *J Biomed Opt* 2009;14(5):054008.
397. Ozawa N, Sumi Y, Shimozato K, Chong C, Kurabayashi T. *In vivo* imaging of human labial glands using advanced optical coherence tomography. *Oral Surg Oral Med Oral Pathol Oral Radiol Endod* 2009;108(3):425–9.
398. Fujimoto JG. Optical coherence tomography for ultrahigh resolution *in vivo* imaging. *Nat Biotechnol* 2003;21(11):1361–7.
399. Brezinski ME, Tearney GJ, Boppart SA, Swanson EA, Southern JF, Fujimoto JG. Optical biopsy with optical coherence tomography: feasibility for surgical diagnostics. *J Surg Res* 1997;71(1):32–40.
400. Alawi SA, Kuck M, Wahrlich C et al. Optical coherence tomography for presurgical margin assessment of non-melanoma skin cancer—a practical approach. *Exp Dermatol* 2013;22(8):547–51.
401. Pelosini L, Smith HB, Schofield JB, Meeckings A, Dhital A, Khandwala M. *In vivo* optical coherence tomography (OCT) in periocular basal cell carcinoma: correlations between *in vivo* OCT images and postoperative histology. *Br J Ophthalmol* 2013;97(7):890–4.
402. Savastru D, Chang EW, Miclos S, Pitman MB, Patel A, Iftimia N. Detection of breast surgical margins with optical coherence tomography imaging: a concept evaluation study. *J Biomed Opt* 2014;19(5):056001.
403. Skarecky DW, Brenner M, Rajan S et al. Zero positive surgical margins after radical prostatectomy: is the end in sight. *Expert Rev Med Devices* 2008;5(6):709–17.
404. South FA, Chaney EJ, Marjanovic M, Adie SG, Boppart SA. Differentiation of *ex vivo* human breast tissue using polarization-sensitive optical coherence tomography. *Biomed Opt Express* 2014;5(10):3417–26.
405. Wessels R, De Bruin DM, Faber DJ, Van Leeuwen TG, Van Beurden M, Ruers TJ. Optical biopsy of epithelial cancers by optical coherence tomography (OCT). *Lasers Med Sci* 2014;29(3):1297–305.
406. Hamdoon Z, Jerjes W, Al-Delayme R, McKenzie G, Jay A, Hopper C. Structural validation of oral mucosal tissue using optical coherence tomography. *Head Neck Oncol* 2012;4:29. Published online June, 2012. doi: 10.1186/1758-3284-4-29.
407. Jerjes W, Upile T, Conn B et al. *In vitro* examination of suspicious oral lesions using optical coherence tomography. *Br J Oral Maxillofac Surg* 2010;48(1):18–25.
408. Wessels R, van Beurden M, de Bruin DM et al. The value of optical coherence tomography in determining surgical margins in squamous cell carcinoma of the vulva: a single-center prospective study. *Int J Gynecol Cancer* 2015;25(1):112–8. doi: 10.1097/IGC.0000000000000310.

409. Wilder-Smith P, Lee K, Guo S et al. *In vivo* diagnosis of oral dysplasia and malignancy using optical coherence tomography: preliminary studies in 50 patients. *Lasers Surg Med* 2009;41(5):353–7.
410. Hamdoon Z, Jerjes W, McKenzie G, Jay A, Hopper C. Optical coherence tomography in the assessment of oral squamous cell carcinoma resection margins. *Photodiagnosis Photodyn Ther* 2016;13:211–7. doi: 10.1016/j.pdpdt.2015.07.170. Epub July 22, 2015.
411. Davies K, Connolly JM, Dockery P, Wheatley AM, Olivo M, Keogh I. Point of care optical diagnostic technologies for the detection of oral and oropharyngeal squamous cell carcinoma (SCC). *Surgeon* 2015;13(6):321–9.
412. Lee AM, Cahill L, Liu K, MacAulay C, Poh C, Lane P. Wide-field *in vivo* oral OCT imaging. *Biomed Opt Express* 2015;6(7):2664–74.
413. Pande P, Shrestha S, Park J et al. Automated classification of optical coherence tomography images for the diagnosis of oral malignancy in the hamster cheek pouch. *J Biomed Opt* 2014;19(8):086022.
414. Pyhtila JW, Chalut KJ, Boyer JD et al. *In situ* detection of nuclear atypia in Barrett's esophagus by using angle-resolved low-coherence interferometry. *Gastrointest Endosc* 2007;65(3):487–91.
415. Terry NG, Zhu Y, Rinehart MT et al. Detection of dysplasia in Barrett's esophagus with *in vivo* depth-resolved nuclear morphology measurements. *Gastroenterology* 2011;140(1):42–50.
416. Kelloff GJ, Sigman CC. Assessing intraepithelial neoplasia and drug safety in cancer-preventive drug development. *Nat Rev Cancer* 2007;7(7):508–18.
417. Backman V, Wallace MB, Perelman LT et al. Detection of preinvasive cancer cells. *Nature* 2000;406(6791):35–6.
418. Nwaneshiudu A, Kuschal C, Sakamoto FH, Anderson RR, Schwarzenberger K, Young RC. Introduction to confocal microscopy. *J Invest Dermatol* 2012;132(12):e3.
419. Wright SJ, Wright DJ. Introduction to confocal microscopy. *Methods Cell Biol.* 2002;70:1–85.
420. White WM, Baldassano M, Rajadhyaksha M et al. Confocal reflectance imaging of head and neck surgical specimens. A comparison with histologic analysis. *Arch Otolaryngol* 2004;130(8):923–8.
421. Rajadhyaksha M, Gonzalez S, Zavislan JM, Anderson RR, Webb RH. *In vivo* confocal scanning laser microscopy of human skin II: advances in instrumentation and comparison with histology. *J Invest Dermatol* 1999;113(3):293–303.
422. El Hallani S, Poh CF, Macaulay CE, Follen M, Guillaud M, Lane P. *Ex vivo* confocal imaging with contrast agents for the detection of oral potentially malignant lesions. *Oral Oncol* 2013;49(6):582–90.
423. Clark AL, Gillenwater AM, Collier TG, Alizadeh-Naderi R, El-Naggar AK, Richards-Kortum RR. Confocal microscopy for real-time detection of oral cavity neoplasia. *Clin Cancer Res* 2003;9(13):4714–21.
424. Contaldo M, Agozzino M, Moscarella E, Esposito S, Serpico R, Ardigo M. *In vivo* characterization of healthy oral mucosa by reflectance confocal microscopy: a translational research for optical biopsy. *Ultrastruct Pathol* 2013;37(2):151–8.
425. Maher NG, Collgros H, Uribe P, Ch'ng S, Rajadhyaksha M, Guitera P. *In vivo* confocal microscopy for the oral cavity: current state of the field and future potential. *Oral Oncol* 2016;54:28–35.
426. Gonzalez Segura I, Secchi D, Carrica A et al. Exfoliative cytology as a tool for monitoring pre-malignant and malignant lesions based on combined stains and morphometry techniques. *J Oral Pathol Med* 2015;44(3):178–84.
427. Bocking A, Sproll C, Stocklein N et al. Role of brush biopsy and DNA cytometry for prevention, diagnosis, therapy, and followup care of oral cancer. *J Oncol* 2011;2011:875959.
428. Peacock ZS, Pogrel MA, Schmidt BL. Exploring the reasons for delay in treatment of oral cancer. *J Am Dent Assoc* 2008;139(10):1346–52.
429. Navone R. Cytology of the oral cavity: a re-evaluation. *Pathologica* 2009;101(1):6–8.
430. Pentenero M, Carrozzo M, Pagano M et al. Oral mucosal dysplastic lesions and early squamous cell carcinomas: underdiagnosis from incisional biopsy. *Oral Dis* 2003;9(2):68–72.
431. Fuller C, Camilon R, Nguyen S, Jennings J, Day T, Gillespie MB. Adjunctive diagnostic techniques for oral lesions of unknown malignant potential: systematic review with meta-analysis. *Head Neck* 2015;37(5):755–62.
432. Sandler HC. Oral cytology. *CA Cancer J Clin* 1966;16(3):97–101.
433. Sridharan G, Shankar AA. Toluidine blue: a review of its chemistry and clinical utility. *J Oral Maxillofac Pathol* 2012;16(2):251–5.
434. Warnakulasuriya KA, Johnson NW. Sensitivity and specificity of OraScan® toluidine blue mouthrinse in the detection of oral cancer and precancer. *J Oral Pathol Med* 1996;25(3):97–103.
435. Su WW, Yen AM, Chiu SY, Chen TH. A community-based RCT for oral cancer screening with toluidine blue. *J Dent Res* 2010;89(9):933–7.
436. Omar E. Future imaging alternatives: the clinical non-invasive modalities in diagnosis of oral squamous cell carcinoma (OSCC). *Open Dent J* 2015;9:311–8.
437. Chhabra N, Chhabra S, Sapra N. Diagnostic modalities for squamous cell carcinoma: an extensive review of literature-considering toluidine blue as a useful adjunct. *J Maxillofac Oral Surg* 2015;14(2):188–200.

438. Ogden GR, Cowpe JG, Green M. Cytobrush and wooden spatula for oral exfoliative cytology. A comparison. *Acta Cytol* 1992;36(5):706–10.
439. Coskun S, Can H, Turan S. Knowledge about cervical cancer risk factors and pap smear testing behavior among female primary health care workers: a study from south Turkey. *Asian Pac J Cancer Prev* 2013;14(11):6389–92.
440. Papanicolaou GN. A new procedure for staining vaginal smears. *Science* 1942;95(2469):438–9.
441. Ahmed HG, Ebnoof SO, Hussein MO, Gbreel AY. Oral epithelial atypical changes in apparently healthy oral mucosa exposed to smoking, alcohol, peppers and hot meals, using the AgNOR and Papanicolaou staining techniques. *Diagn Cytopathol* 2010;38(7):489–95.
442. Derenzini M, Pession A, Trere D. Quantity of nucleolar silver-stained proteins is related to proliferating activity in cancer cells. *Lab Invest* 1990;63(1):137–40.
443. Mansoor Samadi F, Thattil Sebastian B, Singh A, Chandra S. Silver binding nucleolar organizer regions dots in oral leukoplakia with epithelial dysplasia and oral squamous cell carcinoma: an *in vivo* study. 2014;2014:479187.
444. Nanayakkara PG, Dissanayaka WL, Nanayakkara BG, Amaratunga EA, Tilakaratne WM. Comparison of spatula and cytobrush cytological techniques in early detection of oral malignant and premalignant lesions: a prospective and blinded study. *J Oral Pathol Med* 2016;45(4):268–74. doi: 10.1111/jop.12357. Epub September 25, 2015.
445. Queiroz JB, Lima CF, Burim RA, Brandao AA, Cabral LA, Almeida JD. Exfoliative cytology of the oral mucosa: comparison of two collection methods. *Gen Dent* 2010;58(5):e196–9.
446. Koch FP, Kunkel M, Biesterfeld S, Wagner W. Diagnostic efficiency of differentiating small cancerous and precancerous lesions using mucosal brush smears of the oral cavity—a prospective and blinded study. *Clin Oral Investig* 2011;15(5):763–9.
447. Poate TW, Buchanan JA, Hodgson TA et al. An audit of the efficacy of the oral brush biopsy technique in a specialist oral medicine unit. *Oral Oncol* 2004;40(8):829–34.
448. Remmerbach TW, Mathes SN, Weidenbach H, Hemprich A, Bocking A. Noninvasive brush biopsy as an innovative tool for early detection of oral carcinomas. *Dtsch Z Mund Kiefer Gesichtschir* 2004;8(4):229–36.
449. Divani S, Exarhou M, Theodorou LN, Georgantzis D, Skoulakis H. Advantages and difficulties of brush cytology in the identification of early oral cancer. *Arch Oncol* 2009;17(1–2):11–2.
450. Scheifele C, Schmidt-Westhausen AM, Dietrich T, Reichart PA. The sensitivity and specificity of the OralCDx technique: evaluation of 103 cases. *Oral Oncol* 2004;40(8):824–8.
451. Mehrotra R, Mishra S, Singh M, Singh M. The efficacy of oral brush biopsy with computer-assisted analysis in identifying precancerous and cancerous lesions. *Head Neck Oncol* 2011;3:39.
452. Seijas-Naya F, Garcia-Carnicero T, Gandara-Vila P et al. Applications of OralCDx(R) methodology in the diagnosis of oral leukoplakia. *Med Oral Patol Oral Cir Bucal* 2012;17(1):e5–9.
453. Kujan O, Desai M, Sargent A, Bailey A, Turner A, Sloan P. Potential applications of oral brush cytology with liquid-based technology: results from a cohort of normal oral mucosa. *Oral Oncol* 2006;42(8):810–8
454. Alves MG, Perez-Sayans M, Padin-Iruegas ME et al. Comparison of RNA extraction methods for molecular analysis of oral cytology. *Acta Stomatol Croat* 2016;50(2):108–15.
455. Abram TJ, Floriano PN, Christodoulides N et al. "Cytology-on-a-chip" based sensors for monitoring of potentially malignant oral lesions. *Oral Oncol* 2016;60:103–11.
456. Hayama FH, Motta AC, Silva Ade P, Migliari DA. Liquid-based preparations versus conventional cytology: specimen adequacy and diagnostic agreement in oral lesions. *Med Oral Patol Oral Cir Bucal* 2005;10(2):115–22.
457. Sun W, Zaboli D, Wang H et al. Detection of *TIMP3* promoter hypermethylation in salivary rinse as an independent predictor of local recurrence-free survival in head and neck cancer. *Clin Cancer Res* 2012;18(4):1082–91.
458. Reboiras-López MD, Perez-Sayans M, Somoza-Martin JM et al. Comparison of three sampling instruments, Cytobrush, Curette and OralCDx, for liquid-based cytology of the oral mucosa. *Biotech Histochem* 2012;87(1):51–8.
459. Reboiras-López MD, Perez-Sayans M, Somoza-Martin JM et al. Comparison of the Cytobrush®, dermatological curette and oral CDx® brush test as methods for obtaining samples of RNA for molecular analysis of oral cytology. *Cytopathology* 2012;23(3):192–7.
460. Navone R, Burlo P, Pich A et al. The impact of liquid-based oral cytology on the diagnosis of oral squamous dysplasia and carcinoma. *Cytopathology* 2007;18(6):356–60.
461. Delavarian Z, Mohtasham N, Mosannen-Mozafari P, Pakfetrat A, Shakeri MT, Ghafoorian-Maddah R. Evaluation of the diagnostic value of a modified liquid-based cytology using OralCDx brush in early detection of oral potentially malignant lesions and oral cancer. *Med Oral Patol Oral Cir Bucal* 2010;15(5):e671–6.
462. Marsico A, Demurtas A, Rostan I, Pentenero M, Gandolfo S, Navone R. Flow cytometric analysis of DNA ploidy in potentially malignant oral lesions (PMLS). *Cytopathology* 2008;19(Suppl 1):64.

463. McCullough MJ, Farah CS. The assessment of the DNA content of oral cytology *via* virtual microscopy for the early detection of epithelial dysplasia and neoplasia in oral mucosal lesions. *Oral Oncol* 2009;45(9):e114–5.
464. Kämmerer PW, Koch FP, Santoro M et al. Prospective, blinded comparison of cytology and DNA-image cytometry of brush biopsies for early detection of oral malignancy. *Oral Oncol* 2013;49(5):420–6.
465. Navone R, Pentenero M, Rostan I et al. Oral potentially malignant lesions: first-level micro-histological diagnosis from tissue fragments sampled in liquid-based diagnostic cytology. *J Oral Pathol Med* 2008;37(6):358–63.
466. Ye X, Zhang J, Tan Y, Chen G, Zhou G. Meta-analysis of two computer-assisted screening methods for diagnosing oral precancer and cancer. *Oral Oncol* 2015;51(11):966–75.
467. Santos AP, Sugaya NN, Pinto Junior Ddos S, Lemos Junior CA. Fine needle aspiration biopsy in the oral cavity and head and neck region. *Braz Oral Res* 2011;25(2):186–91.
468. Batra M, Wadhwa N, Mishra K. Cytologic diagnosis in benign odontogenic tumor with abundant calcification: a case report. *Acta Cytol* 2009;53(4):460–2.
469. Saleh HA, Clayman L, Masri H. Fine needle aspiration biopsy of intraoral and oropharyngeal mass lesions. *Cytojournal* 2008;5:4.
470. Shah SB, Singer MI, Liberman E, Ljung BM. Transmucosal fine-needle aspiration diagnosis of intraoral and intrapharyngeal lesions. *Laryngoscope* 1999;109(8):1232–7.
471. The 1988 Bethesda System for reporting cervical/vaginal cytologic diagnoses. Developed and approved at the national cancer institute workshop, Bethesda, maryland, USA, December 12–13, 1988. *Acta Cytol.* 1989;33(5):567–74.
472. Smith JH. Bethesda 2001. *Cytopathology* 2002;13(1):4–10.
473. Scher RL, Oostingh PE, Levine PA, Cantrell RW, Feldman PS. Role of fine needle aspiration in the diagnosis of lesions of the oral cavity, oropharynx, and nasopharynx. *Cancer* 1988;62(12):2602–6.
474. Solomon D, Davey D, Kurman R et al. The 2001 Bethesda system: terminology for reporting results of cervical cytology. *JAMA* 2002;287(16):2114–9.
475. Macey R, Walsh T, Brocklehurst P et al. Diagnostic tests for oral cancer and potentially malignant disorders in patients presenting with clinically evident lesions. *Cochrane Database Syst Rev* 2015;5:CD010276.
476. Mehrotra R. *Oral Cytology: a Concise Guide.* New York: Springer New York: Imprint: Springer, 2013.
477. Egger G, Liang G, Aparicio A, Jones PA. Epigenetics in human disease and prospects for epigenetic therapy. *Nature* 2004;429(6990):457–63.
478. Gasche JA, Goel A. Epigenetic mechanisms in oral carcinogenesis. *Future Oncol* 2012;8(11):1407–25.
479. Feinberg AP, Ohlsson R, Henikoff S. The epigenetic progenitor origin of human cancer. *Nat Rev Genet* 2006;7(1):21–33.
480. Nagpal JK, Das BR. Oral cancer: reviewing the present understanding of its molecular mechanism and exploring the future directions for its effective management. *Oral Oncol* 2003;39(3):213–21.
481. Arantes LM, de Carvalho AC, Melendez ME, Carvalho AL, Goloni-Bertollo EM. Methylation as a biomarker for head and neck cancer. *Oral Oncol* 2014;50(6):587–92. doi: 10.1016/j.oraloncology.2014.02.015. Epub March 20, 2014.
482. Lingen MW, Szabo E. Validation of LOH profiles for assessing oral cancer risk. *Cancer Prev Res* 2012;5(9):1075–7.
483. Cruz IB, Meijer C, Snijders PJF, Snow GB, Walboomers JMM, van der Waal I. P53 immunoexpression in non-malignant oral mucosa adjacent to oral squamous cell carcinoma: potential consequences for clinical management. *J Pathol* 2000;191(2):132–7.
484. Bilde A, von Buchwald C, Dabelsteen E, Therkildsen MH, Dabelsteen S. Molecular markers in the surgical margin of oral carcinomas. *J Oral Pathol Med* 2009;38(1):72–8.
485. Partridge M, Li SR, Pateromichelakis S et al. Detection of minimal residual cancer to investigate why oral tumors recur despite seemingly adequate treatment. *Clin Cancer Res* 2000;6(7):2718–25.
486. Bergshoeff VE, Hopman AHN, Zwijnenberg IR et al. Chromosome instability in resection margins predicts recurrence of oral squamous cell carcinoma. *J Pathol* 2008;215(3):347–8.
487. Tunca B, Erisen L, Coskun H, Cecener G, Ozuysal S, Egeli U. P53 gene mutations in surgical margins and primary tumor tissues of patients with squamous cell carcinoma of the head and neck. *Tumori* 2007;93(2):182–8.
488. Graveland AP, Golusinski PJ, Buijze M et al. Loss of heterozygosity at 9p and p53 immunopositivity in surgical margins predict local relapse in head and neck squamous cell carcinoma. *Int J Cancer* 2011;128(8):1852–9.
489. Graveland AP, Bremmer JF, de Maaker M et al. Molecular screening of oral precancer. *Oral Oncol* 2013;49(12):1129–35.
490. Nathan CAO, Amirghahri N, Rice C, Abreo FW, Shi RH, Stucker FJ. Molecular analysis of surgical margins in head and neck squamous cell carcinoma patients. *Laryngoscope* 2002;112(12):2129–40.

491. Martone T, Gillio-Tos A, De Marco L et al. Association between hypermethylated tumor and paired surgical margins in head and neck squamous cell carcinomas. *Clin Cancer Res* 2007;13(17):5089–94.
492. Sinha P, Bahadur S, Thakar A et al. Significance of promoter hypermethylation of p16 gene for margin assessment in carcinoma tongue. *Head Neck* 2009;31(11):1423–30.
493. Wong TS, Man MW, Lam AK, Wei WI, Kwong YL, Yuen AP. The study of p16 and p15 gene methylation in head and neck squamous cell carcinoma and their quantitative evaluation in plasma by real-time PCR. *Eur J Cancer.* 2003;39(13):1881–7.
494. Nathan CAO, Franklin S, Abreo FW, Nassar R, De Benedetti A, Glass J. Analysis of surgical margins with the molecular marker eIF4E: a prognostic factor in patients with head and neck cancer. *J Clin Oncol* 1999;17(9):2909–14.
495. Aguilar-Ramirez P, Reis ES, Florido MP et al. Skipping of exon 30 in C5 gene results in complete human C5 deficiency and demonstrates the importance of C5d and CUB domains for stability. *Mol Immunol* 2009;46(10):2116–23.
496. Roh JL, Westra WH, Califano JA, Sidransky D, Koch WM. Tissue imprint for molecular mapping of deep surgical margins in patients with head and neck squamous cell carcinoma. *Head Neck* 2012;34(11):1529–36.
497. Supic G, Kozomara R, Jovic N, Zeljic K, Magic Z. Prognostic significance of tumor-related genes hypermethylation detected in cancer-free surgical margins of oral squamous cell carcinomas. *Oral Oncol* 2011;47(8):702–8.
498. Santhi WS, Prathibha R, Charles S et al. Oncogenic microRNAs as biomarkers of oral tumorigenesis and minimal residual disease. *Oral Oncol* 2013;49(6):567–75.
499. Calin GA, Dumitru CD, Shimizu M et al. Frequent deletions and down-regulation of micro- RNA genes miR15 and miR16 at 13q14 in chronic lymphocytic leukemia. *Proc Natl Acad Sci USA* 2002;99(24):15524–9.
500. Bremmer JF, Braakhuis BJM, Brink A et al. Comparative evaluation of genetic assays to identify oral pre-cancerous fields. *J Oral Pathol Med* 2008;37(10):599–606.
501. Stafford ND, Ashman JNE, MacDonald AW, Ell SR, Monson JRT, Greenman J. Genetic analysis of head and neck squamous cell carcinoma and surrounding mucosa. *Arch Otolaryngol* 1999;125(12):1341–8.
502. Preuss SF, Brieger J, Essig EK, Stenzel MJ, Mann WJ. Quantitative DNA measurement in oropharyngeal squamous cell carcinoma and surrounding mucosa. *ORL J Otorhinolaryngol Relat Spec* 2004;66(6):320–4.
503. Szukala K, Sowinska A, Wierzbicka M, Biczysko W, Szyfter W, Szyfter K. Does loss of heterozygosity in critical genome regions predict a local relapse in patients after laryngectomy? *Mutat Res* 2006;600(1–2):67–76.
504. Brieger J, Kastner J, Gosepath J, Mann WJ. Evaluation of microsatellite amplifications at chromosomal locus 3q26 as surrogate marker for premalignant changes in mucosa surrounding head and neck squamous cell carcinoma. *Cancer Genet Cytogenet* 2006;167(1):26–31.
505. Chin D, Boyle GM, Theile DR, Parsons PG, Coman WB. Molecular introduction to head and neck cancer (HNSCC) carcinogenesis. *Br J Plast Surg* 2004;57(7):595–602.
506. Choi S, Myers JN. Molecular pathogenesis of oral squamous cell carcinoma: implications for therapy. *J Dent Res* 2008;87(1):14–32.
507. Kim MM, Califano JA. Molecular pathology of head-and-neck cancer. *Int J Cancer* 2004;112(4):545–53.
508. Mirzayans R, Andrais B, Scott A, Murray D. New insights into p53 signaling and cancer cell response to DNA damage: implications for cancer therapy. *J Biomed Biotechnol* 2012;2012:170325.
509. Nathan CO, Liu L, Li BD, Abreo FW, Nandy I, De Benedetti A. Detection of the proto-oncogene eIF4E in surgical margins may predict recurrence in head and neck cancer. *Oncogene* 1997;15(5):579–84.
510. Sunavala-Dossabhoy G, Palaniyandi S, Clark C, Nathan CO, Abreo FW, Caldito G. Analysis of eIF4E and 4EBP1 mRNAs in head and neck cancer. *Laryngoscope* 2011;121(10):2136–41.
511. Mascolo M, Siano M, Ilardi G et al. Epigenetic disregulation in oral cancer. *Int J Mol Sci* 2012;13(2):2331–53.
512. Roh JL, Wang XV, Manola J, Sidransky D, Forastiere AA, Koch WM. Clinical correlates of promoter hypermethylation of four target genes in head and neck cancer: a cooperative group correlative study. *Clin Cancer Res* 2013;19(9):2528–40.
513. Goldenberg D, Harden S, Masayesva BG et al. Intraoperative molecular margin analysis in head and neck cancer. *Arch Otolaryngol Head Neck Surg* 2004;130(1):39–44.
514. Perez-Sayans M, Pilar GD, Barros-Angueira F et al. Current trends in miRNAs and their relationship with oral squamous cell carcinoma. *J Oral Pathol Med* 2012;41(6):433–43.
515. Kato K, Hara A, Kuno T et al. Aberrant promoter hypermethylation of p16 and MGMT genes in oral squamous cell carcinomas and the surrounding normal mucosa. *J Cancer Res Clin Oncol* 2006;132(11):735–43.
516. Rainsbury JW, Ahmed W, Williams HK, Roberts S, Paleri V, Mehanna H. Prognostic biomarkers of survival in oropharyngeal squamous cell carcinoma: systematic review and meta-analysis. *Head Neck* 2013;35(7):1048–55.
517. Calin GA, Croce CM. MicroRNA signatures in human cancers. *Nat Rev Cancer* 2006;6(11):857–66.

518. Clague J, Lippman SM, Yang H et al. Genetic variation in microRNA genes and risk of oral premalignant lesions. *Mol Carcinog* 2010;49(2):183–9.
519. Gorenchtein M, Poh CF, Saini R, Garnis C. MicroRNAs in an oral cancer context—from basic biology to clinical utility. *J Dent Res* 2012;91(5):440–6.
520. Barker EV, Cervigne NK, Reis PP et al. MicroRNA evaluation of unknown primary lesions in the head and neck. *Mol Cancer* 2009;8.
521. John K, Wu J, Lee BW, Farah CS. MicroRNAs in head and neck cancer. *Int J Dent* 2013;2013:650218.
522. Denaro N, Merlano MC, Russi EG, Lo Nigro C. Non coding RNAs in head and neck squamous cell carcinoma (HNSCC): a clinical perspective. *Anticancer Res* 2014;34(12):6887–96.
523. Jamali Z, Asl Aminabadi N, Attaran R, Pournagiazar F, Ghertasi Oskouei S, Ahmadpour F. MicroRNAs as prognostic molecular signatures in human head and neck squamous cell carcinoma: a systematic review and meta-analysis. *Oral Oncol* 2015;51(4):321–31.
524. Kang H, Kiess A, Chung CH. Emerging biomarkers in head and neck cancer in the era of genomics. *Nat Rev Clin Oncol* 2015;12(1):11–26.
525. Malumbres M. miRNAs and cancer: an epigenetics view. *Mol Aspects Med* 2012;34(4):863–74.
526. Scapoli L, Palmieri A, Lo Muzio L et al. MicroRNA expression profiling of oral carcinoma identifies new markers of tumor progression. *Int J Immunopathol Pharmacol* 2010;23(4):1229–34.
527. Calin GA, Sevignani C, Dan Dumitru C et al. Human microRNA genes are frequently located at fragile sites and genomic regions involved in cancers. *Proc Natl Acad Sci USA* 2004;101(9):2999–3004.
528. Childs G, Fazzari M, Kung G et al. Low-level expression of microRNAs let-7d and miR-205 are prognostic markers of head and neck squamous cell carcinoma. *Am J Pathol* 2009;174(3):736–45.
529. Kozaki K-i, Imoto I, Mogi S, Omura K, Inazawa J. Exploration of tumor-suppressive microRNAs silenced by DNA hypermethylation in oral cancer. *Cancer Res* 2008;68(7):2094–105.
530. Abdulhameed Abdulmajeed A, Farah CS. Intra-oral calibre persistent artery. *J Craniomaxillofac Surg* 2010;38(5):331–3.
531. Lajer CB, Garnaes E, Friis-Hansen L et al. The role of miRNAs in human papilloma virus (HPV)-associated cancers: bridging between HPV-related head and neck cancer and cervical cancer. *Br J Cancer* 2012;106(9):1526–34.
532. Lajer CB, Nielsen FC, Friis-Hansen L et al. Different miRNA signatures of oral and pharyngeal squamous cell carcinomas: a prospective translational study. *Br J Cancer* 2011;104(5):830–40.
533. Babu JM, Prathibha R, Jijith VS, Hariharan R, Pillai MR. A miR-centric view of head and neck cancers. *Biochim Biophys Acta* 2011;1816(1):67–72.
534. Xiao W, Bao ZX, Zhang CY et al. Upregulation of miR-31* is negatively associated with recurrent/newly formed oral leukoplakia. *PLoS One* 2012;7(6):e38648.
535. Lingen MW, Pinto A, Mendes RA et al. Genetics/epigenetics of oral premalignancy: current status and future research. *Oral Dis* 2011;17(Suppl 1):7–22.
536. Califano J, Westra WH, Meininger G, Corio R, Koch WM, Sidransky D. Genetic progression and clonal relationship of recurrent premalignant head and neck lesions. *Clin Cancer Res* 2000;6(2):347–52.
537. Sidransky D. Molecular markers in cancer diagnosis. *J Natl Cancer Inst Monographs* 1995;(17):27–9.
538. Mao L, Lee JS, Fan YH et al. Frequent microsatellite alterations at chromosomes 9p21 and 3p14 in oral premalignant lesions and their value in cancer risk assessment. *Nat Med* 1996;2(6):682–5.
539. Lippman SM, Sudbo J, Hong WK. Oral cancer prevention and the evolution of molecular-targeted drug development. *J Clin Oncol* 2005;23(2):346–56.
540. Hong WK, Spitz MR, Lippman SM. Cancer chemoprevention in the 21st century: genetics, risk modeling, and molecular targets. *J Clin Oncol* 2000;18(21 Suppl):9S–18S.
541. Califano J, van der Riet P, Westra W et al. Genetic progression model for head and neck cancer: implications for field cancerization. *Cancer Res* 1996;56(11):2488–92.
542. Tabor MP, Braakhuis BJ, van der Wal JE et al. Comparative molecular and histological grading of epithelial dysplasia of the oral cavity and the oropharynx. *J Pathol* 2003;199(3):354–60.
543. Tsui IF, Rosin MP, Zhang L, Ng RT, Lam WL. Multiple aberrations of chromosome 3p detected in oral premalignant lesions. *Cancer Prev Res* 2008;1(6):424–9.
544. Tabor MP, Brakenhoff RH, van Houten VM et al. Persistence of genetically altered fields in head and neck cancer patients: biological and clinical implications. *Clin Cancer Res* 2001;7(6):1523–32.
545. Rosin MP, Cheng X, Poh C et al. Use of allelic loss to predict malignant risk for low-grade oral epithelial dysplasia. *Clin Cancer Res* 2000;6(2):357–62.
546. Rosin MP, Lam WL, Poh C et al. 3p14 and 9p21 loss is a simple tool for predicting second oral malignancy at previously treated oral cancer sites. *Cancer Res* 2002;62(22):6447–50.
547. Wong DT. Salivary extracellular noncoding RNA: emerging biomarkers for molecular diagnostics. *Clin Ther* 2015;37(3):540–51.
548. Yoshizawa JM, Schafer CA, Schafer JJ, Farrell JJ, Paster BJ, Wong DT. Salivary biomarkers: toward

future clinical and diagnostic utilities. *Clin Microbiol Rev* 2013;26(4):781–91.
549. Wong DT. Salivaomics. *J Am Dent Assoc* 2012;143(10 Suppl):19s–24s.
550. Yakob M, Fuentes L, Wang MB, Abemayor E, Wong DT. Salivary biomarkers for detection of oral squamous cell carcinoma—current state and recent advances. *Curr Oral Health Rep* 2014;1(2):133–41.
551. Wong DT. Salivary diagnostics: amazing as it might seem, doctors can detect and monitor diseases using molecules found in a sample of spit. *Am Sci* 2008;96(1):37–43.
552. Zimmermann BG, Park NJ, Wong DT. Genomic targets in saliva. *Ann NY Acad Sci* 2007;1098:184–91.
553. Zimmermann BG, Wong DT. Salivary mRNA targets for cancer diagnostics. *Oral Oncol* 2008;44(5):425–9.
554. Wong DT. Salivary diagnostics powered by nanotechnologies, proteomics and genomics. *J Am Dent Assoc* 2006;137(3):313–21.
555. Park NJ, Li Y, Yu T, Brinkman BM, Wong DT. Characterization of RNA in saliva. *Clin Chem* 2006;52(6):988–94.
556. Lau C, Kim Y, Chia D et al. Role of pancreatic cancer-derived exosomes in salivary biomarker development. *J Biol Chem* 2013;288(37):26888–97.
557. Lee YH, Wong DT. Saliva: an emerging biofluid for early detection of diseases. *Am J Dent* 2009;22(4):241–8.
558. Segal A, Wong DT. Salivary diagnostics: enhancing disease detection and making medicine better. *Eur J Dent Educ* 2008;12(Suppl 1):22–9.
559. Schafer CA, Schafer JJ, Yakob M, Lima P, Camargo P, Wong DT. Saliva diagnostics: utilizing oral fluids to determine health status. *Monogr Oral Sci* 2014;24:88–98.
560. Zhang Y, Sun J, Lin CC, Abemayor E, Wang MB, Wong DT. The emerging landscape of salivary diagnostics. *Oral Health Dent Manag* 2014;13(2):200–10.
561. Spielmann N, Ilsley D, Gu J et al. The human salivary RNA transcriptome revealed by massively parallel sequencing. *Clin Chem* 2012;58(9):1314–21.
562. Orozco AF, Lewis DE. Flow cytometric analysis of circulating microparticles in plasma. *Cytometry A* 2010;77(6):502–14.
563. Michael A, Bajracharya SD, Yuen PS et al. Exosomes from human saliva as a source of microRNA biomarkers. *Oral Dis* 2010;16(1):34–8.
564. Ogawa Y, Taketomi Y, Murakami M, Tsujimoto M, Yanoshita R. Small RNA transcriptomes of two types of exosomes in human whole saliva determined by next generation sequencing. *Biol Pharm Bull* 2013;36(1):66–75.
565. Majem B, Rigau M, Reventos J, Wong DT. Non-coding RNAs in saliva: emerging biomarkers for molecular diagnostics. *Int J Mol Sci* 2015;16(4):8676–98.
566. Polanska H, Raudenska M, Gumulec J et al. Clinical significance of head and neck squamous cell cancer biomarkers. *Oral Oncol* 2014;50(3):168–77.
567. Weber JA, Baxter DH, Zhang S et al. The microRNA spectrum in 12 body fluids. *Clin Chem* 2010;56(11):1733–41.
568. Patel RS, Jakymiw A, Yao B et al. High resolution of microRNA signatures in human whole saliva. *Arch Oral Biol* 2011;56(12):1506–13.
569. Park NJ, Zhou H, Elashoff D et al. Salivary microRNA: discovery, characterization, and clinical utility for oral cancer detection. *Clin Cancer Res* 2009;15(17):5473–7.
570. Hanson EK, Lubenow H, Ballantyne J. Identification of forensically relevant body fluids using a panel of differentially expressed microRNAs. *Anal Biochem* 2009;387(2):303–14.
571. Wiklund ED, Gao S, Hulf T et al. MicroRNA alterations and associated aberrant DNA methylation patterns across multiple sample types in oral squamous cell carcinoma. *PLoS One* 2011;6(11):e27840.
572. Liu CJ, Lin SC, Yang CC, Cheng HW, Chang KW. Exploiting salivary miR-31 as a clinical biomarker of oral squamous cell carcinoma. *Head Neck J Sci Spec* 2012;34(2):219–24.
573. Yang Y, Li YX, Yang X, Jiang L, Zhou ZJ, Zhu YQ. Progress risk assessment of oral premalignant lesions with saliva miRNA analysis. *BMC Cancer* 2013;13:129.
574. Momen-Heravi F, Trachtenberg AJ, Kuo WP, Cheng YS. Genomewide study of salivary microRNAs for detection of oral cancer. *J Dent Res* 2014;93(7 Suppl):86s–93s.
575. Salazar C, Nagadia R, Pandit P et al. A novel saliva-based microRNA biomarker panel to detect head and neck cancers. *Cell Oncol (Dordr)* 2014;37(5):331–8.
576. Xiao H, Langerman A, Zhang Y et al. Quantitative proteomic analysis of microdissected oral epithelium for cancer biomarker discovery. *Oral Oncol* 2015;51(11):1011–9. doi: 10.1016/j.oraloncology.2015.08.008. Epub August 29, 2015.
577. de Jong EP, Xie H, Onsongo G et al. Quantitative proteomics reveals myosin and actin as promising saliva biomarkers for distinguishing premalignant and malignant oral lesions. *PLoS One* 2010;5(6):e11148.
578. Bagan L, Saez GT, Tormos MC, Labaig-Rueda C, Murillo-Cortes J, Bagan JV. Salivary and serum interleukin-6 levels in proliferative verrucous leukoplakia. *Clin Oral Investig* 2016;20(4):737–43. doi: 10.1007/s00784-015-1551-z. Epub August 9, 2015.
579. Rajkumar K, Nandhini G, Ramya R, Rajashree P, Kumar AR, Anandan SN. Validation of the diagnostic utility of salivary interleukin 8 in the differentiation of potentially malignant oral lesions and oral

squamous cell carcinoma in a region with high endemicity. *Oral Surg Oral Med Oral Pathol Oral Radiol* 2014;118(3):309–19.
580. Yang CY, Brooks E, Li Y et al. Detection of picomolar levels of interleukin-8 in human saliva by SPR. *Lab Chip* 2005;5(10):1017–23.
581. St John MA, Li Y, Zhou X et al. Interleukin 6 and interleukin 8 as potential biomarkers for oral cavity and oropharyngeal squamous cell carcinoma. *Arch Otolaryngol* 2004;130(8):929–35.
582. Wang Y, Springer S, Mulvey CL et al. Detection of somatic mutations and HPV in the saliva and plasma of patients with head and neck squamous cell carcinomas. *Sci Transl Med* 2015;7(293):293ra104.
583. Rettori MM, de Carvalho AC, Bomfim Longo AL et al. Prognostic significance of *TIMP3* hypermethylation in post-treatment salivary rinse from head and neck squamous cell carcinoma patients. *Carcinogenesis* 2013;34(1):20–7.

4

Histopathology

PAUL M. SPEIGHT

ORAL POTENTIALLY MALIGNANT DISORDERS

The term "oral potentially malignant disorder" refers to a state of precancer in the oral cavity represented by a clinical presentation that carries an increased risk of progression to squamous cell carcinoma (1,2). This definition allows for the fact that cancer may not necessarily arise at the site of a specific lesion, but may be associated with a generalized state or "condition" or may arise in altered but clinically normal epithelium. Nevertheless, the most common disorders recognized as potentially malignant are *leukoplakia* and *erythroplakia* (3), which are clinical lesions with characteristic histopathological features. Although these disorders have a statistically increased risk of progression to cancer (2,4), at the present time, the prognostic significance of an individual lesion is difficult to determine. None of the currently available molecular markers have proved to be predictive and none have yet been evaluated in large prospective studies (5).

At the present time, therefore, microscopic evaluation of hematoxylin and eosin-stained sections for the presence of *epithelial dysplasia* remains the gold standard for the assessment of oral potentially malignant disorders (3).

HISTOPATHOLOGY OF ORAL EPITHELIAL DYSPLASIA

Overall, the assessment of altered cytological features in epithelium is similar regardless of the anatomical site, but there are variations in terminology. In the head and neck, the terms "squamous intraepithelial neoplasia" or "squamous intraepithelial lesions" (6) have been suggested, but these are usually used only in the context of laryngeal lesions (3,6). The diagnostic criteria used in each scheme are similar, but the terminology is not exactly the same. In lesions from the oral cavity, therefore, *oral epithelial dysplasia* is regarded as the standard terminology (1–5).

The diagnosis and grading of oral epithelial dysplasia is based on an assessment of the presence or absence of up to 17 architectural and cytological features (3,4) (Table 4.1).

Depending on the presence, severity or extent of each of these features, a lesion can be graded into one of four categories: hyperplasia (no dysplasia), mild dysplasia, moderate dysplasia or severe dysplasia (including carcinoma *in situ*). There has been an attempt to more carefully define the criteria for grading of epithelial dysplasia (3,5). Largely, this has involved an adaptation of the scheme used in cervical pathology where cervical intraepithelial neoplasia (CIN) is graded according to the thickness or levels of involved epithelium. It should be noted, however, that full-thickness change analogous to CIN3 (carcinoma *in situ*) is rarely seen in the mouth. Nevertheless, the latest World Health Organization (WHO) classification (3) now recommends a more objective grading that does, to some extent, take account of levels of involvement.

The criteria for grading of oral epithelial dysplasia can be summarized as follows (1,3–5):

Mild dysplasia. Architectural and cellular changes are minimal and are limited to the lower third of the epithelium (Figure 4.1). There may be proliferation or hyperplasia of the basal and parabasal layers associated with only slight cytological atypia with mild pleomorphism of cells or nuclei. Mitoses are not prominent and, when present, are usually basally located and normal.

Moderate dysplasia. Architectural changes may be seen up to the middle third of the epithelium with loss of polarity and hyperplasia of basal cells leading to bulbous or drop-shaped rete pegs (Figure 4.2). Stratification and maturation are usually normal, although hyperkeratosis is common. The cytological changes are more severe than in mild dysplasia with atypical cells extending into the middle third of the epithelium. Changes such as nuclear hyperchromatism and prominent cell and nuclear pleomorphism may be seen. Mitoses may be increased and some may be abnormal, but they are usually located in the basal layers.

Severe dysplasia. Architectural changes are extensive and extend into the upper third of the epithelium (Figure 4.3). There is often irregular or loss of stratification, with deep abnormal keratinization and even formation of keratin pearls (dyskeratosis). Abnormal rete pegs are usually evident and bulbous rete pegs are particularly significant in the diagnosis of severe dysplasia. Abnormal rete pegs with lateral extensions or nodules may be seen and may represent the earliest signs of invasion (4). There is obvious loss of polarity of basal cells, which may proliferate into the upper third of the epithelium. All the changes seen in mild and moderate dysplasia are seen, but pleomorphism is much more

Table 4.1 Cytological and architectural features of oral epithelial dysplasia

Architectural (tissue) changes
- Irregular epithelial stratification
- Loss of polarity of basal cells
- Drop-shaped rete ridges
- Increased number of mitotic figures
- Abnormally superficial mitotic figures
- Premature keratinization in single cells
- Keratin pearls in the rete pegs
- Loss of epithelial cell cohesion
- Secondary extensions or nodules on rete tips[a]

Cellular changes
- Abnormal variation in nuclear size
- Abnormal variation in nuclear shape
- Abnormal variation in cell size
- Abnormal variation in cell shape
- Increased nuclear–cytoplasmic ratio
- Abnormal mitotic figures
- Increased number and size of nucleoli
- Hyperchromatic nuclei

Source: Based on Reibel J et al. In: El-Naggar AK et al. (eds). *WHO Classification of Head and Neck Tumours* (4th Edition). Lyon: IARC Press, 2017, 112–5 (3).

[a] An additional feature suggested by Bouquot J et al. (4).

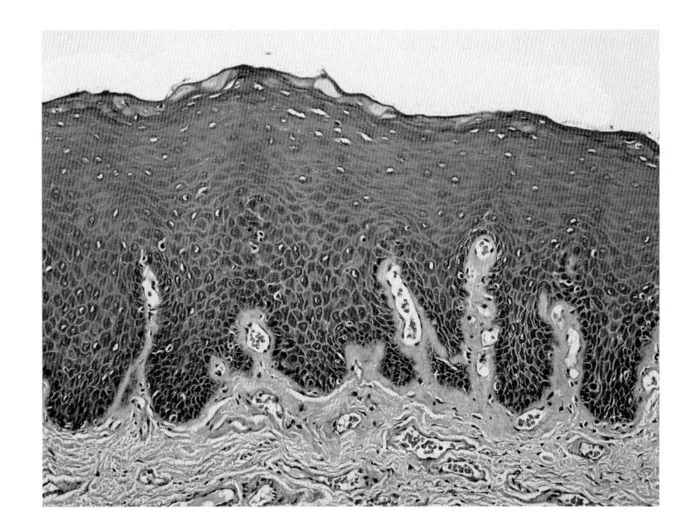

Figure 4.1 Mild epithelial dysplasia. There are minimal architectural and cellular changes, limited to the lower third of the epithelium.

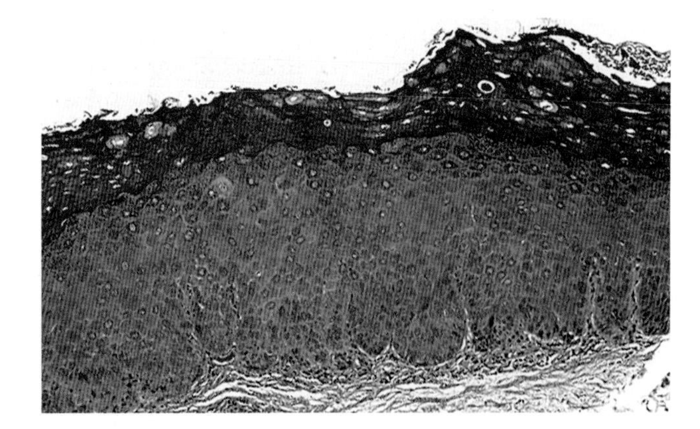

Figure 4.2 Moderate epithelial dysplasia. More marked changes are seen extending into the middle third of the epithelium.

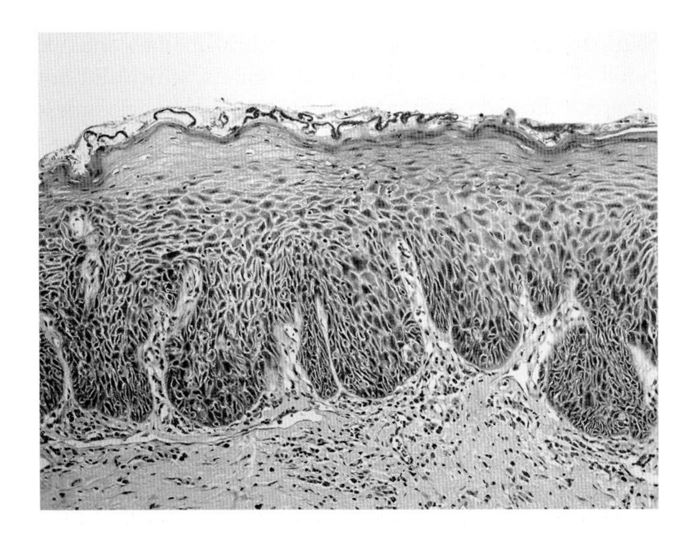

Figure 4.3 Severe epithelial dysplasia. Cellular changes extend into the upper third of the epithelium. Architectural changes may be marked, especially bulbous rete pegs.

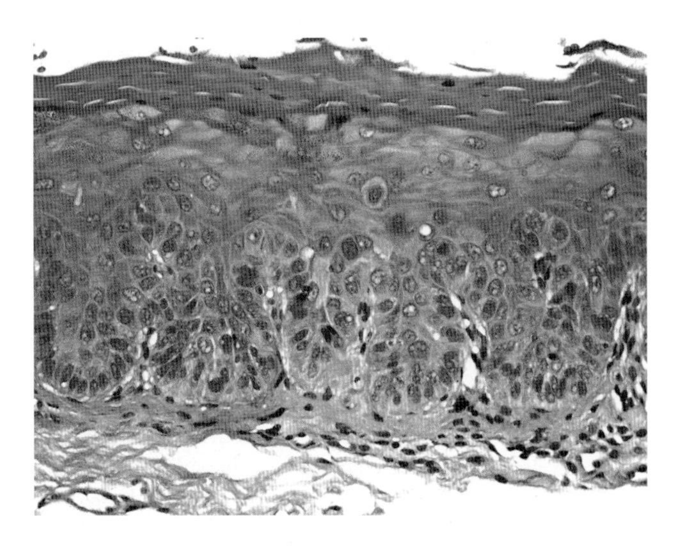

Figure 4.5 Severe epithelial dysplasia. In this example, the changes only reach the middle third of the epithelium, but they are sufficiently severe to warrant "upgrading" to severe dysplasia.

marked, often with abnormally large nuclei with prominent or even multiple nucleoli. Prominent and suprabasal mitoses are usually evident and abnormal tripolar or star-shaped forms may be seen. Apoptotic bodies may also be prominent. Acantholysis may sometimes be seen with severe disruption of the architecture. The epithelium is often thickened, but in severe dysplasia there may be marked epithelial atrophy, especially in lesions from the floor of the mouth, ventral tongue or soft palate. These thin lesions may have presented clinically as erythroplakia. In these cases, however, although there may be disrupted stratification, there is usually still evidence of a thin superficial layer of keratin.

Carcinoma in situ is the most severe form of epithelial dysplasia and is characterized by full-thickness cytological and architectural changes (Figure 4.4), but without evidence of invasion or disruption of the basement membrane. Carcinoma *in situ* is thought by some to be a premalignancy, but others regard it as evidence of actual malignant change but without invasion. Full-thickness changes are rare in oral lesions and even in the presence of the most severe atypia there is often an intact keratinized surface layer. "Carcinoma *in situ*" is therefore not used as a diagnostic term for oral lesions and is regarded as synonymous with severe epithelial dysplasia (3), indicating the need to manage both lesions in a similar manner, usually by excision.

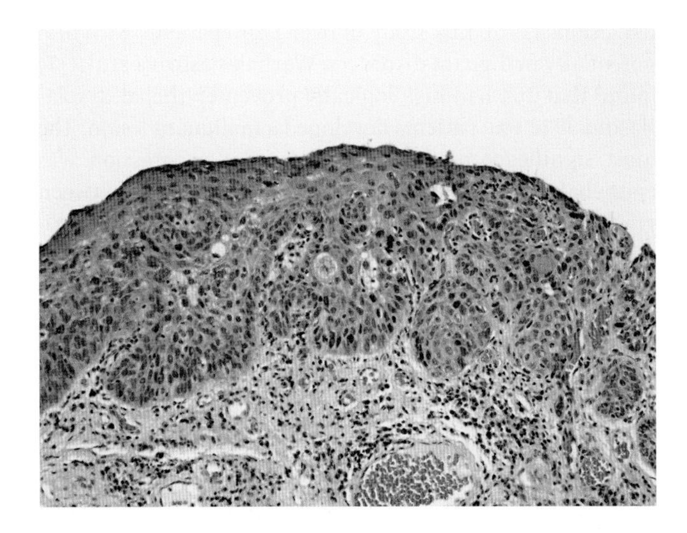

Figure 4.4 Carcinoma *in situ*. There are very severe architectural and cellular changes that extend through the full thickness of the epithelium. Note, however, that there is still evidence of maturation, with a thin layer of parakeratin on the surface.

When grading epithelial dysplasia, the pathologist must consider both the architectural and cytological changes. Lesions may be upgraded, such as from moderate to severe dysplasia if the cytological changes are particularly marked even if they remain in the lower thirds (Figure 4.5). Changes regarded as particularly significant, which may be most predictive of progression to cancer, have been shown to include loss of polarity of basal cells, drop-shaped rete pegs, abnormal or superficial mitoses, nuclear or cellular pleomorphism and increased number of nucleoli.

GRADING OF EPITHELIAL DYSPLASIA

The grading scheme outlined is used to classify oral potentially malignant lesions into four categories (Table 4.2), which is thought to provide good discrimination, but evaluation of the features is subjective and has been subject to considerable inter- and intra-observer variations in the grading of lesions (5,7–11). This is in part due to the problem of defining artificial boundaries to try to classify changes that take place along a continuum of biological change, but also because strict criteria for classification systems have never been agreed. In general, grading systems work quite well when classifying lesions with severe dysplasia or

Table 4.2 Classification of oral potentially malignant lesions into four categories

Epithelial hyperplasia or keratosis without dysplasia
Mild dysplasia
Moderate dysplasia
Severe dysplasia (Including Carcinoma *in situ*)

Source: Based on Reibel J et al. Oral potentially malignant disorders and oral epithelial dysplasia. In: El-Naggar AK, Chan JKC, Grandis JR, Takata T, Sootweg P (eds). WHO Classification of Head and Neck Tumours (4th Edition). Lyon: IARC Press, 2017, 112–5 (3).

actual malignancy, but are much less accurate for low-grade dysplastic lesions, where changes may be subtle and there is considerable overlap with inflammatory and reactive histologic changes (12,13).

In their review, Fleskens and Slootweg (13) noted that interobserver agreement of oral dysplasia showed κ values that varied from only 0.17 (poor) to 0.78 (good). As long ago as 1995, Abbey et al. (8) studied the degree of agreement between six pathologists grading 120 lesions and showed that the average interobserver agreement for the presence or absence of dysplasia was only 81.8%, with κ values ranging from fair to moderate (0.29–0.57). The intraobserver agreement by pathologists with their own previous grading of dysplasia was 81.4% (κ values from 0.31 to 0.71). A number of more recent studies have confirmed these findings (9–11) (Table 4.3).

In light of this, the WHO guidelines have attempted to more carefully define the criteria for grading of epithelial dysplasia as described above (3). Largely this was by an adaptation of the scheme used to grade CIN, so that the three grades of mild, moderate and severe dysplasia depend to some extend on the levels of involvement of the epithelium.

In a further attempt to improve reproducibility, Kujan et al. (14) have suggested a binary grading scheme, which used the WHO morphological criteria to categorize dysplastic lesions into either low grade or high grade (3). They evaluated the histological features of 28 cases of oral dysplastic lesions with a known clinical outcome and were able to define criteria for "high-risk" lesions that progressed and "low-risk" lesions that did not. The high-risk lesions, which subsequently underwent malignant transformation, were characterized by at least four architectural changes and five cytological changes, while low-risk lesions, which did not progress, showed less than four architectural changes or less than five cytological changes. The authors then tested these criteria on 68 lesions that were graded using their binary system and the five-point scheme of the WHO (6). There were good correlations between "low risk" and hyperplasia and mild dysplasia, as well as between "high risk" and severe dysplasia or carcinoma *in situ*. Both schemes were found to predict malignant transformation. The binary scheme was also able to accurately categorize lesions showing moderate dysplasia into high- and low-risk groups, with 14 of 16 cases designated as high risk, actually progressing to cancer. The binary scheme also showed good discrimination for predicting progression-free survival, but the levels of interobserver agreement in both schemes were only fair to moderate (WHO grading system: 0.22; binary grading system: 0.50).

Table 4.3 Four representative studies that have looked at interobserver agreement in the diagnosis of epithelial dysplasia

	κ scores (range)	% agreement, mean (range)
Brothwell et al. (10)	0.51 (0.42–0.58)	77 (75–85)
Karabulut et al. (9)	0.35 (0.27–0.45)	55 (49–69)
Abbey et al. (8)	0.46 (0.29–0.57)	82 (66–86)
Fischer et al. (11)	0.59 (0.45–0.72)	NR

Note: κ values are for a diagnosis of epithelial dysplasia and represent only fair to moderate agreement.
NR = not reported.

MALIGNANT TRANSFORMATION IN POTENTIALLY MALIGNANT DISORDERS

Although it is established that oral potentially malignant disorders are statistically more likely to become malignant, it is not inevitable that each dysplastic lesion will progress to cancer, and non-dysplastic lesions may also progress. In their seminal study in 1984, Silverman et al. (15) showed that 36% of dysplastic lesions progressed to carcinoma, but also that 16% of leukoplakic lesions without evidence of dysplasia progressed. However, there are currently no biomarkers that enable us to distinguish lesions that may progress from those that will not (5,16), and histological examination and grading of dysplasia still remains the most valid method for determining the malignant potential of individual lesions (2–5). In a study of over 1,300 patients with oral potentially malignant disorders, Warnakulasuriya et al. (17) found that 204 had histologically proven epithelial dysplasia and 35 (2.6%) patients developed a malignant lesion. The most significant predictor of malignant progression was epithelial dysplasia with a significant correlation between grade of dysplasia and time to progression. The risks of progression for lesions without dysplasia and for mild, moderate and severe dysplasia were 1.0%, 4.8%, 15.7% and 26.7%, respectively. A review of the literature (4) showed that severe epithelial dysplasia has a malignant transformation rate of about 16%, but with a wide range of 7%–50% (Table 4.4) (15,17–27). Moderate dysplasias have a malignant transformation potential of 3%–15%, and mild epithelial dysplasia shows a very low risk (less than 5%). However, the severity of epithelial dysplasia also correlates with those clinical features known to have the highest risk. For example, Schepman et al. (18) showed that over 60% of non-homogeneous leukoplakias had moderate or severe epithelial dysplasia compared to only 17% of simple or homogeneous lesions. This suggests that dysplasia may not be an independent factor

Table 4.4 Malignant transformation rates (%) for microscopically diagnosed oral carcinoma *in situ* and/or severe epithelial dysplasia

References	Country	Patients (n)	Cumulative follow-up (years)	Mean follow-up (years)	Malignant transformation rate (%)
Gupta et al. (19)	India	90	945	10.5	7.0
Schepman et al. (18)	The Netherlands	166	415	2.5	12.0
Bouquot et al. (20)	USA	32	346	10.8	15.6
Silverman et al. (15)	USA	22	162	7.4	36.0
Banoczy and Csiba (21)	Hungary	23	145	6.3	21.8
Amagasa et al. (22)	Japan	12	120	10.0	50.0
Vedtofte et al. (23)	Denmark	14	55	3.9	35.7
Mincer et al. (24)	USA	16	48	3.0	18.8
Pindborg et al. (25)	India	21	63	3.0	14.3
Lumerman et al. (26)	USA	7	11	1.5	14.3
Jaber et al. (27)	England	480	NR	NR	3.2
Warnakulasuriya et al. (17)	England	8	NR	9.0	26.7

Source: Bouquot J, Speight PM, Farthing PM. *Curr Diagn Pathol* 2006;12:11–22 (4).
NR = not reported.

and some studies have found that dysplasia is not a reliable prognostic indicator. Holmstrup et al. (28) suggested that biopsies are unreliable and that a finding of epithelial dysplasia of any degree did not predict malignant progression. In a similar study of 207 patients, Arduino et al. (29) showed that 7.42% of lesions progressed to cancer, but that neither clinical nor histological factors had any significant association with progression.

Overall, however, a systematic review and meta-analysis (30) has shown that histological grade of dysplasia is significantly associated with malignant transformation. The study showed an overall transformation rate of 12.3%, which increased significantly to 24.1% in lesions with severe dysplasia.

SQUAMOUS CELL CARCINOMA

INTRODUCTION

Over 90% of malignancies in the head and neck region are squamous cell carcinomas arising from the mucosal epithelium. Despite being relatively common, the diagnosis and management of squamous cell carcinoma can still be challenging and difficult. The basis for this difficulty is the subjective nature of diagnosis and grading and the wide range of variants, each with different diagnostic criteria, site predilection and biologic outlook. Although all variants show different histological and clinical features and may require different management approaches, these differences may be subtle. It has become increasingly apparent that "oral cancer" comprises a number of different diseases that should be considered separately, not just on the basis of site, but also etiopathogenesis, prognosis and management. Squamous cell carcinoma of the oral cavity (mouth) should be regarded as a different disease to squamous cell carcinoma arising in the oropharynx. This is based primarily on the etiology, in that oropharyngeal lesions are most often associated with infection by human papillomavirus (HPV), while oral lesions arise in association with the more traditional factors of tobacco and alcohol use. The site distribution of these lesions is shown in Table 4.5, which is based on the International Classification of Disease for Oncology (31). However, there may be crossover in the appearance and cause of lesions and a strict anatomical division is not always easy to apply. Thus, conventional squamous cell carcinoma, associated with tobacco and alcohol and HPV negative, may be encountered in the base of tongue and in overlapping regions between the oral cavity and the oropharynx. Conversely, HPV-positive lesions may occasionally be encountered in the mouth and also in the larynx or elsewhere in the upper aerodigestive tract. The differences, however, and the justification for a division of "oral cancer" into *oral cancer* and *oropharyngeal cancer* will become apparent in subsequent sections where each will be considered separately. We should take note, however, that squamous cell carcinoma of the lip could also be considered as a different disease, as should nasopharyngeal (and sinonasal) cancer. Lip cancer, however, shares many histopathological and prognostic features with oral cancer and will be considered in that category. Nasopharyngeal cancer is a separate disease and will not be considered in detail.

SQUAMOUS CELL CARCINOMA OF THE ORAL CAVITY

These lesions arise from the epithelial lining of the oral cavity, or mouth, and are familiar to most pathologists as

Table 4.5 Sites and ICD codes for oral and oropharyngeal cancers

	Oral carcinoma		Oropharyngeal carcinoma	
Site code	Anatomical sites	ICD-O-03 subcodes	Anatomical sites	ICD-O-03 subcodes
C00	Lips	C00.0–C00.9		
C01			Base of the tongue	C01.9
C02	Tongue	C02.0–C02.9		
C03	Gum	C03.0–C03.9		
C04	Floor of the mouth	C04.0–C04.9		
C05	Palate	C05.0–C05.9		
C06	Other mouth	C06.0–C06.09		
C09			Tonsil	C09.0–C09.9
C10			Oropharynx	C10.0–C10.9
C14			Other sites: pharynx, Waldeyer's ring	C14.0/C14.2
	Other and overlapping sites	C14.8	Other and overlapping sites	C14.8

Source: International Classification of Disease for Oncology. http://codes.iarc.fr/topography (31).

"conventional" squamous cell carcinoma. The defining criterion for a diagnosis of malignancy is invasion of epithelial cells through the basement membrane into the superficial lamina propria. Invasion may be seen as small breaches by a few cells or small islands, to gross infiltration of the underlying connective tissues and submucosa by islands of malignant cells. This permeation of the tissues underlying the surface epithelium gives rise to the classical clinical signs of induration and fixation. The tumor surface is also often ulcerated. All squamous cell carcinomas thus have an endophytic invasive component, where tumor islands can be identified deep to the surface epithelium. Many tumors may also rise above the surface of the mucosa, resulting in an exophytic component that is often associated with hyperkeratosis. This is variable but is most prominent in verrucous carcinoma—a variant characterized by a highly keratinized exophytic component.

HISTOLOGIC GRADING OF ORAL SQUAMOUS CELL CARCINOMA

There are numerous reports in the literature on the histologic grading of oral squamous cell carcinoma and its value in predicting outcomes and metastasis to lymph nodes. The relative significance of individual factors, however, remains uncertain (32). Conventional oral squamous cell carcinoma resembles, at least to some extent, the normal squamous epithelium from which it arises. The degree of resemblance is referred to as "differentiation" and provides the basis for the most widely used grading scheme for squamous cell carcinoma (33), which was first described by Broders in 1920 (reviewed in 34), but has been variably modified subsequently (31–38). Specific histological features that impact on prognosis will be discussed later in this chapter, but here the basic grading scheme is described. Tumors are classified as well, moderately or poorly differentiated depending on the degree of resemblance the tumor has to normal squamous epithelium (Figures 4.6–4.12).

A *well-differentiated squamous cell carcinoma* shows a considerable amount of keratin production and within individual tumor islands there may be evidence of stratification with a quite well polarized basal cell layer. Typically, a well-differentiated lesion shows islands of tumor with central "eddies" of keratin referred to as keratin pearls (Figures 4.6 and 4.7). Elsewhere the tumor cells may be pale, eosinophilic with a glassy or even keratinized cytoplasm, giving the appearance of dyskeratosis (Figure 4.8). The tumor islands are often well defined with a cohesive invasion pattern (Figure 4.7). Special stains may reveal an almost intact basement membrane. In some cases, well-differentiated tumors are clearly continuous with the overlying epithelium and show intact, large, branching rete pegs "pushing" into the underlying connective tissues. Cytological atypia may

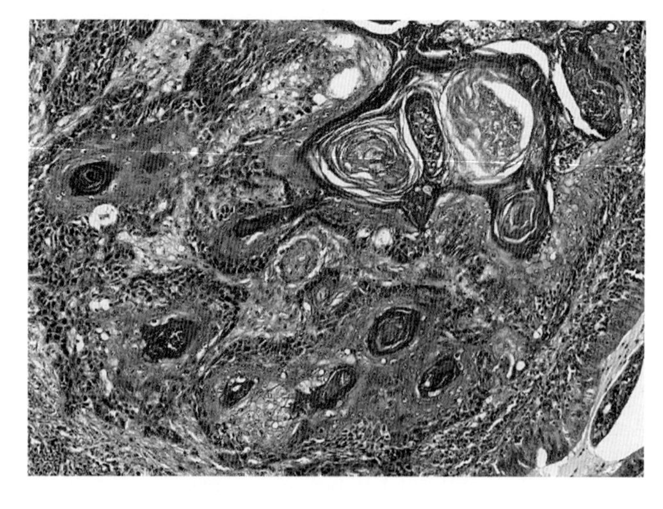

Figure 4.6 Well-differentiated squamous cell carcinoma. The epithelium shows maturation with prominent keratin formation and obvious basal layers.

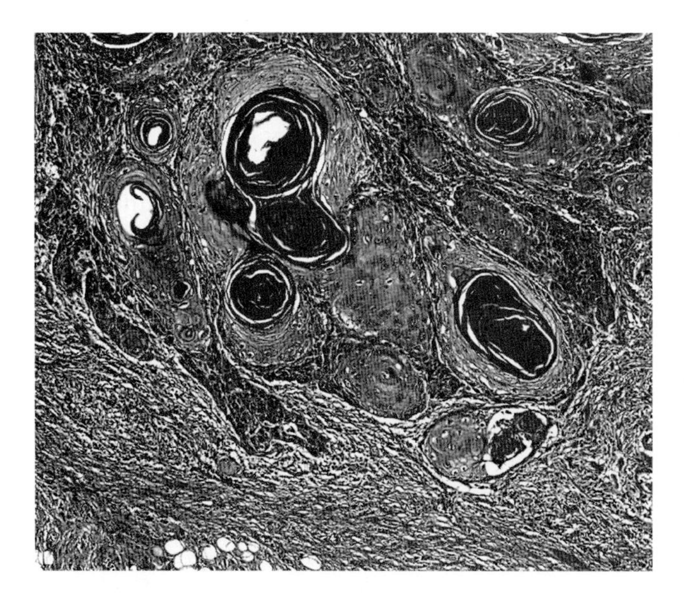

Figure 4.7 Well-differentiated squamous cell carcinoma. Keratin pearls are prominent. The tumor has a cohesive invasion pattern.

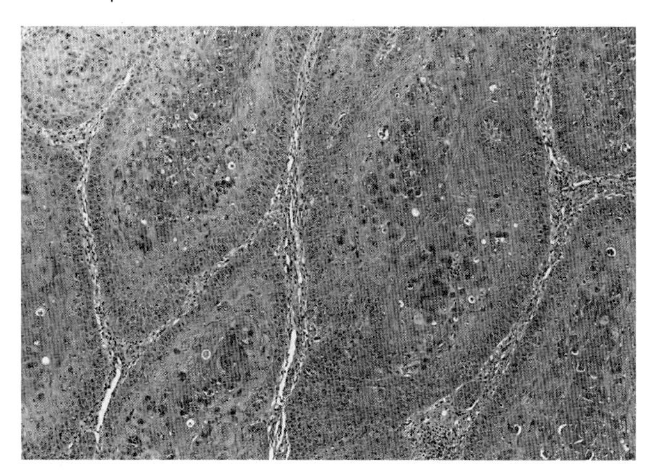

Figure 4.8 Well-differentiated squamous cell carcinoma. Large islands of tumor show marked single-cell keratinization.

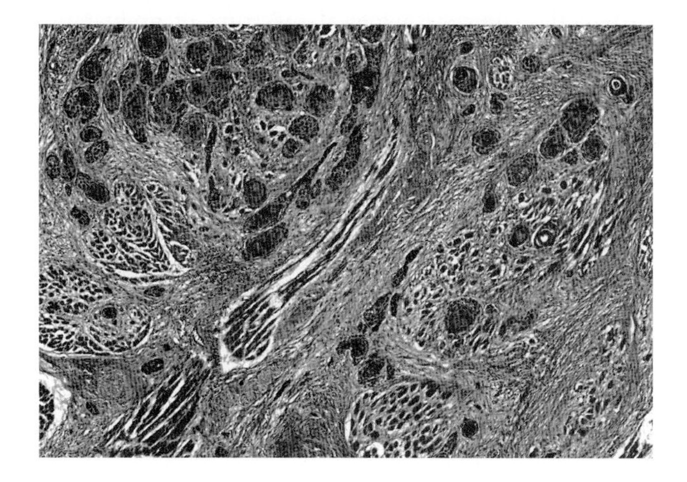

Figure 4.9 Moderately differentiated squamous cell carcinoma. The tumor is composed of small infiltrating islands. Occasional small keratin pearls can be seen.

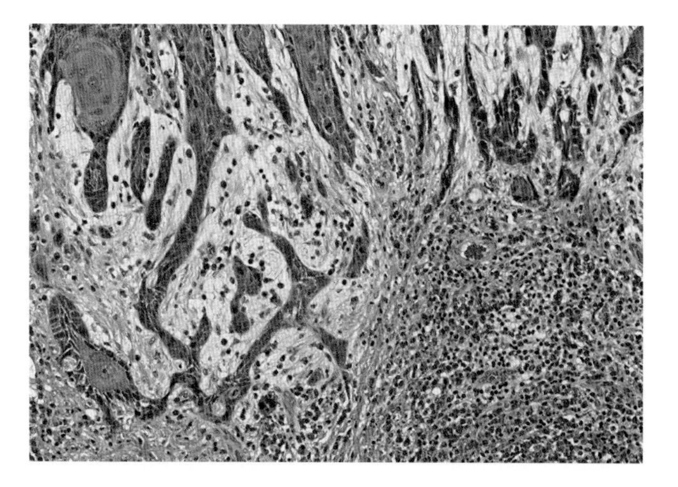

Figure 4.10 Moderately differentiated squamous cell carcinoma. The tumor has a discohesive invasion pattern. Small keratin pearls can be seen (top left).

not be prominent. The most well-differentiated squamous cell carcinomas, with little atypia and a cohesive, pushing, invasive pattern, are typified by verrucous carcinoma (see below).

Moderately differentiated squamous cell carcinomas show a greater degree of atypia and less evidence of keratinization, although keratin pearls and sometimes dyskeratosis are evident (Figure 4.9). The invasive front of the lesion is less cohesive and may be composed of small islands or cords of cells (Figure 4.10). Atypia in the form of nuclear and cellular pleomorphism and hyperchromatic nuclei are consistently seen and may be extensive. Mitotic activity is also prominent and abnormal mitoses may be seen.

Poorly differentiated squamous cell carcinomas show little resemblance to a normal squamous epithelium, but it is important to note that it is still possible to recognize the tissue as being of epithelial origin. Although keratin pearls are unusual, individual keratinizing cells and areas of dyskeratosis may be seen (Figures 4.11 and 4.12). Poorly differentiated

Figure 4.11 Poorly differentiated squamous cell carcinoma. There are sheets of malignant cells with no evidence of differentiation.

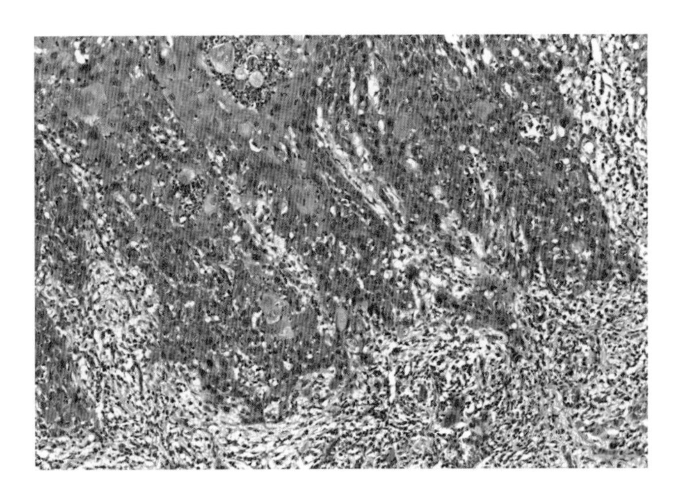

Figure 4.12 Poorly differentiated squamous cell carcinoma. There is considerable cytological atypia. The tumor invades as fine cords and single infiltrating cells.

lesions show considerable atypia, often with bizarre pleomorphic cells. The lesions invade in a less cohesive pattern, with fine cords and small islands infiltrating through the connective tissues (Figure 4.12). Single cells may also be seen at the advancing front. Abnormal mitoses are often prominent. At the worst end of the spectrum, a lesion may be so poorly differentiated that it is not possible to infer its cell of origin on hematoxylin and eosin-stained sections alone. In this case, the tumor is referred to as *anaplastic* or *undifferentiated* and immunocytochemical stains are often needed to confirm an epithelial origin (Figure 4.13).

Overall, about 30% of oral cancers are well differentiated, 60% moderately and only 10% are poorly differentiated. The degree of differentiation may reflect the behavior of a lesion and is used, along with other more refined indictors, to predict the prognosis of individual lesions. These histopathologic prognostic factors are discussed in detail below.

Many workers have attempted to refine this classification, and grading schemes have evolved over the years.

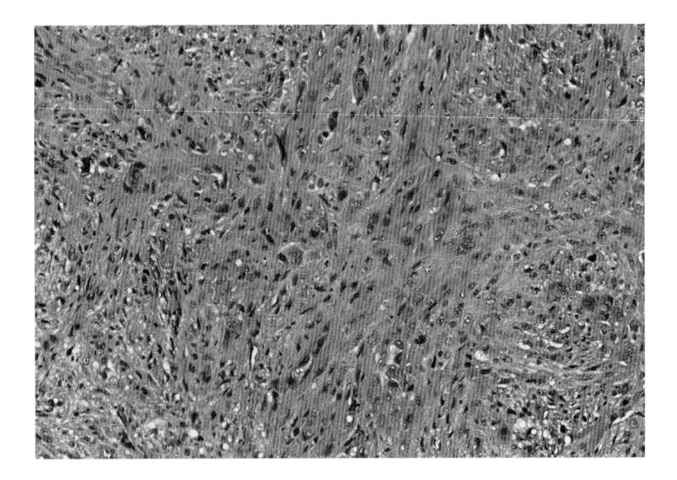

Figure 4.13 Undifferentiated squamous cell carcinoma. There is little evidence that the lesion is of epithelial origin.

Anneroth et al. (34,35) undertook an extensive review of the literature and proposed a modified classification that was further refined by Bryne et al. (36,37) and simplified by Woolgar and Scott (Table 4.6) (38,39). This has become widely used, especially in research and clinical trials. These schemes utilize the degree of differentiation (keratinization), but also take greater account of the tumor–stromal interface, particularly the depth and pattern of invasion.

HISTOPATHOLOGIC VARIANTS OF SQUAMOUS CELL CARCINOMA

Verrucous carcinoma

Verrucous carcinoma was first described by Ackerman in 1948 (40) as a distinctive variant of squamous cell carcinoma with characteristic clinicopathologic features. The lesion's biologic activity places it between conventional squamous cell carcinoma and verrucous hyperplasia of squamous epithelium (41,42).

Predominantly a squamous mucosal lesion, verrucous carcinoma may also be found on cutaneous surfaces, especially in the anogenital region and lower extremities. Whether the carcinomas occur in the upper aerodigestive tract (verrucous carcinoma), on the genitalia (giant condyloma acuminatum) or on the extremities (carcinoma cuniculatum), they are similar.

The mucous membranes of the head and neck are sites of predilection, with the oral cavity and larynx areas especially at risk.

In its early stages, verrucous carcinoma may go unrecognized or be diagnosed as a benign mucosal or cutaneous verruciform growth. The carcinoma may be both persistent and progressive with a clinical phase that lasts several years. In some patients, however, the lesion appears suddenly or a period of slow growth is followed by rapid enlargement. The lesions are often, but not invariably, preceded by a clinical leukoplakia (43), which may be diffuse or focal, but is often part of the clinicopathological spectrum of proliferative verrucous leukoplakia (44,45).

In the head and neck, lesions are most commonly encountered in the oral cavity or the larynx and in males between the ages of 50 and 80 years. At either site, the carcinoma is unusual in a patient younger than 35 years. In the oral cavity, the incidence among all forms of squamous cell carcinoma is between 2% and 4.5% (42,43). Table 4.7 presents the site distribution of 276 oral cavity verrucous carcinomas and indicates that the buccal mucosa accounts for over half of the cases (42,46–48).

The gross appearance of verrucous carcinoma is dependent on several factors: duration of the lesion, degree of keratinization and accompanying changes in the adjacent mucosa. The oral tumors often arise in clinical leukoplakia and are first relatively soft and circumscribed, becoming firmer and more irregular with time. The fully developed carcinoma is an exophytic gray to gray–red bulky lesion

Table 4.6 Histologic malignancy grading system and point scoring criteria

	Point score			
Histologic feature	**1**	**2**	**3**	**4**
Degree of keratinization	High, pearl formation	Moderate	Poor, single cells	None
Nuclear polymorphism	Minimal	Moderate	Numerous	Extreme
Mitotic activity (No./10 HPF)	0–15	16–35	36–55	>55
Invasion pattern	Pushing	Bands	Cord or islands	Single cells, cords/ islands, <15 cells
Stage of invasion	Borderline	Into lamina propria	Into submucosa	Into muscle
Lymphoplasmacytic infiltrate	Continuous rim	Moderate, large patches	Minimal, small patches	Absent

Source: Woolgar JA, Scott J. *Head Neck* 1995;17:463–72 (39).

Table 4.7 Location of verrucous carcinoma of the oral cavity

Oral location	**No. of cases**
Buccal mucosa	147
Gingiva–alveolar	64
Tongue	19
Palate	14
Floor of the mouth	12
Lip	5
Retromolar trigone	2
Too diffuse to localize	13

Source: Data from Batsakis JG et al. *Head Neck Surg* 1982;5:29–38 (42); Medina JE, Dichtel W, Luna MA. *Arch Otolaryngol* 1984;110:437–40 (43).

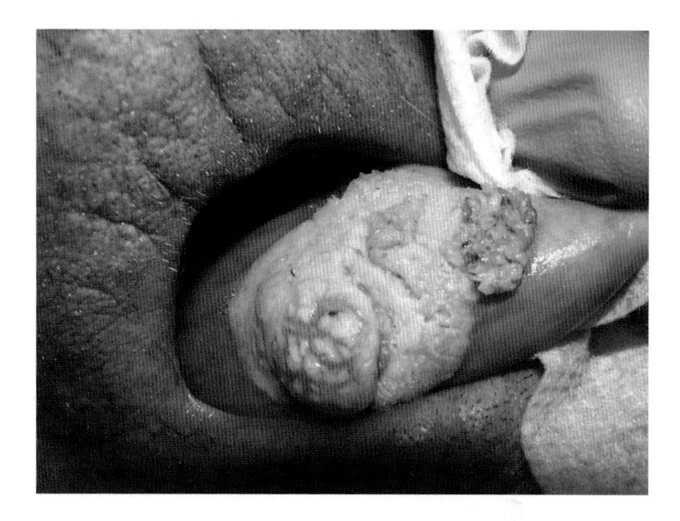

Figure 4.14 Verrucous carcinoma. This clinical lesion is typical, with an exophytic verrucous or papillomatous surface.

presenting as a rough, shaggy, fungating mass with a papillomatous character (Figure 4.14).

Contiguous structures may be involved as tumor growth continues. When the carcinoma arises in the buccal mucosa or extends into the buccal sulcus, it can grow into the soft tissues overlying the mandible and become fixed to the periosteum. With continued growth, it can gradually destroy the periosteum and directly erode and destroy a considerable part of the mandible.

Microscopically, the verrucous carcinoma is broadly based and is exo-endophytic with exophytic papillary fronds and an endophytic element composed of pushing rete pegs (Figures 4.15 and 4.16). It is composed of highly differentiated squamous epithelial cells that lack the usual cytologic criteria of malignancy (Figure 4.16). Mitoses are rare to absent. The surface of the lesion is usually covered by a prominent keratin layer arranged in compressed invaginating folds. The surface has a verruciform pattern, with filiform or broader processes of well-differentiated squamous cells, which have been likened to a series of church spires (Figure 4.17). The diagnosis of malignancy is made

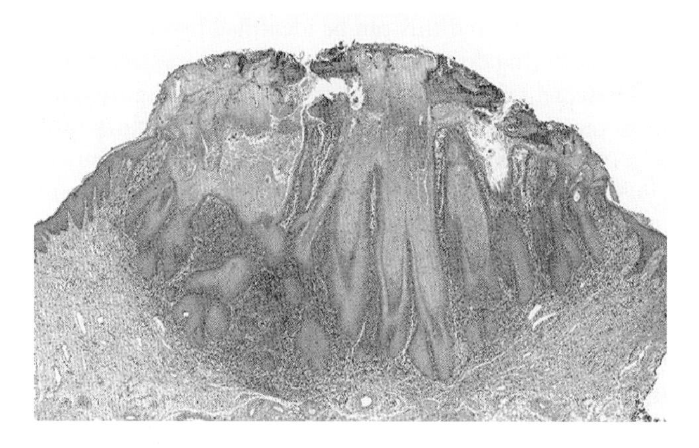

Figure 4.15 Verrucous carcinoma. The lesion is exophytic with a papillary, verruciform surface, but also endophytic, with broad, bulbous rete pegs extending deep to the adjacent epithelium.

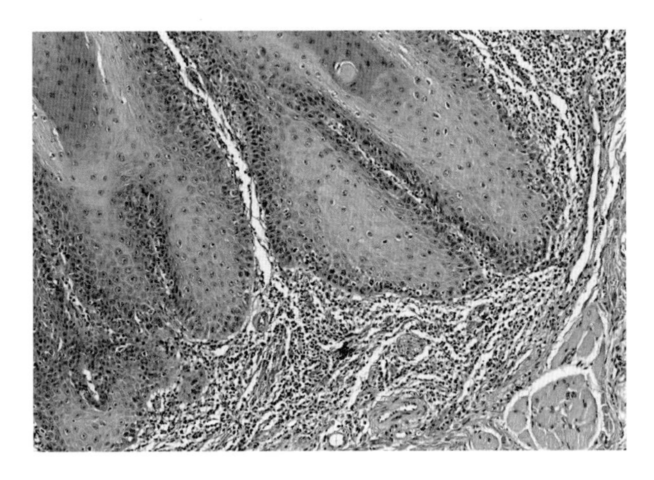

Figure 4.16 Verrucous carcinoma. The broad rete pegs "push" into the connective tissues. There is minimal cytological atypia.

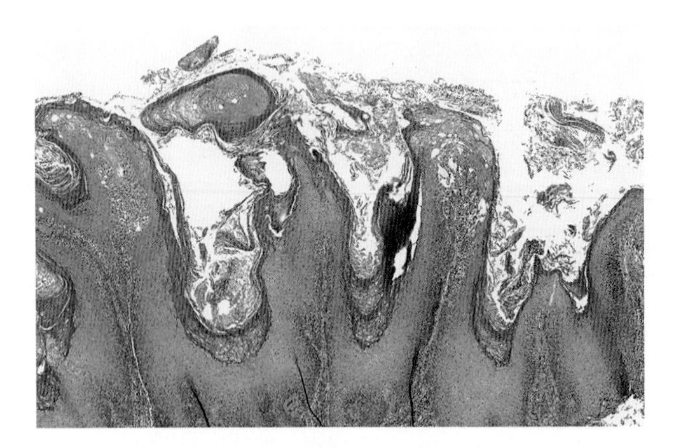

Figure 4.17 Verrucous carcinoma. The surface shows a verrucous pattern with prominent keratosis.

on the invasive quality of the deep parts of the tumor. This infiltrative margin is invariably a blunt "pushing" one usually with good circumscription. This seems to be a point of confusion for pathologists when invasion may be difficult to define. A verrucous squamous cell carcinoma is, by definition, invasive, and this can be identified by the invading tumors growing deep to a plane level with the adjacent normal basement membrane (Figure 4.15; see also Figure 4.46).

In most cases, there is an associated inflammatory reaction in the stroma. This consists predominantly of lymphocytes. The inflammatory layer gives the impression of trying to delimit the carcinoma. Intraneoplastic and stromal reactions to keratin or other cellular debris can be found.

Because of the deceptively benign cytology of the neoplastic cells, an accurate surgical pathologic diagnosis requires a biopsy specimen that includes adjacent normal tissue and shows the invasive depth of the lesion. A full-thickness biopsy plus an appropriate clinical description of the lesion should permit a pathologist to distinguish a verrucous carcinoma from benign hyperplasia or other forms of squamous cell carcinoma. The presence of a regional lymphadenopathy does not help in differential diagnosis and

Table 4.8 Clinicopathologic features of verrucous carcinoma of the oral cavity

Feature	Finding
Site of predilection	Buccal mucosa
Age and sex of patients	Predilection for males older than 50 years
Habits	Tobacco users, poor oral hygiene
Related mucosal changes	Leukoplakia; metachronous or synchronous squamous cell neoplasms
Gross appearance	Exophytic or fungating, usually keratinizing
Differentiation of cells	High degree, uniform; low grade
Cytologic features of malignancy or severe dysplasia	Rare to absent
Mode of invasion	Pushing or blunt and bulbous
Cellular (host) reaction	Usually prominent
Metastatic ability	None in bona fide cases

may be misleading. Bona fide and unperturbed verrucous carcinomas do not metastasize, but can be associated with benign lymph node enlargements secondary to the inflammatory reaction associated with the carcinoma. Table 4.8 summarizes the key features of verrucous carcinoma.

Because they are low grade and often well demarcated, primary treatment for verrucous carcinoma, at any site, is preferably by surgical excision (42,47,48). However, primary radiotherapy has proved to be an effective treatment (49) and for large lesions or in cases where comorbidity limits treatment options chemotherapy with methotrexate has also proved effective (50).

The phenomenon of "anaplastic transformation" following radiation therapy of a verrucous carcinoma has been a factor of contention in the treatment of the neoplasm and has probably been overestimated (42,49). The time interval, or latent period, between radiotherapy and the advent of a more biologically aggressive tumor is short. In five separate reports, the average time interval was 5.4 months, which seems to be too short to be explained by radiotherapy alone (38).

It is probable that lesions may progress to conventional squamous cell carcinoma as part of their normal natural history and conventional squamous cell carcinoma may be found within the lesion (42,43,51). The non-verrucous carcinoma element may be well-differentiated or range to poorly differentiated and non-keratinized. In an MD Anderson series, 20% of oral verrucous carcinomas manifested this hybrid association (43).

CARCINOMA CUNICULATUM

Carcinoma cuniculatum is a rare variant of carcinoma that has been most frequently described on the lower extremities or plantar regions and on the genitals. (Cuniculatum is derived from the Latin "cun- iculus," meaning "rabbit warren" because of the multiple sinuses and crypts found in this tumor.) It has been reported in the oral cavity, but with a total of only about 30 cases up to 2012 (52–56). The true nature of this unusual carcinoma is uncertain and, although it is often regarded as a variant of verrucous carcinoma, it should probably be defined as a distinctive entity. In the oral cavity, it is most common on the maxillary or mandibular gingivae, but cases on the tongue and other sites have been reported (49,52). In the largest series, Sun et al. (56) reviewed 540 cases of oral squamous cell carcinoma and identified 15 cases (2.7%) that met the criteria for carcinoma cuniculatum. Eight (53%) of their cases were found on the tongue and six on the mandible. However, reviews have suggested that more than 50% of cases arise on the gingivae, with the mandible and maxilla being almost equally affected (52–54). The majority of patients have been male with an average age in the sixth decade, but with a wide range from the second to the eighth decades.

Histologically, the tumor is characterized by a complex pattern of folds of keratinized, stratified squamous epithelium that "burrow" into the underlying connective tissues, forming deep, keratin-filled crypts and cystic spaces (Figure 4.18). This has been described as an "inverse architectural epithelial proliferation" (54). The lesions show minimal cytological atypia, are always well differentiated but are associated with considerable local destruction and may permeate deep into muscle or underlying bone. Although primarily endophytic, the lesions are heavily keratinized and may present clinically with an exophytic papillary or verrucous surface resembling verrucous carcinoma. There may be clinical evidence of a large punctum or cavity where the lesion communicates with the surface mucosa. Carcinoma cuniculatum has been reported to have a good prognosis with few reports of metastases and an overall good survival. Of the 15 cases reported by Sun et al. (56), three showed lymph node metastases and only two recurred. The 3- and 5-year disease-free survival rates were 93.3% and 85.7%, respectively.

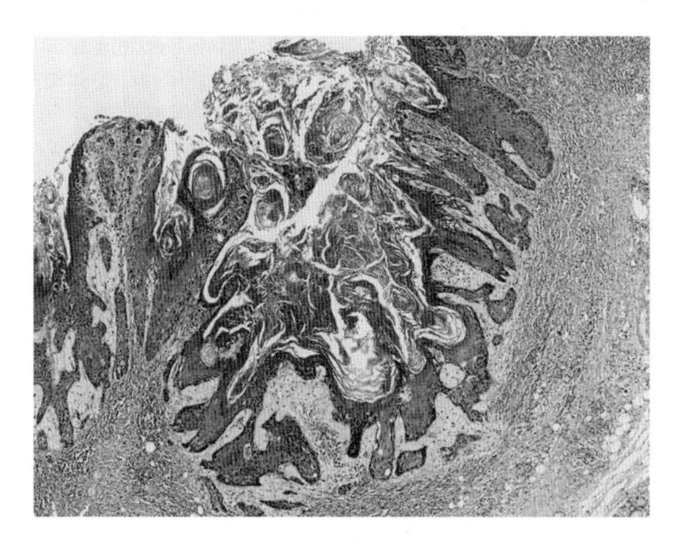

Figure 4.18 Carcinoma cuniculatum. The tumor forms folds of epithelium that permeate into the underlying tissues, forming crypt-like structures.

BASALOID SQUAMOUS CELL CARCINOMA

Basaloid squamous cell carcinoma is an aggressive, histologically distinctive variant of squamous cell carcinoma that has a predilection for the upper aerodigestive tract.

Recently, it has been shown that some basaloid carcinomas are associated with HPV infection (57–59). However, HPV-associated lesions are more often encountered in the oropharynx and may have a better prognosis (see discussion later in this chapter). The term "basaloid squamous cell carcinoma" should therefore only be used for an aggressive basaloid variant of squamous cell carcinoma that is HPV negative and should not be confused with HPV-associated oropharyngeal lesions, which may also have a basaloid morphology, but are regarded as well-differentiated, non-keratinizing lesions (60,61).

Because of the redefinition of these lesions, the clinicopathologic features of basaloid squamous cell carcinoma will need a reappraisal. However, in previous reports of lesions of the head and neck (62), they have been shown to occur in an elderly population with a mean age of 63 years and a male preponderance (82%). They have a predilection for the base of the tongue, pyriform sinus and supraglottic larynx and show an aggressive clinical behavior with a high incidence of metastases to cervical lymph nodes (64%) and distant spread (44%) to lungs, liver, bone, brain and skin. Mortality is high with reported 38% lethality at 17 months' median follow-up. A more recent review of oral lesions found a similar age and gender distribution but noted that the tongue was the most common site followed by the floor of the mouth (59). Few studies, however, have undertaken HPV analyses and further work is needed to clearly distinguish between basaloid variants of oral squamous cell carcinoma and HPV-associated lesions.

Histologically, basaloid squamous cell carcinoma is characterized by the presence of a basaloid and a squamous component (62–65). The basaloid cells are small with hyperchromatic nuclei and little cytoplasm. They are arranged in lobules with a "jigsaw" pattern and with some evidence of palisading of the peripheral cells (Figures 4.19 and 4.20). Cords or trabeculae may also be seen, but prominent mitotic activity with many atypical or bizarre mitoses is typical. Most cases show areas of comedo necrosis in the center of the lobules (Figure 4.21). The squamous component is usually a conventional squamous cell carcinoma that is well to moderately differentiated and invasive. However, in some cases, only surface dysplasia or carcinoma *in situ* is evident (Figure 4.22). It is, however, the basaloid malignancy that sets this carcinoma apart as a distinctive variant of squamous cell carcinoma. The carcinoma may show both deep and lateral invasion at the time of diagnosis and a multifocal origin over a broad area of affected mucosa has been noted (64,65). The diagnosis can be easily made

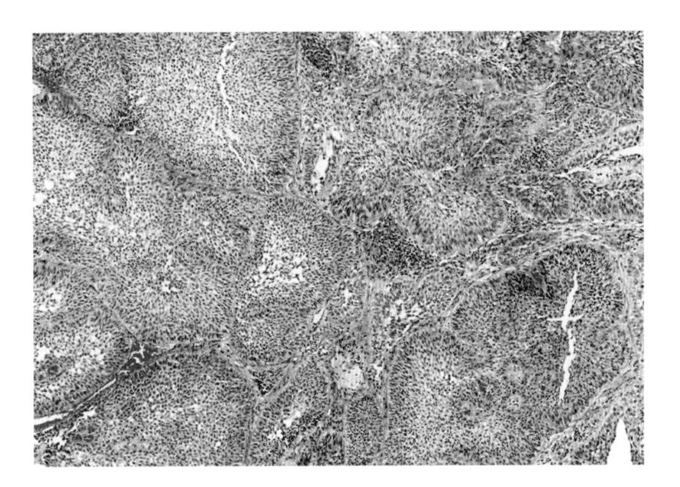

Figure 4.19 Basaloid squamous cell carcinoma. Islands and lobules of basaloid cells with areas of peripheral palisading.

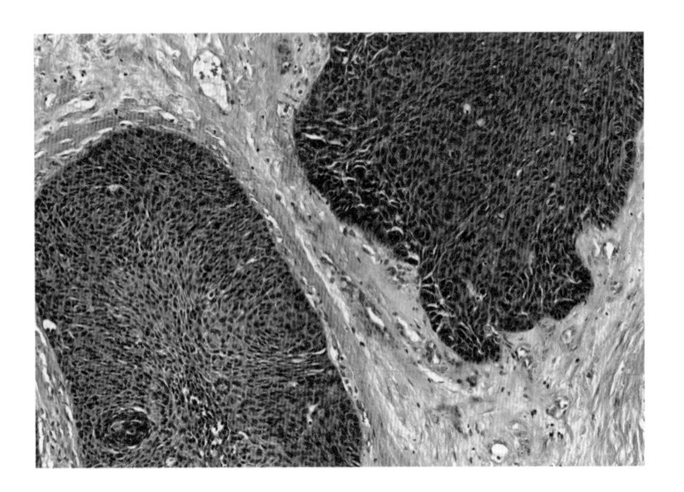

Figure 4.20 Basaloid squamous cell carcinoma. The basaloid cells are small and pleomorphic and have hyperchromatic nuclei.

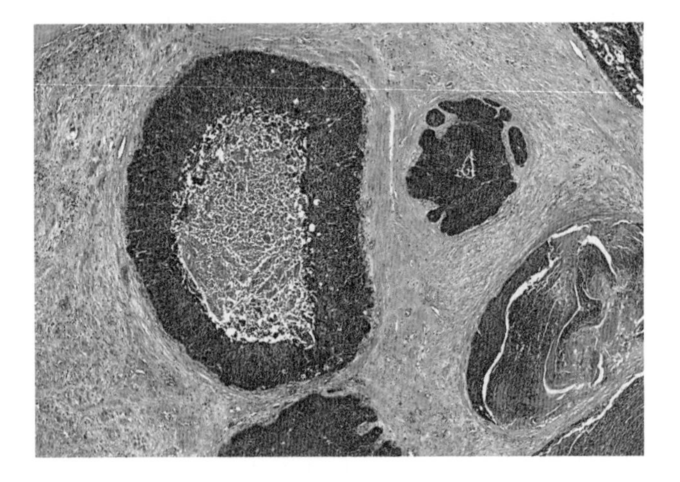

Figure 4.21 Basaloid squamous cell carcinoma. Comedo necrosis is common.

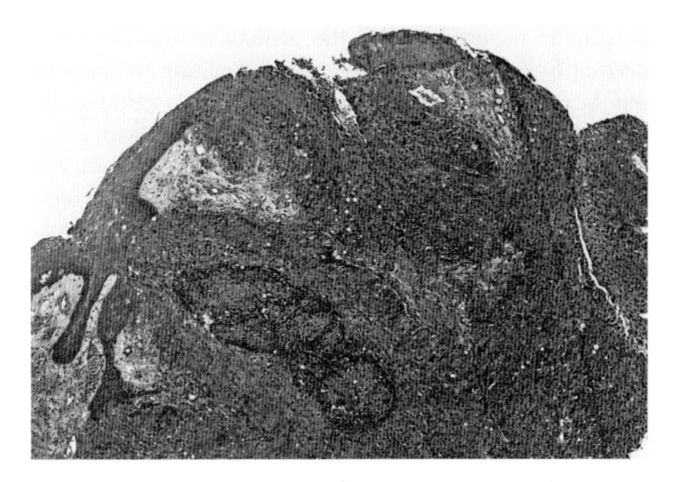

Figure 4.22 Basaloid squamous cell carcinoma. Tumors arise from the overlying epithelium and there may be features of dysplasia and of conventional squamous carcinoma.

when both squamous and basaloid components are present. However, this may depend on an adequate biopsy and careful examination of all the tissue for evidence of a surface origin and both elements. In small biopsies, only the basaloid component may be seen or the surface may be lost or obscured due to ulceration. In these cases, differentiation from other basaloid lesions can be difficult. These include salivary gland tumors, especially basal cell adenocarcinoma or solid adenoid cystic carcinoma, or other small cell carcinomas such as neuroendocrine carcinoma.

Adenoid cystic carcinoma does not show foci of squamous cell carcinoma and there is also no dysplasia or carcinoma *in situ* in the overlying mucosa. Mitoses, nuclear pleomorphism and necrosis are also more conspicuous in basaloid squamous cell carcinoma. Basaloid squamous cell carcinoma is often associated with positive cervical lymph nodes at diagnosis, while adenoid cystic carcinoma is not. Aside from the rarity of neuroendocrine carcinoma in the oral cavity, they can be distinguished from basaloid squamous cell carcinoma by their prominent nuclear molding and the absence of hyalinization and mucinous–myxoid changes in the stroma.

Immunocytochemistry can be useful in excluding these lesions. The immunoprofile is one of an epithelial malignancy (65,66), with positivity for broad-spectrum cytokeratins, but negative for neuroendocrine markers or S100 (66). Neuroendocrine carcinomas also show characteristic paranuclear globular or spot staining for low-molecular-weight keratins, most usefully CK20.

Basaloid squamous cell carcinoma has an overall poor outcome (62–64), but it is possible that the anatomical location of the primary plays a role in prognosis. Luna et al. (64), dealing with basaloid squamous cell carcinomas of the hypopharynx, found no difference in biologic behavior (stage for stage) between conventional squamous cell carcinoma and basaloid squamous cell carcinoma. Basaloid squamous cell carcinomas of the floor of the mouth, on the other hand, have a higher recurrence rate and a worse prognosis than matched groups of conventional squamous cell carcinomas, regardless of the grade of the latter (67), and it is suggested that there is a correlation between the percentage of basaloid components and prognosis; carcinomas with more than 50% basaloid cells have a poorer prognosis (67).

SPINDLE CELL (SARCOMATOID) CARCINOMA

Spindle cell carcinoma is a rare variant of squamous cell carcinoma characterized by a sarcomatoid proliferation of spindled epithelial cells. Molecular studies suggest that the spindled component of the lesion arises due to epithelial–mesenchymal transition from a conventional squamous carcinoma (68–71). There is no evidence for a mixed epithelial and mesenchymal lesion and the term "carcinosarcoma" should no longer be used (71,72).

Clinically, over 90% of spindle cell carcinomas in the head and neck are pedunculated or polypoid masses (73–77) and are often ulcerated and friable. Their size varies from 0.5 to 6.0 cm. If large, they can produce life-threatening obstruction. A large analysis of data from the National Cancer Institute, Surveillance, Epidemiology and End Results (SEER) program shows that, in the head and neck, the larynx is the most common site for spindle cell carcinoma, accounting for 46.4% of cases (78). The oral cavity and oropharynx accounted for 20.4% and 18% of cases, respectively. About half of these cases arise in the tongue, either the mobile tongue or, in the case of oropharyngeal lesions, in the base of the tongue or lingual tonsils (78). Tumors may also occur in the sinonasal tract, pharynx and esophagus (78,79).

The key diagnostic criteria for spindle cell carcinoma is the identification of a biphasic tumor with malignant spindle cells and a malignant epithelial component, which can be identified on microscopy or by immunocytochemistry. The epithelial malignancy may be conventional squamous cell carcinoma or may be dysplasia or carcinoma *in situ* of the overlying epithelium. In most cases, a transition can be seen between the malignant epithelium and the sarcomatoid element (Figure 4.23). However, most lesions are exophytic and ulcerated with widespread loss of surface epithelium so that a conventional epithelial component may not be seen (Figure 4.24). Overall, up to 50% of cases may be composed entirely of spindle cells with no evidence of conventional carcinoma (73,74). However, if multiple sections are examined and carefully searched, evidence of squamous carcinoma or dysplastic epithelium can be found in over 80% of cases (75). It is most reliably found at the base or the margins of the spindle cell proliferation. In most cases, the carcinoma is demarcated and does not exhibit an intermingling with the spindle cell component.

The sarcomatoid component is composed of malignant spindle cells, which are most often arranged in fascicles, but a storiform or streaming growth pattern may also be seen (Figures 4.25 and 4.26). Edema may be prominent, giving

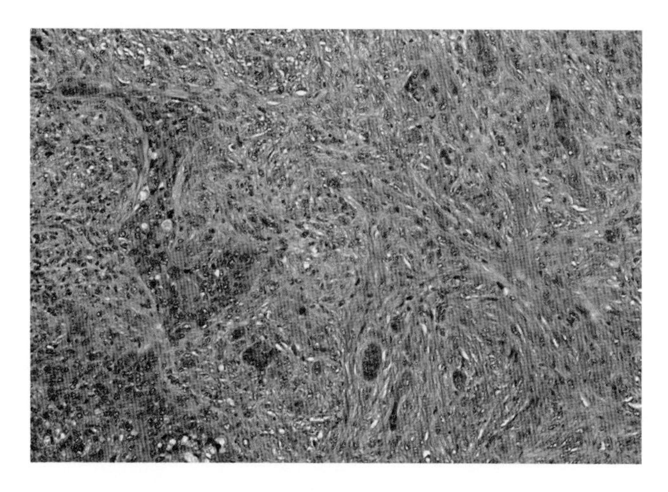

Figure 4.23 Spindle cell carcinoma usually shows areas of transition between areas of malignant epithelium and the spindle cells.

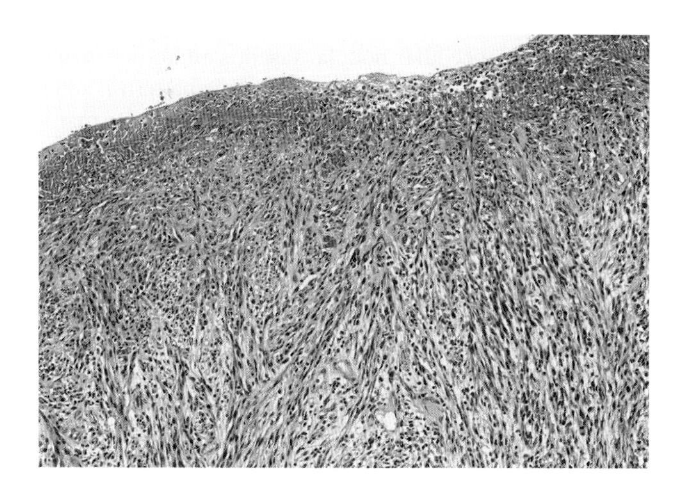

Figure 4.24 Most spindle cell carcinomas are ulcerated and the epithelial component may not be evident.

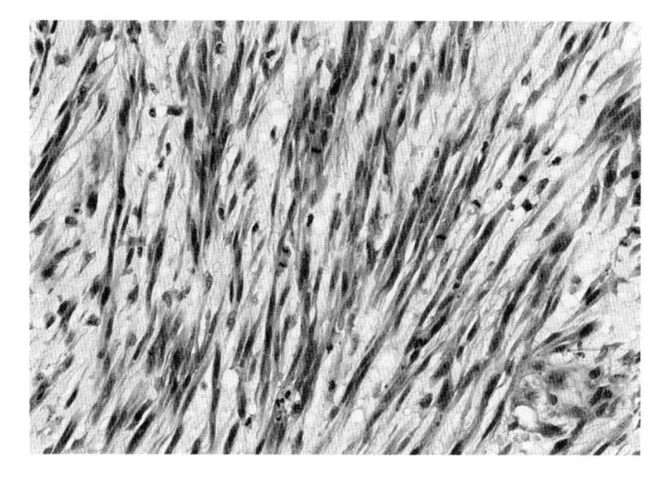

Figure 4.25 Spindle cell carcinoma. Sheets of malignant spindle cells with obvious atypia and mitotic figures.

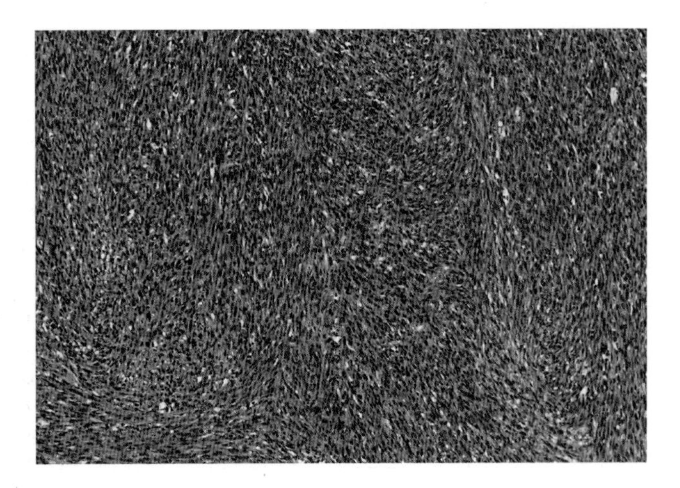

Figure 4.26 Spindle cell carcinoma with densely packed spindle cells resembling fibrosarcoma.

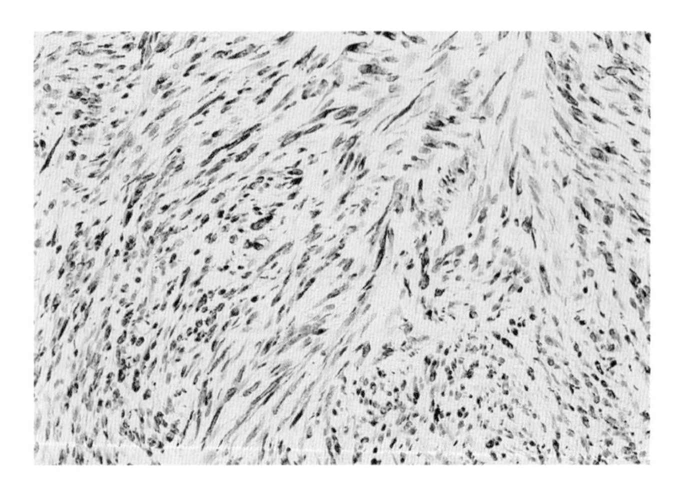

Figure 4.27 A pan-cytokeratin (AE1/AE3) may show the epithelial phenotype of the spindle cells.

the lesion a myxomatous appearance. These patterns may mimic fibrosarcoma, synovial sarcoma, leiomyosarcoma, malignant fibrous histiocytoma or even benign stromal lesions such as a cellular nodular fasciitis and other myofibroblastic proliferations (Figure 4.26). One pattern is often dominant in a given tumor, but most of the tumors manifest a combination. Cellular density and cytological atypia are variable, but most tumors are regarded as high grade or poorly differentiated (78). Multinucleated giant cells of either foreign body type or bizarre neoplastic forms are common (73,75). A very small number of lesions have been reported to show foci of metaplastic malignant mesenchymal elements in the form of osteosarcoma or chondrosarcoma (75,80). These are frequently associated with prior ionizing radiation to the site of the tumor.

Immunocytochemistry for pan-cytokeratins can help identify small areas of squamous carcinoma or may identify an epithelial phenotype in the spindle cell component. In most studies, the spindle cell component is positive for broad-spectrum cytokeratins in 50%–80% of cases (73–77,80,81), with antibody AE1/AE3 proving to be the most sensitive and useful marker (73,75,76,81) (Figure 4.27).

The spindle cells often also co-express mesenchymal markers (73–76,80,81), almost always vimentin (75), and muscle actins in about 20% (73,75,82). Viswanathan et al. (73) describe a very useful algorithm for the diagnosis of spindle cell lesions and show that a malignant epithelial component can be found either by microscopy or by immunocytochemistry in 80% of cases. It is essential to use appropriate markers to exclude other possible spindle cell neoplasms including melanoma, leiomyosarcoma, neural tumors and myofibroblastic lesions (73), including inflammatory pseudotumors (83,84).

Although uncommon in absolute terms, spindle cell carcinomas are nevertheless the most common spindle cell malignancy affecting the mucosa of the head and neck (72,75,79) and, if all markers are negative, the lesion should be diagnosed as a spindle cell carcinoma unless it can be proved otherwise (73).

An issue that still remains unresolved is whether the spindle cells that are negative for epithelial markers are always part of the spectrum of a mesenchymal transition by the carcinoma or whether they may be reactive fibroblast-like cells with a pseudosarcomatous appearance (80,85). The problem is heightened when only mesenchymal differentiation (e.g. vimentin and smooth muscle actin) is demonstrated in the spindle cells (with or without an accompanying squamous cell carcinoma). In the absence of carcinoma, a myofibroblastic tumor becomes a diagnostic consideration and, in the presence of a carcinoma, the possibility of a reactive myofibroblastic proliferation to the carcinoma cannot be completely excluded.

The behavior of a spindle cell carcinoma is biologically like that of a conventional squamous cell carcinoma. Once defined as a carcinoma, the entire lesion should be treated as an epithelial malignancy and managed by surgery as the primary mode of treatment, as with any squamous cell carcinoma of similar stage, location and size. Early-stage (T1, T2) lesions have a better overall survival, disease-free interval and local control. However, overall survival from spindle cell carcinomas is worse than conventional squamous carcinomas (86). At all sites, disease-specific survival at 5 years was about 60% for conventional squamous carcinoma compared to 40% for spindle cell lesions. Similar differences were found for oral lesions, but oropharyngeal lesions fared even worse, with corresponding figures of about 70% and 30%. In the larynx, squamous and spindle cell lesions had similar survival rates of about 45% (86). These data agree with a previous study of Batsakis et al. (79), who reviewed 154 cases and reported a lethality of 42% for all aerodigestive tract sites, but with significant differences by specific sites: 34% for laryngeal spindle cell carcinomas and 60% and 70%, respectively, for those of the oral cavity and sinonasal tract. The more favorable outlook for tumors of the larynx is attributed to their glottic location and exophytic growth, leading to earlier diagnosis and easier treatment. In general, endophytic spindle cell carcinomas have a worse prognosis. This may be related to a greater depth of invasion and its association with a higher frequency of nodal metastases. Prior radiation therapy has also been associated with a poorer prognosis (79).

Very few studies have attempted to determine the prognostic significance of the carcinoma's cytomorphology or keratin immunoreactive status. Olsen et al. (87) found the survival rate of patients with cytokeratin-negative tumors to be significantly greater than that of patients with positive staining. Ploidy analysis has shown the spindle cells to be non-diploid in most laryngeal tumors studied and their DNA profile to be similar to the co-existent squamous cell carcinoma (80). As yet, however, the number of cases is too small to judge the prognostic significance of DNA ploidy.

Table 4.9 summarizes the outcome of 59 spindle cell carcinomas of the oral cavity, studied by Ellis and Corio (88). The oral carcinomas exhibited a 2:1 male predilection and an age range at the time of diagnosis of 29–93 years (mean, 56.6 years). The neoplasms were nearly equally represented in polypoid, exophytic growth against an endophytic sessile and nodular appearance. Tumor size varied from 0.5 to 5.0 cm (mean, 2.1 cm). 45 of the 59 patients had follow-up information. Of these, 59% were dead of their disease and only 31% were alive without residual or recurrent carcinomas. The mean survival time of patients dead of disease was 1.9 years. Recurrences were noted in 12 patients and metastases in 16. The cervical lymph nodes were the most frequent site of metastasis, seen in 11 cases (24%). This is to be compared to sarcomatoid carcinomas arising in the glottis (15%), supraglottis (30%) and hypopharynx (60%). Distant spread occurred in nine patients.

While the outlook is not good for any oral spindle cell carcinoma, those of the lower lip have the best survival rate. Mortality in the Ellis and Corio (88) series was not influenced by size of tumor, gross configuration, history of prior radiation or any histomorphologic characteristic. Surgical resection, with or without neck dissection, resulted in a better survival rate than radiation alone or the combination of radiation and surgery.

Table 4.9 Spindle cell carcinoma of the oral cavity

Oral location	No. of cases	Dead of disease
Lower lip	25	10
Tongue	12	4
Alveolar ridge/ gingiva	11	3
Floor of the mouth	3	2
Maxillary antrum	2	2
Tonsillar pillar/ retromolar	2	2
Buccal mucosa	2	0
Upper lip	1	1
Hard palate	1	1

Source: Modified from Ellis GL, Corio RL. *Oral Surg Oral Med Oral Pathol* 1980;50:523–34 (88).

SQUAMOUS CELL CARCINOMA WITH GLANDULAR FEATURES

Squamous cell carcinomas of the mucous membranes may occasionally contain mucous cells or may contain entrapped ducts due to invasion of glandular tissue. Occasionally, however, carcinomas may display either a real or pseudoglandular architecture (89,90) that can lead to diagnostic difficulties, particularly in differentiating such lesions from adenocarcinoma or mucoepidermoid carcinoma arising from minor salivary glands. Of far more importance is the prognostic significance of these variants and, since most of these carcinomas occur in the skin and mucous membranes of the head and neck, this is especially pertinent to the head and neck surgeon. There are two variants of oral squamous cell carcinoma that may show glandular features. The first, *adenosquamous carcinoma*, is a specific entity, while the second, *acantholytic (adenoid) squamous cell carcinoma*, is a morphological variation of conventional squamous carcinoma. Both, however, may have prognostic significance.

Adenosquamous carcinoma

Adenosquamous carcinoma is regarded as a true variant of squamous cell carcinoma and is defined as a malignant tumor with histological features of both adenocarcinoma and squamous cell carcinoma (90). The glandular and squamous components occur in close proximity, but are generally distinct and easily discernable. Adenosquamous carcinoma is rare, but has been reported in many body sites, including gastrointestinal and genitourinary tracts as well as the upper and lower respiratory tract. It is very rare in the head and neck; in a review in 2011, only 75 cases had been recorded in the head and neck region (91). Of these, about half (48%) arose in the larynx and only 28 (30%) had been reported in the oral cavity.

In the oral cavity, the majority (more than 80%) of cases have arisen in the tongue (91,92), with the floor of the mouth being the second most common site. Other sites include the lip, tonsillar–palatine region and the alveolus (91–94). Patients have an age range from 40 to 75 years (average 57 years). Most reports have described adenosquamous carcinoma as an aggressive neoplasm with a high rate of regional or distant metastases and a poor outcome for individual patients (92–94). A review of all reported cases in 2011 (91) showed that almost 50% of cases had regional metastases at presentation and 25% had distant metastases. Kass et al. (95) have recently added a further 42 cases to the literature and were able to compare 32 cases to a matched cohort of conventional squamous cell carcinomas. They showed overall and disease-free survival for adenosquamous carcinoma to be 42% and 36%, respectively. This did not differ from the squamous cell carcinomas. It must be noted, however, that in this study the adenosquamous carcinoma patients had more aggressive therapy because of the historically poor prognosis of this lesion and, although not significantly different, the survival rates and median survival time were

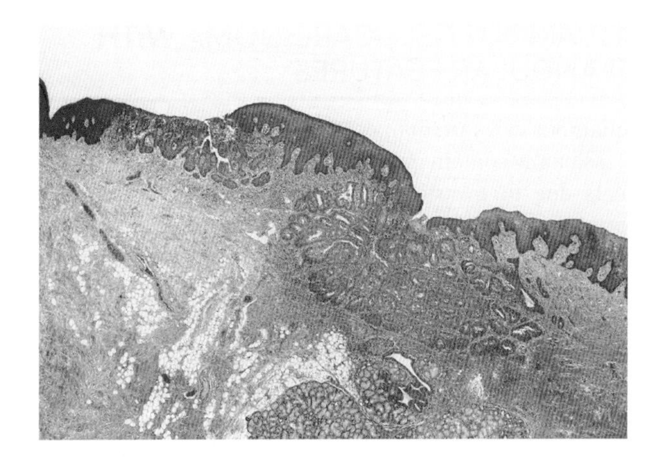

Figure 4.28 Adenosquamous carcinoma arising on the tongue. The squamous (left) and adenocarcinomatous components (right) are clearly separated by the plane of section.

worse than for squamous carcinomas (95). Previous studies have suggested determinate 5-year survival rates as low as 25% (93,94).

Adenosquamous carcinoma is histologically characterized by an association of an adenocarcinoma and a squamous cell carcinoma growing in separate or mixed patterns (Figure 4.28). In most cases, transition zones are found and the two lesions are clearly discernable. The adenocarcinoma component presents with tubular, alveolar or ductal structures that are lined by cuboidal, mucous-containing or poorly differentiated cells with evidence of mucin in the ducts (Figure 4.29). The squamous component is typical squamous cell carcinoma and, in most cases, there is evidence of an origin from the mucosal epithelium.

Mucoepidermoid carcinoma is said to be a difficult differential diagnosis. This should not be if careful attention to cytoarchitecture is followed. The growth pattern of the two neoplasms is quite different. Mucoepidermoid carcinoma rarely has readily recognizable squamous features or demonstrable keratinizing elements, except in some high-grade forms. Mucoepidermoid carcinoma also shows a characteristic admixture of epidermoid (or intermediate) cells with mucous cells, whereas in adenosquamous carcinoma, the glandular and squamous components are separate and distinct. Adenosquamous carcinoma also shows transition from the overlying oral epithelium (Figures 4.28 and 4.29), which is often dysplastic and tends to spread throughout the duct system in a vertical and horizontal fashion (89,92). A recent molecular analysis of 20 cases (95) has also shown that all cases of adenosquamous carcinoma were negative for the *CRTC-MAML* translocation. This may be a useful diagnostic test for difficult cases, but also confirms that adenosquamous carcinoma and mucoepidermoid carcinoma are distinct entities.

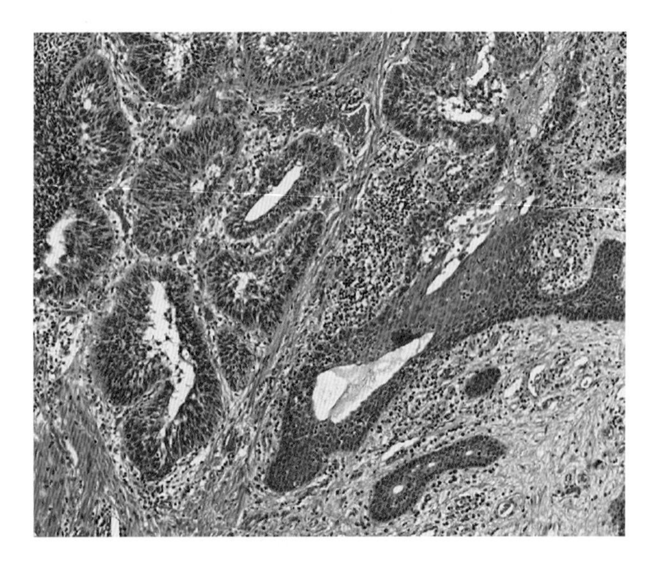

Figure 4.29 The adenocarcinoma component of adenosquamous carcinoma is associated with a salivary duct and shows malignant ductal structures.

Acantholytic (adenoid) squamous carcinoma

Acantholytic squamous cell carcinoma is a morphologic variant of squamous cell carcinoma, usually of the skin, especially of the sun-exposed areas of the head and neck (96). Rare cases have also been reported at mucosal sites, including the vermilion borders of the lips and the tongue and sites in the nasopharynx, sinonasal tract and larynx (97–100).

The histological appearance is caused by widespread acantholysis of the epithelial islands to produce a pseudoglandular appearance (Figures 4.30 and 4.31). The duct-like structures are usually found deep in the lesion and often contain acantholytic or degenerate cells and necrotic cellular debris. True ducts or glands are not seen and there is no evidence of mucin production. The squamous cell carcinoma is nearly always moderately differentiated. In the majority of these carcinomas, the adenoid feature is initiated in the basal layer of the squamous epithelium, with suprabasal clefting and acantholysis followed by a downward rather

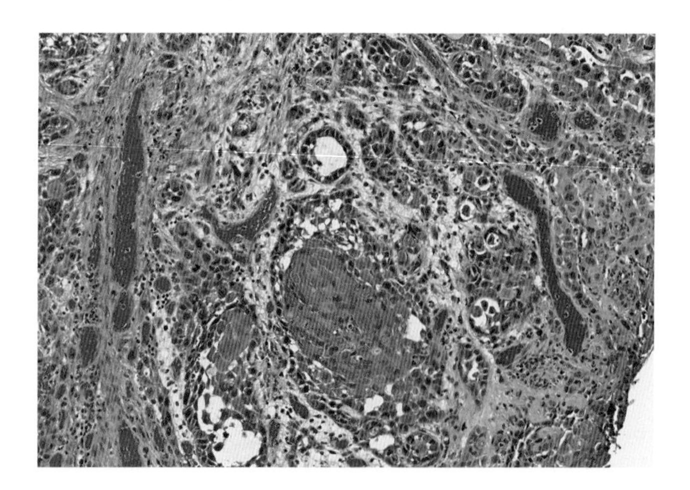

Figure 4.30 Acantholytic carcinoma is a conventional carcinoma with obvious epidermoid areas (center) and duct-like structures.

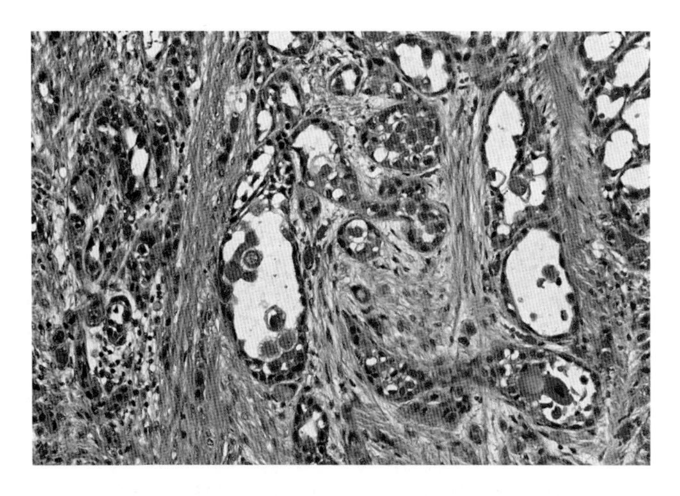

Figure 4.31 Acantholysis forms prominent duct-like structures, many of which contain degenerate acantholytic cells.

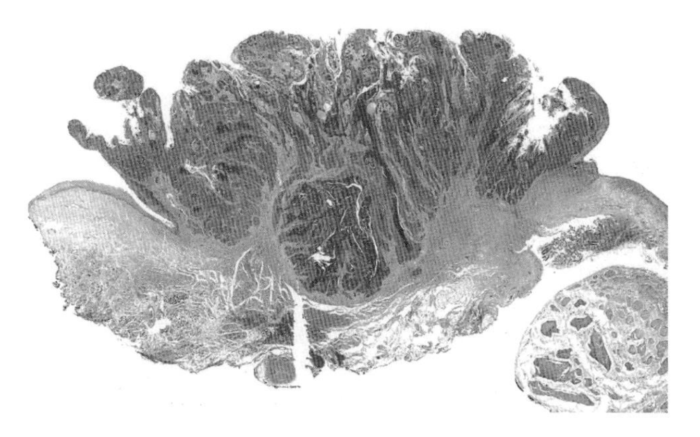

Figure 4.32 Papillary squamous cell carcinoma is characterized by a pedunculated exophytic papillary lesion, but with invasion into the underlying tissues.

than upward progression. The end result is a seemingly biphasic carcinoma (Figure 4.30).

Occasionally, the carcinoma may be less differentiated and can be clear cell or sarcomatoid in appearance. Areas of hemorrhage and anastomosing channels may give the appearance of vascular channels and may be mistaken for angiosarcoma (101,102). Immunocytochemistry for epithelial markers and stains for mucins may be helpful to establish the correct diagnosis.

A number of reports have suggested that acantholytic lesions (89,99) have a worse prognosis than conventional squamous carcinoma, but this has not been substantiated in any large series.

PAPILLARY SQUAMOUS CARCINOMA

Papillary squamous cell carcinoma is a rare variant of squamous cell carcinoma, characterized by an exophytic papillary growth pattern. It is important because it must be differentiated from common benign squamous papillomas. It is thought to have a better prognosis, but in part this may be due to early presentation and ease of removal. In the head and neck, the larynx and hypopharynx are the most common sites of involvement (about 40% of all lesions) (103,104), but the prevalence in the oral cavity and oropharynx varies between series. Mehrad et al. (103) reported 40% of lesions in the oropharynx and 14% in the oral cavity, while Russell et al. (104) found the opposite with 35% oral lesions and 14% in the oropharynx. When they do arise in the mouth, the gingivae and buccal mucosa appear to be the most common sites (105–107). Most reports show an overall male predilection with a male:female ratio of between 2:1 and 3:1 (103,104), but oral lesions may show a more equal distribution between the genders (103,106,108).

Papillary squamous cell carcinoma must be distinguished from other exophytic variants of squamous carcinoma such as verrucous carcinoma and from benign squamous papillomas (105,109). The characteristic features are of an exophytic lesion with a papillary architecture, but with clear evidence of malignancy and invasion into the deeper connective tissues (Figure 4.32). There is cytological atypia resembling severe dysplasia and mitoses and areas of necrosis may be prominent (103–107). Unlike verrucous carcinoma or lesions of proliferative verrucous leukoplakia, which have a wide base, papillary squamous carcinoma is more pedunculated and may have a well-defined papillary stalk (Figure 4.32) (106,107). Stromal invasion may be seen at the base of the lesion, but this is often not prominent.

Occasionally, the papillary processes are non-keratinized and are composed of immature basaloid cells. It has been reported that this morphological pattern is more often seen in the oropharynx (109) and a recent study has shown that about 70% are positive for p16 and almost 80% contained transcriptionally active HPV (103). HPV positivity was found in 66% of oral lesions. This suggests that oropharyngeal lesions, and especially those with a basaloid morphology, may be associated with HPV infection. The role of HPV in oral lesions is less certain; in a study by Mehrad et al. (103), fewer oral lesions were HPV positive, but Argyris et al. (108) showed that all oral lesions were negative for HPV by polymerase chain reaction (PCR), even though 56% were p16 positive.

Little is known about the biologic course of papillary squamous carcinoma of the oral cavity. Mehrad et al. (103) followed 48 cases for a mean of 32.5 months and showed that 33% of patients overall developed lymph node metastases. Two lesions (29%) from the oral cavity metastasized, but the oropharynx showed the highest rate of metastases at 61%. Overall and disease-specific survival (about 52% and 80%, respectively) did not differ from conventional squamous cell carcinoma. They also found that HPV-associated lesions (p16 positive) were more likely to be found in the oropharynx and had a slightly better prognosis.

LYMPHOEPITHELIAL CARCINOMA

Lymphoepithelial carcinoma is an undifferentiated carcinoma with a prominent lymphoplasmacytic infiltrate that is identical to nasopharyngeal carcinoma (110). A number of terms are still used for this lesion, including: undifferentiated or non-keratinizing carcinoma of nasopharyngeal type; undifferentiated carcinoma with lymphoid stroma; lymphoepithelioma; and lymphoepithelial-like carcinoma. While morphologically similar, the non-nasopharyngeal lymphoepithelial carcinoma of the upper aerodigestive tract is not associated with Epstein–Barr virus (EBV) infection (111–113).

Lymphoepithelial carcinoma most commonly arises in the larynx and hypopharynx and in the major salivary glands. Oral lesions are rare, but when encountered may be found in the tongue, soft palate or floor of the mouth (114). Lesions may also be found in the oropharynx, including the base of the tongue and tonsils, where they are associated with HPV infection (115) and represent a variant of non-keratinizing HPV-associated oropharyngeal carcinoma.

The gross appearance of the carcinoma varies from deeply ulcerated to primarily submucosal masses. Microscopically, the carcinoma is composed, either partially or totally, of undifferentiated epithelial cells with large, round, vesicular, sometimes clear nuclei (Figure 4.33). Each nucleus usually has a single large, basophilic to deep red nucleolus. Cell cytoplasm is poorly defined, therefore often imparting a syncytial growth pattern to the neoplasm. The stroma is composed of small, mature lymphoid cells and occasionally plasma cells that surround and extend into the syncytial aggregates. Focal areas of squamous differentiation with keratin formation may occasionally be seen.

Because lymphoepithelial carcinomas are rare and studies have all been retrospective and deal with different sites of involvement, it is not possible to compare, stage for stage, the prognosis of lymphoepithelial carcinomas with conventional squamous cell carcinoma. Also, recent awareness of the role of HPV in some of these lesions means that further studies are needed to determine the prognosis of lesions with differing etiologies. It does appear, however, that the carcinoma is more aggressive with a greater tendency for cervical lymph node involvement and, perhaps, also for distant metastases (111,113,114). It has been suggested that HPV-associated lesions may have a better prognosis than HPV-negative lesions (114,116).

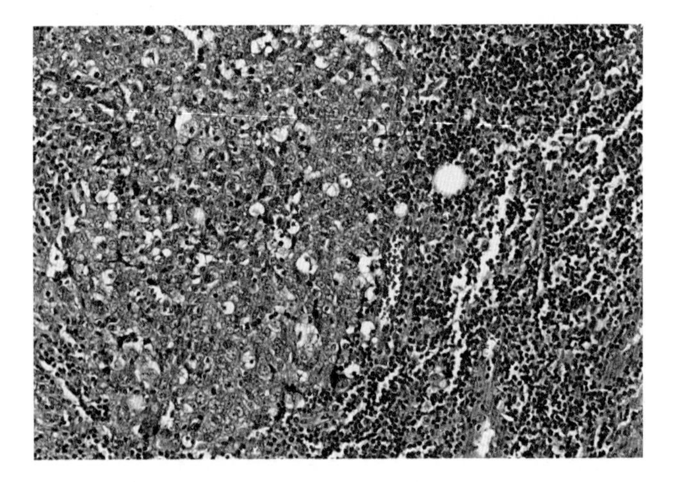

Figure 4.33 Lymphoepithelial carcinoma comprises undifferentiated epithelial cells in a stroma of mature lymphoid cells.

SQUAMOUS CELL CARCINOMA OF THE OROPHARYNX

The rationale for considering oropharyngeal lesions as a separate entity is now well established, as are the association with HPV as a causative agent and the distinctive biological and histological features. These lesions arise primarily in those areas of the oropharyngeal mucosa where tonsillar tissue is present. Essentially, this is represented by Waldeyer's ring, which comprises the palatine tonsils of the fauces and the tonsillar tissue of the base of the tongue. There is also tonsillar tissue in the nasopharynx and associated with the Eustachian tubes, but these areas are rarely affected by HPV-associated carcinomas. Oropharyngeal squamous cell carcinomas are characterized by being non-keratinized with a basaloid morphology (60). Previously, this has been regarded as an indication that they are poorly differentiated, but it is now appreciated that this characteristic morphology actually recapitulates the non-keratinizing tonsillar crypt epithelium from which the tumors arise. In contradistinction to conventional squamous cell carcinoma, this lack of keratinization appears to represent a well-differentiated morphology (61). The Broders type of grading scheme described above cannot be used for these lesions and pathologists should not attempt to grade HPV-associated carcinomas.

Apart from site and characteristic clinical and histological features, oropharyngeal lesions are defined by the presence of high-risk HPV. They thus contain active E6 and E7 proteins, which bind and degrade p53 and Rb, respectively. Degradation of Rb is particularly important because it results in accumulation and overexpression of the tumor suppressor protein, p16. Immunohistochemical expression of p16 protein is therefore an excellent surrogate marker for HPV infection and can be used in routine clinical practice as a diagnostic marker. Conventional squamous cell carcinomas of the oral cavity are not associated with HPV and are usually p16 negative by immunohistochemistry.

The gold standard for the diagnosis of HPV-associated oropharyngeal carcinomas is demonstration of transcriptionally active, high-risk HPV (primarily HPV-16) (117). The most sensitive test for this is reverse transcription PCR (RT-PCR), but DNA *in situ* hybridization (ISH) can be used and commercial probes are available for generic HPV DNA, as well as for the most common subtypes (118). ISH for E6/E7 mRNA has also been shown to be a valuable method for use on routine paraffin-embedded sections. Using a commercially available kit for RNA detection, Schache et al. (118) showed that ISH for high-risk HPV mRNA had a sensitivity of 97% and a specificity of 93% against the gold standard of

RT-PCR. This was better than for DNA detection methods. A variety of antibodies to HPV proteins, including E6 and E7, are also available for immunohistochemistry, ELISA or Western blotting, but in general these are much less specific or sensitive.

In practice, however, these molecular techniques may not be available to all pathologists or may be expensive. HPV positivity is associated with aberrant increased expression of p16 and immunohistochemistry for p16 has been shown to be a valuable surrogate marker for the presence of transcriptionally active HPV, with sensitivity and specificity rates of about 97% and 83%, respectively (117–119). However, results of p16 staining must be interpreted with care and only in the context of the clinical findings. Normal tonsillar crypt epithelium may express low levels of p16 (116) and small numbers of conventional squamous cell carcinomas may express p16 in the absence of any evidence of HPV infection. For example, Begum et al. (120) found that although 82% of HPV-positive tumors expressed p16, expression was also found in 7% (9/131) of HPV-negative, non-oropharyngeal lesions. Harris et al. (121) showed p16 expression in 11 of 25 (44%) tongue cancers from young patients, only two of which were positive for HPV. They also found that p16 was an independent predictor of good prognosis. These findings have been confirmed in a number of studies. Chung et al. (122) also showed that p16 expression may be independent of HPV positivity, but confirmed patients with p16-positive oropharyngeal tumors had better overall survival than those who were p16 negative. Zafereo et al. (123) prospectively analyzed 460 cases of oral cavity squamous cell carcinoma, taking particular care to only include oral lesions and exclude any lesions that may encroach on the oropharynx. They found that of 210 cases tested, 30% were p16 positive, but they were only able to confirm an association with HPV in 3.9% of cases. In this study, neither p16 nor HPV status was associated with survival. In a study of 409 cases of oral cavity lesions, Lingen et al. (124) applied strict criteria for p16 positivity (125) (see below) and found that only 11.2% were positive, but only 5.9% were associated with HPV infection. They also suggested that p16 has poor positive predictive value for HPV status and therefore should not be relied upon as a surrogate marker in oral lesions.

p16 may be expressed in the nucleus and/or in the cytoplasm and the intensity of expression is variable. The criteria for positive staining associated with HPV are that there should be strong, diffuse nuclear and cytoplasmic staining in over 70% of tumor cells (117–119,126). Based on these criteria, Jordan et al. (125) proposed a scoring system for p16 immunohistochemistry for use in clinical trials.

Until now, therefore, this group of tumors has been defined by the clinical site and the presence of HPV or p16 positivity, but the basaloid, non-keratinizing phenotype has led to them being regarded as "poorly differentiated" and similar to basaloid variants of conventional squamous cell carcinoma (33). This has led to confusion and possibly also to inappropriate management. A careful re-evaluation of the characteristic morphological features of these lesions has resulted in a proposed terminology and classification scheme for oropharyngeal squamous cell carcinomas that can be used by pathologists (61,127–130) and has been adopted in the latest WHO classification (131). The word "basaloid" should be avoided as a diagnostic term and lesions should be referred to as HPV-associated squamous cell carcinomas of oropharyngeal type (131). Three types or patterns of oropharyngeal carcinoma have been described and are summarized in Table 4.10 (128–131).

Non-keratinizing squamous cell carcinoma. This type would be regarded as the archetypical HPV-associated oropharyngeal squamous cell carcinoma (131). They are composed of sheets or islands of basaloid or spindled epithelial cells with pale hematoxyphilic ("blue") cytoplasm. Cell borders are poorly defined and desmosomes are not evident. The nuclei are hyperchromatic and mitotic activity is prominent (Figure 4.34). Areas of comedo-like necrosis are common. Although non-keratinizing, areas of obvious epidermoid or squamous cells may be seen and occasional keratin pearls may be evident, but these should comprise less than 10% of the tumor (129) (Figure 4.35). Stromal desmoplasia is not evident and there may be prominent inflammatory change, sometimes giving an appearance similar to lymphoepithelial carcinoma (61,115). Virtually all of these

Table 4.10 Key features of the three types of oropharyngeal squamous cell carcinoma

Histological type	Frequency[a]	Features	p16 positivity	HPV positivity
Non-keratinizing	52%	Sheets of basaloid or spindle "blue" cells. Comedo necrosis. Mitoses. Squamous areas <10%	99%	100%
Hybrid	11%	Non-keratinizing carcinoma with 10% or more showing squamous differentiation with keratin	92%	83%
Keratinizing	26%	Islands of squamous cells. Desmosomes obvious. Keratin variable from isolated cells to keratin pearls. May be poorly to well-differentiated	23%	9%

Source: Adapted from Chernock RD. *Head Neck Pathol* 2012;6(Suppl 1):S41–7 (128); Lewis JS Jr et al. *Histopathology* 2012;60(3): 427–36 (129). Data also from Gondim DD et al. *Am J Surg Pathol* 2016; 40:1117–24 (130).

[a] Approximately 10% of oropharyngeal lesions were of variant morphology.

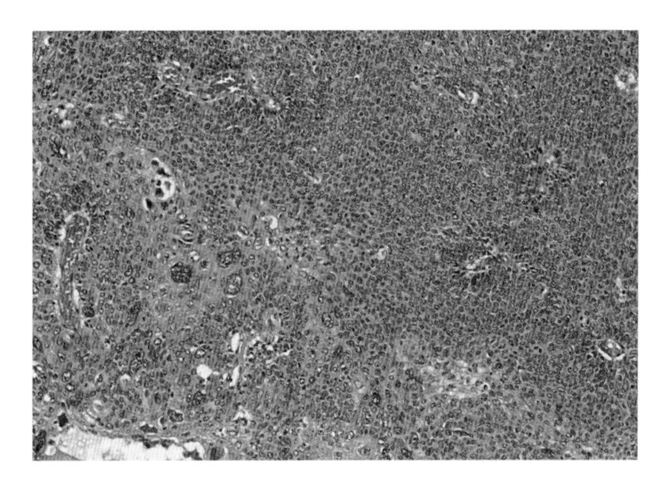

Figure 4.34 HPV-associated carcinoma. The lesion is non-keratinizing with sheets of pale basaloid cells with focal areas of prominent atypia.

lesions (99%) are positive for p16 (129,130) and 100% were positive for HPV by RT-PCR (130) (Table 4.10, Figure 4.36).

This type of HPV-associated oropharyngeal carcinoma must be distinguished from basaloid variants of conventional squamous cell carcinoma (see above) (60,61,129). Basaloid squamous cell carcinoma may arise at any site in the head and neck, but does have a predilection for the oropharynx and base of the tongue, as well as the larynx and hypopharynx. They are not associated with HPV and are regarded as poorly differentiated, aggressive lesions with a poor prognosis. Although differences may be subtle, basaloid carcinomas can be distinguished from HPV-associated non-keratinizing carcinomas based on morphology and, if necessary, p16 staining. Basaloid carcinomas more often have a lobular architecture with molding of the islands into a "jigsaw" pattern and a hyalinized stroma. Cystic areas may be noted and it is often also possible to identify an origin from the overlying dysplastic epithelium or an association with a conventional squamous carcinoma (Figures 4.16 and 4.22) (59).

Keratinizing squamous cell carcinoma. This type of lesion may arise in the oropharynx and the overall histology is similar to conventional oral squamous cell carcinoma. Tumor islands may be irregular or angular, but are well defined and are composed of polygonal epithelial cells with eosinophilic cytoplasm and easily identifiable intercellular bridges (desmosomes). Nuclei may be pale with open chromatin and prominent or multiple nucleoli. Keratin formation is variable, but may be prominent with formation of keratin pearls or may be minimal, but intracellular keratinization is usually clearly evident (Figure 4.37). The stroma is collagenous or desmoplastic and inflammatory changes need not be prominent. This type of oropharyngeal carcinoma may be graded in a similar manner to conventional squamous cell carcinoma as poorly to well differentiated based on the extent of keratinization. Only about 25% of these lesions were positive for p16 and less than 10% contain HPV (129,130) (Table 4.10).

Hybrid lesions (non-keratinizing squamous cell carcinoma with maturation). As the name suggests, this type

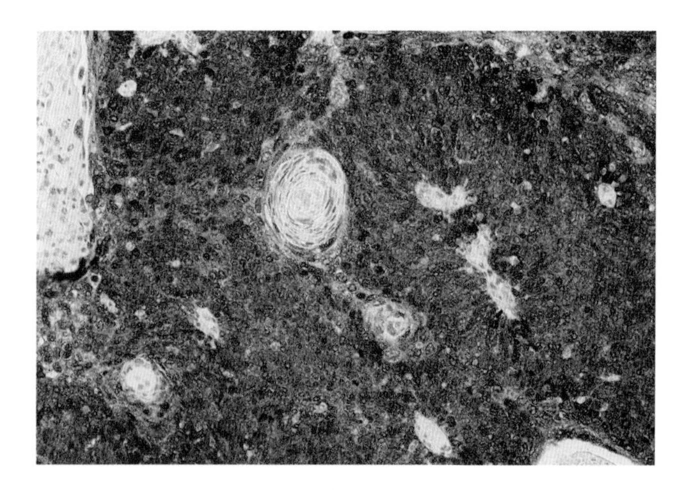

Figure 4.36 Immunohistochemistry of HPV-associated lesions shows positive staining for p16. True-positive lesions show diffuse staining in nuclei and cytoplasm in over 70% of the cells. In this field there is a small, negative keratin pearl.

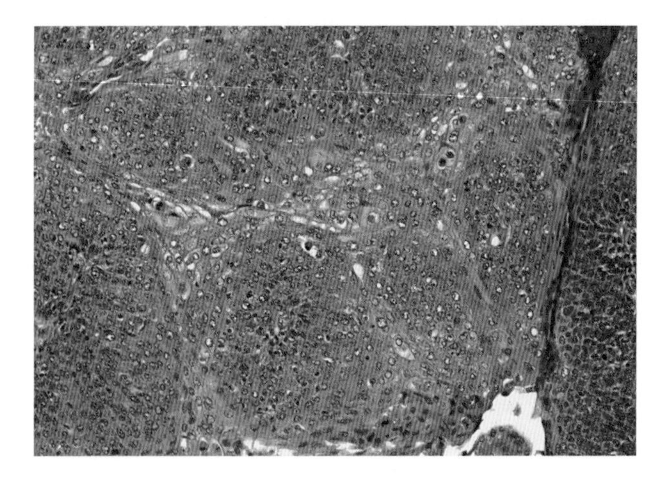

Figure 4.35 Small focal areas of keratinization may be seen, even in non-keratinizing HPV-associated lesions.

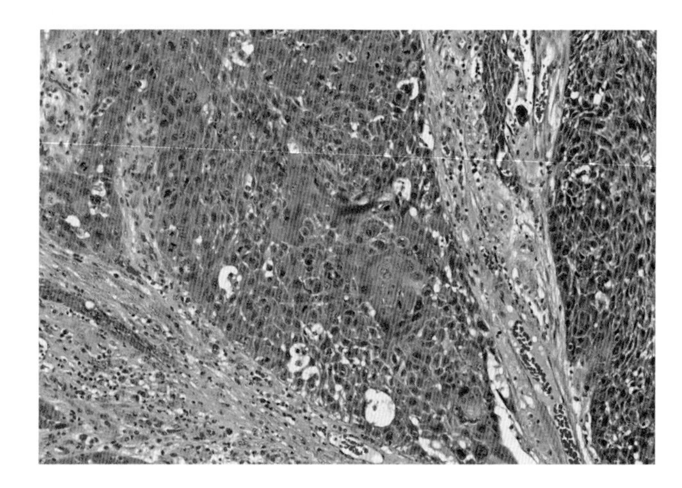

Figure 4.37 HPV-associated keratinizing carcinoma shows features similar to a conventional moderately differentiated squamous cell carcinoma.

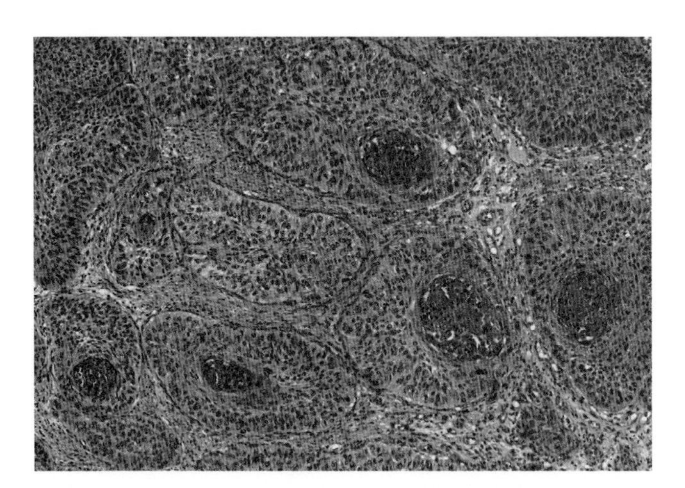

Figure 4.38 A hybrid HPV lesion. Islands of basaloid cells contain areas of maturation with squamous differentiation and keratin formation.

shows features of the non-keratinizing type, but also has areas of squamous differentiation with keratin production (Figure 4.38). In this case, the "mature" or squamous component may comprise greater than 10% of the lesion (122,123). Almost all lesions (90%–95%) of this type are positive for p16 and most (83%) contained HPV (129,130) (Table 4.10).

At the present time, the prognostic significance of these variants is uncertain and it has been unclear how this terminology should be used in diagnostic reporting. The WHO now suggest that the most appropriate terminology for HPV-positive lesions should be "HPV-associated squamous cell carcinoma" (131). However, this should only be used when the HPV status has been confirmed. In the context of a lesion from the oropharyngeal region, the WHO suggest that p16 expression is a satisfactory surrogate for confirmation of HPV association. Care must be taken in interpretation of the staining and only those lesions with strong diffuse expression in the nuclei and cytoplasm and in 70% or more of the cells should be regarded as positive (Figure 4.36) (117–119,125). In other situations, including oral cavity lesions, HPV association must be confirmed by ISH or PCR.

Immunohistochemistry is useful for the identification of small areas of tumor in tonsillar biopsies (Figure 4.39) and may also help identify the source of metastatic lesions in cervical lymph nodes with occult primary lesions. Metastatic lesions of HPV-associated carcinomas are often cystic in nature (Figure 4.40) and strong positive staining for p16 (Figure 4.41) is strongly suggestive of an origin from a primary lesion in the oropharynx.

HISTOPATHOLOGIC VARIANTS OF HPV-ASSOCIATED OROPHARYNGEAL CARCINOMA

The vast majority of HPV-associated carcinomas in the head and neck are found in the oropharynx. Over 90% are one

(a)

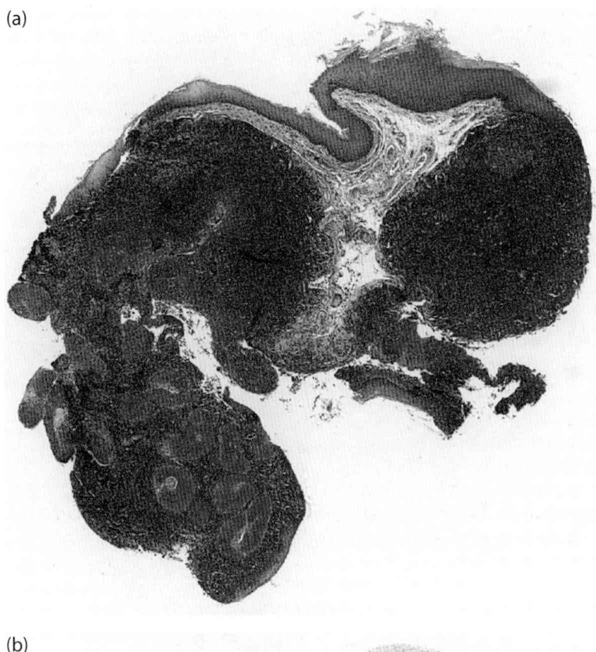

(b)

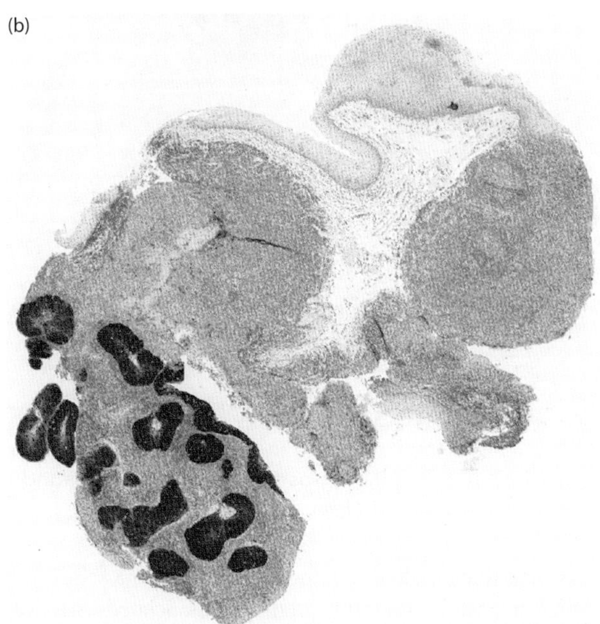

Figure 4.39 **(a)** A small tonsil biopsy contains small islands of malignant epithelial cells (bottom left). **(b)** The carcinoma is strongly positive for p16. Note pale, focal staining in the normal crypt epithelium.

of the three types shown in Table 4.10 and about 55% are non-keratinizing (128–131). However, about 10% of HPV-associated oropharyngeal lesions may be another morphological variant (130) and HPV is increasingly being reported in a variety of oral and other non-oropharyngeal lesions (59,60,103,115,123,130,132). The common variants are summarized in Table 4.11.

Basaloid squamous cell carcinoma may be encountered at any site in the head and neck region. As described above, basaloid variants of squamous cell carcinoma should be distinguished from HPV-associated non-keratinizing carcinomas. Apart from histological differences, the key defining

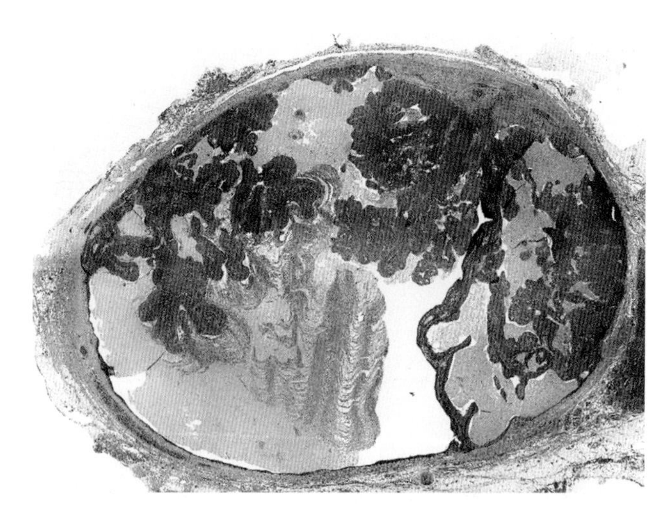

Figure 4.40 A metastatic carcinoma in a cervical node has a prominent cystic morphology.

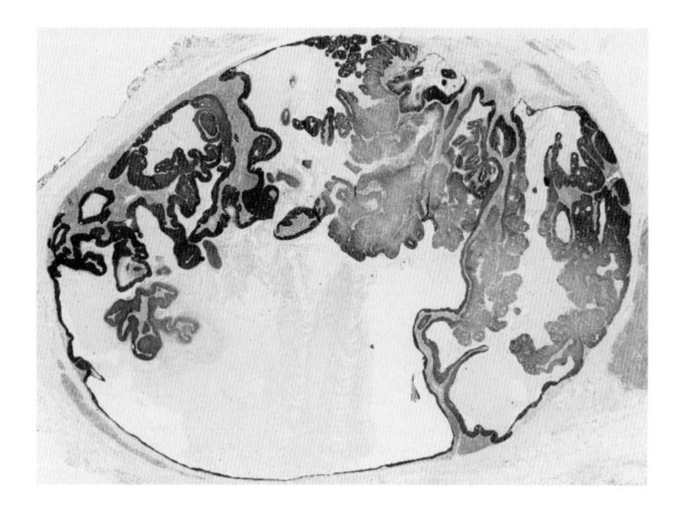

Figure 4.41 p16 staining is positive, strongly suggesting an origin from a primary lesion in the oropharynx.

criterion is that basaloid squamous cell carcinoma arises from surface mucosal epithelium and may be associated with overlying dysplastic epithelium or with conventional squamous cell carcinoma (58,132). Nevertheless, it has been shown that basaloid squamous cell carcinomas that arise in the oropharynx may be HPV positive in up to 75% of cases and that this may be associated with a better prognosis (59,132). Chernock et al. (59) showed that 75% (9/12) of basaloid squamous cell carcinomas in the oropharynx were positive for HPV by ISH compared to 0% of 16 lesions from non-oropharyngeal sites. In a study by Begum and Westra (132), HPV-16 was detected (by ISH) in 16 of 21 (76%) basaloid squamous cell carcinomas of the oropharynx compared to only 2 of 32 (6%) lesions from non-oropharyngeal sites. Both studies showed better overall survival in HPV-positive lesions.

Papillary squamous cell carcinoma is an unusual variant of squamous cell carcinoma with an exophytic papillary surface pattern. The most common sites are the larynx and hypopharynx, but lesions may also arise in the oropharynx and (more rarely) in the oral cavity. Mehrad et al. (103) showed that 54% of papillary squamous cell carcinomas overall may be HPV positive, but that oropharyngeal lesions had the highest prevalence, with 68% and 78% of lesions being positive for p16 or HPV (by ISH), respectively.

Lymphoepithelial carcinoma is an undifferentiated carcinoma that is most often encountered in the nasopharynx, where it may be associated with EBV infection. Morphologically similar lesions, however, may be encountered in the oropharynx (110–114). At this site, Singhi et al. (115) showed that lesions were positive for p16 (100%; 22/22) and 86% showed HPV by ISH. All lesions were negative for EBV.

Adenosquamous carcinoma is most common in the larynx and is rare in the oral cavity and oropharynx. In a study of 18 cases, Masand et al. (91) found that three cases (16%) were positive for p16 and for HPV by ISH. Two cases (2/3; 33%) were from the oropharynx and one from the nasal cavity (1/3).

Other variants that may be associated with HPV include *small cell neuroendocrine carcinoma* and *spindle cell carcinoma*. Two studies (133,134) have reported HPV-associated neuroendocrine carcinomas in the oropharynx. Unlike typical non-keratinizing HPV-associated lesions, these neuroendocrine lesions had an aggressive course and a poor prognosis. El-Mofty (58) noted that this was similar to HPV-positive small cell neuroendocrine carcinomas of the cervix, which are also aggressive with a high incidence of distant metastases and a poor outcome. Spindle cell carcinomas have been shown to be positive for HPV in less than 10% of cases (135).

Table 4.11 Histological variants found in the oropharynx that may be HPV positive

Histological type	Frequency[a] (n = 435)	Features	p16 positivity[b]	HPV positivity[b]
Basaloid	3.4%	Basaloid variant of conventional squamous cell carcinoma	87%	75%
Papillary	3.2%	Exophytic, papillary squamous cell carcinoma. Most common in the larynx	68%	78%
Lymphoepithelial	2.3%	Undifferentiated carcinoma, nasopharyngeal-like. EBV negative	100%	86%
Adenosquamous	0.7%	Mixed adeno- and squamous carcinoma	33%	33%

[a] Data from Reference 130 (n = 435).
[b] Data from References 60,91,103,115,130 (see text for details).

It is likely that as further studies are undertaken, HPV will be found in a greater range of lesions. However, it should be noted that the clinical significance of HPV positivity is still uncertain. In oropharyngeal lesions, there is good evidence that patients with HPV-positive lesions have a better prognosis and that treatment can be de-escalated (136), whereas at non-oropharyngeal sites, HPV may have no significance or may be associated with more aggressive lesions (137). Clinical trials are still ongoing (136) and there is still much important research to be undertaken. It has recently been reported, for example, that there are geographic variations in HPV-associated oropharyngeal lesions, with a greater prevalence of HPV positivity in Western Europe compared to Eastern Europe or Asia (138).

HISTOPATHOLOGIC PROGNOSTIC FACTORS

Over the years, surgical pathologists and clinicians have sought reliable and reproducible histopathologic factors with possible prognostic implications. The goal has been to find factors that will allow the pathologist to predict metastasis or recurrence and thus assist the clinician in staging lesions and planning appropriate management. Much work has also been done on biomarkers and molecular changes, but with the exception of HPV testing discussed previously, few have found their way into routine clinical practice (139). Histopathologic assessment of routinely processed tissue samples remains the standard for diagnostic reporting. In recent years, national guidelines have been developed to provide standardized protocols or minimum datasets for pathology reporting (140,141). Standard criteria for tumor staging (TNM) are also published by the International Union Against Cancer (UICC) (142) and the American Joint Committee on Cancer (143,144). In most countries, the minimum standard of care also includes multidisciplinary meetings or tumor boards to discuss all aspects of a patient's disease and plan appropriate management. As a minimum, the U.K. and U.S. guidelines (140,141) require the pathologist to record the histopathologic parameters listed in Table 4.12, each of which is thought to have some prognostic value. This section will provide an overview of the most important factors.

Table 4.12 Histopathologic parameters of the primary tumor with potential prognostic significance

Parameter
Type of carcinoma
Histologic grade (differentiation)
Pattern of invasion
Tumor size (diameter of the tumor [pT])
Tumor thickness or depth of invasion
Distance to surgical margins
Perineural invasion
Bone invasion
Lymphatic/vascular invasion

Of these histologic features, Woolgar and co-workers have found that the two with most value in predicting metastasis were the pattern of invasion and degree of keratinization (38,39,145,146). Both are easily observed, readily reproduced by different observers and, for pattern of invasion, show a correlation with *in vitro* markers of malignancy such as loss of contact inhibition, tumor cell mobility and secretion of proteolytic enzymes. There is, in addition, a positive correlation between pattern of invasion and the presence of both vascular and perineural invasion.

HISTOLOGIC GRADING

Histologic grading and point scoring criteria of oral squamous cell carcinoma have been described above (Table 4.6). There is good evidence that the conventional three-point grading scheme shows a significant correlation to survival. Rogers et al. (146) showed that 5-year disease-specific survival rates were 89%, 68% and 45% for well, moderately and poorly differentiated tumors, respectively. However, grading is subjective and the majority of cases are moderately differentiated. This means that the system lacks discriminatory power for prediction of prognosis for individual patients (145).

PATTERN OF INVASION

Of all the parameters used, Woolgar and Scott (39) and Odell et al. (32) have suggested that pattern of invasion is the most important. This was also highlighted as an important factor in the invasive front point scoring schemes developed by Anneroth and Bryne and colleagues (34–37) (Table 4.6). Four patterns of invasion have been described (32–37), which overall depend on the degree of cellular discohesion. This may vary throughout any individual tumor, but the score is recorded from the worst area at the advancing front of the lesion.

Type I pattern shows cohesive cells with a pushing invasive front composed of broad, bulbous rete pegs that tend to infiltrate to the same level. The base of the tumor is therefore well defined and expansive (Figure 4.42). This pattern is typically seen in verrucous carcinoma (Figures 4.15 and 4.16). The *type II pattern* shows infiltrating cords, bands or strands of epithelium (Figure 4.43) that tend to be continuous with the main tumor mass, but penetrate at different levels and permeate through collagen and muscle fibers. In the *type III pattern*, there is discohesion with small islands and cords of cells separating from the main tumor and infiltrating through the adjacent tissues (Figure 4.44). These islands tend to contain fewer than 15 cells (32,37). The *type IV pattern* is the worst and is characterized by marked discohesion with small islands and single cells that infiltrate widely (Figure 4.45). In tumors showing patterns III and IV, it is often possible to find islands or individual cells as separate satellites of tumor at some distance from the main advancing front.

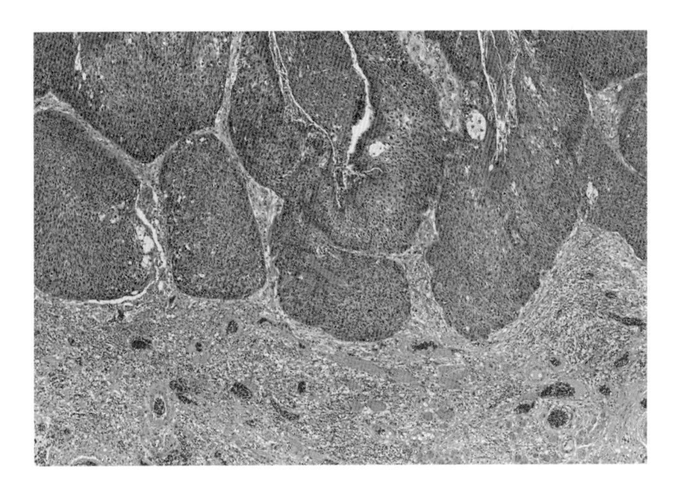

Figure 4.42 Type I pattern of invasion shows cohesive islands of tumor "pushing" into the connective tissues.

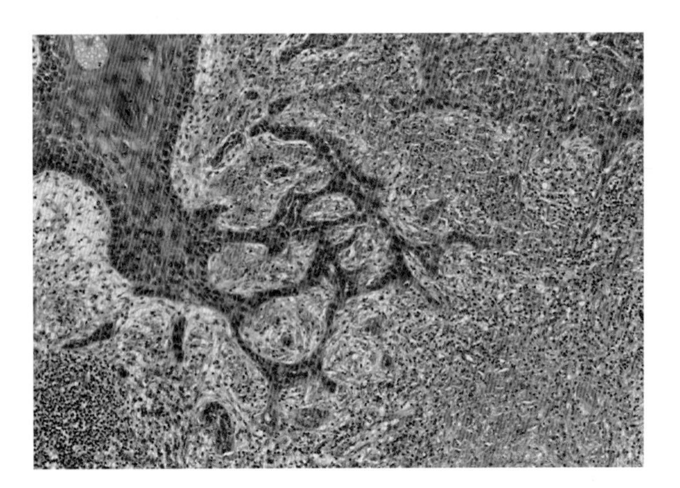

Figure 4.43 Type II pattern of invasion shows fine branching cords of tumor forming a reticular pattern.

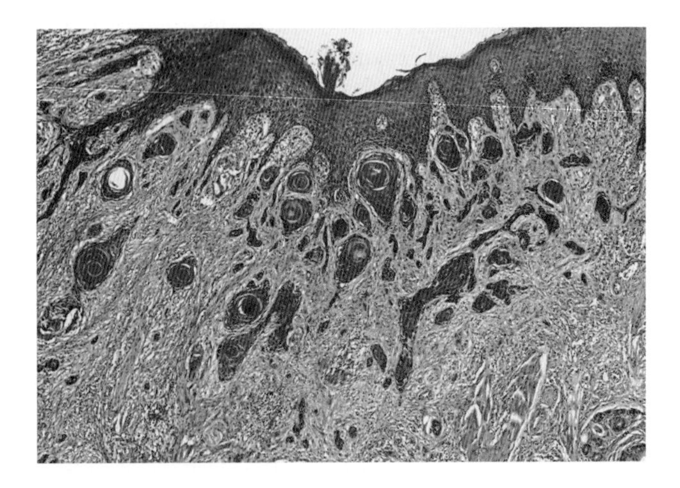

Figure 4.44 Type III pattern of invasion is discohesive with fine strands and small islands of tumor.

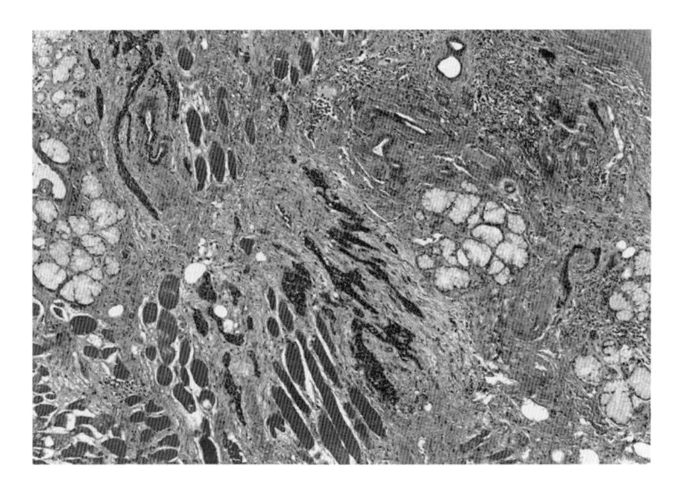

Figure 4.45 Type IV pattern of invasion is characterized by small islands and single cells infiltrating widely through the connective tissues, here involving the muscle and salivary gland.

Studies using the multifactorial scoring system (Table 4.6), which utilizes pattern of invasion, have consistently shown it to have good prognostic value (33,35–39), especially for prediction of lymph node metastases (146). In most studies, the pattern of invasion has been shown to be the most significant parameter (28,35,141). For example, Odell et al. (32) studied 47 carcinomas of the mobile tongue and showed that both grading and invasive front scoring correlated with recurrence and metastases. However, the pattern of invasion at the invasive front was the most useful factor and had the closest correlation with both recurrence and metastasis. They showed that 14 of 19 (74%) carcinomas with a discohesive pattern (patterns III and IV) metastasized compared to only 4 of 25 (16%) with patterns I and II. It has been suggested that for prognostic purposes, in everyday clinical practice, tumors can be graded simply into two patterns: cohesive (patterns I and II) or non-cohesive (patterns III and IV) (140,141,147).

TUMOR SIZE (DIAMETER) AND STAGING

The maximum diameter of the tumor contributes to the TNM classification (142,143), which is widely used to stage tumors and inform management. The maximum diameter of the tumor should be measured macroscopically and is best done on a slice through the tumor, since the widest element may be deep to the surface (140,145). The histologic size of the lesion is used to determine the pT value for final staging, and it is well established that TNM staging correlates with overall survival. It has also been shown that the size of a tumor significantly affects the ability of the surgeon to obtain tumor-free margins (38,148,149) and therefore pT stage significantly correlates with recurrence, metastases and survival. In the previous (seventh edition) staging schemes, squamous carcinomas from the oral cavity and oropharynx were treated as the same. However, there is good evidence than HPV-associated lesions have a better prognosis and in the new eighth editions (142–144), a new staging scheme for HPV-associated oropharyngeal carcinoma has been introduced that is similar to that used in the nasopharynx (150,151). This new scheme takes account of the fact that patients with HPV-associated lesions often present with more advanced disease, but have better survival. In the new scheme, p16-positive and p16-negative tumors are staged differently. Small (T1, T2) p16-positive tumors with a 6 cm or less unilateral metastasis are stage I, whereas a p16-negative lesion would be stage III. Similarly, if p16 positive, only patients with distant metastases (M1) are allocated to stage IV, and even advanced pT4 lesions are stage III (142–144).

DEPTH OF INVASION AND TUMOR THICKNESS

Many studies have identified tumor thickness or depth of invasion as an important prognostic indicator, especially as a predictor of regional metastasis, and it is felt that this may be more important than diameter (38,152–157). There is much controversy in the literature regarding the meaning of depth or thickness and different studies have used different measurements. A clear distinction needs to be made between depth of invasion (neoplastic penetration) and tumor thickness. Depth means the extent of growth into tissues beneath an epithelial surface, whereas thickness measures the full thickness of the tumor. This can be best illustrated using verrucous carcinoma as an example (Figure 4.46).

In the U.K., the Royal College of Pathologists (140) recommends measuring depth of invasion by extrapolating an imaginary line across the tumor from the adjacent normal epithelium. The depth is measured perpendicularly from this line to the deepest point of the tumor cells. Measured in this way, depth of invasion allows for the fact that some tumors may be exophytic and others may be ulcerated or endophytic. This is not the same as tumor thickness, which will be larger than depth of invasion in exophytic tumors and smaller in ulcerated tumors (Figure 4.46).

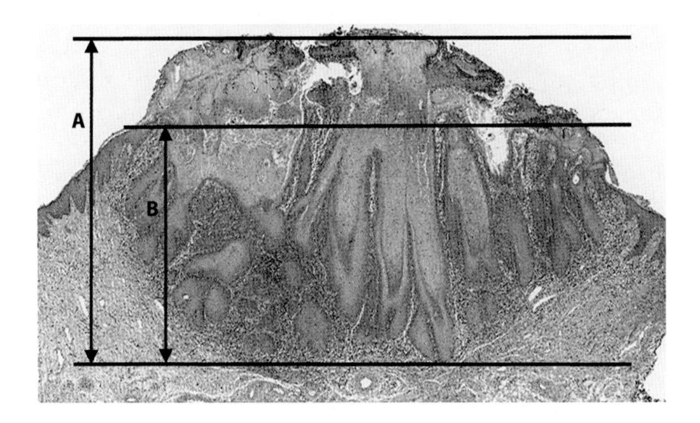

Figure 4.46 A verrucous carcinoma is both exophytic and endophytic. In this example, arrow A represents the thickness of the lesion, which is greater than arrow B, which is the depth of invasion measured from the adjacent normal epithelium.

Depth of invasion has been shown to have significant prognostic value in predicting lymph node metastases and survival (38,152,153), but the actual cut-off value is debated. O-charoenrat et al. (153) measured from the surface of adjacent epithelium and showed that a cut-off of 5 mm had predictive value and recommended an elective neck dissection for T1 and T2 tongue tumors if they were deeper than 5 mm. In a similar study on tongue lesions, Gonzales-Moles et al. (152) recommended a cut-off of 3 mm and showed that patients with thin lesions (3 mm or less) had a 5-year survival rate of 86% compared to 58% or less for lesions 4 mm or greater. However, in this study, they measured depth from a line joining adjacent normal basement membrane.

Ambrosch et al. (158) used depth of invasion as a potential indicator of micrometastasis and found that the depth was the only significant risk factor for metastasis. Logistic regression analysis revealed a depth of invasion of 4 mm as the most valuable cut-off point. The risk of metastasizing in oral, oropharyngeal and hypopharyngeal tumors with a depth of invasion greater than 4 mm compared with less than 4 mm was more than fourfold greater ($p = .0001$). A meta-analysis of all studies to date suggested that a value of 4 mm is the optimal cut-off for prediction of cervical node metastases (159) and this depth is recommended in the U.K. guidelines (38,140).

Tumor thickness is essentially a different value and measures the full thickness from the surface of the tumor to the maximum depth of penetration of malignant cells. This measure is recommended by the guidelines of the American College of Pathologists (141). Account must be taken of hyperkeratinized or ulcerated lesions. If heavily keratinized, the keratin layer is excluded, and if ulcerated, the ulcer surface is used as the tumor surface. As noted (Figure 4.46), this means that exophytic, nodular or verruciform lesions will show greater thickness than depth and, conversely, ulcerated lesions will be thinner. Moore et al. (160) found that thickness and depth are both good general indicators of neoplastic aggressiveness, with good correlation with survival and regional lymph node metastasis. However, they and others (161) agreed with Ambrosch et al. (158) that exophytic or verrucous tumors behave like thin tumors and that, for these lesions, depth of invasion from a reconstructed mucosal line is the better measure.

At non-keratinized sites, however, measurement of tumor thickness has been shown to be valuable. Spiro et al. (154) found a statistically significant association between an increasing thickness of tumor and treatment failure in lesions of the tongue and floor of mouth. Tumors greater than 2 mm thick were noted to have the best correlation with regional neck metastases and to be a better predictor than T stage. They concluded that patients with primary carcinomas greater than 2 mm thick should be treated with elective therapy to the N0 neck regardless of tumor size. Mohit-Tabatabai et al. (155) examined the relationship between stage I and II cancers from the floor of the mouth and regional metastasis. They too showed a strong correlation between metastasis and tumor thickness. Primary lesions were divided into three groups with tumor thickness of less than or equal to

1.5 mm, 1.6–3.5 mm or greater than 3.5 mm. These groups had corresponding regional metastasis rates of 2%, 33% and 60%, respectively. Similar findings have been presented by Baredes et al. (162) who showed that a cut-off point of 2.86 mm was predictive of metastases in soft palate lesions.

There is good evidence from these and other studies that the cut-off point for tumor thickness or depth of invasion should be different at different sites. Balasubramanian et al. (163) determined the prognostic value of "tumor thickness" in the tongue and floor of the mouth. However, they actually measured depth of invasion, defined as the measure from the level of adjacent mucosa to the deepest point of invasion. In this study, the authors found that nodal metastases were found in 41.7% of floor of the mouth tumors with a depth of between 2.1 and 4 mm, but in only 11.2% of tongue cancers of the same depth. Furthermore, they found that floor of the mouth cancers cross the 20% threshold for nodal metastases between 1 and 2 mm, whereas tongue cancers cross this threshold at about 4 mm. They recommended that an elective neck dissection was indicated for floor of the mouth tumors of 2 mm or greater depth and for tongue cancers of 4 mm or greater.

Although either depth of invasion or tumor thickness may be used by individual pathologists, it is essential that terminology is better defined and that there is a clear understanding of the significance of the measurements at local tumor multidisciplinary meetings. From a research perspective, it would be helpful to have international standards so that studies can be properly compared and agreed values used in core outcome measures for clinical trials. Recently, the eighth edition of the TNM classification has adopted depth of invasion as the standard prognostic indicator for lesions of the oral cavity (142–144). Depth is measured from the level of the basement membrane (not the surface) of the adjacent normal mucosal epithelium. A pT1 tumor is less than 2 cm in diameter and 5 mm or less in depth. Small tumors, which were previously T1, are now T2 if the depth of invasion is between 5 and 10 mm. Tumors penetrating greater than 10 mm are T3.

PERINEURAL INVASION

Perineural invasion by squamous cell carcinoma is considered an ominous prognostic sign and has been shown to correlate with an increased incidence of local recurrence and regional lymph node metastasis and decreased survival (39,164–169). Once the carcinoma enters a perineural space, it is possible for it to spread proximally or distally. Extension along the nerve can be for long distances, but in necropsy studies, Carter et al. (164) have shown that the tumor tends to remain localized to the terminal 1 or 2 cm of the nerve. In a clinicopathologic study of perineural spread in squamous cell carcinoma of the head and neck, this same group (165) also demonstrated spread in 24% of an unselected series of 70 patients treated by surgery.

The trigeminal nerve, particularly its mandibular division, was most commonly affected. The perineural invasion was more likely with large carcinomas, moderately or poorly differentiated and also showing lymphatic/vascular invasion. These findings have been supported by more recent studies, which confirm that perineural invasion is associated with both locoregional recurrence and distant metastases (145,166–168).

As with most histopathologic factors relating to prognosis, the status of perineural invasion as an independent prognostic factor remains unclear. Two recent reviews (169,170) discuss these issues and describe great variation in the incidence of perineural infiltration and the problems in its definition and identification. Roh et al. (170) show that the incidence varies from 14% to 63% of cases and illustrate how it is difficult to differentiate between perineural infiltration and perineural spread. They suggest that perineural infiltration involves microscopic infiltration of tumor cells into a nerve (Figure 4.47), while perineural spread may be associated with larger islands of tumor permeating along the nerve (Figure 4.48) or neurovascular bundles. Perineural spread is often therefore a gross finding and may

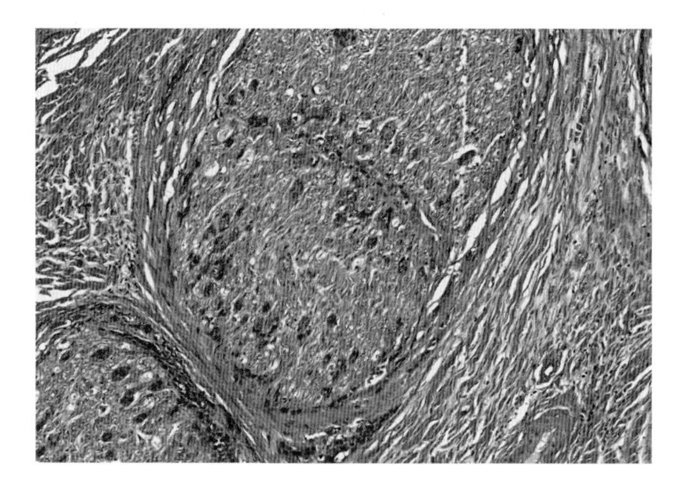

Figure 4.47 Perineural (intraneural) infiltration shows tumor islands within the body of the nerve.

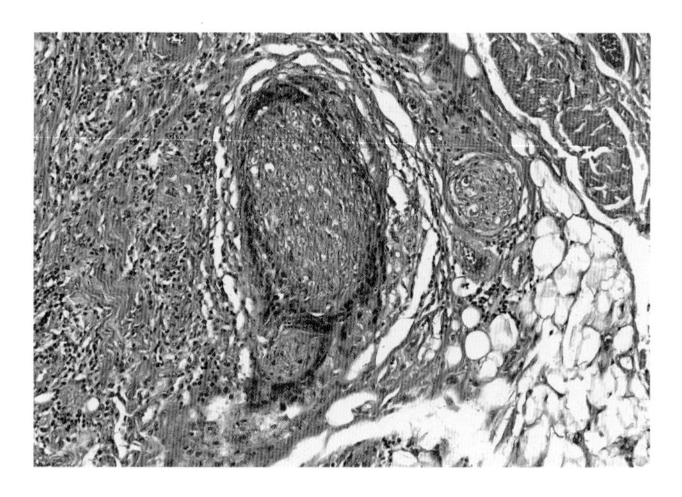

Figure 4.48 Perineural spread of carcinoma. The tumor is seen within the perineural space and may extend along neurovascular bundles.

be more easily detecting on magnetic resonance imaging. Both reviews (169,170) agreed however that perineural infiltration is associated with a poor prognosis. In adenoid cystic carcinomas, it has been shown that involvement of larger or named nerves is of most significance and that perineural infiltration within the tumor mass is of little significance (171). This is likely to also be the case in squamous cell carcinomas and attention should be paid to careful examination of the advancing front of the tumor (38,145,147).

LESIONS MIMICKING INVASION OF NERVES

Remnants of persistent vestigial or rudimentary epithelial structures are common in the oral region and include those of both odontogenic and non-odontogenic origin (145,172). These benign epithelial remnants can occasionally be juxtaneural, perineural or intraneural (173,174) and are often incidental findings in the microscopic study of other lesions (172). Most commonly, they are associated with periapical granulomas or cysts (145) and should not cause confusion with perineural infiltration in carcinomas.

A potential cause of misdiagnosis is the juxtaoral organ of Chievitz (175). This is found deep to the medial pterygoid muscle, at the level of the pterygomandibular raphe, and is associated with the long buccal nerve. It is not normally palpable and measures from 0.5 to 2 mm, except when hyperplastic. Histologically, it is characterized by squamous epithelial islands and duct-like structures set in a fibrous connective tissue stroma that contains numerous myelinated and non-myelinated nerves in close association with the epithelial elements. The function of the organ remains unknown, although it is thought to have both a neuroreceptor and a secretory function. Occasionally, this structure may be found at the margins of mandibular resection specimens and care must be taken not to confuse it with islands of residual or recurrent squamous carcinoma.

The neuroepithelial hamartoma (176) may also be encountered. This is a gingival lesion composed of round to oval and irregular squamous islands within a collagenized stroma. Small bundles of non-myelinated nerves either collide with the epithelial islands or surround them.

LYMPHOVASCULAR INVASION

The finding of squamous cell carcinoma within small blood or lymphatic vessels (Figure 4.49) has been linked to regional lymph node metastasis (39,177–179), but it is probably not an independent indicator since it also correlates with tumor size, perineural invasion and depth and pattern of invasion (38,39). Close et al. (177) studied 43 primary (T2 or greater) carcinomas, most of which were oral, and found vascular invasion in 35 (81%). Of these, 27 (77%) were found to have nodal metastases. Of the eight tumors in which vascular invasion was absent, only two had histologically confirmed cervical metastases.

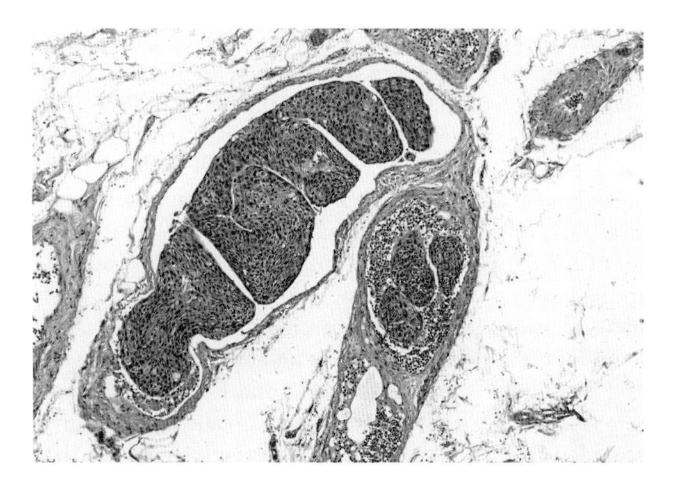

Figure 4.49 Lymphovascular invasion by islands of squamous cell carcinoma.

Neoplastic extension into large vessels is an indicator of extremely poor prognosis. In a review of 4,300 radical neck dissections, Djalilian et al. (180) found invasion of the jugular vein in 48 cases (1.1%). Forty-four of the patients died (72%) within the first 2 years after the neck dissection. Of these, 13 had metastases to the lungs.

DUCTAL INVASION

The frequency of involvement of adjacent salivary ducts by oral dysplastic or malignant epithelium has rarely been reported, but at certain sites, especially the floor of the mouth, it may be quite common. Daley et al. (181) screened routine tissue sections of 1216 cases of oral epithelial dysplasia and squamous cell carcinoma and found 26 (2.14%) that exhibited unequivocal ductal involvement, with floor of the mouth lesions especially likely to manifest this finding. Follow-up on 23 cases indicated an association with increased risk of recurrence. They found that the recurrence rate of pre-invasive lesions with ductal involvement was equal to that of the squamous cell carcinomas. The depth of the ductal dysplasia, however, did not correlate with recurrence rate. Even though uncommon, the involvement of salivary ducts is nonetheless significant. Surgical stripping or ablation of such lesions should extend at least 3 mm below the surface to ensure eradication of these reservoirs of dysplastic cells.

SURGICAL MARGINS IN SQUAMOUS CELL CARCINOMAS

There is considerable evidence that the status of the surgical resection margins is an important and valuable prognostic indicator (145,146,148,182,183). One of the putative indicators of completeness of surgical removal is the size of the histological margin of uninvolved tissue around the excised neoplasm (38,145,182). How generous the margin should be has not, and likely cannot, be defined for all forms of cancer or for selected classes or sites of malignancy. Tumor site, anatomic restrictions, presumed biologic characteristics of the cancer and the respective advantages of conservative and extended surgery are just some of the factors in the determination of adequate margins of resection (182). There is little doubt, however, that gross residual cancer will yield local persistence and nearly always increased mortality (148). For squamous cell carcinomas of the upper aerodigestive tract, there is a site dependency, not only in the ability of the surgeon to obtain tumor-free margins, but also in the biologic significance of involved or uninvolved limits of excision (182,183). For carcinomas of the oral cavity, a cut-off of 5 mm is regarded as an adequate margin (184) and this figure is used in the U.K. and U.S. national datasets (140,141). A histological margin greater than 5 mm is regarded as clear, between 1 and 5 mm is close and less than 1 mm should be recorded as involved (140). At sites outside of the oral cavity, such as the larynx, smaller margins are appropriate (141,183,184). In one study that applied these guidelines (148), only 11% of patients with an involved margin were alive at 5 years compared to 47% of patients with close margins and 78% with clear margins.

A major problem for pathologists, however, remains the definition and measurement of positive and negative surgical margins since there is a lack of standardization and precision. There must be irrefutable microscopic evidence of the presence or absence of invasive carcinoma at the line of resection, but carcinoma may be difficult to see at the margin, especially after laser resection. The pathologist must also measure the distance from the putative margin to the closest islands of tumor, and although this should be objective, its reliability varies with the conditions of measurement. Post-removal artefacts and fixation shrinkage renders these measurements inherently inaccurate. Beaumont and Hains (185) studied squamous cell carcinomas from the anterior oral cavity and showed significant changes in the longitudinal diameter of the whole specimen between the *in situ* and the fresh state ($p < .004$) and again between the fresh and the fixed state ($p < .0002$). The most significant alteration was in the measured diameter of the tumor, with a mean shrinkage of 4.82 mm from the fresh to the fixed state. Of surgical significance were the changes in the surgical margin. The minimal measured surgical margin *in situ* was 10 mm and, following fixation, this became an average of 5.8 mm. When examined microscopically, the average clearance of tumor was 5.4 mm. There was therefore a reduction of 46% from the planned surgical margin before resection to the assessed measurement of microscopic clearance in the surgical pathology laboratory. These data were confirmed in a study of canine oral mucosal margin shrinkage, which showed strikingly similar results, with shrinkage of about 40% (186).

Given optimum conditions (surgical and pathologic), what are the prognostic implications of the microscopic measurement of surgical margins in squamous cell carcinomas of the oral cavity and pharynx? Table 4.13 shows that clinical stage and T-stage have a major influence on local recurrences and on 2- and 5-year survival, even when there are surgically free margins (187,188). The available evidence suggests that lesional tissue within 5 mm of a surgical margin is associated with a nearly 80% incidence of recurrent disease. In a study by Looser et al. (187), 71% of patients with positive margins manifested recurrence at the primary site compared with only 32% of patients with negative margins. Byers et al. reported similar findings (188). Furthermore, it is to be accepted that a rather constant number of carcinomas (5%–10%) will resist the surgical goal of clear margins, regardless of their apparent T stage (182).

Table 4.13 Influence of clinical stage and T stage on local control and survival, in cases with free surgical margins

Clinical stage	Local control (%)	5-year survival (%)
I	85.5	61
II	72.6	46
III	64.8	32
IV	47.3	9.3
T stage	**Local control (%)**	**2-year survival (%)**
T1	95	86
T2	88	79
T3	86	59
T4	60	25

Source: Data from Looser KG, Shah JP, Strong EW. *Head Neck Surg* 1978;1:107–11 (clinical stage) (187); Byers RM et al. *Am J Surg* 1978;136:525–8 (T stage) (188).

Loree and Strong (189) analyzed the significance of positive margins on survival in a large group of patients ($n = 398$) with primary oral cavity carcinomas. The margin was classified as positive according to four criteria: (1) close (within 5 mm) margins; (2) dysplasia at the margin; (3) *in situ* carcinoma at the margin; and (4) invasive carcinoma at the margin. The incidence of positive margins was directly proportional to the increasing size of the tumor, but also varied between sites (Table 4.14). There was little difference in recurrence rates between the four groups (Table 4.15), but the overall local recurrence rate in the entire positive margin group was twice that of the negative margin group: 36% versus 18%, respectively. Positive margins also adversely affected survival: the 5-year survival rates of the positive and negative

Table 4.14 Positive margins in relation to site of primary oral cavity carcinomas

Oral site	No. of carcinomas	No. with positive margins (%)
Buccal	12	7 (58)
Maxillary gingiva	19	8 (42)
Mandibular gingiva	57	22 (39)
Hard palate	17	6 (35)
Floor of the mouth	137	43 (31)
Tongue	137	37 (27)
Retromolar trigone	25	6 (24)

Source: Modified from Loree TR, Strong EW. *Am J Surg* 1990;160:410–4 (189).

Table 4.15 The relationship between margin histopathology and local recurrence or survival

Margin	No. of recurrences (%)	5-year survival (%)
1. Close	29/83 (35)	51
2. Dysplasia	3/9 (33)	94
3. *In situ* carcinoma	4/9 (44)	71
4. Carcinoma	10/28 (36)	43
All positives	46/129 (36)	52
All negatives	49/209 (18)	60

Source: Data from Loree TR, Strong EW. *Am J Surg* 1990;160: 410–4 (189).

margin groups were 52.7% and 60%, respectively—a statistically significant difference. When the impact of postoperative adjuvant therapy was examined, none of the observed differences in survival rates between patients with surgery alone and those with combined therapy were significant. A major finding in the study was that, whereas postoperative radiation therapy to 6000 cGy successfully reduced the local recurrence rate in patients with positive margins, this benefit did not translate to an improved 5-year survival. The patterns of recurrence may change, but the overall risk of failure is increased. Adjuvant postoperative radiation therapy does not appear to decrease the risk of local recurrence in patients with positive margins to a level similar to patients with negative margins not treated with radiation therapy.

Scholl et al. (149) investigated the value of intraoperative frozen sections for the determination of margin status. They studied 268 patients with squamous carcinoma of the tongue treated by glossectomy and showed that 54 (20%) had positive margins on the first frozen section evaluation and 41 were rendered negative at the completion of surgery. Although the frozen sections were valuable in assisting complete excision, it was found that the local recurrence rate in these 41 patients was still significantly worse than in patients who had been negative at the first frozen section evaluation. More recently, Du et al. (190) confirmed the accuracy of frozen sections for intraoperative evaluation of margins. They showed that frozen section evaluation had sensitivity and specificity rates of 83.1% and 97.9%, respectively, against the gold standard of a positive margin on final paraffin sections. The positive and negative predictive values were 77.9% and 98.5%, respectively, with an overall accuracy of 96.7%. Although positive margin groups showed a greater local recurrence, they could not find any differences in disease-specific or overall survival. They concluded that frozen sections are accurate at detecting positive margins, but negative margins do not guarantee a margin-free resection.

An additional finding in the study of Scholl et al. (149) was that positive mucosal margins were more often seen in T1 or T2 tumors, whereas positive deep or soft tissue margins were more common in T3 and T4 lesions. The authors indicate that when dealing with carcinoma of the tongue, the guiding principle is the surgeon's ability to adequately remove all macroscopic disease. If margins are also microscopically negative, the patient probably does not need any additional adjunctive treatment to improve local control. This is echoed by van Es et al. (191), who state that when excision of a small squamous cell carcinoma (T1 and T2) of the mobile tongue or floor of the mouth is histologically complete (all margins are negative), other histopathologic variables are irrelevant in predicting recurrence at the primary site.

From the foregoing, the impact of positive margins on survival is clear. These data are confirmed by larger national studies. The Head and Neck Intergroup found a 16% incidence of positive surgical margins in patients with operable head and neck carcinomas from all sites (192). However, the highest rates were found in the oropharynx (37%) and the oral cavity (27%) and were also higher in larger tumors (T3 and T4: 36% and 32%, respectively). As expected, patients with positive margins experienced a significantly higher local failure rate (21% versus 9%, $p = 0.003$) and a similar incidence of regional failure relative to the negative margin population. The incidence of distant failure was also significantly higher in the positive margin group (20% versus 12%, $p = 0.42$). The addition of chemotherapy did not change survival. The survival of the patients was approximately half that of the corresponding negative margin group. With a median survival of only 19 months, the expectation of the positive margin group is not much better than that of the inoperable population.

Overall, these data are summarized in Table 4.16, which shows that positive margins are a significant prognostic

Table 4.16 Published recurrence and survival rates

References	Local recurrence (%)		3-year survival (%)	
	+ Margins	− Margins	+ Margins	− Margins
Byers et al. (188)	80	16	5	66
Looser et al. (187)	71	32	31	36
Chen et al. (193)	55	20	7	39
Loree and Strong (189)	36	18	52	60
Beaumont and Hains (194)	55	35	63	51
Sutton et al. (148)[a]	55	12	11	60

[a] Sutton et al. reported 5-year survival.

factor, but even if the surgical margins are negative, there is no assurance of successful local control (148,187–189,193,194).

ORAL CARCINOMAS AND BONE INVASION

Of the various oral carcinoma subsites, carcinomas related to the mandibular region (alveolar ridge, floor of the mouth, lower buccal sulcus and lower retromolar area) are among those with the highest rate of recurrence. Neoplastic invasion of the mandible is one of the factors promoting recurrence. It is therefore critical to determine the presence and extent of bony involvement in the management of patients (195,196).

Because the limits of resection of the mandible are often determined by the soft tissue extent of the carcinoma, there is the untoward result of a high percentage of resected mandibles with no evidence of carcinomatous invasion. Clinical examination, however, may be misleading. Weisman and Kimmelman (197) have indicated that a third of carcinomas with histological evidence of invasion of the mandible did not show clinical signs of preoperative bone invasion.

There are two basic types of involvement of the mandible (198–200). The first is an erosive form in which the bone recedes before a pushing tumor margin, such as that seen in verrucous carcinoma. Here, there is a loss of cortical continuity with a U-shaped or scalloped excavation of medullary bone. Radiologically, there is a well-defined radiolucency with no spicules of bone. The second type is infiltrative, in which there is neoplastic spread through the cortical plate into cancellous bone. An ill-defined and irregular lesion is seen on radiographs. Occasionally, a third type may be seen, with spread through the cancellous bone into bone marrow without any marked destruction and minimal radiographic changes. This is rare in squamous cell carcinomas, but is most often seen with adenoid cystic carcinomas.

The invaded bone surface is rarely if ever normal. It shows irregular pitting and various degrees of new bone formation (manifested by spurs and ridges, lined by osteoblasts). The crevices and pits on the bone's surface contain vascular granulation tissue and it is through these defects that the carcinoma begins its penetration. Perimandibular soft tissues also show various amounts of fibrosis and an active, chronic inflammation, all obscuring periosteal and fascial planes. The difficulty of visualizing bone involvement may be further compounded by prior irradiation.

In the great majority of non-irradiated mandibles, squamous cell carcinomas enter the medullary cavity through the upper borders of the mandible, either through the occlusal ridge alone or in combination with a penetration of either the buccal or lingual plates (201,202). This mode of invasion confirms the importance of cortical bone defects in the edentulous alveolus as a principal route for direct spread into the mandible. Size of the carcinoma does not appear to influence the incidence of bone involvement, but proximity of the tumor to bone does, and carcinomas involving the gingival margins appear to have a particularly high incidence of bone involvement.

Having breached the cortex, the carcinoma can extend vertically and laterally and there may be a superficial extension beneath a relatively intact cortex and periosteum (201). Additional spread into the bone is accompanied by a rather consistent and prominent response among bone cells. Carter (201) divides the response into an osteoclast-dependent phase and an osteoclast-independent phase of bone destruction. Each of these responses occurs in advance of the invading carcinoma and so it should be noted that malignant epithelial cells are rarely seen in actual contact with bone. The osteoclastic reaction is always greater than the osteoblastic response and is accentuated with rapidly growing, poorly differentiated carcinomas. Most of the destruction of bone is actually done by the host's cells, particularly osteoclasts. Destruction of bone by the carcinoma itself is a relatively minor late event. Neither the osteoclastic nor osteoblastic responses are particularly affected by prior irradiation of the bone. New bone formation, mediated by osteoblasts, is most prominent in association with slowly advancing and indolent carcinomas. Periosteal new bone formation is usually seen in front of the neoplastic spread. So, too, is marrow fibrosis.

The presence of teeth significantly influences the pattern of bone invasion and involvement of the inferior alveolar nerve. McGregor and MacDonald (202,203) found a fourfold increase of neoplastic invasion of the inferior alveolar nerve in edentulous, mandibles as opposed to partially dentate, mandibles. In nearly every instance, however, nerve involvement was also associated with an extensive spread of the carcinoma in the medullary parts of the bone. Skip areas of nerve involvement were unusual. Irradiation did not appear to affect the frequency or extent of nerve involvement.

The difference in nerve-related spread between dentate and non-dentate mandibles was attributable to the difference in vertical height of the occlusal border above the mandibular canal. The progressive resorption of the alveolar surfaces seen in the edentulous mandible brings the alveolar nerve much closer to the mucosa and hence more vulnerable to a direct vertical spread of the carcinoma. The incomplete remodeling of cortical bone and multiple cortical defects associated with alveolar resorption allows direct continuity between the medullary cavity and the overlying mucoperiosteum (202). Furthermore, the bone changes associated with loss of teeth greatly reduces the distance a floor of mouth carcinoma needs to invade to reach the occlusal ridge.

Spread of the carcinoma, either erosive or infiltrative, is nearly always through cancellous bone and its marrow spaces (203). There is little spread deep to an intact overlying mucosa or intact cortex.

Predicting invasion of the mandible is difficult, with computed tomography only showing a sensitivity of 52% and magnetic resonance imaging of 74% (204). In a prospective study, Brown et al. (205) concluded that while orthopantomograms, bone scans, computed tomography and magnetic resonance imaging were helpful, it was periosteal stripping with direct inspection that was the better predictor of invasion (accurate in all instances in the authors' study). In post-irradiated cortical bone, it may not be possible to separate the periosteum, even in the absence of neoplastic invasion, and that can thwart the inspection of the cortex that is the key.

It is likely that no single method will suffice in the determination of invasion of the mandible by oral squamous cell carcinomas. A combination of available techniques, tempered by clinical judgment, will produce the best result.

REFERENCES

1. Warnakulasuriya S, Johnson NW, van der Waal I. Nomenclature and classification of potentially malignant disorders of the oral mucosa. *J Oral Pathol Med* 2007;10:575–80.
2. Napier SS, Speight PM. Natural history of potentially malignant oral lesions and conditions: an overview of the literature. *J Oral Pathol Med* 2008;37:1–10.
3. Reibel J, Gale N, Hille J et al. Oral potentially malignant disorders and oral epithelial dysplasia. In: El-Naggar AK, Chan JKC, Grandis JR, Takata T, Sootweg P (eds). *WHO Classification of Head and Neck Tumours* (4th Edition). Lyon: IARC Press, 2017, 112–5.
4. Bouquot J, Speight PM, Farthing PM. Epithelial dysplasia of the oral mucosa—diagnostic problems and prognostic features. *Current Diagnostic Pathology* 2006;12:11–22.
5. Warnakulasuriya S, Reibel J, Bouquot J, Dabelsteen E. Oral epithelial dysplasia classification systems: predictive value, utility, weaknesses and scope for improvement. *J Oral Pathol Med* 2008;3:127–33.
6. Gale N, Pilch BZ, Sidransky D et al. Tumours of the hypopharynx, larynx and trachea. Epithelial precursor lesions. In: Barnes L, Eveson JW, Reichart P, Sidransky D (eds). *World Health Organization Classification of Tumours: Pathology and Genetics of Head and Neck Tumours 2005*. Lyon: IARC Press, 2005, Ch3, 140–3.
7. Bosman FT. Dysplasia classification: pathology in disgrace? *J Pathol* 2001;194(2):143–4.
8. Abbey LM, Kaugers GE, Gunsolley JC et al. Intraexaminer and interexaminer reliability in the diagnosis of oral epithelial dysplasia. *Oral Surg Oral Med Oral Pathol Oral Radiol Endod* 1995;80:188–91.
9. Karabulut A, Reibel J, Therkildsen MH, Praetorius F, Nielsen HW, Dabelsteen E. Observer variability in the histologic assessment of oral premalignant lesions. *J Oral Pathol Med* 1995;24:198–200.
10. Brothwell DJ, Lewis DW, Bradley G, Leong I, Jordan RC, Mock D, Leake JL. Observer agreement in the grading of oral epithelial dysplasia. *Commun Dent Oral Epidemiol* 2003;31:300–5.
11. Fischer DJ, Epstein JB, Morton TH, Schwartz SM. Interobserver reliability in the histopathologic diagnosis of oral pre-malignant and malignant lesions. *J Oral Pathol Med* 2004;33(2):65–70.
12. Montgomery E. Is there a way for pathologists to decrease interobserver variability in the diagnosis of dysplasia? *Arch Pathol Lab Med* 2005;129(2):174–6.
13. Fleskens S, Slootweg P. Grading systems in head and neck dysplasia: their prognostic value, weaknesses and utility. *Head Neck Oncol* 2009;1:11.
14. Kujan O, Oliver RJ, Khattab A, Roberts SA, Thakker N, Sloan P. Evaluation of a new binary system of grading oral epithelial dysplasia for prediction of malignant transformation. *Oral Oncol* 2006;42:987–93.
15. Silverman S, Gorsky M, Lozada F. Oral leukoplakia and malignant transformation. A follow up study of 257 patients. *Cancer* 1984;53:563–8.
16. Pitiyage G, Tilakaratne WM, Tavassoli M, Warnakulasuriya S. Molecular markers in oral epithelial dysplasia: review. *J Oral Pathol Med* 2009;38(10):737–52.
17. Warnakulasuriya S, Kovacevic T, Madden P, Coupland VH, Sperandio M, Odell E, Muller H. Factors predicting malignant transformation in oral potentially malignant disorders among patients accrued over a 10-year period in South East England. *J Oral Pathol Med* 2011;40(9):677–83.
18. Schepman KP, van der Meij EH, Smeele LE, van der Waal I. Malignant transformation of oral leukoplakia: a follow-up study of a hospital-based population of 166 patients with oral leukoplakia from The Netherlands. *Oral Oncol* 1998:34:270–5.
19. Gupta PC, Mehta FS, Daftary DK et al. Incidence rates of oral cancer and natural history of oral precancerous lesions in a 10-year follow-up study of Indian villagers. *Commun Dent Oral Epidemiol* 1990;8:287–333.
20. Bouquot JE, Kurland LT, Weiland LH. Carcinoma *in situ* of the upper aerodigestive tract: incidence, time trends and follow-up in Rochester, Minnesota, 1935–1984. *Cancer* 1988;61:1691–8.
21. Bánóczy J, Csiba A. Occurrence of epithelial dysplasia in oral leukoplakia. Analysis and follow-up study of 120 cases. *Oral Surg Oral Med Oral Pathol* 1976;42:766–74.
22. Amagasa T, Yakoo E, Sato K et al. A study of the clinical characteristics and treatment of oral carcinoma *in situ*. *Oral Surg Oral Pathol Oral Pathol* 1985;60:50–5.
23. Vedtofte P, Holmstrup P, Hjorting-Hansen E et al. Surgical treatment of premalignant lesions of the oral mucosa. *Int J Oral Maxillofac Surg* 1987;16:656–64.
24. Mincer HH, Coleman SA, Hopkins KA. Observations on the clinical characteristics of oral lesions showing histologic epithelial dysplasia. *Oral Surg Oral Med Oral Pathol* 1972;33:389–99

25. Pindborg JJ, Daftary DK, Mehta FS. A follow-up study of 61 oral dysplastic precancerous lesions in Indian villagers. *Oral Surg Oral Med Oral Pathol* 1977;43:383–90.
26. Lumerman H, Freedman P, Kerpel S. Oral epithelial dysplasia and the development of invasive squamous cell carcinoma. *Oral Surg Oral Med Oral Pathol* 1995;79:321–9.
27. Jaber MA, Porter SR, Speight PM et al. Oral epithelial dysplasia: Clinical characteristics of western European residents. *Oral Oncol* 2003;39:589–96.
28. Holmstrup P, Vedtofte P, Reibel J, Stoltze K. Oral premalignant lesions: is a biopsy reliable? *J Oral Pathol Med* 2007;36(5):262–6.
29. Arduino PG, Surace A, Carbone M, Elia A, Massolini G, Gandolfo S, Broccoletti R. Outcome of oral dysplasia: a retrospective hospital-based study of 207 patients with a long follow-up. *J Oral Pathol Med* 2009;38(6):540–4.
30. Mehanna HM, Rattay T, Smith J, McConkey CC. Treatment and follow-up of oral dysplasia—a systematic review and meta-analysis. *Head Neck* 2009;31(12):1600–9.
31. International Classification of Disease for Oncology. http://codes.iarc.fr/topography.
32. Odell EW, Jani P, Sherriff M et al. The prognostic value of individual grading parameters in small lingual squamous cell carcinomas. The importance of the pattern of invasion. *Cancer* 1994;74:789–94.
33. Sloan P, Gale N, Hunter K et al. Malignant surface epithelial tumours. In: El-Naggar AK, Chan JKC, Grandis JR, Takata T, Sootweg P (eds). *WHO Classification of Head and Neck Tumours* (4th Edition). Lyon: IARC Press, 2017, 109–11.
34. Anneroth G, Batsakis J, Luna M. Review of the literature and a recommended system of malignancy grading in oral squamous cell carcinomas. *Scand J Dent Res* 1987;95(3):229–49.
35. Anneroth G, Hansen LS. A methodologic study of histologic classification and grading of malignancy in oral squamous cell carcinoma. *Scand J Dent Res* 1984;92(5):448–68.
36. Bryne M, Koppang HS, Lilleng R, Stene T, Bang G, Dabelsteen E. New malignancy grading is a better prognostic indicator than Broders' grading in oral squamous cell carcinomas. *J Oral Pathol Med* 1989;18(8):432–7.
37. Bryne M, Koppang HS, Lilleng R, Kjaerheim A. Malignancy grading of the deep invasive margins of oral squamous cell carcinomas has high prognostic value. *J Pathol* 1992;166(4):375–81.
38. Woolgar JA. Histopathological prognosticators in oral and oropharyngeal squamous cell carcinoma. *Oral Oncol* 2006;42(3):229–39.
39. Woolgar JA, Scott J. Prediction of cervical lymph node metastases in squamous cell carcinoma of the tongue/floor of mouth. *Head Neck* 1995;17:463–72.
40. Ackerman LV. Verrucous carcinoma of the oral cavity. *Surgery* 1948;23(4):670–8.
41. Ackerman LV, Hermann P. Verrucous cancer of the oral cavity. *Proc Int Acad Oral Pathol* 1969:7–13.
42. Batsakis JG, Hybels R, Crissman JD et al. The pathology of head and neck tumors: verrucous carcinoma, part 15. *Head Neck Surg* 1982;5:29–38.
43. Medina JE, Dichtel W, Luna MA. Verrucous-squamous carcinomas of the oral cavity. A clinicopathologic study of 104 cases. *Arch Otolaryngol* 1984;110:437–40.
44. Bagan J, Scully C, Jimenez Y, Martorell M. Proliferative verrucous leukoplakia: a concise update. *Oral Dis* 2010;16(4):328–32.
45. Abadie WM, Partington EJ, Fowler CB, Schmalbach CE. Optimal management of proliferative verrucous leukoplakia: a systematic review of the literature. *Otolaryngol Head Neck Surg* 2015;153(4):504–11.
46. Koch BB, Trask DK, Hoffman HT et al. National survey of head and neck verrucous carcinoma. Patterns of presentation, care and outcome. *Cancer* 2001;92:110–20.
47. McDonald JS, Crissman JD, Gluckman JL. Verrucous carcinoma of the oral cavity. *Head Neck Surg* 1982;5:22–8.
48. Walvekar RR, Chaukar DA, Deshpande MS, Pai PS, Chaturvedi P, Kakade A, Kane SV, D'Cruz AK. Verrucous carcinoma of the oral cavity: a clinical and pathological study of 101 cases. *Oral Oncol* 2009;45(1):47–51.
49. Jyothirmayi R, Sankaranarayanan R, Varghese C, Jacob R, Nair MK. Radiotherapy in the treatment of verrucous carcinoma of the oral cavity. *Oral Oncol* 1997;33(2):124–8.
50. Karagozoglu KH, Buter J, Leemans CR, Rietveld DH, van den Vijfeijken S, van der Waal I. Subset of patients with verrucous carcinoma of the oral cavity who benefit from treatment with methotrexate. *Br J Oral Maxillofac Surg* 2012;50(6):513–8.
51. Terada T. Squamous cell carcinoma arising within verrucous carcinoma of the oral cavity: a case report. *Int J Clin Exp Pathol* 2012;5(4):363–6.
52. Allon D, Kaplan I, Manor R, Calderon S. Carcinoma cuniculatum of the jaw: a rare variant of oral carcinoma. *Oral Surg Oral Med Oral Pathol Oral Radiol Endod* 2002;94(5):601–8.
53. Thavaraj S, Cobb A, Kalavrezos N, Beale T, Walker DM, Jay A. Carcinoma cuniculatum arising in the tongue. *Head Neck Pathol* 2012;6(1):130–4.
54. Pons Y, Kerrary S, Cox A, Guerre A, Bertolus C, Gruffaz F, Capron F, Goudot P, Ruhin-Poncet B. Mandibular cuniculatum carcinoma: apropos of 3 cases and literature review. *Head Neck* 2012;34(2):291–5.
55. Suzuki J, Hashimoto S, Watanabe K, Takahashi K, Usubuchi H, Suzuki H. Carcinoma cuniculatum mimicking leukoplakia of the mandibular gingiva. *Auris Nasus Larynx* 2012;39(3):321–5.

56. Sun Y, Kuyama K, Burkhardt A, Yamamoto H. Clinicopathological evaluation of carcinoma cuniculatum: a variant of oral squamous cell carcinoma. *J Oral Pathol Med* 2012;41(4):303–8.
57. Shah AA, Jeffus SK, Stelow EB. Squamous cell carcinoma variants of the upper aerodigestive tract: a comprehensive review with a focus on genetic alterations. *Arch Pathol Lab Med* 2014;138(6):731–44.
58. El-Mofty SK. Human papillomavirus-related head and neck squamous cell carcinoma variants. *Semin Diagn Pathol* 2015;32(1):23–31.
59. Chernock RD, Lewis JS Jr, Zhang Q, El-Mofty SK. Human papillomavirus positive basaloid squamous cell carcinoma of the upper aerodigestive tract: a distinct clinicopathologic and molecular subtype of basaloid squamous cell carcinoma. *Hum Pathol* 2010;41(7):1016–23.
60. El-Mofty SK, Patil S. Human papillomavirus (HPV)-related oropharyngeal nonkeratinizing squamous cell carcinoma: characterization of a distinct phenotype. *Oral Surg Oral Med Oral Pathol Oral Radiol Endod* 2006;101(3):339–45.
61. Westra WH. The pathology of HPV-related head and neck cancer: implications for the diagnostic pathologist. *Semin Diagn Pathol* 2015;32(1):42–53.
62. Raslan WF, Barnes L, Krause JR et al. Basaloid squamous cell carcinoma of the head and neck: a clinicopathologic and flow cytometric study of 10 new cases with review of the English literature. *Am J Otolaryngol* 1994;15:204–11.
63. Wieneke JA, Heffner DK. Basaloid squamous cell carcinoma: an aggressive variant of squamous cell carcinoma of the head and neck region. *Pathol Case Rev* 2000;5:200–5.
64. Luna MA, El-Naggar A, Parichatikanond P et al. Basaloid squamous carcinoma of the upper aerodigestive tract. *Cancer* 1990;66:537–42.
65. Banks ER, Frierson HF, Mills SE et al. Basaloid squamous cell carcinoma of the head and neck: a clinicopathologic and immunohistochemical study of 40 cases. *Am J Surg Pathol* 1992;16:939–46.
66. Morice WG, Ferreiro JA. Distinction of basaloid squamous cell carcinoma from adenoid cystic and small cell undifferentiated carcinoma by immunohistochemistry. *Hum Pathol* 1998;29(6):609–12.
67. Coppola D, Catalano E, Tang C-K et al. Basaloid squamous cell carcinoma of floor of mouth. *Cancer* 1993;72:2299–305.
68. Thompson L, Chang B, Barsky SH. Monoclonal origin of malignant mixed tumors (carcinosarcomas). Evidence for a divergent histogenesis. *Am J Surg Pathol* 1996;20:277–85.
69. Ansari-Lari MA, Hoque MO, Califano J, Westra WH. Immunohistochemical p53 expression patterns in sarcomatoid carcinomas of the upper respiratory tract. *Am J Surg Pathol* 2002;26(8):1024–31.
70. Choi HR, Sturgis EM, Rosenthal DI, Luna MA, Batsakis JG, El-Naggar AK. Sarcomatoid carcinoma of the head and neck: molecular evidence for evolution and progression from conventional squamous cell carcinomas. *Am J Surg Pathol* 2003;27(9):1216–20.
71. Zidar N, Boštjančič E, Gale N, Kojc N, Poljak M, Glavač D, Cardesa A. Down-regulation of microRNAs of the miR-200 family and miR-205, and an altered expression of classic and desmosomal cadherins in spindle cell carcinoma of the head and neck—Hallmark of epithelial–mesenchymal transition. *Hum Pathol* 2011;42(4):482–8.
72. Wick MR, Swanson PE. Carcinosarcomas: current perspectives and an historical review of nosological concepts. *Semin Diagn Pathol* 1993;10:118–27.
73. Viswanathan S, Rahman K, Pallavi S, Sachin J, Patil A, Chaturvedi P, D'Cruz A, Agarwal J, Kane SV. Sarcomatoid (spindle cell) carcinoma of the head and neck mucosal region: a clinicopathologic review of 103 cases from a tertiary referral cancer centre. *Head Neck Pathol* 2010;4(4):265–75.
74. Zarbo RJ, Crissman JD, Venkat H et al. Spindle-cell carcinoma of the upper aerodigestive tract mucosa. *Am J Surg Pathol* 1986;10:741–53.
75. Thompson LD, Wieneke JA, Miettinen M, Heffner DK. Spindle cell (sarcomatoid) carcinomas of the larynx: a clinicopathologic study of 187 cases. *Am J Surg Pathol* 2002;26:153–70.
76. Romañach MJ, Azevedo RS, Carlos R, de Almeida OP, Pires FR. Clinicopathological and immunohistochemical features of oral spindle cell carcinoma. *J Oral Pathol Med* 2010;39(4):335–41.
77. Gupta R, Singh S, Hedau S, Nigam S, Das BC, Singh I, Mandal AK. Spindle cell carcinoma of head and neck: an immunohistochemical and molecular approach to its pathogenesis. *J Clin Pathol* 2007;60(5):472–5.
78. Gerry D, Fritsch VA, Lentsch EJ. Spindle cell carcinoma of the upper aerodigestive tract: an analysis of 341 cases with comparison to conventional squamous cell carcinoma. *Ann Otol Rhinol Laryngol* 2014;123(8):576–83.
79. Batsakis JG, Rice DH, Howard DR. The pathology of head and neck tumors: spindle cell lesions (sarcomatoid carcinomas, nodular fasciitis and fibrosarcoma) of the aerodigestive tracts. *Head Neck Surg* 1982;4:499–513.
80. Lewis JE, Olsen KD, Sebo TJ. Spindle cell carcinoma of the larynx: review of 26 cases including DNA content and immunohistochemistry. *Hum Pathol* 1997;28:664–73.
81. Ogawa K, Kim Y-C, Nakashima Y et al. Expression of epithelial markers in sarcomatoid carcinoma: an immunohistochemical study. *Histopathology* 1987;11:511–22.

82. Nakhleh RE, Zarbo RJ, Ewing S et al. Myogenic differentiation in spindle cell (sarcomatoid) carcinomas of the upper aerodigestive tract. *Appl Immunohistochem* 1993;1:58–68.
83. Batsakis JG, Luna MA, El-Naggar AK. "Inflammatory pseudotumor": What is it? How does it behave? *Ann Otol Rhinol Laryngol* 1995;104:329–31.
84. Coffin CM, Watterson J, Priest JR, Dehner LP. Extrapulmonary inflammatory myofibroblastic tumor (inflammatory pseudotumor): a clinicopathologic and immunohistochemical study of 84 cases. *Am J Surg Pathol* 1995;19:859–72.
85. Batsakis JG. "Pseudosarcoma" of the mucous membrane in the head and neck. *J Laryngol Otol* 1981;95:311–6.
86. Bice TC, Tran V, Merkley MA, Newlands SD, van der Sloot PG, Wu S, Miller MC. Disease-specific survival with spindle cell carcinoma of the head and neck. *Otolaryngol Head Neck Surg* 2015;153:973–80.
87. Olsen KD, Lewis JE, Suman VJ. Spindle cell carcinoma of the larynx and hypopharynx. *Otolaryngol Head Neck Surg* 1997;116:47–52.
88. Ellis GL, Corio RL. Spindle cell carcinoma of the oral cavity. A clinicopathologic assessment of fifty-nine cases. *Oral Surg Oral Med Oral Pathol* 1980;50:523–34.
89. Batsakis JG, Huser J. Squamous carcinomas with glandlike (adenoid) features. *Ann Otol Rhinol Laryngol* 1990;99:87–8.
90. Schick U, Pusztaszeri M, Betz M et al. Adenosquamous carcinoma of the head and neck: report of 20 cases and review of the literature. *Oral Surg Oral Med Oral Pathol Oral Radiol* 2013;116:313–20.
91. Masand RP, El-Mofty SK, Ma XJ, Luo Y, Flanagan JJ, Lewis JS Jr. Adenosquamous carcinoma of the head and neck: relationship to human papillomavirus and review of the literature. *Head Neck Pathol* 2011;5(2):108–16.
92. Scully C, Porter SR, Speight PM, Eveson JW, Gale D. Adenosquamous carcinoma of the mouth: a rare variant of squamous cell carcinoma. *Int J Oral Maxillofac Surg* 1999;28(2):125–8.
93. Napier SS, Gormley JS, Newlands C et al. Adenosquamous carcinoma. A rare neoplasm with an aggressive course. *Oral Surg Oral Med Oral Pathol Oral Radiol Endod* 1995;79:607–11.
94. Martinez-Madrigal F, Baden E, Casiraghi O et al. Oral and pharyngeal adenosquamous carcinoma. A report of four cases with immunohistochemical studies. *Eur Arch Otorhinolaryngol* 1991;248:255–8.
95. Kass JI, Lee SC, Abberbock S, Seethala RR, Duvvuri U. Adenosquamous carcinoma of the head and neck: molecular analysis using CRTC-MAML FISH and survival comparison with paired conventional squamous cell carcinoma. *Laryngoscope* 2015;125(11):E371–6.
96. Nappi O, Pettinato G, Wick MR. Adenoid (acantholytic) squamous cell carcinoma of the skin. *J Cutan Pathol* 1989;16:114–21.
97. Jones AC, Freedman PD, Kerpel SM. Oral adenoid squamous cell carcinoma: a report of three cases and review of the literature. *J Oral Maxillofac Surg* 1993;51:676–81.
98. Takagi M, Sakato Y, Takayama S et al. Adenoid squamous carcinoma of the oral mucosa. *Cancer* 1977;40:2250–5.
99. Ferlito A, Devany KO, Rinaldo A et al. Mucosal adenoid squamous cell carcinoma of the head and neck. *Ann Otol Rhinol Laryngol* 1996;105:409–13.
100. Terada T. Adenoid squamous cell carcinoma of the oral cavity. *Int J Clin Exp Pathol* 2012;5(5):442–7.
101. Zidar N, Gale N, Zupevc A, Dovsak D. Pseudovascular adenoid squamous-cell carcinoma of the oral cavity—a report of two cases. *J Clin Pathol* 2006;59(11):1206–8.
102. Vidyavathi K, Prasad C, Kumar HM, Deo R. Pseudovascular adenoid squamous cell carcinoma of oral cavity: a mimicker of angiosarcoma. *J Oral Maxillofac Pathol* 2012;16(2):288–90.
103. Mehrad M, Carpenter DH, Chernock RD, Wang H, Ma XJ, Luo Y, Luo J, Lewis JS Jr, El-Mofty SK. Papillary squamous cell carcinoma of the head and neck: clinicopathologic and molecular features with special reference to humanpapillomavirus. *Am J Surg Pathol* 2013;37(9):1349–56.
104. Russell JO, Hoschar AP, Scharpf J. Papillary squamous cell carcinoma of the head and neck: a clinicopathologic series. *Am J Otolaryngol* 2011;32(6):557–63.
105. Bao Z, Yang X, Shi L, Feng J, Liu W, Zhou Z. Clinicopathologic features of oral squamous papilloma and papillary squamous cell carcinoma: a study of 197 patients from eastern China. *Ann Diagn Pathol* 2012;16(6):454–8.
106. Ding Y, Ma L, Shi L, Feng J, Liu W, Zhou Z. Papillary squamous cell carcinoma of the oral mucosa: a clinicopathologic and immunohistochemical study of 12 cases and literature review. *Ann Diagn Pathol* 2013;17(1):18–21.
107. Takeda Y, Satoh M, Nakamura S, Yamamoto H. Papillary squamous cell carcinoma of the oral mucosa: immunohistochemical comparison with other carcinomas of oral mucosal origin. *J Oral Sci* 2001;43(3):165–9.
108. Argyris PP, Kademani D, Pambuccian SE, Nguyen R, Tosios KI, Koutlas IG. Comparison between p16 INK4A immunohistochemistry and human papillomavirus polymerase chain reaction assay in oral papillary squamous cell carcinoma. *J Oral Maxillofac Surg* 2013;71(10):1676–82.
109. Suarez PA, Adler-Storthz K, Luna MA, El-Naggar AK, Abdul-Karim FW, Batsakis JG. Papillary squamous cell carcinomas of the upper aerodigestive tract: a clinicopathologic and molecular study. *Head Neck* 2000;22(4):360–8.

110. Tsang WYW, Chan JKC. Lymphoepithelial carcinoma. In: Barnes L, Eveson JW, Reichart P, Sidransky D (eds). *World Health Organization Classification of Tumours: Pathology and Genetics of Head and Neck Tumours 2005*. Lyon: IARC Press, 2005, Ch 3, 132.
111. MacMillan C, Kapadia SM, Finkelstein SD et al. Lymphoepithelial carcinoma of the larynx and hypopharynx: study of eight cases with relationship to Epstein–Barr virus and p53 gene alterations, and review of the literature. *Hum Pathol* 1996;27:1172–9.
112. Frank DK, Cheron F, Costanzo D et al. Non-nasopharyngeal lymphoepitheliomas (undifferentiated carcinomas) of the upper aerodigestive tract. *Ann Otol Rhinol Laryngol* 1995;104:305–10.
113. Bansberg SF, Olsen KD, Gafey TA. Lymphoepithelioma of the oropharynx. *Otolaryngol Head Neck Surg* 1989;100:303–7.
114. Wenig BM. Lymphoepithelial-like carcinomas of the head and neck. *Semin Diagn Pathol* 2015;32:74–6.
115. Singhi AD, Stelow EB, Mills SE, Westra WH. Lymphoepithelial-like carcinoma of the oropharynx. A morphologic variant of HPV-related head and neck cancer. *Am J Surg Pathol* 2010;34:800–5.
116. Carpenter DH, El-Mofty SK, Lewis JS Jr. Undifferentiated carcinoma of the oropharynx: a human papilloma virus—associated tumor with a favorable prognosis. *Mod Pathol* 2011;24:1306–12.
117. Westra WH. Detection of human papillomavirus (HPV) in clinical samples: evolving methods and strategies for the accurate determination of HPV status of head and neck carcinomas. *Oral Oncol* 2014;50(9):771–9.
118. Schache AG, Liloglou T, Risk JM et al. Validation of a novel diagnostic standard in HPV-positive oropharyngeal squamous cell carcinoma. *Br J Cancer* 2013;108(6):1332–9.
119. Lewis JS Jr. p16 immunohistochemistry as a standalone test for risk stratification in oropharyngeal squamous cell carcinoma. *Head Neck Pathol* 2012;6(Suppl 1):S75–82.
120. Begum S, Cao D, Gillison M, Zahurak M, Westra WH. Tissue distribution of human papillomavirus 16 DNA integration in patients with tonsillar carcinoma. *Clin Cancer Res* 2005;11(16):5694–9.
121. Harris SL, Thorne LB, Seaman WT, Hayes DN, Couch ME, Kimple RJ. Association of p16(INK4a) overexpression with improved outcomes in young patients with squamous cell cancers of the oral tongue. *Head Neck* 2011;33(11):1622–7.
122. Chung CH, Zhang Q, Kong CS et al. p16 protein expression and human papillomavirus status as prognostic biomarkers of nonoropharyngeal head and neck squamous cell carcinoma. *J Clin Oncol* 2014;32(35):3930–8.
123. Zafereo ME, Xu L, Dahlstrom KR, Viamonte CA, El-Naggar AK, Wei Q, Li G, Sturgis EM. Squamous cell carcinoma of the oral cavity often overexpresses p16 but is rarely driven by human papillomavirus. *Oral Oncol* 2016;56:47–53.
124. Lingen MW, Xiao W, Schmitt A, Jiang B, Pickard R, Kreinbrink P, Perez-Ordonez B, Jordan RC, Gillison ML. Low etiologic fraction for high-risk human papillomavirus in oral cavity squamous cell carcinomas. *Oral Oncol* 2013;49(1):1–8.
125. Jordan RC, Lingen MW, Perez-Ordonez B, He X, Pickard R, Koluder M, Jiang B, Wakely P, Xiao W, Gillison ML. Validation of methods for oropharyngeal cancer HPV status determination in US cooperative group trials. *Am J Surg Pathol* 2012;36(7):945–54.
126. Schache A, Croud J, Robinson M, Thavaraj S. Human papillomavirus testing in head and neck squamous cell carcinoma: best practice for diagnosis. *Methods Mol Biol* 2014;1180:237–55.
127. Chernock RD, El-Mofty SK, Thorstad WL, Parvin CA, Lewis JS Jr. HPV-related nonkeratinizing squamous cell carcinoma of the oropharynx: utility of microscopic features in predicting patient outcome. *Head Neck Pathol* 2009;3(3):186–94.
128. Chernock RD. Morphologic features of conventional squamous cell carcinoma of the oropharynx: "keratinizing" and "nonkeratinizing" histologic types as the basis for a consistent classification system. *Head Neck Pathol* 2012;6(Suppl 1):S41–7.
129. Lewis JS Jr, Khan RA, Masand RP et al. Recognition of nonkeratinizing morphology in oropharyngeal squamous cell carcinoma—a prospective cohort and interobserver variability study. *Histopathology* 2012;60(3):427–36.
130. Gondim DD, Haynes W, Wang X, Chernock RD, El-Mofty SK, Lewis JS Jr. Histologic typing in oropharyngeal squamous cell carcinoma: a 4-year prospective practice study with p16 and high-risk HPV mRNA testing correlation. *Am J Surg Pathol* 2016; 40:1117–24.
131. Westra WH, Boy S, El-Mofty SK et al. Squamous cell carcinoma, HPV positive. In: El-Naggar AK, Chan JKC, Grandis JR, Takata T, Sootweg P (eds). *WHO Classification of Head and Neck Tumours* (4th Edition). Lyon: IARC Press, 2017, 136–8.
132. Begum S, Westra WH. Basaloid squamous cell carcinoma of the head and neck is a mixed variant that can be further resolved by HPV status. *Am J Surg Pathol* 2008;32(7):1044–50.
133. Bishop JA, Westra WH. Human papillomavirus-related small cell carcinoma of the oropharynx. *Am J Surg Pathol* 2011;35(11):1679–84.
134. Kraft S, Faquin WC, Krane JF. HPV-associated neuroendocrine carcinoma of the oropharynx: a rare new entity with potentially aggressive clinical behavior. *Am J Surg Pathol* 2012;36(3):321–30.

135. Watson RF, Chernock RD, Wang X, Liu W, Ma XJ, Luo Y, Wang H, El-Mofty SK, Lewis JS Jr. Spindle cell carcinomas of the head and neck rarely harbor transcriptionally-active human papillomavirus. *Head Neck Pathol* 2013;7(3):250–7.
136. Bhatia A, Burtness B. Human papillomavirus-associated oropharyngeal cancer: defining risk groups and clinical trials. *J Clin Oncol* 2015;33(29):3243–50.
137. Isayeva T, Li Y, Maswahu D, Brandwein-Gensler M. Human papillomavirus in non-oropharyngeal head and neck cancers: a systematic literature review. *Head Neck Pathol* 2012;6(Suppl 1):S104–20.
138. Mehanna H, Franklin N, Compton N et al. Geograph ic variation in human papillomavirus-related oropharyngeal cancer: data from 4 multinational randomized trials. *Head Neck* 2016;38(Suppl 1): E1863–9.
139. Hunt JL, Barnes L, Lewis JS Jr et al. Molecular diagnostic alterations in squamous cell carcinoma of the head and neck and potential diagnostic applications. *Eur Arch Otorhinolaryngol* 2014;271(2):211–23.
140. Helliwell T, Woolgar JA. *Dataset for Histopathology Reporting of Mucosal Malignancies of the Oral Cavity*. London: Royal College of Pathologists: 2013. https://www.rcpath.org/profession/publications/cancer-datasets.html.
141. Seethala RR, Weinreb I, Carlson DL et al. *Protocol for the Examination of Specimens from Patients with Carcinomas of the Lip and Oral Cavity*. American College of Pathologists, 2016. http://www.cap.org/ShowProperty?nodePath=/UCMCon/Contribution%20Folders/WebContent/pdf/liporalca-version-16 protocol.pdf.
142. Brierley JD, Gospodarowicz MK, Wittekind C (eds) *UICC. TNM Classification of Malignant Tumours* (8th Edition). Oxford: Wiley Blackwell, 2017.
143. Amin MB, Edge S, Greene F (eds). *AJCC Cancer Staging Manual* (8th Edition). New York: Springer, 2017.
144. Lydiatt WM, Patel SG, O'Sullivan B et al. Head and neck cancers—major changes in the American Joint Committee on Cancer eighth edition cancer staging manual. *CA Cancer J Clin* 2017;67:122–7.
145. Woolgar JA, Triantafyllou A. Pitfalls and procedures in the histopathological diagnosis of oral and oropharyngeal squamous cell carcinoma and a review of the role of pathology in prognosis. *Oral Oncol* 2009;45(4–5):361–85.
146. Rogers SN, Brown JS, Woolgar JA, Lowe D, Magennis P, Shaw RJ, Sutton D, Errington D, Vaughan D. Survival following primary surgery for oral cancer. *Oral Oncol* 2009;45(3):201–11.
147. Sawair FA, Irwin CR, Gordon DJ, Leonard AG, Stephenson M, Napier SS. Invasive front grading: reliability and usefulness in the management of oral squamous cell carcinoma. *J Oral Pathol Med* 2003;32(1):1–9.
148. Sutton DN, Brown JS, Rogers SN, Vaughan ED, Woolgar JA. The prognostic implications of the surgical margin in oral squamous cell carcinoma. *Int J Oral Maxillofac Surg* 2003;32(1):30–4.
149. Scholl P, Byers RM, Batsakis JG et al. Microscopic cut-through of cancer in the surgical treatment of squamous carcinoma of the tongue. Prognostic and therapeutic implications. *Am J Surg* 1986;152:354–60.
150. Dahlstrom KR, Garden AS, William WN Jr, Lim MY, Sturgis EM. Proposed staging system for patients with HPV-related oropharyngeal cancer based on nasopharyngeal cancer N categories. *J Clin Oncol* 2016;34(16):1848–54.
151. O'Sullivan B, Huang SH, Su J et al. Development and validation of a staging system for HPV-related oropharyngeal cancer by the International Collaboration on Oropharyngeal Cancer Network for Staging (ICON-S): a multicentre cohort study. *Lancet Oncol* 2016;17(4):440–51.
152. Gonzalez-Moles MA, Esteban F, Rodriguez-Archilla A, Ruiz-Avila I, Gonzalez-Moles S. Importance of tumour thickness measurement in prognosis of tongue cancer. *Oral Oncol* 2002;38(4):394–7.
153. O-charoenrat P, Pillai G, Patel S, Fisher C, Archer D, Eccles S, Rhys-Evans P. Tumour thickness predicts cervical nodal metastases and survival in early oral tongue cancer. *Oral Oncol* 2003;39(4):386–90.
154. Spiro RH, Huvos AG, Wong GY et al. Predictive value of tumor thickness in squamous carcinoma confined to the tongue and floor of mouth. *Am J Surg* 1986;152:345–50.
155. Mohit-Tabatabai MA, Sobel HJ, Rush BF et al. Relation of thickness of floor of mouth stage I and II cancers to regional metastasis. *Am J Surg* 1986;152:351–3.
156. Shah JP, Cendon RA, Farr HW et al. Carcinoma of the oral cavity. Factors affecting treatment failure at the primary site and neck. *Am J Surg* 1976;132:504–7.
157. Fukano H, Matsuura H, Hasegawa Y et al. Depth of invasion as a predictive factor for cervical lymph node metastasis in tongue carcinoma. *Head Neck* 1997;19:205–10.
158. Ambrosch P, Kron M, Fischer G et al. Micrometastases in carcinoma of the upper aerodigestive tract: detection, risk of metastasizing, and prognostic value of depth of invasion. *Head Neck* 1995;17:473–9.
159. Huang SH, Hwang D, Lockwood G, Goldstein DP, O'Sullivan B. Predictive value of tumor thickness for cervical lymph-node involvement in squamous cell carcinoma of the oral cavity: a meta-analysis of reported studies. *Cancer* 2009;115:1489–97.
160. Moore C, Kuhns JG, Greenberg RA. Thickness as prognostic aid in upper aerodigestive tract cancer. *Arch Surg* 1986;121:1410–4.

161. Thompson SH. Cervical lymph node metastases in oral carcinoma related to the depth of invasion of the primary lesion. *J Surg Oncol* 1986;31:120–2.
162. Baredes S, Leeman DJ, Chen TS. Significance of tumor thickness in soft palate carcinoma. *Laryngoscope* 1993;103:389–93.
163. Balasubramanian D, Ebrahimi A, Gupta R, Gao K, Elliott M, Palme CE, Clark JR. Tumour thickness as a predictor of nodal metastases in oral cancer: comparison between tongue and floor of mouth subsites. *Oral Oncol* 2014;50(12):1165–8.
164. Carter RL, Tanner NSB, Clifford P et al. Perineural spread in squamous cell carcinomas of the head and neck: a clinicopathological study. *Clin Otolaryngol* 1979;4:271–81.
165. Soo K, Carter RL, O'Brien CJ. Prognostic implications of perineural spread in squamous carcinomas of the head and neck. *Laryngoscope* 1986;96:1145–8.
166. Tarsitano A, Tardio ML, Marchetti C. Impact of perineural invasion as independent prognostic factor for local and regional failure in oral squamous cell carcinoma. *Oral Surg Oral Med Oral Pathol Oral Radiol* 2015;119(2):221–8.
167. Fagan JJ, Collins B, Barnes L, D'Amico F, Myers EN, Johnson JT. Perineural invasion in squamous cell carcinoma of the head and neck. *Arch Otolaryngol Head Neck Surg* 1998;124:637–40.
168. Rahima B, Shingaki S, Nagata M, Saito C. Prognostic significance of perineural invasion in oral and oropharyngeal carcinoma. *Oral Surg Oral Med Oral Pathol Oral Radiol Endod* 2004;97:423–31.
169. Binmadi NO, Basile JR. Perineural invasion in oral squamous cell carcinoma: a discussion of significance and review of the literature. *Oral Oncol* 2011;47(11):1005–10.
170. Roh J, Muelleman T, Tawfik O, Thomas SM. Perineural growth in head and neck squamous cell carcinoma: a review. *Oral Oncol* 2015;51(1):16–23.
171. Barrett AW, Speight PM. Perineural invasion in adenoid cystic carcinoma of the salivary glands: a valid prognostic indicator? *Oral Oncol* 2009;45:936–40.
172. Dunlap CL, Barker B. Diagnostic problems in oral pathology. *Semin Diagn Pathol* 1985;2:16–30.
173. Wysocki GP, Wright BA. Intraneural and perineural epithelial structures. *Head Neck Surg* 1981;4:69–71.
174. Lutman GB. Epithelial nests in intraoral sensory nerve endings simulating perineural invasion in patients with oral carcinoma. *Am J Clin Pathol* 1974;61:275–84.
175. Miko T, Molnar P. The juxtaoral organ: a pitfall for pathologists. *J Pathol* 1981;133:17–23.
176. Mesa M, Baden E, Grodjesk J et al. Neuroepithelial hamartoma of the oral cavity. *Oral Surg Oral Med Oral Pathol* 1994;78:627–30.
177. Close LG, Burns DK, Reisch J et al. Microvascular invasion in cancer of the oral cavity and oropharynx. *Arch Otolaryngol Head Neck Surg* 1987;113:1191–5.
178. Poleksic S, Kalwaic HJ. Prognostic value of vascular invasion in squamous cell carcinoma of the head and neck. *Plast Reconstr Surg* 1978;61:234–40.
179. Batsakis JG. Invasion of the microcirculation in head and neck cancer. *Ann Otol Rhinol Laryngol* 1984;93:646–7.
180. Djalilian M, Weiland LH, Devine KD et al. Significance of jugular vein invasion by metastatic carcinoma in radical neck dissection. *Am J Surg* 1973;126:566–9.
181. Daley TD, Lovas JGL, Peters E et al. Salivary gland duct involvement in oral epithelial dysplasia and squamous cell carcinoma. *Oral Surg Oral Med Oral Pathol Oral Radiol Endod* 1996;81:186–92.
182. Batsakis JG. Surgical excision margins: a pathologist's perspective. *Adv Anat Pathol* 1999;6:140–8.
183. Lee JG. Detection of residual carcinoma of the oral cavity, oropharynx, hypopharynx, and larynx: a study of surgical margins. *Trans Am Acad Ophthalmol Otolaryngol* 1974;78:49–53.
184. Hinni ML, Ferlito A, Brandwein-Gensler MS et al. Surgical margins in head and neck cancer: a contemporary review. *Head Neck* 2013;35(9):1362–70.
185. Beaumont DG, Hains JD. Changes in surgical margins in vivo following resection and after fixation. *Aust J Otolaryngol* 1992;1:51–2.
186. Johnson RE, Sigman JD, Funk GF et al. Quantification of surgical margin shrinkage in the oral cavity. *Head Neck* 1997;19:281–6.
187. Looser KG, Shah JP, Strong EW. The significance of "positive" margins in surgically resected epidermoid carcinomas. *Head Neck Surg* 1978;1:107–11.
188. Byers RM, Bland KI, Borlase B et al. Prognostic and therapeutic value of frozen section determinations in the surgical treatment of squamous carcinoma of the head and neck. *Am J Surg* 1978;136:525–8.
189. Loree TR, Strong EW. Significance of positive margins in oral cavity squamous carcinoma. *Am J Surg* 1990;160:410–4.
190. Du E, Ow TJ, Lo YT, Gersten A, Schiff BA, Tassler AB, Smith RV. Refining the utility and role of frozen section in head and neck squamous cell carcinoma resection. *Laryngoscope* 2016;126:1768–75.
191. van Es RJJ, Amerongen NN, Slootweg PJ et al. Resection margin as a predictor of recurrence at the primary site for T1 and T2 oral cancers. Evaluation of histopathologic variables. *Arch Otolaryngol Head Neck Surg* 1996;122:521–5.
192. Jacobs JR, Ahmad K, Casiano R et al. Implications of positive surgical margins. *Laryngoscope* 1993;103:64–8.
193. Chen TY, Emrich LJ, Driscoll DL. The clinical significance of pathological findings in surgically resected margins of the primary tumor in head and neck carcinoma. *Int J Rad Oncol Biol Phys* 1987;13:833–7.
194. Beaumont DG, Hains JD. Surgical margins in oral cavity and oropharyngeal cancer. *Aust J Otolaryngol* 1992;1:47–50.

195. Cleary KR, Batsakis JG. Oral squamous cell carcinoma and the mandible. *Ann Otol Rhinol Laryngol* 1995;104:977–9.
196. Haribhakti VV. The dentate adult human mandible: An anatomic basic for surgical decision making. *Plast Reconstr Surg* 1996;97:536–41.
197. Weisman RA, Kimmelman CP. Bone scanning in the assessment of mandibular invasion by oral cavity carcinoma. *Laryngoscope* 1982;92:1–4.
198. Müller H, Slootweg PJ. Mandibular invasion by oral squamous cell carcinoma. Clinical aspects. *J Cranio-Maxillofac Surg* 1990;18:80–4.
199. Slootweg PJ, Müller H. Mandibular invasion by oral squamous cell carcinoma. *J Cranio-Maxillofac Surg* 1989;17:69–74.
200. Shaw RJ, Brown JS, Woolgar JA, Lowe D, Rogers SN, Vaughan ED. The influence of the pattern of mandibular invasion on recurrence and survival in oral squamous cell carcinoma. *Head Neck* 2004;26(10):861–9.
201. Carter RL. Patterns and mechanisms of localized bone invasion by tumors: studies with squamous carcinomas of the head and neck. *Crit Rev Clin Lab Sci* 1985;22:275–315.
202. McGregor AD, MacDonald DG. Routes of entry of squamous cell carcinoma to the mandible. *Head Neck Surg* 1988;10:294–301.
203. McGregor AD, MacDonald DG. Patterns of spread of squamous cell carcinoma within the mandible. *Head Neck* 1989;11:457–61.
204. Silva M, Zambrini EI, Chiari G, Montermini I, Manna C, Poli T, Lanfranco D, Sesenna E, Thai E, Sverzellati N. Pre-surgical assessment of mandibular bone invasion from oral cancer: comparison between different imaging techniques and relevance of radiologist expertise. *Radiol Med* 2016; 121:704–10.
205. Brown JS, Griffith JF, Phelps PD et al. A comparison of different imaging modalities and direct inspection after periosteal stripping in predicting the invasion of the mandible by oral squamous cell carcinoma. *Br J Oral Maxillofac Surg* 1994;32:347–59.

5

Molecular pathology

RIFAT HASINA, NISHANT AGRAWAL, AND MARK W. LINGEN

INTRODUCTION

Approximately 95% of malignant neoplasms of the oral and oropharyngeal region are represented by the histologic diagnosis of squamous cell carcinoma (SCC), with the remainder largely consisting of salivary gland neoplasms. Epithelial carcinogenesis is thought to be a multistep process involving the sequential activation of oncogenes and the inactivation of tumor suppressor genes in a clonal population of cells. These genetic and epigenetic changes generate concomitant phenotypic changes in the tumor cells that promote their survival and proliferation (1). A number of reproducible molecular alterations, some definitively characterized and some inferred, have been identified in both oral potentially malignant disorders (OPMDs) and SCC. This chapter will summarize the currently available data with respect to the molecular changes observed in OPMDs and SCC. Importantly, rather than merely providing a list of individual genetic alterations observed with some varying incidence/prevalence within small cohorts of patients, this chapter will instead focus on studies that have investigated entire classes of genetic changes at a global level. Where possible, it will also seek to correlate these molecular changes with potential improvements in the areas of diagnosis, prognosis and prediction.

MOLECULAR CHANGES IN OPMD

As described in Chapter 4, a definition and diagnosis of an OPMD that is based solely upon histopathologic evaluation is problematic. Currently, lesions are considered to be precancerous based on morphologic changes in individual epithelial cells and epithelial tissues. However, the criteria for diagnosing and grading dysplasia are subjective and open to a wide range of interpretations, even among highly qualified pathologists (2–8). In addition, validated histologic prognostic criteria do not exist for predicting the risk of malignant transformation of a given dysplastic lesion, and even severely dysplastic oral lesions can undergo spontaneous regression (9–11). Furthermore, as outlined in Figure 5.1, contrary to conventional wisdom, oral mucosal lesions do not follow a linear pattern of biological/clinical progression. For example, a clinically and histologically benign lesion may be biologically reactive in nature or it may represent a molecularly altered lesion that carries some risk for progressing to SCC. Our ability to improve on this prognostication is further compounded by the fact that only ~15% of histologically dysplastic lesions will progress to SCC over some period of time (9,12–17). Finally, there is evidence for lesions that are not readily visible on conventional visual tactile examination that are in fact histologically and partly

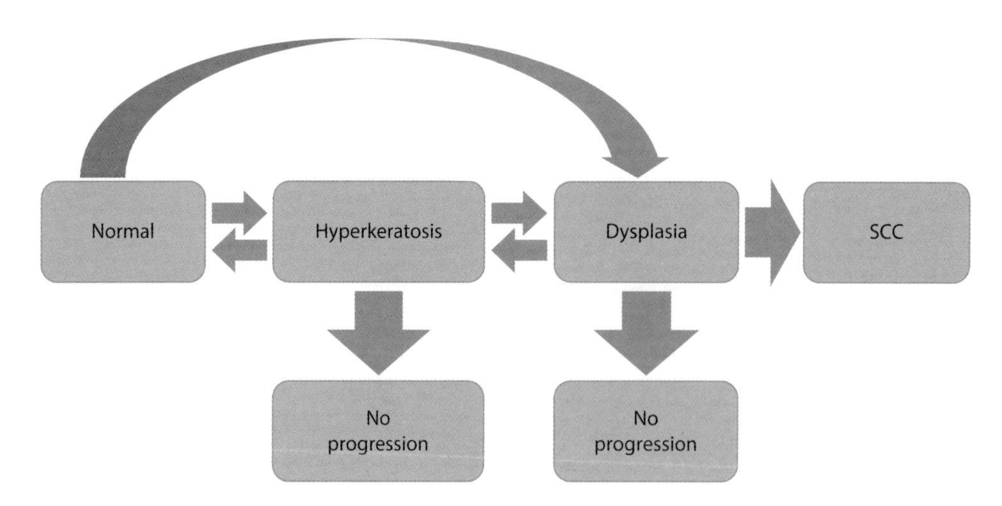

Figure 5.1 Squamous cell carcinoma (SCC) progression. Mucosal lesions do not follow a linear progression pattern to SCC. While a small percentage of dysplastic lesions will progress to SCC, the majority will either remain quiescent or regress. Similarly, mucosal lesions lacking histologic atypia at the time of biopsy may represent molecularly premalignant lesions.

committed to malignant transformation from a molecular perspective (18–22). Therefore, histological findings can only be used to indicate that a particular lesion has an undetermined malignant potential and cannot be used for the prediction of malignant transformation. These findings also underscore that, at the present time, we are unable to accurately prognosticate on the basis of histologic changes and point to the need for protocols that address these diagnostic/prognostic challenges. Therefore, the development of molecularly based approaches to identifying predictive genetic changes prior to and after the development of cytologic atypia and/or tissue dysplasia would greatly improve the potential for early detection, prognostication and intervention.

As will be discussed in the Section titled DNA Alterations in SCC, a number of recurring somatic alterations have been identified in SCC. However, while there has been considerable focus on the mutational landscape of SCC, biomarker discovery for premalignant lesions has largely focused on alternative molecular aberrations. In general, these have included loss of heterozygosity (LOH), aneuploidy, methylation and expression changes in RNA molecules (mRNA, microRNA [miRNA] and long noncoding RNA [lncRNA]).

DNA ALTERATIONS IN ORAL PREMALIGNANCY

LOSS OF HETEROZYGOSITY

LOH can be defined as an event in which large portions of a chromosome(s) are lost (Figure 5.2). This is a common occurrence in cancer development and the repeated loss of a specific chromosomal region is often associated with the presence of a tumor suppressor gene. Over the last two decades, a large body of literature has demonstrated LOH at 3p and 9p as a common event in both malignant and potentially malignant oral lesions (17–20,22–41). In addition, alterations at 3p and 9p have been associated with increased disturbances in cellular organization and architecture (18,23,25,37,38,42–46). There is also evidence that LOH at 3p and 9p can be observed in histologically normal-appearing lesions (18,19,22,29). The relationship between LOH and risk of progression has also been investigated in a number of important publications. In a retrospective analysis of OPMDs, the Rosin group demonstrated that 96% of low-grade lesions (mild and moderate dysplasia) with LOH at 3p and 9p progressed to cancer over 15 years of follow-up.

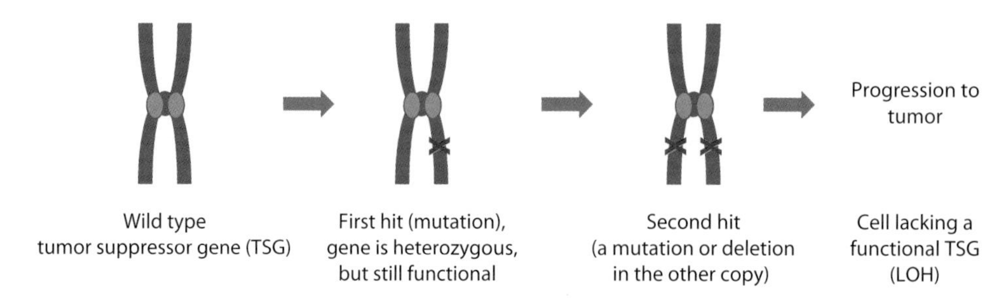

Figure 5.2 Loss of heterozygosity (LOH). Some genes may contain one normal and one mutated allele—that is, be heterozygous—and still function normally. When a chromosomal event causes the cell to lose that normal allele (LOH), it also loses its normal function. If this happens in a tumor suppressor gene, it predisposes the cell to turn malignant.

Overall, 3p and/or 9p LOH demonstrated a 20-fold increased risk in dysplastic lesions progressing to SCC (33). In another retrospective study, Partridge et al. reported that LOH at 3p and 9p occurred in 90% of cases that progressed to SCC (285). A subsequent prospective study validated the predictive value of 3p and/or 9p LOH. Moreover, it also demonstrated that the inclusion of two additional markers, 4q/17p, improved the risk prediction. Using a three-tier prediction model, the authors were able to demonstrate 5-year progression rates of 4.8%, 22.9% and 65.4% for low-, intermediate- and high-risk groups, respectively (17).

Summary and clinical significance: While these findings highlight promising prognostic value in testing for LOH in premalignant lesions, a number of unanswered questions remain when considering the utility of this as a diagnostic platform. First, as is often the case with three-tiered risk classifications, it is unclear how intermediate-risk patients would be managed. Given the 5% chance of progression to SCC over a 5-year period of time, one might envision that patients falling into the low-risk group would not require aggressive treatment or monitoring. On the other hand, high-risk patients, with a 65% risk of progression over 5 years, would likely require aggressive treatment and monitoring (47,48). However, the management of patients characterized as intermediate risk is less clear. Patients falling into this category have a 22.9% risk of developing cancer over a 5-year period. This risk is considerably different from both the low- and high-risk groups and these patients may benefit from a different and as-yet undefined preventive and surveillance strategy. It may be possible to include an additional type of molecular test. For example, Graveland et al. demonstrated that testing of TP53 point mutations, in conjunction with 9p LOH, increased the diagnostic accuracy for predicting progression of dysplastic lesions (49). It is also unclear if low- and intermediate-risk lesions that do progress to SCC maintain their initial LOH profile. If these low-risk lesions change their profiles with progression, one might be able to monitor lesions by way of sequential sampling. Alternatively, if the low-risk lesion LOH profiles remain the same during progression, this may suggest alternative pathways to SCC progression that are independent of the proposed LOH model. However, as with conventional histopathologic evaluation, the risk of sampling error will always be a confounder when incisional biopsies are performed. Further work is likely needed before one can develop monitoring and treatment protocols. Finally, recent data have suggested that OPMDs, like their malignant counterparts, demonstrate inter- and intra-lesional heterogeneity. Specifically, Gomes et al. (50) found that individual dysplastic lesions demonstrated unique patterns of allelic loss for chromosomes 3, 9, 11 and 17. Importantly, they found that there were different LOH patterns within different areas of the same lesion. While this was a small study requiring further validation, the implications of the findings are important as they raise the possibility of inaccurate diagnostic/prognostic tests as a result of sampling error.

ANEUPLOIDY

Aneuploidy can be defined as abnormal DNA content that arises as a result of chromosomal instability (Figure 5.3). The mechanisms of aneuploidy development and the biologic implications of these chromosomal abnormalities are actively being pursued, but are out of the realm of this discussion (51–53). Aneuploidy can be measured using a number of different methods including DNA flow cytometry (FCM) and DNA image cytometry (ICM). While there is some evidence suggesting variable diagnostic accuracy among techniques measuring ploidy in oral lesions (54), we will collectively consider all the methods for determining ploidy status.

Because chromosomal instability and DNA aneuploidy are considered to be hallmarks of malignant cells, there has been considerable interest in investigating the landscape of copy number alterations (CNAs) observed in cancer, including in SCC (55–58). Several studies have also investigated

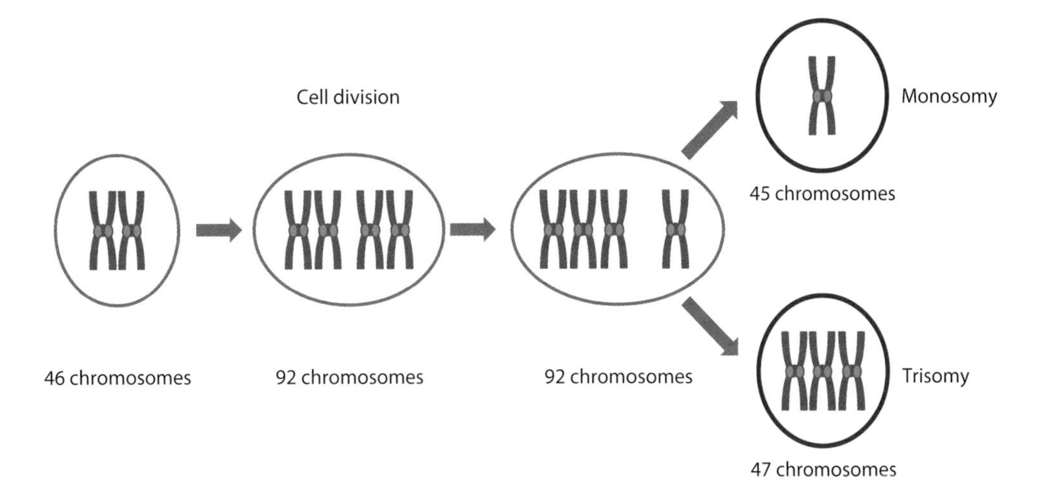

Figure 5.3 Aneuploidy. Aneuploidy is the situation in which a cell has an abnormal number of chromosomes instead of 46. This can be as a result of either chromosomal loss or gain.

the relationship between oral dysplasia and aneuploidy. Overall, the published data suggest that approximately 20%–45% of oral tissues exhibiting dysplasia are aneuploid, with one study reporting a frequency of 83% (57,59,60). In addition, aneuploidy has been reported to be significantly associated with the histologic grade of dysplasia (59–61).

Torres-Rendon et al. (57) performed ICM on a retrospective cohort of 86 dysplastic lesions that did ($n = 42$) or did not ($n = 44$) progress to cancer within a 5-year minimum follow-up. They found that aneuploid lesions were more likely to progress to SCC than diploid lesions (74% versus 42%). While statistically significant, the data suggest that ploidy status alone lacked sufficient diagnostic accuracy to predict whether an individual lesion was more likely to progress to SCC in a manner that would aid the clinician in determining appropriate monitoring and treatment. However, it was observed that the rate of progression to SCC for aneuploid lesions was significantly greater than for diploid lesions (52% versus 25%), suggesting that the presence of aneuploidy might trigger the need for shorter follow-up intervals. Similarly, Bradley et al. (62) performed ICM on a retrospective case–control study to investigate the association between aneuploidy and progression to SCC. A total of 1,313 patients and 1,477 biopsies with a diagnosis of dysplasia were initially included in the study. In total, 8% of the lesions progressed to cancer over an interval of 6–131 months. Of the evaluable cases, 28% (28/99) demonstrated abnormal DNA content and 78% of these (22/28) progressed to SCC. Furthermore, multivariate analysis revealed that abnormal DNA content was a significant predictor of malignant transformation with a hazard ratio of 3.3 (95% confidence interval: 1.5–7.4). The proportions of subjects who were cancer free at 5 years were 75% for patients with normal DNA content and 44% for those with aneuploidy. Similar to the Torres-Rendon et al. study, the authors found that the median time to cancer for aneuploid lesions was 49 months versus 130 months for diploid lesions. Bremmer et al. employed ICM in a cohort of 62 leukoplakias to assess the value of ploidy status for predicting progressing to SCC (63). During a median follow-up period of 69 months, 21% (13/62) of patients progressed to SCC. Overall, 44% (27/62) of the biopsies demonstrated aneuploidy. Of the lesions that progressed, 54% (7/13) of the lesions were aneuploid and 46% (6/13) were diploid. In addition, Sperandio et al. sought to determine the value of ICM analysis in predicting malignant transformation (64). This retrospective analysis was performed on 273 patients and the results were correlated with histopathology and outcome. In total, 12% (32/273) of the patients underwent malignant transformation during the follow-up period, which ranged from 5 to 15 years. Of the lesions that progressed to SCC, 63% (20/32) were aneuploid. Conversely, of the 241 that did not progress, 16% (39/273) were aneuploid. As a standalone prognostic marker, the positive predictive value (PPV) of aneuploidy for transformation was 38.5%, with sensitivity and specificity rates of 65% and 75%, respectively. The negative predictive values (NPVs) for diploid or tetraploid lesions were 90% and 96%, respectively. Finally, the combination of histology and ploidy was found to have the highest PPV. In a retrospective study, Siebers et al. (65) investigated the prognostic value of chromosomal instability, measured by both ICM and FISH (Fluorescent in situ Hybridization) for chromosomes 1 and 7, in predicting the transformation of 102 oral leukoplakias with a minimum of 6 months follow-up (median 91.5 months). Malignant transformation occurred in ~16% of the lesions (16/102). Aneuploidy was observed in 23% (23/102) and 16% (17/102) as determined by ICM and FISH, respectively. For the aneuploid lesions detected by ICM, 43.5% (10/23) progressed to SCC, while 47% (8/17) of the lesions detected by FISH progressed. Conversely, only 7.6% (6/79) and 9.4% (8/85) of the diploid lesions, as determined by ICM or FISH for chromosomes 1 and 7, progressed to SCC. The authors found that both tests were able to provide prognostic information that was independent of the histopathological diagnosis. In addition, they found that the combination of tests allowed for the stratification of patients into three different risk groups for progression to cancer.

Summary and clinical significance: Aneuploidy is observed in a large proportion of oral dysplastic lesions and there is some correlation between aneuploidy and histologic grade. In addition, the data indicate that aneuploid lesions may progress to cancer at a significantly faster rate than diploid lesions (i.e. the presence of aneuploidy may suggest a more aggressive biologic course). However, cumulatively, the data have shown that the prognostic value for aneuploidy testing lacks sufficient diagnostic accuracy to reliably stratify patients into appropriate risk cohorts that could be used for monitoring and treatment.

METHYLATION

Epigenetic modifications are a group of dynamic and reversible changes that can affect DNA function. These include DNA methylation, histone modifications and alterations in chromatin conformation (66). DNA methylation involves the addition of methyl groups to cytosine bases by the enzyme DNA methyltransferase (67). In normal tissues, unmethylated cytosine residues are found in high densities within CpG islands (areas with high concentrations of cytosine and guanine) that map close to the promoter region in approximately 40% of mammalian genes (68). A hypomethylated state is associated with a higher rate of transcriptional activity, while the hypermethylated state is associated with a reduction or silencing of transcription (Figure 5.4). While aberrant DNA methylation has been shown to be important in a number of different disease states, considerable attention has been placed on the role of methylation in the dysregulation of cancer-related genes (69–71). Hypermethylation of tumor suppressor gene promoter regions is thought to play a significant role in cell cycle control, DNA damage repair, apoptosis, angiogenesis, invasion and metastasis. In fact, there is evidence to suggest that gene silencing, by way of promoter hypermethylation, is a more common mechanism of gene inactivation than

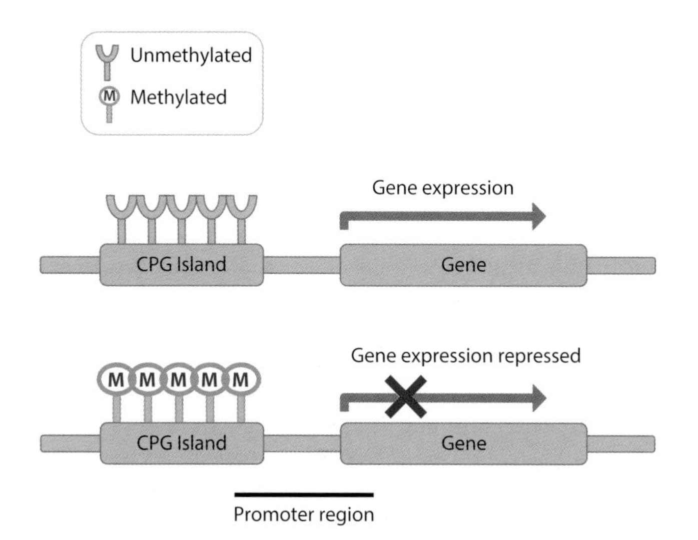

Figure 5.4 DNA methylation. DNA methylation is the process of epigenetic modification of gene expression. These have wide effects, including on DNA repair, and can contribute to genomic stability.

other mechanisms, such as somatic mutations and deletions in some cancers (72,73).

Hypermethylation of specific tumor-associated genes is often observed in dysplasia and is thought to be an early event in the development of SCC (74,75). As a result, there has been considerable interest in determining the methylation status of SCC-associated genes in OPMDs. For example, several cross-sectional studies have reported increased methylation of the p16 promoter region in dysplastic lesions (76,77). Similarly, two cross-sectional studies found higher degrees of methylation of the p16 promoter in dysplastic lesions that progressed to SCC when compared to lesions that did not progress (78,79). In addition, Shridhar et al. performed a critical review summarizing the evidence regarding aberrant DNA methylation patterns as a potential predictive biomarker for the progression of OPMDs (75). From a total of 21 eligible studies, the authors found that the most commonly reported hypermethylated loci were p16, p14, MGMT and DAPK. However, to date, there are limited data regarding genome-wide methylation patterns of OPMDs. Towle et al. performed a global analysis of DNA methylation using 30 paired tissues (adjacent normal, dysplasia and CIS [Carcinoma-in-situ]/oral SCC [OSCC]) from 10 patients (80). They reported increased methylation of CpG islands in the CIS/OSCC samples when compared to the adjacent normal regions. However, there were no differences in methylation patterns between the adjacent normal and dysplasia groups. These preliminary findings suggest that changes in CpG methylation patterns may be prominent in the later stages of progression.

Summary and clinical significance: Hypermethylation of cancer-associated genes has been observed in dysplastic oral lesions with variable frequencies. These include p16, p14, MGMT and DAPK, suggesting the potential importance of inactivation of these genes at early stages of carcinogenesis. Importantly, longitudinal studies have suggested a correlation between increased methylation of the p16 promoter region in dysplastic lesions that progress to SCC. However, there has been only one genome-wide study that has characterized the hypermethylation landscape of dysplastic oral lesions. Therefore, a considerable amount of additional research is necessary to determine the utility of specific gene methylation patterns before hypermethylation can be used to identify patients at risk for developing SCC or as a predictive biomarker for the progression of dysplastic lesions.

COPY NUMBER ALTERATIONS

CNAs represent another type of genetic abnormality where large or small segments of the genome are lost or gained and have been associated with cancer development (1,81). CNA analysis has been found to have diagnostic and predictive utility in the oncology field. For example, amplification of the epidermal growth factor receptor 2 (HER2) gene can dictate specific types of treatment (82). Similarly, gains in 14q32.33 can be predictive of response to therapy and progression in a subset of ovarian cancers (83). There are many different methods for determining CNAs, including fluorescence *in situ* hybridization (84), multiplex ligation-dependent probe amplification (MLPA), array comparative genomic hybridization (aCGH) arrays, single-nucleotide polymorphism arrays, next-generation sequencing (85), quantitative polymerase chain reaction (PCR), digital PCR and droplet digital PCR (86–94). For this discussion, we will not stratify observations of CNAs based upon the various methods of detection.

There are a limited number of genome-wide CNA studies focusing on OPMDs. Tsui et al. applied a whole-genome analysis to a panel of high-grade lesions and identified chromosomal loci 7p11.2 and 11q13 as the most frequently occurring regions of amplification in oral dysplasia (37). The region of 7p11.2 is worth particular consideration as it spans the region of the epidermal growth factor receptor (EGFR) gene, a member of the receptor tyrosine kinase family, which is overexpressed or amplified in a number of cancers, including OSCC (37,85,95–99). Furthermore, EGFR amplification has been shown to be of both prognostic and predictive value in SCC of the lung (100–102). Importantly, amplification of EGFR has been shown to be of prognostic value in terms of predicting increased risk of progression to oropharyngeal SCC (OPSCC) (103–106).

Cha and colleagues performed aCGH and MLPA on seven primary SCCs as well as the adjacent areas of dysplastic and normal mucosa (107). The dysplastic lesions contained frequent copy number gains (>70%) in 3q, 5p, 6p, 7p, 8q and Xq. Conversely, frequent copy number losses (>70%) were identified for 1p, 2p, 3p, 5q, 9q, 12q, 17q and 22q. With respect to individual genes, high amplification frequencies were detected in *RNF36* (100%), *CYP26B1* (86%), *PIK3CA* (86%) and *NLGN1* (86%), while the highest deletion frequencies were observed in *CKAP2l* (100%) and *TCF8* (100%). Similarly, Cervigne and colleagues performed aCGH analysis on 25 sequential, progressive potentially malignant lesions from five patients in order to identify CNAs associated with malignant transformation (108). Recurrent DNA copy number gains were observed for a number of genes, including 1p (80%), 11q13.4 (68%), 9q34.13 (64%), 21q22.3 (60%), 6p21 (56%), 6q25 (56%) and 10q24, 19q13.2, 22q12, 5q31.2, 7p13, 10q24 and 14q22 (48%). Recurrent DNA copy number losses included 5q31.2 (35%), 16p13.2 (30%), 9q33.1 and 9q33.29 (25%) and 17q11.2, 3p26.2, 18q21.1, 4q34.1 and 8p23.2 (20%). A subset of amplified genes within the recurrent CNAs (*KHDRBS1*, *PARP1*, *RAB1A*, *HBEGF*, *PAIP2* and *BTBD7*) were subsequently validated *via* real-time PCR in an independent cohort of 32 progressing dysplasias, 21 non-progressing dysplasias and 32 SCCs. Of those, amplification of *KHDRBS1*, *HBEGF*, *PAIP2* and *BTBD7* was exclusively detected in dysplastic lesions that progressed to SCC. Finally, a recent review by Salahshourifar et al. summarized the common genomic CNAs and their frequencies for oral OPMDs and cancer as determined by aCGH. Drawing on data from a total of 12 studies, the authors observed that gains in 3q (36.5%), 5p (23%), 7p (21%), 8q (47%), 11q (45%) and 20q (31%) were most common, while losses in 3p (37%), 8p (18%), 9p (10%) and 18q (11%) were most common (109).

Summary and clinical significance: Recurrent CNAs are observed in oral OPMDs with considerable frequency. Some regions, such as 7p11.2 spanning the EGFR, are well known and show considerable promise in terms of screening, prognosis and prediction. To date, EGFR amplification has not been incorporated into clinical practice. Prior to this, additional large, multi-institutional, prospective studies are required. Several other frequent alterations have been observed in novel chromosomal regions of unknown biologic or clinical significance. Future studies of these chromosomal amplifications may identify key molecular changes and pathways critical for the progression of oral dysplasias and elucidate novel diagnostic and therapeutic strategies.

RNA ALTERATIONS IN OPMDs

mRNA EXPRESSION

Gene expression profiling using high-density microarrays (both cDNA and oligonucleotide-based arrays) allows for the rapid and comprehensive determination of mRNA transcript expression. These technologies allow for the comparison of entire transcriptomes between multiple samples of diseased and normal biospecimens. The development of these high-throughput platforms has garnered considerable interest from both basic science and clinical practice disciplines. It is anticipated that mRNA expression profiling can aid in cancer diagnosis, prognosis and prediction in response to treatment. A number of validated commercial biomarker gene sets are currently in clinical practice. For example, several gene signature tests are available for predicting metastasis-free survival and determining adjuvant therapies for breast cancer, including Oncotype DX, Mammaprint and Breast Cancer Index.

Although several expression profiling studies have been performed on OSCC (93,110–119), there has been a limited number of global gene expression profiling studies on dysplastic oral lesions. In a systematic review, AbdulMajeed and Farah identified a total of 15 studies that performed expression profiling on dysplastic or potentially malignant lesions (120). Of those, they were able to obtain data for dysregulated gene sets from nine studies. They identified a total of 31 genes that had common expression changes in at least two independent studies. The gene categories that were consistently overexpressed included components of the keratinocyte cytoskeleton network (loricrin, calmodulin-like skin protein and keratins 1, 10 and 19) and those related to immunological response (*CXCL9*, *CXCL10*, *CXCL13*, *USP18*, *IFI44* and *EVA1*). Interestingly, this expression set is composed of genes that are not generally considered to be traditional biomarkers for oral dysplasia or SCC. Whether altered expression of these genes has biologic significance or simply represents candidate surrogate biomarkers will require further investigation. In addition, a recent pilot study by Zhang et al. performed RNA sequencing (RNA-seq) on three paired cases of normal and moderately dysplastic oral mucosa. The authors identified 346 differentially expressed genes, of which 132 demonstrated upregulation while 214 were downregulated. Subsequent validation experiments suggested that interferon-stimulated gene 15 (*ISG15*) may be a candidate biomarker predicting the progression of oral dysplasia to SCC (286).

Summary and clinical significance: To date, there are limited data regarding the gene expression profiles of potentially malignant oral lesions. There are even fewer data regarding sequential changes in gene expression profiles when comparing paired samples of normal and diseased mucosa. Therefore, at this time, there are no gene panels currently available that can be used in a diagnostic, prognostic or predictive fashion for OPMDs. However, the common gene list identified by AbdulMajeed and Farah and Zhang et al. may serve to identify a cohort of genes that can be used to interrogate lesions in a more focused manner with the goal of identifying novel diagnostic or predictive biomarkers.

miRNAs

Traditionally, the non-coding regions of the human genome were classified as "junk DNA" that had little to no functional importance. However, while only 2% of the genome is ultimately translated into functional proteins, we now appreciate that 70%–75% of the human genome can be transcribed into RNA (121). Collectively, RNA molecules lacking the ability to code for proteins are referred to as non-coding (ncRNAs). This group can be further sub-classified into lncRNAs and small ncRNAs, including miRNAs and small interfering RNA. miRNAs are single-stranded RNA molecules initially described in the nematode *Caenorhabditis elegans* and are typically 20–22 nucleotides in length (122). They may be present as intergenic transcription units or found in the intronic sequences of protein-coding genes. Initially, miRNAs are transcribed as short hairpin precursors that are processed by the ribonuclease Dicer into sequences that are 20–22 nucleotides in length capable of interacting with mRNA *via* conventional base pairing interactions. miRNAs regulate gene expression *via* a number of different mechanisms, including degradation or repression of target mRNAs, binding to non-complementary regions and binding to sites located within the coding regions of transcripts. The miRBase Release 21 now contains 1881 annotated human miRNA loci (www.mirbase.org). miRNAs play an important role in a variety of physiologic and pathologic processes, including apoptosis, development and differentiation. Importantly, in the context of cancer biology, functional studies have demonstrated that miRNAs can act as conventional tumor suppressors or as oncogenes. The potential importance of miRNAs in cancer biology was first demonstrated by Calin et al., who characterized the frequent loss and downregulation of miR-15 and miR-16 in the majority of cases of chronic lymphocytic leukemia (123). An increasing number of studies have characterized the expression of miRNAs in SCC. However, the majority of these studies have employed cell lines and the candidate gene approach rather than a global approach on tissue specimens (124–130).

Cervigne et al. sought to identify changes in miRNA expression in sequential samples from 12 patients with progressive leukoplakias compared to four non-progressive leukoplakias (124). The initial expression profiles were validated in an independent cohort of progressive and non-progressive leukoplakias. In total, 109 miRNAs were identified that were exclusively expressed at high levels in the progressive leukoplakias. Of those, miR-21, miR-181b and miR-345 demonstrated consistent overexpression. Elevated expression of these miRNAs, particularly miR-21 and miR-345, was also associated with increasing grades of dysplasia as well as individual cytologic features of atypia.

Similarly, Yang et al. performed global profiling of mammalian miRNAs on tissue from eight progressing and seven non-progressing low-grade dysplasias (131). From the 754 miRNAs initially screened, 25 differentially expressed transcripts were identified in the progressing lesions when compared to the non-progressing lesions. From these, 13 were downregulated and 12 upregulated in the progressing lesions. Specifically, they observed upregulation of miR-708, miR-10b, miR-19a, miR-30e, miR-26a and miR-660 and downregulation of miR-99, miR-15a, miR-197, miR-145 and miR-150. To explore the potential diagnostic utility of miRNAs, the authors validated the expression of a subset of the differentially expressed transcripts in saliva from the same patients and demonstrated that expression of miR-10b, miR-145, miR-99b, miR-708 and miR-181c was significantly different in the saliva of progressive leukoplakia patients compared to that of non-progressive leukoplakia patients. These results show promise for using saliva miRNA signatures for monitoring of OPMDs and early detection of disease progression. Using a bioinformatics approach, Maimaiti et al. (132) searched the Gene Expression Omnibus (GEO) and ArrayExpress datasets to identify miRNA expression profiles. Unsupervised hierarchical clustering and principal component analysis identified 38 candidates that were associated with malignant transformation of oral leukoplakias. Further validation is still required to determine the diagnostic utility of this platform.

Towle et al. investigated the miRNA expression profile in a cohort of nine non-smokers who developed SCC (287). For each patient, areas of SCC, dysplasia and adjacent normal were obtained from the same contiguous disease field. These 27 samples were arrayed for the expression of 742 miRNAs. They found that some of the miRNA changes occurred across various stages of histologic progression, while other changes occurred specific to different histologic stages. This observation is particularly important when considering diagnostic markers and targeted therapies, as one would prefer to have a biomarker or target for therapy that was expressed across all stages of progression. The authors identified miR-155 as one such candidate and demonstrated that its expression was altered in the majority of dysplasia and SCC samples in a validation cohort.

Maclellan et al. (133) sought to examine the serum miRNA expression profiles in 30 patients with high-risk oral lesions compared to normal controls. They found that 15 miRNAs were upregulated while five were downregulated by a minimum of twofold change in a least 50% of the samples. Further, receiver operating characteristic (ROC) analysis demonstrated that five of these transcripts (miR-16, let-7b, miR-338-3p, miR-223 and miR-29a) had an area under the curve (AUC) >0.8, suggesting their potential utility as oral cancer screening biomarkers.

Using an 847 human miRNA array, Xiao and colleagues (134) interrogated 20 non-progressing and seven progressing oral leukoplakias for alterations in miRNA expression. In total, there were 72 upregulated and 50 downregulated miRNAs found in the progressing leukoplakias. Unsupervised hierarchical clustering analyses of the 122-miRNA subset identified 25 upregulated and nine downregulated miRNAs that could be used to discriminate between progressing and non-progressing oral leukoplakias. In particular, the authors demonstrated that upregulation of miR-31* may play an important role in progression of leukoplakias to OSCC *via* its regulation of the FGF3 pathway. Similarly, Maimaiti and colleagues (132) utilized the GEO miRNA expression database to identify miRNA profiles that might aid in the prediction of leukoplakia transformation. Using unsupervised hierarchical clustering and principal component analyses, the authors identified a panel of 38 miRNAs that were capable of discriminating between progressing and non-progressing lesions. Ultimately, a three-miRNA signature (miR-129-5p, miR-339-5p and miR-31*) was found to be a hub that mediated initiation and progression.

Zahran and colleagues demonstrated that salivary miR-184 was able to distinguish between potentially malignant oral lesions and SCC with a specificity of 75% and a sensitivity of 80%. These findings support the hypothesis that salivary miRNAs may be a rapid and non-invasive screening adjunct to aid in the delineation of dysplastic lesions versus overt SCC (135). Hung et al. demonstrated that the saliva of patients with potentially malignant lesions had significantly increased levels of miR-21 and miR-31 compared to controls, underscoring their potential in the screening setting. In addition, they demonstrated that the combination of histopathologic evidence of dysplasia, in conjunction with increased miR-31 expression, improved prognostication for predicting which lesions were likely to undergo malignant transformation (136). Finally, Philipone et al. (137) sought to identify an miRNA profile capable of identifying non-dysplastic and low-grade dysplastic oral lesions at risk of progressing to SCC. The authors determined that the combination of miR-208b-3p, miR-204-5p, miR-129-2-3p and miR-3065-5p, along with other clinical parameters, had an AUC predictive value of 0.792, a sensitivity of 76.9% and a specificity of 73.7% to accurately identify non-dysplastic and low-grade dysplastic lesions at risk of cancer progression.

Summary and clinical significance: Current data demonstrate that altered expression of miRNAs can be observed in OPMDs. A number of studies have suggested that a set of miRNAs may also have prognostic utility in predicting which OPMDs will progress to cancer. In addition, the use of a saliva-based platform for screening for OPMDs/cancer is very attractive from a clinical perspective and holds great promise. However, there is considerable variability among studies with respect to the specific miRNAs that demonstrate dysregulated expression. Therefore, larger prospective clinical trials will be required to validate the utility of miRNAs in both the diagnostic and screening realms.

LONG NON-CODING RNAs

lncRNAs are ncRNAs that are arbitrarily categorized as being longer than 200 nucleotides in length. The most recent dataset of the GENECODE project contains approximately 30,000 lncRNAs (https://www.gencodegenes.org/releases/current.html). These RNAs are thought to play critical regulatory roles in both physiologic and pathologic conditions (Figure 5.5) (138,139). Furthermore, aberrant lncRNA expression may play an important role in cancer biology and may have diagnostic/prognostic utility (140–148). There is a growing body of evidence that lncRNAs may play an important role in SCC of the oral and oropharyngeal region. A comprehensive review by Gomes et al. (149) summarized our current knowledge of lncRNAs with respect to their expression profiles, biological roles, clinicopathologic parameters and potential as biomarkers in SCC. In addition, Nohata et al. utilized the TCGA (The Cancer Genome Atlas) sequencing data to identify lncRNAs that correlated with prognosis and patient survival (150). They found 728 transcripts that were significantly and differentially expressed in SCC when compared to adjacent normal tissue. Importantly, 55 of those lncRNAs were significantly associated with decreased disease-free survival or overall survival. In addition, they identified a total of 140 lncRNA transcripts that were differentially expressed between human papillomavirus (HPV)-positive and HPV-negative SCC. These findings highlight the potential of lncRNAs in the context of

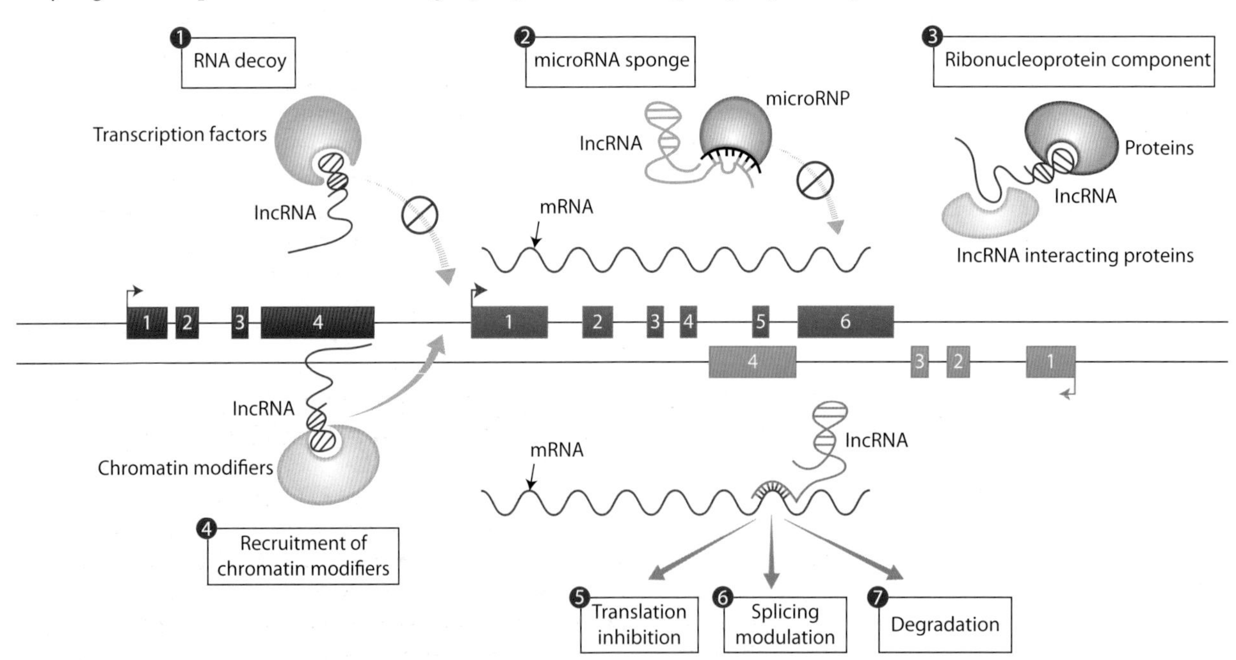

Figure 5.5 Mechanisms of long non-coding RNA (lncRNA) function. The mechanisms by which lncRNAs regulate their targets are many and varied. These include acting as RNA decoys, as microRNA target site decoys, titrating microRNA effector complexes away from their mRNA targets, binding to regulatory proteins, recruiting chromatin-modifying complexes and modulating mRNA processing. (From https://www.ncbi.nlm.nih.gov/pmc/articles/PMC3492712; reprinted with permission from John Wiley & Sons, Inc.)

diagnostic and prognostic biomarkers. Taken together, these two manuscripts underscore the importance of lncRNAs in the context of SCC and highlight the need for future studies that will further elucidate the biologic and prognostic implications of the differentially expressed lncRNAs.

Data regarding alterations of lncRNA expression in oral OPMDs are limited. Using serial analysis of gene expression, Gibb et al. sought to establish a preliminary expression map of lncRNAs in dysplastic and normal oral mucosa (151). The authors initially identified 325 unique lncRNAs that were expressed in normal oral mucosa. In dysplastic tissue, 50% (164/325) of the transcripts demonstrated a twofold or greater differential expression compared to normal. Interestingly, 12 of the lncRNAs were found only to be expressed in dysplastic mucosa. Similarly, in an effort to identify biomarkers of early disease, Conway et al. (152) sought to identify markers of early disease by performing RNA-seq on 19 matched oral mucosa samples with a diagnosis of normal, dysplasia and SCC. The authors found differences in immune cell signatures at different stages of the histologic progression. In addition, they were able to distinguish potentially early progression events, including upregulation of HOX family genes, as well as events that may be critical later in progression, such as downregulation of adherens genes. Finally, using lncRNA profile datasets from the GEO, Han et al. (153) discovered a total of 409 and 108 differentially expressed mRNAs and lncRNAs, respectively. A total of 38 potential regulatory relationships between lncRNAs and mRNAs were identified.

Summary and clinical significance: lncRNAs can exert their biological effects *via* a number of different mechanisms, including transcriptional and post-transcriptional regulation, RNA processing and epigenetic modification. Current evidence suggests that dysregulation of lncRNAs may play a central role in carcinogenesis, including SCC. Further investigation is required to better understand the specific mechanisms by which these nucleotides alter critical tumor phenotypes. In addition, it will be important that future translational research efforts investigate the utility of developing biomarker panels of lncRNAs for screening, diagnosis, prognosis and prediction.

MOLECULAR CHANGES IN SCC

Traditionally, "classical" SCC has been associated with older individuals who were chronic abusers of tobacco and alcohol. This is still largely true for the oral cavity (oral tongue, floor of the mouth, buccal mucosa and gingiva). Conversely, OPSCC (base of the tongue, tonsils and pharynx) has undergone a dramatic etiologic shift away from a carcinogen-based etiology. Today, upwards of 80% of OPSCCs in North America and Western Europe are associated with HPV infection, while other regions of the world appear to have lower incidence rates of HPV-positive tumors (154–158). Additional subsets of SCC exist, including users of betel quid and areca nut, verrucous carcinoma (VC) and individuals with no known risk factors. These are discussed in greater detail in Chapter 4. When appropriate, molecular alterations to these unique SCC variants will be compared to those observed in both the "classical" and HPV-positive SCC.

DNA ALTERATIONS IN SCC

SOMATIC MUTATIONS

The development of multiple large-scale genomic analysis platforms, including next-generation sequencing, has resulted in the generation of unprecedented datasets detailing global changes in the cancer genomic landscape. As a result, we have a markedly improved understanding of the types and frequencies of genetic alterations observed in cancer (159,160). These include changes from single-nucleotide variations to large structural rearrangements. When combined with high-level bioinformatics analyses, the interrogation of these sizable and complex datasets has led to more refined understanding of cancer drivers and their roles in tumor biology. From a clinical perspective, it is hoped that this information will aid in the identification of novel biomarkers that can improve screening, diagnosis, prognosis and treatment. Many of these data are now freely available on a number of websites, including the TCGA Data Portal (http://cancergenome.nih.gov/abouttcga), the Cancer Genomics Hub (https://cghub.ucsc.edu) and the Genomic Data Commons (https://gdc.cancer.gov).

In 2011, two research groups published the first exome sequencing results on a total of 124 unique HNSCC (head and neck squamous cell carcinoma) tumor samples (161,162). A number of important observations were made from these initial efforts. First, both studies reported that *TP53* is the most frequently mutated gene in HNSCC. Secondly, HPV-negative tumors harbored more somatic mutations than HPV-positive tumors. However, in additional studies, the mutational burden in HPV-negative and HPV-positive tumors was similar (163,164). This apparent discrepancy is likely related to the extent of sequencing, depth of sequencing and bioinformatics. Furthermore, HPV-positive patients with a history of significant tobacco use have significantly higher mutational burdens compared to non-smoking HPV-positive patients (163,164). Third, several genes previously proposed as playing critical roles in SCC (*TP53*, *CDKN2A* and *PIK3CA*) were found to be mutated with sufficient frequency to support their potential role as drivers in cancer development. Lastly, a number of novel and potentially targetable genetic alterations were identified, particularly *NOTCH1* and its associated pathways and *FAT1* (165). These findings were also observed in a number of subsequent studies (166–168).

Subsequently, the Cancer Genome Atlas Network (163) published their large-scale sequencing of 275 tumors that provided the most comprehensive picture of the mutational

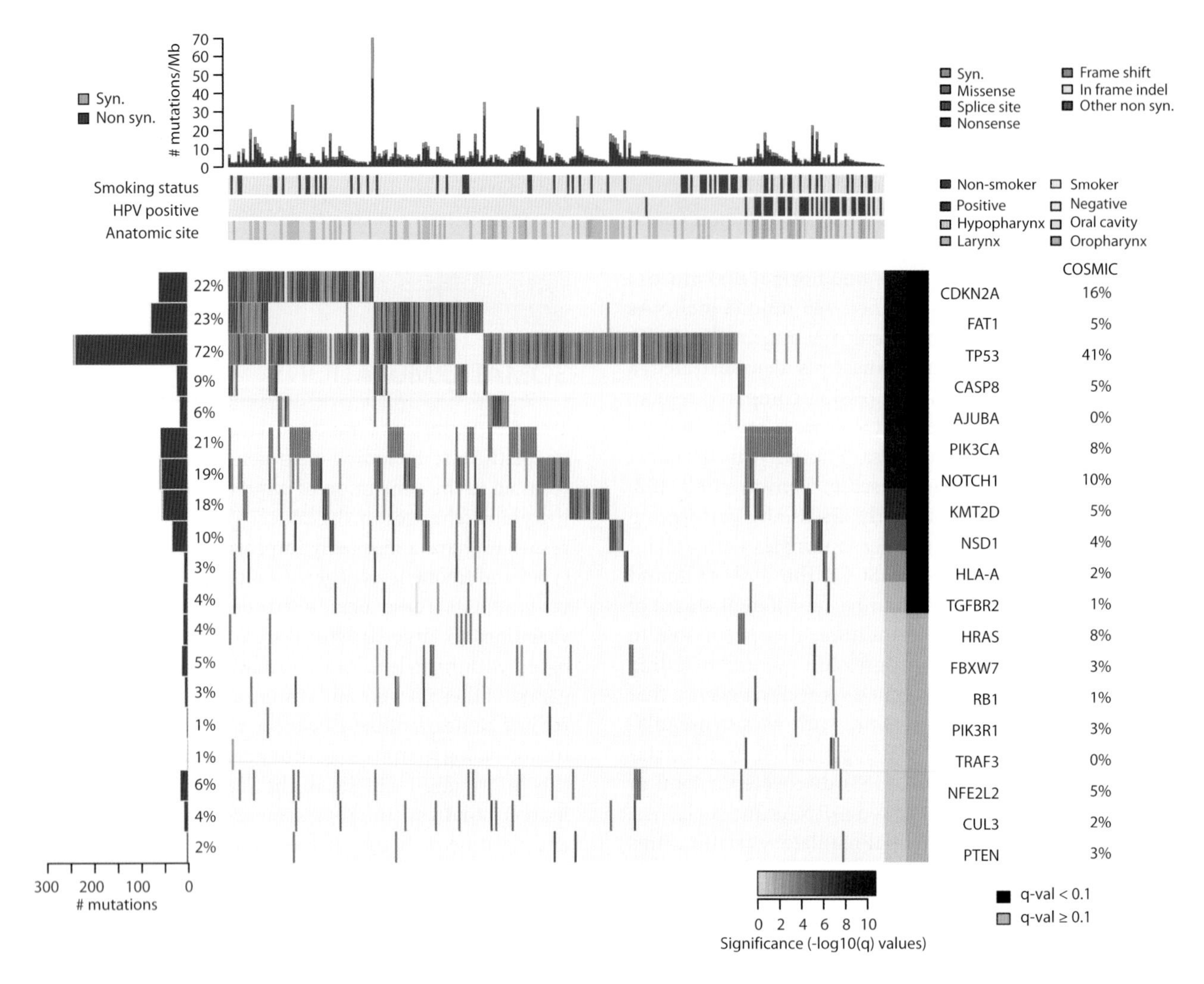

Figure 5.6 Somatic gene mutations in squamous cell carcinoma. Data from the head and neck cancer The Cancer Genome Atlas (TCGA) project underscore the considerable intratumoral genetic variability among tumors as demonstrated by the variable somatic gene mutation rates. In addition, clear differences in genetic alterations are observed when comparing human papillomavirus (HPV)-positive and HPV-negative tumors. (From https://www.ncbi.nlm.nih.gov/pubmed/25631445; reprinted with permission from SpringerNature.)

landscape of SCC. Several important points regarding this study require emphasis. First, as demonstrated in Figure 5.6, aside from the high incidence of *TP53* mutations, the mutational frequency for the next most common genes ranged from 1% to 23%. These findings suggest that, while the histopathologic diagnosis is the same (SCC), there is considerable intertumoral variability with respect to the specific mutations harbored in a given tumor. Second, the alterations observed between HPV-positive and HPV-negative tumors were considerably different. For example, HPV-negative tumors often harbored *TP53* mutations, *CCND1*, *PIK3CA*, *EGFR* and *FGFR1* amplifications and *CDKN2A* deletions. Conversely, HPV-positive tumors typically demonstrated *PIK3CA* amplifications/deletions and *FGFR3* mutations. These observations may have some generalizability across the world, as many of these mutations have also been identified in patient cohorts from a number of different countries, including, Taiwan, China and India (169–171). However, Vettore et al. (171) found that SCC samples from Singapore demonstrated frequent mutations in *DST* and *RNF213* and had less frequent alterations in *CDKN2A* and *NOTCH1*.

In general, tobacco-associated SCC of the oral cavity is occurring with decreasing frequency, while HPV-associated OPSCC is dramatically increasing (155). One exception to this generalization appears to be restricted to SCC of the oral tongue in younger individuals (172–174). This cohort of patients tends to be non-smokers with HPV-negative tumors. There has been considerable interest in whether this group demonstrates a unique genomic profile that might provide implications for etiology as well as for identifying novel therapeutic opportunities. Recently, Pickering et al. performed whole-exome sequencing and CNA analysis on tongue SCCs from non-smoking patients under the age of 45 and compared these findings to an independent cohort of older smoking SCC patients (175). Surprisingly, the genomic profiles of the two cohorts were very similar in terms of the number and types of mutations, including *TP53* alterations. However, caution should be exercised, as the sample size was limited. To emphasize this point, Pickering et al.'s findings are at odds with those of Li et al. (176), who observed the opposite when performing exome sequencing on patients with SCC who were non-smokers. For example, they found that non-smoker patients had fewer *TP53* mutations.

VC is a diagnostically challenging subset of SCC. Its diagnosis has important clinical implications as VC is thought to have a less aggressive clinical course, as these tumors rarely develop regional or distant metastases. Samman et al. (177) compared the molecular signature of VC to SCC. Exome sequencing of VC tumors found a lack of mutation in genes that are commonly mutated in SCC, including *TP53*, *NOTCH1*, *CDKN2a* and *FAT1*. Conversely, there were a number of genes (*DSPP*, *MUC4* and *ANP32E*) harboring mutations in VC that were rarely found in SCC. These findings suggest that while possessing obvious histopathological similarities, SCC and VC are different on a molecular level, supporting the hypothesis that SCC and VC should be considered distinct entities.

There has been considerable interest in identifying cancer-associated genes that have "druggable" potential (178). EGFR is overexpressed in 80%–90% of HNSCCs and cetuximab is the only U.S. Food and Drug Administration (FDA)-approved targeted agent of use against HNSCC, with modest overall impact. As additional examples of research evaluating targeted therapy in HNSCC, Lui et al. (179) sought to identify mutational events in the major mitogenic pathways that are thought to play a role in SCC. The PI3K pathway was found to be mutated ~30% of the time, particularly in advanced (stage IV) tumors. Importantly, tumor cells harboring a PI3K mutation demonstrated enhanced *in vivo* sensitivity to PI3K inhibition, suggesting that targeting of this pathway may have therapeutic benefit. Similarly, Sun et al. investigated the comprehensive molecular alterations of the *NOTCH1* signaling pathway in a cohort of 44 HNSCC tumors. They found a bimodal pattern of alteration in HNSCC. One subgroup of tumors was found to have inactivating loss of function mutations in the NOTCH pathway. Conversely, a larger group of tumors was found to demonstrate an increase/gain of NOTCH function by way of ligand receptor copy number increases, increased expression and downstream pathway activation (180). Similarly, analysis of whole-exome sequencing and reverse-phase protein array data by Lui et al. (181) demonstrated that receptor-like protein tyrosine phosphatases (PTPRT) were frequently (30%) mutated in SCC. Importantly, these mutations were associated with increased STAT3 signaling. Activation of STAT3 signaling is regularly observed in many cancers, including SCC, and is associated with reduced survival. The oncogenic importance of constitutive STAT3 expression and the identification of a high PTPRT mutation rate suggest that patients with PTPRT mutations may be responsive to STAT3 pathway inhibitors.

There is also an increasing number of publications that have identified classes or panels of mutations that may have prognostic and diagnostic utility. For example, Tinhofer et al. (182) performed targeted next-generation sequencing of locally advanced HPV-positive and HPV-negative SCC and found that activating mutations in *PIK3CA*, *KRAS*, *NRAS* and *HRAS* identified a subgroup of patients with HPV-positive SCC that are associated with reduced overall survival after adjuvant chemoradiation. Seeking to define the mutational landscape of recurrent and metastatic SCC, Morris et al. (165) performed next-generation sequencing on advanced treatment-resistant head and neck cancers. The genetic profiles of the tumors were quite distinct when compared to the matched primary tumors. For example, recurrent and metastatic HPV-positive tumors exhibited profiles that were more similar to HPV-negative tumors as characterized by *TP53* mutations, whole-genome duplications and chromosome 3p deletions. These findings suggest that the molecular landscape of recurrent and metastatic SCC can be quite variable and this may influence how one approaches treatment in the advanced stage/recurrent setting. In addition, Chen et al. (183) performed next-generation sequencing on 345 patients with advanced-stage oral cavity SCC (OCSCC), focusing on 45 cancer-related genes. A mutation-based signature of 10 genes (*HRAS*, *BRAF*, *FGFR3*, *SMAD4*, *KIT*, *PTEN*, *NOTCH1*, *AKT1*, *CTNNB1* and *PTPN11*) was found to be an independent predictor of decreased disease-free survival. Similarly, Gross et al. (184) reported that the combination of a *TP53* mutation and loss of chromosome 3p was associated with a significantly decreased survival time. Finally, using whole-exome sequencing, Hedberg et al. (185) examined the intertumoral genetic heterogeneity in synchronous nodal metastasis and metachronous recurrent SCC across 23 patients. They found that there was a greater degree of intertumoral genetic heterogeneity in metachronous recurrence versus synchronous nodal metastasis. These findings support the concept of field cancerization (186).

Tumor heterogeneity is essential for the development of critical tumor phenotypes such as metastasis and drug resistance but it is a poor prognostic indicator and a major therapeutic challenge (187–191). The significant genomic alterations and instability observed in SCC further signify the possibility of extensive molecular heterogeneity among and within individual tumors. Mroz et al. (192) determined the Mutant-Allele Tumor Heterogeneity (MATH) score in a cohort of 74 SCC samples and compared this to clinical, pathological and overall survival data. High MATH scores were significantly associated with tumor progression, adverse treatment outcomes and decreased overall survival, supporting the hypothesis that tumors with a greater degree of heterogeneity result in poor clinical outcome. Using the same dataset, Mroz et al. (192) identified three different subgroups with poor prognosis that had high MATH scores: tumors with disruptive *TP53* mutations, tumors negative for HPV and smokers with HPV-negative tumors. In a follow-up study of whole-exome sequencing data on 305 patients from the TCGA project, Mroz et al. (193) calculated MATH scores to determine whether intratumoral heterogeneity affected patient mortality. As in their previous study, the authors found that high MATH values correlated with decreased overall survival. They also demonstrated that the relationship between intratumoral heterogeneity and survival was not associated with other factors, including patient age, HPV status, *TP53* mutation, tumor grade or N classification. These findings suggest that MATH scores may be of prognostic value. However, additional prospective studies are required, as this study utilized a retrospective dataset. Using an alternative novel computational approach termed "evolutionary action" (EAp53), Neskey et al. (194) sought to stratify survival and risk of distant metastasis based on the specific type of *TP53* mutation present in the patient's primary tumor. Similarly, Osman et al. (195) used EAp53 to identify a subset of *TP53* mutations that were associated with decreased sensitivity to cisplatin, suggesting that EAp53 may aid in defining the most appropriate treatment.

In addition to therapeutic and prognostic utility, somatic mutations may also play a role in diagnostic assays. To explore the potential of using tumor-specific DNA as a biomarker for SCC, Wang et al. (196) interrogated DNA samples that were derived from saliva or plasma from 93 SCC patients for somatic mutations, including HPV. Saliva-derived DNA was most accurate for detecting OCSCC, while plasma-derived DNA was more useful for detecting oropharynx, larynx and hypopharynx SCC. Importantly, tumor DNA was identified in some patients post-surgically prior to any clinical evidence of recurrence. These findings suggest that saliva and plasma tumor DNA may be useful for HNSCC screening, monitoring during treatment as a marker of tumor burden and surveillance after completion of treatment to detect persistent or recurrent minimal residual disease.

Summary and clinical significance: Genetic alterations are characteristics of human cancers, including HNSCC. DNA alterations, including somatic mutations, CNAs, LOH and epigenetic changes, characterize the genome of cancer cells. Beyond the contribution of somatic mutations to HNSCC pathogenesis, somatic mutations play a role in the development of targeted therapy, prognostication and the development of diagnostics assays in HNSCC.

LOSS OF HETEROZYGOSITY

As discussed above, LOH profiles have been extensively characterized in potentially malignant oral lesions. In the context of SCC, LOH at several regions (2q, 3p, 4q, 6q25–27, 8p, 8p21.2, 8p23, 9p21–22, 10q, 11q23, 13q, 14q, 17p and 18q) is associated with poor prognosis, including increased risk of recurrence and decreased survival (29,197–204).

Summary and clinical significance: LOH is a common genetic event in cancer development, including HNSCC, and most importantly indicates the loss of tumor suppressor genes, which are discussed above.

METHYLATION

Aberrant gene promoter methylation is considered to be an early event and a required event for the development of SCC, as altered methylation patterns are both persistent and increase during progression from dysplasia to SCC. As with "premalignant" disease, many methylation studies have focused on individual or small subsets of genes. A recent review of these studies by Koffler and colleagues (205) summarized the literature with respect to the predictive value of gene promoter methylation in SCC. They identified different methylation patterns associated with a number of pathologic features including lymph node metastasis (*CDKN2A*, *DAPK1*, *MGMT* and *MLH1*), treatment response (*CHD1*, *DAPK1*, *NEFL* and *TIMP3*), progression-free survival (*CCNA1*, *MGMT*, *GAL*, *GALR1*, *TAC*, *TACR1* and *TIMP3*) and overall survival (*CDH1*, *CDKN2A*, *CSPG4*, *DCC*, *MGMT* and *MINT31*). Overall, the predictive value of these methylation patterns appears to be related to a significant correlation between promoter methylation and resistance to either radiation or specific chemotherapies such as cisplatin, cetuximab and erlotinib.

Several global methylation studies have also been recently performed. Using restriction landmark genomic scanning, Bennett et al. identified a number of genes (Septin 9, *SLCFA8*, *FUSSEL18*, *EBF3* and *IRX1*) that were hypermethylated in as many as 67% of the samples examined (206,207). These genes are involved in the TGF-β pathway and their disruption appears to be associated with malignant transformation as determined by reduced apoptosis and increased proliferation (208,209). Carvalho et al. (210) demonstrated that detection of hypermethylated DNA for a subset of genes (*DAPK*, *DCC*, *MINT31*, *TIMP3*, *p16*, *MGMT* and *CCNA1*) in pretreatment saliva samples was predictive of local recurrence and overall survival. Jithesh et al. (211) employed the Illumnia GoldenGate high-throughput array to assay the methylation patterns of 44 SCCs and their matched normal control tissues. Significant epigenetic downregulation of the NOTCH signaling pathway was observed, suggesting there may be several mechanisms by which NOTCH is downregulated in SCC. In addition, differential methylation patterns were observed and putative methylation signatures for extracapsular lymph node extension and recurrence were identified. Using discovery and validation cohorts of 91 and 101 patients, respectively, Poage et al. (212) used an array-based approach to determine if methylation profiles of sets of phenotypically characterized DNA sequence elements were associated with survival. They found that hypermethylation associated with the *TAP1* and *ALDH3A1* genes was associated with reduced survival, suggesting that methylation patterns have prognostic value. Guerrero-Preston et al. (213) determined global methylation patterns in SCC compared to matched normal tissue samples. They identified 186 downregulated genes, including known as well as novel tumor suppressor genes. These findings support the contention that, in addition to somatic mutations, promoter methylation of important tumor suppressor genes may play a significant role in the mechanism of SCC development.

However, there is also evidence of variability in methylation patterns in SCC. For example, several studies have reported differences in methylation patterns when comparing HPV-positive and HPV-negative SCC (214,215). Similarly, methylation patterns have been shown to vary significantly across different anatomic subsites of SCC (216). Conversely, Basu et al. (217) determined the global methylation patterns of SCC patients in India and found that they were approximately 95% similar to those found in the TCGA data. Of note was that approximately 5% of the genes were uniquely different in the Indian population. This might be attributable to differences in oral habits in the Indian population.

Summary and clinical significance: Promoter methylation is an important physiologic and pathologic mechanism of gene regulation. Therefore, methylation profiling of tumor samples may provide important diagnostic, predictive and prognostic information. However, most studies have investigated only a small number of candidate genes.

COPY NUMBER ALTERATIONS

As with potentially malignant lesions, a number of studies have investigated the CNA landscape for SCC. In general, copy number gains have been observed in 3p, 6p, 8q, 11q, 16p and 17q. Conversely, reproducible losses are observed in 2q, 3p, 4q, 8p, 9p, 11q and 18q (163,164,203,218–221). Salahshourifar et al. (109) summarized 12 studies that had interrogated SCC samples *via* aCGH. The most common gains were at 3q (36%), 5p (23%), 7p (21%), 8q (47%), 11q (45%) and 20q (31%), while the most common losses were at 3p (37%), 8p (18%) and 18q (11%). Similar CNAs were also observed by Pickering et al. as part of the integrative genomic characterization of SCC (203). HPV-negative and HPV-positive SCCs have been shown to have both similar and unique CNAs. However, some differences do exist. For example, loss of 14q32 and 11q has been observed with far greater frequency in HPV-positive tumors (163).

From a diagnostic perspective, CNAs have also been reported to be of prognostic value in predicting recurrence and/or decreased overall survival (222–225).

In addition, in order to investigate the mechanisms of metastasis, Morita et al. (226) compared the genetic profiles of paired primary and metastatic SCC of the tongue using high-density single-nucleotide polymorphism microarrays. The authors found considerable similarity between the primary and metastatic lesions. However, 20q11.2 gain, which codes for the *E2F1* gene, was only observed in metastatic lesions, suggesting that overexpression of this gene may be critical for the metastatic phenotype in SCC.

CNAs have also been used to investigate the differences between SCC and VC. Samman et al. (177) found that VC did not demonstrate the typical alterations found in SCC, such as gains of 3q and losses of 3p. Therefore, as with the somatic mutation findings described above, the CNA data suggest that VC may be a unique type of malignancy that is biologically and clinically distinct from SCC.

Summary and clinical significance: Most HNSCCs demonstrate CNAs, including losses of 3p and 8p and gains of 3q, 5p, 8q and 11q. The oncogene and tumor suppressor gene targets and functional roles of these CNAs will further elucidate their critical roles in oncogenesis, diagnostics and therapeutics.

RNA ALTERATIONS IN SCC

mRNA EXPRESSION

Alterations at the genomic level, owing to mutations or large structural rearrangements, ultimately lead to extensive changes in the expression profile of mRNA transcripts in SCC. Changes at the transcript levels are thus indicative of the clinical relevance of the genomic changes and their significance in the carcinogenic process. Chung et al. (227) determined the gene expression profiles of 60 SCC samples, allowing for the categorization of tumors into four independent subtypes that demonstrated differences in recurrence-free survival. In addition, supervised analyses were able to predict lymph node metastasis with 80% accuracy. Similarly, Liu et al. (228) identified differential gene expression profiles of primary and metastatic SCCs. Upregulation of *CCL19*, *CD2*, *EGR2*, *FUCA1*, *RGS1*, *SELL*, *MMPs*, *uPA*, *TNC* and Integrin-α and downregulation of *IGFBP6* and *KLK8* were subsequently validated to be associated with the presence of lymph node metastasis. Nguyen et al. (229) identified an eight-gene panel (*DCTD*, *IL15*, *THBD*, *GSDML*, *SH3GL3*, *PTHLH*, *RP5-1022P6* and *C9irf46*) that was predictive of cervical lymph node metastasis in OCSCC. Gene expression profiles have also been utilized to identify genes that were predictive of T stage, depth of invasion, progression and survival (230). Similarly, using integrated genomic analysis, Walter et al. (231) identified four gene expression subtypes of SCC characterized as basal, mesenchymal, atypical and classical. Importantly, they demonstrated that these subtypes had biological and clinical relevance. In SCC of the tongue, profiling of responder versus non-responder patients has identified a potential gene panel (*COL5A1*, *HBB*, *IGLA* and *TSC*) that may be predictive of treatment response (232).

Expression profiling has also been used to stratify tumors based upon different etiologies. For example, profiling has identified that multiple subtypes of HPV-positive and HPV-negative SCC may exist (233–235). Similarly, Farshadpour et al. sought to identify differences in genetic profiles between patients who were either smokers/drinkers or non-smokers/non-drinkers (236). Analysis of the microarray data revealed 49 differentially expressed genes. In the non-smoking/non-drinking group, there were seven genes associated with the interferon-γ (IFN-γ) pathway that were activated. Unfortunately, the HPV status of the non-smoker/non-drinker cohort was not determined. This is particularly relevant in this study as HPV infection is known to induce the secretion of various inflammatory cytokines, including IFN-γ. The largest percentage of SCC occurs in Asia, where habits such as betel quid chewing are somewhat unique when compared to North America and Western Europe. As such, observations made regarding the SCC mRNA expression alterations may be different. Saeed et al. compared the gene expression profiles of SCC samples from the U.K. and Sri Lanka (237). In many respects, the gene expression profiles were very similar. However, the

U.K. tumors demonstrated expression patterns that were more associated with tumor invasion and metastases, while the Sri Lanka tumors demonstrated a more activated cell-mediated immune response. This is in keeping with the accepted clinical course of SCCs in Asian countries, which tend to be more exophytic with local extension compared to SCCs of Western countries, often being more invasive and with a greater propensity for regional and distant metastasis.

Roepman et al. (238) demonstrated that expression profiling improved the prediction of lymph node metastasis in the clinical N0 neck when compared to standard methods. Importantly, no false-negative predictions were made in this study. In a follow-up to their initial study, van Hooff et al. (239) sought to validate their gene expression profile in a larger cohort of node-positive and node-negative disease in OCSCC and OPSCC. They found that incorporation of the panel with current clinical assessment protocols decreased the rate of undetected nodal metastasis from 28% to 11% in early-stage OCSCC. While these findings were preliminary in nature, they do underscore the potential for incorporating molecular diagnostics into the treatment decision process with respect to managing patients with clinical N0 necks.

Summary and clinical significance: We now have a wealth of mRNA expression data that will be used to distinguish subclasses of HNSCC with different biologies and different clinical properties to stratify prognostic, diagnostic and therapeutic information and deliver personalized care.

miRNAs

Similar to OPMDs, altered miRNA expression has been observed in SCC (127,240–243). In general, downregulated miRNAs act as tumor suppressor genes, while upregulated miRNAs typically act as oncogenes. A number of publications have investigated the global expression changes of miRNA in SCC patient samples (244–252). In summary, these reports have identified several hundred different miRNAs that have aberrant expression in SCC. However, while there is some overlap, there is considerable variability among the different profiles reported. The variability among these signatures is likely multifactorial, including variable etiologies. For example, HPV-positive SCC miRNA profiles are closer to those of cervical cancers than HPV-negative SCC miRNA profiles (129). Other differences are likely attributable to additional variables, including different platforms used (TaqMan, Affymetrix and Illumina), differences in patient populations and quality/composition of specimens. Similarly, Towle et al. evaluated the expression of 742 miRNAs in tissue samples from non-smokers who had developed SCC of the oral cavity. Many of the same miRNAs with altered expression in this study are found to be dysregulated in the SCC samples derived from patients who are smokers, suggesting that the mechanisms of inactivation/activation may have mechanistic similarities (287).

A number of studies have investigated the diagnostic utility of miRNA panels. For example, Ries et al. (253) identified a 21-miRNA panel that could differentiate between normal oral mucosa and OCSCC. Similarly, Maclellan et al. (133) demonstrated that differential expression of miR-16, let-7b, miR-338-3p, miR-223 and miR-29a in the serum of patients with high-risk oral lesions was a useful biomarker for identifying patients with SCC. Lin et al. (254) reported that plasma levels of miR-24 were significantly higher in patients with OCSCC when compared to healthy controls. Zahran et al. (135) sought to identify the diagnostic utility of miRNAs for identifying malignant transformation in a cohort of patients with OPMDs and SCC. When compared to controls and OPMDs, increased expression of miR-184 was observed in SCC, suggesting its potential in screening for SCC. Importantly, the authors also demonstrated that while miR-21 was significantly overexpressed in OPMDs and SCC, there were no increased levels in healthy controls of individuals with inflammatory lesions. This is an important preliminary finding as it suggests that expression of salivary miR-21 may help the general dentist/primary care physician in discriminating between common inflammatory lesions and OPMDs/early SCCs. Finally, there are limited data regarding the potential utility of miRNAs to improve the diagnosis of surgical margins. Santhi et al. (255) reported increased expression of miR-96 and decreased expression of miR-16, miR-125a and miR-184 at the surgical margins of recurrent lesions.

miRNA expression profiles are also being investigated for their prognostic utility and have been reported to correlate with certain clinical features, including clinical stage, metastasis and survival. For example, expression of miR-21 has been associated with advanced clinical stage, nodal disease and survival (256,257). In addition, altered expression of a number of other miRNAs, including let-7, miR-31, miR-17, miR-125b, miR-155, miR-181, miR-205, miR-375 and miR-491, has been found to be associated with poor survival (125,258–263).

Peng et al. (264) evaluated the expression of 760 miRNAs for prognostic significance in OCSCC. They found that differential expression of miR-218, miR-125b and let-7g held prognostic significance for disease-free survival, suggesting that reduced expression of these miRNAs may improve prognostic stratification. Ganci et al. (265) determined that increased expression of miR-21-3p, miR-96-5p, miR-141-3p and miR-130-3p was associated with shorter recurrence-free survival. Wong et al. (266) utilized the TCGA data to identify a set of prognostic biomarkers of OPSCC and OCSCC. They identified increased expression of miR-193b-3pj and miR-455-5p as being positively associated with OPSCC survival and miR-92a-39 and miR-497-5p as being negatively associated with OPSCC survival. Importantly, this model was able to further stratify HPV-positive patients into low-risk and high-risk cohorts. This is an important observation. In general, HPV-positive patients have a better prognosis. However, there is growing appreciation of survival heterogeneity among HPV-positive patients. Therefore, further validation of the risk stratification by Wong and colleagues may provide us with improved prognostic capabilities and treatment options for HPV-positive patients. Scapoli et al. further identified an association with progression and metastasis in OCSCC and the downregulation of miR-155, miR-146a and let-7i (267). Li et al. (257) demonstrated that upregulation of miR-21 was positively correlated with advanced clinical stage, lymph node metastasis and decreased overall survival. A panel of 12 miRNAs has also been identified that is an independent prognosticator of recurrence-free survival and a panel of four miRNAs that correlates with cancer-specific survival (268).

There is also evidence that changes in miRNA expression patterns may correlate with resistance to therapy. For example, Dai et al. (269) reported that upregulation of miR-101, miR-181a, miR-181d and miR-195, combined with the downregulation of miR-100, miR-130a and miR-197, was consistent with resistance to chemotherapy. Similarly, Sun et al. (270) found that decreased expression of miR-15b and miR-200b was associated with radioresistance. Finally, chemoradioresistance has been associated with increased expression of miR-196a (271).

Similar to OPMDs, there is considerable interest in the possibility of detecting salivary miRNAs in the context of cancer screening and monitoring of disease. Park et al. (272) characterized the profile of miRNA in saliva and evaluated its potential as an oral cancer biomarker. From a total of 314 miRNAs measured, miR-125a and miR-200a were found to be significantly lower in the saliva of patients with cancer when compared to normal controls. In addition, aberrant methylation of miR-375, miR-200a and miR-200c-141 could distinguish oral cancer patients using oral rinses as well as saliva, suggesting a potential clinical application (273). Further, Liu et al. (261) determined that increased levels of salivary miR-31 were detectable at all clinical stages of SCC. Similarly, increased levels of salivary miR-27b have also been identified in patients with SCC (274). Using a genome-wide approach, Momen-Heravi et al. (274) examined the differential expression of more than 700 miRNAs in saliva from patients categorized into four different groups: healthy controls, lichen planus, SCC and in remission following treatment for SCC. The authors identified a panel of 13 miRNAs that were significantly downregulated and two miRNAs that were significantly upregulated in SCC when compared to healthy controls. Importantly, miR-27b was significantly upregulated in SCC when compared to each of the other three groups (healthy controls, lichen planus and SCC in remission). These findings suggest that salivary miR-27b may have clinical utility in both screening and monitoring. In most studies, miR-31 has been found to be upregulated in SCC, suggesting that it may have screening/detection utility. Liu et al. (261) analyzed salivary levels of miR-31 in patients with SCC. Relative to control patient saliva, miR-31 was significantly higher at all stages of SCC. In addition, salivary levels of miR-31 were significantly reduced following excision of the tumor. These findings suggest that salivary miR-31 is an additional candidate biomarker for screening and monitoring.

Summary and clinical significance: Current data demonstrate that there are numerous miRNAs whose expression is altered in SCC. A number of studies have suggested that a set of miRNAs may also have prognostic and predictive utility. In addition, the use of a saliva-based platform for screening for OPMDs/cancer is very attractive from a clinical perspective and holds great promise. However, there is considerable variability among studies with respect to the specific miRNAs that demonstrate dysregulated expression. Therefore, larger prospective clinical trials will be required in order to validate the utility of miRNAs in both the diagnostic and screening realms.

LONG NON-CODING RNA

There is a growing body of evidence that lncRNAs may play an important role in SCC of the oral and oropharyngeal region. A comprehensive review by Gomes et al. (149) summarized our current knowledge of lncRNAs with respect to their expression profiles, biological roles, clinicopathologic parameters and potential as biomarkers. Some of these include *HOTAIR*, *NEAT1*, *UCA1*, *MALAT1*, *MBL2-4:3* and *AL355149.1-1*. In addition, by using the Atlas of Noncoding RNAs in Cancer (TANRIC) to obtain lncRNA expression data from the TCGA HNSCC database, Nohata et al. sought to identify dysregulated expression of lncRNAs during SCC progression by comparing sequence data from 42 adjacent normal oral tissues and 426 SCCs (150). They identified a total of 728 lncRNA transcripts that were significantly and differentially expressed in SCC. Of those, 55 lncRNAs were significantly associated with decreased disease-free survival and/or overall survival. Many of these were linked to important cellular events such as the cell cycle, spliceosome, endocytosis, actin cytoskeleton regulation and several important genetic signaling pathways, including Wnt, VEGF, neurotrophin and NOTCH. In addition, 140 lncRNA transcripts were found to be differentially expressed between HPV-positive and HPV-negative SCCs. Taken together, these two manuscripts underscore the importance of lncRNAs in the context of SCC and highlight the need for future studies that will further elucidate the biologic and prognostic implications of the differentially expressed lncRNAs.

Summary and clinical significance: The investigation of lncRNAs in SCC is still at the initial stages of inquiry and considerably more work regarding their biological roles as well as their potential utility as diagnostic/prognostic markers is required. Further investigation in order to understand their mechanisms of action during the development of SCC and whether they also have potential as biomarkers is necessary.

PROTEIN ALTERATIONS IN SCC

Proteomic profiling using advanced technologies such as mass spectrometry, isobaric tagging for relative and absolute protein quantification (iTRAQ)-liquid chromatography–tandem mass spectrometry (LC–MS/MS) and Matrix Assisted Laser Desorption/Ionization Time of Flight (MALDI-TOF) have allowed for the global characterization of protein profiles of SCC. In general, there has been considerable variability among multiple studies regarding the profiles of differentially expressed proteins and none have been sufficiently validated for their diagnostic utility or in the point-of-care setting.

Ralhan et al. (275,276) identified several candidate biomarkers when comparing inflamed oral mucosa, dysplasia and SCC. Patel et al. (173) performed laser capture microdissection and proteomic analyses to identify novel SCC molecular targets and candidate biomarkers. The authors identified ~100 proteins in tumor tissues that were involved in cell migration, signaling, proteolysis, DNA synthesis, metabolism and cell signaling. Wang et al. (277) determined differences in protein expression in paired SCC and control samples. Using two-dimensional electrophoresis and mass spectrometry, the authors identified a total of 85 proteins that demonstrated twofold or greater changes in the samples. In this group, 53 were upregulated and 32 were downregulated. The proteins were involved in various tumor-associated pathways including apoptosis, proliferation and metabolism, supporting the hypothesis that these proteins were important for malignant transformation. Similarly, Xiao et al. (278) sought to identify cancer biomarkers for oral epithelium utilizing liquid chromatography-mass spectrometry on laser capture microdissected tissue samples. Of the 500 proteins identified, 17 were consistently up- or down-regulated in SCC when compared to normal oral mucosa. Of these candidate biomarkers, a significant decrease in cornulin protein expression was observed in both tissue and saliva samples from patients with SCC.

As one would expect, there appears to be a number of proteomic differences when comparing HPV-positive and HPV-negative tumors. For example, Melle et al. (279) performed peptide fingerprint mapping and surface-enhanced laser desorption/ionization mass spectrometry (SELDI-MS) on proteins isolated from microdissected cells from HPV-positive and HPV-negative tumors. They identified thioredoxin and epidermal fatty acid binding proteins as being differentially regulated in HPV-positive SCC. In addition, Slebos et al. (280) performed a proteomic analysis on HPV-positive and HPV-negative OPSCC samples. For HPV-negative tumors, analysis revealed an enrichment of proteins involved in epithelial cell development and extracellular matrix organization. Conversely, HPV-positive tumors demonstrated enrichment for DNA initiation and replication and cell cycle control such as E2F1 and E2F4.

Given the long-standing use of immunohistochemistry in diagnostic pathology, there has been considerable interest in identifying biomarkers that could be easily added to this existing laboratory platform and provide prognostic and predictive information. Harris et al. (281) sought to identify differentially expressed proteins that were associated with poor outcome in patients with OCSCC. Using two-dimensional gel electrophoresis, the authors identified 72 peptide features that were associated with either disease-specific death, distant metastasis or locoregional recurrence. In particular, reduced expression of *DSP*, *PKP1* and *TRIM29* was associated with a significantly increased risk of distant metastasis. In addition, reduced expression of *PKP1* and *TRIM29* correlated with decreased disease-free survival. Skinner et al. (282) performed a systematic proteomic analysis in order to identify markers of radioresistance in HPV-negative SCC. Focusing specifically on proteins having the potential to be targeted with agents currently undergoing investigation in clinical trials, the authors identified several proteins that were associated with radioresistance. These included FGFR1, ERK1, EGFR and FAK. Experimental inhibition of FAK resulted in significant radiosensitization of SCC tumor cell lines. Furthermore, FAK expression was significantly associated with outcome in patients with locally advance SCC who were treated with radiation. Further, Chauhan et al. (283) sought to identify protein-based prognostic biomarkers for SCC. Using a discovery cohort ($n = 282$) from India and a validation cohort ($n = 135$) from Canada, the authors sought to correlate the expression of candidate proteins in order to develop a predictive model of recurrence. The expression of PTMA, S100A7 and hnRNPK was strongly associated with prediction of 3-year recurrence-free survival. Finally, Schaaij-Visser et al. (284) sought to discover and validate protein biomarkers capable of predicting local relapse. The authors performed proteomic analysis on paired normal, dysplastic and tumor tissues. The diagnostic utility of candidate biomarkers was evaluated *via* immunohistochemistry on 222 surgical margins from 46 patients who underwent excisions for SCC that were either disease free or had relapsed. Expression of both cornulin and keratin 4 at the surgical margins was found to be significantly predictive of relapse.

Summary and clinical significance: Validation of these markers/pathways in patient cohorts is essential to establishing their clinical benefit and thereby adopting them into the concept of personalized medicine. Randomized patient trials that enable administration of drugs based on molecular profile and observational studies that correlate the marker status with the clinical outcome will help establish a panel of clinically viable biomarkers.

REFERENCES

1. Hanahan D, Weinberg RA. Hallmarks of cancer: the next generation. *Cell* 2011;144(5):646–74.
2. Abbey LM, Kaugars GE, Gunsolley JC et al. The effect of clinical information on the histopathologic diagnosis of oral epithelial dysplasia. *Oral Surg Oral Med Oral Pathol Oral Radiol Endod* 1998;85(1):74–7.
3. Abbey LM, Kaugars GE, Gunsolley JC et al. Intraexaminer and interexaminer reliability in the diagnosis of oral epithelial dysplasia. *Oral Surg Oral Med Oral Pathol Oral Radiol Endod* 1995;80(2):188–91.
4. Fischer DJ, Epstein JB, Morton TH, Schwartz SM. Interobserver reliability in the histopathologic diagnosis of oral pre-malignant and malignant lesions. *J Oral Pathol Med* 2004;33(2):65–70.

5. Karabulut A, Reibel J, Therkildsen MH, Praetorius F, Nielsen HW, Dabelsteen E. Observer variability in the histologic assessment of oral premalignant lesions. *J Oral Pathol Med* 1995;24(5):198–200.
6. Kujan O, Khattab A, Oliver RJ, Roberts SA, Thakker N, Sloan P. Why oral histopathology suffers inter-observer variability on grading oral epithelial dysplasia: an attempt to understand the sources of variation. *Oral Oncol* 2007;43(3):224–31.
7. Kujan O, Oliver RJ, Khattab A, Roberts SA, Thakker N, Sloan P. Evaluation of a new binary system of grading oral epithelial dysplasia for prediction of malignant transformation. *Oral Oncol* 2006;42(10): 987–93.
8. Pindborg JJ, Reibel J, Holmstrup P. Subjectivity in evaluating oral epithelial dysplasia, carcinoma *in situ* and initial carcinoma. *J Oral Pathol* 1985;14(9):698–708.
9. Arduino PG, Surace A, Carbone M et al. Outcome of oral dysplasia: a retrospective hospital-based study of 207 patients with a long follow-up. *J Oral Pathol Med* 2009;38(6):540–4.
10. Holmstrup P, Vedtofte P, Reibel J, Stoltze K. Oral premalignant lesions: is a biopsy reliable? *J Oral Pathol Med* 2007;36(5):262–6.
11. Silverman S Jr, Gorsky M, Lozada F. Oral leukoplakia and malignant transformation. A Follow-up Study of 257 Patients. *Cancer* 1984;53(3):563–8.
12. Arnaoutakis D, Bishop J, Westra W, Califano JA. Recurrence patterns and management of oral cavity premalignant lesions. *Oral Oncol* 2013;49(8):814–7.
13. Brouns E, Baart J, Karagozoglu K, Aartman I, Bloemena E, van der Waal I. Malignant transformation of oral leukoplakia in a well-defined cohort of 144 patients. *Oral Dis* 2014;20(3):e19–24.
14. Mehanna HM, Rattay T, Smith J, McConkey CC. Treatment and follow-up of oral dysplasia—a systematic review and meta-analysis. *Head Neck* 2009;31(12):1600–9.
15. Napier SS, Speight PM. Natural history of potentially malignant oral lesions and conditions: an overview of the literature. *J Oral Pathol Med* 2008;37(1):1–10.
16. van der Waal I. Oral lichen planus and oral lichenoid lesions; a critical appraisal with emphasis on the diagnostic aspects. *Med Oral Patol Oral Cir Bucal* 2009;14(7):E310–4.
17. Zhang L, Poh CF, Williams M et al. Loss of heterozygosity (LOH) profiles—validated risk predictors for progression to oral cancer. *Cancer Prev Res (Phila Pa)* 2012;5(9):1081–9.
18. Mao L, Lee JS, Fan YH et al. Frequent microsatellite alterations at chromosomes 9p21 and 3p14 in oral premalignant lesions and their value in cancer risk assessment. *Nat Med* 1996;2(6):682–5.
19. Partridge M, Li SR, Pateromichelakis S et al. Detection of minimal residual cancer to investigate why oral tumors recur despite seemingly adequate treatment. *J Oral Pathol Med* 2000;6(7):2718–25.
20. Partridge M, Pateromichelakis S, Phillips E, Emilion G, Langdon J. Profiling clonality and progression in multiple premalignant and malignant oral lesions identifies a subgroup of cases with a distinct presentation of squamous cell carcinoma. *J Oral Pathol Med* 2001;7(7):1860–6.
21. Thomson PJ, Soames JV, Booth C, O'Shea JA. Epithelial cell proliferative activity and oral cancer progression. *Cell Prolif* 2002;35(Suppl 1):110–20.
22. Jiang WW, Fujii H, Shirai T, Mega H, Takagi M. Accumulative increase of loss of heterozygosity from leukoplakia to foci of early cancerization in leukoplakia of the oral cavity. *Cancer* 2001;92(9):2349–56.
23. Califano J, van der Riet P, Westra W et al. Genetic progression model for head and neck cancer: implications for field cancerization. *Cancer Res* 1996;56(11):2488–92.
24. Cheng YS, Wright JM. Oral and maxillofacial pathology case of the month. focal cemento-osseous dysplasia. *Tex Dent J* 2005;122(9):986–7, 90–1.
25. Epstein JB, Zhang L, Poh C, Nakamura H, Berean K, Rosin M. Increased allelic loss in toluidine blue-positive oral premalignant lesions. *Oral Surg Oral Med Oral Pathol Oral Radiol Endod* 2003;95(1):45–50.
26. Garnis C, Chari R, Buys TP et al. Genomic imbalances in precancerous tissues signal oral cancer risk. *Mol Cancer* 2009;8:50.
27. Garnis C, Coe BP, Ishkanian A, Zhang L, Rosin MP, Lam WL. Novel regions of amplification on 8q distinct from the MYC locus and frequently altered in oral dysplasia and cancer. *Genes Chromosomes Cancer* 2004;39(1):93–8.
28. Ha PK, Pilkington TA, Westra WH, Sciubba J, Sidransky D, Califano JA. Progression of microsatellite instability from premalignant lesions to tumors of the head and neck. *Int J Cancer* 2002;102(6):615–7.
29. Kayahara H, Yamagata H, Tanioka H, Miki T, Hamakawa H. Frequent loss of heterozygosity at 3p25–p26 is associated with invasive oral squamous cell carcinoma. *J Hum Genet* 2001;46(6):335–41.
30. Partridge M, Emilion G, Pateromichelakis S, A'Hern R, Phillips E, Langdon J. Allelic imbalance at chromosomal loci implicated in the pathogenesis of oral precancer, cumulative loss and its relationship with progression to cancer. *Oral Oncol* 1998;34(2):77–83.
31. Partridge M, Emilion G, Pateromichelakis S, Phillips E, Langdon J. Field cancerisation of the oral cavity: comparison of the spectrum of molecular alterations in cases presenting with both dysplastic and malignant lesions. *Oral Oncol* 1997;33(5):332–7.
32. Poh CF, Zhang L, Lam WL et al. A high frequency of allelic loss in oral verrucous lesions may explain malignant risk. *Lab Invest* 2001;81(4):629–34.
33. Rosin MP, Cheng X, Poh C et al. Use of allelic loss to predict malignant risk for low-grade oral epithelial dysplasia. *Clin Cancer Res* 2000;6(2):357–62.

34. Rosin MP, Epstein JB, Berean K et al. The use of exfoliative cell samples to map clonal genetic alterations in the oral epithelium of high-risk patients. *Cancer Res* 1997;57(23):5258–60.
35. Rosin MP, Lam WL, Poh C et al. 3p14 and 9p21 loss is a simple tool for predicting second oral malignancy at previously treated oral cancer sites. *Cancer Res* 2002;62(22):6447–50.
36. Tabor MP, Brakenhoff RH, Ruijter-Schippers HJ, Kummer JA, Leemans CR, Braakhuis BJ. Genetically altered fields as origin of locally recurrent head and neck cancer: a retrospective study. *Clin Cancer Res* 2004;10(11):3607–13.
37. Tsui IF, Rosin MP, Zhang L, Ng RT, Lam WL. Multiple aberrations of chromosome 3p detected in oral premalignant lesions. *Cancer Prev Res (Phila Pa)* 2008;1(6):424–9.
38. Zhang L, Cheung KJ Jr, Lam WL et al. Increased genetic damage in oral leukoplakia from high risk sites: potential impact on staging and clinical management. *Cancer* 2001;91(11):2148–55.
39. Zhang L, Rosin MP. Loss of heterozygosity: a potential tool in management of oral premalignant lesions? *J Oral Pathol Med* 2001;30(9):513–20.
40. Bremmer JF, Braakhuis BJ, Brink A et al. Comparative evaluation of genetic assays to identify oral pre-cancerous fields. *J Oral Pathol Med* 2008;37(10):599–606.
41. Bremmer JF, Braakhuis BJ, Ruijter-Schippers HJ et al. A noninvasive genetic screening test to detect oral preneoplastic lesions. *Lab Invest* 2005;85(12):1481–8.
42. Califano J, Westra WH, Meininger G, Corio R, Koch WM, Sidransky D. Genetic progression and clonal relationship of recurrent premalignant head and neck lesions. *Clin Cancer Res* 2000;6(2):347–52.
43. Roz L, Wu CL, Porter S et al. Allelic imbalance on chromosome 3p in oral dysplastic lesions: an early event in oral carcinogenesis. *Cancer Res* 1996;56(6):1228–31.
44. Tabor MP, Braakhuis BJ, van der Wal JE et al. Comparative molecular and histological grading of epithelial dysplasia of the oral cavity and the oropharynx. *J Pathol* 2003;199(3):354–60.
45. Tabor MP, Brakenhoff RH, van Houten VM et al. Persistence of genetically altered fields in head and neck cancer patients: biological and clinical implications. *Clin Cancer Res* 2001;7(6):1523–32.
46. Zhang L, Tang ZG, Zhou ZG, Tong XJ, Li XL. The expression of maspin and VEGF gene in oral squamous cell carcinoma and its significance. *Shanghai Kou Qiang Yi Xue* 2005;14(6):557–60.
47. Thomson PJ, McCaul JA, Ridout F, Hutchison IL. To treat…or not to treat? clinicians' views on the management of oral potentially malignant disorders. *Br J Oral Maxillofac Surg* 2015;53(10):1027–31.
48. Zhang L, Lubpairee T, Laronde DM, Rosin MP. Should severe epithelial dysplasia be treated? *Oral Oncol* 2016;60:125–9.
49. Graveland AP, Bremmer JF, de Maaker M et al. Molecular screening of oral precancer. *Oral Oncol* 2013;49(12):1129–35.
50. Gomes CC, Fonseca-Silva T, Galvao CF, Friedman E, De Marco L, Gomez RS. Inter-and intra-lesional molecular heterogeneity of oral leukoplakia. *Oral Oncol* 2015;51(2):178–81.
51. Gordon DJ, Resio B, Pellman D. Causes and consequences of aneuploidy in cancer. *Nat Rev Genet* 2012;13(3):189–203.
52. Ricke RM, van Ree JH, van Deursen JM. Whole chromosome instability and cancer: a complex relationship. *Trends Genet* 2008;24(9):457–66.
53. Teixeira MR, Heim S. Multiple numerical chromosome aberrations in cancer: what are their causes and what are their consequences? *Semin Cancer Biol* 2005;15(1):3–12.
54. Brouns ER, Bloemena E, Belien JA, Broeckaert MA, Aartman IH, van der Waal I. DNA ploidy measurement in oral leukoplakia: different results between flow and image cytometry. *Oral Oncol* 2012;48(7):636–40.
55. Abou-Elhamd KE, Habib TN. The role of chromosomal aberrations in premalignant and malignant lesions in head and neck squamous cell carcinoma. *Eur Arch Otorhinolaryngol* 2008;265(2):203–7.
56. Beroukhim R, Mermel CH, Porter D et al. The landscape of somatic copy-number alteration across human cancers. *Nature* 2010;463(7283):899–905.
57. Torres-Rendon A, Stewart R, Craig GT, Wells M, Speight PM. DNA ploidy analysis by image cytometry helps to identify oral epithelial dysplasias with a high risk of malignant progression. *Oral Oncol* 2009;45(6):468–73.
58. Diwakar N, Sperandio M, Sherriff M, Brown A, Odell EW. Heterogeneity, histological features and DNA ploidy in oral carcinoma by image-based analysis. *Oral Oncol* 2005;41(4):416–22.
59. Donadini A, Maffei M, Cavallero A et al. Oral cancer genesis and progression: DNA near-diploid aneuploidization and endoreduplication by high resolution flow cytometry. *Cell Oncol* 2010;32(5–6):373–83.
60. Pentenero M, Giaretti W, Navone R et al. DNA aneuploidy and dysplasia in oral potentially malignant disorders: association with cigarette smoking and site. *Oral Oncol* 2009;45(10):887–90.
61. Saito T, Yamashita T, Notani K et al. Flow cytometric analysis of nuclear DNA content in oral leukoplakia: relation to clinicopathologic findings. *Int J Oral Maxillofac Surg* 1995;24(1 Pt 1):44–7.
62. Bradley G, Odell EW, Raphael S et al. Abnormal DNA content in oral epithelial dysplasia is associated with increased risk of progression to carcinoma. *Br J Cancer* 2010;103(9):1432–42.

63. Bremmer JF, Brakenhoff RH, Broeckaert MA et al. Prognostic value of DNA ploidy status in patients with oral leukoplakia. *Oral Oncol* 2011;47(10): 956–60.
64. Sperandio M, Brown AL, Lock C et al. Predictive value of dysplasia grading and DNA ploidy in malignant transformation of oral potentially malignant disorders. *Cancer Prev Res (Phila Pa)* 2013;6(8):822–31.
65. Siebers TJ, Bergshoeff VE, Otte-Holler I et al. Chromosome instability predicts the progression of premalignant oral lesions. *Oral Oncol* 2013; 49(12):1121–8.
66. Baylin SB, Jones PA. A decade of exploring the cancer epigenome—biological and translational implications. *Nat Rev Cancer* 2011;11(10):726–34.
67. Schubeler D. Function and information content of DNA methylation. *Nature* 2015;517(7534):321–6.
68. Egger G, Liang G, Aparicio A, Jones PA. Epigenetics in human disease and prospects for epigenetic therapy. *Nature* 2004;429(6990):457–63.
69. Berdasco M, Esteller M. Aberrant epigenetic landscape in cancer: how cellular identity goes awry. *Dev Cell* 2010;19(5):698–711.
70. Feinberg AP, Koldobskiy MA, Gondor A. Epigenetic modulators, modifiers and mediators in cancer aetiology and progression. *Nat Rev Genet* 2016;17(5): 284–99.
71. Feinberg AP, Ohlsson R, Henikoff S. The epigenetic progenitor origin of human cancer. *Nat Rev Genet* 2006;7(1):21–33.
72. Azad N, Zahnow CA, Rudin CM, Baylin SB. The future of epigenetic therapy in solid tumours—lessons from the past. *Nat Rev Clin Oncol* 2013;10(5):256–66.
73. Rodriguez-Paredes M, Esteller M. Cancer epigenetics reaches mainstream oncology. *Nat Med* 2011;17(3):330–9.
74. D'Souza W, Saranath D. Clinical implications of epigenetic regulation in oral cancer. *Oral Oncol* 2015;51(12):1061–8.
75. Shridhar K, Walia GK, Aggarwal A et al. DNA methylation markers for oral pre-cancer progression: a critical review. *Oral Oncol* 2016;53:1–9.
76. Kresty LA, Mallery SR, Knobloch TJ et al. Alterations of p16(INK4a) and p14(ARF) in patients with severe oral epithelial dysplasia. *Cancer Res* 2002;62(18):5295–300.
77. Takeshima M, Saitoh M, Kusano K et al. High frequency of hypermethylation of p14, p15 and p16 in oral pre-cancerous lesions associated with betel-quid chewing in Sri Lanka. *J Oral Pathol Med* 2008;37(8): 475–9.
78. Cao J, Zhou J, Gao Y et al. Methylation of p16 CpG island associated with malignant progression of oral epithelial dysplasia: a prospective cohort study. *Clin Cancer Res* 2009;15(16):5178–83.
79. Hall GL, Shaw RJ, Field EA et al. P16 promoter methylation is a potential predictor of malignant transformation in oral epithelial dysplasia. *Cancer Epidemiol Biomarkers Prev* 2008;17(8):2174–9.
80. Towle R, Truong D, Hogg K, Robinson WP, Poh CF, Garnis C. Global analysis of DNA methylation changes during progression of oral cancer. *Oral Oncol* 2013;49(11):1033–42.
81. Zack TI, Schumacher SE, Carter SL et al. Pan-cancer patterns of somatic copy number alteration. *Nat Genet* 2013;45(10):1134–40.
82. Hurvitz SA, Hu Y, O'Brien N, Finn RS. Current approaches and future directions in the treatment of HER2-positive breast cancer. *Cancer Treat Rev* 2013;39(3):219–29.
83. Despierre E, Moisse M, Yesilyurt B et al. Somatic copy number alterations predict response to platinum therapy in epithelial ovarian cancer. *Gynecol Oncol* 2014;135(3):415–22.
84. Clough AR, Fitts MS, Robertson JA et al. Study protocol—alcohol management plans (AMPs) in remote indigenous communities in queensland: their impacts on injury, violence, health and social indicators and their cost-effectiveness. *BMC Public Health* 2014;14:15.
85. Ryott M, Wangsa D, Heselmeyer-Haddad K et al. EGFR protein overexpression and gene copy number increases in oral tongue squamous cell carcinoma. *Eur J Cancer* 2009;45(9):1700–8.
86. D'Haene B, Vandesompele J, Hellemans J. Accurate and objective copy number profiling using real-time quantitative PCR. *Methods* 2010;50(4):262–70.
87. Hu L, Ru K, Zhang L et al. Fluorescence in situ hybridization (FISH): an increasingly demanded tool for biomarker research and personalized medicine. *Biomark Res* 2014;2(1):3.
88. Hughesman CB, Lu XJ, Liu KY, Zhu Y, Poh CF, Haynes C. A robust protocol for using multiplexed droplet digital PCR to quantify somatic copy number alterations in clinical tissue specimens. *PLoS One* 2016;11(8):e0161274.
89. Kallioniemi A, Kallioniemi OP, Sudar D et al. Comparative genomic hybridization for molecular cytogenetic analysis of solid tumors. *Science* 1992;258(5083):818–21.
90. Peiffer DA, Le JM, Steemers FJ et al. High-resolution genomic profiling of chromosomal aberrations using infinium whole-genome genotyping. *Genome Res* 2006;16(9):1136–48.
91. Scheinin I, Sie D, Bengtsson H et al. DNA copy number analysis of fresh and formalin-fixed specimens by shallow whole-genome sequencing with identification and exclusion of problematic regions in the genome assembly. *Genome Res* 2014;24(12):2022–32.

92. Snijders AM, Nowak N, Segraves R et al. Assembly of microarrays for genome-wide measurement of DNA copy number. *Nat Genet* 2001;29(3):263–4.
93. Ylstra B, van den Ijssel P, Carvalho B, Brakenhoff RH, Meijer GA. BAC to the future! or oligonucleotides: a perspective for micro array comparative genomic hybridization (array CGH). *Nucleic Acids Res* 2006;34(2):445–50.
94. Vogelstein B, Kinzler KW. Digital PCR. *Proc Natl Acad Sci U S A* 1999;96(16):9236–41.
95. Garnis C, Campbell J, Zhang L, Rosin MP, Lam WL. OCGR array: an oral cancer genomic regional array for comparative genomic hybridization analysis. *Oral Oncol* 2004;40(5):511–9.
96. Grandis JR, Drenning SD, Chakraborty A et al. Requirement of Stat3 but not Stat1 activation for epidermal growth factor receptor-mediated cell growth In vitro. *J Clin Invest* 1998;102(7):1385–92.
97. Grandis JR, Tweardy DJ. Elevated levels of transforming growth factor alpha and epidermal growth factor receptor messenger RNA are early markers of carcinogenesis in head and neck cancer. *Cancer Res* 1993;53(15):3579–84.
98. Sheu JJ, Hua CH, Wan L et al. Functional genomic analysis identified epidermal growth factor receptor activation as the most common genetic event in oral squamous cell carcinoma. *Cancer Res* 2009;69(6):2568–76.
99. Temam S, Kawaguchi H, El-Naggar AK et al. Epidermal growth factor receptor copy number alterations correlate with poor clinical outcome in patients with head and neck squamous cancer. *J Clin Oncol* 2007;25(16):2164–70.
100. Hirsch FR, Varella-Garcia M, Bunn PA Jr et al. Epidermal growth factor receptor in non-small-cell lung carcinomas: correlation between gene copy number and protein expression and impact on prognosis. *J Clin Oncol* 2003;21(20):3798–807.
101. Nicholson RI, Gee JM, Harper ME. EGFR and cancer prognosis. *Eur J Cancer* 2001;37(Suppl 4):S9–15.
102. Takano T, Ohe Y, Sakamoto H et al. Epidermal growth factor receptor gene mutations and increased copy numbers predict gefitinib sensitivity in patients with recurrent non-small-cell lung cancer. *J Clin Oncol* 2005;23(28):6829–37.
103. Bates T, Kennedy M, Diajil A et al. Changes in epidermal growth factor peceptor gene copy number during oral carcinogenesis. *Cancer Epidemiol Biomarkers Prev* 2016;25(6):927–35.
104. Poh CF, Zhu Y, Chen E et al. Unique FISH patterns associated with cancer progression of oral dysplasia. *J Dent Res* 2012;91(1):52–7.
105. William WN Jr, Papadimitrakopoulou V, Lee JJ et al. Erlotinib and the risk of oral cancer: the erlotinib prevention of oral cancer (EPOC) randomized clinical trial. *JAMA Oncol* 2016;2(2):209–16.
106. Taoudi Benchekroun M, Saintigny P, Thomas SM et al. Epidermal growth factor receptor expression and gene copy number in the risk of oral cancer. *Cancer Prev Res (Phila Pa)* 2010;3(7):800–9.
107. Cha JD, Kim HJ, Cha IH. Genetic alterations in oral squamous cell carcinoma progression detected by combining array-based comparative genomic hybridization and multiplex ligation-dependent probe amplification. *Oral Surg Oral Med Oral Pathol Oral Radiol Endod* 2011;111(5):594–607.
108. Cervigne NK, Machado J, Goswami RS et al. Recurrent genomic alterations in sequential progressive leukoplakia and oral cancer: drivers of oral tumorigenesis? *Hum Mol Genet* 2014;23(10):2618–28.
109. Salahshourifar I, Vincent-Chong VK, Kallarakkal TG, Zain RB. Genomic DNA copy number alterations from precursor oral lesions to oral squamous cell carcinoma. *Oral Oncol* 2014;50(5):404–12.
110. Belbin TJ, Singh B, Barber I et al. Molecular classification of head and neck squamous cell carcinoma using cDNA microarrays. *Cancer Res* 2002;62(4):1184–90.
111. Ibrahim SO, Aarsaether N, Holsve MK et al. Gene expression profile in oral squamous cell carcinomas and matching normal oral mucosal tissues from black africans and white caucasians: the case of the Sudan vs. Norway. *Oral Oncol* 2003;39(1):37–48.
112. Leethanakul C, Knezevic V, Patel V et al. Gene discovery in oral squamous cell carcinoma through the head and neck cancer genome anatomy project: confirmation by microarray analysis. *Oral Oncol* 2003;39(3):248–58.
113. Mendez E, Cheng C, Farwell DG et al. Transcriptional expression profiles of oral squamous cell carcinomas. *Cancer* 2002;95(7):1482–94.
114. Saintigny P, Zhang L, Fan YH et al. Gene expression profiling predicts the development of oral cancer. *Cancer Prev Res (Phila Pa)* 2011;4(2):218–29.
115. Sok JC, Kuriakose MA, Mahajan VB, Pearlman AN, DeLacure MD, Chen FA. Tissue-specific gene expression of head and neck squamous cell carcinoma *in vivo* by complementary DNA microarray analysis. *Arch Otolaryngol Head Neck Surg* 2003;129(7):760–70.
116. Sumino J, Uzawa N, Okada N et al. Gene expression changes in initiation and progression of oral squamous cell carcinomas revealed by laser microdissection and oligonucleotide microarray analysis. *Int J Cancer* 2013;132(3):540–8.
117. Tomioka H, Morita K, Hasegawa S, Omura K. Gene expression analysis by cDNA microarray in oral squamous cell carcinoma. *J Oral Pathol Med* 2006;35(4):206–11.
118. Tsai WC, Tsai ST, Ko JY et al. The mRNA profile of genes in betel quid chewing oral cancer patients. *Oral Oncol* 2004;40(4):418–26.

119. Chen C, Mendez E, Houck J et al. Gene expression profiling identifies genes predictive of oral squamous cell carcinoma. *Cancer Epidemiol Biomarkers Prev* 2008;17(8):2152–62.
120. AbdulMajeed AA, Farah CS. Gene expression profiling for the purposes of biomarker discovery in oral potentially malignant lesions: a systematic review. *Clin Med Insights Oncol* 2013;7:279–90.
121. Djebali S, Davis CA, Merkel A et al. Landscape of transcription in human cells. *Nature* 2012;489(7414):101–8.
122. Lee RC, Feinbaum RL, Ambros V. The *C. elegans* heterochronic gene *lin-4* encodes small RNAs with antisense complementarity to *lin-14*. *Cell* 1993;75(5): 843–54.
123. Calin GA, Dumitru CD, Shimizu M et al. Frequent deletions and down-regulation of micro-RNA genes miR15 and miR16 at 13q14 in chronic lymphocytic leukemia. *Proc Natl Acad Sci U S A* 2002;99(24):15524–9.
124. Cervigne NK, Reis PP, Machado J et al. Identification of a microRNA signature associated with progression of leukoplakia to oral carcinoma. *Hum Mol Genet* 2009;18(24):4818–29.
125. Childs G, Fazzari M, Kung G et al. Low-level expression of microRNAs let-7d and miR-205 are prognostic markers of head and neck squamous cell carcinoma. *Am J Pathol* 2009;174(3):736–45.
126. Clague J, Lippman SM, Yang H et al. Genetic variation in microRNA genes and risk of oral premalignant lesions. *Mol Carcinog* 2010;49(2):183–9.
127. Gorenchtein M, Poh CF, Saini R, Garnis C. MicroRNAs in an oral cancer context—from basic biology to clinical utility. *J Dent Res* 2012;91(5): 440–6.
128. Kozaki K, Imoto I, Mogi S, Omura K, Inazawa J. Exploration of tumor-suppressive microRNAs silenced by DNA hypermethylation in oral cancer. *Cancer Res* 2008;68(7):2094–105.
129. Lajer CB, Garnaes E, Friis-Hansen L et al. The role of miRNAs in human papilloma virus (HPV)-associated cancers: bridging between HPV-related head and neck cancer and cervical cancer. *Br J Cancer* 2012;106(9):1526–34.
130. Lajer CB, Nielsen FC, Friis-Hansen L et al. Different miRNA signatures of oral and pharyngeal squamous cell carcinomas: a prospective translational study. *Br J Cancer* 2011;104(5):830–40.
131. Yang Y, Li YX, Yang X, Jiang L, Zhou ZJ, Zhu YQ. Progress risk assessment of oral premalignant lesions with saliva miRNA analysis. *BMC Cancer* 2013;13:129.
132. Maimaiti A, Abudoukeremu K, Tie L, Pan Y, Li X. MicroRNA expression profiling and functional annotation analysis of their targets associated with the malignant transformation of oral leukoplakia. *Gene* 2015;558(2):271–7.
133. Maclellan SA, Lawson J, Baik J, Guillaud M, Poh CF, Garnis C. Differential expression of miRNAs in the serum of patients with high-risk oral lesions. *Cancer Med* 2012;1(2):268–74.
134. Xiao W, Bao ZX, Zhang CY et al. Upregulation of miR-31* is negatively associated with recurrent/newly formed oral leukoplakia. *PLoS One* 2012;7(6):e38648.
135. Zahran F, Ghalwash D, Shaker O, Al-Johani K, Scully C. Salivary microRNAs in oral cancer. *Oral Dis* 2015;21(6):739–47.
136. Hung KF, Liu CJ, Chiu PC et al. MicroRNA-31 upregulation predicts increased risk of progression of oral potentially malignant disorder. *Oral Oncol* 2016;53:42–7.
137. Philipone E, Yoon AJ, Wang S et al. MicroRNAs-208b-3p, 204-5p, 129-2-3p and 3065-5p as predictive markers of oral leukoplakia that progress to cancer. *Am J Cancer Res* 2016;6(7):1537–46.
138. Geisler S, Coller J. RNA in unexpected places: long non-coding RNA functions in diverse cellular contexts. *Nat Rev Mol Cell Biol* 2013;14(11):699–712.
139. Quinodoz S, Guttman M. Long noncoding RNAs: an emerging link between gene regulation and nuclear organization. *Trends Cell Biol* 2014;24(11):651–63.
140. Gibb EA, Enfield KS, Stewart GL et al. Long non-coding RNAs are expressed in oral mucosa and altered in oral premalignant lesions. *Oral Oncol* 2011;47(11):1055–61.
141. Gupta RA, Shah N, Wang KC et al. Long non-coding RNA HOTAIR reprograms chromatin state to promote cancer metastasis. *Nature* 2010;464(7291): 1071–6.
142. Huarte M. The emerging role of lncRNAs in cancer. *Nat Med* 2015;21(11):1253–61.
143. Kunej T, Obsteter J, Pogacar Z, Horvat S, Calin GA. The decalog of long non-coding RNA involvement in cancer diagnosis and monitoring. *Crit Rev Clin Lab Sci* 2014;51(6):344–57.
144. Ling H, Vincent K, Pichler M et al. Junk DNA and the long non-coding RNA twist in cancer genetics. *Oncogene* 2015;34(39):5003–11.
145. Meseure D, Drak Alsibai K, Nicolas A, Bieche I, Morillon A. Long noncoding RNAs as new architects in cancer epigenetics, prognostic biomarkers, and potential therapeutic targets. *Biomed Res Int* 2015;2015:320214.
146. Pichler M, Calin GA. MicroRNAs in cancer: from developmental genes in worms to their clinical application in patients. *Br J Cancer* 2015;113(4):569–73.
147. Prensner JR, Chinnaiyan AM. The emergence of lncRNAs in cancer biology. *Cancer Discov* 2011;1(5):391–407.
148. Prensner JR, Iyer MK, Balbin OA et al. Transcriptome sequencing across a prostate cancer cohort identifies PCAT-1, an unannotated lincRNA implicated in disease progression. *Nat Biotechnol* 2011;29(8):742–9.

149. Gomes CC, de Sousa SF, Calin GA, Gomez RS. The emerging role of long noncoding RNAs in oral cancer. *Oral Surg Oral Med Oral Pathol Oral Radiol* 2017;123(2):235–41.
150. Nohata N, Abba MC, Gutkind JS. Unraveling the oral cancer lncRNAome: identification of novel lncRNAs associated with malignant progression and HPV infection. *Oral Oncol* 2016;59:58–66.
151. Gibb EA, Vucic EA, Enfield KS et al. Human cancer long non-coding RNA transcriptomes. *PLoS One* 2011;6(10):e25915.
152. Conway C, Graham JL, Chengot P et al. Elucidating drivers of oral epithelial dysplasia formation and malignant transformation to cancer using RNAseq. *Oncotarget* 2015;6(37):40186–201.
153. Han X, Wei YB, Tian G, Tang Z, Gao JY, Xu XG. Screening of crucial long non-coding RNAs in oral epithelial dysplasia by serial analysis of gene expression. *Genet Mol Res* 2015;14(4):11729–38.
154. Abogunrin S, Di Tanna GL, Keeping S, Carroll S, Iheanacho I. Prevalence of human papillomavirus in head and neck cancers in european populations: a meta-analysis. *BMC Cancer* 2014;14:968.
155. Chaturvedi AK, Engels EA, Pfeiffer RM et al. Human papillomavirus and rising oropharyngeal cancer incidence in the United States. *J Clin Oncol* 2011;29(32):4294–301.
156. Jiron J, Sethi S, Ali-Fehmi R et al. Racial disparities in human papillomavirus (HPV) associated head and neck cancer. *Am J Otolaryngol* 2014;35(2):147–53.
157. Lopez RV, Levi JE, Eluf-Neto J et al. Human papillomavirus (HPV) 16 and the prognosis of head and neck cancer in a geographical region with a low prevalence of HPV infection. *Cancer Causes Control* 2014;25(4):461–71.
158. Oga EA, Schumaker LM, Alabi BS et al. Paucity of HPV-related head and neck cancers (HNC) in Nigeria. *PLoS One* 2016;11(4):e0152828.
159. Kandoth C, McLellan MD, Vandin F et al. Mutational landscape and significance across 12 major cancer types. *Nature* 2013;502(7471):333–9.
160. Lawrence MS, Stojanov P, Mermel CH et al. Discovery and saturation analysis of cancer genes across 21 tumour types. *Nature* 2014;505(7484):495–501.
161. Agrawal N, Frederick MJ, Pickering CR et al. Exome sequencing of head and neck squamous cell carcinoma reveals inactivating mutations in NOTCH1. *Science* 2011;333(6046):1154–7.
162. Stransky N, Egloff AM, Tward AD et al. The mutational landscape of head and neck squamous cell carcinoma. *Science* 2011;333(6046):1157–60.
163. Lawrence MS, Sougnez C, Lichtenstein L et al. Comprehensive genomic characterization of head and neck squamous cell carcinomas. *Nature* 2015;517(7536):576–82.
164. Seiwert TY, Zuo Z, Keck MK et al. Integrative and comparative genomic analysis of HPV-positive and HPV-negative head and neck squamous cell carcinomas. *Clin Cancer Res* 2015;21(3):632–41.
165. Morris LG, Chandramohan R, West L et al. The molecular landscape of recurrent and metastatic head and neck cancers: insights from a precision oncology sequencing platform. *JAMA Oncol* 2016.
166. Gaykalova DA, Mambo E, Choudhary A et al. Novel insight into mutational landscape of head and neck squamous cell carcinoma. *PLoS One* 2014;9(3):e93102.
167. Lechner M, Frampton GM, Fenton T et al. Targeted next-generation sequencing of head and neck squamous cell carcinoma identifies novel genetic alterations in HPV+ and HPV− tumors. *Genome Med* 2013;5(5):49.
168. Rizzo G, Black M, Mymryk JS, Barrett JW, Nichols AC. Defining the genomic landscape of head and neck cancers through next-generation sequencing. *Oral Dis* 2015;21(1):e11–24.
169. Er TK, Wang YY, Chen CC, Herreros-Villanueva M, Liu TC, Yuan SS. Molecular characterization of oral squamous cell carcinoma using targeted next-generation sequencing. *Oral Dis* 2015;21(7):872–8.
170. Song X, Xia R, Li J et al. Common and complex Notch1 mutations in Chinese oral squamous cell carcinoma. *Clin Cancer Res* 2014;20(3):701–10.
171. Vettore AL, Ramnarayanan K, Poore G et al. Mutational landscapes of tongue carcinoma reveal recurrent mutations in genes of therapeutic and prognostic relevance. *Genome Med* 2015;7:98.
172. Joseph LJ, Goodman M, Higgins K et al. Racial disparities in squamous cell carcinoma of the oral tongue among women: a SEER data analysis. *Oral Oncol* 2015;51(6):586–92.
173. Patel V, Hood BL, Molinolo AA et al. Proteomic analysis of laser-captured paraffin-embedded tissues: a molecular portrait of head and neck cancer progression. *Clin Cancer Res* 2008;14(4):1002–14.
174. Tota JE, Anderson WF, Coffey C et al. Rising incidence of oral tongue cancer among white men and women in the United States, 1973–2012. *Oral Oncol* 2017;67:146–52.
175. Pickering CR, Zhang J, Neskey DM et al. Squamous cell carcinoma of the oral tongue in young non-smokers is genomically similar to tumors in older smokers. *Clin Cancer Res* 2014;20(14):3842–8.
176. Li R, Faden DL, Fakhry C et al. Clinical, genomic, and metagenomic characterization of oral tongue squamous cell carcinoma in patients who do not smoke. *Head Neck* 2015;37(11):1642–9.
177. Samman M, Wood HM, Conway C et al. A novel genomic signature reclassifies an oral cancer subtype. *Int J Cancer* 2015;137(10):2364–73.

178. Chen Y, Azman SN, Kerishnan JP et al. Identification of host-immune response protein candidates in the sera of human oral squamous cell carcinoma patients. *PLoS One* 2014;9(10):e109012.
179. Lui VW, Hedberg ML, Li H et al. Frequent mutation of the PI3K pathway in head and neck cancer defines predictive biomarkers. *Cancer Discov* 2013;3(7):761–9.
180. Sun W, Gaykalova DA, Ochs MF et al. Activation of the NOTCH pathway in head and neck cancer. *Cancer Res* 2014;74(4):1091–104.
181. Lui VW, Peyser ND, Ng PK et al. Frequent mutation of receptor protein tyrosine phosphatases provides a mechanism for STAT3 hyperactivation in head and neck cancer. *Proc Natl Acad Sci U S A* 2014;111(3):1114–9.
182. Tinhofer I, Budach V, Saki M et al. Targeted next-generation sequencing of locally advanced squamous cell carcinomas of the head and neck reveals druggable targets for improving adjuvant chemoradiation. *Eur J Cancer* 2016;57:78–86.
183. Chen SJ, Liu H, Liao CT et al. Ultra-deep targeted sequencing of advanced oral squamous cell carcinoma identifies a mutation-based prognostic gene signature. *Oncotarget* 2015;6(20):18066–80.
184. Gross AM, Orosco RK, Shen JP et al. Multi-tiered genomic analysis of head and neck cancer ties *TP53* mutation to 3p loss. *Nat Genet* 2014;46(9):939–43.
185. Hedberg ML, Goh G, Chiosea SI et al. Genetic landscape of metastatic and recurrent head and neck squamous cell carcinoma. *J Clin Invest* 2016;126(1):169–80.
186. Slaughter DP, Southwick HW, Smejkal W. Field cancerization in oral stratified squamous epithelium; clinical implications of multicentric origin. *Cancer* 1953;6(5):963–8.
187. Bedard PL, Hansen AR, Ratain MJ, Siu LL. Tumour heterogeneity in the clinic. *Nature* 2013;501(7467): 355–64.
188. Burrell RA, McGranahan N, Bartek J, Swanton C. The causes and consequences of genetic heterogeneity in cancer evolution. *Nature* 2013;501(7467):338–45.
189. Fidler IJ, Kripke ML. Metastasis results from preexisting variant cells within a malignant tumor. *Science* 1977;197(4306):893–5.
190. Hiley C, de Bruin EC, McGranahan N, Swanton C. Deciphering intratumor heterogeneity and temporal acquisition of driver events to refine precision medicine. *Genome Biol* 2014;15(8):453.
191. Nowell PC. The clonal evolution of tumor cell populations. *Science* 1976;194(4260):23–8.
192. Mroz EA, Tward AD, Pickering CR, Myers JN, Ferris RL, Rocco JW. High intratumor genetic heterogeneity is related to worse outcome in patients with head and neck squamous cell carcinoma. *Cancer* 2013;119(16):3034–42.
193. Mroz EA, Tward AD, Hammon RJ, Ren Y, Rocco JW. Intra-tumor genetic heterogeneity and mortality in head and neck cancer: analysis of data from the cancer genome atlas. *PLoS Med* 2015;12(2):e1001786.
194. Neskey DM, Osman AA, Ow TJ et al. Evolutionary action score of TP53 identifies high-risk mutations associated with decreased survival and increased distant metastases in head and neck cancer. *Cancer Res* 2015;75(7):1527–36.
195. Osman AA, Neskey DM, Katsonis P et al. Evolutionary action score of TP53 coding variants is predictive of platinum response in head and neck cancer patients. *Cancer Res* 2015;75(7):1205–15.
196. Wang Y, Springer S, Mulvey CL et al. Detection of somatic mutations and HPV in the saliva and plasma of patients with head and neck squamous cell carcinomas. *Sci Transl Med* 2015;7(293): 293ra104.
197. Beder LB, Gunduz M, Ouchida M et al. Genome-wide analyses on loss of heterozygosity in head and neck squamous cell carcinomas. *Lab Invest* 2003;83(1):99–105.
198. Chen C, Zhang Y, Loomis MM et al. Genome-wide loss of heterozygosity and DNA copy number aberration in HPV-negative oral squamous cell carcinoma and their associations with disease-specific survival. *PLoS One* 2015;10(8):e0135074.
199. Chen Y, Chen C. DNA copy number variation and loss of heterozygosity in relation to recurrence of and survival from head and neck squamous cell carcinoma: a review. *Head Neck* 2008;30(10):1361–83.
200. el-Naggar AK, Hurr K, Batsakis JG, Luna MA, Goepfert H, Huff V. Sequential loss of heterozygosity at microsatellite motifs in preinvasive and invasive head and neck squamous carcinoma. *Cancer Res* 1995;55(12):2656–9.
201. Lazar AD, Winter MR, Nogueira CP et al. Loss of heterozygosity at 11q23 in squamous cell carcinoma of the head and neck is associated with recurrent disease. *Clin Cancer Res* 1998;4(11):2787–93.
202. Mavros A, Hahn M, Wieland I et al. Infrequent genetic alterations of the tumor suppressor gene *PTEN/MMAC1* in squamous cell carcinoma of the oral cavity. *J Oral Pathol Med* 2002;31(5):270–6.
203. Pickering CR, Zhang J, Yoo SY et al. Integrative genomic characterization of oral squamous cell carcinoma identifies frequent somatic drivers. *Cancer Discov* 2013;3(7):770–81.
204. Waber PG, Lee NK, Nisen PD. Frequent allelic loss at chromosome arm 3p is distinct from genetic alterations of the Von-hippel lindau tumor suppressor gene in head and neck cancer. *Oncogene* 1996;12(2):365–9.
205. Koffler J, Sharma S, Hess J. Predictive value of epigenetic alterations in head and neck squamous cell carcinoma. *Mol Cell Oncol* 2014;1(2):e954827.

206. Bennett KL, Karpenko M, Lin MT et al. Frequently methylated tumor suppressor genes in head and neck squamous cell carcinoma. *Cancer Res* 2008;68(12):4494–9.
207. Bennett KL, Lee W, Lamarre E et al. HPV status-independent association of alcohol and tobacco exposure or prior radiation therapy with promoter methylation of *FUSSEL18*, *EBF3*, *IRX1*, and *SEPT9*, but not *SLC5A8*, in head and neck squamous cell carcinomas. *Genes Chromosomes Cancer* 2010;49(4):319–26.
208. Bennett KL, Romigh T, Eng C. Disruption of transforming growth factor-beta signaling by five frequently methylated genes leads to head and neck squamous cell carcinoma pathogenesis. *Cancer Res* 2009;69(24):9301–5.
209. Xavier FC, Destro MF, Duarte CM, Nunes FD. Epigenetic repression of *HOXB* cluster in oral cancer cell lines. *Arch Oral Biol* 2014;59(8):783–9.
210. Carvalho AL, Henrique R, Jeronimo C et al. Detection of promoter hypermethylation in salivary rinses as a biomarker for head and neck squamous cell carcinoma surveillance. *Clin Cancer Res* 2011;17(14):4782–9.
211. Jithesh PV, Risk JM, Schache AG et al. The epigenetic landscape of oral squamous cell carcinoma. *Br J Cancer* 2013;108(2):370–9.
212. Poage GM, Butler RA, Houseman EA et al. Identification of an epigenetic profile classifier that is associated with survival in head and neck cancer. *Cancer Res* 2012;72(11):2728–37.
213. Guerrero-Preston R, Michailidi C, Marchionni L et al. Key tumor suppressor genes inactivated by "greater promoter" methylation and somatic mutations in head and neck cancer. *Epigenetics* 2014;9(7):1031–46.
214. Parfenov M, Pedamallu CS, Gehlenborg N et al. Characterization of HPV and host genome interactions in primary head and neck cancers. *Proc Natl Acad Sci U S A* 2014;111(43):15544–9.
215. Sartor MA, Dolinoy DC, Jones TR et al. Genome-wide methylation and expression differences in HPV(+) and HPV(−) squamous cell carcinoma cell lines are consistent with divergent mechanisms of carcinogenesis. *Epigenetics* 2011;6(6):777–87.
216. Poage GM, Houseman EA, Christensen BC et al. Global hypomethylation identifies loci targeted for hypermethylation in head and neck cancer. *Clin Cancer Res* 2011;17(11):3579–89.
217. Basu B, Chakraborty J, Chandra A et al. Genome-wide DNA methylation profile identified a unique set of differentially methylated immune genes in oral squamous cell carcinoma patients in India. *Clin Epigenetics* 2017;9:13.
218. Chung CH, Guthrie VB, Masica DL et al. Genomic alterations in head and neck squamous cell carcinoma determined by cancer gene-targeted sequencing. *Ann Oncol* 2015;26(6):1216–23.
219. Peng CH, Liao CT, Peng SC et al. A novel molecular signature identified by systems genetics approach predicts prognosis in oral squamous cell carcinoma. *PLoS One* 2011;6(8):e23452.
220. Ribeiro IP, Marques F, Caramelo F et al. Genetic gains and losses in oral squamous cell carcinoma: impact on clinical management. *Cell Oncol (Dordr)* 2014;37(1):29–39.
221. Smeets SJ, Braakhuis BJ, Abbas S et al. Genome-wide DNA copy number alterations in head and neck squamous cell carcinomas with or without oncogene-expressing human papillomavirus. *Oncogene* 2006;25(17):2558–64.
222. Ashman JN, Patmore HS, Condon LT, Cawkwell L, Stafford ND, Greenman J. Prognostic value of genomic alterations in head and neck squamous cell carcinoma detected by comparative genomic hybridisation. *Br J Cancer* 2003;89(5):864–9.
223. Bockmuhl U, Schluns K, Kuchler I, Petersen S, Petersen I. Genetic imbalances with impact on survival in head and neck cancer patients. *Am J Pathol* 2000;157(2):369–75.
224. Wreesmann VB, Shi W, Thaler HT et al. Identification of novel prognosticators of outcome in squamous cell carcinoma of the head and neck. *J Clin Oncol* 2004;22(19):3965–72.
225. Zhang X, Huang M, Wu X et al. *GSTM1* copy number and promoter haplotype as predictors for risk of recurrence and/or second primary tumor in patients with head and neck cancer. *Pharmgenomics Pers Med* 2013;6:9–17.
226. Morita T, Uzawa N, Mogushi K et al. Characterizing genetic transitions of copy number alterations and allelic imbalances in oral tongue carcinoma metastasis. *Genes Chromosomes Cancer* 2016;55(12):975–86.
227. Chung CH, Parker JS, Karaca G et al. Molecular classification of head and neck squamous cell carcinomas using patterns of gene expression. *Cancer Cell* 2004;5(5):489–500.
228. Liu CJ, Liu TY, Kuo LT et al. Differential gene expression signature between primary and metastatic head and neck squamous cell carcinoma. *J Pathol* 2008;214(4):489–97.
229. Nguyen ST, Hasegawa S, Tsuda H et al. Identification of a predictive gene expression signature of cervical lymph node metastasis in oral squamous cell carcinoma. *Cancer Sci* 2007;98(5):740–6.
230. Estilo CL, O-Charoenrat P, Talbot S et al. Oral tongue cancer gene expression profiling: identification of novel potential prognosticators by oligonucleotide microarray analysis. *BMC Cancer* 2009;9:11.
231. Walter V, Yin X, Wilkerson MD et al. Molecular subtypes in head and neck cancer exhibit distinct patterns of chromosomal gain and loss of canonical cancer genes. *PLoS One* 2013;8(2):e56823.

232. Suresh A, Vannan M, Kumaran D et al. Resistance/response molecular signature for oral tongue squamous cell carcinoma. *Dis Markers* 2012;32(1):51–64.
233. Keck MK, Zuo Z, Khattri A et al. Integrative analysis of head and neck cancer identifies two biologically distinct HPV and three non-HPV subtypes. *Clin Cancer Res* 2015;21(4):870–81.
234. Pyeon D, Newton MA, Lambert PF et al. Fundamental differences in cell cycle deregulation in human papillomavirus-positive and human papillomavirus-negative head/neck and cervical cancers. *Cancer Res* 2007;67(10):4605–19.
235. Zhang Y, Koneva LA, Virani S et al. Subtypes of HPV-positive head and neck cancers are associated with HPV characteristics, copy number alterations, *PIK3CA* mutation, and pathway signatures. *Clin Cancer Res* 2016;22(18):4735–45.
236. Farshadpour F, Roepman P, Hordijk GJ, Koole R, Slootweg PJ. A gene expression profile for non-smoking and non-drinking patients with head and neck cancer. *Oral Dis* 2012;18(2):178–83.
237. Saeed AA, Sims AH, Prime SS, Paterson I, Murray PG, Lopes VR. Gene expression profiling reveals biological pathways responsible for phenotypic heterogeneity between UK and Sri Lankan oral squamous cell carcinomas. *Oral Oncol* 2015;51(3):237–46.
238. Roepman P, Wessels LF, Kettelarij N et al. An expression profile for diagnosis of lymph node metastases from primary head and neck squamous cell carcinomas. *Nat Genet* 2005;37(2):182–6.
239. van Hooff SR, Leusink FK, Roepman P et al. Validation of a gene expression signature for assessment of lymph node metastasis in oral squamous cell carcinoma. *J Clin Oncol* 2012;30(33):4104–10.
240. John K, Wu J, Lee BW, Farah CS. MicroRNAs in head and neck cancer. *Int J Dent* 2013;2013:650218.
241. Koshizuka K, Hanazawa T, Fukumoto I, Kikkawa N, Okamoto Y, Seki N. The microRNA signatures: aberrantly expressed microRNAs in head and neck squamous cell carcinoma. *J Hum Genet* 2017;62(1):3–13.
242. Min A, Zhu C, Peng S, Rajthala S, Costea DE, Sapkota D. MicroRNAs as important players and biomarkers in oral carcinogenesis. *Biomed Res Int* 2015;2015:186904.
243. Tu HF, Lin SC, Chang KW. MicroRNA aberrances in head and neck cancer: pathogenetic and clinical significance. *Curr Opin Otolaryngol Head Neck Surg* 2013;21(2):104–11.
244. Fukumoto I, Kinoshita T, Hanazawa T et al. Identification of tumour suppressive microRNA-451a in hypopharyngeal squamous cell carcinoma based on microRNA expression signature. *Br J Cancer* 2014;111(2):386–94.
245. Hui AB, Lenarduzzi M, Krushel T et al. Comprehensive microRNA profiling for head and neck squamous cell carcinomas. *Clin Cancer Res* 2010;16(4):1129–39.
246. Kikkawa N, Hanazawa T, Fujimura L et al. miR-489 is a tumour-suppressive miRNA target *PTPN11* in hypopharyngeal squamous cell carcinoma (HSCC). *Br J Cancer* 2010;103(6):877–84.
247. Liu CJ, Tsai MM, Hung PS et al. miR-31 ablates expression of the HIF regulatory factor FIH to activate the HIF pathway in head and neck carcinoma. *Cancer Res* 2010;70(4):1635–44.
248. Nohata N, Hanazawa T, Kikkawa N et al. Tumour suppressive microRNA-874 regulates novel cancer networks in maxillary sinus squamous cell carcinoma. *Br J Cancer* 2011;105(6):833–41.
249. Severino P, Bruggemann H, Andreghetto FM et al. MicroRNA expression profile in head and neck cancer: HOX-cluster embedded microRNA-196a and microRNA-10b dysregulation implicated in cell proliferation. *BMC Cancer* 2013;13:533.
250. Soga D, Yoshiba S, Shiogama S, Miyazaki H, Kondo S, Shintani S. MicroRNA expression profiles in oral squamous cell carcinoma. *Oncol Rep* 2013;30(2):579–83.
251. Wang F, Lu J, Peng X et al. Integrated analysis of microRNA regulatory network in nasopharyngeal carcinoma with deep sequencing. *J Exp Clin Cancer Res* 2016;35:17.
252. Zhang Y, Chen Y, Yu J, Liu G, Huang Z. Integrated transcriptome analysis reveals miRNA–mRNA crosstalk in laryngeal squamous cell carcinoma. *Genomics* 2014;104(4):249–56.
253. Ries J, Vairaktaris E, Kintopp R, Baran C, Neukam FW, Nkenke E. Alterations in miRNA expression patterns in whole blood of OSCC patients. *In Vivo* 2014;28(5):851–61.
254. Lin SC, Liu CJ, Lin JA, Chiang WF, Hung PS, Chang KW. miR-24 up-regulation in oral carcinoma: positive association from clinical and in vitro analysis. *Oral Oncol* 2010;46(3):204–8.
255. Santhi WS, Prathibha R, Charles S et al. Oncogenic microRNAs as biomarkers of oral tumorigenesis and minimal residual disease. *Oral Oncol* 2013;49(6):567–75.
256. Jung HM, Phillips BL, Patel RS et al. Keratinization-associated miR-7 and miR-21 regulate tumor suppressor reversion-inducing cysteine-rich protein with kazal motifs (RECK) in oral cancer. *J Biol Chem* 2012;287(35):29261–72.
257. Li J, Huang H, Sun L et al. MiR-21 indicates poor prognosis in tongue squamous cell carcinomas as an apoptosis inhibitor. *Clinical Cancer Research: an Official Journal of the American Association for Cancer Res* 2009;15(12):3998–4008.
258. Chang CC, Yang YJ, Li YJ et al. MicroRNA-17/20a functions to inhibit cell migration and can be used a

prognostic marker in oral squamous cell carcinoma. *Oral Oncol* 2013;49(9):923–31.

259. Harris T, Jimenez L, Kawachi N et al. Low-level expression of miR-375 correlates with poor outcome and metastasis while altering the invasive properties of head and neck squamous cell carcinomas. *Am J Pathol* 2012;180(3):917–28.
260. Huang WC, Chan SH, Jang TH et al. miRNA-491-5p and GIT1 serve as modulators and biomarkers for oral squamous cell carcinoma invasion and metastasis. *Cancer Res* 2014;74(3):751–64.
261. Liu CJ, Lin SC, Yang CC, Cheng HW, Chang KW. Exploiting salivary miR-31 as a clinical biomarker of oral squamous cell carcinoma. *Head Neck* 2012;34(2):219–24.
262. Shi LJ, Zhang CY, Zhou ZT et al. MicroRNA-155 in oral squamous cell carcinoma: overexpression, localization, and prognostic potential. *Head Neck* 2015;37(7):970–6.
263. Yang CC, Hung PS, Wang PW et al. miR-181 as a putative biomarker for lymph-node metastasis of oral squamous cell carcinoma. *J Oral Pathol* 2011;40(5):397–404.
264. Peng SC, Liao CT, Peng CH et al. MicroRNAs miR-218, miR-125b, and let-7g predict prognosis in patients with oral cavity squamous cell carcinoma. *PLoS One* 2014;9(7):e102403.
265. Ganci F, Sacconi A, Manciocco V et al. MicroRNA expression as predictor of local recurrence risk in oral squamous cell carcinoma. *Head Neck* 2016;38(Suppl 1):E189–97.
266. Wong N, Khwaja SS, Baker CM et al. Prognostic microRNA signatures derived from The cancer genome atlas for head and neck squamous cell carcinomas. *Cancer Med* 2016;5(7):1619–28.
267. Scapoli L, Palmieri A, Lo Muzio L et al. MicroRNA expression profiling of oral carcinoma identifies new markers of tumor progression. *Int J Immunopathol Pharmacol* 2010;23(4):1229–34.
268. Ganci F, Sacconi A, Bossel Ben-Moshe N et al. Expression of *TP53* mutation-associated microRNAs predicts clinical outcome in head and neck squamous cell carcinoma patients. *Ann Oncol* 2013;24(12):3082–8.
269. Dai Y, Xie CH, Neis JP, Fan CY, Vural E, Spring PM. MicroRNA expression profiles of head and neck squamous cell carcinoma with docetaxel-induced multidrug resistance. *Head Neck* 2011;33(6):786–91.
270. Sun L, Yao Y, Liu B et al. MiR-200b and miR-15b regulate chemotherapy-induced epithelial–mesenchymal transition in human tongue cancer cells by targeting BMI1. *Oncogene* 2012;31(4):432–45.
271. Suh YE, Raulf N, Gaken J et al. MicroRNA-196a promotes an oncogenic effect in head and neck cancer cells by suppressing annexin A1 and enhancing radioresistance. *Int J Cancer* 2015;137(5):1021–34.
272. Park NJ, Zhou H, Elashoff D et al. Salivary microRNA: discovery, characterization, and clinical utility for oral cancer detection. *Clin Cancer Res* 2009;15(17):5473–7.
273. Wiklund ED, Gao S, Hulf T et al. MicroRNA alterations and associated aberrant DNA methylation patterns across multiple sample types in oral squamous cell carcinoma. *PLoS One* 2011;6(11):e27840.
274. Momen-Heravi F, Trachtenberg AJ, Kuo WP, Cheng YS. Genomewide study of salivary microRNAs for detection of oral cancer. *J Dent Res* 2014;93(Suppl 7):86s–93s.
275. Ralhan R, Desouza LV, Matta A et al. Discovery and verification of head-and-neck cancer biomarkers by differential protein expression analysis using iTRAQ labeling, multidimensional liquid chromatography, and tandem mass spectrometry. *Mol Cell Proteomics* 2008;7(6):1162–73.
276. Ralhan R, Desouza LV, Matta A et al. iTRAQ-multidimensional liquid chromatography and tandem mass spectrometry-based identification of potential biomarkers of oral epithelial dysplasia and novel networks between inflammation and premalignancy. *J Proteome Res* 2009;8(1):300–9.
277. Wang Z, Feng X, Liu X et al. Involvement of potential pathways in malignant transformation from oral leukoplakia to oral squamous cell carcinoma revealed by proteomic analysis. *BMC Genomics* 2009;10:383.
278. Xiao H, Langerman A, Zhang Y et al. Quantitative proteomic analysis of microdissected oral epithelium for cancer biomarker discovery. *Oral Oncol* 2015;51(11):1011–9.
279. Melle C, Ernst G, Winkler R et al. Proteomic analysis of human papillomavirus-related oral squamous cell carcinoma: identification of thioredoxin and epidermal-fatty acid binding protein as upregulated protein markers in microdissected tumor tissue. *Proteomics* 2009;9(8):2193–201.
280. Slebos RJ, Jehmlich N, Brown B et al. Proteomic analysis of oropharyngeal carcinomas reveals novel HPV-associated biological pathways. *Int J Cancer* 2013;132(3):568–79.
281. Harris TM, Du P, Kawachi N et al. Proteomic analysis of oral cavity squamous cell carcinoma specimens identifies patient outcome-associated proteins. *Arch Pathol Lab Med* 2015;139(4):494–507.
282. Skinner HD, Giri U, Yang L et al. Proteomic profiling identifies PTK2/FAK as a driver of radioresistance in HPV-negative head and neck cancer. *Clin Cancer Res* 2016;22(18):4643–50.
283. Chauhan SS, Kaur J, Kumar M et al. Prediction of recurrence-free survival using a protein expression-based risk classifier for head and neck cancer. *Oncogenesis* 2015;4:e147.

284. Schaaij-Visser TB, Graveland AP, Gauci S et al. Differential proteomics identifies protein biomarkers that predict local relapse of head and neck squamous cell carcinomas. *Clin Cancer Res* 2009;15(24):7666–75.
285. Partridge M, Emilion G, Langdon JD. LOH at 3p correlates with a poor survival in oral squamous cell carcinoma. *Br J Cancer* 1996;73(3):366–71.
286. Zhang J, Chen SI, Yin L, Chen X. Transcriptome profiles of moderate dysplasia in oral mucosa associated with malignant conversion. *Int J Clin Exp Pathol.* 2016;9(6):6107–16.
287. Towle R, Gorenchtein M, Dickman C, Zhu Y, Poh CF et al. Dysregulation of microRNAs across oral squamous cell carcinoma fields in non-smokers. *J Interdiscip Med Dent Sci* 2014;2:131. doi:10.4172/2376-032X.1000131.

PART II

Clinical management

6

Clinical evaluation and differential diagnosis

LAURA WANG AND JATIN P. SHAH

Clinical evaluation of head and neck cancer patients requires eliciting a complete history and a physical examination requiring a thorough assessment of the tumor, the patient and the social milieu in which the patient lives. The clinician is expected to establish a preliminary diagnosis, develop a relationship of trust with the patient and family members, initiate additional diagnostic investigations, formulate a treatment plan and coordinate patient care with a multidisciplinary team. This chapter will address the anatomy of the oral cavity and oropharynx as well as the required components of initial in-office assessment of the patient and the key differential diagnoses to consider.

ANATOMY

Knowledge of anatomy is essential for accurate clinical evaluation, but is also crucial to formulating a treatment plan to achieve best oncologic and functional outcomes. The designated anatomic sites in the oral cavity described by the International Union Against Cancer (UICC)/American Joint Committee on Cancer (AJCC) staging system for oral and oropharyngeal cancer is demonstrated in Figure 6.1a and b (1).

Anatomical components such as fascial planes, neurovascular bundles and lymphatic drainage pathways directly impact on tumor spread, clinical presentation, treatment selection and prognosis. Understanding of the functional relationships of the oral cavity and oropharynx subsites, overlying skin, underlying bones (maxilla and mandible) and dentition, which play important roles in articulation, mastication, deglutition and facial expression as well as cosmesis, is central to achieving eventual best quality of life outcomes.

The oral cavity is the beginning of the upper aerodigestive tract that extends from the mucocutaneous junction of the vermilion border to the junction of the hard–soft palate, laterally to the anterior tonsillar pillars and onto the circumvallate papillae and linea terminalis of the tongue. The oropharynx is the posterior continuation of the oral cavity to the hypopharynx. Superiorly, the oropharynx extends to the lower border of the soft palate and inferiorly to the tip of the epiglottis. Apart from the lips, the mucosa is lined by non-keratinized, squamous epithelium and the submucosa is interspersed with minor salivary glands. The oral cavity is divided into multiple sites consisting of the lips, upper and lower alveolar ridges (with upper and lower dentition), oral tongue, retromolar trigone, floor of the mouth, buccal mucosa and hard palate (Figure 6.1a). The oropharynx is composed of four sites: the base of the tongue, tonsils, soft palate and posterior pharyngeal wall (Figure 6.1b). Primary tumors of the oral cavity and oropharynx may arise from the surface epithelium, minor salivary glands or submucosal soft tissues, as well as from dental structures, bone or neurovascular tissues.

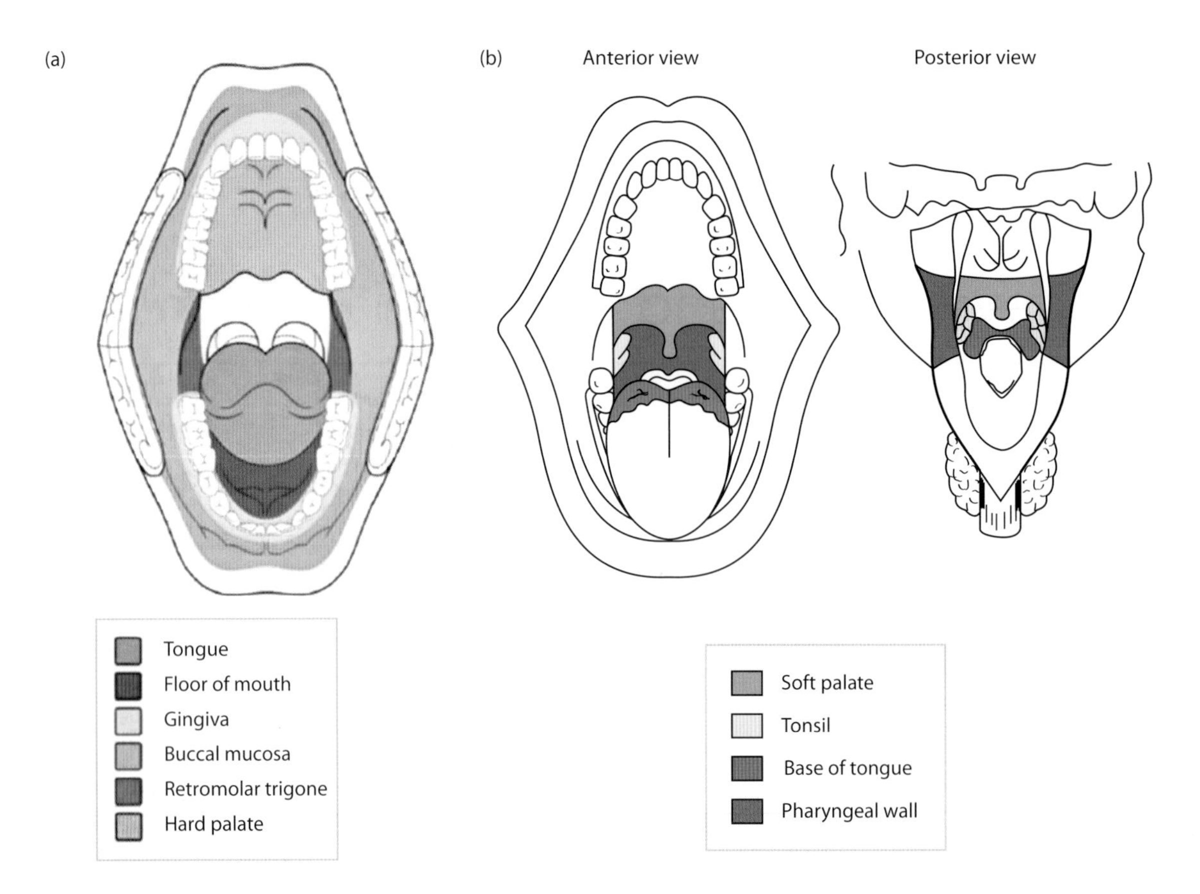

Figure 6.1 Anatomical sites in the oral cavity and oropharynx **(a)** oral cavity, **(b)** oropharynx—anterior and posterior views.

LIPS

The lips are limited laterally by the oral commissures and the vermillion borders superiorly and inferiorly. They serve as a transitional zone between the skin of the face to the internal mucous membrane. They are supported by the sphincter-like orbicularis oris muscle, which is innervated by the terminal branches of the lower division of the facial nerve (CN VII). Upper lip sensation is supplied by branches of the infraorbital nerve (CN V2), while lower lip sensation is provided by the mental nerve branches from the inferior alveolar nerve (CN V3). Most malignancies of the lips arise due to excessive UV light exposure and hence arise predominately on the lower lip. While both upper and lower lip lesions preferentially drain to the ipsilateral submandibular lymph node basins (level IB), lower lip lesions may drain to submental lymphatics (level 1A) and cross the midline.

BUCCAL MUCOSA

The buccal mucosa is a mucosal surface situated between the oral commissure and posterior surface of the lips, the alveolar ridges medially and the pterygomandibular raphe posteriorly. The surface is pierced by the papule of Stensen's (parotid) duct opposite the second maxillary molar. The layers underlying the mucosa are the pharyngobasilar fascia, the buccinator muscles (innervated by buccal branches of CN VII), the buccal fat pad and finally the subcutaneous tissue and the overlying skin of the cheek. Sensation is supplied by CN V2 and CN V3 and initial lymphatic drainage is to the level IB regions. The pre-vascular facial lymph nodes accompanying the facial artery and overlying the body of the mandible are at particular risk and are considered the first-echelon nodes for this primary site. Notably, the lack of bony or fascial planes leads to relatively fast and uninhibited tumor spread, particularly to the masticator space, making buccal mucosal cancer more aggressive with poorer prognosis (2,3).

ALVEOLAR RIDGES

The upper and lower alveolar ridges provide structural support for dentition and are composed of mucosa overlying the alveolar process of the maxilla and mandible, respectively. Laterally, the ridges form a gingivobuccal sulcus that transitions to the buccal and labial mucosa. The lower alveolar ridge transitions to the floor of the mouth medially, while the posterior margin borders the retromolar trigone and ascending ramus of the mandible. The medial margin of the upper alveolar ridge borders the hard palate, while the posterior margin is the maxillary tuberosity, which lies adjacent to the pterygopalatine arch. The tight adherence of thin mucosa to underlying bone leads to early bone invasion by malignant tumors arising at these sites. However, cortical bone acts as a barrier to tumor invasion early on, but the lack of cortex in an empty tooth socket permits entry of cancer into the marrow space. Deep extension in the marrow space involves the mandibular canal, causing anesthesia or paresthesia of the distal teeth and skin of the chin and potential for perineural spread of tumor to the skull base.

Retromolar trigone

The retromolar trigone is a small, triangular mucosal space bordered by the last lower molar tooth, the ascending mandibular ramus and the maxillary tuberosity. It connects with the buccal mucosa laterally and the anterior tonsillar pillar medially. Similar to the alveolar ridge, the mucosa is very thin and early bone invasion is common. Sensation is provided by the lesser palatine nerve (CN V2) and branches of the glossopharyngeal nerve (CN IX). Patients may present with referred otalgia from CN IX impingement or lower lip paresthesias from inferior alveolar nerve involvement. Lymphatics preferentially drain to level II lymph nodes in the neck.

FLOOR OF THE MOUTH

This space is located between the lower alveolar ridge and oral tongue and is bisected by the lingual frenulum. Wharton's (submandibular) ducts and the sublingual gland openings pierce the mucosa of the floor of the mouth and drain saliva on either side of the frenulum. These structures are supported by the underlying musculature (mylohyoid and hyoglossus muscles, as well as the genioglossus muscle). The hypoglossal (CN XI) and lingual nerves (CN V3) travel through this region and are commonly at risk of invasion by tumor. Sensation is provided by the lingual nerve. Lymphatic drainage tends to be bilateral (levels IA and IB) for anterior floor of the mouth lesions and ipsilateral (level II) for posterior lesions.

HARD PALATE

The palatine process of the maxilla and the horizontal plate of the palatine bone form the hard palate. The overlying mucosa is supported by thick mucoperiosteum. Both the hard and soft palates contain numerous minor salivary glands. At the junction of the hard and soft palates are located the foramina through which the greater and lesser palatine nerves and vessels traverse. The incisive foramen, posterior to the maxillary incisors, conveys the nasopalatine vessels and nerve. Lesions spread easily through these foramina into the nasal vault or maxillary sinus. Posterior hard palate lesions that extend to the soft palate drain to level II, but also to retropharyngeal lymph node basins.

TONGUE

The oral tongue (anterior two-thirds) is embryologically distinct from the tongue base (posterior third) and is separated by the linea terminalis. It is divided at the midline by the median fibrous raphe and is composed of paired intrinsic and extrinsic tongue musculature. The four paired intrinsic muscles (superior longitudinal, inferior longitudinal, verticalis and transversus) originate and insert within the tongue and are responsible for the dexterity of the tongue. The four paired extrinsic muscles (genioglossus, hyoglossus, styloglossus and palatoglossus) are anchored to bone and adjust tongue position. The absence of fascial planes between these muscles enables tumors to easily penetrate and infiltrate among the various muscles.

Motor innervation is supplied by the hypoglossal nerve (CN XI), except for the palatoglossus muscle, which is supplied by the vagus nerve (CN X). Sensory innervation for the oral tongue is supplied by the lingual nerve (CN V3), which also carries the chorda tympani branches (CN VII) that convey taste. Because CN V3 simultaneously covers sensation for the external auditory canal and tympanic membrane, referred otalgia is a common presenting complaint. Both sensory and taste innervation to the base of the tongue is by the glossopharyngeal nerve (CN IX). Lymphatic drainage importantly depends on the tongue site. The tongue tip primarily drains into the submental (level IA) lymphatics, while the lateral borders drain into ipsilateral levels IB and II. The antero-lateral tongue has drainage to level III lymph nodes, thus explaining the presence of mid-neck metastasis among some patients with primary tumors arising in this location. The base of the tongue has rich lymphatic drainage and, as a result, many patients will have early nodal involvement. The most frequent site of nodal metastases is in ipsilateral level II; however, levels III and IV as well as retropharyngeal nodal groups may also be involved. In contrast to the oral tongue, there is often spread of disease across the midline. The contralateral neck therefore requires consideration in treatment planning.

TONSILS

The palatine tonsils are almond-shaped lymphoid tissues encapsulated in a fibrous capsule within the tonsilar fossa. The lower portion of the fossa is crossed by the glossopharyngeal nerve (CN IX) as it crosses the inferior portion of the superior constrictor and then passes under its inferior boarder. The tonsillar pillars are formed by mucosal folds over two small muscles; the palatoglossus muscle raises a fold of mucosa anterior to the tonsils, forming the anterior pillar at the lateral junction between the oral and oropharyngeal cavities. The posterior pillar is formed by raised mucosa from the superior fibers of the palatopharyngeus muscle.

SOFT PALATE

The soft palate hangs down as an extension of the hard palate. This mobile myomucosal fold fuses at the sides with the lateral wall of the pharynx and is essential for velopharyngeal competency and for opening of the estuation tubes. It is composed of an aponeurosis and five paired muscles that act upon it to alter its shape. These are the tensor veli palatini, levator veli palatini, palatoglossus, palatopharyngeus and muscle of the uvula (musculus uvulae). Innervation of the soft palate musculature is by the pharyngeal plexus (CN X and XI), except for the tensor veli palatini, which is supplied by a branch from the nerve to the medial pterygoid muscle (CN V3). Sensation is conveyed by CN V2 with overlapping contributions from CN IX at the lateral boarder with the pharyngeal wall. The greater petrosal nerve conveys taste from the soft palate. Lymphatics drain from these structures into the retropharyngeal and upper deep cervical nodal basins. Tumors almost exclusively arise from the oropharyngeal surface of the soft palate. Lesions near the uvula are at higher risk of bilateral nodal spread.

PHARYNGEAL WALL

The pharyngeal wall forms the postero-lateral aspects of the oropharynx. It consists of mucous membrane, submucosal layer, muscular layer and thin buccopharyngeal fascia. Immediately posterior to it lies the prevertebral fascia, separated by a potential space. The pharyngeal muscular wall is thin and consists of three curved, overlapping muscle sheets: the superior, middle and inferior constrictor muscles. Structures passing between the superior and middle constrictors include the glossopharyngeal nerve (CN IX), providing sensory supply, and the lingual nerve (CN V3). The pharyngeal wall is rich in lymphatics and drains to the retropharyngeal, level II and III nodal basins.

CLINICAL EVALUATION

All patients with head and neck tumors should undergo a comprehensive history and physical examination. Clinical assessment should include:

- Detailed description of all symptoms leading up to presentation
- Profile of the patient for risk factors for head and neck cancer
- Assessment of functional status and medical comorbidities
- Detailed physical examination, including adjunct instrumentation
- Obtaining of an in-office tissue sample where possible for histologic diagnosis

Additional investigations and referrals to members of the multidisciplinary head and neck team are discussed in Chapter 7.

HISTORY

Presenting symptom

Specific questions should be asked about a sore in the mouth (ulceration), dysphagia, odynophagia, dysarthria, cough, bleeding episodes, excessive salivation, facial numbness, referred otalgia, trismus, obstructive sleep apnea, snoring, a neck mass or weight loss. Superficial, early-stage tumors most often present as non-healing ulcers or exophytic growths, with varying degrees of pain and occasional episodes of bleeding from the lesion. These tumors are usually present for several weeks to a few months before most patients seek medical attention. Occasionally, a suspicious lesion may be identified by the dentist during routine dental examination in asymptomatic patients. Superficial ulcerations and early tumors are often assumed to be non-neoplastic lesions and are treated with oral rinses, topical therapy or antibiotics. In contrast to ulceration, some tumors present as exophytic growths that may be white to pink in color. Friability and surface bleeding are often prominent features of malignancy. Some white lesions present as papillary growths characteristic of a verrucous carcinoma. Halitosis secondary to a fungating necrotic tumor is present in some patients with massive lesions. Presentation can also be due to mass symptoms causing sleep apnea, snoring or a neck lump.

Other presenting symptoms depend on the location and extent of the primary tumor. Lip cancer usually presents as an ulcerative or proliferative lesion of the lower lip. This can be associated with numbness of the skin of the chin due to mental nerve involvement. Assessment of the length of lip involvement is important for surgical treatment planning. Figures 6.2 through 6.11 demonstrate examples of malignant and non-malignant lip lesions. Buccal mucosal lesions can occasionally present with parotitis secondary to a blocked Stensen's duct. Figures 6.12 through 6.15 demonstrate images of varying extents of buccal mucosa squamous cell carcinoma (SCC) lesions. Lesions of the anterior floor of the mouth may cause obstruction of the opening of the Wharton's ducts, leading to obstructive submandibular sialadenitis and a palpable mass in the submandibular region, which may be the presenting symptom (4). Examples of benign and malignant lesions involving the floor of the mouth are shown in Figures 6.16 through 6.26. Very early lesions on the gum or the alveolar process can often be

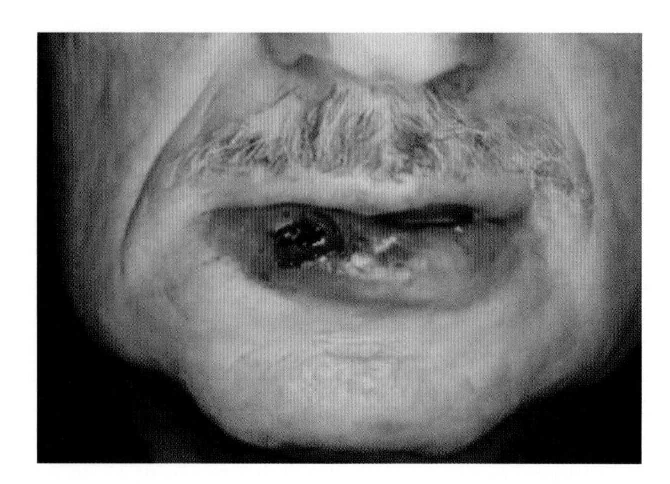

Figure 6.2 Squamous cell carcinoma of lower lip with invasion of deep musculature.

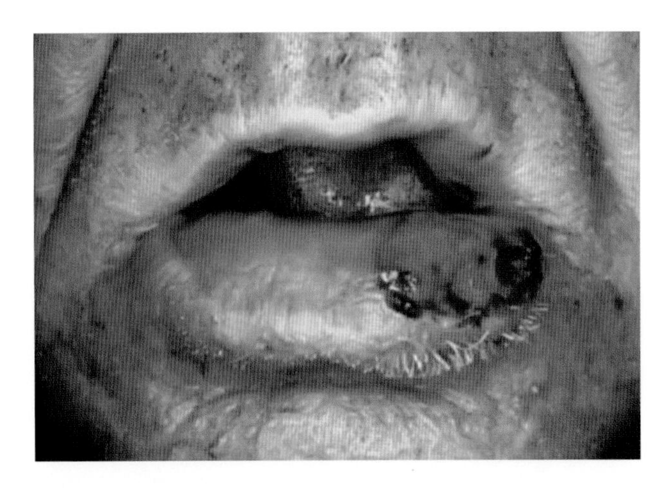

Figure 6.3 Chronic inflammatory ulceration of the vermilion border of the lower lip.

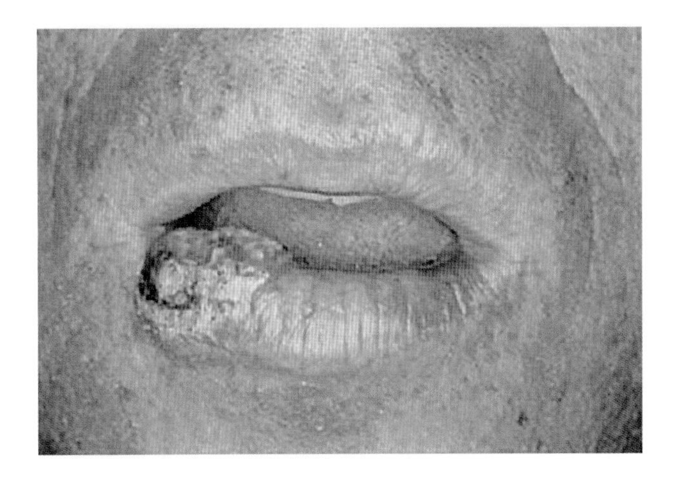

Figure 6.4 Exophytic, well-differentiated, keratinizing squamous cell carcinoma of the lower lip adjacent to the commissure.

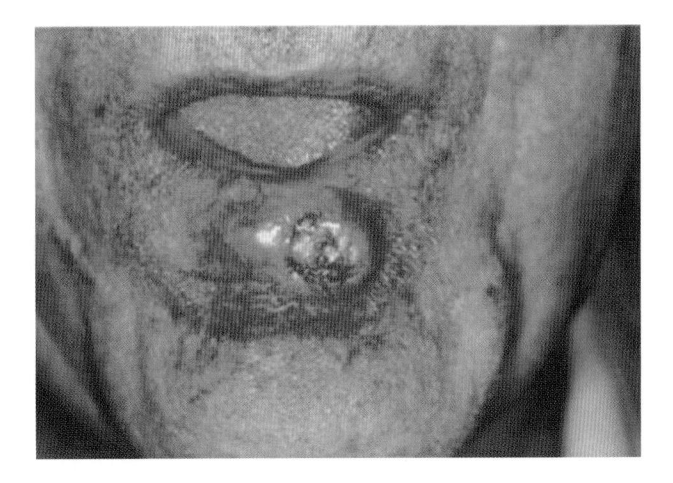

Figure 6.5 Squamous cell carcinoma of the lower lip with invasion of the deep musculature.

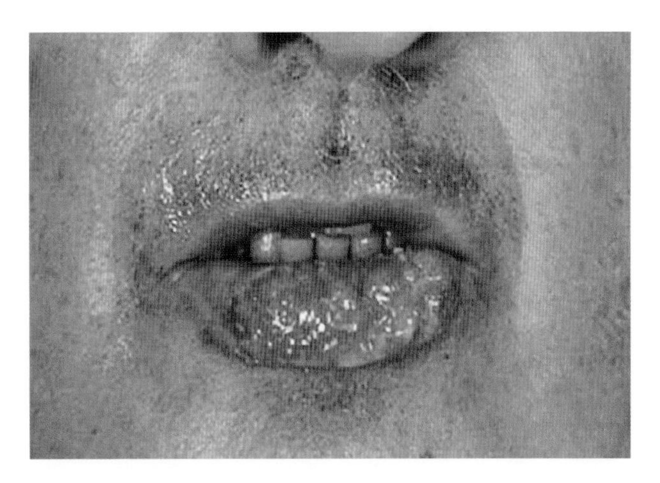

Figure 6.6 Superficial extensive carcinoma of the vermilion border of the lower lip.

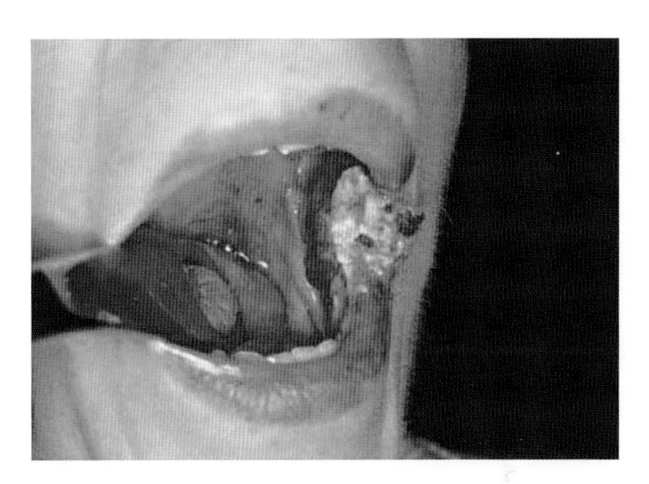

Figure 6.7 Squamous cell carcinoma of the oral commissure extending to the cheek mucosa.

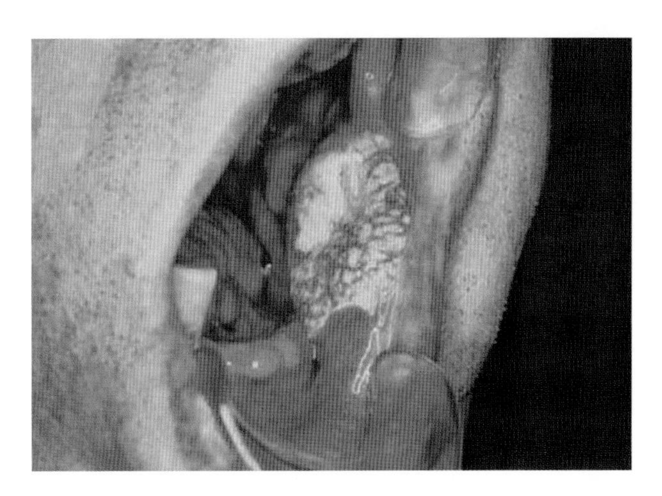

Figure 6.8 Papillary verrucous carcinoma of the oral commissure with extension to the cheek mucosa.

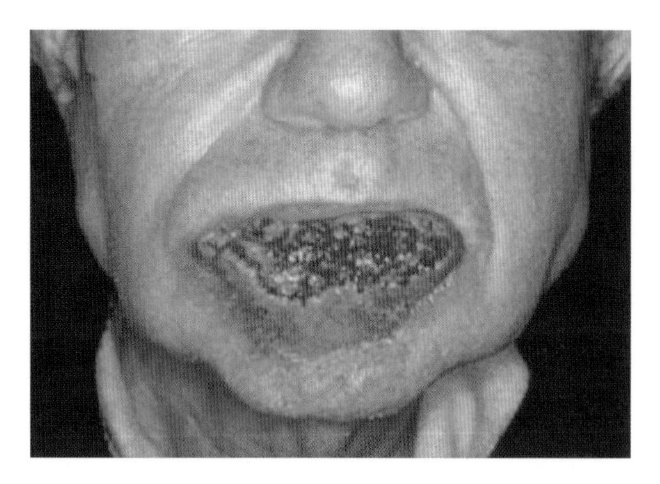

Figure 6.9 Massive carcinoma of the lower lip with invasion of the skin, soft tissues and mandible.

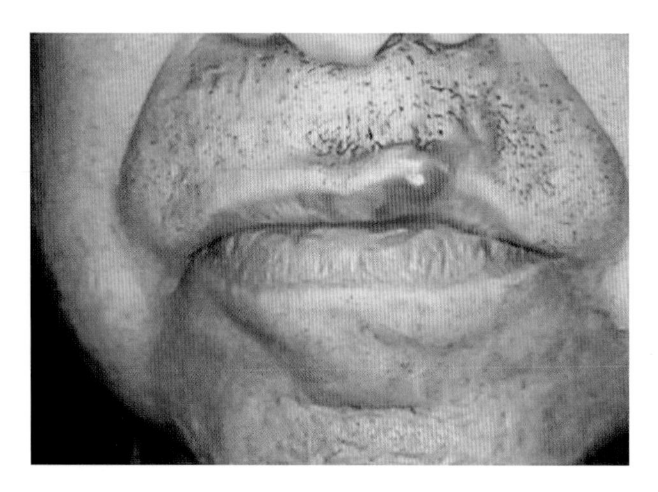

Figure 6.10 Adnexal carcinoma of sweat gland origin involving the vermilion border of the upper lip and adjacent skin.

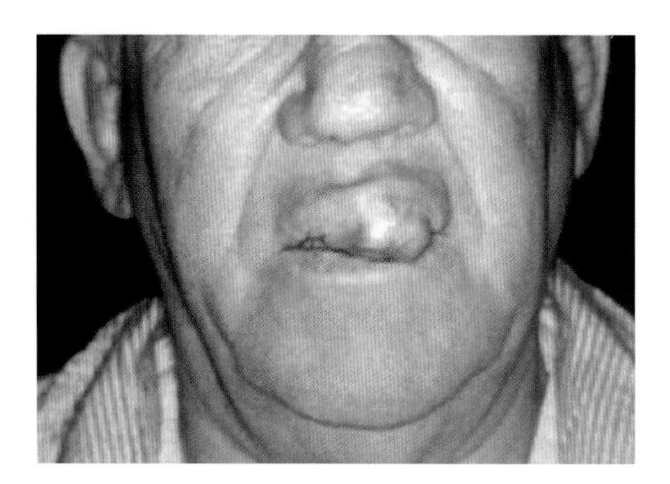

Figure 6.11 Adenoid cystic carcinoma of minor salivary gland origin involving the upper lip.

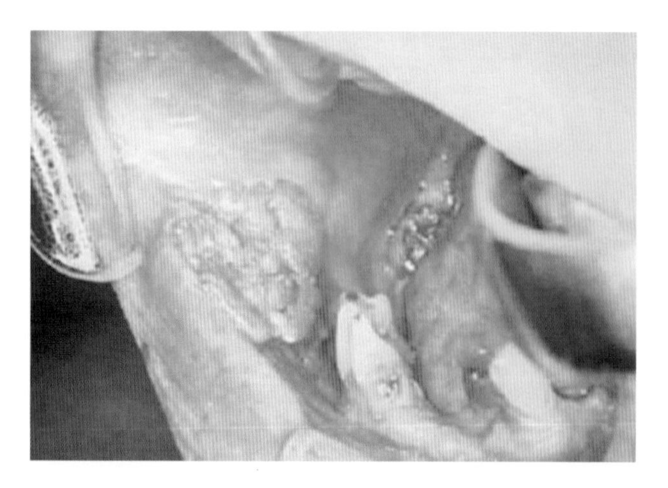

Figure 6.12 Papillary squamous cell carcinoma of the right cheek mucosa.

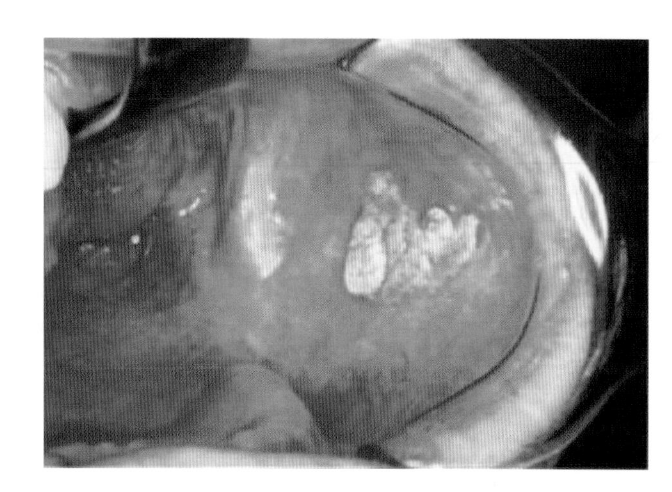

Figure 6.13 Superficially invasive squamous cell carcinoma of the right cheek mucosa.

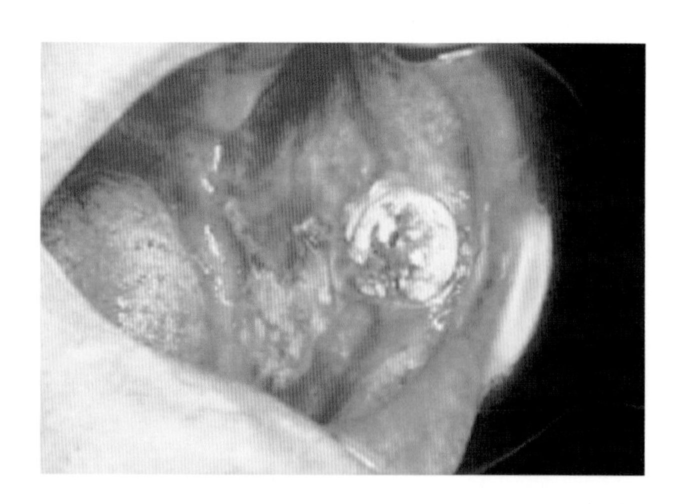

Figure 6.14 Squamous cell carcinoma of the left cheek mucosa with superficial areas of hyperkeratosis.

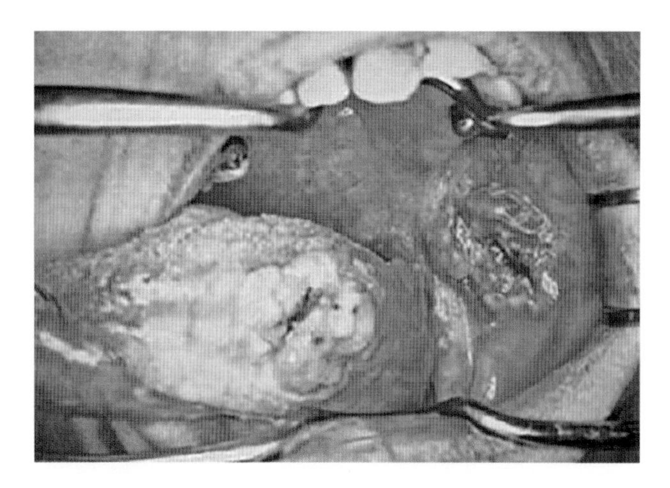

Figure 6.15 Synchronous squamous cell carcinomas of the lateral border of the tongue and buccal mucosa.

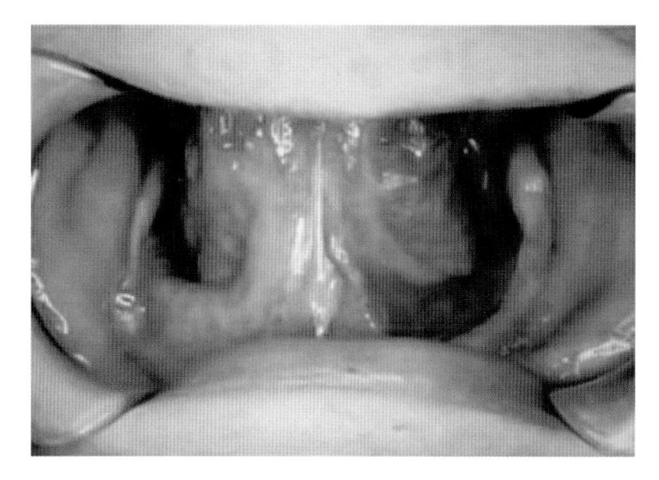

Figure 6.16 Erythroplakia of the anterior floor of the mouth. (*Note:* No treatment was given to this patient at this juncture.)

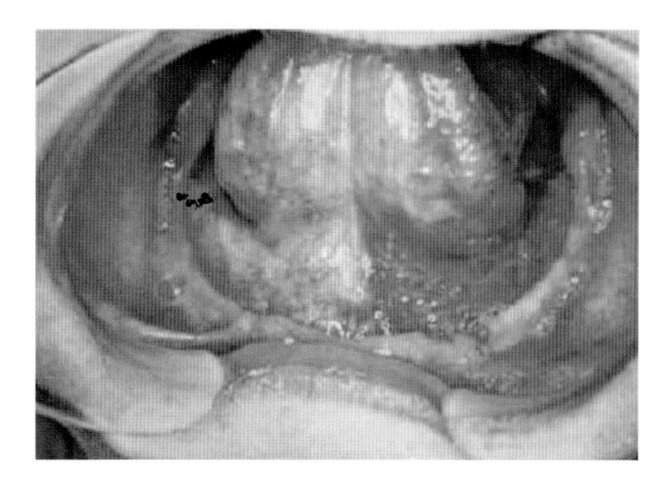

Figure 6.17 Three years later, the patient shown in Figure 6.16 has superficially invasive squamous cell carcinoma arising in an area of pre-existing erythroplakia.

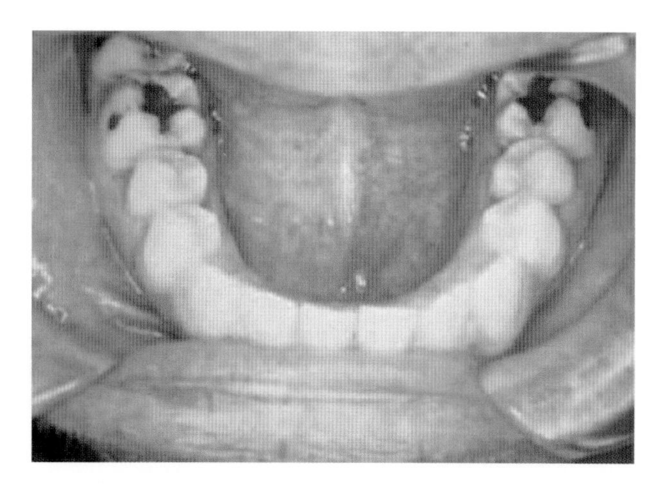

Figure 6.18 Impacted calculus at the opening of left Wharton's duct.

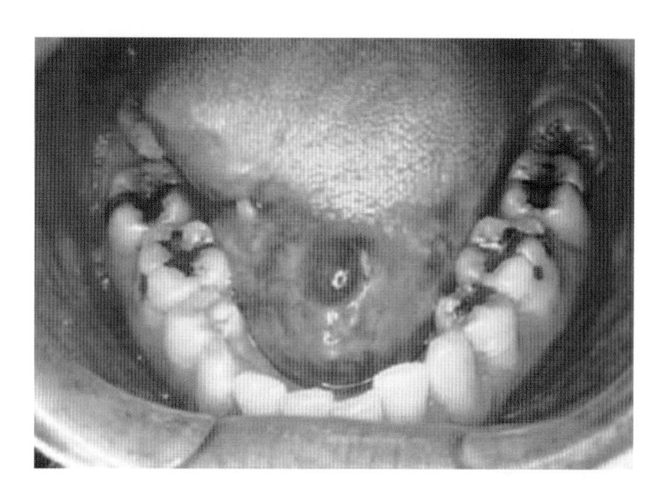

Figure 6.19 Ranula of the floor of the mouth post-previous partial glossectomy.

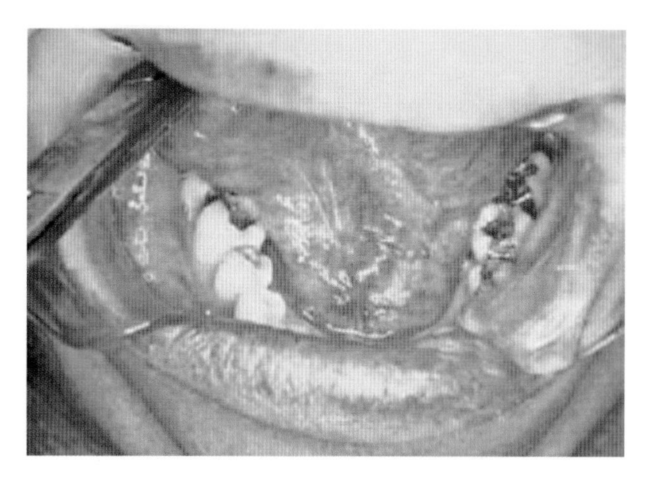

Figure 6.20 Squamous cell carcinoma in a pre-existing area of leukoplakia

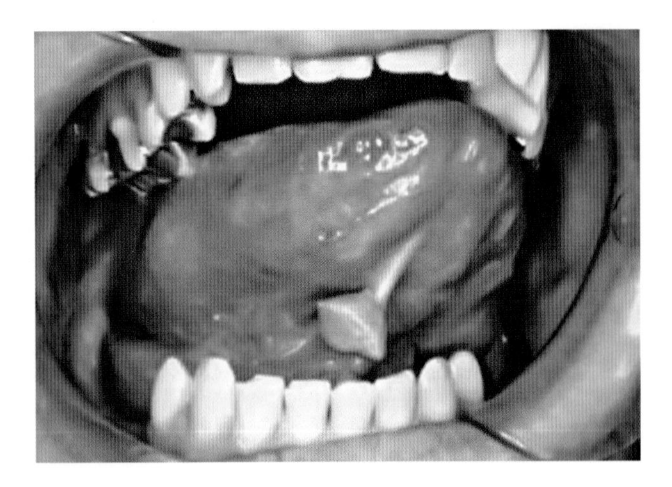

Figure 6.21 Squamous cell papilloma of the anterior floor of the mouth.

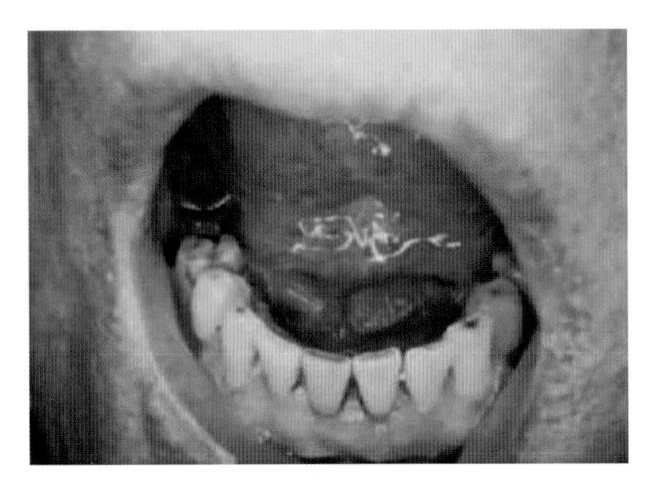

Figure 6.22 Squamous cell carcinoma of the anterior floor of the mouth and ventral tongue.

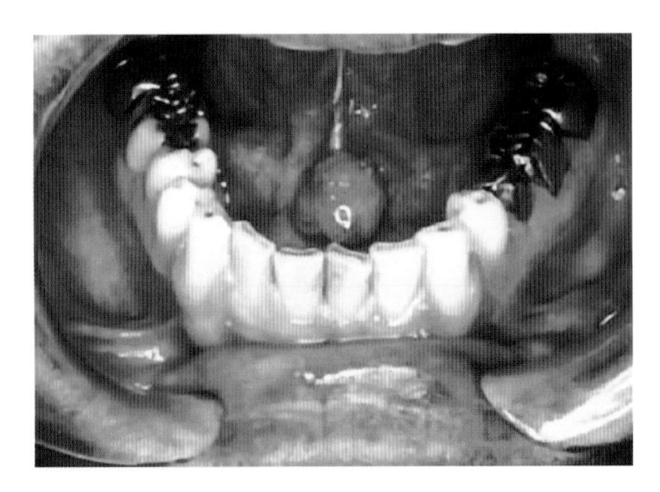

Figure 6.23 Squamous cell carcinoma of the anterior floor of the mouth.

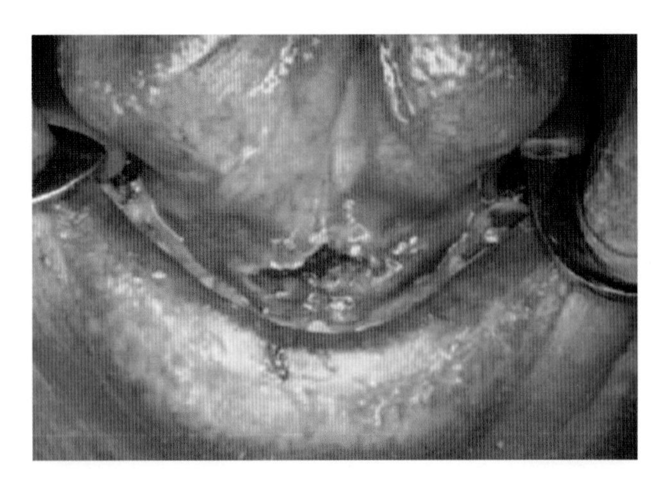

Figure 6.24 Ulcerated infiltrating squamous cell carcinoma of the anterior floor of the mouth.

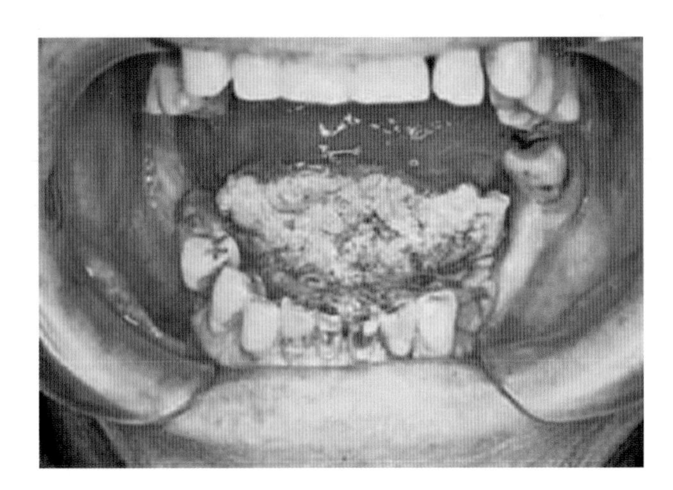

Figure 6.25 Deeply invasive squamous cell carcinoma of the anterior floor of the mouth involving the lingual gingiva.

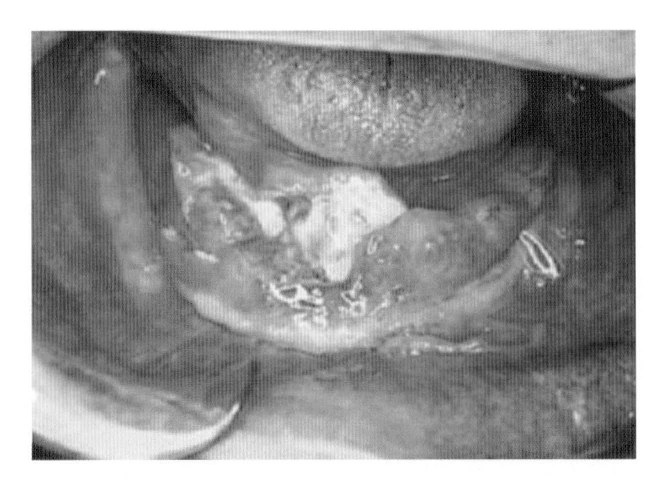

Figure 6.26 Verrucoid deeply invasive squamous cell carcinoma of the anterior floor of the mouth with extension to lower gingiva.

mistaken for sepsis around a tooth socket and treated as gingivitis or dental infection. Lack of response to conservative treatment or the presence of a loose tooth, however, should immediately raise suspicion of a malignant process necessitating biopsy to establish tissue diagnosis. Similarly, changes to dentition or an ill-fitting denture should also raise suspicion in some patients with cancer of the gum or palate (5). The presence of an exophytic lesion associated with several contiguous loose teeth should raise the index of suspicion for a locally advanced malignant tumor of the gum. A history of a non-healing extraction site should also raise the suspicion of a neoplastic process in a patient who has undergone recent tooth extraction. Advanced lesions with invasion of the mandible and the inferior alveolar nerve may produce anesthesia of the skin of the chin. Figures 6.27 through 6.34 demonstrate a variety of oral lesions involving the alveolar ridge with or without local extension into adjacent oral subsites. Tonsillar cancers account for an increased proportion of oropharyngeal disease, particularly in the younger patients (Figures 6.35 through 6.37).

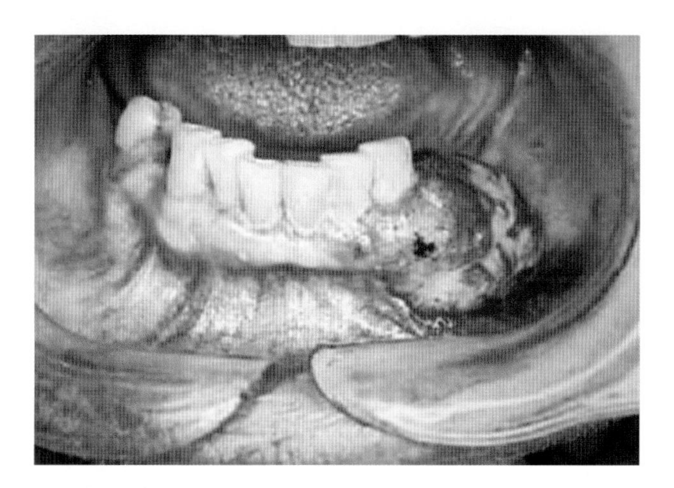

Figure 6.27 Squamous cell carcinoma of the lower gum with invasion of the underlying mandible.

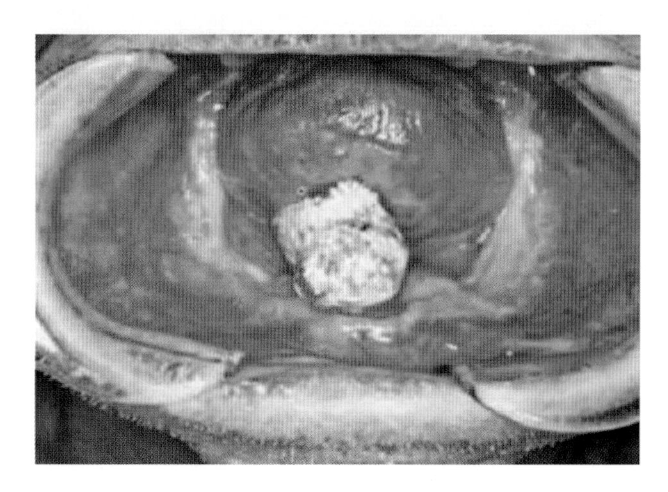

Figure 6.28 Exophytic verrucous carcinoma of the lower gum in the midline extending to the floor of the mouth.

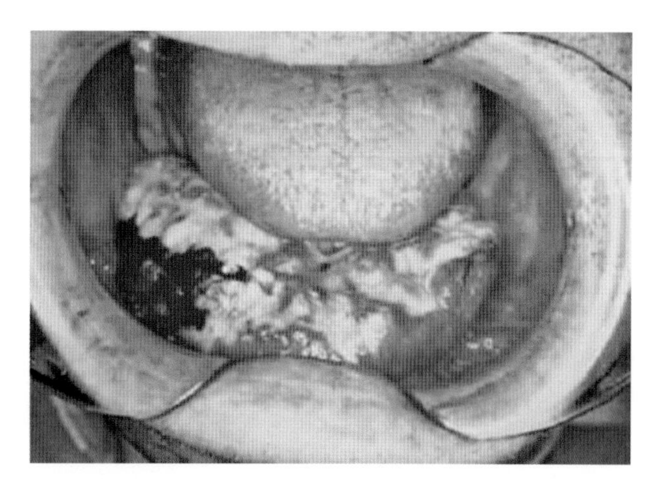

Figure 6.29 Extensive squamous cell carcinoma of the lower gum.

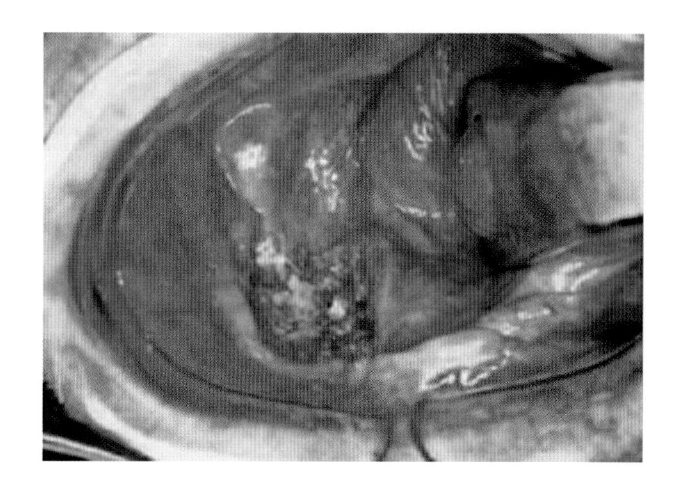

Figure 6.30 Squamous cell carcinoma of the edentulous lower gum with extension to the floor of the mouth.

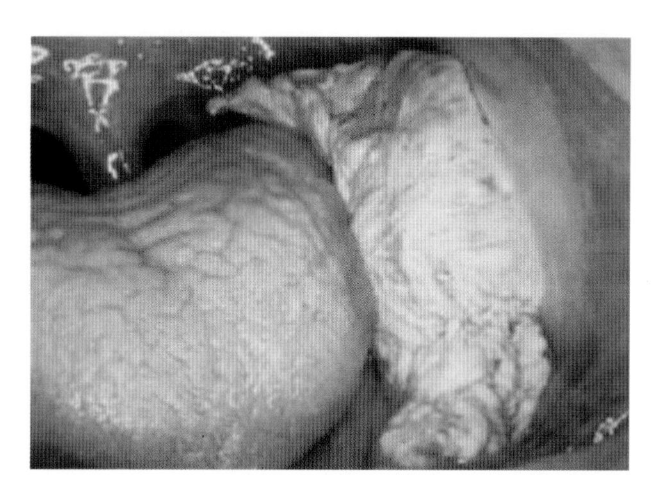

Figure 6.31 Verrucous carcinoma of the left lower gum with extension to the retromolar gingiva.

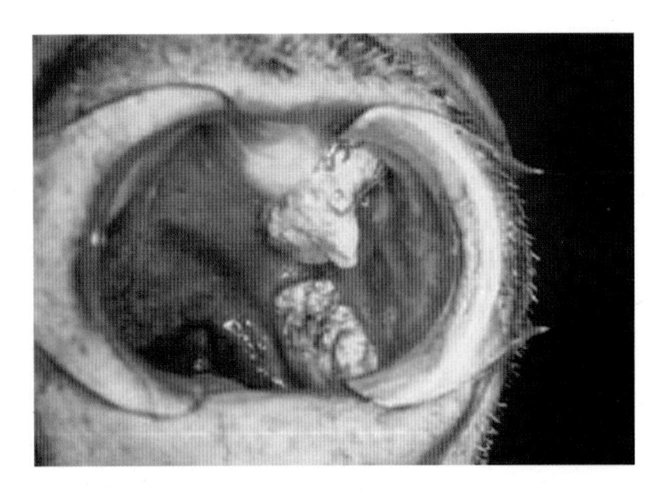

Figure 6.32 Multifocal squamous cell carcinomas involving the lower and upper gum.

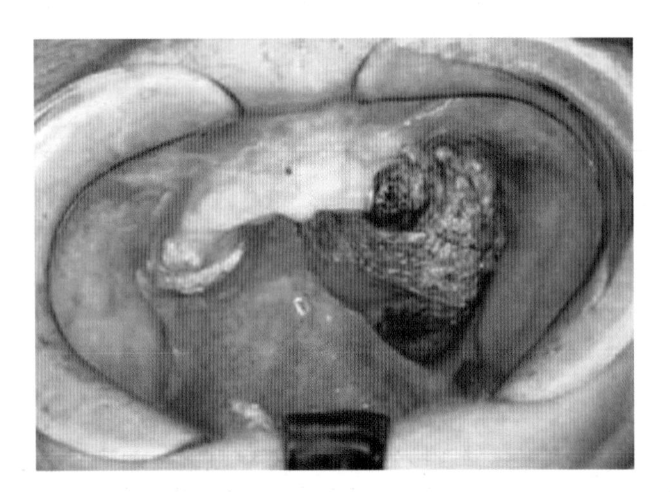

Figure 6.33 Squamous cell carcinoma of the upper gum with extension to the buccal mucosa and hard palate.

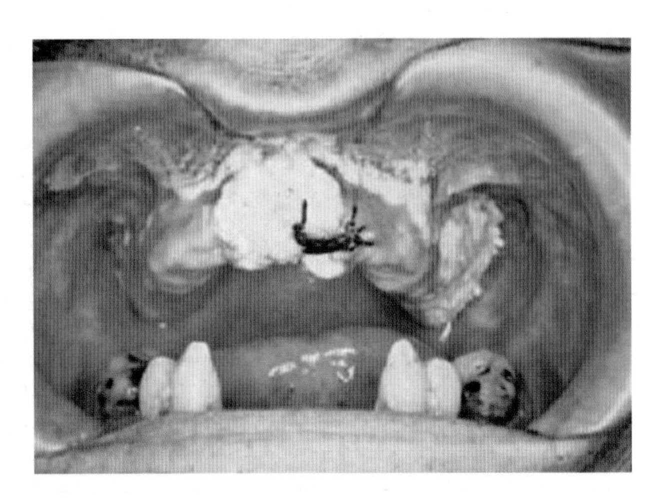

Figure 6.34 Verrucous carcinoma of the upper gum with extensive areas of hyperkeratosis.

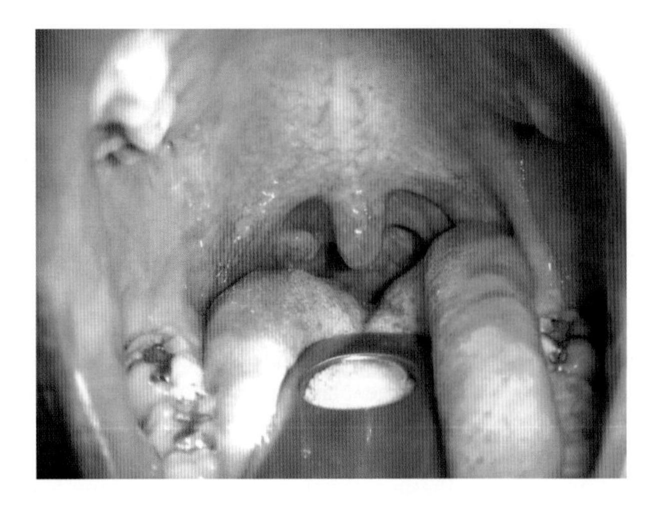

Figure 6.35 Small exophytic tonsilar squamous cell carcinoma.

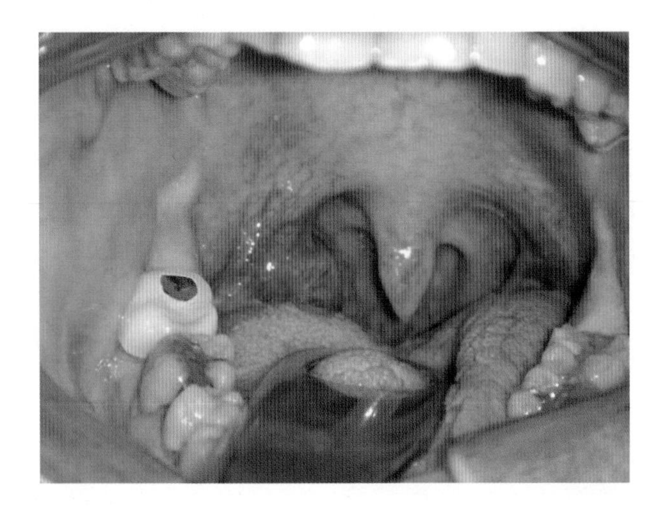

Figure 6.36 Ulcerated tonsilar squamous cell carcinoma.

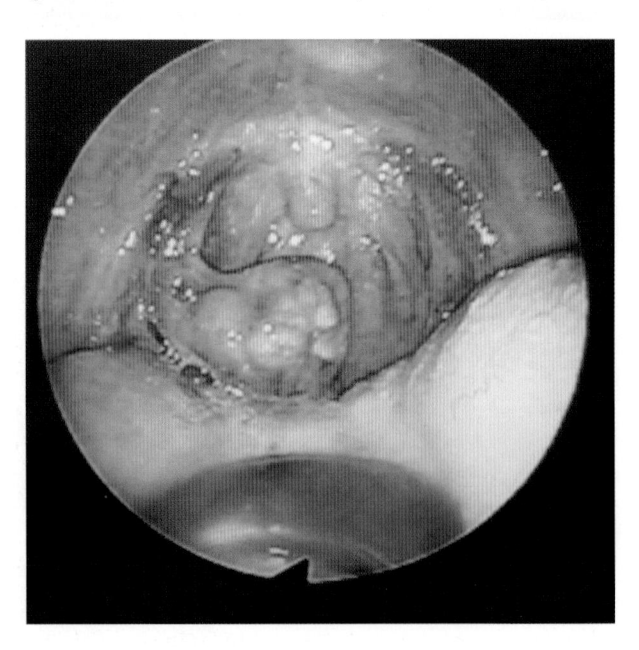

Figure 6.37 Tonsilar squamous cell carcinoma extending to base of tongue.

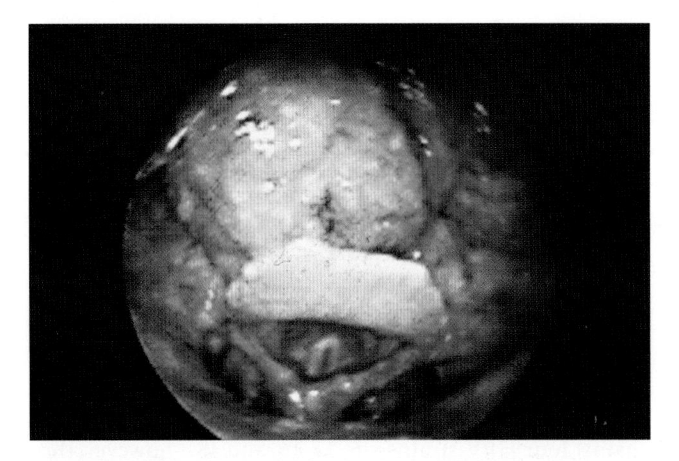

Figure 6.38 Base of tongue squamous cell carcinoma extending to valeculla.

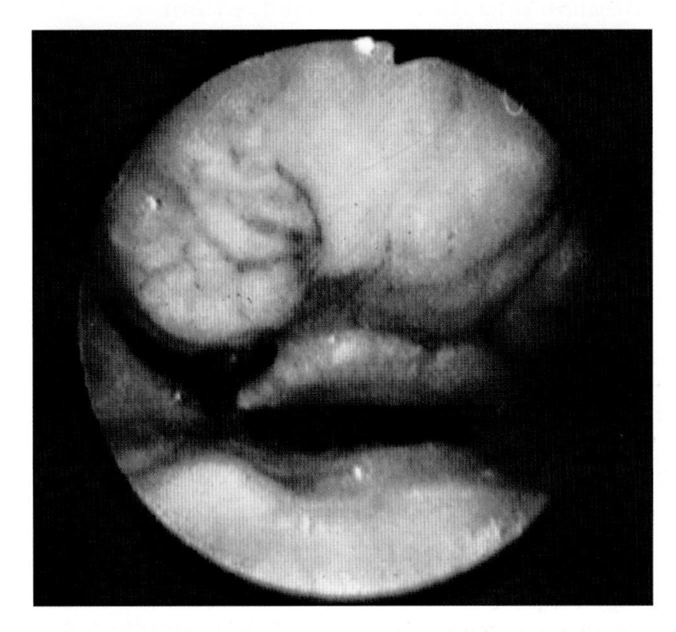

Figure 6.39 Squamous cell carcinoma presenting as a submucosal mass with mucosal vascularity.

Progressive trismus is a manifestation of local progression of tumor in the masticator space and pterygomaxillary region, particularly from posterior extension of buccal mucosa or tonsilar tumors with invasion of the pterygoid muscles. However, trismus may also be related to chronic submucous fibrosis in patients with a habit of chewing areca (betel) nuts (6). Extension into the parapharyngeal space toward the base of skull can affect cranial nerve function. Base of the tongue and pharyngeal wall lesions are insidious and frequently asymptomatic until significant disease progression has ensued (Figures 6.38 through 6.40). Very advanced lesions can cause significant local and referred pain (otalgia) and restriction in the mobility of the tongue. Excessive salivation with reduced mobility of the tongue is an ominous sign and usually suggests advanced disease. Impairment in the oral phase of swallowing with the resultant pooling of saliva and distortion of speech may also result from the continued growth. With further progression

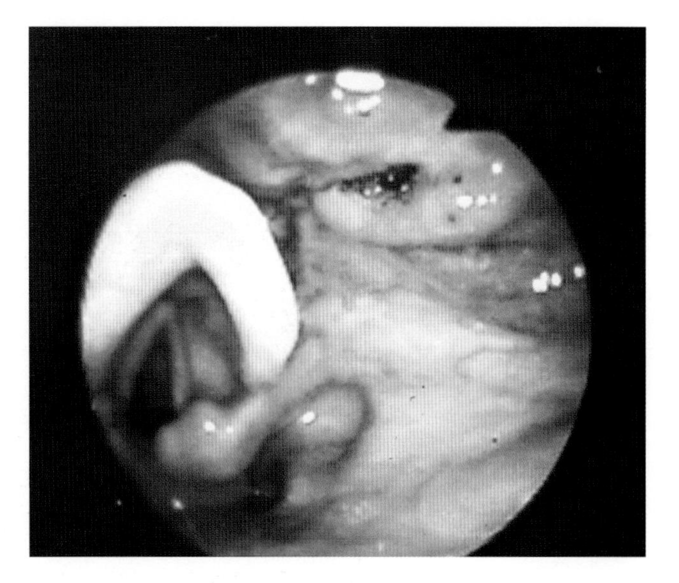

Figure 6.40 Mostly submucosal carcinoma of the base of the tongue with central ulceration.

and delay of treatment, tumor growth can result in impairment of mastication and deglutition. Oral consumption of food may be restricted to soft foods and patients may lose significant weight.

Particularly in human papillomavirus (HPV)-positive oropharyngeal cancer patients, initial presentation can be with ipsilateral or bilateral nodal metastases. Such adults presenting with nodal masses that are cystic clinically or radiologically can be mistaken as having branchial cleft cyst carcinomas. They need metastatic cystic SCC to be strongly considered and excluded.

Risk profile

An accurate history about tobacco and alcohol use should be elicited. The risk of cancer is increased from about 1.5-fold for light smokers (<10 pack-years) to fourfold for heavy smokers (>30 pack-years). Alcohol alone imparts a risk of oral SCC (OSCC) of threefold with >15 units per week (7). The synergistic impact of smoking with alcohol imparting a multiplied risk of OSCC is well documented. The use of tobacco in the form of snuff and chewing is associated with the development of mucosal dysplasia and an increased risk of developing OSCC. A history of areca (betel) nut use is associated with development of a unique case of premalignancy typified by labial and buccal mucosal atrophy, palpable submucosal fibrosis and progressive trismus.

Numerous additional etiologic factors may contribute to oral and oropharyngeal carcinogenesis. Assessment of such risk factors can facilitate diagnosis and contribute to devising an appropriate treatment plan. A history of prior skin cancers or extensive sun exposure is significant for lip cancer. Prior premalignant oral/oropharyngeal lesions such as leukoplakia or erythroplakia may be indicative of field cancerization for mucosal lesions (Figures 6.16 and 6.41 through 6.43). History of poor oral hygiene has been

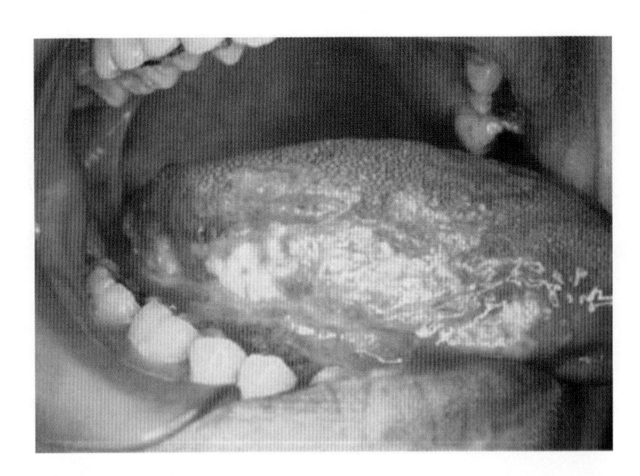

Figure 6.41 Multifocal areas of hyperkeratosis involving the lateral border of the tongue. (*Note:* No treatment was given to this patient at this juncture.)

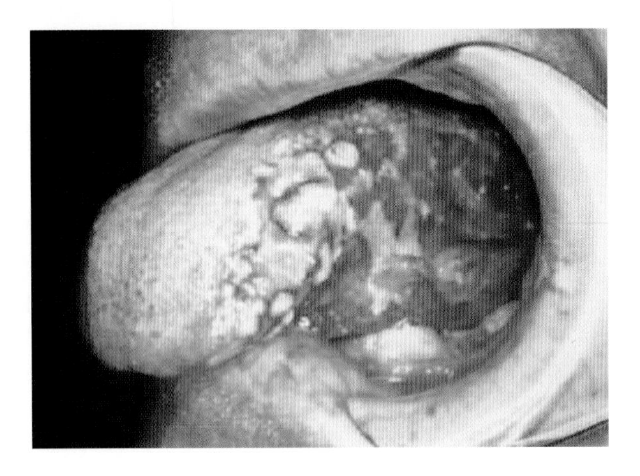

Figure 6.42 Speckled leukoplakia involving the lateral border of the oral tongue.

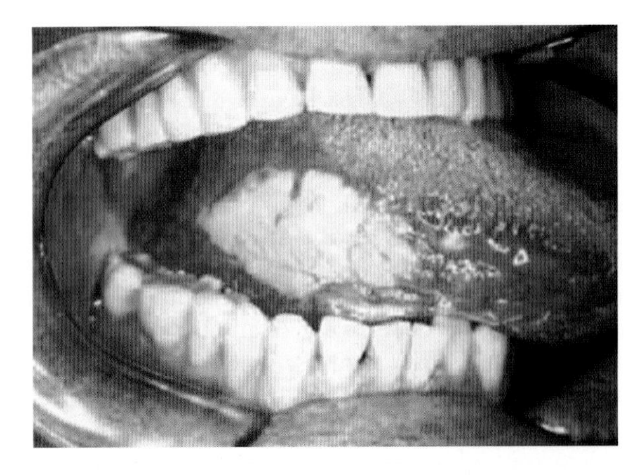

Figure 6.43 Discoid hyperkeratosis involving the lateral border of the oral tongue.

associated with oral cavity disease. Lichen planus, an autoimmune disease, causes lacy leukoplakia that has a small potential for malignant transformation. Genetic predisposition to oral tongue cancer is seen in patients with Fanconi's anemia, a rare recessive condition that leads to leukemia and also development of oral tongue cancer at a young age. Furthermore, such patients are at high risk of secondary malignancies from radiation therapy. Immunosuppressed patients, most commonly following bone marrow transplant, are more likely to develop OSCC in the setting of graft-versus-host disease. This condition leads to chronic inflammation of mucosal surfaces and may lead to OSCC after 2–10 years. Whole-body irradiation following treatment for leukemia will similarly cause increased incidence of secondary cancers. HPV is an established causative agent of oropharyngeal cancers, most commonly arising from the tonsils. Its role in oral cancer, however, is less established. Patients who have received the HPV vaccine are protected against four HPV strains—6, 11, 16, and 18—however, they are still vulnerable to other strains.

Medical and functional assessment

Assessment of the patient's overall medical and functional status is important to formulating an appropriate treatment strategy and establishing a realistic likelihood of treatment completion. Patients with a history of heavy alcohol use and smoking are at significant risk for chronic cardiac, respiratory, liver, renal and peripheral vascular diseases, as well as malnutrition. Pre-existing comorbidities should be identified and optimized before institution of cancer therapy. Critical information regarding previous cancers, particularly head and neck cancers, and their treatment should be collected. Previous treating physicians or institutions should be contacted for medical records regarding key elements of radiotherapy, chemotherapy or surgery. A thorough psychosocial history should be taken. Referral to smoking and alcohol cessation programs, as appropriate, should be offered.

DIFFERENTIAL DIAGNOSIS

The tumor may be ulcerative, exophytic, endophytic or a superficial proliferative lesion. The visible features of the lesion are usually sufficient to raise the index of suspicion regarding the need for a biopsy to establish tissue diagnosis. It is important to note that the appearances of HPV-positive and HPV-negative oropharyngeal lesions are similar and cannot be differentiated on clinical examination alone.

Ulcerative or endophytic lesions are usually accompanied by an irregular edge and induration of the underlying soft tissues (Figures 6.44 and 6.45). On the other hand, exophytic lesions may present either as a cauliflower-like irregular growths (Figures 6.28 and 6.46) or they may be flat, pink to pinkish-white proliferative lesions. Occasionally, a red to pink, velvety, flat lesion is the only manifestation of superficially invasive cancer or carcinoma *in situ*. Bleeding from the surface of the lesion should raise the suspicion of a neoplasm. Squamous carcinoma with excessive keratin production and verrucous carcinoma present as white, heaped-up lesions with varying degrees of keratin debris on the surface (Figures 6.31, 6.34, and 6.47). Papillary projections are often seen in lesions that are accompanied or preceded by a squamous papilloma (Figures 6.48 and 6.49). Endophytic lesions have a very small surface component but have a substantial amount of soft tissue involvement beneath the surface (Figures 6.44 and 6.50). Palpation should be performed to assess depth of invasion and fixation to adjacent bone. Leukoplakia and erythroplakia have a varying incidence of malignancy (8,9). Speckled leukoplakia (Figure 6.42) has

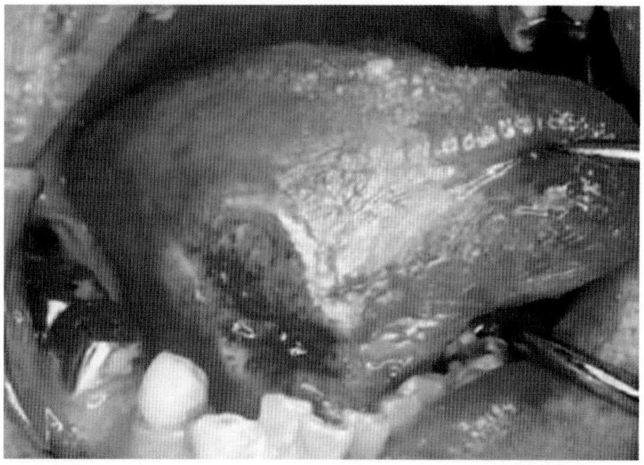

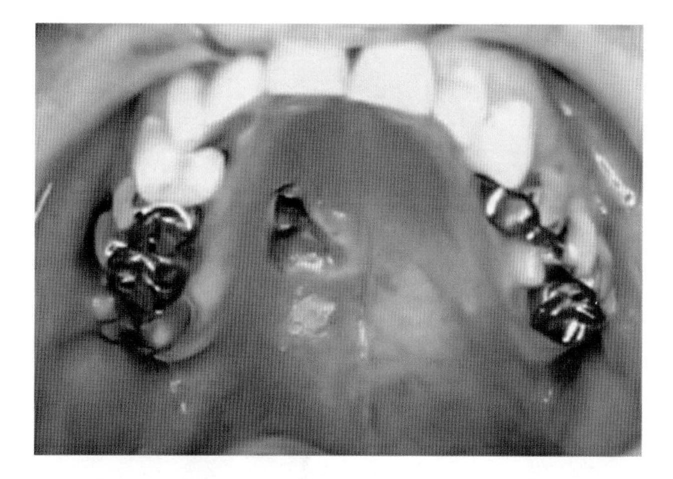

Figure 6.44 Ulcerated endophytic squamous cell carcinoma of the right lateral border of the tongue.

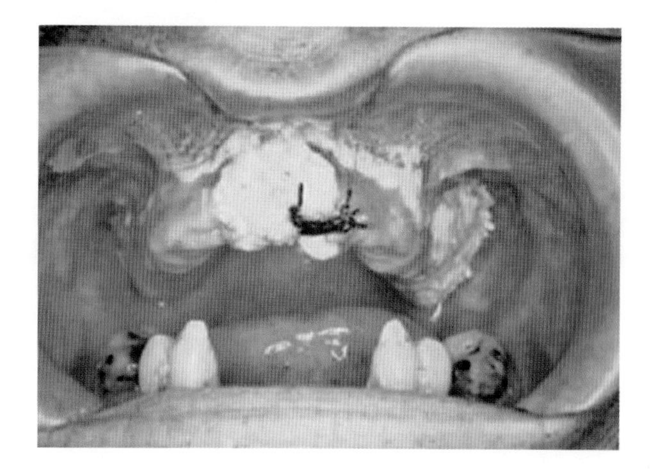

Figure 6.47 Verrucous carcinoma of the upper gum with extensive areas of hyperkeratosis.

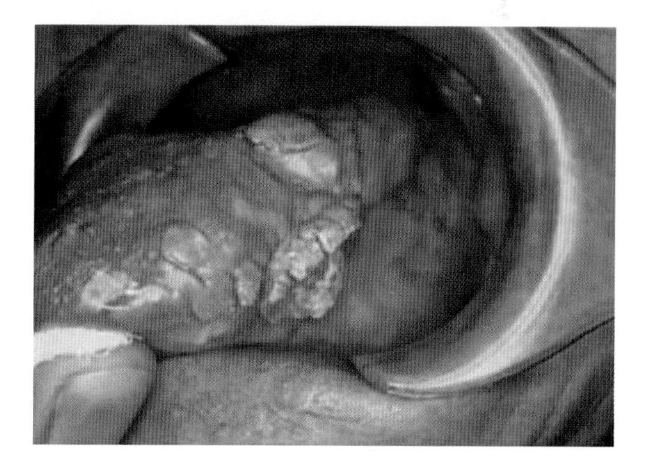

Figure 6.48 Multifocal papillomas of the lateral border of the oral tongue.

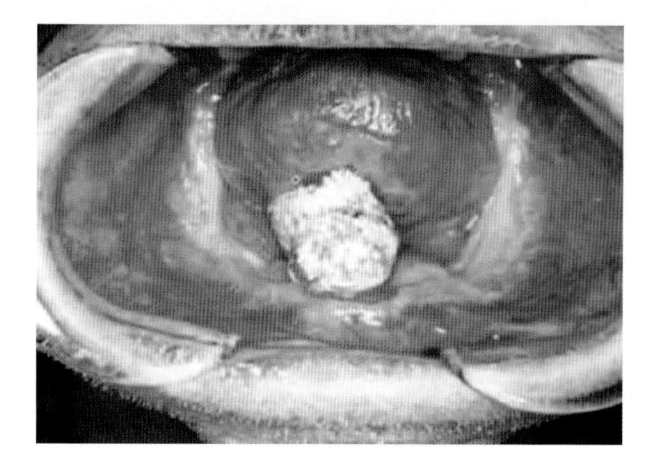

Figure 6.46 Exophytic verrucous carcinoma of the lower gum in the midline extending to the floor of the mouth.

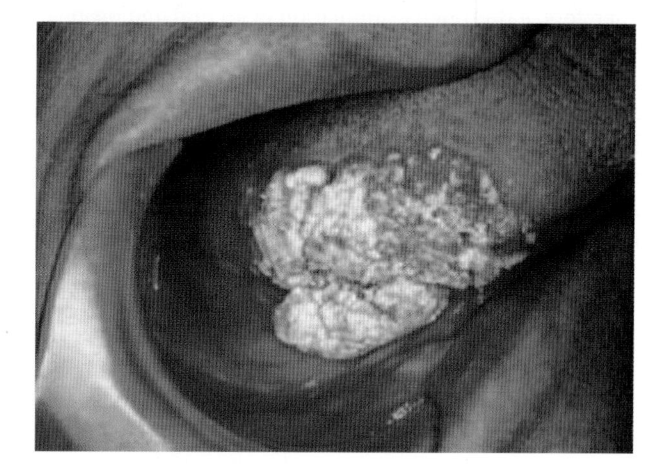

Figure 6.49 Papillary squamous cell carcinoma of the right lateral border of the tongue.

Figure 6.45 Mostly endophytic ulcerated squamous cell carcinoma of the hard palate.

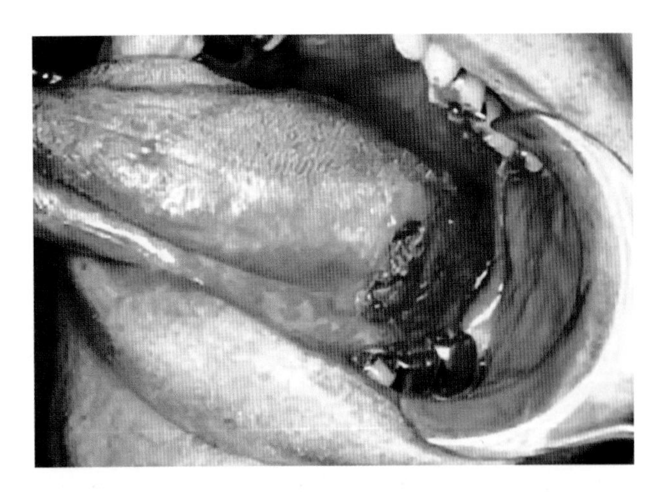

Figure 6.50 Ulcerated endophytic squamous cell carcinoma of the lateral border of the tongue adjacent to the retromolar region.

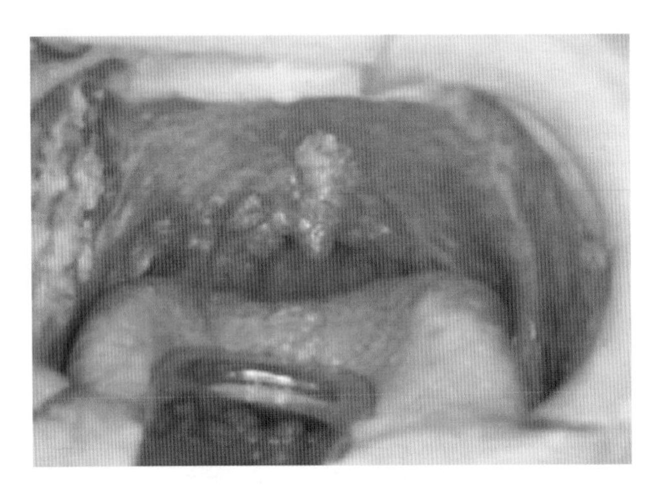

Figure 6.51 Multifocal hyperkeratotic superficially invasive squamous cell carcinoma involving the right cheek mucosa and soft palate.

a particularly high incidence of malignant transformation (10). Synchronous primary cancers occur in approximately 2% of patients with oral cancers (11) (Figures 6.15 and 6.51). Therefore, a thorough examination of all oral and oropharynx structures should be performed in every case.

SCCs, whether exophytic or endophytic, arise from or are intimately related to the surface epithelium. Whenever a lesion is encountered that is below the epithelium, other entities should be considered in the differential diagnosis. These tumors may arise from structures beneath the mucosa or represent metastatic disease from other sites. Tumors of minor salivary origin present as submucosal masses and most commonly occur in the hard or soft palate (12) (Figures 6.52 through 6.54). When these lesions become large, however, the overlying mucosa may ulcerate, making it difficult to determine their submucosal origin. Sarcomas may also arise from the soft tissues beneath the mucosa, thus presenting as a submucosal mass. Finally, lesions may occasionally involve the epithelium, but arise from structures not normally found in the mucosa lining the oral cavity.

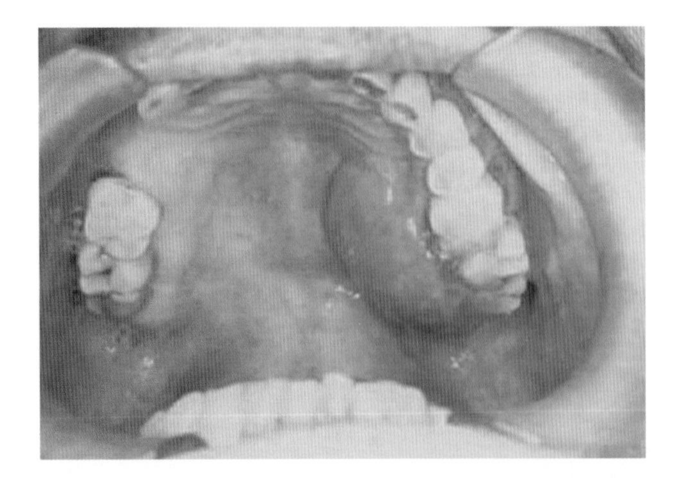

Figure 6.52 Adenoid cystic carcinoma of the hard palate.

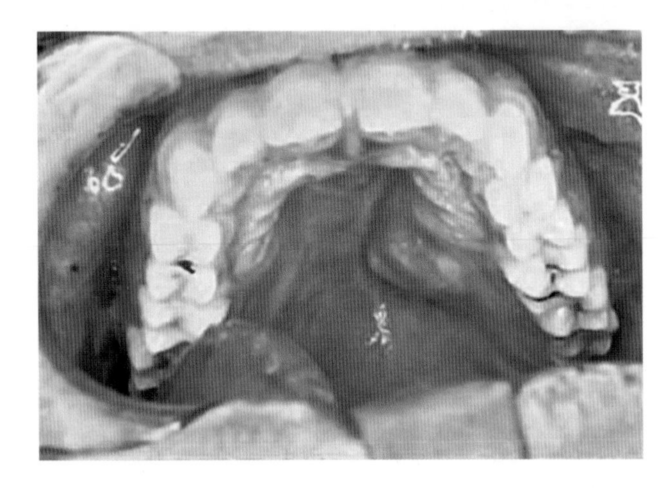

Figure 6.53 Mucoepidermoid carcinoma of the hard palate.

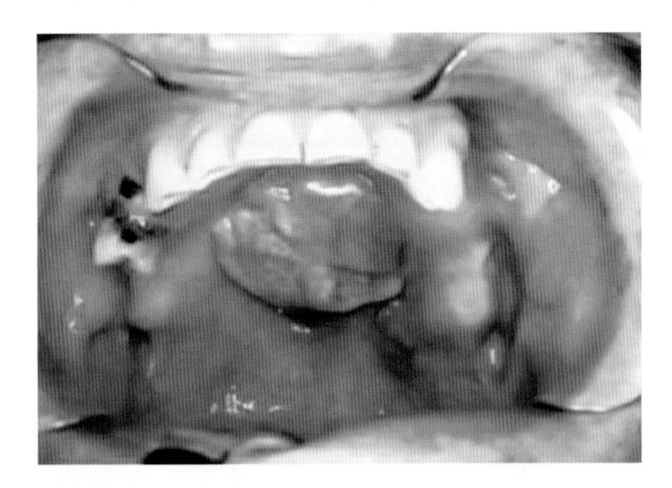

Figure 16.54 Adenocarcinoma of minor salivary gland origin of the hard palate.

One example is mucosal melanoma, which may present as a pigmented or non-pigmented lesion of the oral cavity mucosa. Brownish-black pigmented lesions are very characteristic of mucosal melanoma, as demonstrated in Figure 6.55. However, it must be borne in mind that melanosis is quite common in patients of African and Asian descent.

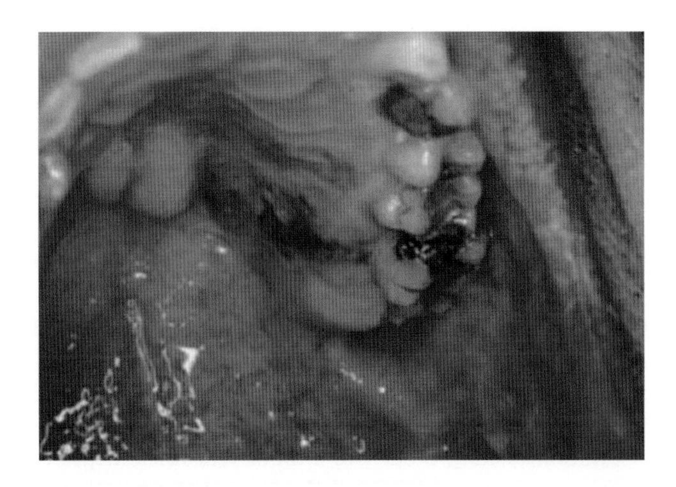

Figure 6.55 Mucosal melanoma involving the hard palate.

PHYSICAL EXAMINATION

A complete examination of the head and neck region should be performed in all patients with tumors of the oral cavity. This includes searching for and assessment of the primary tumor in the upper aerodigestive tract as well as regional lymph nodes.

Extraoral examination

In assessing patients with tumors of the oral cavity and oropharynx, full inspection and palpation of the skin of the face and scalp and evaluation of the major salivary glands and neck for lymph node metastases should be performed. The nasal cavity and nasopharynx, the hypopharynx and larynx, the auditory canal and the cranial nerves should also be assessed for second primaries.

In particular, an evaluation of sensation of the skin of the forehead, cheek, upper lip, chin and lower lip should be performed to assess for clinical evidence of perineural involvement. Invasion of CN V2 from primary tumors of the upper alveolus and palate may cause anesthesia of the skin of the cheek and upper lip. Similarly, anesthesia of the skin of the chin and lower lip signifies invasion of the inferior alveolar nerve (CN V3).

The major salivary glands (parotid, submandibular and sublingual) should be carefully examined by bimanual palpation for any masses or lesions. Openings of the Stensen's and Wharton's ducts should be inspected for free flow of saliva. Function of the facial nerve should be documented.

Examination of the nasal cavity with a speculum for any visible or obstructing lesions should be documented. Tumors of the palate or oropharynx may produce secondary nasal obstruction. Similarly, apparent oral cavity or oropharynx tumors may be from inferior extension of tumors arising from the nasal cavity or nasopharynx.

The status of regional cervical lymph nodes should be carefully evaluated by systematic palpation of accessible cervical lymph nodes including preauricular, periparotid, submental, prevascular facial, submandibular, deep jugular and posterior triangle lymph nodes. Nodal levels I, II, and III are most commonly involved by regional metastasis from oral cavity cancers (13–15). Occasionally, it is difficult to distinguish an enlarged submandibular salivary gland from an enlarged metastatic level I lymph node. Bimanual palpation through the floor of the mouth may assist in differentiating these. Levels II, III, and IV are most commonly involved in tumors of the oropharynx. If cervical lymph nodes are enlarged, they should be appropriately described as to their location and level, size, number and clinical signs of extranodal spread. Appropriate "N" staging should be assigned at this time according to the UICC/AJCC staging system (1).

The skin of the external ear canal should also be examined. Examination of the proximal ear canal and tympanic membrane should be performed, particularly for patients presenting with otalgia. An adult with a finding of serous otitis media should have fiber-optic endoscopy to exclude Eustachian tube obstruction by a tumor.

Intraoral examination

Examination of the oral cavity and oropharynx requires systematic inspection and palpation of the vermilion surface of the lips, labial and buccal mucosa, upper and lower alveolus, as well as mucosa of the gingiva, floor of the mouth, oral tongue and base of tongue, hard and soft palates, retromolar trigone, tonsils and pharyngeal wall. Figures 6.16, 6.42 through 6.44, 6.46 through 6.50 and 6.41 through 6.43, 6.56 through 6.59 demonstrate a variety of malignant and premalignant lesions of the oral tongue. Presence of trismus should be looked for and, in such instances, the inter incisor distance should be measured and documented. Extreme trismus will significantly affect the ability to do a thorough intraoral examination. Trismus

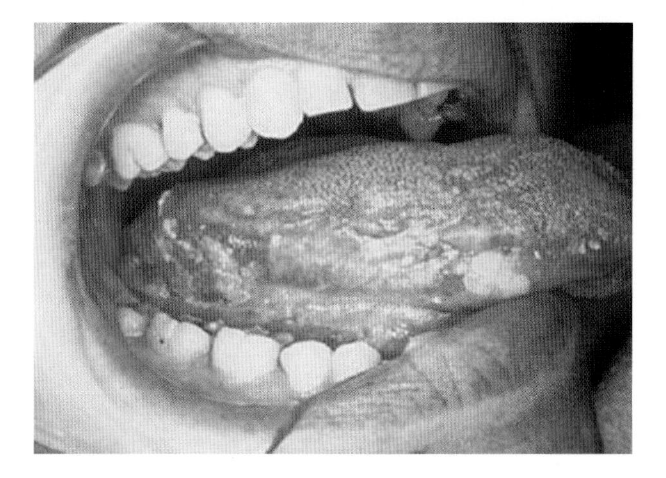

Figure 6.56 Eight months later, the patient shown in Figure 6.41 has developed two synchronous primary squamous cell carcinomas of the lateral border of the oral tongue involving the junction of the anterior and middle third of the tongue as well as the junction of the middle and posterior third of the tongue on the right-hand side

may be related to deep infiltration of masticator muscles by the primary tumor or by submucous fibrosis. Presence of submucous fibrosis should be noted. A tongue depressor and satisfactory lighting, preferably with a head light, provide visualization of the accessible sites in the oral cavity and oropharynx. The examination findings of the primary tumor arising on the mucosal surface of the oral cavity and oropharynx are variable. Inspect the size and character of the lesion, including its degree of infiltration (endophytic or exophytic) and its potential involvement of adjacent structures. Lesions involving the retromolar trigone and maxillary tubercle involve underlying bone early (Figures 6.60 through 6.62). Palpation of the lesion allows assessment of the third dimension or depth of infiltration of the tumor. An estimate of the depth of invasion in millimeters should be recorded, since that will be required for assigning appropriate T stage of the primary oral cancer. The lesion should be described as "thin" (depth of invasion <5 mm), "thick" (depth of invasion >5 but <10 mm) or very thick (depth of invasion >10 mm). Lesions of the floor of the mouth and cheek mucosa should be palpated bimanually. Proximity of the primary tumor to the adjacent bone (mandible or maxilla) should be carefully evaluated and documented to assess the need for bone imaging studies, in preparation for bone resection in conjunction with excision of the primary tumor. Palpation of the base of the tongue is essential to

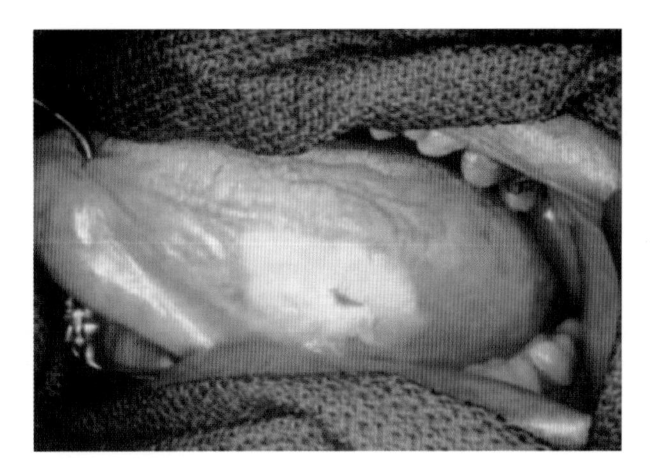

Figure 6.57 Squamous cell carcinoma arising in a preexisting area of hyperkeratosis.

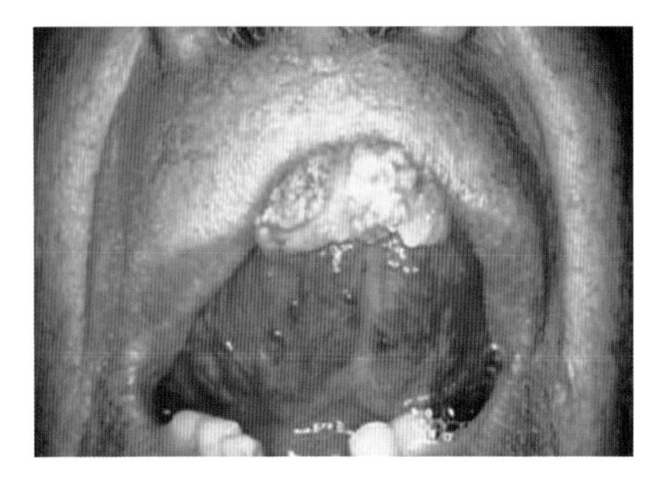

Figure 6.58 Exophytic cauliflower-like squamous cell carcinoma of the tip of the tongue.

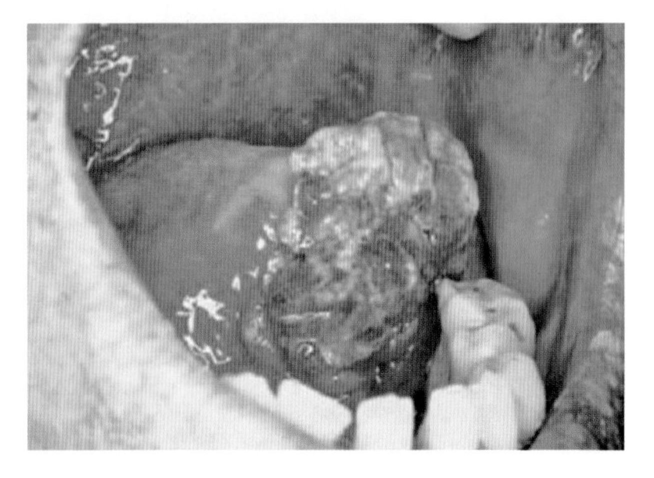

Figure 6.59 Squamous cell carcinoma of the lateral border of the tongue and floor of the mouth.

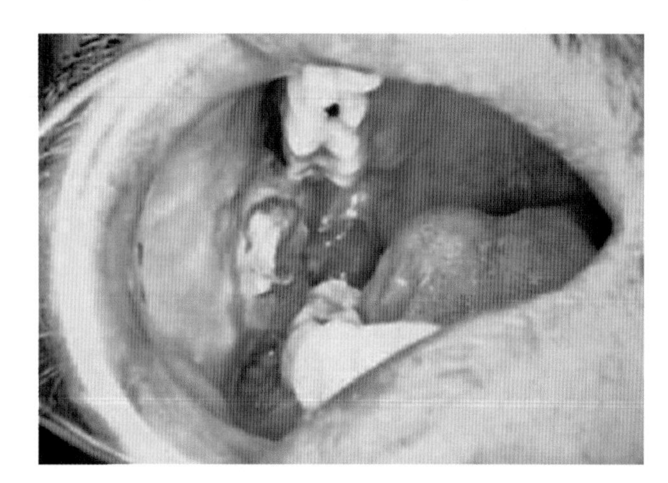

Figure 6.60 Squamous cell carcinoma of the retromolar gingiva.

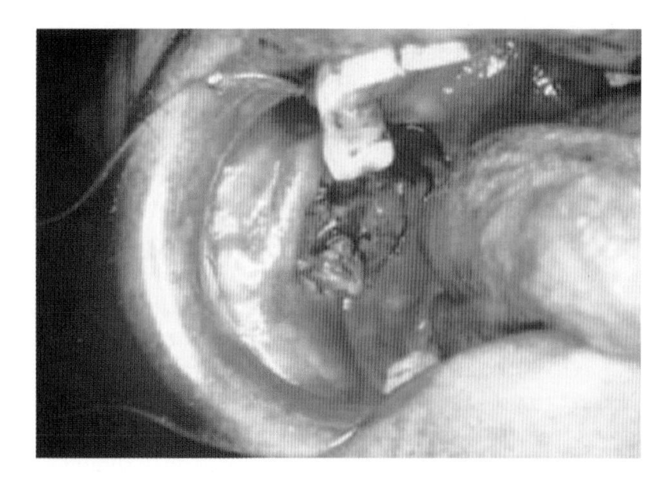

Figure 6.61 Squamous cell carcinoma of the retromolar gingiva with extension to the lower gum and the maxillary tubercle.

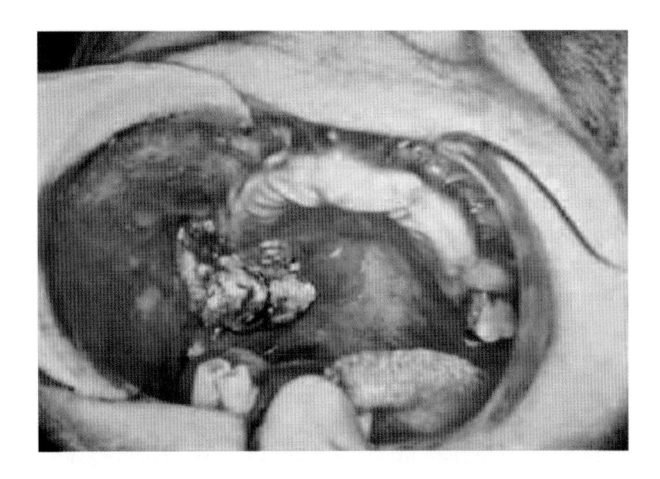

Figure 6.62 Squamous cell carcinoma of the maxillary tubercle and adjacent hard palate.

rule out a submucosal tumor mass. Mobility of the tongue should be evaluated to assess deep infiltration of the musculature of the tongue or invasion of the hypoglossal nerve by the tumor. Fixation of the tongue (ankyloglossia) will result in incomplete protrusion or deviation of the tongue toward the side of the lesion. Numbness of the oral tongue signifies invasion of the lingual nerve (CN V3), numbness of the posterior tongue signifies involvement of the glossopharyngeal nerve (CN IX) and numbness of the lower teeth and gingiva signifies invasion of the inferior alveolar branch of the mandibular nerve (CN V3). Vitality of the teeth should be checked, particularly in lesions of the lower or upper gum. Grossly septic teeth that are unlikely to survive radiation therapy should be evaluated for extraction. Conversely, loose teeth at the tumor site should be retained, as premature removal opens dental sockets and potentially leads to tumor implantation into the mandibular canal. Finally, surgical access options to the lesion should be considered, as well as potential reconstruction options.

Mirror examination

A dental mirror should be used for careful evaluation of the lingual gingivae of the upper and lower alveolar processes, particularly in the anterior aspect of the oral cavity. With appropriate technique in a cooperative patient, the dental mirror can also be used to examine the nasopharynx, base of the tongue, hypopharynx and larynx. The patient is instructed to breathe at a normal rate "through the mouth." This automatically moves the soft palate cephalad, allowing good mirror examination. The mirror is used in such a way that the shaft of the mirror is stabilized by pressure contact against the oral commissure. This avoids tremor-like movement of the mirror in the oropharynx causing tickling and coughing. The back of the mirror is used to push the soft palate up, giving an excellent view of the oropharynx, hypopharynx and larynx. The presence of any mucosal lesions should be noted, with accurate description of their visual characteristics. The mucosal surface of the posterior third of the tongue (posterior to the circumvallate papillae) should be carefully scrutinized and the presence of any lesions in the hypopharynx and larynx should be recorded. Adequacy of airway and mobility of the vocal cords should be recorded.

Flexible laryngoscopy

If adequate examination of the oropharynx, hypopharynx and larynx is not feasible with a dental mirror, then a fiberoptic flexible laryngoscope should be used. Figures 6.38 through 6.40 demonstrate base of the tongue lesions visualized on flexible laryngoscopy. This may be done without any anesthetic. However, topical anesthetic may be used in the nasal cavity. The added advantage of using the flexible laryngoscope is that it provides good visual examination of the nasal cavity and nasopharynx and a detailed survey of the base of the tongue, hypopharynx and larynx for tumor extension or presence of synchronous lesions. Video recording or photography are also possible for documenting the findings.

TISSUE DIAGNOSIS

For the oral cavity and oropharynx, tissue diagnosis is usually confirmed by a wedge or punch biopsy obtained from the periphery of the lesion or from the center of the lesion. Biopsies of lesions of the oral cavity can generally be obtained in-office with topical or local anesthetic. Grossly visible lesions of the oropharynx are also suitable for biopsy with a topical anesthetic; however, subtle lesions may require general anesthetic due to difficult access. An adequate volume of viable tumor tissue should be retrieved. Highly keratinizing SCCs and verrucous carcinomas may not provide satisfactory representative tissue from the surface of the lesion and the diagnosis of invasive carcinoma can be missed from a superficial biopsy. Therefore, where excessive keratin deposits are seen on the surface of an exophytic lesion, the biopsy should be obtained from an adjacent invasive zone or from the depth of the lesion rather than the surface. Similarly, areas of necrotic tumor should be avoided for biopsy. Harvesting of viable tissue in a biopsy is generally confirmed if some bleeding occurs at the biopsy site. If a biopsy fails to show carcinoma in a clinically suspicious lesion, then the biopsy should be repeated until the tissue diagnosis is confirmed. A fine needle aspiration of suspicious neck lymphadenopathy is also useful for diagnosis and staging. Occasionally, tissue biopsy may require imaging guidance, such as ultrasound-guided needle biopsy of a neck node or endoscopy under general anesthesia for biopsy of a lesion of the base of the tongue.

DOCUMENTATION

Surface measurements of the tumor as well as estimated depth of invasion should be documented for accurate T staging (1). Accurate clinical description of the lesion should include the specific primary site, size, its depth and appearance (such as ulcerative, fungating, exophytic or endophytic) and the presence of associated features (such as leukoplakia or erythroplakia). The presence of multiple primary tumors should be carefully checked. Documentation of the surface characteristics of the mucosa of the oral cavity and oropharynx not involved by the tumor is also important. Photography or video recording prior to biopsy is useful in most patients. Such records document baseline findings for comparison in future examinations. In the absence of photographic documentation, a diagram of the lesion on anatomic stamp drawings is recommended.

ADJUNCT SCREENING TOOLS

A wide range of commercially available clinical diagnostic aids in the detection of potentially malignant mucosal lesions are available. These include supravital staining, brush biopsy/cytology and numerous light-based technologies, used independently or in combination. Adjunct methods aim to either improve the visibility of oral mucosal lesions or provide non-invasive, real-time information in order to determine the malignant potential of mucosal lesions beyond conventional visual examination alone. The benefit of each adjunct test differs based on the patient's pre-test probability as well as the clinician's expertise. At present, there is limited evidence to draw definitive conclusions regarding their routine clinical use and cost-effectiveness (16–19).

SUPRAVITAL STAINING

Toluidine blue (TB) is one of the oldest clinical diagnostic aids for visualization of oral premalignant lesions and cancer and is widely used in many parts of the world. TB is a vital stain that can color malignant or premalignant tissues to facilitate diagnosis. However, studies have found wide-ranging sensitivity and specificity associated with the stain. Consequently, it is not recommended for use as a standalone test in the United States (16).

EXFOLIATIVE CYTOLOGY

Current general perception among both dentists and oral physicians and surgeons is that the sensitivity of oral cytology in collected sputum or oral rinse specimens is not sufficiently reliable to warrant its widespread use as a screening modality for visible lesions.

Autofluorescence

VELscope® is a device that uses tissue autofluorescence for direct visualization of the oral mucosa for subtle lesions. Oral neoplasias are associated with a loss of stromal collagen and hence have reduced autofluorescence compared to normal mucosa. This, however, is also present in benign inflammatory lesions, which significantly limits its diagnostic specificity. Numerous studies have yielded inconclusive or inconsistent results (20–22). Rana et al. suggested that using the autofluorescence device leads to higher sensitivity (but lower specificity) compared to clinical examination alone (21). Sweeny et al., however, did not find the technology to add additional information to standard clinical examination (22).

CHEMILUMINESCENCE

ViziLite® is an optic-based test originally developed for use by gynecologists for examination of the cervix. When used alone, numerous studies found a very low specificity of 0%–20%, but good sensitivity (23). With added TB, the specificity improves. In a recent meta-analysis by Kämmerer et al., who evaluated the role of a chemiluminescent light system in combination with TB, the authors concluded that the ViziLite system could not discriminate between inflammatory or premalignant lesions (18).

REFERENCES

1. Sobin L, Gospodarowicz M, Wittekind C. *International Union Against Cancer (UICC) TNM Classification of Malignant Tumors* (7th Edition). New York, NY: Wiley-Liss, 2009.
2. Inagi K, Takahashi H, Okamoto M, Nakayama M, Makoshi T, Nagai H. Treatment effects in patients with squamous cell carcinoma of the oral cavity. *Acta Otolaryngol Suppl* 2002;547:25–9.
3. Lin CS, Jen YM, Cheng MF et al. Squamous cell carcinoma of the buccal mucosa: an aggressive cancer requiring multimodality treatment. *Head Neck* 2006;28:150–7.
4. Mashberg A, Meyers H. Anatomical site and size of 222 early asymptomatic oral squamous cell carcinomas: a continuing prospective study of oral cancer. *II. Cancer* 1976;37:2149–57.
5. Shah JP, Patel SG, Singh B. *Jatin Shah's Head and Neck Surgery and Oncology* (4th Edition). Philadelphia, PA: Elsevier Mosby, 2012.
6. Norton S. Betel: consumption and consequences. *J Am Acad Dermatol* 1998;38:81–8.
7. Franceschi S, Bidoli E, Herrero R, Munoz N. Comparison of cancers of the oral cavity and pharynx worldwide: etiological clues. *Oral Oncol* 2000;36:106–15.
8. Waldron C, Shafer W. Leukoplakia revisited. A clinicopathologic study of 3,256 oral leukoplakias. *Cancer* 1975;36:1386–92.
9. Mashberg A. Erythroplasia vs. leukoplasia in the diagnosis of early asymptomatic oral squamous carcinoma. *N Engl J Med* 1977;297:109–10.
10. Craig R. 1981. Speckled leukoplakia of the floor of the mouth. *J Am Dent Assoc* 102:690–2.

11. de Vries N, Van der Waal I, Snow G. Multiple primary tumours in oral cancer. *Int J Oral Maxillofac Surg* 1986;15:85–7.
12. Spiro R. Salivary neoplasms: overview of a 35-year experience with 2,807 patients. *Head Neck Surg* 1986;8:177–84.
13. Shah J. Patterns of cervical lymph node metastasis from squamous carcinomas of the upper aerodigestive tract. *Am J Surg* 1990;160:405–9.
14. Shaha A, Spiro R, Shah J, Strong E. Squamous carcinoma of the floor of the mouth. *Am J Surg* 1984;148:455–9.
15. Franceschi D, Gupta R, Spiro R, Shah J. Improved survival in the treatment of squamous carcinoma of the oral tongue. *Am J Surg* 1993;166:360–5.
16. Rethman M, Carpenter W, Cohen E et al. Evidence-based clinical recommendations regarding screening for oral squamous cell carcinomas. *Tex Dent J* 2012;129:491–507.
17. Çankaya H, Guneri P, Epstein JB. Adjunctive methods and devices for clinical detection of oral squamous cell carcinoma. *Oral Health Prev Dent* 2014;13:29–39.
18. Kämmerer P, Rahimi-Nedjat R, Ziebart T, Bemsch A, Walter C, Al-Nawas B, Koch F. A chemiluminescent light system in combination with Toluidine blue to assess suspicious oral lesions—clinical evaluation and review of the literature. *Clin Oral Invest* 2015;19:459–66.
19. Rashid A, Warnakulasuriya S. The use of light-based (optical) detection systems as adjuncts in the detection of oral cancer and oral potentially malignant disorders: a systematic review. *J Oral Pathol Med* 2015;44:307–28.
20. Hanken H, Kraatz J, Smeets R et al. The detection of oral pre-malignant lesions with an autofluorescence based imaging system (VELscope)—a single blinded clinical evaluation. *Head Face Med* 2013;9:23.
21. Rana M, Zapf A, Kuehle M, Gellrich N, Eckardt A. Clinical evaluation of an autofluorescence diagnostic device for oral cancer detection: a prospective randomized diagnostic study. *Eur J Cancer Prev* 2012;21:460–6.
22. Sweeny L, Dean N, Magnuson J, Carroll W, Clemons L, Rosenthal E. Assessment of tissue autofluorescence and reflectance for oral cavity cancer screening. *Otolaryngol Head Neck Surg* 2011;145:956–60.
23. Vashisht N, Ravikiran A, Samatha Y, Rao P, Naik R, Vashisht D. Chemiluminescence and Toluidine blue as diagnostic tools for detecting early stages of oral cancer: an *in vivo* study. *J Clin Diagn Res* 2014;8:ZC35–8.

7

Workup and staging

LAURA WANG AND JATIN P. SHAH

Cancers of the oral cavity and oropharynx are a heterogeneous group of pathologic entities with variations in preoperative imaging requirements, optimal treatment selection, prognosis and quality of life repercussions. Given such complexities, the best oncologic and functional outcomes require a concerted multidisciplinary approach. In addition to the head and neck surgeon, input from radiation and medical oncologists and a full team of medical, dental and allied health specialists is required before selection and institution of therapy. Further workup requirements include obtaining appropriate radiographic imaging for clinical tumor staging, determining human papillomavirus (HPV) status and assessment and optimization of the general physical status of the patient. This includes assessment of general medical conditions, nutritional status, smoking and alcohol habits, dental health and available psychosocial supports. Postoperative complications and likely outcomes should be anticipated and their prevention and management should be prepared for in advance.

RADIOGRAPHIC EVALUATION

The use of complementary imaging modalities is an essential adjunct to a comprehensive physical examination in evaluating oral and oropharyngeal lesions for staging and treatment planning.

RADIOGRAPHIC ASSESSMENT OF DISEASE CHARACTERISTICS

Primary tumor

The new American Joint Committee on Cancer (AJCC) staging system (8th edition) measures tumor (T) status by greatest surface dimension and estimated tumor depth (1,2). Accurate clinical assessment of tumor depth can be challenging. Careful palpation of the lesion should be able to describe the lesion as thin, thick or very thick. However, superficial lesions, particularly within the oropharyngeal lymphoid tissue, cannot be reliably detected, even on computed tomography (CT) or magnetic resonance imaging (MRI). Though not commonly used, studies suggest that intraoral ultrasound can be useful in determining depth of primary oral cavity tumors. Ota et al. showed that preoperative ultrasound measured buccal squamous cell carcinoma (SCC) depth, guided extent of local surgical resection and could improve outcomes (3). Other studies similarly demonstrated that depth of tumor invasion on ultrasound was a significant prognosticator for presence of nodal metastasis (4).

Once the tumor infiltrates into the deep soft tissue planes, both CT and MRI can document extension into adjacent structures. Axial and sagittal MRI scans can vividly demonstrate tumor depth (Figure 7.1a and b).

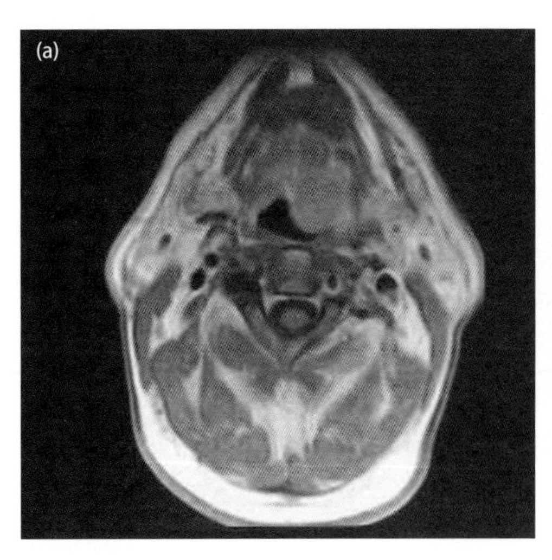

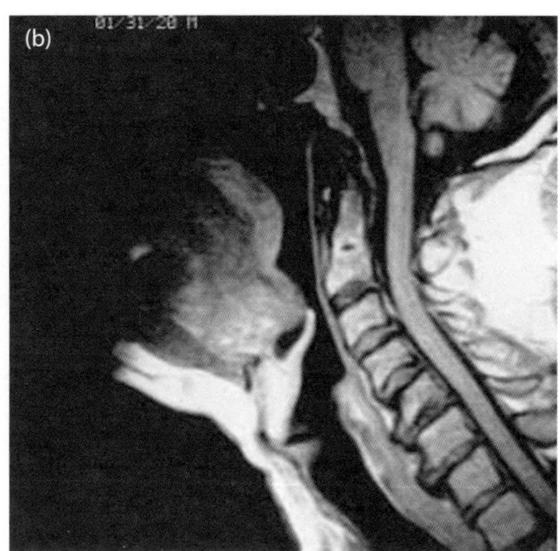

Figure 7.1 **(a)** Axial and **(b)** sagittal MRI scans can vividly demonstrate tumor depth.

Bone involvement

While the absence of radiographic findings does not rule out bone invasion, bone erosion or destruction as seen on radiological studies confirms tumor invasion. Plain radiographs of the mandible in anteroposterior and oblique views are not satisfactory as a routine screening procedure to establish or rule out bone invasion. Nevertheless, a panoramic view of the mandible (orthopantomogram) is perhaps the most commonly used radiographic study to assess the general architecture of the mandible in relation to the dentoalveolar structures and invasion by tumor (Figure 7.2). It should, however, be appreciated that, due to technical reasons, the midline of the mandible near the symphysis is not adequately evaluated by a panoramic view. While involvement of the alveolar process is readily assessable, early erosion of the lingual or buccal cortex is not assessable on the panoramic X-ray. Thus, for evaluation of early invasion of the cortex or the medullary bone, CT or MRI is generally required.

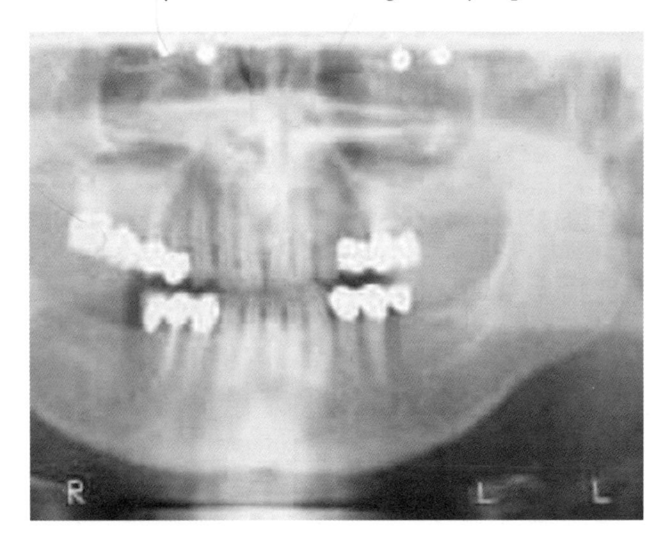

Figure 7.2 Panoramic X-ray (Panorex, orthopantomogram) of the mandible.

Thin-section CT can provide finer details and enables three-dimensional modeling that is excellent for detection of subtle cortical bone erosions. However, MRI is preferred for medullary bone extension. A CT scan with contrast can be particularly valuable for evaluating lesions that arise from the palate, alveolar ridge or floor of the mouth due to proximity of maxillary and mandibular cortical bone. It is important to obtain coronal cuts with bone windows and soft tissue windows to adequately assess the extent of tumor involving the hard palate and upper alveolus (Figure 7.3a–c). In the coronal plane, tumor and involvement of the palatal foramina and extension into adjacent areas such as the maxillary sinus antrum are clearly assessed. MRI, however, may have important advantages over CT in the presence of significant dental filling artifacts and for soft tissue invasion into the masticator or parapharyngeal spaces.

Radionucleotide bone scans are often positive prior to radiographic appearance of bone destruction, but they seldom provide accurate information regarding the extent of bone invasion. Bone scans may also be positive in non-neoplastic conditions, such as inflammatory lesions, thus leading to false-positive results. In one study, the false-positive rate of bone scans for detecting mandible invasion in oral cavity tumors exceeded 50% (5).

Perineural spread

Perineural spread is identified on imaging through a loss of fat planes, enlargement and enhancement of nerves and expansion of bony foramina through which nerves traverse. It is also worth noting that tumors can similarly spread along blood vessels and muscle fascia. Invasion of a vessel can be assumed if tumor surrounds it by more than 270°. In general, MRI is superior to CT for imaging of perineural spread of disease, with coronal fat-suppressed post-gadolinium T1-weighted MRI best demonstrating perineural spread (6).

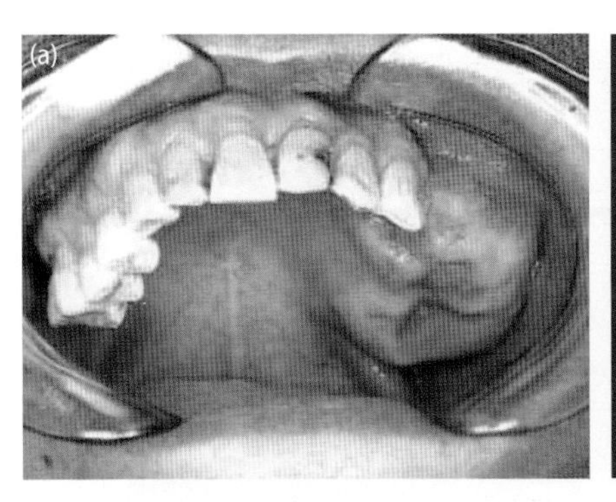

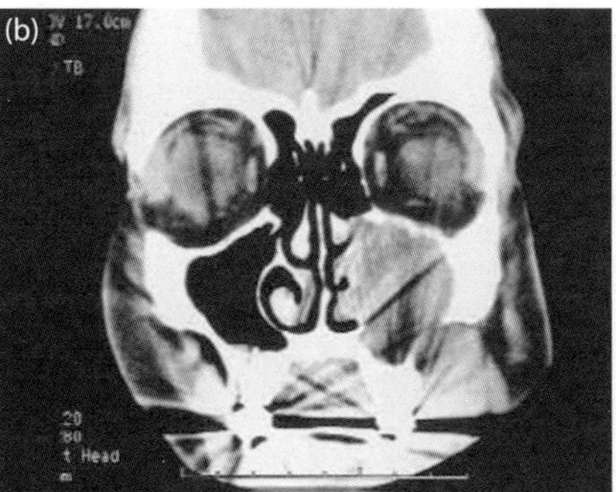

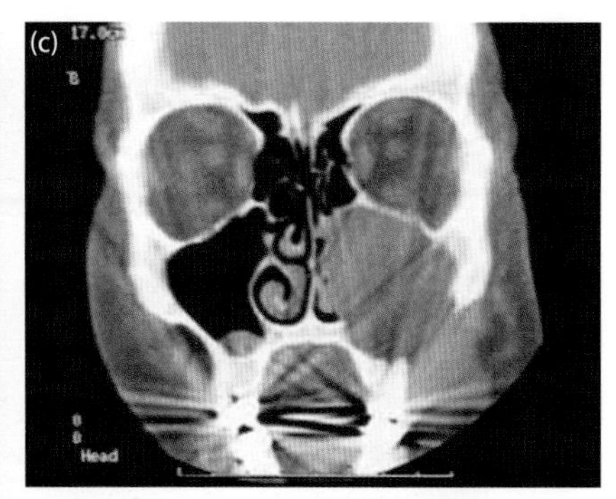

Figure 7.3 **(a)** Intraoral view of a patient with myxoma of the left maxilla with involvement of the left upper gum. **(b)** Coronal view of the CT scan of the paranasal sinuses with a soft tissue window and **(c)** bone window of the patient shown in **(a)**.

Nodal metastases

Modern CT scans appear equally effective as MRI for staging of nodal disease and with regard to the presence of extranodal spread (7–9). Indistinct peripheral boarders suggest the presence of extranodal spread (Figure 7.4). The latter characteristic has staging, prognostic and treatment implications (10). Enlarged nodes, rounded nodes, rim enhancement and the presence of central necrosis are suggestive of metastatic involvement (Figure 7.5). It should be noted that a careful evaluation of the retropharyngeal space should be performed for metastatic nodal disease, particularly for primary tumors of the oropharynx. Such disease is not apparent on clinical examination and would not be included in a routine selective neck dissection for clinically N0 patients. Both CT and MRI are good at characterizing nodal disease; choice of imaging modality should therefore be based on other management concerns.

Distant metastases

For the evaluation of distant metastases in patients with clinically advanced locoregional disease, a positron emission tomography (PET)/CT scan should be performed. If this shows evidence of fluorodeoxyglucose (FDC) uptake in the lungs, then a chest CT scan should be done for further evaluation.

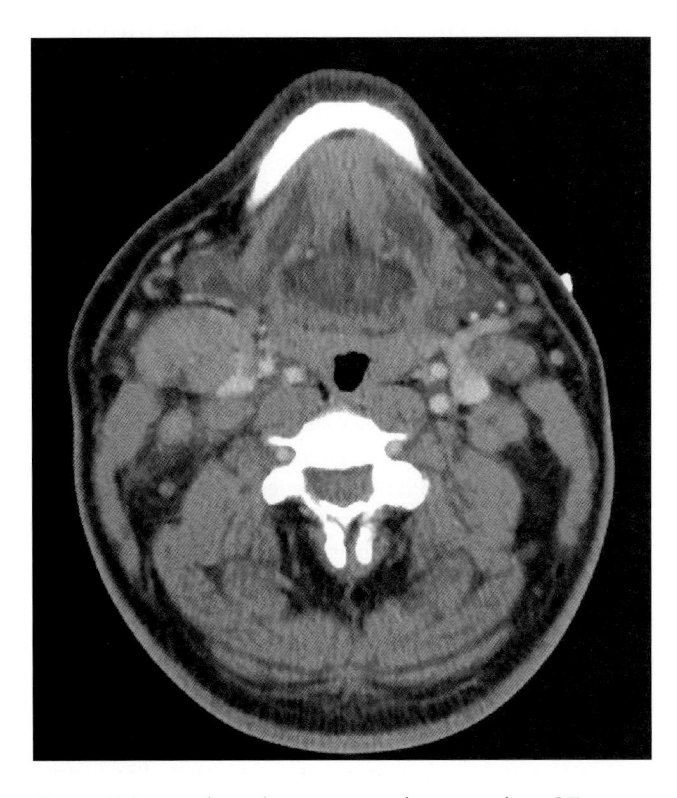

Figure 7.4 Lymph node extracapsular spread on CT

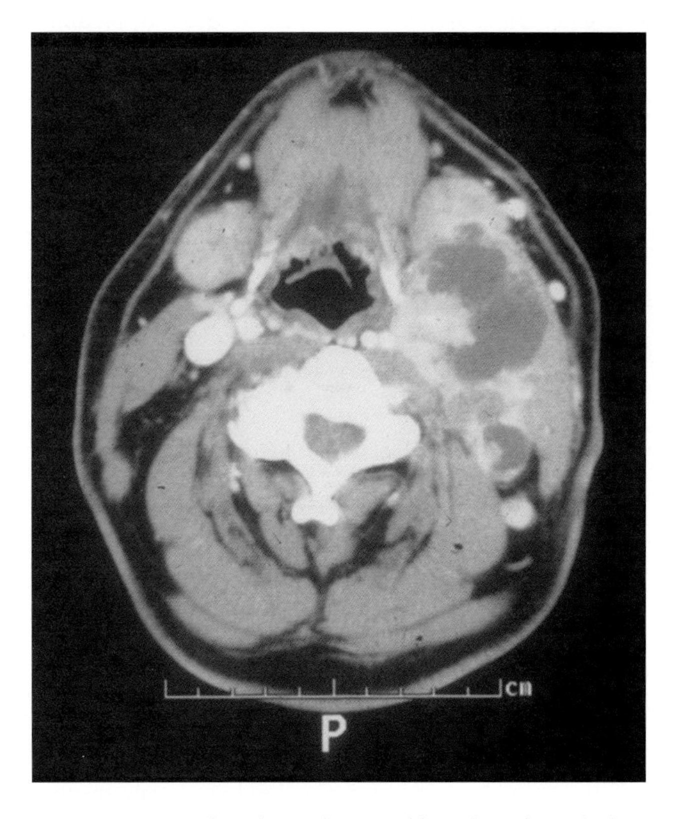

Figure 7.5 Grossly enlarged cervical lymph node with the presence of central necrosis on CT.

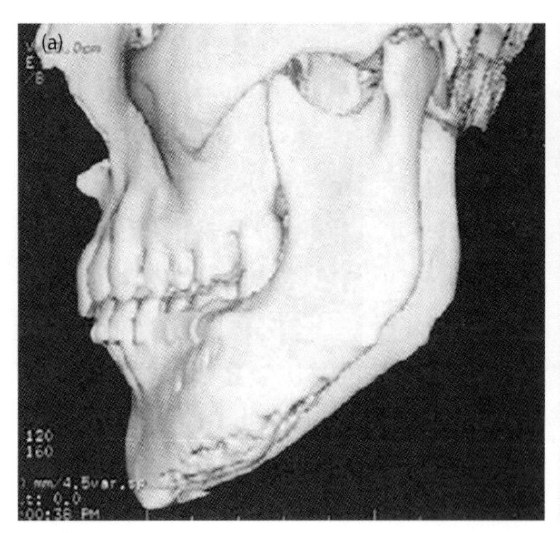

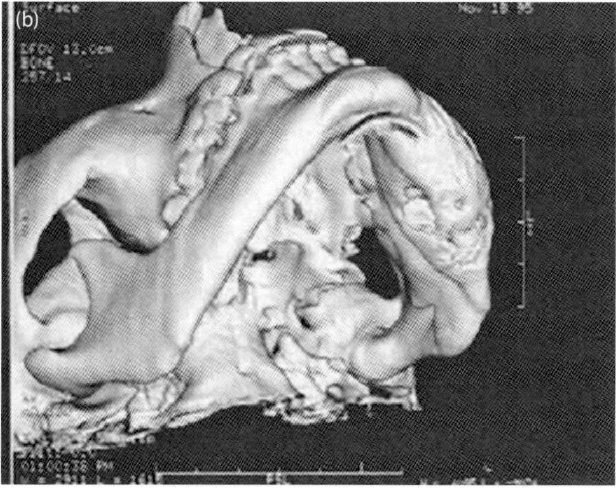

Figure 7.6 **(a)** Lateral view of three-dimensional reconstruction of the CT scan of the mandible of a patient with sarcoma. **(b)** Oblique inferior view of three-dimensional reconstruction of the mandible of the same patient.

Reconstruction

As previously mentioned, panoramic X-ray is useful to grossly evaluate the dentoalveolar structures in relation to the mandible. In addition, three-dimensional reconstructions of CT images provide an excellent overview of the mandible or maxilla from any desired angle (Figure 7.6a and b). Mandibular height can be assessed with CT images in the coronal views when evaluating the need for marginal or segmental mandibulectomy. A three-dimensional CT scan or DentaScan is of great value to the surgeon for planning mandible reconstruction with a microvascular free flap. These images are also essential in fabricating a graft that matches the resected portion of the mandible. Commercial software programs are available to prefabricate free vascularized bone grafts to accurately replace the resected portion of the mandible for reconstruction. Detailed assessment of the circulation of the donor site is essential in patients with peripheral vascular disease or diabetes. Angiograms or magnetic resonance angiograms of the lower extremity may be required in some patients with heavy smoking history or peripheral vascular disease who require fibula-free flap reconstruction.

Indications for CT

CT with contrast is generally the initial imaging modality of choice in oral and oropharyngeal cancers. Its rapid image acquisition, ready availability and low cost compared to MRI or PET are significant advantages. It is an invaluable adjunct to mucosal assessment *via* endoscopy of oropharyngeal tumors, depicting deep tissue extent of disease and involvement of adjacent structures. Soft tissue and bone windows should be acquired to demonstrate contrast enhancement of soft tissue and bone invasion. Cortical bone involvement of the mandible or maxilla is particularly well identified with a CT scan in bone windows.

Indications for MRI

Compared to CT, MRI has superior soft tissue definition and is more sensitive for perineural, medullary bone and intracranial extension. In situations when extensive soft tissue invasion in the masticator or parapharyngeal space is suspected, an MRI scan may be desirable. MRI has greater sensitivity and accuracy in the detection of perineural extension (11). While CT is good for cortical bone involvement, early marrow space involvement is clearly depicted on MRI. However, limitations are limited access and higher cost in comparison to CT, as well as prolonged imaging time associated with motion artifact, which is particularly frequent due to involuntary movements of the tongue and swallowing motions.

Indications for PET

PET scans provide imaging details based the increased metabolic activity of cancers and resultant increased absorption of ^{18}F-flourodeoxyglucose. PET alone does not allow for clear evaluation of the primary tumor due to limited resolution. This is improved with the use of PET in combination with CT. PET/CT scans are often useful in localizing a primary in the oropharynx that is not readily visible on clinical examination and in patients with equivocal CT or MRI (Figure 7.7). A PET-positive lesion is thus helpful in directing appropriate biopsies to confirm tissue diagnosis. PET/CT scans can also be helpful in determining the presence of disease in a suspicious lymph node and can very effectively rule out metastases and secondary primaries. However, it is associated with a low sensitivity to small-volume disease, including those with cystic metastases, as well as a high false-positive rate (12). Thus, its pretreatment use may be justified in patients with advanced locoregional oral and oropharyngeal cancer (13). Recent studies suggest that tumor volume and total glycolytic activity measured

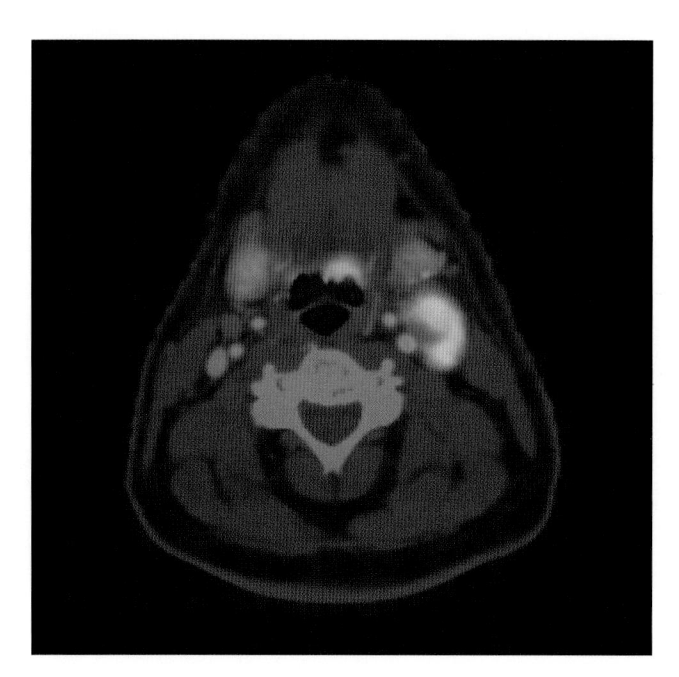

Figure 7.7 PET scan demonstrating enhancing cervical nodal disease.

on PET scan may be of prognostic importance in patient outcomes (14,15).

HPV STATUS

HPV infection is now well accepted as a risk factor for the development of SCC of the oropharynx, particularly those affecting the lingual and palatine tonsils and base of the tongue. The incidence of HPV-related oropharyngeal SCC is approximately 62%–71% in the United States, depending on inclusion criteria and method of diagnosis (16, 17). HPV-16, -18, -31 and -33 genotypes have been identified as causative agents in pathogenesis (18–20). The prognostic impact of HPV in non-oropharyngeal SCC is, however, less certain. The incidence of HPV-positive oral cavity SCC is approximately 6% (21), with some evidence to suggest that HPV-positive non-oropharyngeal cancers are similarly associated with improved prognosis in a subgroup of patients (22). However, the role of HPV in non-oropharyngeal cancers at this time requires further investigation.

Two HPV diagnostic tests are commonly used for its detection in oropharyngeal cancers: HPV DNA *in situ* hybridization and immunohistochemistry for p16 expression, a surrogate marker of HPV status. Fresh tissue samples or paraffin-fixed blocks can be used for analysis. Studies using p16 have demonstrated similar prognostic impact on survival to direct measurements of HPV DNA when positivity is defined as diffuse staining in >70% (16,23,24). Examples of p16 staining positive for HPV are demonstrated in Figure 7.8a–c.

In general, HPV positivity portends better prognosis; however, at present, there is insufficient evidence to alter management based on HPV status in oropharyngeal cancers (10). Prospective studies are currently in progress to evaluate the validity of de-intensification in the treatment of HPV-positive disease. Nevertheless, HPV status may be important for prognostic assessment and patient counseling. Patients and their partners can often be anxious regarding past and future potential HPV transmission. Despite the recognized association between sexual behavior and HPV status, studies suggest that long-term partners of individuals with HPV cancer have a similar rate of oral HPV infection compared to the general population. Such findings suggest that, despite exposure, most partners can effectively clear an active infection (25).

MULTIDISCIPLINARY TEAM ASSESSMENT

Comprehensive management of head and neck cancer patients requires a range of specialists, including:

- Head and neck surgeons
- Radiation oncologists
- Medical oncologists
- Neuroradiologists
- Head and neck pathologists
- Microvascular reconstructive surgeons

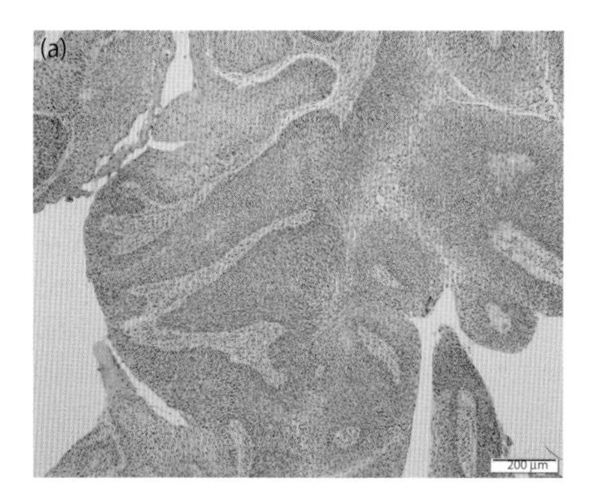

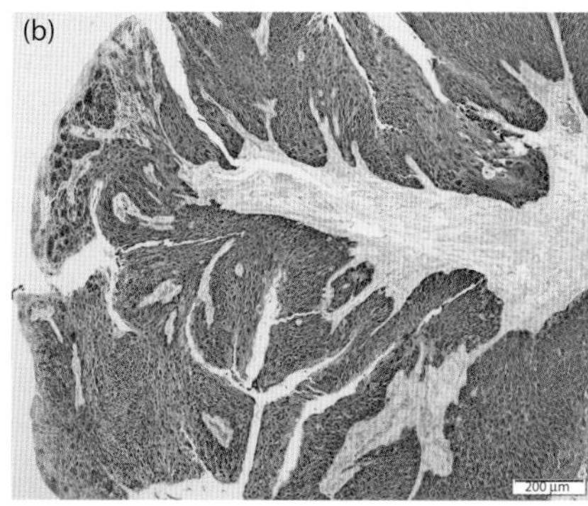

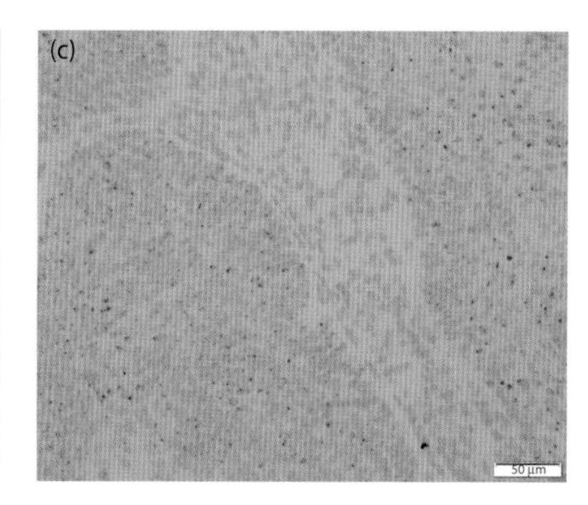

Figure 7.8 **(a)** Hematoxylin and eosin stain **(b)** p16 positive for HPV and **(c)** p16 staining negative for HPV.

- Dentists and prosthodontists
- Speech pathologists, nutritionists, social workers and nursing coordinators

Coordinating such interdisciplinary care can be challenging, but is necessary for delivering optimal patient care and achieving the desired outcome. In addition to the advantage of having radiology and pathology services aid in treatment planning, a tumor board allows discussion by different experts to facilitate treatment consensus. Care outside a tertiary care multidisciplinary setting has been shown to produce staging inaccuracies, inadequate or incomplete treatments, non-adherence to management guidelines and non-enrollment into suitable clinical trials. Importantly, these inaccuracies collectively have been shown to lead to decreased survival (26–28). In head and neck cancer, a treatment time of less than 100 days from surgery to completion of radiation therapy is associated with improved locoregional control and survival (29). This finding highlights the importance of pretreatment patient optimization to minimize the risk of complications that lead to potential delays in therapy.

BASELINE PHYSICAL CONDITION

A complete assessment of the general physical condition of the patient is essential to establishing baseline measurements (30, 31). Anesthetic workup to assess fitness for various therapies needs to be conducted. Head and neck cancer patients can often be anemic; thus, a complete blood cell count is required. Coagulation studies are required as part of the surgical workup. Alcohol intake and nutritional status can be assessed with markers such as albumin, prealbumin and Fe. Baseline liver, kidney and thyroid functions are also useful to obtain prior to initiation of therapy. Causes of biochemical deficiencies should be diagnosed and reversible causes corrected prior to definitive treatment. In particular, cardiorespiratory health assessment is required, including pulmonary function tests, chest X-rays and cardiac stress tests as indicated.

TOBACCO/ALCOHOL ABUSE AND PSYCHIATRIC CONDITIONS

Preoperative counseling in patients with a history of tobacco/alcohol abuse and psychiatric disorders is vitally important to reduce postoperative morbidity. Studies have demonstrated smoking cessation in the perioperative period can improve outcomes. High alcohol intake patients are at significant risk of alcohol withdrawal symptoms in the postoperative period. They need to be seen preoperatively by psychiatric and rehabilitation specialists to facilitate perioperative management of alcoholism. Cessation of smoking and alcohol also offers long-term benefits by reducing the risk of multiple primary tumors. Head and neck cancer patients have been shown to have higher rates of depression and suicide (32). These are likely to be premorbid risk factors compounded by the postoperative impact on speech, swallowing and cosmesis. The presence of these risk factors and comorbid conditions can significantly impact on postoperative complications and overall prognosis (30).

ORAL HYGIENE

Many patients with primary carcinomas of particularly the oral cavity have poor oral hygiene (33). Dental prophylaxis prior to surgery or radiation therapy can prevent local sepsis following surgery. Deposits of tartar need to be removed and all grossly septic teeth should be extracted, either preoperatively or intraoperatively. However, it is important to emphasize that teeth, whether loose or immobile within the tumor or in its vicinity, should not be extracted prior to the definitive surgical resection. Extraction of teeth near a tumor opens up dental sockets that are vulnerable to implantation of tumor. The efficacy of a satisfactory surgical procedure may be seriously jeopardized under these circumstances (34). Similarly, any restorative dental work should be postponed until treatment of the primary oral cancer is completed.

DENTAL PROSTHESIS

If the contemplated surgical procedure requires resection of any part of the mandible or maxilla, dental consultation for consideration of either a mandibular splint or a palatal obturator fabrication should be obtained. If a postoperative splint, obturator or dental prosthesis is needed, then it is imperative that dental impressions prior to surgery are obtained to allow fabrication of an appropriate prosthesis.

SPEECH AND SWALLOWING

A formal baseline speech and swallowing evaluation may be beneficial for patients with preoperative speech and/or swallowing dysfunction, as well as in whom treatment is likely to result in speech and/or swallowing impediment. Clinical swallowing assessments or videofluoroscopic swallowing studies can assess dysphagia and swallowing function. Patient quality of life evaluations should also include baseline assessment of speech and communication, taste, xerostomia, pain and trismus.

NUTRITION ASSESSMENT

Patients may be malnourished due to a combination of pre-existing chronic conditions or acutely due to the local/systemic effects of the cancer. Patients who manifest signs of chronic malnutrition, significant weight loss or difficulty in swallowing because of pain or tumor involvement prior to treatment require nutritional evaluation and intervention, since this may profoundly impact on post-treatment recovery (35). Nutrition counseling by a registered dietitian and, if indicated, treatment with various interventions, such as feeding tubes (nasogastric or percutaneous endoscopic gastrostomy [PEG]) may be required. At this time, no recommendation can be made regarding the indications for prophylactic PEG insertion (36).

RECONSTRUCTION

For complex resections of oral cancers and oropharynx tumors, adequate reconstruction is essential to achieving optimal function and cosmesis. If involvement of reconstructive surgeons is anticipated and such reconstruction is to be done by a second surgical team, then free flap selection should be planned preoperatively with the reconstructive team. This would entail review of applicable and available free flaps, appropriate imaging (discussed earlier) and patient discussion of donor site sequelae and disability.

STAGING

Clinical staging for primary tumors of the oral cavity and oropharynx by the AJCC and the union for international cancer control (UICC) is based on the TNM system (37). There has been significant change in the latest revision (8th edition) of the AJCC/UICC staging system between oral cavity and oropharynx cancers. Therefore, the staging for these two sites is described separately.

ORAL CAVITY

The new 8th edition staging system for oral cancer is shown in Tables 7.1–7.3. The clinical staging for oropharyngeal cancer is separate for HPV-positive and HPV-negative cancers. The T staging for the oropharynx is similar to the previous editions and is different from the T staging for oral cancers, which now includes tumor depth (Table 7.1). The following section is in reference to mucosal SCC and is not for staging of cancers arising from non-epithelial tumors of the oral cavity or oropharynx and mucosal melanomas.

After clinical examination, appropriate imaging and biopsy, it is usually possible to accurately stage the patient without the need for further endoscopy under general anesthesia. In the past, panendoscopy (i.e. direct laryngoscopy, bronchoscopy and esophagoscopy) was routinely performed to exclude the possibility of a synchronous cancer. However,

Table 7.1 AJCC tumor (T) staging for lip and oral cavity (8th edition)

TX—Primary tumor cannot be assessed
Tis—Carcinoma *in situ*
T1—Tumor ≤2 cm, ≤5 mm depth of invasion (DOI; not tumor thickness)
T2—Tumor ≤2 cm, DOI >5 mm and ≤10 mm or tumor >2 cm but ≤4 cm and ≤10 mm DOI
T3—Tumor >4 cm or any tumor >10 mm DOI
T4—Moderately advanced or very advanced local disease
T4a—Moderately advanced local disease
(Lip): Tumor invades through cortical bone or involves inferior alveolar nerve, floor of the mouth or skin of the face; that is, chin or nose
(Oral cavity): Tumor invades adjacent structures only (e.g. through cortical bone [mandible or maxilla], maxillary sinus and skin of the face). *Note:* superficial erosion of bone/tooth socket (alone) by a gingival primary is not sufficient to classify a tumor as T4
T4b—Very advanced local disease. Tumor invades masticator space, pterygoid plates or the skull base and/or encases the internal carotid artery

Table 7.2 AJCC regional lymph node (N) staging for oral cavity (8th edition)

NX—Regional lymph nodes cannot be assessed
N0—No regional lymph node metastasis
N1—Metastasis in a single ipsilateral lymph node, 3 cm or smaller in greatest dimension and extranodal extension (ENE) negative
N2—Metastasis in a single ipsilateral lymph node, larger than 3 cm but not larger than 6 cm in greatest dimension and ENE negative; *or* metastases in multiple ipsilateral lymph nodes, none larger than 6 cm in greatest dimension and ENE negative; *or* in bilateral or contralateral lymph modes, none larger than 6 cm in greatest dimension and ENE negative
N2a—Metastasis in a single ipsilateral lymph node, larger than 3 cm but not larger than 6 cm in greatest dimension and ENE negative
N2b—Metastasis in multiple ipsilateral lymph nodes, none larger than 6 cm in greatest dimension and ENE negative
N2c—Metastasis in bilateral or contralateral lymph nodes, none larger than 6 cm in greatest dimension and ENE negative
N3—Metastasis in a lymph node larger than 6 cm in greatest dimension and ENE negative; *or* metastasis in any node(s) with clinically overt ENE positivity
N3a—Metastasis in a lymph node larger than 6 cm in greatest dimension and ENE negative
N3b—Metastasis in any node(s) and clinically overt ENE positivity

Table 7.3 AJCC TNM stage groupings for oral cancers

When T is...	And N is...	And M is...	Then the stage group is...
T1	N0	M0	I
T2	N0	M0	II
T3	N0	M0	III
T1, T2 or T3	N1	M0	III
T4a	N0,1	M0	IVA
T1, T2, T3 or T4a	N2	M0	IVA
Any T	N3	M0	IVB
T4b	Any N	M0	IVB
Any T	Any	M1	IVC

with advances in imaging and office flexible endoscopy, most institutions now reserve bronchoscopy and esophagoscopy for cases with worrisome imaging or with symptoms such as dysphagia, hemoptysis or odynophagia.

Primary tumor (T stage)

The T stage of oral cancer is defined by the maximal diameter of the lesion and its depth of invasion, which are the most important parameters for determining tumor staging (37). The AJCC primary tumor (T) staging for oral cancer is shown in Table 7.1. For lip cancer, T4 disease specifies tumor involving cortical bone, the inferior alveolar nerve, the floor of the mouth or the skin of the face. For other oral cavity subsites, T4a disease signifies moderately advanced local disease, with involvement of adjacent structures or skin. T4b disease, however, represents very advanced local disease, with involvement of the masticator space, pterygoid muscles or plates, skull base or internal carotid artery encasement and involvement of the nasopharynx for oropharyngeal disease. One significant deficiency of the staging of the primary tumor in the past was the omission of the third dimension of the lesion, since it reflects the depth of infiltration. This has now been addressed and incorporated into the latest version (8th edition). It is well known that deeply infiltrating but clinically early-staged primary tumors of the tongue and floor of the mouth have an increased risk of regional metastasis and death due to disease compared to superficial tumors of the same T stage (1). Thus, a more aggressive therapeutic approach may have to be considered, including elective treatment of regional lymph nodes for patients with early-staged but deeply infiltrating tumors. In contrast, lesions that are at an advanced T stage but are relatively superficial have a better prognosis. The new AJCC staging system has addressed these issues and thus the new T staging for oral cancers will facilitate appropriate treatment planning as well as assessment of prognosis.

Regional lymph nodes (N stage)

The N staging system for regional cervical lymph nodes is uniform for all epithelial tumors of the upper aerodigestive tract (37). The nodal staging system in the past took into account only the size and multiplicity as well as the unilateral or bilateral presence of metastatic nodes as the parameters for N staging. Important prognostic parameters such as the location of the metastatic lymph node as well as the presence of capsular penetration and extranodal extension were not used as parameters in the N staging system. However, it is well known that the presence of metastatic lymph nodes beyond the first-echelon locations and the presence of extranodal soft tissue extensions of metastatic tumor carry a significant negative impact on prognosis (38,39). The new nodal staging system (8th edition) has addressed these issues and included extranodal extension in upstaging the N stage. Nodal staging (N0/1/2/3) is shown in Table 7.2.

Distant metastases (M stage)

The presence or absence of distant metastasis is documented as M0/M1. A routine chest radiograph and serum chemistries, if normal, are generally considered sufficient to rule out distant metastasis in patients with early locoregional disease in the absence of other specific symptoms. PET/CT may be helpful in patients with advanced T or N status. Specific clinical symptoms or physical findings indicative of distant metastasis require additional investigation, including radiographic studies such as bone scans and CT scans of brain, chest, abdomen or pelvis. The most frequently involved sites for distant metastasis are the lungs, liver and bones (40). The new stage groupings for the TNM system classification for oral cancer (8th edition) are shown in Table 7.3.

OROPHARYNX

Due to the significant rise in the incidence of HPV-positive cancers of the tonsils and oropharynx and their unique biological behavior, a separate staging system is proposed for HPV-positive and HPV-negative oropharyngeal cancers in the latest revision (8th edition) of the AJCC/UICC staging manual. However, the T staging criteria for both HPV-positive and HPV-negative primary tumors remain the same (Table 7.4). The impact of nodal metastasis and the extent of metastatic disease in lymph nodes has very diverse impacts on prognosis in HPV-positive and HPV-negative patients. Therefore, new nodal staging for HPV-positive patients is developed and is shown in Table 7.5. On the other

Table 7.4 AJCC TNM staging for primary tumors of the oropharynx (both HPV positive and HPV negative)

TX—Primary tumor cannot be assessed
Tis—Carcinoma *in situ*
T1—Tumor 2 cm or smaller in greatest dimension
T2—Tumor larger than 2 cm but not larger than 4 cm in greatest dimension
T3—Tumor larger than 4 cm in greatest dimension or extension to lingual surface of epiglottis
T4—Moderately advanced or very advanced local disease
T4a—Moderately advanced local disease. Tumor invades the larynx, extrinsic muscle of the tongue, medial pterygoid, hard palate or mandible
T4b—Very advanced local disease. Tumor invades lateral pterygoid muscle, pterygoid plates, lateral nasopharynx or the skull base or encases the carotid artery

Table 7.5 AJCC TNM staging for nodal metastasis for HPV-positive oropharynx cancers

NX—Regional lymph nodes cannot be assessed
N0—No regional lymph node metastasis
N1—One or more ipsilateral lymph nodes, none larger than 6 cm
N2—Contralateral or bilateral lymph nodes, none larger than 6 cm
N3—Lymph node(s) larger than 6 cm

Table 7.6 AJCC TNM stage groupings for HPV-positive oropharynx cancer

When T is...	And N is...	And M is...	Then the stage group is...
T0, T1 or T2	N0 or N1	M0	I
T0, T1 or T2	N2	M0	II
T3	N0, N1 or N2	M0	II
T0, T1, T2, T3 or T4	N3	M0	III
T4	N0, N1, N2 or N3	M0	III
Any T	Any N	M1	IV

Table 7.7 AJCC TNM stage groupings for HPV-negative oropharynx cancer

When T is...	And N is...	And M is...	Then the stage group is...
Tis	N0	M0	0
T1	N0	M0	I
T2	N0	M0	II
T3	N0	M0	III
T1, T2 or T3	N1	M0	III
T4a	N0,1	M0	IVA
T1, T2, T3 or T4a	N2	M0	IVA
Any T	N3	M0	IVB
T4b	Any N	M0	IVB
Any T	Any N	M1	IVC

hand, nodal staging for HPV-negative oropharynx cancer is similar to that for oral cavity primary tumors (Table 7.2).

Because of the separate classification systems for HPV-positive and HPV-negative oropharyngeal carcinomas, the stage groupings have changed. The prognostic stage groups for HPV-positive oropharynx carcinoma are shown in Table 7.6 and those for HPV-negative oropharynx cancer are shown in Table 7.7.

REFERENCES

1. Amin MB, Edge S, Greene F (eds). *AJCC Cancer Staging Manual*. 8th ed. New York, NY: Springer International Publishing, 2017.
2. Spiro R, Huvos A, Wong G, Spiro J, Gnecco C, Strong E. Predictive value of tumor thickness in squamous carcinoma confined to the tongue and floor of the mouth. *Am J Surg* 1986;152(4):345–50.
3. Ota Y, Aoki T, Karakida K et al. Determination of deep surgical margin based on anatomical architecture for local control of squamous cell carcinoma of the buccal mucosa. *Oral Oncol* 2009;45(7):605–9.
4. Shinozaki Y, Jinbu Y, Ito H et al. Relationship between appearance of tongue carcinoma on intraoral ultrasonography and histopathologic findings. *Oral Surg Oral Med Oral Pathol Oral Radiol* 2014;117(5):634–9.
5. Weisman R, Kimmelman C. Bone scanning in the assessment of mandibular invasion by oral cavity carcinomas. *Laryngoscope* 1982;92(1):1–4.
6. Ong C, Chong V. Imaging of perineural spread in head and neck tumours. *Cancer Imaging* 2010;10(Spec no A):S92–8.
7. King A, Tse G, Ahuja A et al. Necrosis in metastatic neck nodes: diagnostic accuracy of CT, MR imaging, and US. *Radiology* 2004;230(3):720–6.
8. King A, Tse G, Yuen E et al. Comparison of CT and MR imaging for the detection of extranodal neoplastic spread in metastatic neck nodes. *Eur J Radiol* 2004;52(3):264–70.
9. Adams S, Baum R, Stuckensen T, Bitter K, Hor G. Prospective comparison of ^{18}F-FDG PET with conventional imaging modalities (CT, MRI, US) in lymph node staging of head and neck cancer. *Eur J Nucl Med* 1998;25(9):1255–60.
10. NCCN NCCN. NCCN Clinical Practice Guidelines in Oncology—Head and Neck (Ver. 2.2014) 2014 (cited November 15, 2014). Available from: http://www.nccn.org/professionals/physician_gls/pdf/head-and-neck.pdf.
11. Arya S, Rane P, Deshmukh A. Oral cavity squamous cell carcinoma: role of pretreatment imaging and its influence on management. *Clin Radiol* 2014;69(9):916–30.
12. O'Neill J, Moynagh M, Kavanagh E, O'Dwyer T. Prospective, blinded trial of whole-body magnetic resonance imaging versus computed tomography positron emission tomography in staging primary and recurrent cancer of the head and neck. *J Laryngol Otol* 2010;124(12):1274–7.
13. Johnson J, Branstetter BT. PET/CT in head and neck oncology: state-of-the-art 2013. *Laryngoscope* 2014;124(4):913–5.
14. Romesser P, Lim R, Spratt D et al. The relative prognostic utility of standardized uptake value, gross tumor volume, and metabolic tumor volume in oropharyngeal cancer patients treated with platinum based concurrent chemoradiation with a pre-treatment [^{18}F] fluorodeoxyglucose positron emission tomography scan. *Oral Oncol* 2014;50(9):802–8.

15. Dibble E, Alvarez A, Truong M, Mercier G, Cook E, Subramaniam R. ^{18}F-FDG metabolic tumor volume and total glycolytic activity of oral cavity and oropharyngeal squamous cell cancer: adding value to clinical staging. *J Nucl Med* 2012;53(5):709–15.
16. Ang K, Harris J, Wheeler R et al. Human papillomavirus and survival of patients with oropharyngeal cancer. *N Engl J Med* 2010;363(1):24–35.
17. Chaturvedi A, Engels E, Pfeiffer R et al. Human papillomavirus and rising oropharyngeal cancer incidence in the United States. *J Clin Oncol* 2011;29(32):4294–301.
18. Sturgis E, Ang K. The epidemic of HPV-associated oropharyngeal cancer is here: is it time to change our treatment paradigms? *J Natl Compr Canc Netw* 2011;9(6):665–73.
19. Gillison M, D'Souza G, Westra W et al. Distinct risk factor profiles for human papillomavirus type 16-positive and human papillomavirus type 16-negative head and neck cancers. *J Natl Cancer Inst* 2008;100(6):407–20.
20. Isayeva T, Li Y, Maswahu D, Brandwein-Gensler M. Human papillomavirus in non-oropharyngeal head and neck cancers: a systematic literature review. *Head Neck Pathol* 2012;6(Suppl 1):104–20.
21. Lingen M, Xiao W, Schmitt A et al. Low etiologic fraction for high-risk human papillomavirus in oral cavity squamous cell carcinomas. *Oral Oncol* 2013; 49(1):1–8.
22. Chung C, Zhang Q, Kong C et al. p16 protein expression and human papillomavirus status as prognostic biomarkers of nonoropharyngeal head and neck squamous cell carcinoma. *J Clin Oncol* 2014;32(35):3930–8.
23. Rischin D, Young R, Fisher R et al. Prognostic significance of p16INK4A and human papillomavirus in patients with oropharyngeal cancer treated on TROG 02.02 phase III trial. *J Clin Oncol* 2010;28(27):4142–8.
24. Weinberger P, Yu Z, Haffty B et al. Molecular classification identifies a subset of human papillomavirus-associated oropharyngeal cancers with favorable prognosis. *J Clin Oncol* 2006;24(5):736–7.
25. D'Souza G, Gross N, Pai S et al. Oral human papillomavirus (HPV) infection in HPV-positive patients with oropharyngeal cancer and their partners. *J Clin Oncol* 2014;32(23):2408–15.
26. Chen AY, Fedewa S, Pavluck A, Ward EM. Improved survival is associated with treatment at high-volume teaching facilities for patients with advanced stage laryngeal cancer. *Cancer* 2010;116(20):4744–52.
27. Lassig AA, Joseph AM, Lindgren BR et al. The effect of treating institution on outcomes in head and neck cancer. *Otolaryngol Head Neck Surg* 2012;147(6):1083–92.
28. Chen AY, Pavluck A, Halpern M, Ward E. Impact of treating facilities' volume on survival for early-stage laryngeal cancer. *Head Neck* 2009;31(9):1137–43.
29. Rosenthal DI, Liu L, Lee JH et al. Importance of the treatment package time in surgery and postoperative radiation therapy for squamous carcinoma of the head and neck. *Head Neck* 2002;24(2):115–26.
30. Piccirillo J. Inclusion of comorbidity in a staging system for head and neck cancer. *Oncology (Williston Park)* 1995;9(9):831–6; discussion 41.
31. Singh B, Bhaya M, Stern J et al. Validation of the Charlson comorbidity index in patients with head and neck cancer: a multi-institutional study. *Laryngoscope* 1997;107(11 Pt 1):1469–75.
32. Lydiatt W, Moran J, Burke W. A review of depression in the head and neck cancer patient. *Clin Adv Hematol Oncol* 2009;7(6):397–403.
33. Maier H, Zoller J, Herrmann A, Kreiss M, Heller W. Dental status and oral hygiene in patients with head and neck cancer. *Otolaryngol Head Neck Surg* 1993;108(6):655–61.
34. Soo K, Spiro R, King W, Harvey W, Strong E. Squamous carcinoma of the gums. *Am J Surg* 1988;156(4):281–5.
35. Ondrey F, Hom D. Effects of nutrition on wound healing. *Otolaryngol Head Neck Surg* 1994;110(6):557–9.
36. Locher J, Bonner J, Carroll W et al. Prophylactic percutaneous endoscopic gastrostomy tube placement in treatment of head and neck cancer: a comprehensive review and call for evidence-based medicine. *JPEN J Parenter Enteral Nutr* 2011;35(3):365–74.
37. Sobin L, Gospodarowicz M, Wittekind C. *International Union Against Cancer (UICC) TNM Classification of Malignant Tumors.* 7th ed New York, NY: Wiley-Liss, 2009.
38. Farr H, Arthur K. Epidermoid carcinoma of the mouth and pharynx 1960–1964. *J Laryngol Otol* 1972;86(3):243–53.
39. Spiro R, Alfonso A, Farr H, Strong E. Cervical node metastasis from epidermoid carcinoma of the oral cavity and oropharynx. A critical assessment of current staging. *Am J Surg* 1974;128(4):562–7.
40. Nishijima W, Takooda S, Tokita N, Takayama S, Sakura M. Analyses of distant metastases in squamous cell carcinoma of the head and neck and lesions above the clavicle at autopsy. *Arch Otolaryngol Head Neck Surg* 1993;119(1):65–8.

8

Factors affecting choice of treatment

LAURA WANG AND JATIN P. SHAH

TREATMENT INTENT

Treatment of oral cavity and oropharyngeal cancers can be broadly divided into therapies with curative or palliative intent. Traditionally, the two categories have been considered distinct entities (Figure 8.1a); however, it is preferable to integrate these treatment objectives at all cancer stages. With progression of disease, the likelihood of success and cost-effectiveness of curative therapy diminishes and palliation and quality of life issues become increasingly important (Figure 8.1b). Palliative treatment options are discussed in detail in Chapter 18. Integration of the totality of treatment intentions is a concept that has not been paid attention to in the past. With advancing stage of the disease at presentation or with recurrent disease, the probability of cure diminishes and the need for addressing the issues pertaining to quality of life and symptomatic palliation becomes increasingly important. Thus, covering all bases at the outset allows smooth transition from curative, invasive and expensive therapies into cost-effective symptomatic care with control of pain, nutrition and overall optimization of quality of life and eventually quality of death. This approach allows delivery of value-based care, with optimal utilization of available resources.

TREATMENT OPTIONS

The currently available life-prolonging therapeutic modalities for tumor control include surgery, radiotherapy, chemotherapy and combinations of these treatments. Primary and secondary prevention strategies including lifestyle changes are also important to address. Single-modality treatment is effective and preferred in early-stage disease. Due to the acute short-term as well as long-term sequelae of multimodal therapy, such strategies are generally reserved for advanced-stage disease, where single-modality treatments are not effective in controlling the disease.

Surgery remains central in the management of oral cavity cancers and is sometimes required in oropharyngeal cancer patients. For oral cavity lesions, most small tumors (T1 and T2) can be accessed *via* a transoral approach with retention of function. Advancements in minimally invasive options such as transoral robotic surgery (TORS) and transoral laser microsurgery (TLM) now offer wider options for definitive management of oropharyngeal cancers. Surgical resection is preferred for tumors of salivary, soft tissue and bone origin, as well as squamous cell carcinoma (SCC) with evidence of bone invasion. Surgical resection is further required in salvage treatment after persistent or recurrent disease after failing primary radiation or chemoradiation therapy.

The benefits of radiation therapy as the initial definitive treatment are primarily anatomical organ preservation, coverage of a wider treatment field and its use in patients who cannot tolerate surgery for medical reasons. Radiation is preferred for patients in whom surgical resection would result in irreversible morbidity, including total glossectomy or laryngectomy. Due to the sensitivity of surrounding normal tissues exposed to ionizing radiation, several factors need to be considered during the treatment selection process. Long-term sequelae of radiation therapy are common, particularly in tissues with low radiation tolerance, such as the salivary glands (leading to xerostomia), dentoalveolar structures (increasing the risk of osteoradionecrosis) and neural tissues as a result of ischemic nerve injury. Re-irradiation in a previously treated area is poorly

(a)

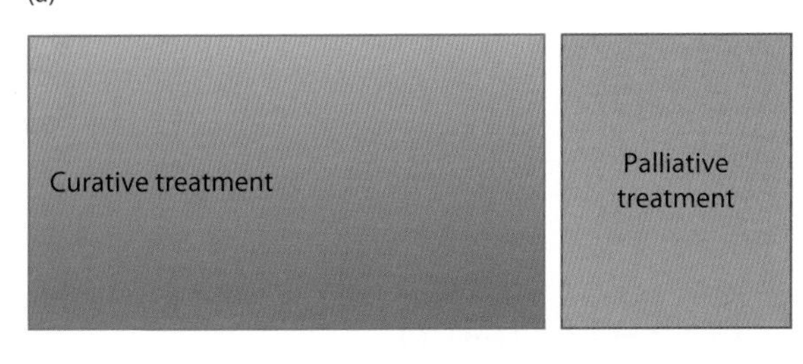

(b)

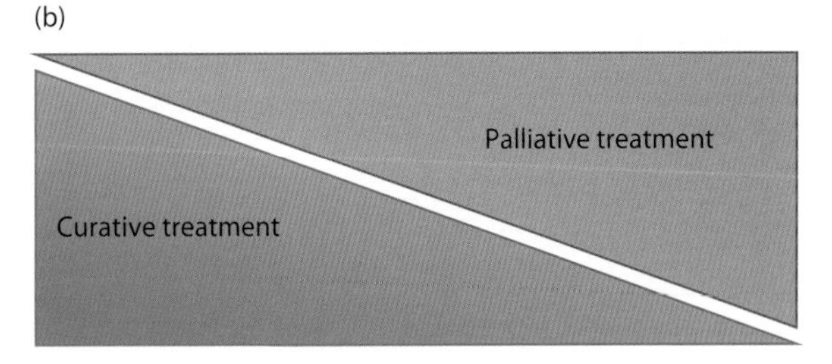

Figure 8.1 **(a)** Conventional dichotomous model. **(b)** Integrated treatment model.

tolerated, limiting the use of radiation for subsequent treatment. The rate of second primary cancers is high, nearing 30% in head and neck cancer patients who continue to smoke and drink. Thus, in such high-risk patients, surgery is preferred for early-stage oral cancer in order to avoid the use of radiotherapy, which may be required for a future second primary cancer.

In the past, the role of chemotherapy in the management of oral and oropharyngeal cancer was limited to the palliative setting. With improved understanding of the role of multimodal therapy and the enhanced efficacy of radiation combined with chemotherapy, this combination has become the standard of care in select advanced cancers of both of the oral cavity and most tumors of the oropharynx (1–3). The rationale for the addition of chemotherapy to radiotherapy is twofold: chemotherapy adds an independent mechanism of cancer cell death for locoregional as well as distant disease control; and a secondary radiosensitizing effect further contributes to improved locoregional control at the irradiated site. Use of induction chemotherapy has not demonstrated an overall survival benefit in randomized prospective trials (4). Thus, concurrent chemoradiotherapy is currently considered the standard of care for advanced cancers of the oropharynx and advanced unresectable cancers of the oral cavity. The role of biological agents is emerging; epidermal growth factor receptor (EGFR) antagonists and second-generation EGFR tyrosine kinase inhibitors are being explored to provide less morbid alternatives to concomitant chemoradiation therapy. Cetuximab has been demonstrated to improve treatment response to radiotherapy without increasing the severe adverse effects observed with the use of cisplatin (5). Radiation with cetuximab may be an alternative in patients who are not fit for chemoradiation with cisplatin (5,6). The role of immunotherapy is currently being investigated in clinical trials with the introduction of anti-PD1 and PDL1 drugs, nivolumab and pembrolizumab. However, at this juncture, it is premature to draw any conclusions as to their role pending the outcomes from ongoing clinical trials.

FACTORS AFFECTING TREATMENT SELECTION

The ultimate goal in cancer treatment is to balance long-term disease control with good quality of life whilst minimizing potential sequelae of treatment. In selecting appropriate treatments or combinations of therapies, disease control at the primary site, draining nodal basins and distant sites needs to be considered. Functional outcomes, particularly speech, swallowing and esthetics, are central to a patient's quality of life. Minimizing potential treatment sequelae is an increasingly important variable to be considered during treatment selection as patient demographics evolve. Additional considerations in treatment selection should also include salvage options in case of disease recurrence or persistence, treatment options for second primary cancers, cost-effectiveness of therapy (value-based care) and eligibility for prospective clinical trials.

Treatment selection should be evidence-based but also personalized depending on the characteristics and the extent of the disease (tumor factors), the patient's constitution and wishes (patient factors) and the expertise of the physicians and treatment delivery teams at large (physician factors). The clinical characteristics and histopathological parameters of the primary tumor, such as location of primary disease, size, depth, histological grade, surgical access, proximity to bone, radiosensitivity, lymphatic density and drainage basins, functional impact and treatment sequelae, are all important factors that impact upon treatment selection (Table 8.1). For example, primary carcinomas of minor salivary gland origin, soft tissue and bone tumors are considered radio-resistant and are best treated by surgical resection. The proximity of the primary tumor to bone increases the risk of bone exposure and subsequent development of osteoradionecrosis; therefore, radiotherapy is not preferred in that setting. It may also reduce the likelihood of a favorable response to ionizing radiation. Positive human papillomavirus (HPV) status has been associated with improved outcomes in oropharyngeal cancers, regardless of the treatment chosen; however, at present, HPV

Table 8.1 Tumor factors influencing choice of treatment

Site of the primary tumor
Location in the oral cavity (anterior versus posterior)
Size and Depth of Invasion (T stage)
Proximity to bone (mandible or maxilla)
Status of cervical lymph nodes
Histology (type, grade and depth of invasion)
Previous treatment

Table 8.2 Patient factors influencing choice of treatment

Age
General medical condition
Tolerance
Occupation
Acceptance and compliance
Lifestyle, smoking/drinking status
Socioeconomic and geographic considerations

status does not impact on treatment intensity, but may do in the near future, pending the outcomes from ongoing clinical trials.

The selected therapy also must be tolerated by the patient. This is influenced by pretreatment baseline function. These patient characteristics are listed in Table 8.2. Multimodal treatment has significant potential sequelae for the patient both acutely and in the long term. In general, older age is not considered to be a contraindication for appropriate surgical treatment for cancer. However, advancing age, concurrent disease and debility due to associated cardiopulmonary conditions increase the risk of a major adverse perioperative event. The patient's occupation and acceptance of and compliance with the proposed treatment are similarly important considerations when the optimal treatment program is designed. The patient's lifestyle, particularly with reference to smoking and drinking, impacts heavily on the selection of and tolerance to treatment offered. Willingness on the part of the patient to abstain from tobacco and alcohol will greatly reduce the rate of therapy-related complications and reduce the risk of subsequent primary tumors (7). Previous treatment of another head and neck cancer will significantly impact on treatment selection. Patients with previous radiotherapy to the oral cavity or oropharynx are generally not the best candidates for definitive radiotherapy for a second primary tumor within the irradiated field. On the other hand, all options remain open for patients in whom initial treatment was surgery, including further surgery and radiotherapy alone or in combination with chemotherapy (8). Treatment selection, however, needs to be tailored depending on the location, size of the lesion and extent of previous excision. For example, a patient with a significant partial glossectomy in the past is generally not considered a good candidate for a further glossectomy due to significant loss of function in relation to speech and deglutition. Alternative treatment with radiation therapy programs should be considered in that setting. Use of chemotherapy has been shown to induce responses in salvage cases; however, no overall survival advantage has been demonstrated (9). Similarly, if the patient is at a significant risk of developing multiple primary tumors, then radiotherapy may be reserved for its potential use in the future for subsequent primary tumors and may not be the ideal choice of therapy in early-stage oral carcinoma. Patient preference regarding the balance of oncologic, functional and esthetic outcomes should also be incorporated into the treatment selection process. Within reason, treatment selection should consider government, insurance or healthcare provider regulations for cost-effective delivery of therapies. The geographic location of the patient in relation to the treatment facility and the fiscal impact of the proposed treatment on the patient and their family are also important factors to consider, as these may impact on compliance with the recommended treatment.

Table 8.3 Physician factors influencing choice of treatment

Surgical skills
Access to minimally invasive surgical technology
Radiotherapy skills
Chemotherapy expertise
Dental and prosthetic services
Rehabilitation services
Support services

In addition to tumor and patient variables, treatment selection should also be based on the expertise of the treating medical team and facility (Table 8.3). A multidisciplinary team approach has been demonstrated to yield improved patient outcomes and therefore management of head and neck cancers should be within such a context. Access to and experience with various surgical modalities such as TORS and TLM differ across institutions within the United States and around the world. The learning curve for these minimally invasive treatment modalities is steep and significant experience is required for their routine application. Treatment selection should be affected by the expertise of the treating institution. However, it is important to note that there is no demonstrable improvement in oncological outcomes with the aid of modern surgical technology. Thus, the lack of availability of such technology does not necessarily jeopardize treatment outcomes.

ORAL CAVITY CANCER TREATMENT CONSIDERATIONS

Small and superficial tumors of the oral cavity (clinical stage 1 or 2 disease) are equally amenable for cure by single-modality treatment. As the overall outcomes of treatment are comparable by either surgery or radiotherapy alone, treatment selection is largely dictated by site-specific considerations and by anticipated functional and cosmetic results as well as treatment-related sequelae.

In general, primary tumors in the vicinity of bone are less suitable for definitive radiotherapy due to the risk of bone exposure and the greater risk of osteoradionecrosis. Thus, primary tumors of the lower gum, upper gum and hard palate are better treated by surgical resection. On the other hand, primary tumors of the tongue, floor of the mouth or cheek mucosa, as well as the lips, are suitable for radiotherapy or surgery as the definitive treatment. If radiotherapy is selected as the initial definitive treatment, in most instances a combination of external and interstitial irradiation is required. Select small, superficial lesions may be treated by brachytherapy alone. Patients with poor oral hygiene and significant dental sepsis may require total exodontia prior to initiation of radiotherapy to minimize the long-term risks of osteoradionecrosis and dental caries. In addition to the above, the long-term sequelae of radiotherapy such as permanent xerostomia and temporary loss of taste are important issues to be considered in therapy selection. If the patient is at significant risk of developing multiple primary tumors, then radiotherapy may be better reserved for potential future use for subsequent primary tumors and may not be the ideal choice of therapy in early-stage oral carcinoma. Other factors such as the availability of medical expertise, ease of surgical access, length of treatment, convenience to the patient and cost of treatment are also important considerations that will influence selection of initial treatment.

The decision regarding elective treatment of regional lymph nodes is based on the likelihood of nodal involvement. Typically, elective management is considered when the anticipated rate of nodal disease exceeds 20%. Rates of occult nodal involvement increase with increasing T stage and tumor depth. Disease propensity for nodal metastases also varies by oral cavity subsite. Generally, primary tumors located anteriorly in the oral cavity have a lower risk of dissemination to regional lymph nodes compared to similar-staged lesions in the posterior oral cavity and oropharynx. Similarly, tumors of the upper part of the oral cavity, hard palate or upper alveolar ridge have a lower risk of nodal involvement compared to tumors of the floor of the mouth and oral tongue. Thus, more posteriorly and inferiorly located lesions and larger and more infiltrative lesions are more likely to require elective treatment of the clinically negative neck in the initial treatment planning.

For advanced-stage cancers (clinical stage 3 or 4 disease), multimodality treatment options are required. In general, primary treatment of advanced but resectable oral cavity disease is with surgery and adjuvant radiation. Adverse pathology findings, particularly gross extranodal extension (Figure 8.2a and b) and positive surgical margins, portend a poor outcome and require the addition of chemotherapy to postoperative radiation (1,2). The need for adjuvant therapy is less certain when extranodal disease is found only on histopathological examination (microscopic) (Figure 8.3). For lesions that are unresectable or for which resection will lead to major functional debility, concomitant chemoradiation in selected patients has been shown to have a moderate overall survival advantage by meta-analysis (10).

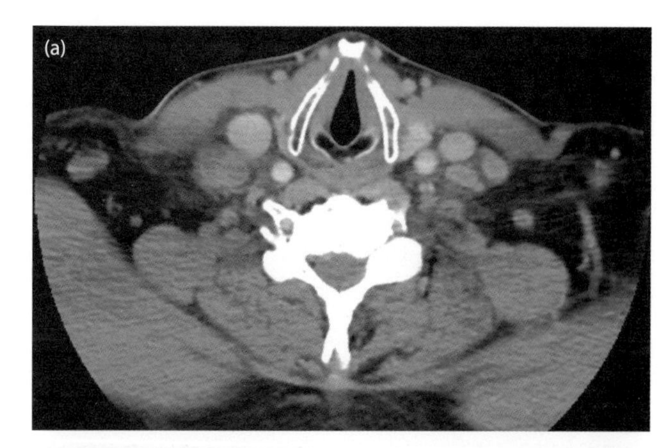

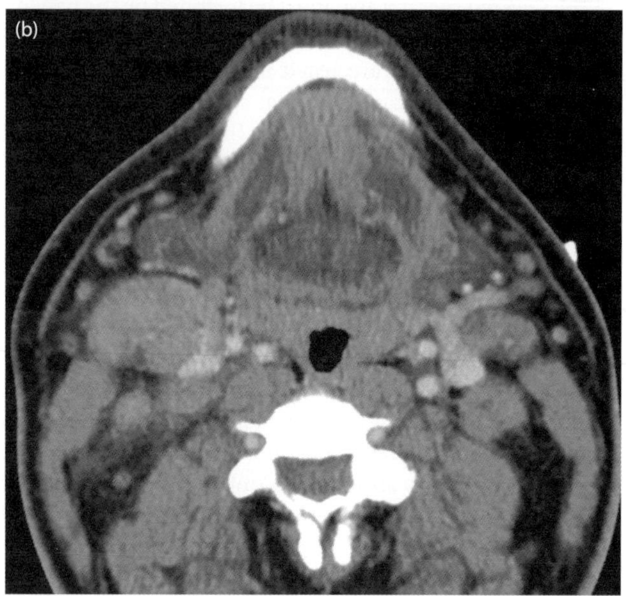

Figure 8.2 **(a)** Cervical lymph node, posterolateral to the right internal jugular vein with no demonstrable extracapsular spread on contrast-enhanced computed tomography scan. **(b)** Cervical lymph node demonstrating extracapsular spread on computed tomography scan, showing invasion of the right internal jugular vein.

OROPHARYNGEAL CANCER TREATMENT CONSIDERATIONS

The realization of HPV's association with oropharyngeal cancers has opened up a whole new paradigm in treatment selection and outcomes in these patients. HPV-positive patients in general have a better prognosis. They are usually young and non-smokers. In recent decades, patients with early oropharyngeal cancers have commonly been treated with primary radiation therapy alone. No randomized data are available to compare surgery or radiation therapy in this setting. The treatment decision is based largely on functional outcomes and side effect profiles of the therapy. Radiation therapy has been advocated due to its ability to treat the primary site, in-transit lymphatics and cervical and retropharyngeal nodal basins (11,12). Intensity modulated radiation therapy techniques are now widely employed to achieve this goal and to minimize the radiation dose to surrounding normal tissues whilst maintaining a therapeutic dose to tumor targets (13). Generally, in patients with early, well-lateralized oropharyngeal tumors, elective irradiation of the ipsilateral nodal basin is adequate (14). For patients who do not respond to initial non-surgical treatment, salvage surgery is the only effective option (8). Management of such patients is difficult given that tumors resistant to chemotherapy or radiotherapy are biologically more aggressive and have limited healing reserves and are therefore at the highest risk of treatment failure and complications after surgery.

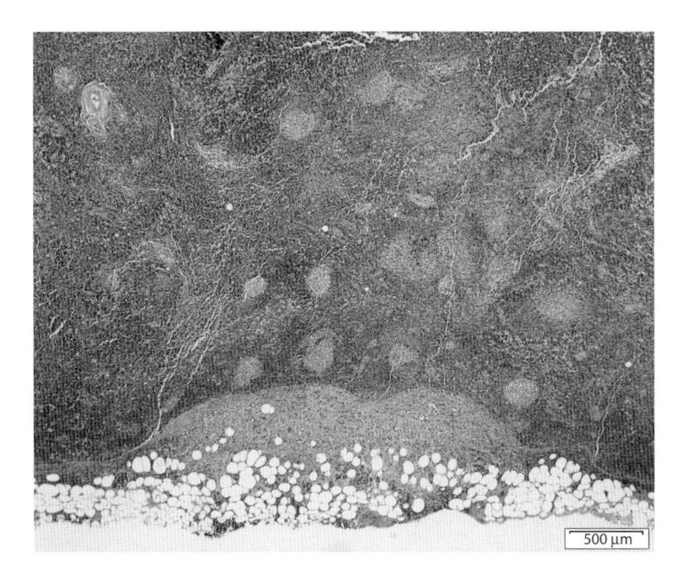

Figure 8.3 Microscopic extranodal spread seen on Haematoxylene/Eosin (H/E).

The role of primary open surgery for T1 and T2 oropharyngeal lesions has been limited largely due to poor surgical access to the oropharynx, requiring large incisions and resulting in poorer functional outcomes. Whilst transoral access to small oropharyngeal tumors of the tonsils, soft palate and pharyngeal wall is often satisfactory, access to larger tumors and lesions located at the base of the tongue have traditionally required mandibulotomy. Alternative access through transhyoid or lateral pharyngotomy is rarely used due to limited exposure and significant postoperative functional morbidity. Technological advances with the development of TORS and TLM has expanded the role of surgery as a management option for early-stage disease. These techniques have greatly improved transoral access to oropharyngeal tumors (Figure 8.4). A secondary surgical procedure for ipsilateral regional nodal dissection, with or without contralateral dissection, is generally required if surgical resection is employed for the primary tumor. The use of minimally invasive surgical approaches has been

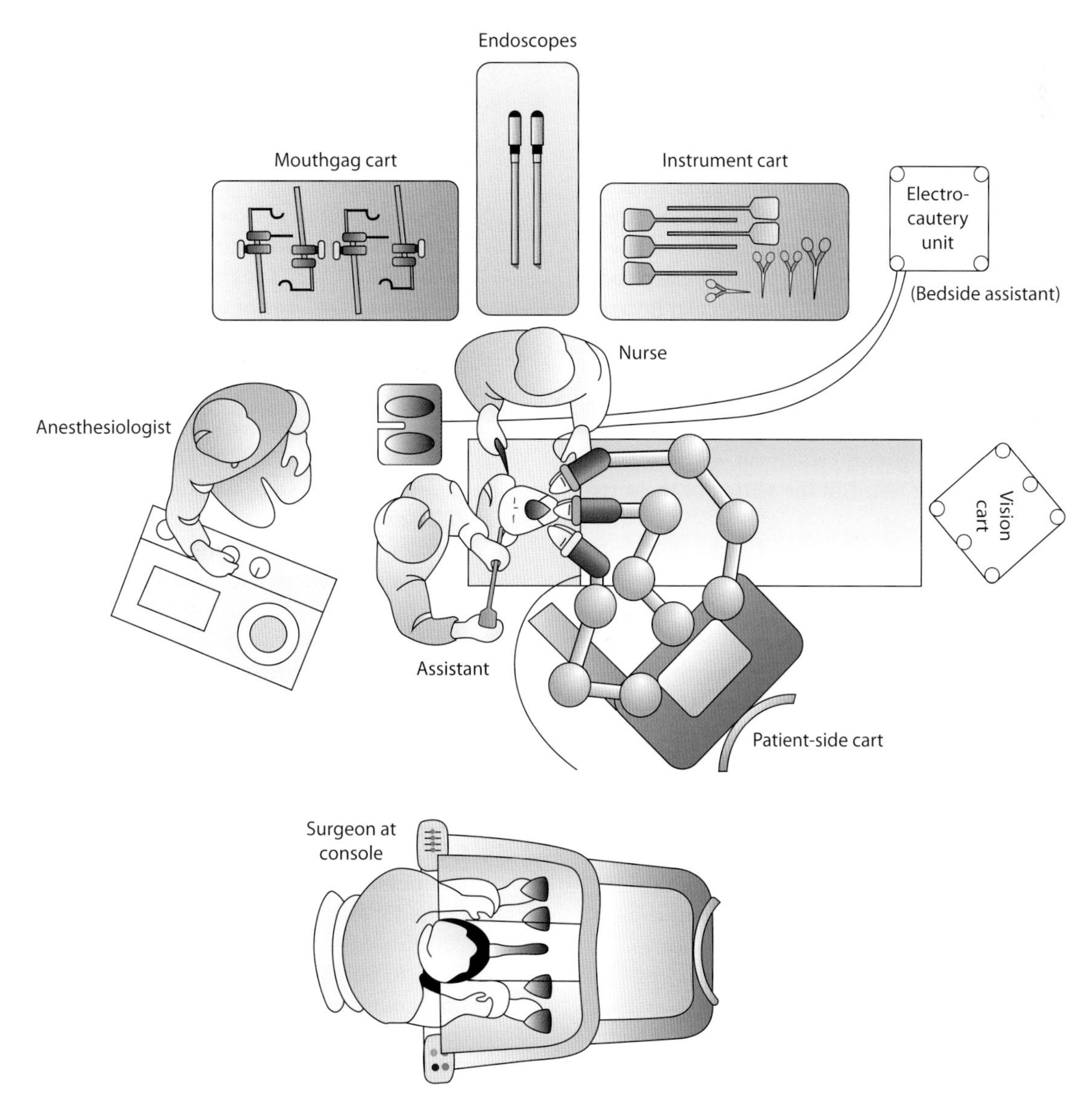

Figure 8.4 Transoral robotic surgery setup for oropharyngeal cancer excision.

reported to show superior quality of life outcomes compared to chemoradiotherapy in non-randomized trials (15). However, these reports should be critically reviewed taking into account the factors of selection bias and the fact that there are no quantitative comparative data of functional outcomes. As the incidence of HPV-positive oropharyngeal cancers increases, avoiding potential adverse sequelae of radiotherapy with or without chemotherapy is increasingly crucial. Younger patients with improved long-term survival have a greater likelihood of experiencing chemoradiation-related complications. Prospective trials are currently underway comparing transoral surgery approaches with definitive non-surgical therapies.

Concomitant chemoradiation is the treatment of choice for advanced-stage oropharyngeal cancers (clinical stage T3 or T4 lesions) (3,16,17). Surgical resection may still be considered in selected patients who are unlikely to harbor adverse pathological features (low-volume stage 3 disease). With increasing T and N stages, however, the likelihood of adverse pathological features increases. In patients in whom primary surgery is employed and found to have adverse pathological features such as positive surgical margins or gross extracapsular nodal spread, postoperative chemoradiotherapy is required (1,2,18,19). These surgical patients received three modalities of treatment instead of two had chemoradiation been selected initially. This gross overtreatment should be avoided, since the functional sequelae of triple-modality treatments are severe and lifelong. Indications for adjuvant chemoradiotherapy in the presence of adverse features such as N2 or greater nodal disease, close margins and perineural or perivascular invasion are less certain; however, radiotherapy is generally warranted. It is therefore important to avoid surgery in patients who are likely to require postoperative chemoradiation therapy, as the associated toxicity of tri-modal therapy is significant. A combination of an EGFR antagonist, cetuximab, with radiation therapy is currently being tested in the setting of these risk factors in an ongoing trial.

REFERENCES

1. Bernier J, Domenge C, Ozsahin M et al. Postoperative irradiation with or without concomitant chemotherapy for locally advanced head and neck cancer. *N Engl J Med* 2004;350:1945–52.
2. Cooper J, Pajak T, Forastiere A et al. Postoperative concurrent radiotherapy and chemotherapy for high-risk squamous-cell carcinoma of the head and neck. *N Engl J Med* 2004;350:1937–44.
3. Calais G, Alfonsi M, Bardet E et al. Randomized trial of radiation therapy versus concomitant chemotherapy and radiation therapy for advanced-stage oropharynx carcinoma. *J Natl Cancer Inst* 1999;91:2081–6.
4. Mazeron J, Martin M, Brun B, et al. Induction chemotherapy in head and neck cancer: results of a phase III trial. *Head Neck* 1992;14:85–91.
5. Bonner J, Harari P, Giralt J, et al. Radiotherapy plus cetuximab for locoregionally advanced head and neck cancer: 5-year survival data from a phase 3 randomised trial, and relation between cetuximab-induced rash and survival. *Lancet Oncol* 2010;11:21–8.
6. Ang K, Zhang Q, Rosenthal D et al. Randomized phase III trial of concurrent accelerated radiation plus cisplatin with or without cetuximab for stage III to IV head and neck carcinoma: RTOG 0522. *J Clin Oncol* 2014;32:2940–50.
7. Browman G, Wong G, Hodson I et al. Influence of cigarette smoking on the efficacy of radiation therapy in head and neck cancer. *N Engl J Med* 1993;328:159–63.
8. Wong L, Wei W, Lam L et al. Salvage of recurrent head and neck squamous cell carcinoma after primary curative surgery. *Head Neck.* 2003;25:953–9.
9. Jacobs C, Lyman G, Velez-Garcia E, Sridhar K, Knight W, Hochster H, Goodnough L, Mortimer J, Einhorn L, Schacter L. A phase III randomized study comparing cisplatin and fluorouracil as single agents and in combination for advanced squamous cell carcinoma of the head and neck. *J Clin Oncol* 1992;10:257–63.
10. Pignon J, Bourhis J, Domenge C, Designe L. Chemotherapy added to locoregional treatment for head and neck squamous-cell carcinoma: three meta-analyses of updated individual data. MACH-NC Collaborative Group. Meta-Analysis of Chemotherapy on Head and Neck Cancer. *Lancet* 2000;355:949–55.
11. Mendenhall W, Morris C, Amdur R et al. Definitive radiotherapy for squamous cell carcinoma of the base of tongue. *Am J Clin Oncol* 2006;29:32–9.
12. Harrison L, Zelefsky M, Armstrong J et al. Performance status after treatment for squamous cell cancer of the base of tongue—a comparison of primary radiation therapy versus primary surgery. *Int J Radiat Oncol Biol Phys* 1994;30:953–7.
13. Eisbruch A, Harris J, Garden A et al. Multi-institutional trial of accelerated hypofractionated intensity-modulated radiation therapy for early-stage oropharyngeal cancer (RTOG 00-22). *Int J Radiat Oncol Biol Phys* 2010;76:1333–8.
14. O'Sullivan B, Warde P, Grice B et al. The benefits and pitfalls of ipsilateral radiotherapy in carcinoma of the tonsillar region. *Int J Radiat Oncol Biol Phys* 2001;51:332–43.
15. Chen A, Daly M, Luu Q et al. Comparison of functional outcomes and quality of life between transoral surgery and definitive chemoradiotherapy for oropharyngeal cancer. *Head Neck* 2015;37(3):381–5. doi: 10.1002/hed.23610.

16. Adelstein D, Li Y, Adams G et al. An intergroup phase III comparison of standard radiation therapy and two schedules of concurrent chemoradiotherapy in patients with unresectable squamous cell head and neck cancer. *J Clin Oncol* 2003;21:92–8.
17. Denis F, Garaud P, Bardet E, Alfonsi M, Sire C, Germain T, Bergerot P, Rhein B, Tortochaux J, Calais G. Final results of the 94-01 French Head and Neck Oncology and Radiotherapy Group randomized trial comparing radiotherapy alone with concomitant radiochemotherapy in advanced-stage oropharynx carcinoma. *J Clin Oncol* 2004;22:69–76.
18. Bernier J, Cooper J, Pajak T et al. Defining risk levels in locally advanced head and neck cancers: a comparative analysis of concurrent postoperative radiation plus chemotherapy trials of the EORTC (#22931) and RTOG (# 9501). *Head Neck* 2005;27:843–50.
19. Cooper J, Zhang Q, Pajak T et al. Long-term follow-up of the RTOG 9501/intergroup phase III trial: postoperative concurrent radiation therapy and chemotherapy in high-risk squamous cell carcinoma of the head and neck. *Int J Radiat Oncol Biol Phys* 2012;84:1198–205.

9

Management of potentially malignant disorders of the mouth and oropharynx

RACHEL A. GIESE, JAY O. BOYLE, AND JATIN P. SHAH

INTRODUCTION

Premalignant lesions of the oral cavity are frequently observed in asymptomatic patients in clinical practice of dentistry, general medicine and otolaryngology head and neck surgery. Patients and clinicians are aware of the finite but low risk of progression to malignancy and are motivated to consider treatment in an attempt to mitigate the risk of future cancer. While excision of a well-defined lesion would eliminate the risk of malignant transformation of that lesion, the overall risk of developing oral cancer is not affected due to the impact of carcinogen exposure to the entire oral mucosa. In addition, surgical intervention is not feasible in people with multifocal lesions.

The World Health Organization (WHO) in 2005 recommended use of the term "potentially malignant disorders" (PMDs) to describe lesions with altered morphology that may or may not progress to carcinoma (1). Pathologically, many PMDs express a degree of epithelial dysplasia and naturally those with severe dysplasia are more likely to progress to carcinoma. Notably, though, not all PMDs exhibit hyperplasia and not all areas of epithelial dysplasia will go on to develop carcinoma. Because of the variety of PMD pathology and the unpredictable behavior of each lesion, determining which lesions require a biopsy or intervention can be challenging. Although there are tools for early detection and emerging alternative therapies, management of PMDs is an evolving field.

INCIDENCE AND EPIDEMIOLOGY

Due to discrepant reporting and uncertain diagnosis, it is unclear what the true incidence of PMDs is in the general population. Most studies report a prevalence between 1% and 5% and most commonly in the fifth decade of life (2). A white patch, generally called leukoplakia, is the most common PMD and has a variety of histological appearances. It is more common over the age of 70 and occurs in 8% of men and 2% of women (3). Although there is a trend toward more malignant transformation in women, the data are not statistically significant between genders (2,4,5). Proliferative verrucous leukoplakia is more commonly seen in women (4:1) and has a higher risk of malignant transformation. Erythroplakia—a red patch—is less common, with a reported incidence of 0.2%, but a much higher risk of malignant transformation (up to 50% for erythroplakia compared to 5%–15% for leukoplakia).

ETIOLOGY

The WHO working group consensus definition for leukoplakia is "white plaques of questionable risk having excluded other known diseases or disorders that carry no increased risk for cancer" (Figure 9.1) (1). Leukoplakia is thought to be a clinical manifestation of the field cancerization process

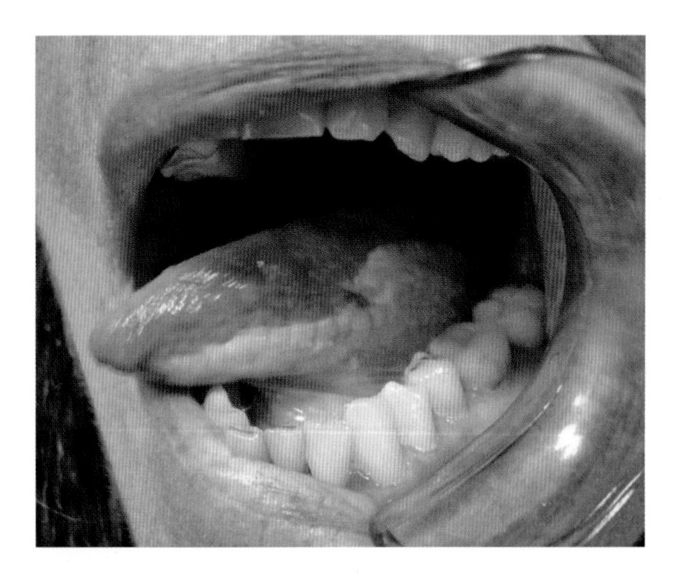

Figure 9.1 Leukoplakia of the tongue.

caused by decades of exposure to carcinogens. The most common carcinogens are from tobacco smoke and alcohol in the Western world and chewing tobacco and areca (betel) nut in Asia. Logically, leukoplakia more often leads to cancer in patients with prolonged exposure to these carcinogens and multifocal lesions carry a higher risk (4).

The risk of oral cancer in the United States has been quantified according to the extent of smoking and the amount of alcohol consumed. Blot et al. have reported that the risk of oral cancer in two packs per day smokers is sixfold higher than never-smokers and similarly it is sixfold higher in people consuming greater than 30 alcoholic drinks per week (6). It is important to note that their data suggest that the risk of smoking and drinking is synergistic. Those individuals drinking more than 30 drinks per week and also smoking two packs of cigarettes or more per day had a 40-fold increase in oral cancer, suggesting strong synergy between alcohol and tobacco exposure and oral cancer risk (6). The molecular mechanisms of alcohol carcinogenesis are unknown but may be related to inflammation or the solubilization of other carcinogens or due to effects on carcinogen-metabolizing enzymes.

Papillomas, a subset of PMDs, are usually caused by human papillomavirus (HPV). The strains of HPV responsible for condylomata are 6, 7, and 11, unlike strains 16 and 18, which are responsible for cervical and oropharyngeal cancer. Over 95% of oropharynx cancers are caused by HPV-16. Most of the rest are caused by HPV-18. In the uterine cervix, it is also known that strains that cause condylomata and cancer are different, but may be transmitted together. Uterine cervical HPV cancer patients often have a history of concurrent or antecedent condylomata. On the other hand, oropharynx cancer patients do not often have known antecedent papillomas.

It is certain that HPV-16 is rarely the cause of oral cancer (7). HPV is usually associated with cancers arising in the mucosa lining Waldeyer's ring. The oropharynx, tonsils and base of the tongue are the most prevalent sites. It is postulated that the predilection of HPV cancer in the mucosa of the tonsils and base of the tongue is related to the immune surveillance function of the lymphoid tissue of Waldeyer's ring. The mucosal cells there have receptors for viral antigens to facilitate immune recognition and affect immunologic response. After the immune system has cleared the HPV infection, DNA integration and expression of E6 and E7 lead to tumorigenesis decades later.

The etiology of oral cancer in patients never exposed to tobacco is unknown. It is rarely related to HPV infection and E6 or E7 overexpression, although it does occur. It is likely that eventually a viral etiology of oral squamous cell carcinoma (SCC; either a different strain of HPV or another virus) may be identified. However, it is presently clear that HPV is not the leading cause of oral cancer. In addition to a viral etiology, there are currently ongoing investigations into the carcinogenic role of bacteria in the oral cavity. Certainly, periodontal disease and poor oral hygiene that elicit a chronic inflammatory state are correlated with increased risk of oral cancer. Even in the absence of overt periodontal disease, there may be an imbalance in the diversity of oral cavity species, which causes a dysbiosis. The oral cavity hosts over 700 bacterial species, a third of which are uncultivated. Such bacteria may produce metabolites (e.g. metabolizing alcohol to acetaldehyde) that are genotoxic. Important genes such as transcriptional regulators and genes altering the growth cycle may be affected. As a result, there is an altered cell phenotype that is considered "initiated" and these cells may have a growth advantage compared to other cells (8). In the right environment, these cells experience clonal outgrowth and a premalignant lesion emerges.

PATHOLOGY

Leukoplakia has been a challenge to classify for over five decades. There are four main types of leukoplakia—thin, thick, verruciform and speckled (erythroleukoplakia)—and many variations of these (Figure 9.2) (2). On a genetic level, erythroleukoplakia shows loss of heterozygosity (LOH) and thus carries the highest risk of malignant transformation and should be excised (Figure 9.3). Leukoplakia should not be confused with candidiasis or thrush. In the oral cavity, clinically white (leukoplakia) or red patches (erythroplakia) with histologically confirmed dysplasia may progress to SCC. The majority of leukoplakias show only hyperplasia in the absence of dysplasia and are not harbingers of carcinoma. Notwithstanding this, a third of oral cancers arise within a pre-existing clinically recognized leukoplakic lesion; thus, they must be carefully followed. Examples of carcinoma arising in a bed of long-standing leukoplakia are seen in Figure 9.4.

Frictional trauma due to dentures, chronic biting or tooth trauma is common and often leads to lesions in the oral cavity and can also lead to lesions such as epulis fissuratum (Figure 9.5). Chronic inflammation can often lead to

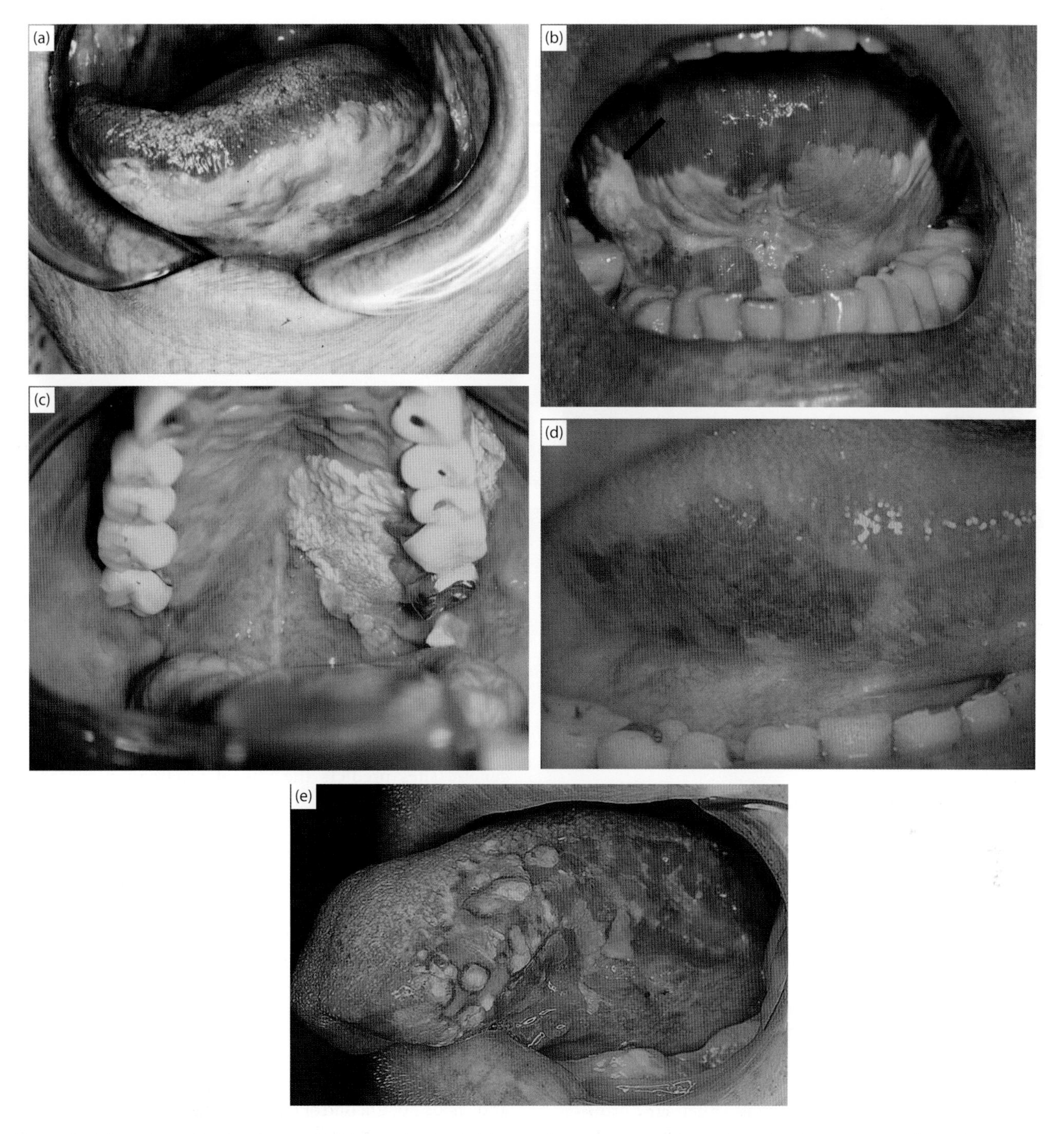

Figure 9.2 **(a)** Discoid leukoplakia. **(b)** Discoid leukoplakia with hyperkeratosis (arrow). **(c)** Leukoplakia with hyperkeratosis of the hard palate and upper gum. **(d)** Erythroplakia of the lateral border of the tongue. **(e)** Speckled leukoplakia (erythroleukoplakia) of lateral tongue.

histologic minimal atypia; however, this does not necessarily equate with cancer risk.

MOLECULAR BIOLOGY OF PROGRESSION

The process of molecular carcinogenesis of tobacco-derived carcinogens is well understood. There are at least 70 individual chemical constituents of tobacco smoke that are proven to cause cancer in animals. Polycyclic aromatic hydrocarbons bind covalently to DNA and cause mutations to occur during DNA replication. Point mutations lead to substitution errors in transcription of mRNA and translation of proteins, leading to dysfunction. Mutation may also lead to translocations, placing genes under expression control of unintended promoter segments and overexpression. Gene amplifications occur in which dozens to thousands of gene copy numbers are generated. Conversely, tobacco

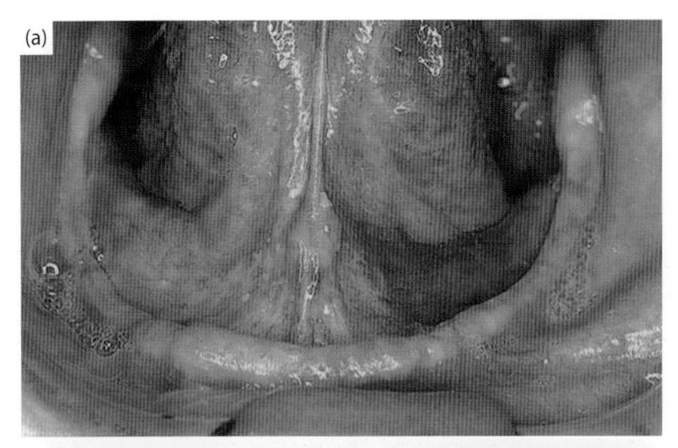

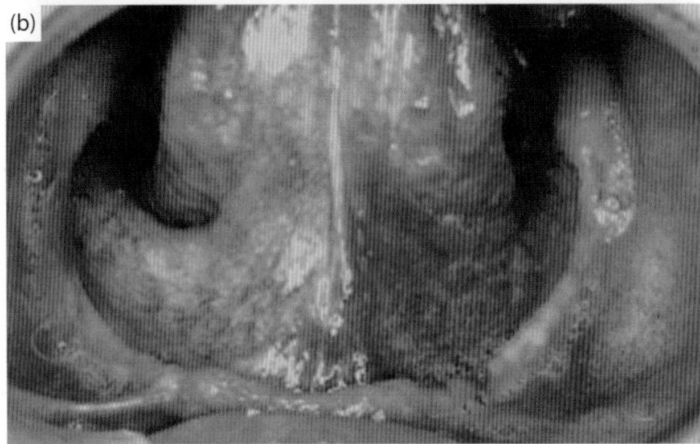

Figure 9.3 **(a)** Erythroplakia of left floor of the mouth. **(b)** Progression of erythroplakia to squamous cell carcinoma in 3 years.

carcinogens often lead to losses of large segments of DNA, detectable as LOH. Some of the earliest clonal genetic events that are detectable in chronically tobacco-exposed mucosa are LOH for important tumor suppressor genes such as the cyclin-dependent kinase inhibitor p16 on chromosome 9p (9).

Decades of carcinogen exposure to oral mucosal cells leads to the accumulation of genetic abnormalities that provide a proliferative advantage. Loss of important tumor suppressor genes such as *CDKN2A* (which encodes p16) or mutations in *TP53* can lead to uncontrolled cellular proliferation. The abnormal clones eventually spread along the basement membrane and exclude other slow-growing clones. There is a typical "survival of the fittest" scenario of evolutionary biology taking place in the mucosal field. Multiple abnormal clones can be detected in the upper aerodigestive tract of smokers (10). Often, baseline genetic changes of distant sites can be correlated, suggesting that there is clonality of the lesions in the mouth and even the lung. On top of this observed clonality is clonal divergence due to the accumulation of further genetic events. Cells with increased proliferation demonstrate less genomic surveillance and apoptosis so the accumulation of genetic events in these cells is exponential with time and continued tobacco exposure. The genetic progression model from normal epithelial mucosa to hyperplasia, dysplasia and ultimately malignancy is shown in Figure 9.6. At each stage of the sequential progression until the development of invasive cancer, specific mutations have been identified. Although these mutational changes are unique for the stage of progression, their ability to predict progressive carcinogenesis remains to be elucidated.

The computational biologist Carlo Maley has described computer models of clonal evolution in the mucosa of the aerodigestive tract (11). By altering rates of mutation and growth, the effect on eventual cancer events (incidence) can be estimated for the mucosal field in the model. The most effective methods of reducing cancer events in these models are to decrease mutation event rates and proliferation. One of the most common themes in cancer prevention is normalizing proliferation rates.

Most known genomic changes in the oral cavity are studied in many sites of head and neck SCC. Investigators have previously identified mutations of *TP53*, *CDKN2A*, *PIK3CA* and *HRAS*. In a study of 32 head and neck tumors, Agrawal et al. described mutations in *NOTCH1* and *FBXW7* (12). In fact, after *p53* mutations, *NOTCH1* is the most common genetic mutation in head and neck carcinoma and it has been correlated with malignant transformation. Next-generation sequencing in head and neck tumors showed that *FAT1* tumor suppressor and *TERT* promoter mutations were identified in a large proportion of oral cavity carcinomas (13). Lastly, cyclin D1 and $p16^{INK4A}$ have been shown to be correlated with worse prognosis in head and neck cancers (14). Experimentally, Zhang and others have shown that LOH for high-risk genetic sites predicts the risk of progression to cancer after resection of leukoplakia. The genetic progression model for head and neck cancer was first described by Califano et al. (15). Zhang and colleagues expanded on Califano et al.'s previous work in the largest longitudinal study to date in PMDs (16). The study suggested LOH, especially 3p and 9p, is the best predictor of progression to malignancy.

Interestingly, overexpression of p16 is one of the immunohistochemical hallmarks of HPV-related carcinogenesis. HPV infection can lead to viral genome integration in oropharynx mucosal cells. Overexpression of the viral proteins E6 and E7 disables the functions of p53 and Rb proteins and leads to uncontrolled proliferation and cancer. The cells overexpress p16 in an attempt to reduce HPV-driven proliferation signals. HPV-related oropharynx cancers are genetically much simpler than tobacco-related cancers. The number and spectrum of mutations are much lower. It is likely that this is why HPV oropharynx cancers are highly curable and responsive to surgery, chemotherapy and radiation treatments.

Unfortunately, most studies are done by comparing genomic changes in tissue at the time of resection after the diagnosis of carcinoma has been made. Accordingly, it is hard to capture genetic changes that occur during carcinogenesis. Ideally, there would be an easily assessed early biomarker to capture PMDs undergoing malignant transformation.

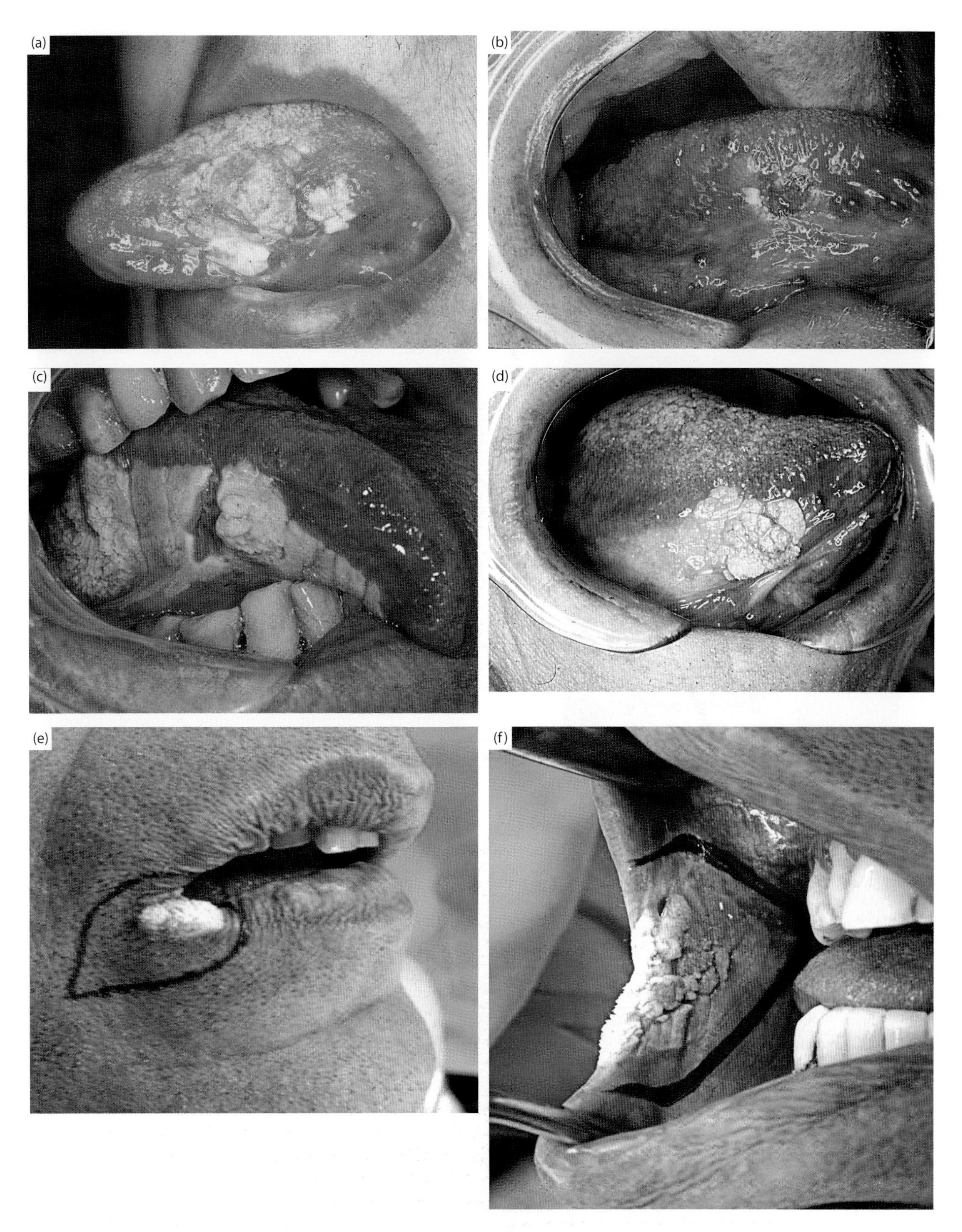

Figure 9.4 **(a)** Well-differentiated squamous cell carcinoma with multifocal hyperkeratosis. **(b)** Squamous cell carcinoma with leukoplakia. **(c)** Carcinoma developing in proliferative verrucous leukoplakia. **(d)** Squamous cell carcinoma with hyperkeratosis. **(e)** Verrucous carcinoma in keratosis (external component). **(f)** Verrucous carcinoma in keratosis (intraoral component).

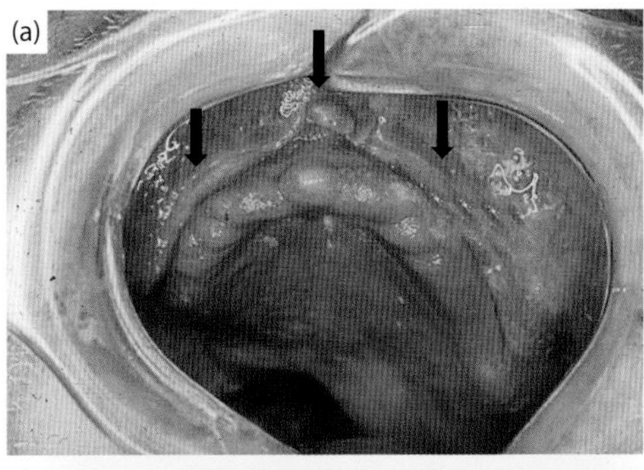

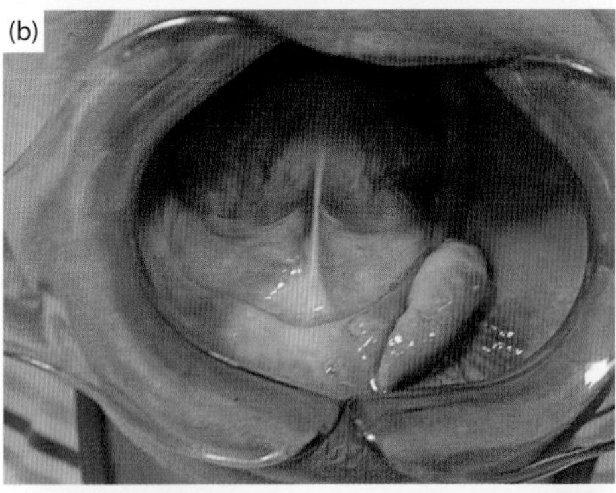

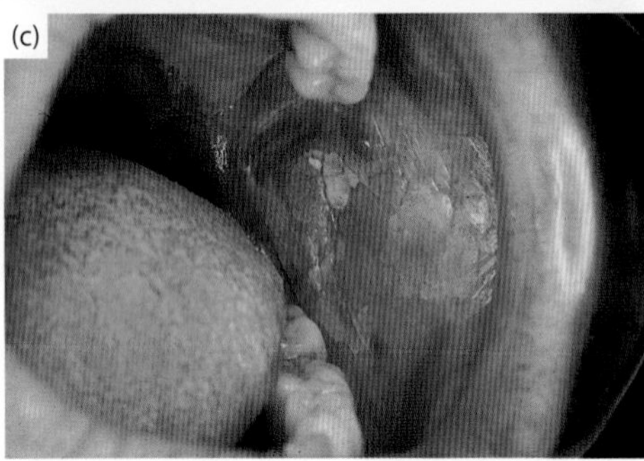

Figure 9.5 **(a)** Epulis fissuratum spanning the upper alveolar arch due to ill-fitting dentures. **(b)** Epulis fissuratum of the lower alveolus. **(c)** Leukoplakia of the buccal mucosa along occlusal line due to bite trauma.

CLINICAL DIAGNOSIS AND EVALUATION

White patches in the mouth are common. Idiopathic and tobacco-related precancerous leukoplakia must be differentiated from many other common non-precancerous lesions. Oral premalignant lesions can be classified based on history, physical examination, appearance, texture and location (Table 9.1). Suspicion for candidiasis should be raised in patients using inhaled corticosteroids in immunosuppressed patients or those undergoing radiation therapy to the oral cavity. Diagnosis of candidiasis can be made clinically (gently scraping the lesion) or with response to anti-fungal therapy. Likewise, periodontal inflammation is extremely common and treated with dental hygiene. In the case of PMDs from frictional lesions or trauma in the oral cavity, patient awareness, tooth guards, bite blocks, adjustment of dentures and regular dental care can often effectively avert the development of these lesions. It is not logical to extract otherwise healthy, functioning teeth to reduce trauma.

History of autoimmune disease such as systemic lupus erythematosus, scleroderma, discoid lupus, Calcinosis, Raynaud's, Esophageal dysmotility, sclerodactyly, telangiectasia (CREST) syndrome and graft-versus-host disease (such as after bone marrow transplant) should raise suspicion of lichen planus and other diseases that involve an immune response to the basement membrane. Lichen planus is a common autoimmune lacy white lesion of the oral cavity, most often seen in the buccal mucosa, which is not precancerous except in its aggressive, ulcerative, highly inflamed form. Notably, lichen planus is a submucosal process and needs to be differentiated from keratosis of the mucosa (Figure 9.7). A variety of chemical agents and metals used in dental treatments, appliances and medications can elicit an oral lichenoid reaction, including

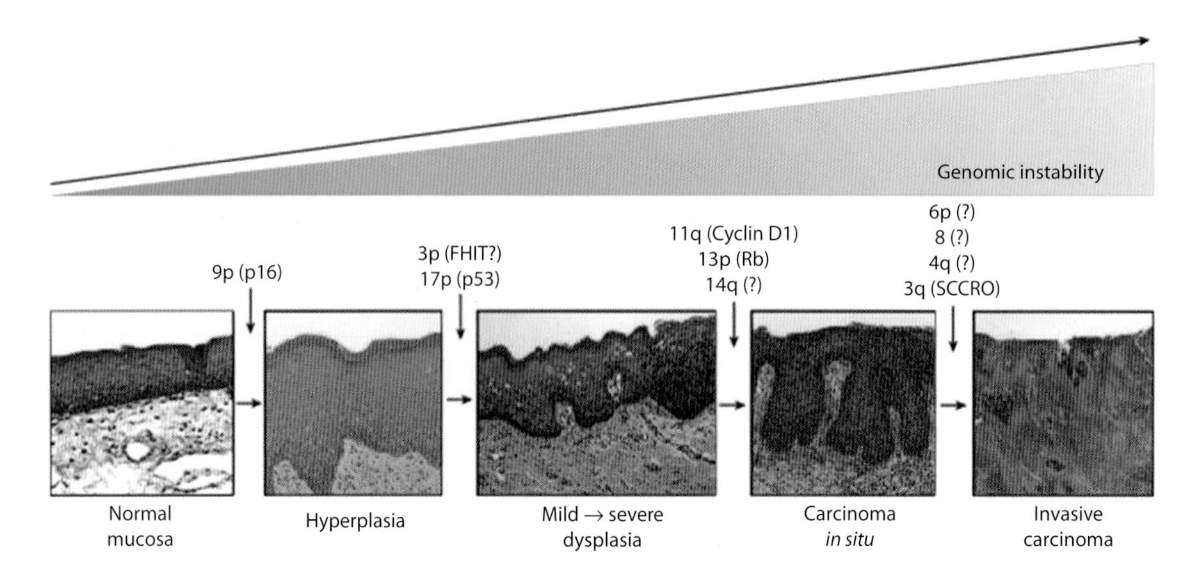

Figure 9.6 Pathologic progression model and genomic changes for squamous cell carcinoma of the oral mucosa.

Table 9.1 Characteristics, location and risk of malignancy in oral PMDs.

Disorders	Clinical features	Locations	Risk of malignancy
Leukoplakia	White plaque	Cheeks, lips, gingivae	15.6%–39.2%
Early (thin)			Not assigned
Homogeneous			1%–7%
Verruciform			4%–15%
Speckled			18%–47%
Erythroplakia	A predominantly red lesion	Floor of the mouth, tongue, retromolar pad, soft palate	51%
Proliferative verrucous leukoplakia	Multifocal white patch or plaque + rough surface projections	Gingivae	63.3%–100%
Viadent leukoplakia	White patch or plaque	Gingivae, buccal and labial vestibule	Not assigned
Candida leukoplakia	Firm, white, leathery plaques	Cheeks, lips, palate	4–5 times more common than leukoplakia
Smokeless tobacco keratosis	White plaque	Buccal or labial vestibule	Not assigned
Palatal keratosis associated with reverse smoking	White patches and plaques	Palate, tongue	83.3% dysplasia, 12.5% SCC
Verrucous hyperplasia	Extensive thick, white plaque	Buccal mucosa	68% dysplasia
Oral verrucous carcinoma	Extensive thick, white plaque	Buccal mucosa	20%
Dyskeratosis congenita	Oral leukoplakia	Buccal mucosa, tongue, oropharynx	Not assigned
Actinic cheilosis	Diffuse, poorly defined atrophic, erosive, ulcerative or keratotic plaques	Lower lip	6%–10%
Keratoacanthoma	Firm, sessile, non-tender nodule + a central plug of keratin	Lips, tongue, sublingual region	24%
Oral submucous fibrosis	Mucosal rigidity	Buccal mucosa, retromolar area, tongue, soft palate	7%–26%
Lichen planus	Reticular, erosive, atrophic, bullous, ulcerative, popular, plaque-like	Posterior buccal mucosa, tongue, gingivae, palate, vermilion border	0.4%–3.7%
Discoid lupus erythematosus	White plaques with elevated borders, radiating white striae and telangiectasia	Cheeks, lips, palate	Not assigned
Epidermolysis bullosa	Bullae and vesicle formation following mild trauma	Cheeks, tongue, palate	25%
Verruciform xanthoma	A well-demarcated mass with a yellow–white or red color and a papillary or verruciform surface	Gingivae, tongue, buccal mucosa, vestibular mucosa, floor of the mouth	Not assigned
Graft-versus-host disease	Atrophy, erythema, erosions, ulcers, lichenoid lesions	Cheeks, tongue, lips, buccal and labial vestibule	Not assigned

Source: Reproduced from Mortazavi, H et al. *J Dent Res Dent Clin Dent Prospects* 2014;8(1):6–14 (2).

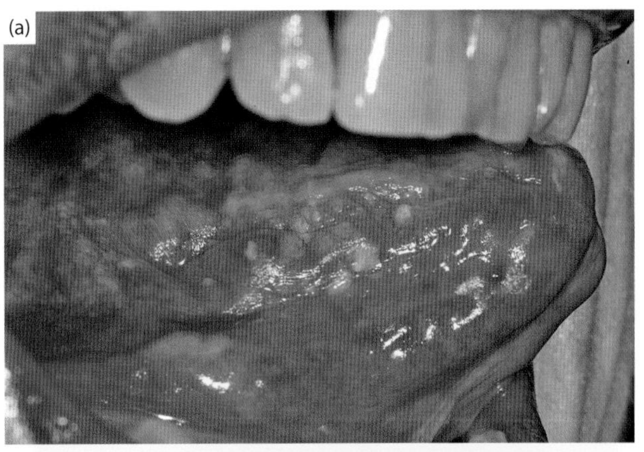

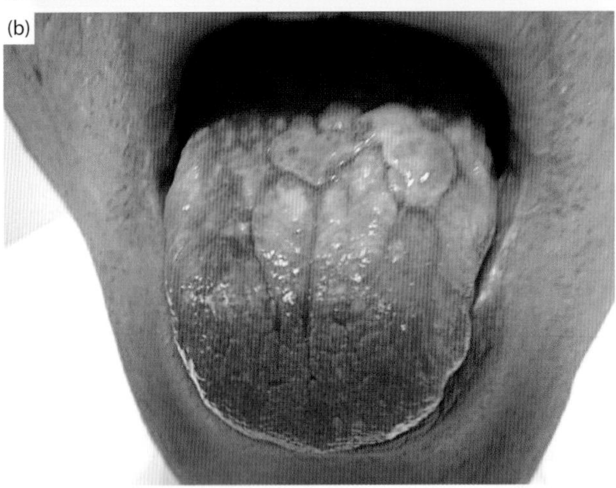

Figure 9.7 **(a)** Diffuse areas of lichen planus of the tongue. **(b)** Lichen planus of the dorsal tongue.

non-steroidal anti-inflammatories, anti-hypertensives, anti-malarials, psychotropic medications and even tartar control toothpaste (17).

The commonly seen papillomas in the oral cavity and oropharynx are seldom premalignant (Figure 9.8). Other more obscure causes of white patches include white sponge nevus, Greenspan's lesion or oral hairy leukoplakia associated with HIV infection, salicylate burns, cheilitis, geographic tongue and other rare conditions (Figure 9.9). Clinical factors that are more concerning for the risk of transformation into malignancy include tongue or floor of the mouth location, long duration, large size (>2 cm), ulceration, non-homogeneous subtype, female gender, red speckles and especially erythroplakia.

All leukoplakias should be measured and photographed when possible and the majority should be biopsied at least once to establish histologic diagnosis. A 3-mm punch biopsy is preferred or excisional biopsy if the lesion is less than 1 cm. Punch biopsy sampling at the area in which the lesion appears to be most invasive into normal tissue (not necessarily thickest) is preferred. This may give a diagnosis of cancer and a preoperative prediction of depth of invasion, which is useful when determining the need for neck dissection at the time of resection (18). For larger lesions, a punch biopsy is preferred rather than excisional biopsy so that the

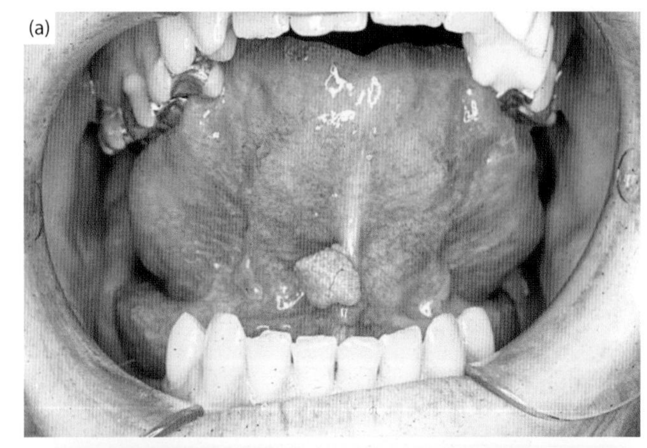

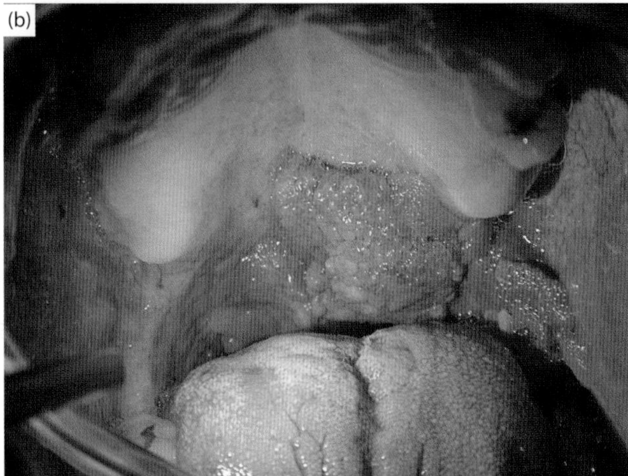

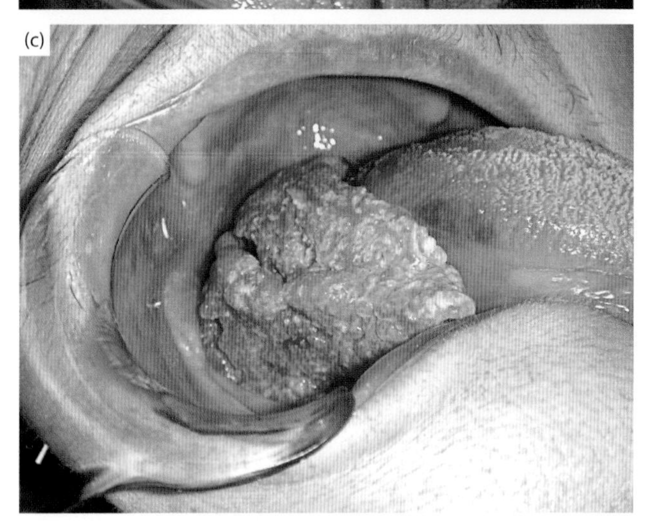

Figure 9.8 **(a)** Papilloma along the lingual frenulum. **(b)** Squamous papilloma of the hard and soft palate extending to the retromolar trigone. **(c)** Squamous cell carcinoma developing in a papilloma.

lesion is apparent and the margins can be adequately managed at the time of definitive excision. Furthermore, brush biopsies (exfoliative cytology) can be useful in suggesting the need for additional biopsy or excision, but have high false-positive results (19).

There is no substitute for a formal biopsy, but there are a variety of non-invasive detection techniques to show

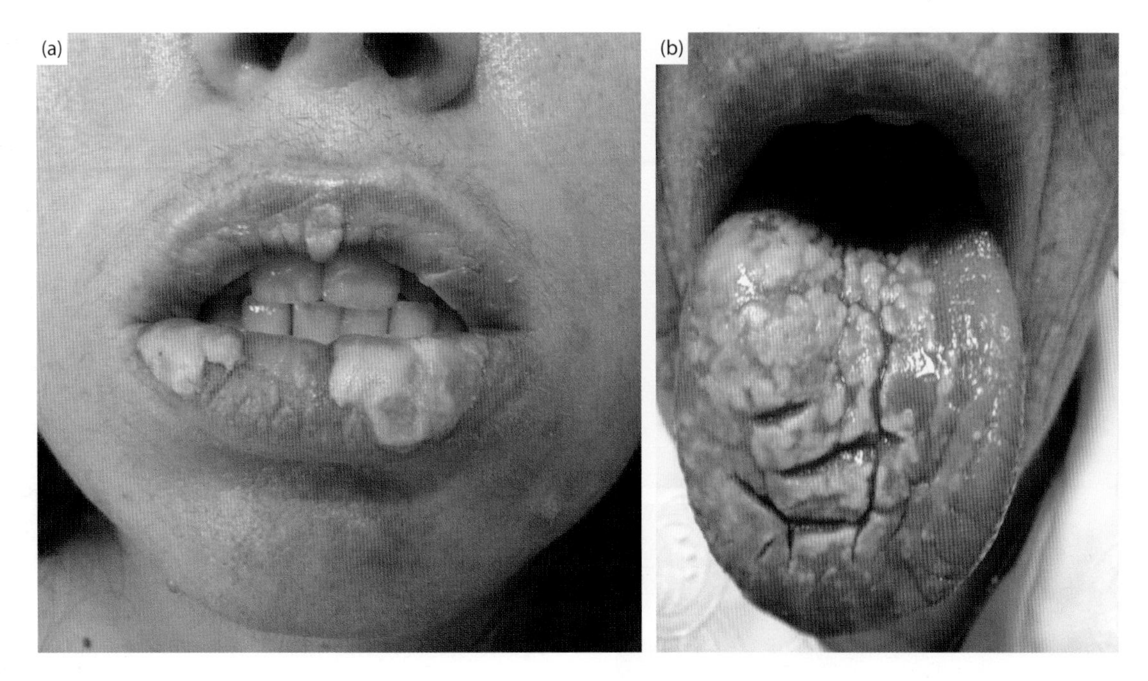

Figure 9.9 **(a)** Cheilitis with keratosis of the lips. **(b)** Geographic tongue with keratosis.

structural abnormalities in the mucosa, including vital staining, brush or exfoliative cytology and light-based detection systems, such as autofluorescence, chemiluminescence and confocal microscopy (20,21). The absorption and reflectance of light are altered in dysplastic mucosa compared to normal. There are commercially available light sources to visually detect alterations in chemiluminescence in oral mucosa. The enhanced visibility more sharply delineates the extent of the lesion and may guide the location of a biopsy. Notably, chemiluminescence recognizes leukoplakia but may not recognize erythroplakia and may be better when combined with Toluidine blue staining (19, 22, 23). In addition, innate tissue autofluorescence of collagen and elastin has been used to identify structural abnormalities in the epithelium using tissue fluorescence imaging (24). While highly sensitive and easily performed, this technique may yield a lot of false positives and biopsy must be performed to confirm diagnosis (23). Lastly, reflectance confocal microscopy can identify aberrations in cellular architecture and keratin pearls in oral cavity lesions and may be helpful in diagnosing SCC *in vivo* with further development (25). The published studies on these imaging techniques indicate that they are not precise enough to make a definitive diagnosis of malignancy (26,27). Thus, they currently do not offer an advantage in reducing the incidence of oral cancer by early diagnosis. Hopefully, with further development, these technologies will lead to improvements in our understanding and assessments of oral PMDs (28).

With regard to staining, a solution (mouthwash or topical) is applied that stains carcinoma, but not hyperplasia or hyperkeratosis. The most common stain is Toluidine blue dye, an acidophilic metachromatic nuclear stain. Staining shows a high correlation with LOH and has a high negative predictive value (22,29). In addition to differentiating benign from malignant lesions, it may be useful at the time of resection to define the extent of the lesion (Figures 9.10 and 9.11). A Cochrane review of vital staining, cytology and light-based detection systems revealed that cytology is the best way to classify lesions in the absence of a formal biopsy (30).

A quantitative staining technique for S100A7 (psoriasin, a biomarker thought to activate the MAPK pathway (31)) is commercially available to predict the 5-year risk of transformation into malignancy (32). This technique is more sensitive than standard dysplasia grading by pathology for determining risk and transformation into malignancy.

Podoplanin, a glycoprotein expressed in epithelial cells that regulates cellular motility, may be another biomarker for lesions at high risk of malignant transformation. One

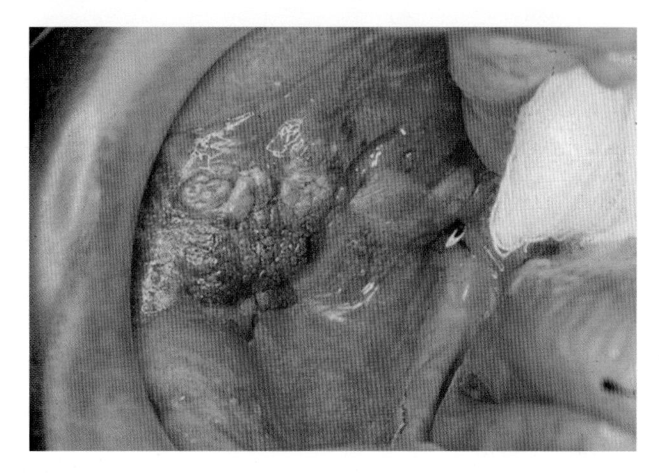

Figure 9.10 Squamous carcinoma of the buccal mucosa in the background of leukoplakia. Areas of dysplasia highlighted by Toluidine blue dye.

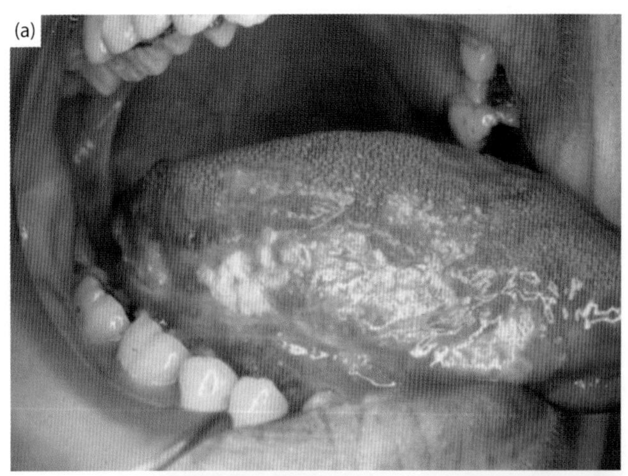

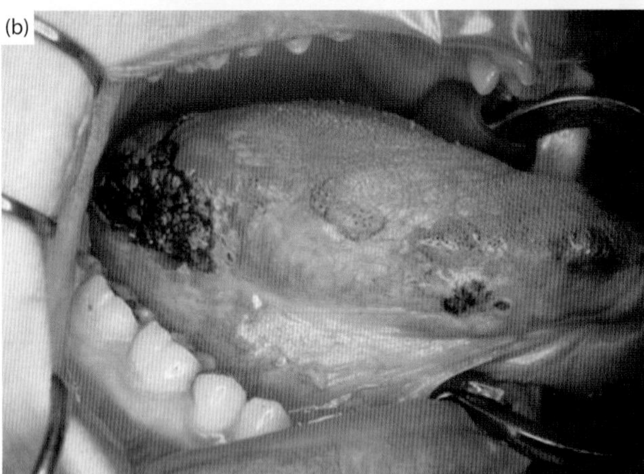

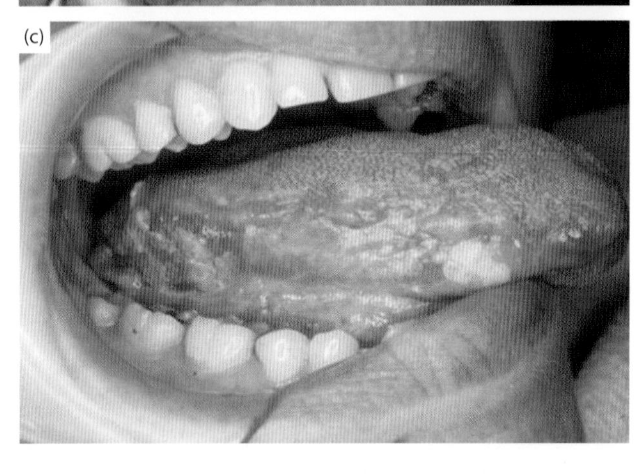

Figure 9.11 Toluidine blue staining to detect progression of benign leukoplakia to carcinoma in 6 months. **(a)** Initial leukoplakia. **(b)** Toluidine blue staining highlighting areas of malignant transformation. **(c)** Unstained lesions after progression to invasive carcinoma at 6 months.

study has shown podoplanin is associated with increased chance of malignant transformation in dysplasia, but further efforts are necessary to validate its use and improve availability (33).

Additional approaches using the salivary proteome are being developed to diagnose oral cancer. Salivary biomarkers are appealing because specimens are stable, more easily collected than a traditional invasive biopsy and highly sensitive. Artificial neural networks using proteomic data from saliva are able to identify the risk of nodal metastases in patients with oral cavity SCC (34). Ultimately, further development of all alternative diagnostic modalities is needed to support the practitioner and the patient in the decision to intervene in a PMD.

RISK OF PROGRESSION

In observation trials conducted on large numbers of patients, the rate of premalignant lesions progressing to SCC is reported in up to 12.1% of subjects and, on average, transformation occurred in 4.3 years (35). Thus, early diagnosis of SCC requires close observation to determine when visual changes in the lesion appear, raising the suspicion of malignant transformation. Dysplastic lesions that express VEGF, cytokeratins, EGFR, integrins, granulocyte colony stimulating factor receptor and p53 may be correlated with a higher rate of transformation into malignancy.

In the era of the HPV-related oropharynx cancer pandemic, there are no known clinical precursor lesions in the oropharynx. There is no effective medical therapy for HPV infection. It is likely that the widespread use of currently available HPV vaccination in children against high-risk strains will be effective in the prevention of HPV-related cancers. Presence of HPV DNA in blood or saliva does not necessarily imply that a patient has a premalignant or malignant lesion (36–38) and, conversely, HPV DNA in a malignancy does not mean the carcinogenesis was driven by the virus (39).

It is now well known that smokers with HPV-related oropharynx cancer have an intermediate cure rate between that of never-smokers with HPV-related cancers and those patients with HPV-negative cancers and heavy tobacco carcinogen exposure (40). Predicting which lesions will progress from dysplasia to carcinoma is difficult and even early intervention in the most suspicious-appearing lesion may not decrease the chance of malignant transformation in other sites in the oral mucosa (41). It is clear that smoking cessation is critically important to preventing malignant transformation of pre-existing PMDs.

OBSERVATION

Fortunately, most PMDs in the oral cavity do not progress to malignancy, but evaluation should be performed by an experienced practitioner to identify high-risk lesions. Many primary care providers should be educated about lesions that require further evaluation (such as persistent ulceration) and a referral should be made for consideration of biopsy. In cases where an experienced practitioner has evaluated the lesion adequately, observation of leukoplakia can be performed at expanding intervals from 1 to 6 months for reliable patients over time. Re-biopsy is indicated for clinical changes. Patients should be made aware that the risk of cancer progression in dysplastic leukoplakia is ~30% in 10 years. Cure rates for stage I oral cancers are typically greater than 95%. It is not reasonable to render the mouth dysfunctional in an attempt to prevent an unlikely oral cancer that is cured at a very high rate. The medical record should reflect a detailed discussion of the risks, benefits and alternatives with the patient.

Recurrence rates of resected oral leukoplakia are high and depend on the size and number of previous resections. In lesions over 2 cm, recurrence risk is in at least a third. After each excision, the chance of recurrence increases. Recurrence rates of 35%, 50% and 75% can be expected for resections after one, two or three recurrences, respectively. It is not appropriate to injure the oral tissues excessively to remove precancerous lesions that are destined to recur and may not represent the site of future oral cavity cancer.

SURGERY

Treatment of oral leukoplakic lesions is based on histologic diagnosis. Carcinoma is resected with 10-mm margins and appropriate consideration of elective neck dissection is given based on the size of the lesion and depth of invasion of the primary tumor. Carcinoma *in situ* is resected with 5–10-mm margins. Severe dysplasia is best resected with 5-mm margins if solitary and resectable. Mild dysplasia and moderate dysplasia lesions are resected if they are solitary and resectable without significant sequelae and they are observed if they are large, multiple or recurrent.

Resection of oral dysplastic leukoplakia is controversial, but it is not proven to reduce oral cancer risk. A meta-analysis of 14 studies suggests that resection of dysplastic lesions may reduce malignant transformation risk (35). A Cochrane review showed that there are no randomized controlled trials for laser excision, cryotherapy or surgical resection of leukoplakia that included a placebo or observation arm; thus, it is difficult to assess the efficacy of early interventions (42). Furthermore, the review highlighted that independent evaluations of systemic vitamin A, systemic β-carotene and topical bleomycin have not been shown to reduce the risk of malignant transformation more than a placebo.

Oral leukoplakia is a marker for diffuse mucosal changes that are subclinical. It is often not possible to estimate if the abnormal cells in the clinical white lesion are the most abnormal cells in the aerodigestive tract. In many reports, the eventual location of oral cancer is different from the previously resected oral leukoplakia. Therefore, surgical resection is not advisable in most cases of leukoplakia because it may cause considerable morbidity without preventing malignancy.

Resection techniques are largely similar to one another with the exception of CO_2 laser ablation. Resection can be well performed with electro-cautery, CO_2 laser or scalpel techniques. Lesions should be sent for complete pathologic analysis to rule out carcinoma. Reconstruction can be accomplished with primary closure, skin graft or by secondary healing. Dysfunction should be avoided with the use of reconstructive techniques, as is employed in the reconstruction of defects after cancer resection. CO_2 laser ablation (vaporization) should be reserved for benign lesions or lesions with mild dysplasia that are less than 10 mm. It is likely that recurrences and transformations in this subset are low. The main disadvantage of laser vaporization is that there is no tissue sample/specimen for pathologic analysis. Larger lesions are heterogeneous and need pathologic assessment. The risk of recurrence and the extent of scarring after CO_2 ablation is the same as for resection.

NON-SURGICAL TREATMENTS

Based on the theory of clonal evolution, it is clear that surgery for tobacco-related precancerous lesions has little hope of eradicating all the abnormal cells. It is possible that surgery can sometimes eradicate the most aggressive clones, but this is not always true. This is illustrated by the high rate of recurrence of clinical precancerous lesions after surgery and by the frequent incidence of oral cancer after resection of precancerous lesions, often at different sites. Systemic treatment theoretically offers the advantage of treating all the mucosa at risk.

Historically, 13-*cis*-retinoic acid has been tried for the treatment of leukoplakia by topical and systemic treatment with oral lozenges. Although excellent response rates are observed during treatment, nearly all leukoplakias returned after cessation of therapy (43). Subsequent to this initial study, larger clinical trials were conducted by Khuri and colleagues, who studied extensively the effects of 13-*cis*-retinoic acid (Accutane) for the treatment of leukoplakia and the prevention of oral precancer (44). The favorable observations in this phase II trial of 100 patients led to a study of over 1000 subjects in a randomized trial. The data, however, suggest no benefit of 13-*cis*-retinoic acid in preventing second primary cancers in oral cancer patients (45). It is likely that the molecular activity of vitamin A derivatives will prove useful in cancer prevention in some settings. Other avenues of research that have not shown efficacy in early clinical trials thus far include bleomycin, herbal tea extracts, selective COX-2 inhibition, non-steroidal anti-inflammatory drugs and PPAR-γ ligands (42). In addition, such an approach is not routinely employed due to the toxicities of such agents and uncertain length of therapy required.

Photodynamic therapy (PDT) involves specifically sensitizing cancerous or precancerous cells with photophores. These chemicals are preferentially taken up by neoplastic cells and then light-mediated activation leads to cell death. PDT has been used in head and neck cancer and premalignant lesions. It is used today in managing Barrett's esophagus lesions. In a systematic review of PDT, most patients showed at least a partial response, but many required multiple treatments and the recurrence rate was 36% (46). The treatment appears to be no different from other tissue-destructive techniques and selectivity, scarring and recurrence are still challenges. Thus, PDT has not yet found a mainstream use in managing oral precancerous lesions (47).

The immune system is capable of identifying genetically altered cells and, in some cases, destroying them. Immunocompromised patients are at elevated risk of oral and skin cancers. Investigators are exploring many different ways to teach the immune system to recognize and eliminate cancer cells. These approaches include tumor vaccines, *ex vivo* sensitization of immune cells, checkpoint blockade and targeting abnormal cell populations with antibodies to enhance immune recognition. Targeted therapies can block molecules that inhibit anticancer immunity. These drugs are widely used in malignant melanoma, for example (48). These immunologic approaches to cancer therapy will likely find applications in treating PMDs in order to prevent malignant transformation.

NOVEL THERAPIES

Today, any cutting-edge cancer treatment approach is also a potential approach for cancer prevention. In the era of targeted therapies and personalized medicine, these themes are also extant in prevention. Recently, William completed a trial using EGFR tyrosine kinase inhibitor-targeted therapy to reduce cancer incidence in high-risk patients with molecular high-risk findings of LOH for important genetic loci (49). Their findings suggest only a trend toward efficacy in the highest-risk subjects with a previous history of oral cancer, but studies like this usher in a new era of investigation in the prevention of oral cancer. Critical areas of discovery that are necessary to move the field forward are the detection and characterization of abnormal clones and the development of new endpoints for interventions with putative cancer-preventing agents.

Because precancerous changes in the aerodigestive tracts of smokers and former smokers are a diffuse process and our present ability to visualize abnormal clones is limited, novel approaches to cancer detection, treatment and prevention are necessary. The quest for a medical treatment to prevent tobacco-related cancers has been ongoing for at least five decades. There is at this time no proven effective therapy to halt or reverse the process of carcinogenesis in the human upper aerodigestive tract. It is important to reflect on the evolution of this field in order to appreciate the shortfalls of early approaches and to envision the promise for new paradigms. In the 1960s and 1970s, it was hoped that presumed-safe and abundant natural vitamins could be used to prevent lung cancer in active smokers or former smokers. For example, several large prospective studies over several decades proved that supplementation of β-carotene in active smokers caused a 25% increase in lung cancer (50–52). These results took the cancer prevention community aback and led to changes in cancer prevention trial design. The early studies were decades long with thousands of patients and cancer incidence as an endpoint.

Modern cancer prevention studies are now different. Importantly, there is much more reliance on a defined mechanism-based hypothesis. The preclinical phase of the hypothesis is carefully evaluated to minimize the risk of harm to the study participants. *In vitro* models are used to generate hypotheses that may be confirmed in biopsies of human tissues. Potential interventions are tested *in vitro* to assess for molecular evidence of efficacy at the proposed molecular targets. Animal models such as carcinogen-induced tumor models are utilized to test the potential cancer prevention efficacy of interventions *in vivo*. The early human studies are now small proof-of-principle studies in high-risk patients using surrogate endpoint biomarkers rather than cancer incidence. This allows preliminary evidence to be developed before large, expensive clinical trials with cancer endpoints are accomplished. Placebo-controlled randomized clinical trials are needed with long-term follow-up to show true efficacy of any intervention to thwart malignant transformation (42).

Similarly, nanoparticles can be targeted to abnormal cells in the body with antibodies or direct application. These particles can be made toxic by attaching chemotherapy molecules or by activating with light, magnets or irradiation. The potential for nanoparticles in the diagnosis and management of cancer and precancer is promising (53).

Because there is a natural selection process and clonal evolution occurring in the mucosal field of the head and neck, it is attractive to consider altering the growth advantages of some cell clones compared to others. It is conceivable that mucosal cells from the mouth could be harvested and characterized. They could be genetically engineered to grow more rapidly than the surrounding precancerous clones and then reintroduced into the oral cavity. The growth advantage could potentially be drug inducible. With drug treatment and by natural selection, the genetically engineered cells could eventually exclude other more dangerous clones with mutations of proto-oncogenes or loss of tumor suppressor gene functions. The engineered cells could later be made quiescent by stopping the drug-inducible treatment. The imagination alone limits the potential of these techniques (54).

CONCLUSIONS

Tobacco-related oral cancers often do present with clinically identifiable premalignant lesions prior to the development of carcinoma. However, oral precancerous dysplasia and oral leukoplakia are markers of diffuse genetic changes in the mucosa of the aerodigestive tract and thus surgical resection of the lesion is not proven to reduce the risk of oral cancer. However, judicious use of surgery in this setting is wise in order to minimize the risk of unnecessary dysfunction. In spite of several chemoprevention trials employing retinoic acid analogues and COX-2 inhibitors, such medical therapies have not been proven to be effective. In addition, the toxicities of such agents and the uncertain length of therapy required mean that such approaches are not routinely employed. Observation of lesions that are low grade, large, multifocal and recurrent is often the optimal approach. Systemic targeted approaches and novel technologies offer hope for halting the progression of tobacco-related premalignant lesions.

REFERENCES

1. Warnakulasuriya S, Johnson NW, van der Waal I. Nomenclature and classification of potentially malignant disorders of the oral mucosa. *J Oral Pathol Med* 2007;36(10):575–80.
2. Mortazavi H, Baharvand M, Mehdipour M. Oral potentially malignant disorders: an overview of more than 20 entities. *J Dent Res Dent Clin Dent Prospects* 2014;8(1):6–14.
3. Neville BW, Day TA. Oral cancer and precancerous lesions. *CA Cancer J Clin* 2002;52(4):195–215.
4. Narayan TV, Shilpashree S. Meta-analysis on clinicopathologic risk factors of leukoplakias undergoing malignant transformation. *J Oral Maxillofac Pathol* 2016;20(3):354–61.
5. Silverman S Jr, Gorsky M, Lozada F. Oral leukoplakia and malignant transformation. A follow-up study of 257 patients. *Cancer* 1984;53(3):563–8.
6. Blot WJ, McLaughlin JK, Winn DM et al. Smoking and drinking in relation to oral and pharyngeal cancer. *Cancer Res* 1988;48(11):3282–7.
7. Scapoli L, Palmieri A, Rubini C et al. Low prevalence of human papillomavirus in squamous-cell carcinoma limited to oral cavity proper. *Mod Pathol* 2009;22(3):366–72.
8. Yuspa SH, Poirier MC. Chemical carcinogenesis: from animal models to molecular models in one decade. *Adv Cancer Res* 1988;50:25–70.
9. Perez-Sayans M, Somoza-Martín JM, Barros-Angueira F et al. Genetic and molecular alterations associated with oral squamous cell cancer (review). *Oncol Rep* 2009;22(6):1277–82.
10. Boyle JO, Lonardo F, Chang JH et al. Multiple high-grade bronchial dysplasia and squamous cell carcinoma: concordant and discordant mutations. *Clin Cancer Res* 2001;7(2):259–66.
11. Reid BJ, Kostadinov R, Maley CC. New strategies in Barrett's esophagus: integrating clonal evolutionary theory with clinical management. *Clin Cancer Res* 2011;17(11):3512–9.
12. Agrawal N, Frederick MJ, Pickering CR et al. Exome sequencing of head and neck squamous cell carcinoma reveals inactivating mutations in NOTCH1. *Science* 2011;333(6046):1154–7.
13. Morris LG et al. The molecular landscape of recurrent and metastatic head and neck cancers: insights from a precision oncology sequencing platform. *JAMA Oncol* 2016;3(2):244–55.
14. Bova RJ, Quinn DI, Nankervis JS et al. Cyclin D1 and p16INK4A expression predict reduced survival in carcinoma of the anterior tongue. *Clin Cancer Res* 1999;5(10):2810–9.
15. Califano J, Van Der Riet P, Westra W et al. Genetic progression model for head and neck cancer: implications for field cancerization. *Cancer Res* 1996;56(11):2488–92.
16. Zhang L, Poh CF, Williams M et al. Loss of heterozygosity (LOH) profiles—validated risk predictors for progression to oral cancer. *Cancer Prev Res (Phila)* 2012;5(9):1081–9.
17. Muller S. Oral lichenoid lesions: distinguishing the benign from the deadly. *Mod Pathol* 2017;30(s1):S54–67.
18. Kuan EC, Clair J M-S, Badran KW et al. How does depth of invasion influence the decision to do a neck dissection in clinically N0 oral cavity cancer? *Laryngoscope* 2016;126(3):547–48.
19. Seoane Leston J, Diz Dios P. Diagnostic clinical aids in oral cancer. *Oral Oncol* 2010;46(6):418–22.
20. Liu D, Zhao X, Zeng X et al. Non-invasive techniques for detection and diagnosis of oral potentially malignant disorders. *Tohoku J Exp Med* 2016;238(2):165–77.
21. Macey R et al. Diagnostic tests for oral cancer and potentially malignant disorders in patients presenting with clinically evident lesions. *Cochrane Database Syst Rev* 2015;29(5).
22. Epstein JB, Silverman S, Epstein JD et al. Analysis of oral lesion biopsies identified and evaluated by visual examination, chemiluminescence and toluidine blue. *Oral Oncol* 2008;44(6):538–44.
23. Spivakovsky S, Gerber MG. Little evidence for the effectiveness of chemiluminescence and autofluorescent imaging devices as oral cancer screening adjuncts. *Evid Based Dent* 2015;16(2):48.
24. Cicciu M, Herford AS, Cervino G et al. Tissue fluorescence imaging (VELscope) for quick non-invasive diagnosis in oral pathology. *J Craniofac Surg* 2017;28(2):e112–5.
25. Karassawa Zanoni D, Migliacci JC, Ghossein R et al. Feasibility study of *in vivo* real-time reflectance confocal microscopy of oral squamous cell carcinoma, unpublished data.
26. Laronde DM, Williams PM, Hislop TG et al. Influence of fluorescence on screening decisions for oral mucosal lesions in community dental practices. *J Oral Pathol Med* 2014;43(1):7–13.
27. Brocklehurst P, Kujan O, Glenny AM et al. Screening programmes for the early detection and prevention of oral cancer. *Cochrane Database Syst Rev* 2013;11:CD004150.

28. Malik BH, Jabbour JM, Cheng S et al. A novel multimodal optical imaging system for early detection of oral cancer. *Oral Surg Oral Med Oral Pathol Oral Radiol* 2016;121(3):290–300.e2.
29. Zhang L, Williams M, Poh CF et al. Toluidine blue staining identifies high-risk primary oral premalignant lesions with poor outcome. *Cancer Res* 2005;65(17):8017–21.
30. Macey R et al. Diagnostic tests for oral cancer and potentially malignant disorders in patients presenting with clinically evident lesions. *Cochrane Database Syst Rev* 2015;5:CD010276.
31. Dey KK, Bharti R, Dey G et al. S100A7 has an oncogenic role in oral squamous cell carcinoma by activating p38/MAPK and RAB2A signaling pathway. *Cancer Gene Ther* 2016;23(11):382–91.
32. Hwang JT, Gu YR, Shen M et al. Individualized five-year risk assessment for oral premalignant lesion progression to cancer. *Oral Surg Oral Med Oral Pathol Oral Radiol* 2017;123(3):374–81.
33. D'Souza B, Nayak R, Kotrashetti VS. Immunohistochemical expression of podoplanin in clinical variants of oral leukoplakia and its correlation with epithelial dysplasia. *Appl Immunohistochem Mol Morphol* 2016;26(2):132–139.
34. Gallo C, Ciavarella D, Santarelli A et al. Potential salivary proteomic markers of oral squamous cell carcinoma. *Cancer Genomics Proteomics* 2016;13(1):55–61.
35. Mehanna HM, Rattay T, Smith J et al. Treatment and follow-up of oral dysplasia—a systematic review and meta-analysis. *Head Neck* 2009;31(12):1600–9.
36. Chaudhary AK, Singh M, Sundaram S et al. Role of human papillomavirus and its detection in potentially malignant and malignant head and neck lesions: updated review. *Head Neck Oncol* 2009;1:22.
37. Smith EM, Ritchie JM, Summersgill KF et al. Human papillomavirus in oral exfoliated cells and risk of head and neck cancer. *J Natl Cancer Inst* 2004;96(6):449–55.
38. Agalliu I et al. Associations of oral alpha-, beta-, and gamma-human papillomavirus types with risk of incident head and neck cancer. *JAMA Oncol* 2016; 2(5):599–606.
39. Hubbers CU, Akgul B. HPV and cancer of the oral cavity. *Virulence* 2015;6(3):244–8.
40. Ang KK, Harris J, Wheeler R et al. Human papillomavirus and survival of patients with oropharyngeal cancer. *N Engl J Med* 2010;363(1):24–35.
41. Brennan M, Migliorati CA, Lockhart PB et al. Management of oral epithelial dysplasia: a review. *Oral Surg Oral Med Oral Pathol Oral Radiol Endod* 2007;103(Suppl):S19.e1–12.
42. Lodi G, Sardella A, Bez C et al. Interventions for treating oral leukoplakia to prevent oral cancer. *Cochrane Database Syst Rev* 2016;7:CD001829.
43. Shah JP, Strong EW, DeCosse JJ et al. Effect of retinoids on oral leukoplakia. *Am J Surg* 1983;146(4):466–70.
44. Lee JJ, Hong WK, Hittelman WN et al. Predicting cancer development in oral leukoplakia: ten years of translational research. *Clin Cancer Res* 2000;6(5):1702–10.
45. Khuri FR, Lee JJ, Lippman SM et al. Randomized phase III trial of low-dose isotretinoin for prevention of second primary tumors in stage I and II head and neck cancer patients. *J Natl Cancer Inst* 2006;98(7):441–50.
46. Vohra F, Al-Kheraif AA, Qadri T et al. Efficacy of photodynamic therapy in the management of oral premalignant lesions. A systematic review. *Photodiagnosis Photodyn Ther* 2015;12(1):150–9.
47. Selvam NP, Sadaksharam J, Singaravelu G et al. Treatment of oral leukoplakia with photodynamic therapy: a pilot study. *J Cancer Res Ther* 2015;11(2):464–7.
48. Ibrahim R, Stewart R, Shalabi A. PD-L1 blockade for cancer treatment: MEDI4736. *Semin Oncol* 2015;42(3):474–83.
49. William WN Jr, Papadimitrakopoulou V, Lee JJ et al. Erlotinib and the risk of oral cancer: the Erlotinib Prevention of Oral Cancer (EPOC) randomized clinical trial. *JAMA Oncol* 2016;2(2):209–16.
50. Liu C, Wang X-D, Mucci L et al. Modulation of lung molecular biomarkers by beta-carotene in the Physicians' Health Study. *Cancer* 2009;115(5):1049–58.
51. The ATBC Cancer Prevention Study Group. The alpha-tocopherol, beta-carotene lung cancer prevention study: design, methods, participant characteristics, and compliance. *Ann Epidemiol* 1994;4(1):1–10.
52. The Alpha-Tocopherol, Beta Carotene Cancer Prevention Study Group. The effect of vitamin E and beta carotene on the incidence of lung cancer and other cancers in male smokers. *N Engl J Med* 1994;330(15):1029–35.
53. Durymanov MO, Rosenkranz AA, Sobolev AS. Current approaches for improving intratumoral accumulation and distribution of nanomedicines. *Theranostics* 2015;5(9):1007–20.
54. Nunney L, Maley CC, Breen M et al. Peto's paradox and the promise of comparative oncology. *Philos Trans R Soc Lond B Biol Sci* 2015;370(1673):pii: 20140177.

10

Cervical lymph nodes

AVIRAM MIZRACHI AND JATIN P. SHAH

Head and neck squamous cell carcinoma cells have the ability to spread along lymphatic channels to regional cervical lymph nodes. The pattern of spread of these cancer cells in the head and neck region has been well studied and is predictable. A sequential dissemination to cervical lymph nodes usually occurs and is almost always consistent. The negative impact of regional lymph node metastases on disease-specific survival cannot be over-emphasized (Figure 10.1) (1–16). While some head and neck cancer types tend to spread to regional lymph nodes at an early stage, others are associated with advanced primary tumor (Figure 10.2). Until recently, the acceptable rule of thumb was that spread of disease to regional lymph nodes decreases 5-year survival by approximately half. While this observation remains true for all mucosal cancers of the upper aerodigestive tract resulting from tobacco and alcohol abuse, in recent years, the human papillomavirus (HPV)-related oropharyngeal cancer epidemic has broken that rule. These HPV-positive tumors may present with bulky nodal disease and still carry a favorable prognosis regardless of treatment modality employed.

The overall risk for lymph node metastasis at presentation is generally site and stage dependent. In the oral cavity, it is grossly estimated as 25%, depending on the subsite, surface dimensions and depth of tumor invasion, both of which are now included in T staging. Nearly half of the patients with oral cancer have metastases to cervical lymph nodes at initial presentation. In the oropharynx, cancers tend to spread to regional lymph nodes at a relatively early stage and sometimes with a small or even occult primary tumor. This pattern is owing to the combination of rich lymphatic drainage of the oropharynx and the less visible anatomic location. It is imperative for the head and neck surgeon to thoroughly evaluate the neck in every patient and appreciate that the management of cervical lymph nodes is an integral component of the overall treatment strategy.

ANATOMY OF CERVICAL LYMPHATICS

Lymphatic drainage of the head and neck region occurs to a specific group of lymph nodes for a specific primary site and in a relatively predictable pattern (3,5,16–27). Thus, specific regional lymph node groups are at risk for initial involvement by metastatic disease. Therefore, these should be appropriately addressed in treatment planning for a given primary site. These include those regional lymph nodes that are accessible for surgical resection and those that are relatively inaccessible for adequate surgical resection such as retropharyngeal nodes and thus are important for inclusion in radiation ports.

Cervical lymph nodes of the head and neck region are shown in Figure 10.3. The relevant lymph nodes that drain the oral cavity are in levels I, II, III and IV and those that drain the oropharynx include levels II, III and IV and the retropharyngeal lymph nodes. The patterns of spread of disease can be further subdivided according to primary sites within the oral cavity. Generally, level IA nodes drain the upper and lower lips, anterior lower gum, anterior floor of the mouth and tip of the oral tongue. Level 1B nodes drain the upper and lower lips, floor of the mouth, oral tongue, upper and lower alveolar ridges, buccal mucosa and hard palate. Level IIA nodes drain the oral tongue, alveolar ridge, buccal mucosa and retromolar trigone. Level IIB nodes are rarely involved in the absence of disease at level IIA and drain the posterior oral tongue and floor of the mouth, buccal mucosa and retromolar

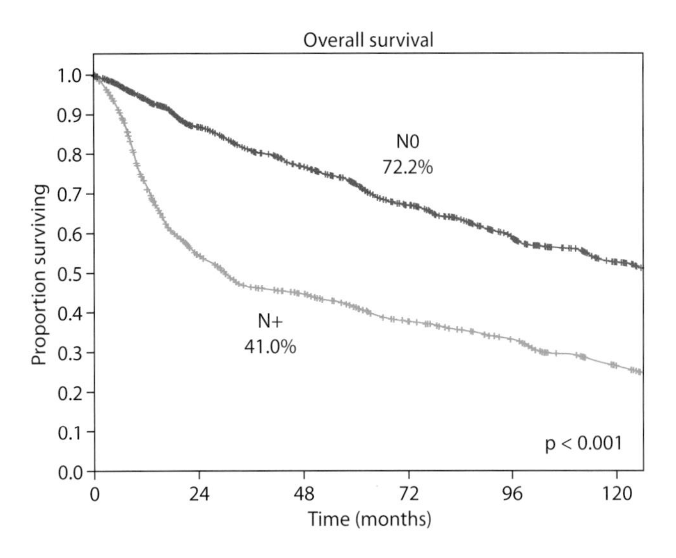

Figure 10.1 Impact of clinically palpable lymph node metastasis on disease-specific survival in squamous cell carcinoma of the oral cavity. (Courtesy of Memorial Sloan-Kettering Cancer Center, New York, 1985–2012.)

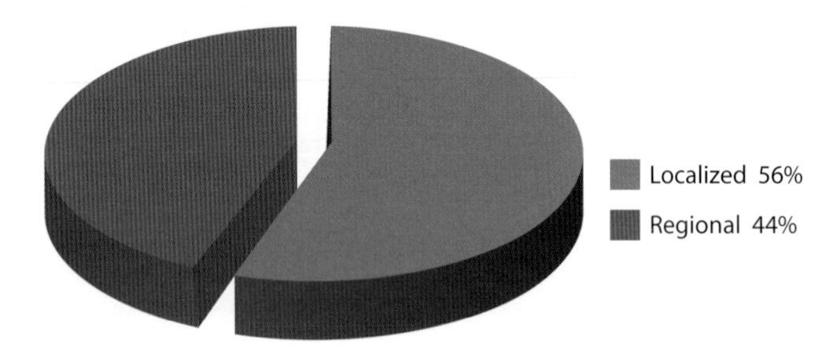

Figure 10.2 Cancer of the oral cavity (Memorial Sloan-Kettering Cancer Center, 1985–2012).

trigone. Level 3 and 4 nodes drain the oral tongue and floor of the mouth. Retropharyngeal nodes drain the posterior part of the hard palate, tonsils, base of the tongue and pharyngeal walls. Oropharyngeal tumors spread in a similar pattern to levels IIA, IIB, III and IV and the retropharyngeal nodes.

The upper lip drains to the submental, peri-facial and submandibular groups of lymph nodes in the submental and submandibular triangles of the neck. Deep jugular lymph nodes include the jugulodigastric, jugulo-omohyoid and supraclavicular groups of lymph nodes adjacent to the internal jugular vein. Lymph nodes in the posterior triangle of the neck include the accessory chain of lymph nodes located along the spinal accessory nerve and the transverse cervical chain of lymph nodes in the floor of the posterior triangle of the neck. Parapharyngeal and retropharyngeal lymph nodes are at risk of metastatic dissemination from tumors of the pharynx (28).

The central compartment of the neck includes the prelaryngeal (Delphian) lymph nodes overlying the thyroid cartilage in the midline draining the larynx and perithyroid lymph nodes adjacent to the thyroid gland. Lymph nodes in the tracheo-esophageal groove provide primary drainage to the thyroid gland as well as the hypopharynx, subglottic larynx and cervical esophagus. Lymph nodes in the anterior superior mediastinum provide drainage to the thyroid gland and cervical esophagus and serve as a secondary lymphatic basin for anatomic structures in the central compartment of the neck. Each anatomic subgroup of lymph nodes described above specifically serves as primary-echelon lymph nodes draining a specific site in the head and neck region. Thus, location of a palpable metastatic lymph node may often indicate the source of a primary tumor. In Figure 10.4 the regional lymph node groups draining a specific primary site as first-echelon lymph nodes are depicted.

In order to establish a consistent and easily reproducible, user-friendly method for description of regional cervical lymph nodes that establishes a common language between the clinician and the pathologist, the Head and Neck Service at Memorial Sloan-Kettering Cancer Center in New York has described a leveling system of cervical lymph nodes. This system divides the lymph nodes in the lateral aspect of the neck into five nodal groups or levels. However, the American Academy of Otolaryngology—Head and Neck Surgery has further subdivided levels I, II, and V into the subcategories a and b (Figure 10.5) (3,22,23).

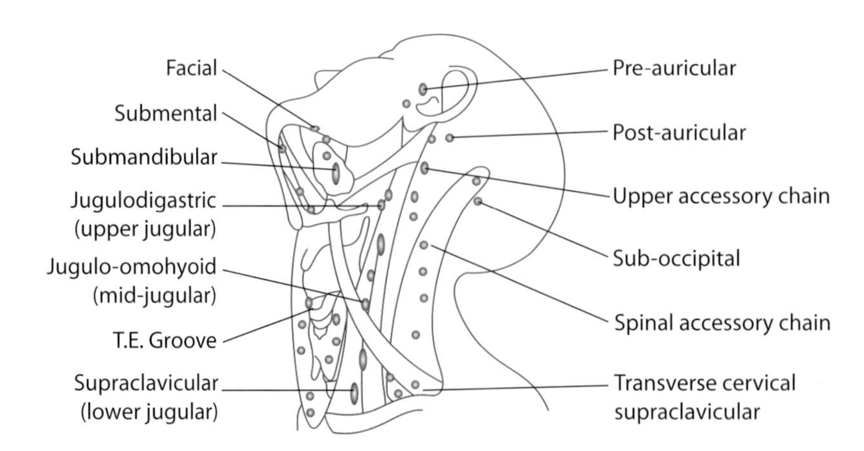

Figure 10.3 Regional cervical lymph nodes. Additional lymph node groups not shown; parapharyngeal, retropharyngeal and superior mediastinal.

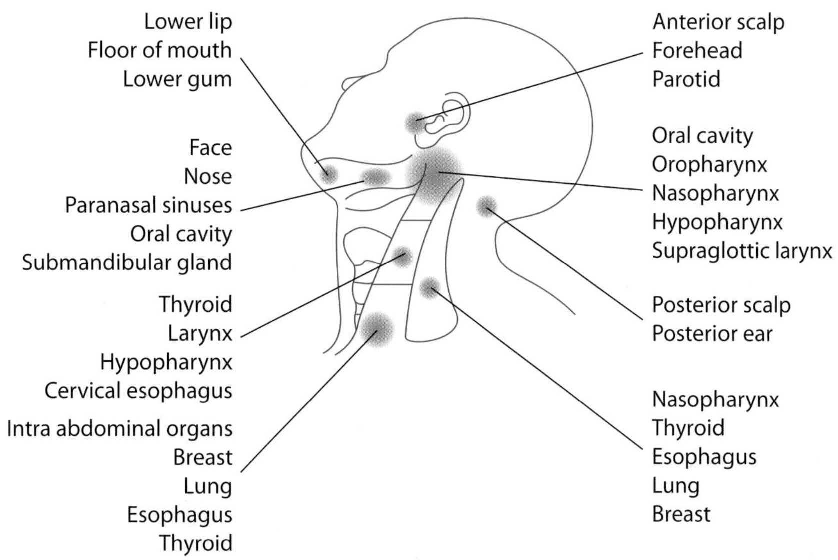

Lower lip
Floor of mouth
Lower gum

Face
Nose
Paranasal sinuses
Oral cavity
Submandibular gland

Thyroid
Larynx
Hypopharynx
Cervical esophagus

Intra abdominal organs
Breast
Lung
Esophagus
Thyroid

Anterior scalp
Forehead
Parotid

Oral cavity
Oropharynx
Nasopharynx
Hypopharynx
Supraglottic larynx

Posterior scalp
Posterior ear

Nasopharynx
Thyroid
Esophagus
Lung
Breast

Figure 10.4 Potential primary sites in relation to the locations of cervical lymph node metastases.

Level I: Lymph nodes at level 1 are divided into two groups: *submental group (level IA)*, the nodal tissue between the anterior belly of the digastric muscles and cephalad to the hyoid bone; and *submandibular group (level IB)*, nodal tissue in the triangular area bounded by the anterior and posterior bellies of the digastric muscle and the inferior border of the body of the mandible. The lymph nodes adjacent to the submandibular salivary gland and along the facial artery are included in this group.

Level II, upper jugular group: Nodal tissue around the upper portion of the internal jugular vein and the upper part of the spinal accessory nerve, extending from the base of the skull up to the bifurcation of the carotid artery or the hyoid bone (clinical landmark). The posterior limit for this level is the posterior border of the sternocleidomastoid muscle and the anterior border is the lateral limit of the sternohyoid muscle. This level is also divided into two subgroups: *Level IIA* are lymph nodes in the jugulodigastrics region, anterior to the accessory nerve; and *level IIB* are lymph nodes at this level posterior to the spinal accessory nerve.

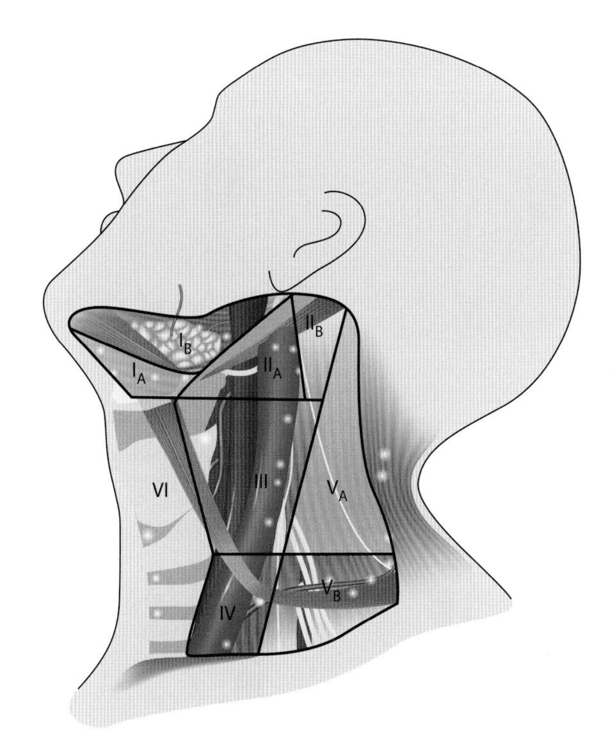

Figure 10.5 Cervical lymph nodes: locations and levels.

Level III, midjugular group: Nodal tissue around the middle third of the internal jugular vein from the inferior border of level II up to the omohyoid muscle or the lower border of the cricoid cartilage (clinical landmark). The anterior and posterior borders are the same as those for level II.

Level IV, lower jugular group: Nodal tissue around the lower third of the internal jugular vein from the inferior border of level III up to the clavicle. The anterior and posterior borders are the same as those for levels II and III.

Level V, posterior triangle group: Nodal tissue around the lower portion of the spinal accessory nerve *(level VA)* and along the transverse cervical vessels (*level VB*). It is bounded by the triangle formed by the clavicle, the posterior border of the sternocleidomastoid muscle and the anterior border of the trapezius muscle.

In addition to the leveling of lymph nodes in the lateral neck, two further levels are described to include lymph nodes in the central compartment of the neck and anterior superior mediastinum.

Level VI, central compartment group: Lymph nodes in the tracheoesophageal grooves and perithyroid region, extending from below the hyoid bone up to the suprasternal notch. These nodes include prelaryngeal (Delphian), pretracheal, paratracheal and paraesophageal lymph nodes in the tracheoesophageal groove.

Level VII, superior mediastinal group. Lymph nodes in the anterior superior mediastinum, extending from the suprasternal notch up to the innominate artery in a cephalocaudal plane and from carotid to carotid artery laterally.

CLINICAL STAGING OF CERVICAL LYMPH NODES (N STAGING)

The American Joint Committee on Cancer (AJCC) and the International Union Against Cancer (UICC) have agreed upon a uniform staging system for metastatic cervical lymph nodes. This nodal staging system up until this year included the nodal parameters such as presence, size, number, levels and laterality of lymph nodes. The latest revision of the nodal staging system (8th edition) includes extranodal extension (ENE) and location of the lymph nodes as well in order to more accurately define the prognostic importance of these features in nodal staging. The new nodal staging is depicted in Figure 10.6. The N stages of lymph node metastasis are described in Chapter 7, Table 7.2.

Several factors pertaining to the characteristics of regional lymph node metastasis directly influence prognosis. These include the presence or absence of clinically palpable cervical lymph node metastasis, the size of the metastatic lymph node, the number of lymph nodes involved, the location of lymph nodes involved by metastatic cancer, the volume of metastatic focus within an enlarged node and the presence of gross ENE (3–5,9,11,14,17,28–30). Involvement of lower cervical lymph nodes (level IV) and lower posterior triangle lymph nodes (level V) by metastatic cancer from a primary cancer in the oral cavity or oropharynx usually implies an ominous prognosis (7). Thus, involvement of lymph nodes in the lateral neck below the lower border of the cricoid cartilage is of serious prognostic significance. In addition to this, the presence of extranodal spread of metastatic disease by capsular rupture of the lymph node with invasion of the soft tissues clearly impacts on prognosis (6,7,11,13,31–35). Lymphovascular and perineural infiltration by tumor as well as the presence of tumor emboli in regional lymphatics also have adverse impacts on prognosis (4,6,29,30,33,36). Therefore, these factors must be considered when developing a treatment strategy for patients in whom regional lymph nodes are involved by metastatic disease, particularly for planning adjuvant therapy and for assessment of prognosis.

RISK OF NODAL METASTASIS

Involvement of regional lymphatics by primary squamous cell carcinomas of the upper aerodigestive tract is dependent on various factors related to the primary tumor, including the site, size, depth of invasion, T stage and location of the primary tumor. The newly revised AJCC staging system (8th edition) includes depth of invasion of the primary tumor in the T staging of oral cancers. In addition, histomorphologic features of the primary tumor also influence the risk of nodal metastasis (3,4,12,21,22,27,37–40). The risk of nodal metastasis increases in relation to the location of

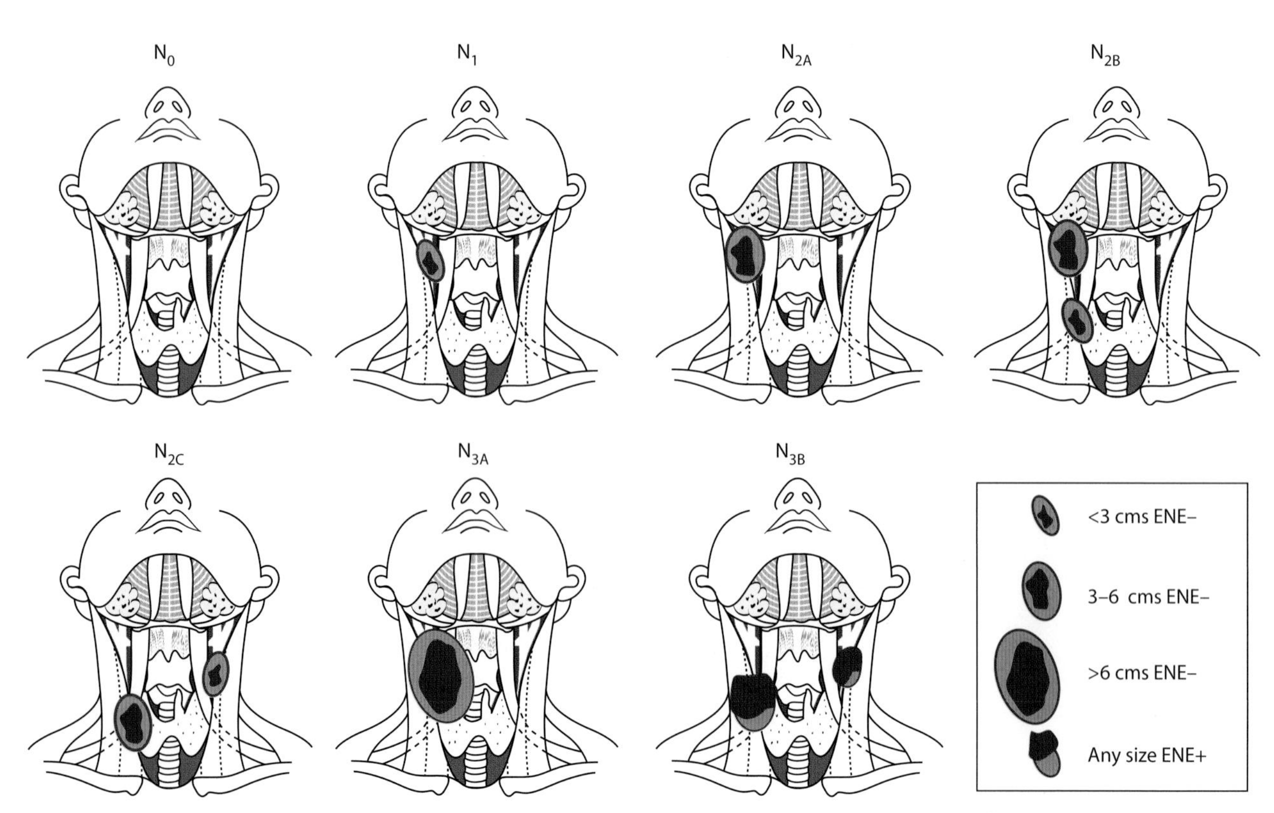

Figure 10.6 American Joint Committee on Cancer/International Union Against Cancer N staging (8th edition).

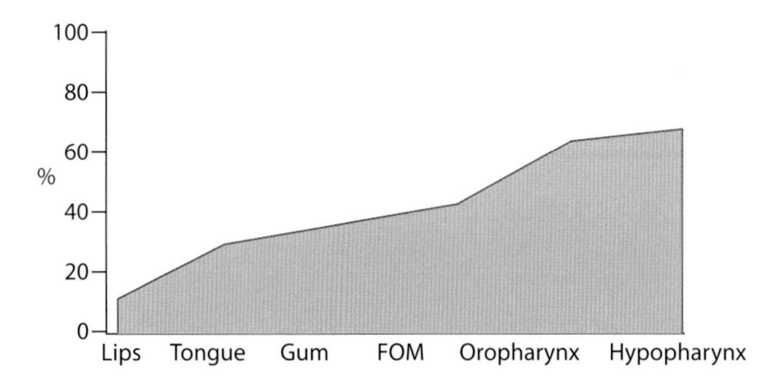

Figure 10.7 Incidence of nodal metastases at presentation in relation to primary site and location. FOM: Floor of Mouth.

the primary tumor as one progresses from the anterior to the posterior aspect of the upper aerodigestive tract (i.e. the lips, oral cavity, oropharynx and hypopharynx) (Figure 10.7) (3,4,21,22,27).

Within the oral cavity, certain primary sites have a significantly increased risk of nodal metastasis compared to the other sites (e.g. floor of the mouth versus hard palate). In general, the T stage usually reflects tumor burden and therefore the risk of nodal metastasis increases with increasing T stage of the primary tumor at any site.

Certain histomorphological features of the primary tumor also increase the risk of nodal metastasis. Thus, endophytic tumors are more inclined to metastasize than exophytic tumors. It has been well documented that for tongue and floor of the mouth cancers, tumor thickness is related to the risk of nodal metastases (Figure 10.8). This feature is now incorporated in the new TNM staging system by the AJCC in the latest revision (8th edition). Poorly differentiated carcinomas have a higher risk of nodal metastases compared to well-differentiated lesions. Finally, HPV-positive oropharyngeal cancers have a significantly higher risk of nodal metastasis at presentation compared to their HPV-negative counterparts. Clinical observations to date, however, indicate that presence of nodal metastasis in HPV-positive oropharyngeal cancers does not have the same degree of negative impact on prognosis as for their HPV-negative counterparts.

PATTERNS OF NECK METASTASIS

Dissemination of metastatic cancer to regional lymph nodes from primary sites in the upper aerodigestive tract occurs in a predictable and sequential fashion (3,4,19,21,22,27). Thus, only select regional lymph node groups are at risk of nodal metastases initially from any primary site in the absence of grossly palpable metastatic lymph nodes. On the other hand, when clinically palpable lymph nodes are present at the time of initial diagnosis, comprehensive clearance of all regional lymph node groups at risk is warranted. Several well-documented studies in the literature have confirmed that select groups of regional lymph nodes are initially at risk for each primary site in the head and neck region. Understanding the sequential patterns of neck metastasis therefore greatly facilitates surgical management of regional lymph nodes in the clinically negative neck where the lymph nodes are at risk of harboring micrometastasis.

For primary tumors in the oral cavity, the regional lymph nodes at highest risk for early dissemination by metastatic cancer are limited to levels I, II, and III (Figure 10.9). Anatomically, this translates into regional lymph node groups contained within the supraomohyoid triangle of the neck, including the submental, submandibular, prevascular facial, jugulodigastric, upper deep jugular and superior spinal accessory chain of lymph nodes, and midjugular lymph nodes. Skip metastasis to levels IV and V in the absence of metastatic disease at levels I, II, or III is exceedingly rare (41). Therefore, if the neck is clinically negative, levels IV and V lymph nodes are generally not considered at risk of harboring micrometastasis from primary squamous carcinomas of the oral cavity. Similarly, metastatic disease at level IIB is almost never present in the absence of metastatic disease at level IIA.

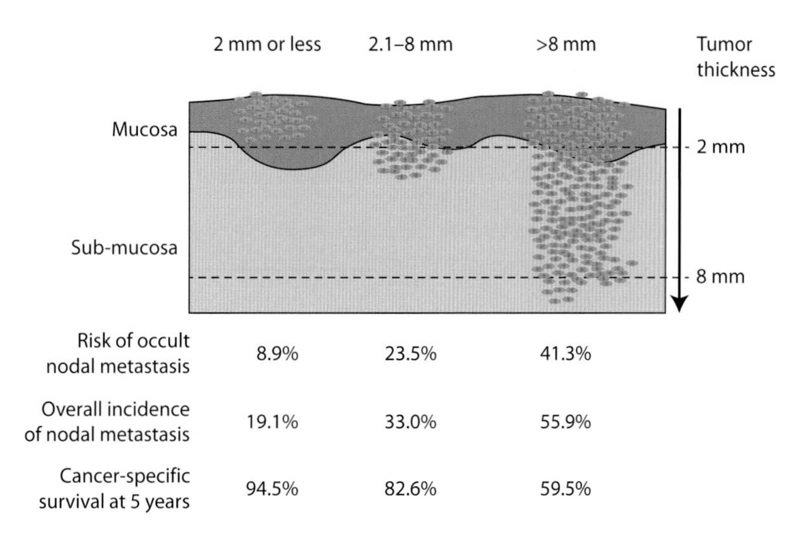

Figure 10.8 Percentages of occult and overt lymph node metastases and percentages dead of disease in relation to tumor thickness for tongue and floor of the mouth cancers.

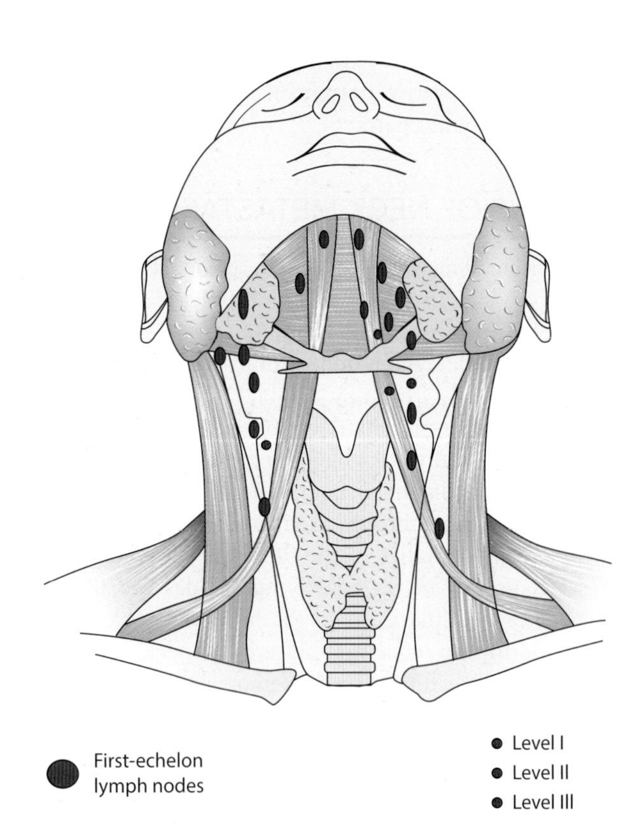

Figure 10.9 Patterns of lymph node metastases for cancer of the oral cavity. First-echelon lymph nodes: levels I, II, and III.

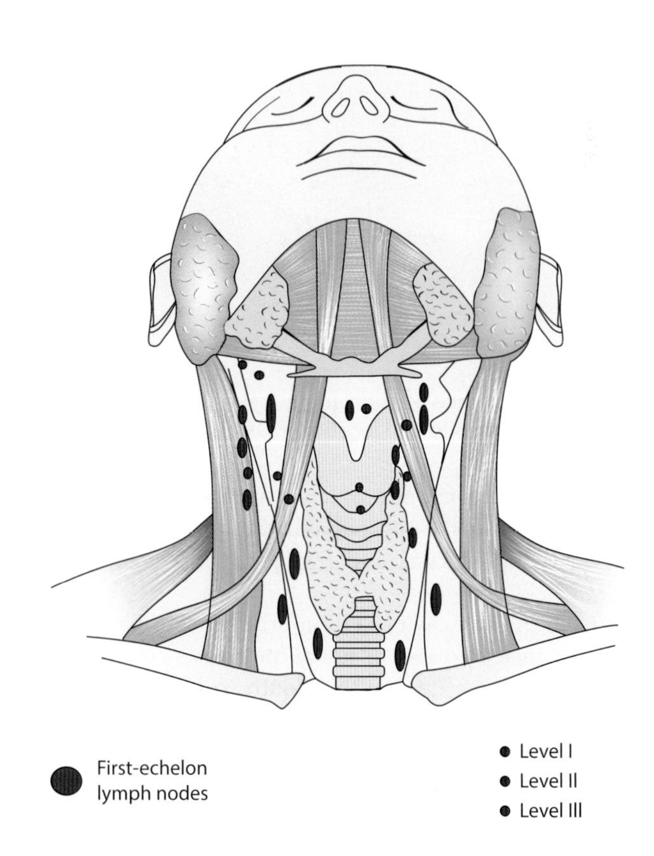

Figure 10.10 Patterns of lymph node metastases for cancer of the larynx and pharynx. First-echelon lymph nodes: levels II, III, and IV.

For tumors on the lateral aspect of the oropharynx, the first-echelon lymph nodes at highest risk of harboring micrometastasis in the clinically negative neck are the deep jugular lymph nodes at levels II, III, and IV on the ipsilateral side (Figure 10.10) (16,22,38). The lymph node groups in the deep jugular chain are the jugulo-digastric, highest spinal accessory chain of lymph nodes, midjugular lymph nodes, jugulo-omohyoid lymph nodes and supraclavicular lymph nodes deep to the sternocleidomastoid muscle. Contiguous lymph nodes lateral to the internal jugular vein overlying the cutaneous roots of the cervical plexus are usually considered a component of levels II, III, and IV. In patients with primary carcinomas of the oropharynx with a clinically negative neck, the risk of micrometastasis to levels I and V is extremely small (16,22,38,42). Skip metastasis to levels I and V in the absence of disease at levels II, III, or IV is usually not seen. Primary tumors that involve both sides of the midline have a potential for microscopic dissemination of metastatic disease to jugular lymph nodes on both sides of the neck.

CLINICAL FEATURES AND DIAGNOSIS

The presence of a clinically palpable, unilateral, firm, enlarged lymph node in the adult should be considered metastatic until proven otherwise. The clinically enlarged lymph node may be present at any of the previously described anatomic locations in the head and neck region. The location of a palpable lymph node may point to the potential site of a primary tumor. The important features to note during examination of the neck for cervical lymph nodes are the location, size, consistency and number of palpable lymph nodes, as well as clinical signs of extracapsular spread such as invasion of the overlying skin, fixation to deeper soft tissues or paralysis of cranial nerves. Histological diagnosis of metastatic carcinoma is usually established by a needle aspiration biopsy and cytological examination of the smears (3,4,14,43,44). An enlarged metastatic cervical lymph node may be the only physical finding present in some patients whose primary tumors are either microscopic or occult at the time of presentation. A systematic search for a primary tumor should be undertaken in these patients prior to embarking upon therapy for the metastatic nodes.

RADIOGRAPHIC EVALUATION

Most patients with palpable cervical lymph node metastasis seldom require radiographic evaluation of the nodes for diagnosis. However, when massive metastatic disease is present, radiographic evaluation by computed tomography (CT) scan with intravenous contrast or magnetic resonance imaging (MRI) scan with gadolinium contrast is desirable to assess the extent of the nodal disease, particularly as it relates to the carotid artery, the skull base and the parapharyngeal space on the ipsilateral side, as well as to evaluate the clinically negative contralateral side

(43,45–49). Several lymph node groups that are not accessible to clinical examination, such as those in the parapharyngeal and retropharyngeal areas, are best assessed by a CT or magnetic resonance imaging (MRI) scan. Similarly, evaluation of lymph nodes in the superior mediastinum is best accomplished with radiographic studies. The radiographic features for diagnosis of a metastatic node are size, rim enhancement, central necrosis and ENE (Figure 10.11) (45). Ultrasound-guided fine needle aspiration biopsy of a small lymph node often helps to establish accurate tissue diagnosis (43).

The role of ^{18}F-fluorodeoxyglucose (FDG) positron emission tomography (PET) in oral and oropharyngeal cancer has been evolving constantly (50). While providing an excellent functional perspective, FDG-PET is inferior to CT and MRI at illustrating the relevant anatomy (51). Initial data showed limited abilities; however, newer-generation equipment is able to increase the potential of FDG-PET for the detection of subclinical primary or simultaneous secondary tumors and of nodal or systemic spread. FDG-PET can also contribute to the detection of residual/early recurrent tumors, leading to the timely institution of salvage therapy or the prevention of unnecessary biopsies of irradiated tissues, which may aggravate injury (52). Certainly, FDG-PET may have potential roles in initial staging, survival prediction and the detection of recurrences and second cancers (53).

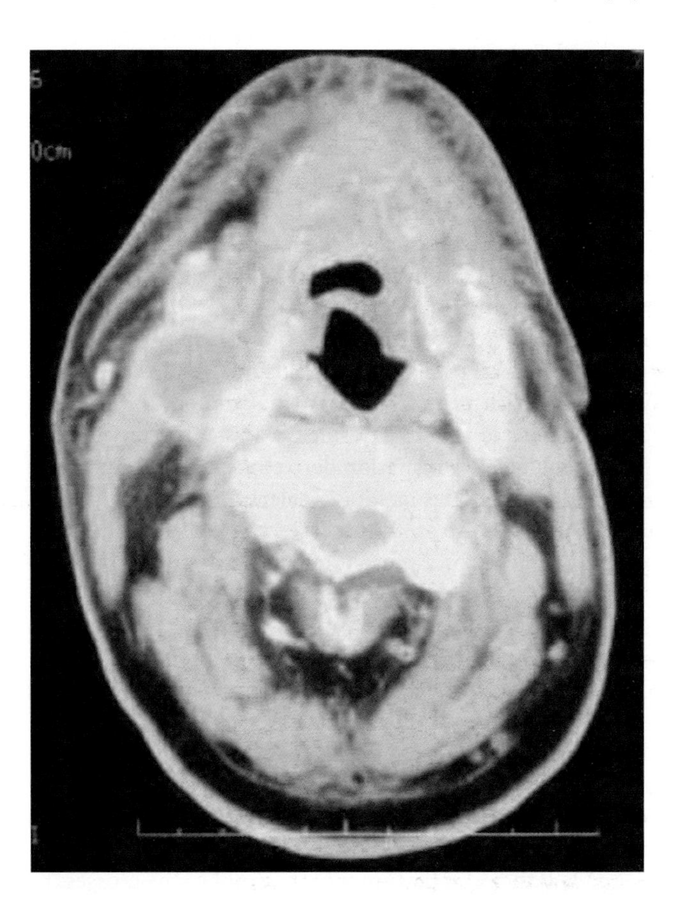

Figure 10.11 CT scan of the neck with contrast showing a metastatic lymph node with central necrosis and rim enhancement.

In patients with advanced Head and Neck Squamous Cell Carcinoma (HNSCC), normal FDG-PET/CT after chemoradiotherapy has a high negative predictive value and specificity for excluding residual locoregional disease. Therefore, in patients without residual lymphadenopathy, neck dissection may be withheld. In patients with residual lymphadenopathy, a lack of abnormal FDG uptake in these nodes also excludes viable tumor with high certainty (53).

GOAL OF TREATMENT

Clearly, the goal of treatment for cervical lymph node metastasis is regional control of disease and improvement in overall cure of cancer. Micrometastases and minimal gross metastases may be controlled by radiotherapy alone. However, surgery remains the mainstay of treatment of cervical lymph node metastases since it provides comprehensive clearance of all grossly enlarged lymph nodes as well as other nodes in that compartment of the neck and offers accurate histological information on lymph nodes at risk of having micrometastasis in the clinically negative neck (1,54,55).

While the indications for comprehensive surgical clearance of regional lymph nodes in the neck for clinically palpable metastatic lymph nodes are obvious, the indications for elective treatment of the N_0 neck are less clear (14,56–59). Statistically, one is unable to document difference in regional control rates or survival between patients undergoing elective neck dissection for micrometastasis or those undergoing therapeutic neck dissection for N_1 disease (14,43,56,57,59). It is presumed that progression of metastatic disease from micrometastasis to gross metastasis occurs in a sequential manner from $N_0 \rightarrow N+$ microscopic $\rightarrow N_1 \rightarrow N_2 \rightarrow N_3$. However, in clinical practice, it is not uncommon to see N_0 patients present with advanced nodal metastasis even during close surveillance (Figure 10.12). Review of a consecutive series of patients whose N_0 neck was observed initially and who subsequently underwent therapeutic neck dissection shows that a significant number of patients had clinically apparent metastatic disease greater than N_1 at the

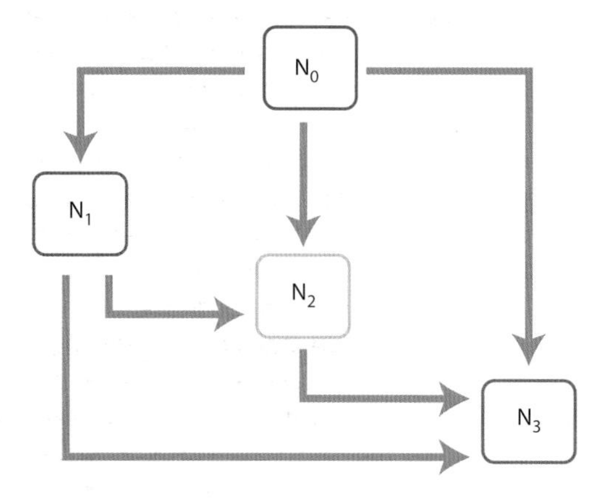

Figure 10.12 Expected disease progression in untreated N_0 necks.

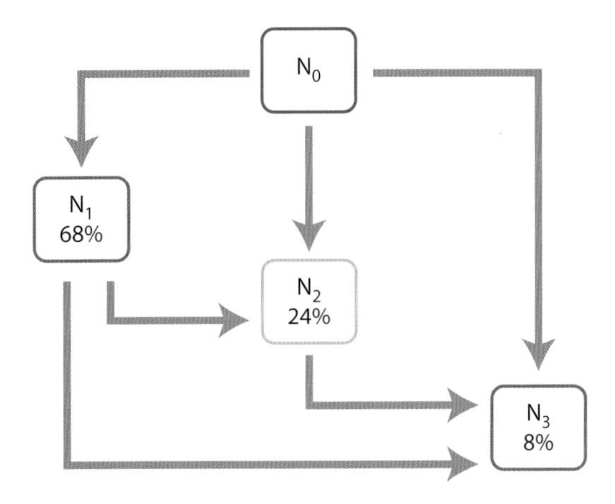

Figure 10.13 Clinical findings at delayed therapeutic neck dissection in untreated N_0 necks.

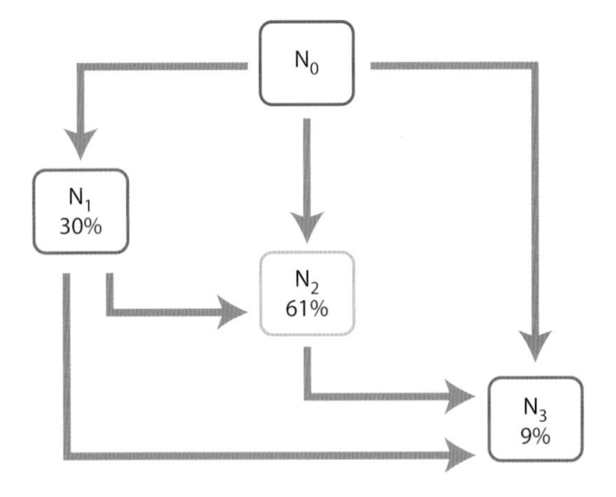

Figure 10.14 Pathologic findings at delayed therapeutic neck dissection in untreated N_0 necks.

time of neck dissection (Figure 10.13) (32,56–58,60–62). This was confirmed on pathological analysis of the neck dissection specimen demonstrating multiple lymph node involvement in a majority of patients (Figure 10.14). It is well known that the prognosis of a patient with metastatic squamous carcinoma to regional cervical lymph nodes is dependent on the extent of nodal disease in the neck. Thus, when a significant risk of micrometastasis to regional lymph nodes is present based on the characteristics of the primary tumor, an elective dissection of regional lymph nodes at risk should be considered.

Another prognostic factor that was found to be of significance is lymph node density or nodal ratio, which is the ratio between the number of metastatic lymph nodes and the total number of excised lymph nodes. Several large-volume retrospective studies concluded that, in squamous cell carcinoma of the oral cavity, an increased nodal ratio is a strong predictor of decreased survival (63,64).

SELECTION OF INITIAL TREATMENT

The surgical treatment of regional lymph nodes for carcinoma of the oral cavity is based on the understanding of the anatomy of the regional lymphatics, the patterns of regional lymph node metastasis and the risk of nodal metastasis depending on the characteristics of the primary tumor. When regional metastases are clinically palpable, comprehensive clearance of all regional lymph nodes at risk is mandatory. Classical radical neck dissection has been the gold standard of surgical management of clinically positive metastatic lymph nodes. However, the morbidity of the operation is significant and therefore it is recommended only under select circumstances where vital anatomic structures are grossly involved by nodal disease and preserving them will compromise the oncologic outcome.

On the other hand, when appropriate indications exist, a function-preserving comprehensive neck dissection sparing one or more vital anatomic structures should be considered as long as it does not compromise satisfactory clearance of metastatic disease. Preservation of the spinal accessory nerve alone significantly reduces the morbidity of neck dissection (65–68). Thus, if the spinal accessory nerve is not involved by metastatic cancer, it should be routinely preserved even in patients with clinically palpable metastatic lymph nodes. Such a surgical approach does not adversely impact on local recurrence or long-term survival (9,19,22,69–71). However, comprehensive clearance of all five cervical lymph node levels should be strongly considered when a neck dissection is undertaken for grossly palpable cervical lymph node metastasis. Limited neck dissection for palpable nodal metastasis is considered risky and is not recommended.

When an elective neck dissection is undertaken to excise cervical lymph nodes at risk of harboring micrometastasis (occult metastasis), it is seldom necessary to perform a comprehensive neck dissection to excise all five levels of lymph nodes. As mentioned earlier, the patterns of cervical lymph node metastasis are predictable and sequential, with involvement of the first-echelon lymph nodes initially before dissemination occurs to other lymph node levels. Thus, an elective neck dissection is usually of limited extent, addressing only the lymph node groups at highest risk for a given primary site. Such a limited dissection of lymph nodes is usually considered a "staging procedure." The histological information derived from the study of the excised lymph nodes facilitates selection of adjuvant therapy in patients who are at increased risk of neck failure and spares the need for a morbid operation or adjuvant radiotherapy in others who are at reduced risk. Thus, an elective operation for primary tumors of the oral cavity with an N_0 neck requires dissection of lymph nodes at levels I, II, and III (19,26,41,72–76). If the primary tumor crosses the midline, bilateral clearance of levels I, II, and III should be undertaken.

For primary tumors of the oropharynx, the elective operation in the neck for clearance of occult metastases requires comprehensive excision of lymph nodes at levels 2, 3, and 4. If the primary tumor of the oropharynx crosses the midline, then elective dissection of regional lymph nodes should include removal of lymph nodes at levels II, III, and IV bilaterally.

The role of sentinel lymph node biopsy (SLNB) has been well established in the management of breast cancer and cutaneous malignant melanoma. However, the role of SLNB in head and neck mucosal squamous cell carcinoma is somewhat controversial. Nevertheless, in some head and neck cancer centers, SLNB is advocated for all clinically N_0 oral cancer patients. Recent studies on the subject in the context of elective neck dissections revealed SLNB detection rates above 95% and negative predictive values for negative sentinel nodes of 95%. According to these studies, SLNB has proven its ability to select patients with occult lymphatic disease for elective neck dissection and to spare the costs and morbidity to patients with negative necks. These centers have abandoned routine elective neck dissection and entered in observational trials. These trials so far were able to confirm the high accuracy of the validation trials, with less than 5% of the patients with negative sentinel nodes developing lymph node metastases during observation (77–79). It is imperative, however, to note that SLNB is feasible only in certain sites in the oral cavity, such as the tongue and floor of the mouth. It has been difficult to perform adequate SLNB at other sites and experience for these is limited. Even the floor of the mouth is a somewhat difficult site due to the "shine through" of the injected radionuclide, obscuring adequate assessment of lymph nodes at level 1B.

CLASSIFICATION OF NECK DISSECTIONS

The understanding of the biological progression of metastatic disease from primary sites in the head and neck region to cervical lymph nodes has allowed the development of several modifications of the classical radical neck dissection in order to reduce morbidity and maintain therapeutic efficacy. In order to standardize the terminology of the various types of neck dissections, the following classification scheme is recommended (19,23–25,75,80).

Comprehensive neck dissection

The term "comprehensive neck dissection" is applied to all surgical procedures on the lateral neck that comprehensively remove cervical lymph nodes from level I through to level V. Under this broad category are included the following operative procedures:

1. *Classical radical neck dissection.*
2. *Extended radical neck dissection* (resection of additional regional lymph nodes, more than those included in the classical radical neck dissection, or sacrifice of other structures such as cranial nerves, muscles, skin, etc.).
3. *Modified radical neck dissection type I (MRND-I).* This procedure selectively preserves the spinal accessory nerve.
4. *Modified radical neck dissection type II (MRND-II).* This procedure preserves the spinal accessory nerve and the sternocleidomastoid muscle, but sacrifices the internal jugular vein.
5. *Modified radical neck dissection type III (MRND-III).* This procedure requires preservation of the spinal accessory nerve, internal jugular vein and sternocleidomastoid muscle.

Selective neck dissection

These operations selectively remove lymph node groups at designated levels only and do not comprehensively dissect all five levels of lymph nodes. Selective neck dissections are usually employed as staging procedures for the clinically negative neck where the lymph nodes are at risk of harboring micrometastasis. These operations include:

1. *Supraomohyoid neck dissection (SOHND).* This procedure encompasses dissection of lymph nodes at levels I, II, and III and is recommended as an elective procedure for primary tumors of the oral cavity.
2. *Jugular node dissection.* This procedure encompasses dissection of lymph nodes at levels II, III, and IV.
3. *Anterior triangle neck dissection.* This procedure encompasses lymph nodes removed in supraomohyoid and jugular neck dissections (levels I, II, III, and IV).
4. *Central compartment neck dissection.* This procedure encompasses clearance of lymph nodes in the central compartment of the neck adjacent to the thyroid gland and in the tracheo-esophageal groove (level VI). This operation is recommended for cancers of the thyroid gland and larynx or hypopharynx.
5. *Posterolateral neck dissection.* This operation encompasses lymph nodes in the occipital triangle, posterior triangle of the neck (level V) and the deep jugular chain of lymph nodes at levels II, III, and IV. This operation is recommended for cutaneous melanomas and squamous carcinomas of the posterior scalp.

PREOPERATIVE PREPARATION

No specific preoperative preparation is required for patients undergoing neck dissection other than planning of the incisions for neck dissection, particularly if the primary tumor is to be resected simultaneously. In addition to this, planning of the neck dissection incisions must take into consideration any reconstructive effort required to repair the surgical defect created following excision of the primary tumor. The most commonly employed incisions for various types of neck dissections for oral and oropharyngeal cancers are shown in Figure 10.15. Nearly all neck dissections can be performed through a single transverse incision in a natural skin crease. The transverse incision used for SOHND (Figure 10.15a) can be extended anteriorly and posteriorly to perform a comprehensive neck dissection, such as modified neck dissection type I or classical radical neck dissection. A vertical incision in the neck for neck dissection should be avoided to minimize esthetic disfigurement.

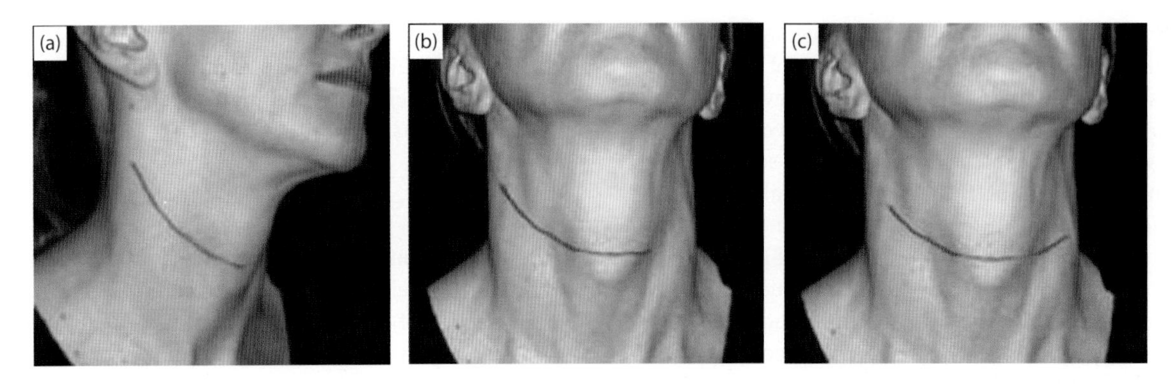

Figure 10.15 Incisions for neck dissections: **(a)** supraomohyoid; **(b)** jugular (pharynx); and **(c)** jugular bilateral.

OPERATIVE TECHNIQUES

Supraomohyoid neck dissection

This operation may be performed in conjunction with excision of the primary tumor from the oral cavity, either in continuity where the primary tumor and lymph nodes at levels I, II, and III are removed in a monobloc fashion or as a discontinuous procedure where the primary tumor in the oral cavity may be excised through a peroral approach and the SOHND is performed through a separate transverse incision in the upper part of the neck (Figure 10.16). The incision is placed in an upper neck skin crease extending from the mastoid process toward the hyoid bone up to the midline. If the primary tumor is to be resected perorally, this incision should be satisfactory. On the other hand, if the primary tumor is not accessible through the open mouth or if the primary tumor of the oral cavity is to be excised en bloc with the contents of the supraomohyoid triangle of the neck, then a lower cheek flap approach will be required. The skin incision therefore is extended cephalad in the midline to divide the lower lip.

The skin incision is outlined in Figure 10.17, with an alternate extension in the midline shown by the dotted line. The patient's neck is extended and rotated to the opposite side to put the skin at the site of surgery under tension.

The skin incision is deepened through the platysma throughout its length (Figure 10.18). Since the incision is quite low in the neck, the use of electrocautery to divide the platysma has no risk of injury to the mandibular branch of the facial nerve. However, in the posterior aspect of the skin incision, attention should be paid to avoid injury to the greater auricular nerve, which can be safely preserved. Similarly, the external jugular vein should be carefully preserved if a microvascular free flap is to be used for reconstructive surgery since it is an excellent recipient vein.

The upper skin flap is elevated first; it remains close to the platysma and the marginal branch of the facial nerve is carefully identified. Posteriorly, the greater auricular nerve and the external jugular vein overlying the sternomastoid muscle come into view as elevation of the flap continues. They should be carefully identified and preserved (Figure 10.19). The nerve is demonstrated here with a hook.

Attention is now focused on careful identification, dissection and preservation of the mandibular branch of the facial nerve, which directly overlies the submandibular salivary gland (Figure 10.20). This dissection should be performed sharply, either by scalpel or scissors, since use of electrocautery in the vicinity of the mandibular branch can produce temporary paralysis of this nerve. In identifying and preserving the mandibular branch of the nerve, it may become necessary to sacrifice the cervical branch of the facial nerve. Once the nerve is identified and dissected along

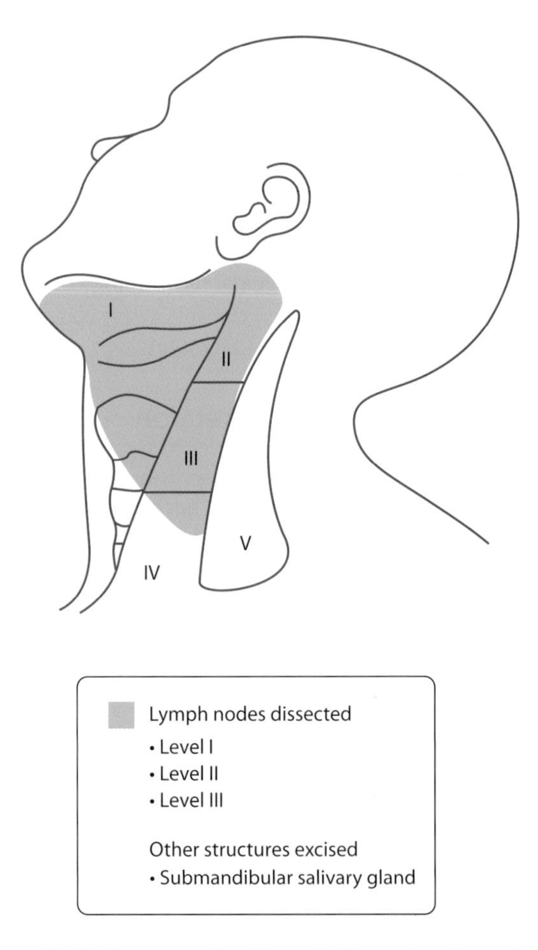

Figure 10.16 Supraomohyoid neck dissection. Lymph nodes dissected: levels I, II, and III. Other structures excised: submandibular salivary gland.

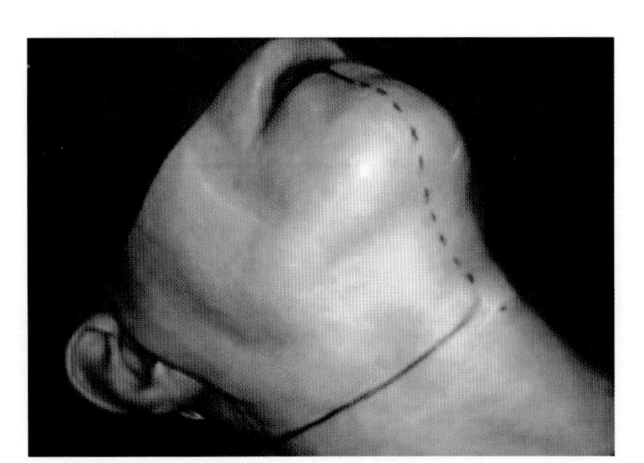

Figure 10.17 Skin incision outlined. Alternate extension for a lower cheek flap is shown with a dotted line.

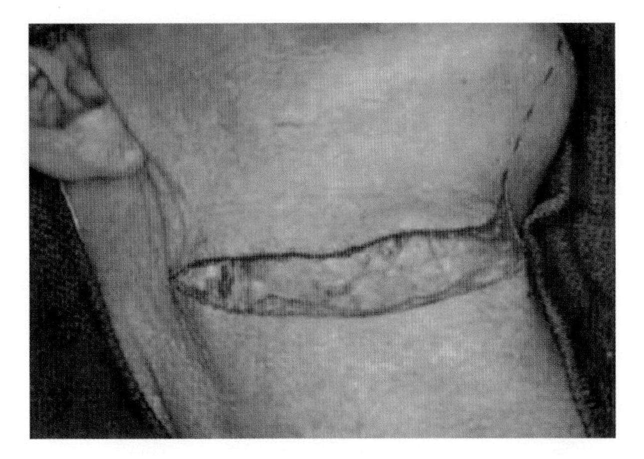

Figure 10.18 Skin incision deepened through platysma.

its course, it is retracted cephalad, along with the upper skin flap, by shifting the nerve with the flap and placing a suture between soft tissues caudad to the nerve and those of the upper cheek flap cephalad to the nerve to form an envelope to protect the nerve. Alternatively, one may elect to identify

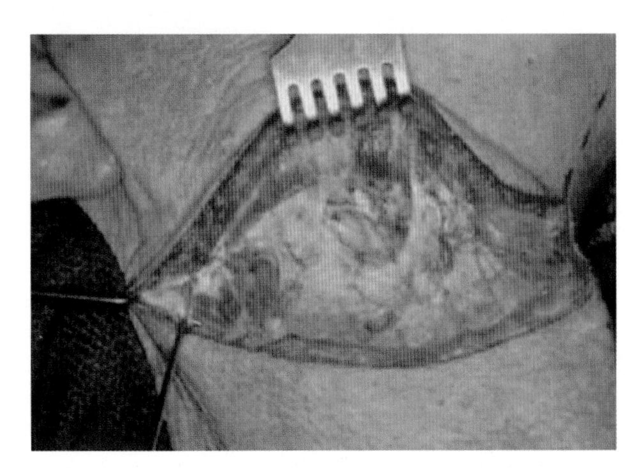

Figure 10.19 Care should be exercised to preserve the greater auricular nerve during elevation of the upper flap.

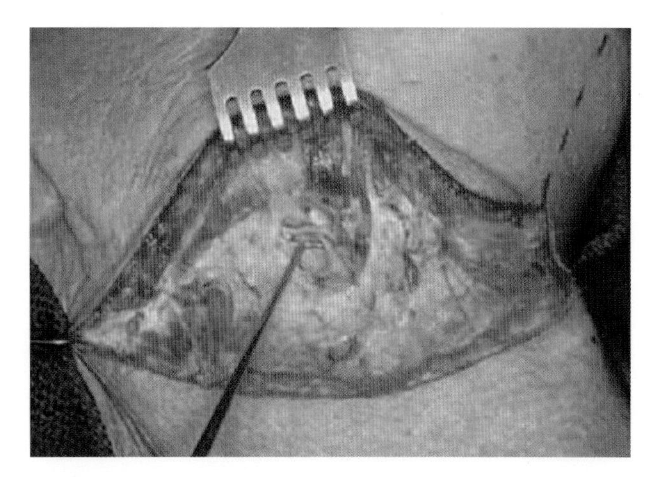

Figure 10.20 The marginal branch of the facial nerve crossing the facial artery and overlying the submandibular salivary gland is preserved.

the posterior facial vein first, as shown in Figure 10.21. The vein is divided and its stump is suture-ligated at its upper end, with the platysma on the upper skin flap carefully preserving the marginal branch of the facial nerve between the stump of the vein and the platysma muscle. Dissection now proceeds along the lower border of the body of the mandible. The fascial attachments between the sternomastoid muscle and the angle of the mandible are divided. Mobilization of soft tissues along the lower border of the body of the mandible exposes the prevascular facial lymph nodes (Figure 10.22). These are meticulously dissected and maintained in continuity with the rest of the specimen. The facial artery and its accompanying veins adjacent to these nodes are divided between clamps and ligated. Dissection now continues anteriorly along the lower border of the body of the mandible up to the attachment of the anterior belly of the digastric muscle. Soft tissues between the mandible and anterior belly of the digastric are separated. At this point, brisk hemorrhage is likely to be encountered from several vessels that provide blood supply to the anterior belly of the

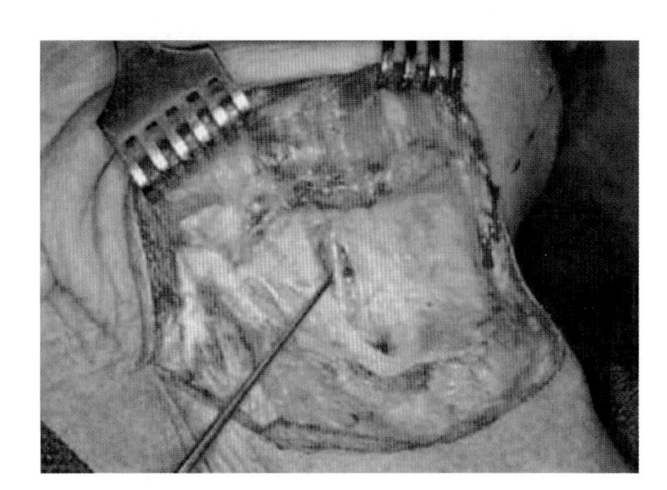

Figure 10.21 Posterior facial vein shown here is divided.

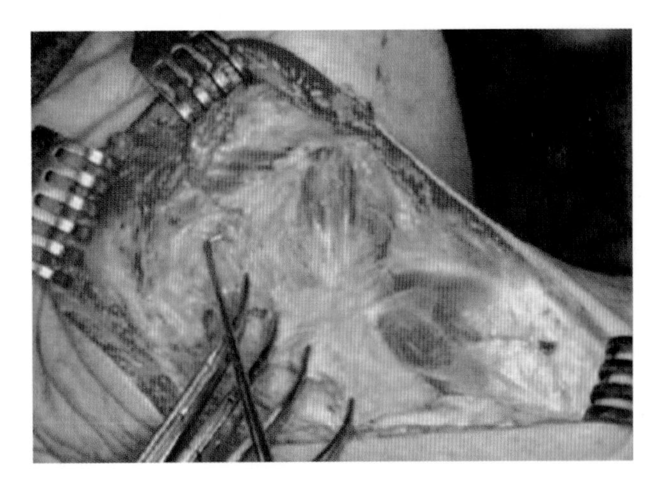

Figure 10.22 The prevascular facial group of lymph nodes adjacent to the body of the mandible are dissected en bloc.

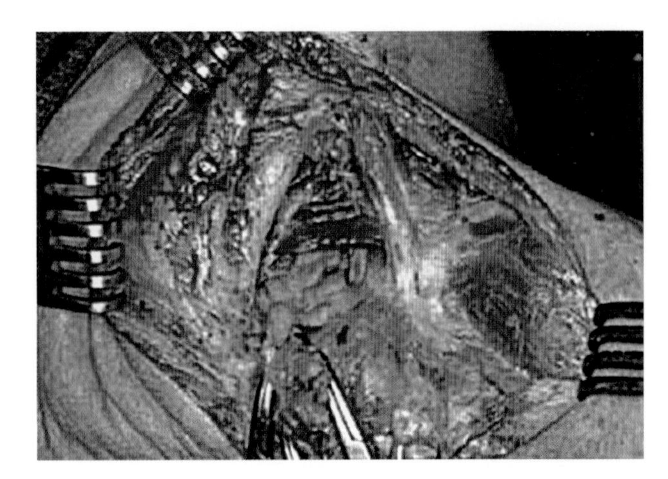

Figure 10.24 The anterior belly of the digastric muscle and mylohyoid muscle are exposed.

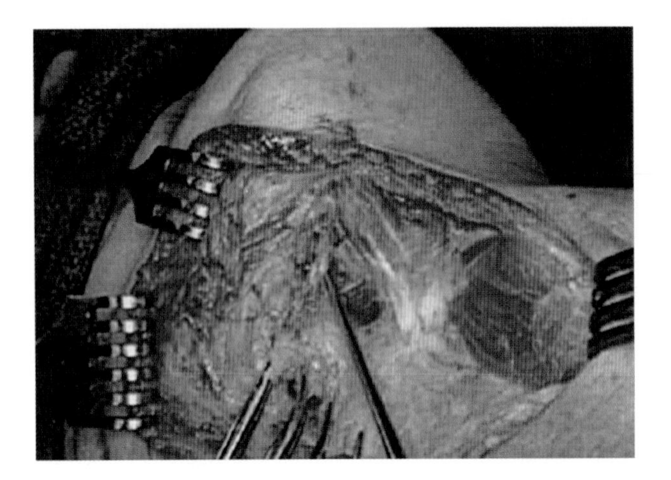

Figure 10.23 The blood vessels to the mylohyoid muscle are divided and ligated.

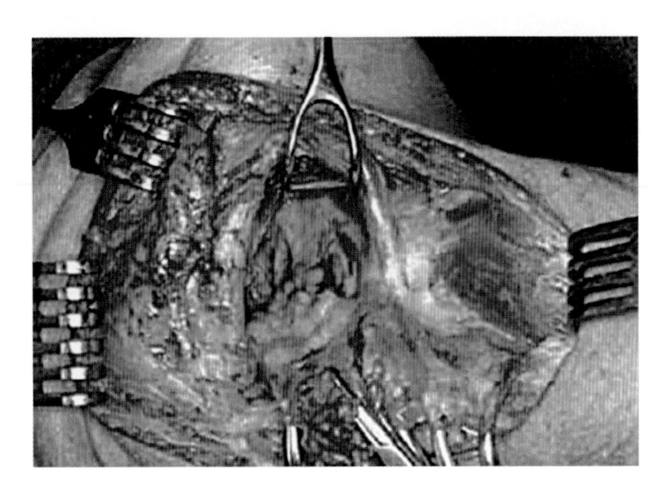

Figure 10.25 The lateral edge of the mylohyoid muscle is retracted medially to expose Wharton's duct.

digastric muscle and the mylohyoid muscle. The nerve and vessels to the mylohyoid muscle, however, enter parallel to each other in a fascial envelope that is identified, clamped, divided and ligated (Figure 10.23). Once all the nerve filaments and vessels along the free border of the mylohyoid muscle are divided, the muscle will come into full view.

Gentle traction on the submandibular salivary gland with several hemostats allows mobilization and delivery of the submandibular gland from its bed (Figure 10.24). A loop retractor is now placed along the lateral border of the mylohyoid muscle, which is retracted medially toward the chin of the patient (Figure 10.25). This exposes the undersurface of the floor of the mouth and brings into view the secretomotor fibers to the submandibular salivary gland as they come off the lingual nerve, as well as Wharton's duct with accessory salivary tissue along the duct. At this juncture, alternate blunt and sharp dissection is necessary to clearly identify Wharton's duct and the lingual and hypoglossal nerves in the floor of the mouth as they enter the tongue.

Both the lingual and the hypoglossal nerves are shown in Figure 10.26, with Wharton's duct in the middle showing small amounts of salivary gland tissues along its length. Once the lingual nerve is clearly identified, the secretomotor fibers to the submandibular gland are divided. The latter are shown in Figure 10.27 as they come off the lingual nerve. There is usually a small blood vessel accompanying this nerve so it is divided between clamps and ligated. Similarly, Wharton's duct is divided between clamps and its distal stump is ligated. The entire submandibular gland is now retracted posteroinferiorly and loose areolar tissue between the salivary gland and the digastric muscle is divided. As one approaches the posterior belly of the digastric muscle, the proximal part of the facial artery as it enters the submandibular salivary gland is exposed (Figure 10.28). It is divided between clamps and ligated. The entire contents of the submandibular triangle are now dissected off and retracted inferiorly.

Attention is now focused on the region of the tail of the parotid gland and the anterior border of the upper part of

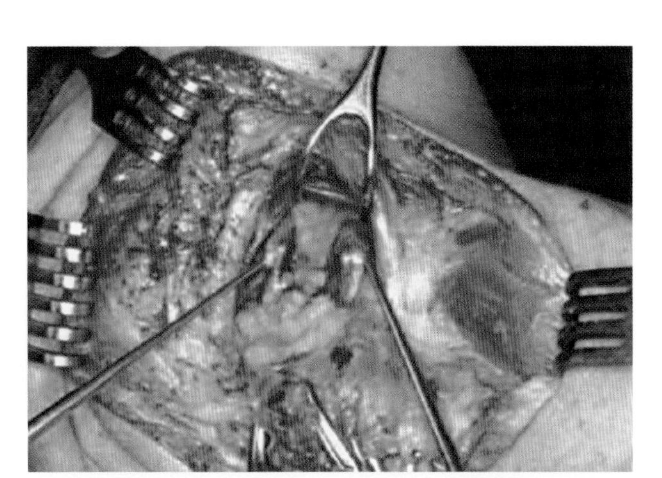

Figure 10.26 The lingual and hypoglossal nerves are identified and protected.

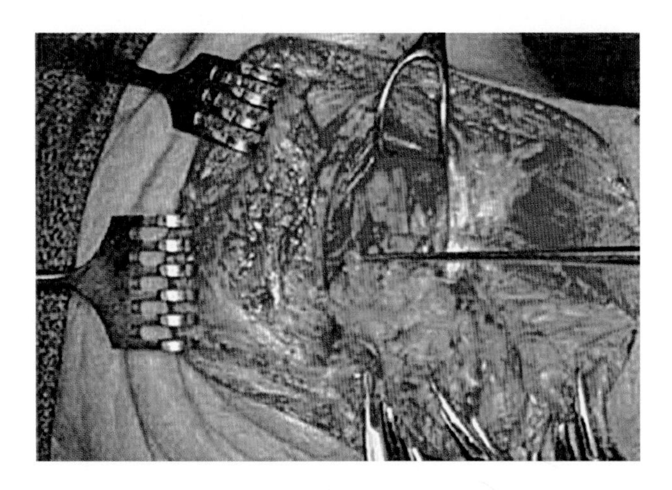

Figure 10.27 The secretomotor fibers to the submandibular salivary gland are divided.

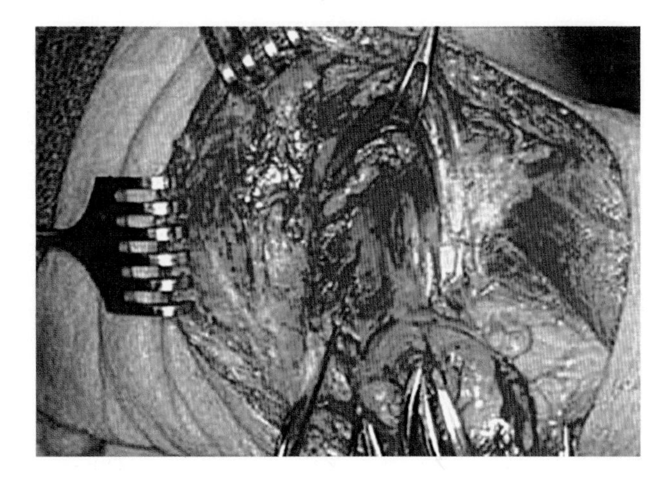

Figure 10.28 The facial artery entering the submandibular salivary gland at its posteroinferior edge is divided and ligated.

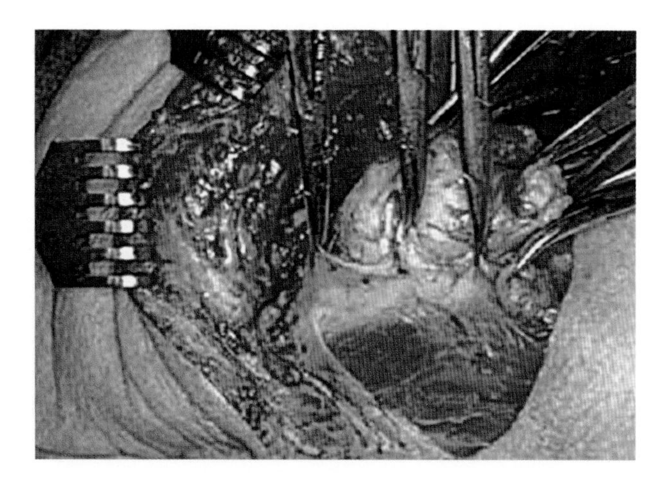

Figure 10.29 The fascia on the anterior border of the sternocleidomastoid muscle is dissected and retracted medially.

the sternomastoid muscle. The fascia along the anterior border of the sternomastoid muscle is grasped with several hemostats and retracted medially to provide traction along its anterior border (Figure 10.29). Electrocautery is used to clear the fascial attachments from the anterior border of the sternomastoid muscle. Several tiny vessels entering the upper part of the sternomastoid muscle (branches from the occipital and superior thyroid arteries) are divided by electrocautery. Further medial retraction of the specimen exposes the carotid sheath, as shown in Figure 10.30. The latter is incised and dissection now proceeds cephalad toward the base of the skull.

A hemostat is used to separate the fascia of the carotid sheath, which is divided and retracted medially (Figure 10.31). This dissection continues cephalad up to the posterior belly of the digastric muscle, which is retracted cephalad to expose the upper end of the jugular vein entering the jugular foramen. Several pharyngeal veins as well

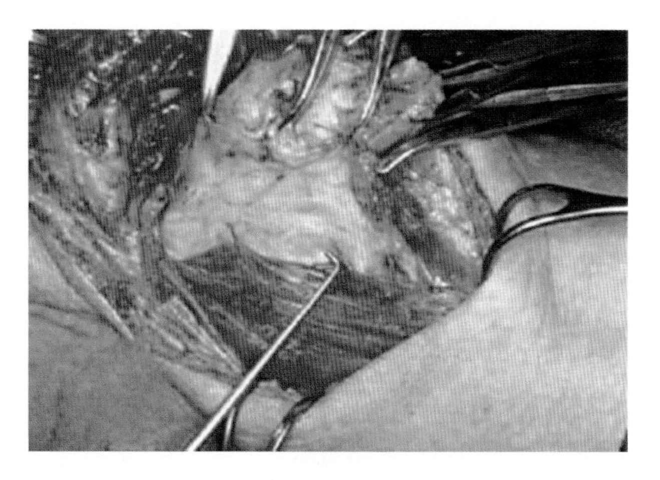

Figure 10.30 Further medial retraction of the fascia provides exposure of the carotid sheath.

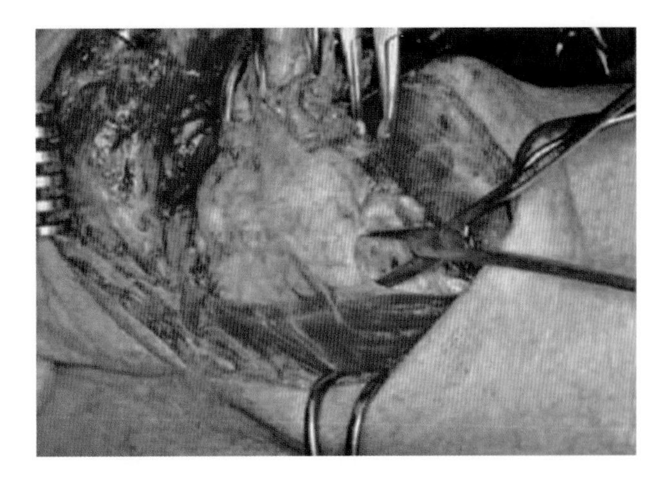

Figure 10.31 The carotid sheath is opened to facilitate its dissection.

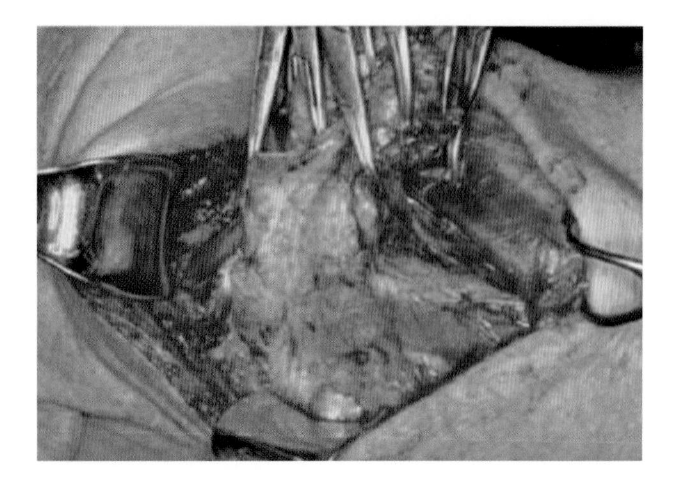

Figure 10.33 Lateral retraction of the sternocleidomastoid muscle exposes the jugulodigastric lymph nodes.

as branches of the superior thyroid vein may have to be divided in order to mobilize the specimen.

One of the pharyngeal veins shown in Figure 10.32 will be divided to facilitate mobilization of the specimen. The sternomastoid muscle is now retracted further posteriorly, exposing the jugular vein in its entirety. The latter is still covered by a fascial envelope containing upper deep jugular and jugulodigastric lymph nodes (Figure 10.33). The sternomastoid muscle is retracted posteriorly to expose lymph nodes in the accessory chain at the apex of the posterior triangle; these are meticulously dissected out and retracted anteriorly with the rest of the surgical specimen.

While the lymph nodes at the apex of the posterior triangle of the neck are dissected, extreme care should be exercised to identify and carefully preserve the accessory nerve as well as the cutaneous and muscular branches of the cervical plexus (Figure 10.34). Once the accessory nerve is identified, the lymph nodes posterolateral to it are dissected and passed beneath the nerve anteriorly to remain in continuity with the rest of the specimen. The upper end of the jugular vein is now nearly fully cleared of deep jugular, jugulodigastric and upper accessory chain lymph nodes.

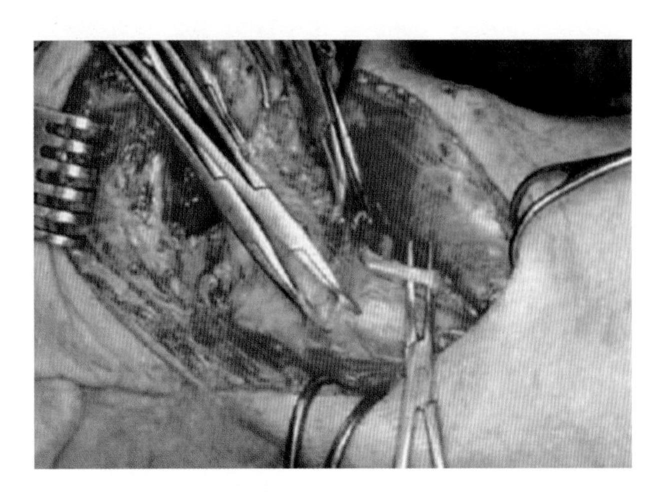

Figure 10.32 The pharyngeal veins are divided and ligated.

Dissection of the apex of the posterior triangle clearly shows the upper end of the internal jugular vein and the occipital artery.

The highest root of the cervical plexus is exposed with further dissection of the 11th nerve and removal of lymph nodes in the jugulodigastric region. The posterior boundary of the SOHND in this area is rather arbitrary, since no specific anatomical landmarks exist to define the extent of posterior triangle lymph node dissection, so clinical judgment must be exercised to decide on the extent of their removal.

Dissection of the accessory chain lymph nodes posterior to the internal jugular vein at the apex of the posterior triangle is now complete (Figure 10.35). The entire jugular vein is exposed with the posterior belly of the digastric muscle retracted cephalad. The common facial vein is now divided as it enters the internal jugular vein and is ligated (Figure 10.36). Dissection continues anteriorly, carefully identifying and preserving the hypoglossal nerve as well as the descendens hypoglossi, the nerve supply to the strap muscles.

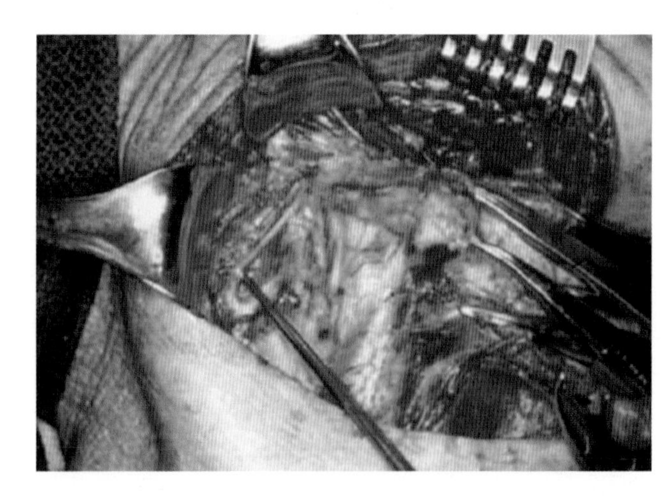

Figure 10.34 The lymph nodes at the apex of the posterior triangle are dissected out, carefully preserving the spinal accessory nerve.

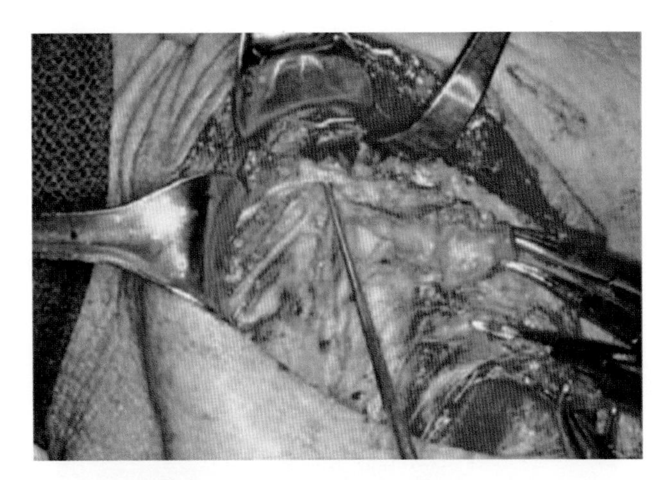

Figure 10.35 The occipital artery is seen crossing the internal jugular vein near its upper end.

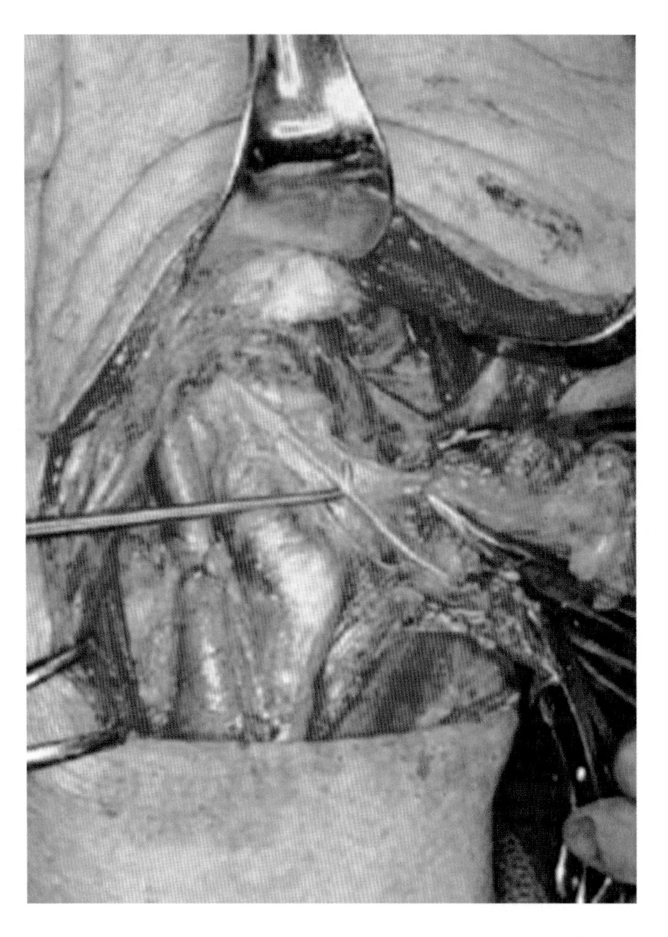

Figure 10.37 The descendens hypoglossi coming off the hypoglossal nerve is preserved.

The descendens hypoglossi is shown in Figure 10.37 as it comes off the hypoglossal nerve and runs anteroinferiorly. Dissection also continues along the medial aspect of the carotid sheath, exposing the carotid bulb. The surgical specimen mobilized so far consists of the contents of the submandibular triangle, lymph nodes from the jugulodigastric region and the apex of the posterior triangle of the neck, as well as the upper deep jugular lymph nodes. The specimen is reflected anteriorly.

Dissection is now continued caudad toward the apex of the supraomohyoid triangle, at the junction where the superior belly of the omohyoid muscle meets the sternomastoid muscle (Figure 10.38). A loop retractor is placed to expose the lower part of the carotid sheath from where midjugular lymph nodes are dissected out and reflected cephalad. Dissection continues further medially, exposing the origin of the superior thyroid artery, which is preserved, but the superior thyroid vein will have to be sacrificed since this was previously divided from the internal jugular vein. The final attachments of the specimen in the region of the thyrohyoid membrane and the insertion of the strap muscles over the hyoid bone are divided by electrocautery.

The surgical field following removal of the specimen shows complete clearance of the supraomohyoid triangle (Figure 10.39). The anatomical structures demonstrated here are the anterior and posterior bellies of the digastric and mylohyoid muscles. The lingual and hypoglossal nerves as well as the marginal branch of the facial nerve

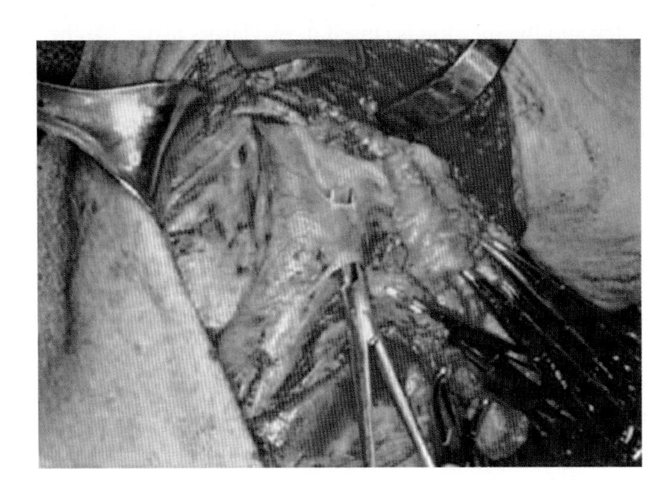

Figure 10.36 The common facial vein is divided and ligated.

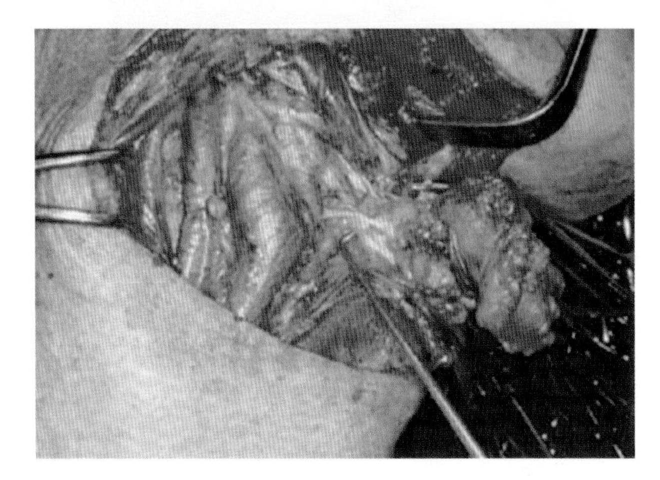

Figure 10.38 The specimen is reflected anteriorly, showing the carotid bifurcation

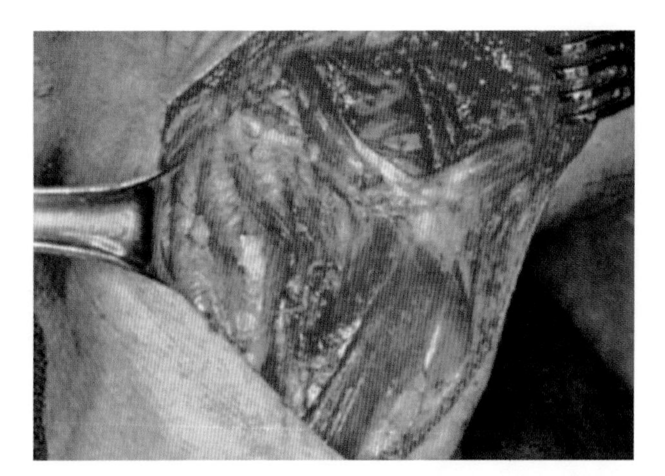

Figure 10.39 The surgical field following removal of the specimen.

are also seen in the submandibular triangle. The superior belly of the omohyoid, sternohyoid and the stylohyoid muscles, as well as the bifurcation of the carotid artery, are also in clear view. Note that the lymph nodes from levels II and III along the internal jugular vein are all dissected off with the specimen. The posterior and inferior views of the surgical field demonstrate the accessory nerve as well as branches of the cervical plexus and the lower end of the supraomohyoid triangle where the sternomastoid and the omohyoid muscles cross each other (Figure 10.40).

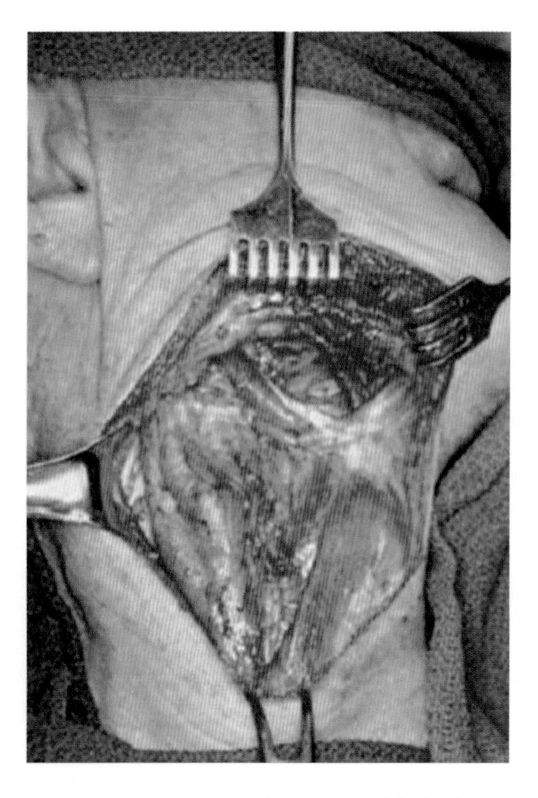

Figure 10.40 Posterior part of the surgical field showing the spinal accessory nerve and the roots of the cervical plexus.

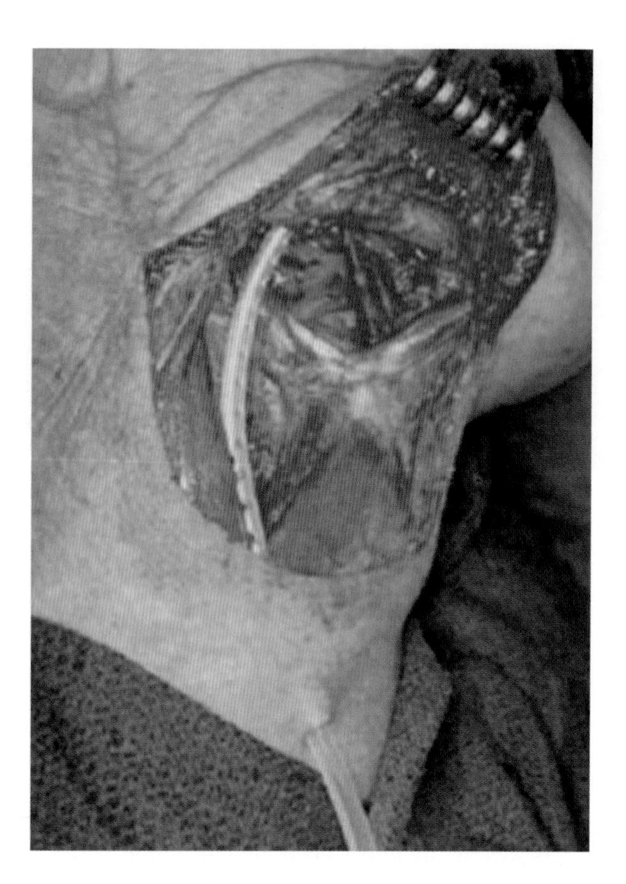

Figure 10.41 A single suction drain is placed parallel to the anterior border of the sternocleidomastoid muscle.

The wound is now irrigated with bacitracin solution. A single suction drain is inserted through a separate stab incision and is placed parallel to the anterior border of the sternomastoid muscle up to the submandibular triangle (Figure 10.41). Occasionally, a hypertrophic scar develops at the site of drain insertion, leading to unsightly esthetic deformity. To avoid this, it is desirable to insert the drain through a stab incision in the post-auricular region overlying the mastoid process with the drain placed anterior to the sternomastoid muscle up to the lower part of the surgical field. The drain is secured in place with a silk suture to the skin at the site of entry and the incision is closed in two layers using 3/0 chromic catgut interrupted sutures for platysma and 5/0 nylon interrupted sutures for skin (Figure 10.42). Blood loss during this operative procedure should be minimal. The postoperative appearance of the patient demonstrates that there is essentially no esthetic or functional deformity following this operation (Figure 10.43).

Jugular node dissection

This operation is usually performed in conjunction with resection of the primary tumor of the oropharynx, larynx or hypopharynx (16,22,38,73). Jugular node dissection may be performed on the ipsilateral side for lesions that are unilateral in their mucosal extent or it may be performed bilaterally for those lesions that cross the midline to involve both sides of the laryngopharyngeal mucosa.

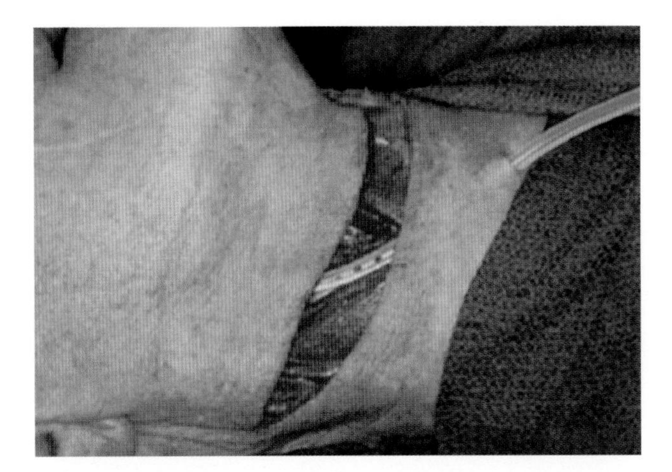

Figure 10.42 The skin incision is closed in two layers.

The operative procedure is usually performed through the same incision employed for resection of the primary tumor, which is usually a transverse incision along an upper neck skin crease in the region of the thyrohyoid membrane, extending from the posterior border of the sternocleidomastoid muscle on one side of the neck to that on the other side of the neck.

Following skin incision, the platysma is divided throughout the entire length of the incision and the upper and lower skin flaps are elevated in the usual fashion, exposing the anterior border of the sternocleidomastoid muscle in its entirety from the region of the posterior belly of the digastric muscle cephalad to the insertion of the sternal head caudad. There is no particular virtue in performing jugular node dissection in continuity with resection of the primary tumor, since technically it may be somewhat awkward to perform. In as much as all internal jugular chains of lymph nodes at levels II, III, and IV are excised in a monobloc fashion, the oncologic purpose of this operation is served. The extent of the nodal tissue to be cleared is shown in Figure 10.44. The internal jugular group of lymph nodes that lie anteriorly, laterally and posteriorly to the internal jugular vein are excised in a monobloc fashion. This, by necessity,

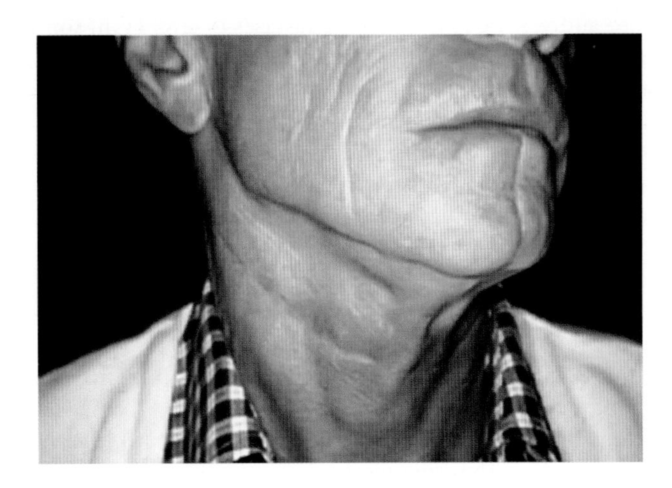

Figure 10.43 Postoperative appearance of the patient after supraomohyoid neck dissection.

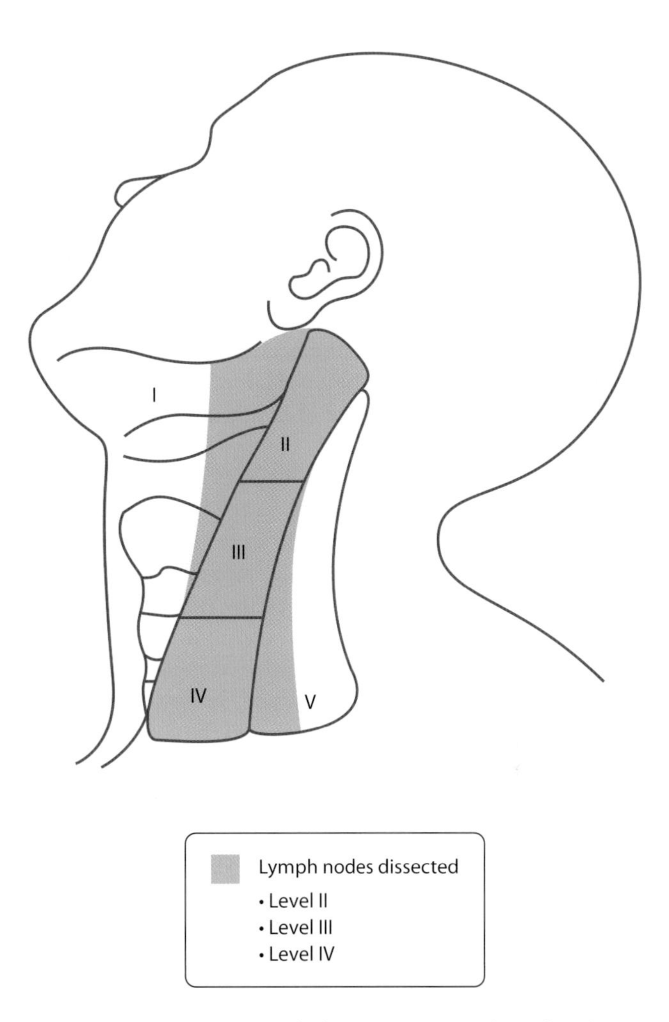

Figure 10.44 Jugular neck dissection. Lymph nodes dissected: levels II, III, and IV.

will require clearance of lymph nodes at least up to the posterior border of the sternocleidomastoid muscle from the internal jugular chain.

The operative procedure begins with incision of the fascia along the anterior border of the sternocleidomastoid muscle, which is grasped with hemostats to permit retraction of the sternomastoid muscle posteriorly. This dissection continues on the undersurface of the sternocleidomastoid muscle all the way up to its posterior border. During the course of this part of the operation, the blood supply to the sternocleidomastoid muscle from branches of the occipital artery and superior thyroid artery will be encountered. These vessels are carefully divided and ligated. Once this is accomplished, the entire sternocleidomastoid muscle can be retracted with Richardson retractors posteriorly, totally exposing the internal jugular lymph nodes from the jugulodigastric region cephalad to the supraclavicular region caudad.

Dissection begins at the upper end, clearing the lymph nodes that are posterior to the accessory nerve as it exits from the jugular foramen. These lymph nodes are covered by the upper end of the sternocleidomastoid muscle and lie over the splenius capitus and levator scapulae muscles in the floor of the posterior triangle of the neck. Meticulous dissection of these lymph nodes allows delivery from beneath the accessory nerve anteriorly to remain in continuity with the jugulodigastric group of lymph nodes. Similarly, dissection of lymph nodes overlying the sensory roots of the cervical plexus is undertaken, exposing the sensory roots, and the dissection is carefully continued up to the lateral border of the internal jugular vein to keep these lymph nodes in continuity with the deep jugular lymph nodes. Clearance of the accessory chain of lymph nodes and exposure of all the cervical roots are essential to provide satisfactory clearance of contiguous lymph nodes in the posterior triangle.

At this juncture, dissection continues anterolaterally to the internal jugular vein, clearing all the lymph nodes and freeing up the internal jugular vein in its entirety from the jugular foramen cephalad and to the supraclavicular region caudad. In so doing, the tendon of the omohyoid muscle is divided. No attempt is made to continue the dissection of lymph nodes in the submandibular triangle, leaving the submandibular salivary gland intact. Several pharyngeal branches of the internal jugular vein and the common facial vein, however, will have to be divided and ligated to facilitate dissection of the upper jugular lymph nodes. By meticulous alternate blunt and sharp dissection, the hypoglossal nerve, the desendens hypoglossi and the branches of the superior thyroid artery are identified and carefully preserved, delivering the specimen.

The specimen shown in Figure 10.45 demonstrates monobloc excision of the bilateral internal jugular group of lymph nodes from levels II, III, and IV. To facilitate accurate description of the excised lymph nodes, it is important to apply numerical tags to the lymph nodes depicting levels II, III, and IV. This would facilitate proper analysis of the surgical specimen to render an accurate histopathologic report. If bilateral jugular node dissection is undertaken, then the surgical specimen should also indicate whether it is from the left- or the right-hand side.

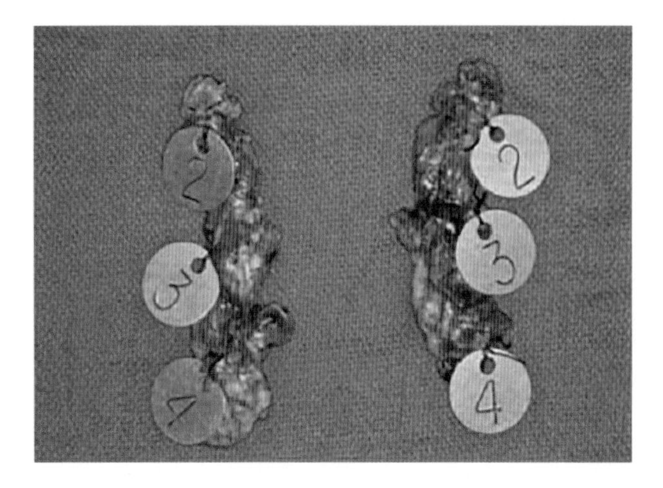

Figure 10.45 Specimen of bilateral jugular lymph node dissections, clearing levels II, III, and IV.

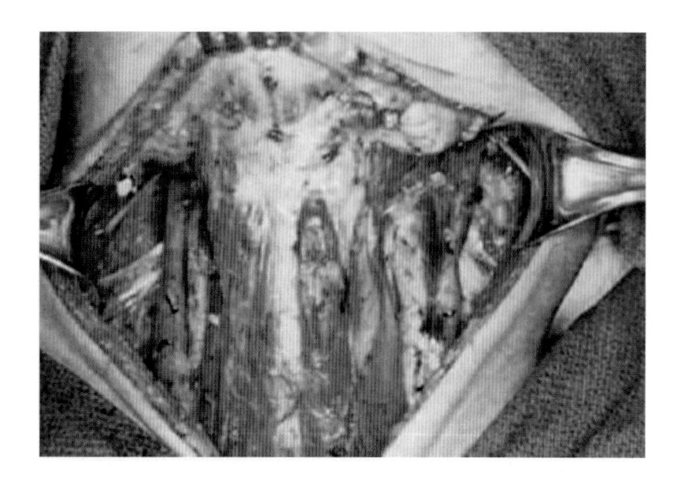

Figure 10.46 Surgical field following bilateral jugular neck dissections.

The surgical field following bilateral jugular neck dissections performed in this patient with carcinoma of the posterior pharyngeal wall is shown in Figure 10.46. Note the complete clearance of internal jugular lymph nodes, exposing the internal jugular vein in its entirety. Roots of the cervical plexus in the posterior triangle are exposed. Submandibular salivary glands are seen cephalad. Suction drains are placed appropriately and the incision is closed in layers in the usual manner. The functional and esthetic impacts of this surgical procedure are essentially nil. However, the histologic information derived from analysis of the surgical specimen allows accurate pathologic staging of the primary tumor to select patients who would require adjuvant postoperative radiation therapy.

Anterior triangle neck dissection (levels I–IV)

This extended selective neck dissection may ultimately prove to be the ideal elective operation for patients at risk of nodal metastases from primary cancers of the oral cavity and oropharynx (Figure 10.47). This operation would also address the risk of skip metastases to level IV in some patients with primary tumors of the oral tongue (41). In fact, this operation may even prove to be equally satisfactory as a therapeutic neck dissection in patients with limited neck disease (N_1). Clearly, the role of anterior triangle neck dissection as a therapeutic procedure for patients with N_1 disease needs to be studied by a prospective randomized trial, comparing it with MRND-I. On observational statistical grounds, it should prove to be satisfactory since the incidence of posterior triangle lymph node metastasis from primary tumors of the oral cavity is exceedingly low (42).

The incision for this operation is usually transverse along a midcervical skin crease. This incision is somewhat lower than that for SOHND to provide access to level IV lymph nodes. The remaining steps of the operation are well described above under supraomohyoid and jugular neck dissections. If the operation is performed in a therapeutic

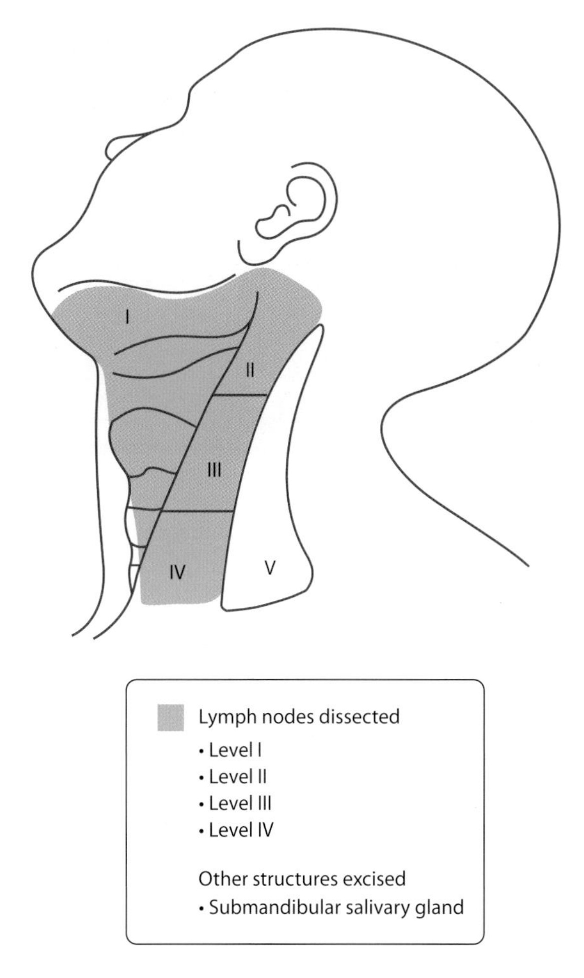

Figure 10.47 Selective anterior triangle neck dissection. Lymph nodes dissected: levels I, II, III, and IV. Other structures excised: submandibular salivary gland.

setting for oral primaries or in an elective setting for laryngopharyngeal primaries, then particular attention should be paid to adequate clearance of jugular lymph nodes lateral to the internal jugular vein, overlying the roots of the cervical plexus (70).

Modified radical neck dissection type I

This operative procedure comprehensively clears cervical lymph nodes at all five levels in the neck, but selectively preserves only one anatomic structure, which is the spinal accessory nerve (Figure 10.48). The patient shown here had a primary carcinoma of the tongue treated previously and he now presents with a clinically apparent metastatic lymph node at level II. The location of the lymph node is shown in relation to the outline of the lower border of the mandible (Figure 10.49). In patients with such a limited extent of metastatic disease or in others with palpable metastatic nodes located in the anterior triangle of the neck, sparing the spinal accessory nerve is considered feasible as long as gross metastatic disease does not involve the accessory nerve. The procedure can be performed through a single transverse incision in a midcervical skin crease or a single trifurcate

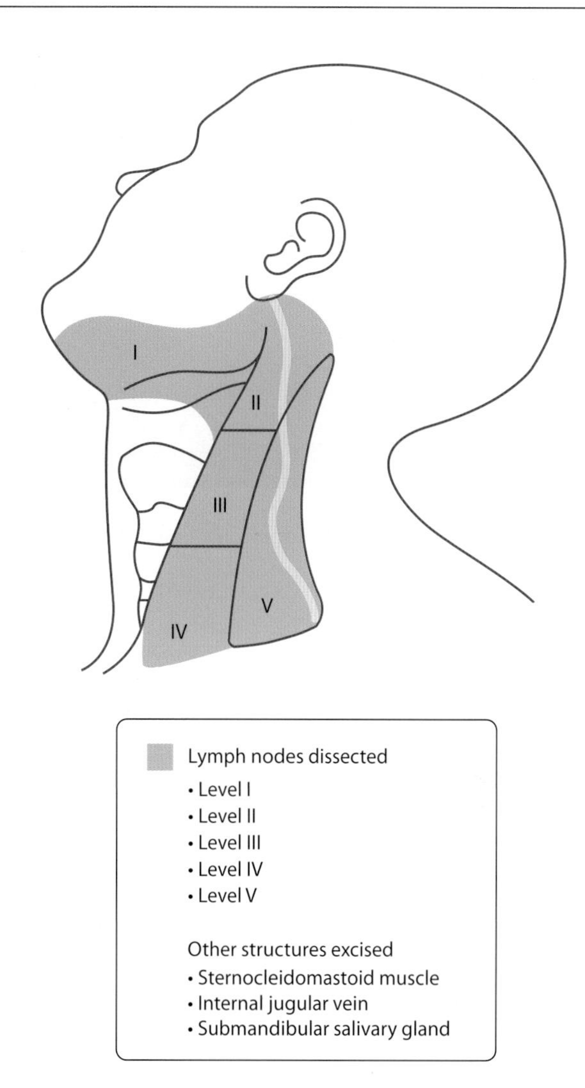

Figure 10.48 Modified radical neck dissection type I. Lymph nodes dissected: levels I, II, III, IV, and V. Other structures excised: sternocleidomastoid muscle, internal jugular vein, and submandibular salivary gland. Preserved: spinal accessory nerve.

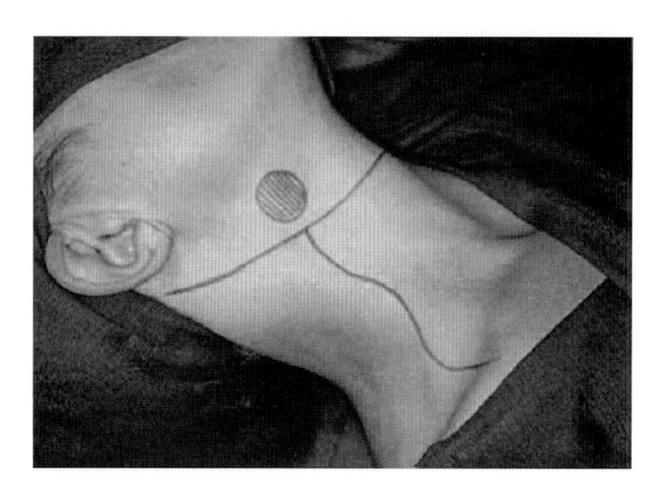

Figure 10.49 Skin incision for modified radical neck dissection type I in a patient with cancer of the tongue

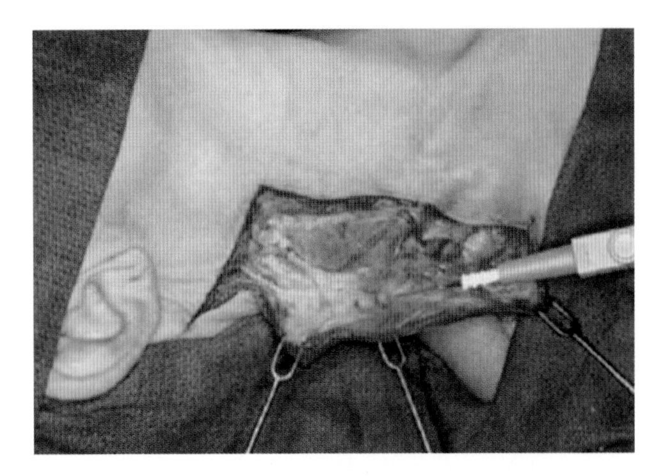

Figure 10.50 The operation begins with elevation of the posterior skin flap.

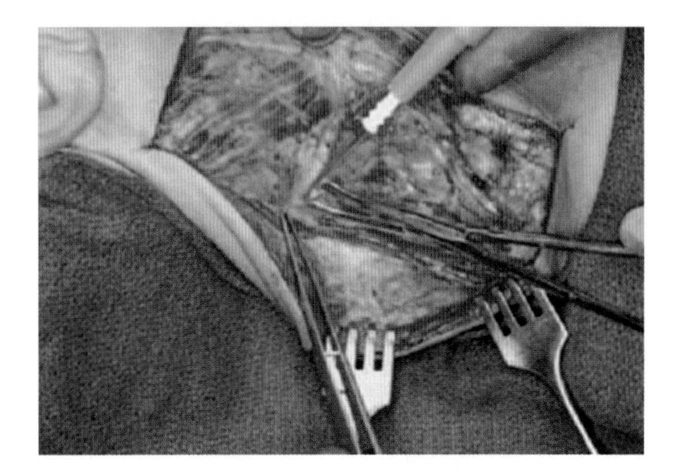

Figure 10.52 The spinal accessory nerve is meticulously dissected through the soft tissues of the posterior triangle.

incision. For a trifurcate incision, the horizontal part of the skin incision is at least two fingerbreadths below the angle of the mandible, with a curvaceous, vertical limb posterior to the carotid artery.

The posterior skin flap is elevated first, keeping it just on the undersurface of the platysma (Figure 10.50). Meticulous attention should be paid as elevation of the lateral aspect of the skin flap approaches the anterior border of the trapezius muscle in the lower part of the neck, since the accessory nerve enters the muscle in this region. The flap is elevated well over the anterior border of the trapezius muscle to expose at least 1 cm of its anterolateral surface. On occasion, elevation of the superior part of the skin flap may have to be withheld if the accessory nerve is found to enter the trapezius muscle high in the neck rather than in its usual lower location. At this point, the accessory nerve is identified as it enters the trapezius muscle, using a hemostat and spreading technique to prevent injury to the nerve (Figure 10.51).

Once identified, the nerve is traced cephalad by careful and meticulous sharp dissection. It becomes necessary to split the contents of the posterior triangle of the neck to dissect the nerve out of the posterior triangle (Figure 10.52). Dissection of the accessory nerve through the posterior triangle continues until the nerve emerges from the posterior border of the sternomastoid muscle (Figure 10.53). At this point, the muscle is divided in order to trace the nerve further cephalad. The posterior half of the upper part of the sternomastoid muscle is divided, with care taken to keep the nerve in view at all times during its division.

The anterior portion of the divided sternomastoid muscle is retracted anteriorly, while the posterior part is retracted posteriorly (Figure 10.54). As dissection of the accessory nerve through the sternomastoid muscle and deep to it proceeds cephalad, the sternomastoid branch of the accessory nerve comes into view. This branch is sacrificed, which facilitates further dissection of the nerve up to the jugular foramen.

Dissection of the nerve continues further cephalad near the upper end of the jugular vein in a plane deep to the posterior

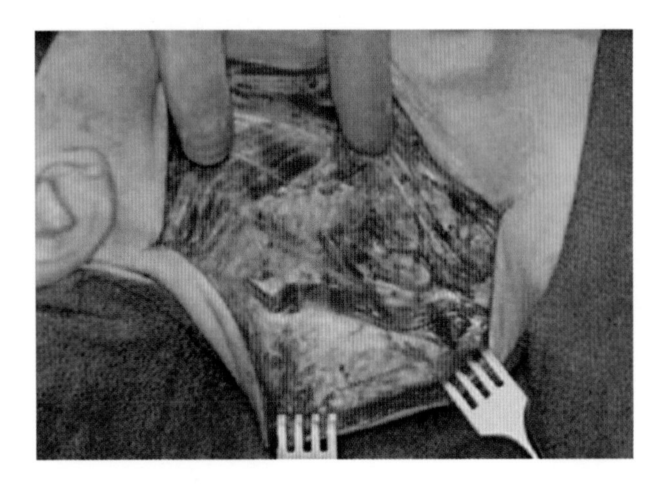

Figure 10.51 The posterior skin flap is elevated until the anterior border of the trapezius muscle.

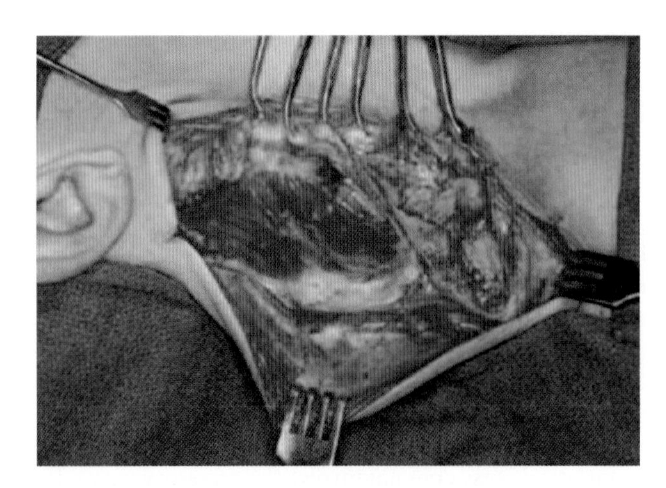

Figure 10.53 The nodal tissue overlying the splenius capitis and levator scapulae muscles is dissected.

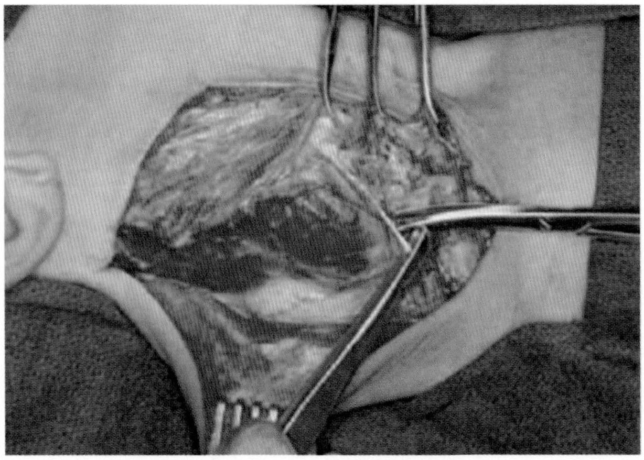

Figure 10.54 The spinal accessory nerve is freed from the nodal tissue in the posterior triangle of the neck.

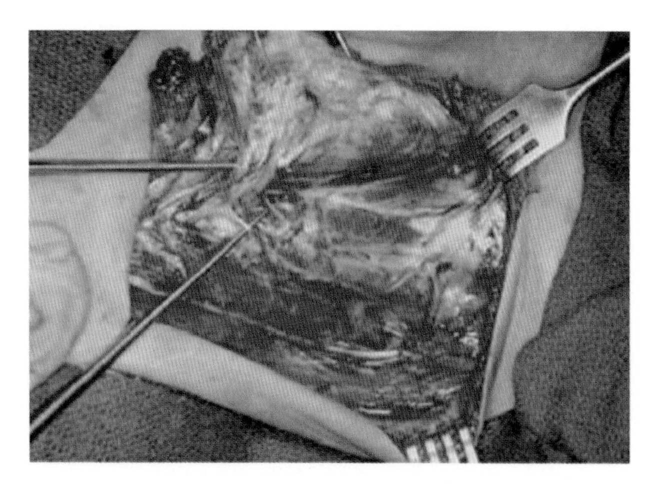

Figure 10.56 Dissected nodal tissue from the posterior triangle is passed under the nerve anteriorly.

belly of the digastric muscle (Figure 10.55). The entire nerve is now exposed from its exit at the skull base up to its entry in the trapezius muscle. Dissection of the nerve, however, requires splitting the specimen in the posterior triangle and the upper half of the sternomastoid muscle in the upper part of the neck. Therefore, if gross metastatic nodes are found adherent to the nerve along its course, it should not be preserved.

The nerve is completely free at this point. Using a nerve hook, it is lifted up and the dissected contents of the posterior triangle of the neck are pushed from behind the nerve and pulled out anteriorly (Figure 10.56). The specimen from the dissected posterior triangle is pushed from behind the nerve into the anterior aspect of the surgical field to remain in continuity with the rest of the specimen. The nerve is allowed to rest on the exposed, clean musculature of the floor of the posterior triangle of the neck.

The rest of the neck dissection continues as described in classical radical neck dissection. All other steps of the operative procedure are exactly the same, removing all other structures as described for a radical neck dissection. The surgical field at the conclusion of the operation is similar to a classical radical dissection, except for the accessory nerve, which is preserved in its entirety as seen in the lower part of the surgical field (Figure 10.57). Suction drains are placed in the wound after irrigation and the incisions are closed in the usual way.

The postoperative appearance of the patient approximately 6 months following MRND-I is shown in Figure 10.58. Note the absence of a dropped shoulder. The contour of the trapezius muscle is preserved, demonstrating that the nerve supply to the muscle is maintained intact, preserving the shoulder function. The patient is able to raise his shoulders all the way up. The only esthetic debility is due to loss of the sternomastoid muscle and soft tissues.

Modified radical neck dissection type II

This operative procedure is similar to MRND-I, preserving the sternocleidomastoid muscle and the spinal accessory nerve, but selectively sacrificing the internal jugular vein

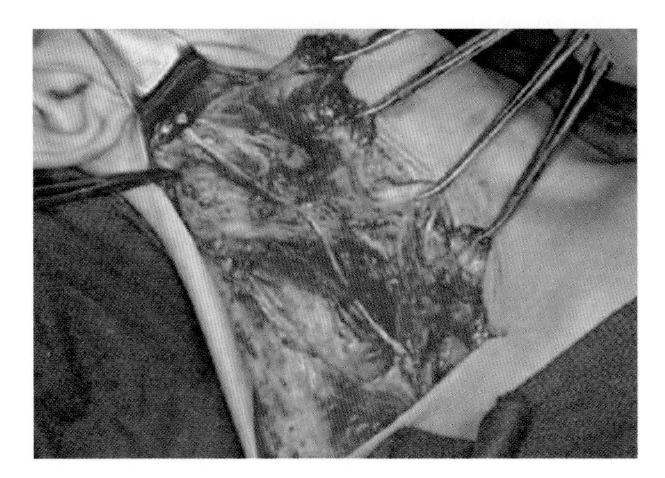

Figure 10.55 The spinal accessory nerve is dissected and freed up throughout its course in the neck.

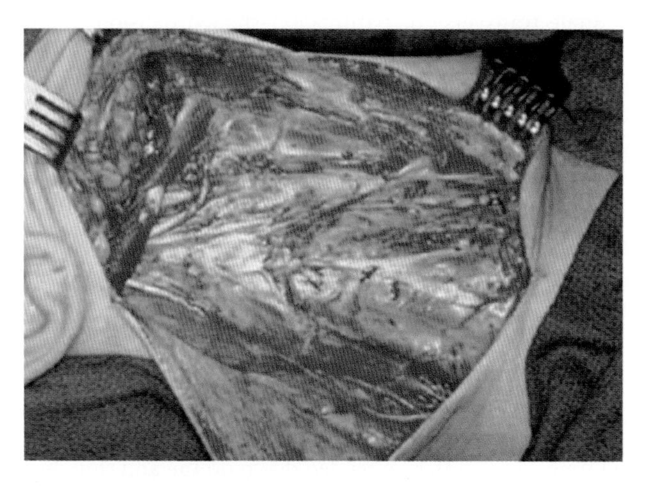

Figure 10.57 Surgical field showing comprehensive clearance of all five levels of lymph nodes with preservation of the spinal accessory nerve.

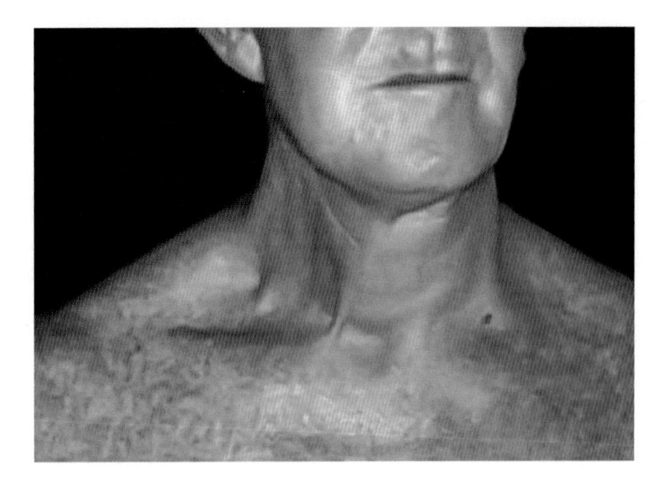

Figure 10.58 Postoperative appearance following modified radical neck dissection, type I. Note the absence of shoulder droop.

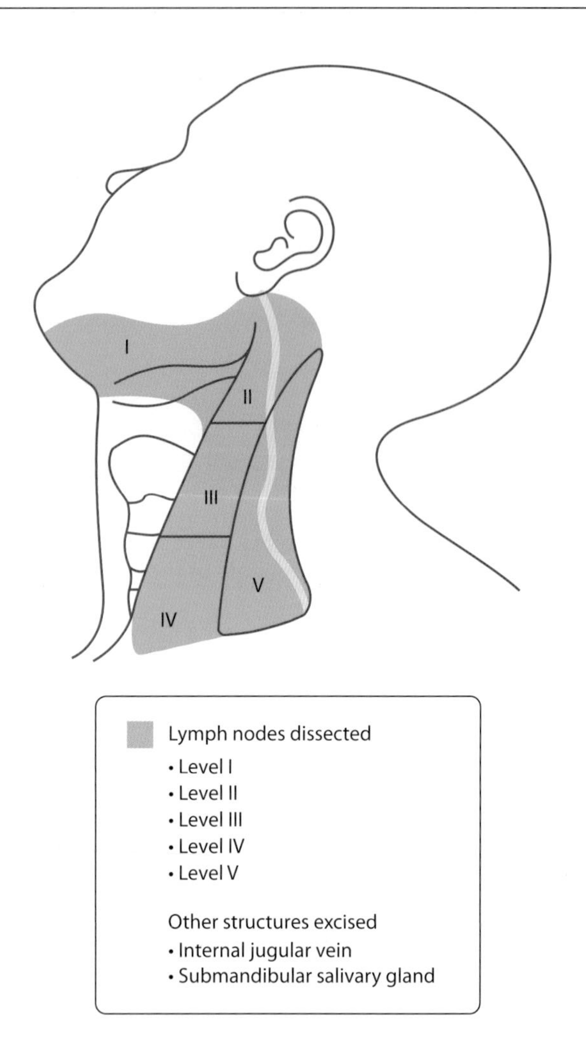

Figure 10.59 Modified radical neck dissection type II. Lymph nodes dissected: levels I, II, III, IV, and V. Other structures excised: internal jugular vein and submandibular salivary gland. Preserved: sternocleidomastoid muscle and spinal accessory nerve.

(Figure 10.59). The indications for this operation are massive metastatic disease grossly involving the internal jugular vein. All the steps of the operative procedure are otherwise essentially similar to those described for other comprehensive neck dissections.

Classical radical neck dissection

The classic radical neck dissection has been the gold standard for the surgical treatment of clinically apparent, metastatic cervical lymph nodes in the past. It comprehensively clears lymph nodes from levels I, II, III, IV, and V, but also requires sacrifice of the sternocleidomastoid muscle, spinal accessory nerve, internal jugular vein and submandibular salivary gland (Figure 10.60). However, due to significant postoperative esthetic deformity and functional disability, the operation is now rarely performed and is currently recommended only when appropriate indications are present, as discussed before. A variety of incisions have been described for completing a radical neck dissection. However, a single transverse or trifurcate T-shaped incision is preferred (Figure 10.61). The transverse limb of the T begins at the mastoid process and follows an upper neck skin crease, remaining at least two fingerbreadths below the angle of the mandible. The incision extends across the midline up to the anterior border of the opposite sternomastoid muscle. At about the midpoint of the transverse incision near the posterior border of the sternomastoid muscle, the vertical limb of the T incision is begun. This vertical limb is curvaceous and ends at the midclavicular point. The incision provides adequate exposure for completion of a radical neck dissection; it is suitable both for bilateral radical neck dissections with a similar incision on the opposite side of the neck and for a pectoralis major myocutaneous flap, since the vertical limb can be safely extended down on the anterior chest wall for elevation of the myocutaneous flap. Since the blood supply to the three skin flaps resulting from this incision is not disturbed, marginal necrosis at the trifurcation of the skin incision is rarely seen. The trifurcation of the incision is shown marked out on the skin here in relation to the carotid artery. The trifurcation point should be kept posterior to the carotid artery when feasible. This incision provides the necessary exposure by elevation of the posterior, anterior and superior skin flaps.

The dissection begins with elevation of the posterior skin flap. The incision begins with the posterior half of the transverse incision at the mastoid process and continues with the vertical incision beyond the trifurcation point (Figure 10.62). The anterior and superior skin flaps are not elevated at this time. The skin incision is made with a scalpel, but the rest of the dissection is carried out with an electrocautery. The skin incision is deepened through the platysma, but if grossly enlarged lymph nodes are present and there is suspicion of extension of disease beyond the capsule of the lymph nodes, then the flap is elevated superficially to the platysma muscle, which is sacrificed. Electrocautery aids rapid elevation of the posterior skin flap. Several skin hooks are employed to retract the posterior skin flap, while

I

II

III

IV

V

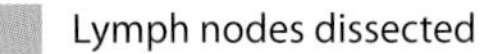
Lymph nodes dissected
- Level I
- Level II
- Level III
- Level IV
- Level V

Other structures excised
- Sternocleidomastoid muscle
- Internal jugular vein
- Spinal accessory nerve
- Submandibular salivary gland

Figure 10.60 Radical neck dissection. Lymph nodes dissected: levels I, II, III, IV, and V. Other structures excised: sternocleidomastoid muscle, internal jugular vein, spinal accessory nerve and submandibular salivary gland.

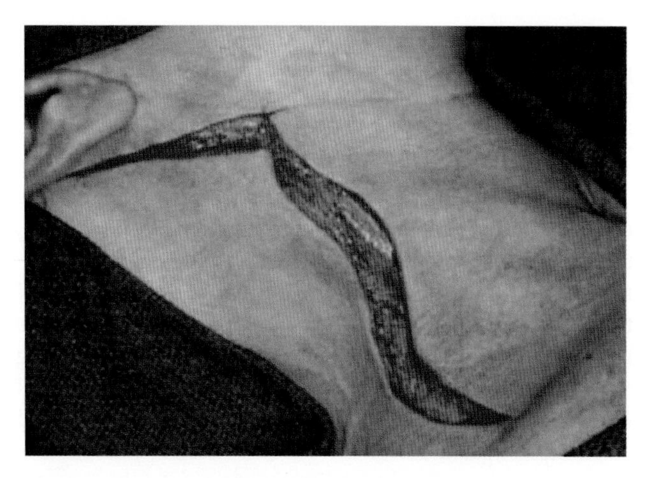

Figure 10.62 The operation is begun with elevation of only the posterior flap and dissection of the posterior triangle of the neck first.

counter-traction is provided by the second assistant over the soft tissues in the neck. The plane of dissection is along the undersurface of the platysma muscle. The posterior skin flap is elevated until the anterior border of the trapezius muscle is identified and exposed all the way from the mastoid process down to the clavicle. It is important to remember that platysma is not present all the way up to the trapezius muscle and therefore meticulous attention should be paid to remain in the proper subcutaneous plane beyond the platysma to maintain uniform thickness of the skin flap.

Rake retractors are now employed to retract the posterior skin flap (Figure 10.63). Soft tissues anterior to the trapezius muscle are now grasped with several hemostats, which are used to provide traction on the surgical specimen. Dissection proceeds along the floor of the posterior triangle of the neck, exposing each successive muscle with anterior elevation of the specimen. The superior attachment of the sternomastoid muscle is detached from the mastoid process

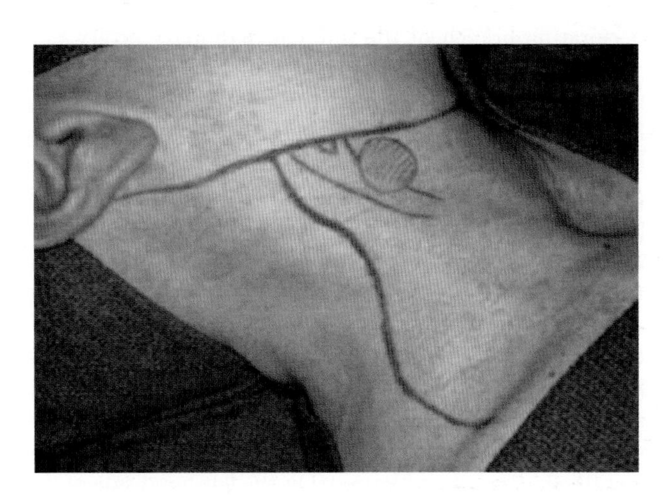

Figure 10.61 A trifurcate incision is outlined; however, a single transverse incision is preferred.

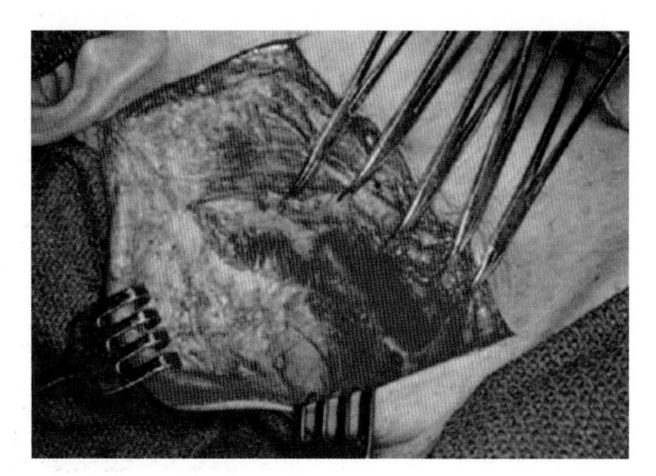

Figure 10.63 Nodal tissue anterior to the trapezius muscle from the posterior triangle is dissected and retracted anteriorly.

and retracted anteriorly. The plane of dissection continues just anterior to the anterior border of each successive muscle in the posterior triangle of the neck. The splenius capitis and levator scapulae muscles are then exposed. Several small veins have to be divided and ligated as this dissection proceeds anteriorly. In the lower part of the neck, the transverse cervical artery and its accompanying vein are identified, divided between clamps and ligated. Likewise, the posterior belly of the omohyoid muscle is divided in the floor of the posterior triangle of the neck and its anterior stump is retracted medially. Dissection continues medially, exposing the posterior scalene muscle. The lower end of the external jugular vein is divided between clamps near the clavicle and its stump is ligated.

As the scalene muscles are exposed, roots of the cervical plexus come into view (Figure 10.64). However, these are left intact until the phrenic nerve is identified lying on the anterior aspect of the scalenus anticus muscle. Similarly, motor branches of the cervical plexus providing nerve supply to the posterior compartment muscles should be carefully preserved. The cutaneous branches of the cervical plexus are transected, leaving short stumps to prevent injury to the phrenic nerve. The cutaneous branches of the cervical roots carry with them small blood vessels and therefore these stumps should be ligated. In the lower part of the posterior triangle of the neck, the brachial plexus comes into view. Dissection over this is easy because there is a plane of loose areolar tissue between the cervical lymph nodes and the supraclavicular fat pad contained within the deep cervical fascia. Dissection of the posterior triangle of the neck is now complete. The specimen mobilized so far is now reflected posteriorly (Figure 10.65). A dry gauze pad is placed on the musculature of the posterior triangle of the neck over which the surgical specimen is allowed to rest.

Attention is now focused on the anterior skin flap. The transverse skin incision is completed by extending it from the trifurcation point up to the medial end, deepening through the platysma. The anterior skin flap is retracted

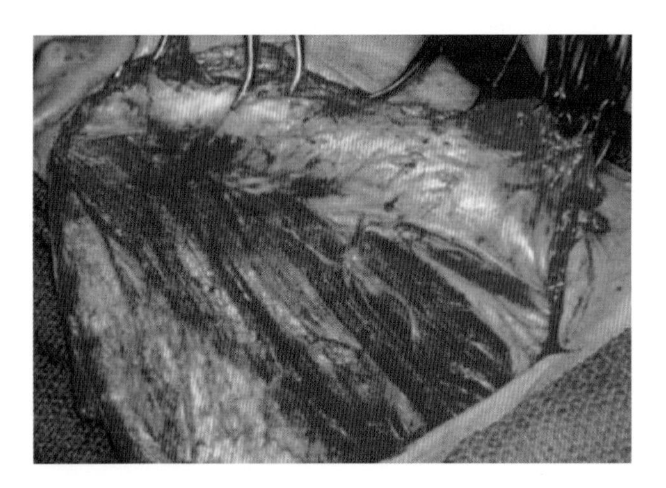

Figure 10.64 Dissection of the posterior triangle is complete with exposure of the cervical roots and brachial plexus.

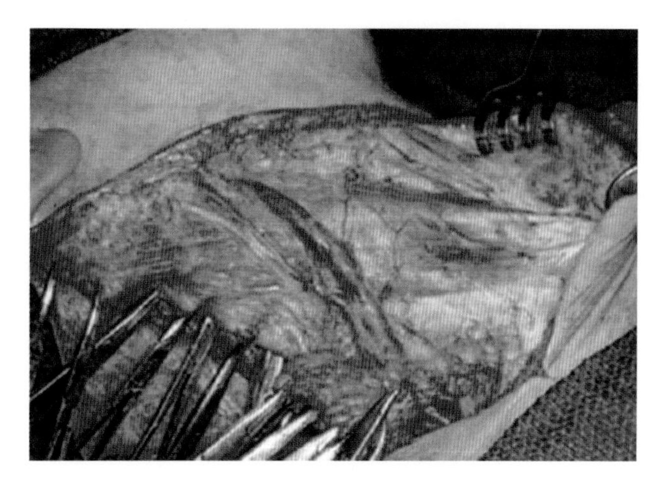

Figure 10.65 The anterior skin flap is elevated to the midline to expose the lower end of the sternocleidomastoid muscle.

medially by the use of skin hooks and rake retractors. The use of electrocautery permits rapid elevation of this skin flap through the loose plane of areolar tissue lying deep to the platysma muscle. Several cutaneous vessels are encountered during elevation and these are electrocoagulated. The skin flap is elevated up to the medial border of the omohyoid muscle superiorly and up to the medial border of the sternomastoid muscle at its attachment to the manubrium sterni inferiorly. A large loop retractor is now used to expose the sternal end of the sternomastoid muscle, which facilitates complete elevation of the anterior skin flap. Using electrocautery with the cutting current, the tendon of the sternomastoid muscle is divided from the sternal end and the rest of the muscular attachment on the manubrium and the clavicle is divided using the coagulating current. There is a plane of loose areolar tissue containing fat between the carotid sheath and the posterior aspect of the sternomastoid muscle, so the latter can be safely divided by electrocautery.

Several small vessels enter the anterior skin flap as it is elevated near the clavicle. These are branches from the first perforating branch of the internal mammary artery that provide blood supply to the lower skin flap. These are carefully preserved. Once the sternomastoid muscle is detached from both its sternal and clavicular ends, it is grasped with hemostats and retracted cephalad. The fascia between the carotid sheath and the strap muscles is incised with a scalpel. A small loop retractor is used to retract the strap muscles medially to expose the common carotid artery and the vagus nerve. By alternate blunt and sharp dissection, the areolar tissue of the carotid sheath is divided circumferentially around the internal jugular vein (Figure 10.66). At this juncture, the proximal ends of the transverse cervical artery and vein are identified, divided and ligated. Lymphatic vessels present in the vicinity of the jugular vein are carefully identified, divided and ligated. On the left-hand side of the neck, the thoracic duct requires special attention. It should be meticulously identified, carefully dissected, divided and

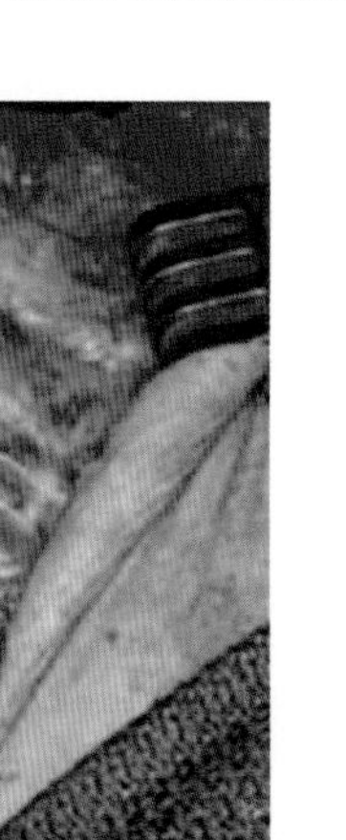

Figure 10.66 The sternocleidomastoid muscle is detached from its lower attachment and retracted cephalad, exposing the carotid sheath.

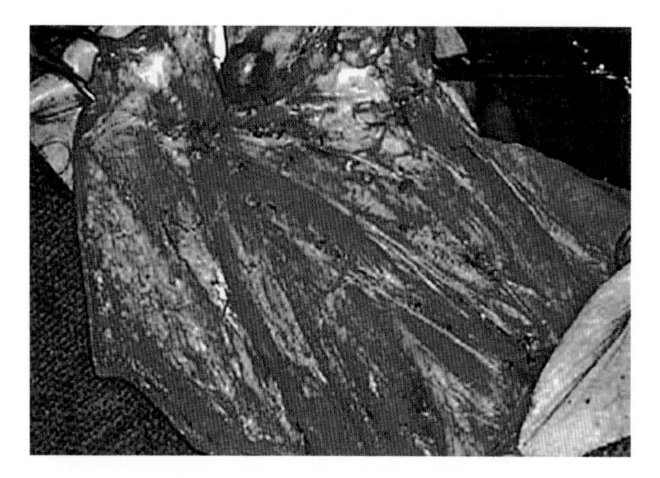

Figure 10.68 Dissection proceeds along the carotid sheath cephalad, protecting the vagus nerve until the hypoglossal nerve is identified.

ligated in order to prevent chyle leak and fistulae. Lymph nodes contained in loose areolar tissue behind the internal jugular vein are dissected and pulled out at this time to remain in continuity with the rest of the specimen. During this dissection, the phrenic nerve should be carefully protected and kept out of harm's way.

The small loop retractor placed on the strap muscles is now pulled to expose the common carotid artery and the vagus nerve (Figure 10.67). The internal jugular vein should not be ligated until after both the carotid artery and nerve are identified and retracted medially. The vein is doubly ligated, divided in between and its proximal stump is suture ligated.

The middle thyroid vein usually seen at this point entering the medial aspect of the internal jugular vein is divided and ligated. Dissection now proceeds along the lateral border of the carotid sheath, remaining posterior to the vein but anterolateral to the vagus nerve. This is a relatively avascular plane and one can safely divide the carotid sheath along this plane all the way up to the base of the skull. As dissection proceeds cephalad, minor vessels in the carotid sheath may cause bleeding, which is easily controlled with electrocoagulation (Figure 10.68).

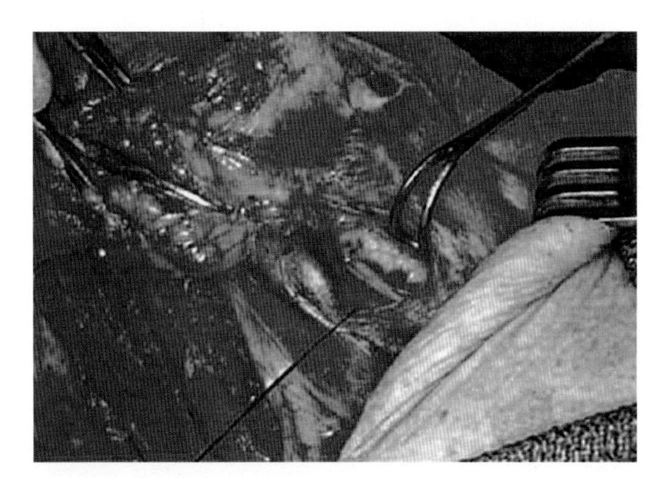

Figure 10.67 The internal jugular vein is divided and ligated after identification of the vagus nerve in the carotid sheath.

Dissection of the lateral aspect of the carotid sheath in the upper part of the neck brings the hypoglossal nerve into view. On the medial aspect of the carotid sheath, the dissection is carried cephalad along the medial border of the superior belly of the omohyoid muscle up to the hyoid bone, from which it is detached. Small blood vessels running along the descendens hypoglossi are divided and ligated. The superior thyroid artery is preserved, but the superior thyroid vein will have to be divided and ligated. A dry gauze pad is now placed on the surgical field and the entire specimen is allowed to rest over the gauze pad.

The superior skin flap is now elevated in the usual fashion and is retained close to the platysma. The mandibular branch of the facial nerve is located in the fascia over the submandibular salivary gland, approximately two fingerbreadths below and two fingerbreadths anterior to the angle of the mandible. The nerve is carefully identified, dissected off the fascia and retracted cephalad with the skin flap. The facial vessels are divided and ligated (Figure 10.69). The contents of the submandibular triangle are dissected off by dividing the secretomotor fibers to the submandibular salivary gland and Wharton's duct, but preserving the lingual and hypoglossal nerves. The submandiblar gland and level I lymph nodes are thus reflected caudad to remain in continuity with the rest of the specimen. Several pharyngeal veins along the digastric tendon and the posterior belly of the digastric muscle are divided and ligated. At this juncture, the hypoglossal nerve should be carefully dissected, protected and preserved. Finally, the tail of the parotid gland is separated or transected along the superior border of the posterior belly of the digastric muscle. During division of the tail of the parotid gland, the posterior facial vein and several arterial branches of the occipital artery have to be divided and ligated.

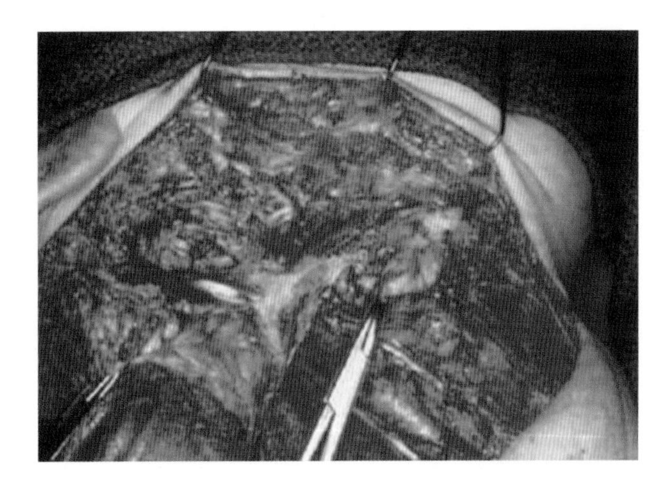

Figure 10.69 The upper skin flap is elevated and dissection of the submandibular triangle completed, carefully preserving the mandibular branch of the facial nerve.

The posterior belly of the digastric muscle is now retracted cephalad with a deep, right-angled retractor, bringing into view the occipital artery, which runs across the internal jugular vein anteriorly at right angles to it. If the occipital artery is high behind the digastric muscle it may be left alone, but if it is quite low it will have to be divided and ligated. The adipose tissue and lymph nodes lateral to the internal jugular vein under the sternomastoid muscle are dissected out. This is easily accomplished once the tendon of the sternomastoid muscle is detached from the mastoid process.

The accessory nerve is divided near the jugular foramen and its proximal stump is ligated as there is a small vessel running with the nerve. Finally, the upper end of the internal jugular vein is skeletonized and the vein is doubly ligated and divided. The surgical specimen is now delivered.

The surgical field following radical neck dissection shows clearance of all five levels of lymph nodes as previously described, along with loss of the sternomastoid muscle, internal jugular vein, spinal accessory nerve and submandibular salivary gland (Figure 10.70). The wound is now irrigated with bacitracin solution. Meticulous hemostasis must be ensured prior to closure of the wound. Two suction drains are now inserted through separate stab incisions (Figure 10.71). One drain overlies the anterior border of the trapezius muscle in the posterior triangle and is retained there through a loop of chromic catgut suture between the skin flap and the trapezius muscle; another is maintained over the strap muscles anteriorly and is retained by a loop of catgut suture. The rest of the skin wound is closed in two layers using 3/0 chromic catgut interrupted sutures for platysma and 5/0 nylon sutures for skin (Figure 10.72). It is vital for the suction drains to be on continuous suction while the wound is being closed.

As soon as the last skin sutures are applied, the wound should be made airtight, allowing the skin flaps to remain completely down and snug to the deeper tissues by suction through the drains. If suction in this manner is not maintained, minor venous oozing will allow the flaps to become lifted, causing collection of hematoma and clotting of blood in drainage tubes that will, in turn, initiate new venous oozing, leading to a larger hematoma. The

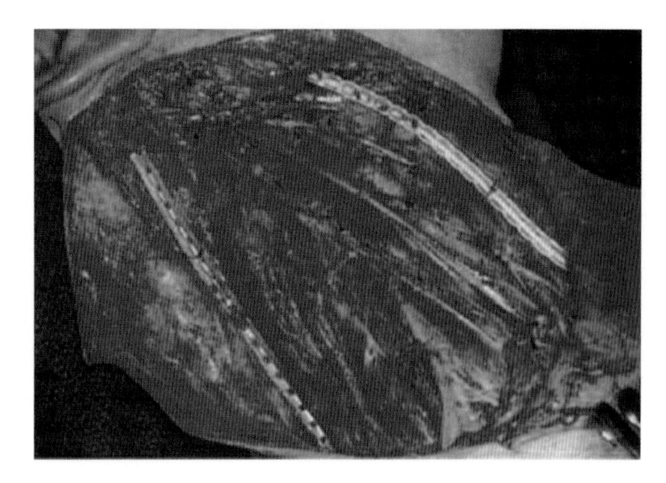

Figure 10.71 Two suction drains are inserted and appropriately positioned.

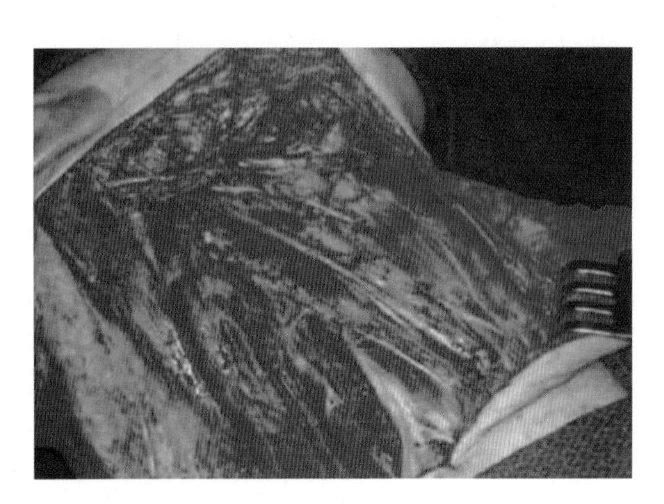

Figure 10.70 The surgical field following removal of the specimen.

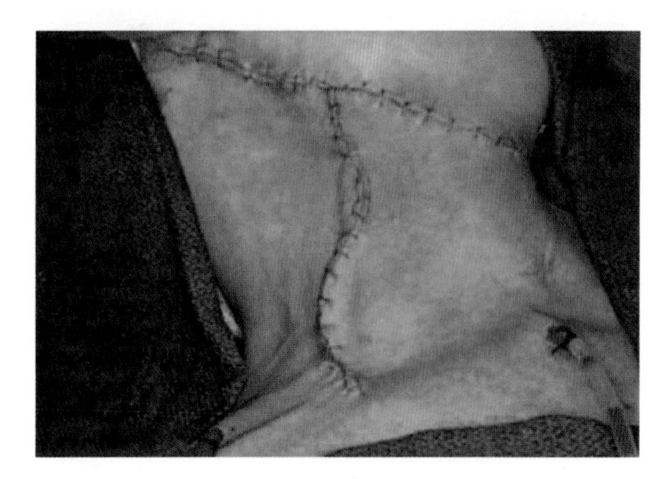

Figure 10.72 The incision is closed in two layers with interrupted sutures.

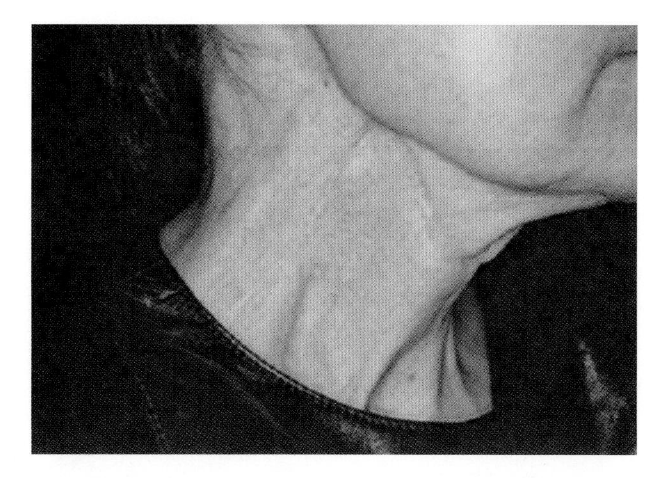

Figure 10.73 Postoperative appearance of the patient 6 months following classical radical neck dissection.

suction drains are retained until the volume of serous drainage is minimal.

The postoperative appearance of the patient approximately 6 months after surgery shows a well-healed scar with esthetic deformity due to loss of sternomastoid muscle (Figure 10.73). The functional disability is due to inability to abduct the shoulder beyond 90° cephalad. This is due to loss of function of the trapezius muscle. In addition to this, the imbalance of shoulder musculature due to the paralyzed trapezius muscle causes drooping of the shoulder (Figure 10.74). When bilateral radical neck dissections are performed with sacrifice of the internal jugular vein on both sides for tumors of the oral cavity or oropharynx, chronic lymphedema of the face and swelling result. Although venous drainage is initially compromised, within a few weeks collateral venous drainage through the pharyngeal veins is restored as long as the anatomy of the central compartment is not disturbed. However, chronic lymphedema of the face with thickening of the subdermal plane and cutaneous telangiectasia remains (Figure 10.75). On the other hand, when simultaneous bilateral radical neck dissections

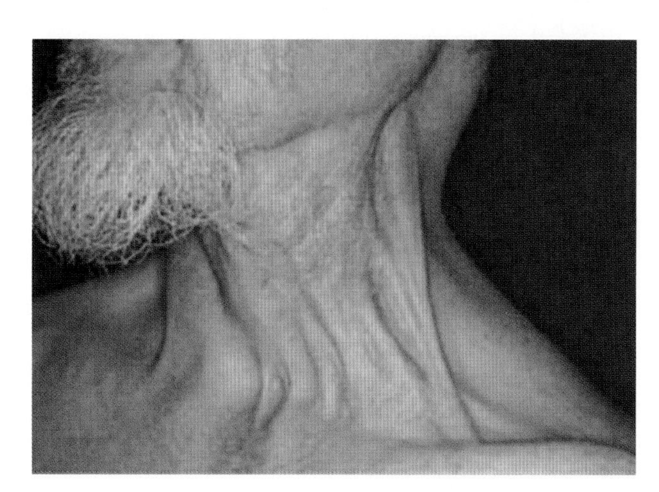

Figure 10.74 Drooping shoulder and fibrotic scar following radical neck dissection.

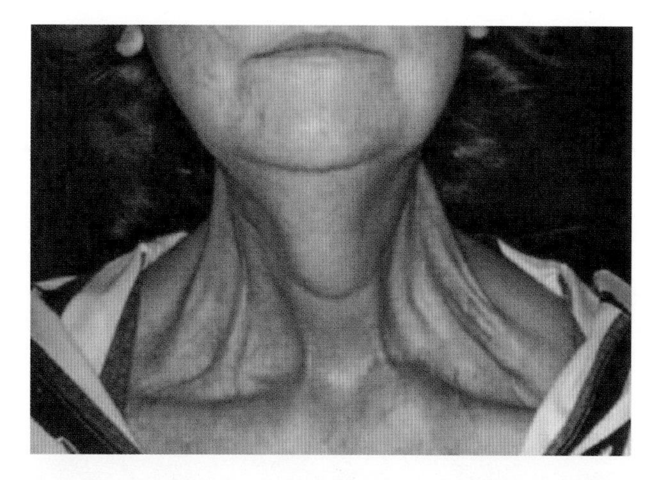

Figure 10.75 Chronic lymphedema and venous telangiectasia following bilateral radical neck dissections for oral cancer.

are performed in conjunction with laryngectomy, acute venous obstruction to intracranial and extracranial venous drainage occurs. This leads to the development of massive venous and lymphatic edema of the face in the postoperative period (Figure 10.76).

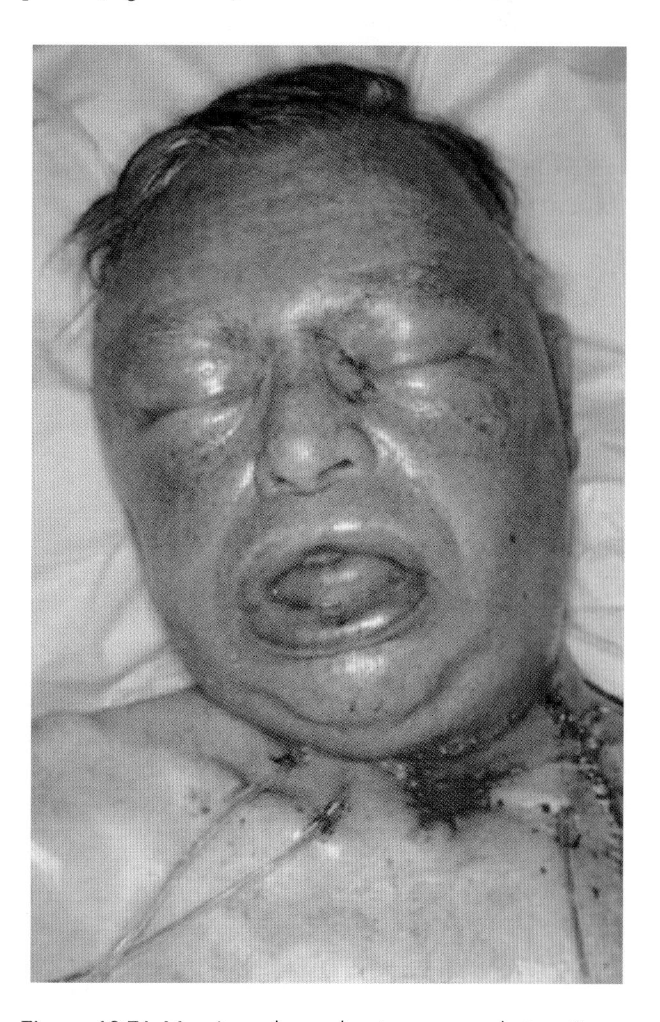

Figure 10.76 Massive edema due to venous obstruction immediately following total laryngectomy and bilateral radical neck dissections.

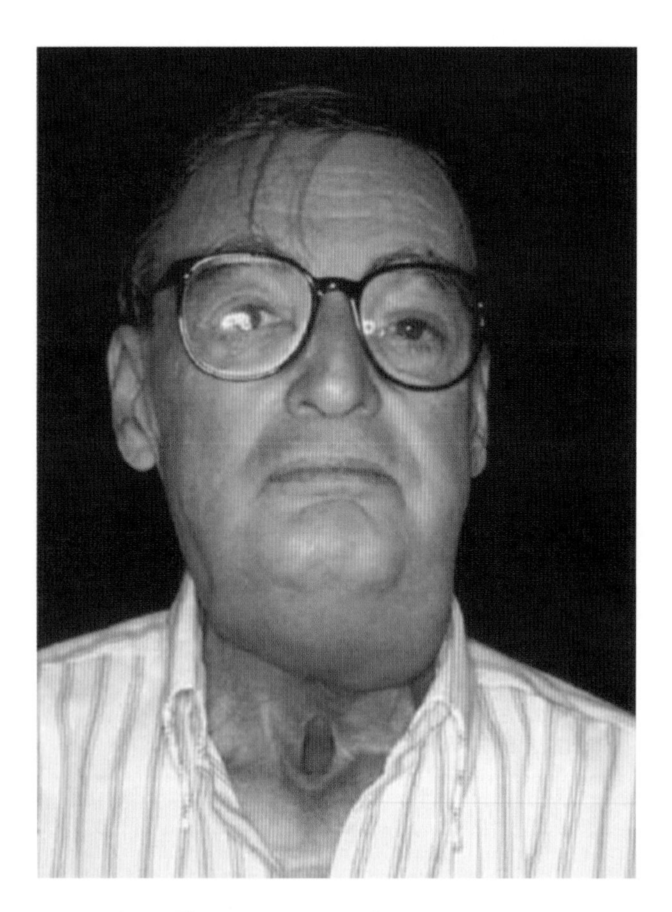

Figure 10.77 The same patient shown in Figure 10.76 at 1 year following surgery.

Although with the passage of time collateral venous drainage is established through Batson's prevertebral venous plexus, the extent of venous and lymphatic edema leaves significant facial swelling for a long time (Figure 10.77). In addition to this, the operative mortality of such a massive resection is significant and therefore, when feasible, bilateral radical neck dissections in conjunction with pharyngolaryngectomy as a single-stage procedure should be avoided. Patients undergoing classic radical neck dissection require an intensive program of postoperative physiotherapy for rehabilitation of shoulder function and to avoid a painful and stiff shoulder joint.

Results of treatment

As indicated earlier, the single most important factor in the prognosis of squamous cell carcinoma of the head and neck is the presence or absence of cervical lymph node metastasis (1–11). Cure rates for patients with cervical lymph node metastasis are nearly half of those achieved in patients who present with tumors localized at the primary site. The extent of nodal metastasis in the neck clearly has an impact on prognosis. Patients with N_1 disease in the neck have a better prognosis compared to those with N_2 and N_3 disease. In addition to this, the presence of capsular rupture and ENE has a significant adverse impact on prognosis (Figure 10.78) (6,7,31–34,81). Thus, regional failure in the dissected neck depends

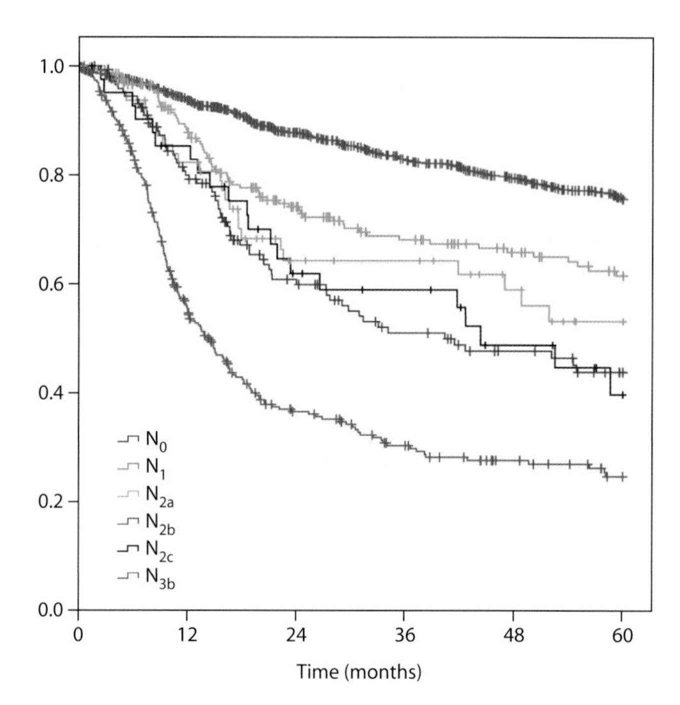

Figure 10.78 Overall survival based on N staging incorporating ENE as a prognostic factor (American Joint Committee on Cancer, 8th edition) in patients with oral cavity cancer (Memorial Sloan-Kettering Cancer Center and PMH data).

on the extent of nodal disease. Patients undergoing neck dissection for an N_0 neck have the lowest risk of local recurrence compared to those with N_1, N_2, and N_3 disease. Patients with multilevel involvement develop recurrence in the dissected neck twice as often as those with single-level involvement. Adjuvant postoperative radiation therapy, however, significantly improves regional control in the dissected neck (62,82–84). This improvement in regional control is seen in patients with limited neck disease (N_1) as well as in patients with extensive nodal disease (N_{2B}) (Figure 10.79). The role

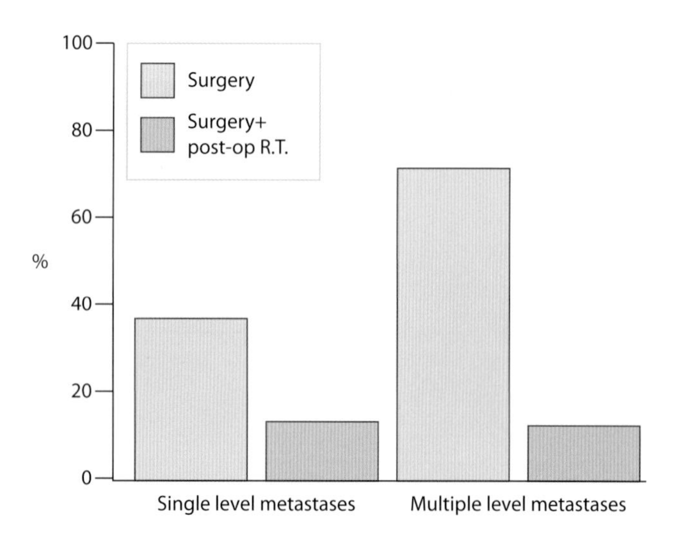

Figure 10.79 Regional failure in the neck after neck dissection with and without postoperative radiotherapy.

of adding chemotherapy to postoperative radiotherapy has been tested in two randomized trials (81,85,86). Based on the results of these studies, postoperative chemoradiotherapy is recommended in patients with ENE and those with positive margins of resection at the primary site. A modest improvement in locoregional control is observed with the addition of chemotherapy. However, it should be remembered that adding chemotherapy to postoperative radiotherapy increases acute and long-term morbidity in a significant number of patients.

Significant functional and esthetic morbidity following classic radical neck dissection led to modification of the operation to reduce morbidity without compromising regional control rates or survival (9,19,22,65–71). MRND-I achieves that goal without an adverse impact on prognosis. Five-year survival rates, regional failure rates in the dissected neck and the location of recurrence are comparable in patients with palpable metastatic disease undergoing classic radical neck dissection and MRND with preservation of the spinal accessory nerve (MRND-I) (Figure 10.80). Regional recurrence rates in the dissected neck following classical radical neck dissection and MRND-I are also comparable (Figure 10.81). The observed difference in neck failure rates seen in Figure 10.81 is not statistically significant. In highly selected patients with limited upper neck metastasis, even a selective neck dissection can be performed without compromise in neck failure or survival (Figure 10.81). These are usually patients with oral cavity primary tumors and low-volume (N_1) disease at level I in the neck. The presence of extranodal spread by metastatic disease does not seem to influence regional recurrence rates following classic radical neck dissection or MRND-I as long as the accessory nerve is not directly involved by cancer. At present, it is felt inadvisable to perform MRND-I for N_3 disease.

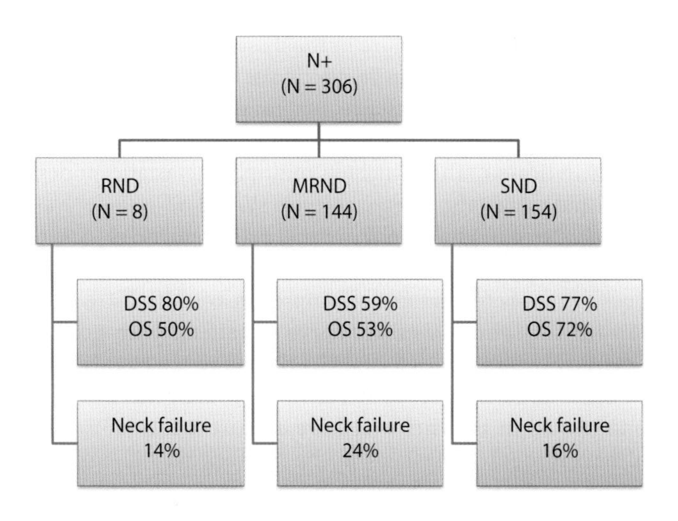

Figure 10.81 Two-year disease-specific survival and regional failure rates following radical neck dissection (RND), modified radical neck dissection (MRND) type I and SND for N+ disease.

Selective neck dissections in patients with an N_0 neck provide accurate pathologic staging of the regional lymph nodes at risk of micrometastasis and offer regional control rates comparable to those obtained with more radical operative procedures. Currently, selective neck dissections based on the primary site and predicted pattern of neck metastasis are considered the standard of care. Clearly, patients with histologically negative nodes in the selective neck dissection specimen enjoy excellent long-term survival and very little risk of regional failure (Figure 10.82). On the other hand, patients proven to have micrometastasis in the selective neck dissection specimen (27%) have a 2-year disease-specific survival that is comparable to more comprehensive

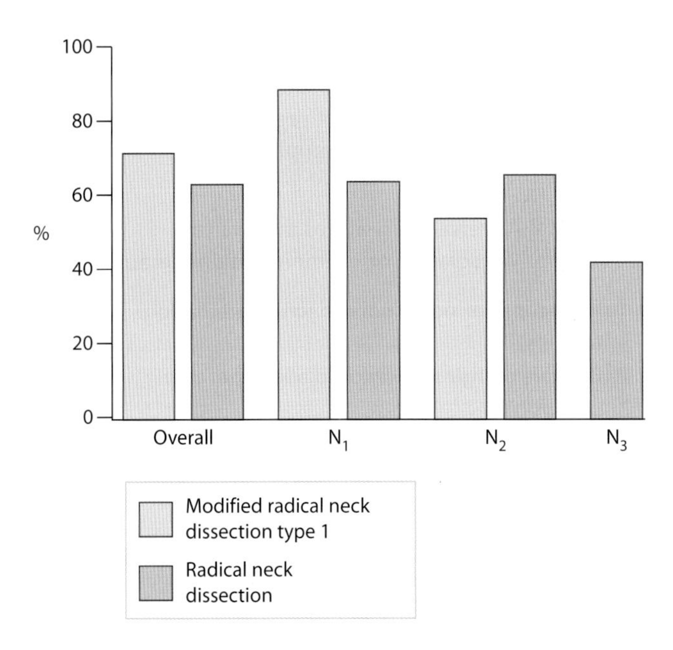

Figure 10.80 Overall 5-year survival after therapeutic neck dissection by N stage.

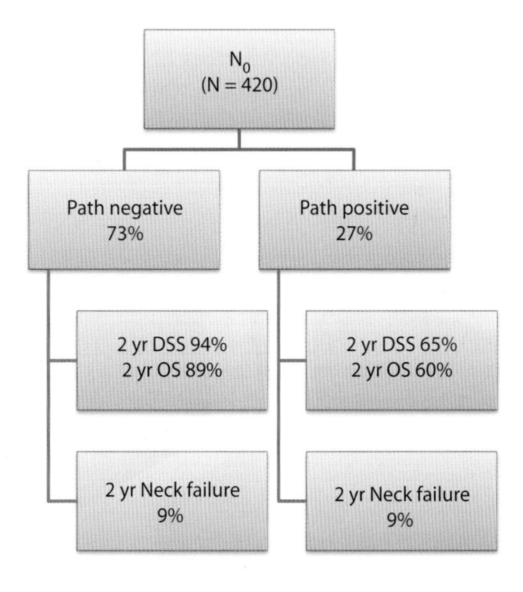

Figure 10.82 Two-year disease-specific and regional failure rates in N_0 patients undergoing selective neck dissection with pathologically negative and positive nodes for metastasis.

operations. Regional failure in the dissected neck following selective neck dissection is also quite low (Figure 10.82). However, in order to achieve comparable regional control rates, postoperative radiation therapy should be employed when indicated. These include multiple metastatic nodes, ENE and metastatic disease at levels IV and V.

The current philosophy in the management of cervical lymph nodes in squamous carcinomas of the head and neck region is to perform a comprehensive MRND-I, preserving the spinal accessory nerve in patients with grossly enlarged lymph nodes as long as the nerve is not involved by metastatic disease. A selective neck dissection is recommended in patients who have at least a 10%–15% risk of having micrometastasis in the N_0 neck on the basis of the characteristics of the primary tumor. Postoperative radiation therapy or chemoradiotherapy is recommended in all patients with multiple metastatic lymph nodes, ENE of tumor or where other ominous histopathologic features are present.

The distributions of various types of neck dissections performed by the Head and Neck Service at Memorial Sloan-Kettering Cancer Center from 1985 to 2012 are shown in Figure 10.83. It is important to note that classical radical neck dissection is now rarely performed. Over the same period, the number of patients undergoing a classic radical neck dissection declined and an increasing number of patients underwent modifications in neck dissection for the management of cervical lymph node metastasis (Figure 10.84).

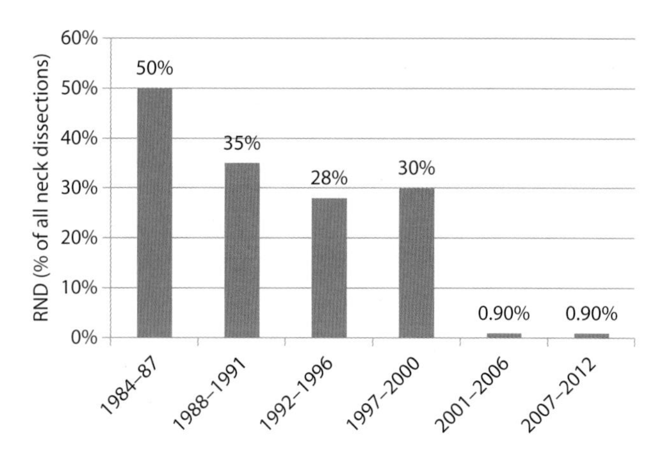

Figure 10.84 Declining incidence of radical neck dissection at Memorial Sloan-Kettering Cancer Center (1984–2012).

Regional recurrence

Regional recurrence of metastatic disease in the dissected neck is dependent on the extent and volume of neck metastasis at the time of neck dissection (29). Regional recurrence following neck dissection for multiple metastatic lymph nodes and in those with gross ENE is prohibitively high (62,82). Therefore, to enhance the regional control rate, postoperative radiation or chemoradiation is recommended. Adding chemotherapy to postoperative radiation therapy alone in patients with ENE and/or positive margins of resection of the primary tumor reduces the hazard ratio to 0.7 compared to radiation therapy alone (86). The need for adjuvant postoperative radiation therapy, however, depends on the extent of disease in the neck. Regional control of metastatic disease in the neck is significantly enhanced with postoperative radiation or chemoradiation therapy (1,62,81–84). Indications for postoperative radiotherapy with or without chemotherapy are listed in Table 10.1.

As for oropharyngeal cancer, there has been a major shift in the treatment paradigm due to the rising incidence of HPV-associated oropharyngeal squamous cell carcinoma. HPV-associated oropharyngeal cancer patients are being treated either with definitive chemoradiation therapy or, more recently, with surgery (usually transoral robotic resection and neck dissection) followed by adjuvant radiation therapy for patients with T1/T2 N0/N1 disease (87). The data collected so far from multiple centers suggest that patients that received chemoradiation and had partial regional responses can be salvaged with subsequent neck dissection. This may result in high rates of regional disease control in patients with HPV-associated oropharyngeal cancer (88).

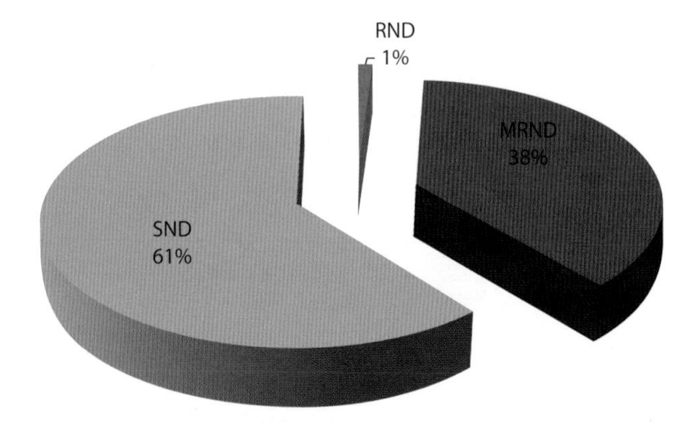

Figure 10.83 Distribution of types of neck dissections currently performed at Memorial Sloan-Kettering Cancer Center.

Table 10.1 Adverse risk features that warrant postoperative radiation or chemoradiation therapy

1. Extracapsular nodal spread (chemoradiation therapy)
2. Positive margins (chemoradiation therapy)
3. pT3 or pT4
4. N2 or N3 nodal disease
5. Nodal disease in levels IV or V
6. Perineural invasion
7. Vascular embolism by tumor
8. Cranial nerve invasion
9. Vascular embolism by tumor
10. Invasion of skull base
11. Gross residual disease following neck dissection

REFERENCES

1. Amin MB, Edge SB, Greene FL et al (eds). AJCC Cancer Staging Manual. 8th ed. New York: Springer; 2017.
2. NCCN clinical practice guidelines in oncology. Head and Neck Cancer. Version 1.2017. National Comprehensive Cancer Network, Inc., 2017. https://www.nccn.org/professionals/physician_gls/pdf/head-and-neck.pdf.
3. Shah J. Cervical lymph nodes. In: Shah J, Patel SG, Singh B (eds). *Jatin Shah's Head and Neck Surgery and Oncology.* (4th Edition). Philadelphia: Elsevier, 2012, 426–70.
4. Shah J, Medina J, Shaha A. Cervical lymph node metastasis. *Curr Probl Surg* 1993;30:284–335.
5. Grandi C, Alloisio M, Moglia D et al. Prognostic significance of lymphatic spread in head and neck carcinomas: therapeutic implications. *Head Neck Surg* 1985;8:67–73.
6. Shah JP, Cendon RA, Farr HW, Strong EW. Carcinoma of the oral cavity. Factors affecting treatment failure at the primary site and neck. *Am J Surg* 1976;132:504–7.
7. Silver CE, Moisa II. Elective treatment of the neck in cancer of the oral tongue. *Semin Surg Oncol* 1991;7:14–9.
8. Snow GB, Annyas AA, van Slooten EA, Bartelink H, Hart AA. Prognostic factors of neck node metastasis. *Clin Otolaryngol* 1982;7:185–92.
9. Houck JR, Medina JE. Management of cervical lymph nodes in squamous carcinomas of the head and neck. *Semin Surg Oncol* 1995;11:228–39.
10. Richard JM, Sancho-Garnier H, Micheau C, Saravane D, Cachin Y. Prognostic factors in cervical lymph node metastasis in upper respiratory and digestive tract carcinomas: study of 1,713 cases during a 15-year period. *Laryngoscope* 1987;97:97–101.
11. Leemans CR, Tiwari R, Nauta JJ, van der Waal I, Snow GB. Regional lymph node involvement and its significance in the development of distant metastases in head and neck carcinoma. *Cancer* 1993;71:452–6.
12. Ho CM, Lam KH, Wei WI, Lau WF. Treatment of neck nodes in oral cancer. *Surg Oncol* 1992;1:73–8.
13. Leemans CR, Tiwari R, Nauta JJ, van der Waal I, Snow GB. Recurrence at the primary site in head and neck cancer and the significance of neck lymph node metastases as a prognostic factor. *Cancer* 1994;73:187–90.
14. Snow GB, Patel P, Leemans CR, Tiwari R. Management of cervical lymph nodes in patients with head and neck cancer. *Eur Arch Otorhinolaryngol* 1992;249:187–94.
15. Snow GB, van den Brekel MW, Leemans CR, Patel P. Surgical management of cervical lymph nodes in patients with oral and oropharyngeal cancer. *Recent Results Cancer Res* 1994;134:43–55.
16. Spiro RH, Alfonso AE, Farr HW, Strong EW. Cervical node metastasis from epidermoid carcinoma of the oral cavity and oropharynx. A critical assessment of current staging. *Am J Surg* 1974;128:562–7.
17. Spiro RH. The management of neck nodes in head and neck cancer: a surgeon's view. *Bull N Y Acad Med* 1985;61:629–37.
18. Shah J, Andersen P. Evolving role of modifications in neck dissections for oral squamous cell carcinoma. *Br J Oral Maxillofac Surg* 1995;33:3–8.
19. Shah JP, Andersen PE. The impact of patterns of nodal metastasis on modifications of neck dissection. *Ann Surg Oncol* 1994;1:521–32.
20. Shah J. Indications, rationale, and techniques in neck dissection. In: Najarian J, Delaney J (eds). *Progress in Cancer Surgery.* St Louis: Mosby Year Book, 1991. 262–73.
21. Shah JP, Candela FC, Poddar AK. The patterns of cervical lymph node metastases from squamous carcinoma of the oral cavity. *Cancer* 1990;66:109–13.
22. Shah JP. Patterns of cervical lymph node metastasis from squamous carcinomas of the upper aerodigestive tract. *Am J Surg* 1990;160:405–9.
23. Robbins KT. Classification of neck dissection: current concepts and future considerations [in process citation]. *Otolaryngol Clin North Am* 1998;31:639–55.
24. Robbins KT, Medina JE, Wolfe GT, Levine PA, Sessions RB, Pruet CW. Standardizing neck dissection terminology. Official report of the Academy's Committee for Head and Neck Surgery and Oncology [see comments]. *Arch Otolaryngol Head Neck Surg* 1991;117:601–5.
25. Medina JE. A rational classification of neck dissections. *Otolaryngol Head Neck Surg* 1989;100:169–76.
26. Medina JE, Byers RM. Supraomohyoid neck dissection: rationale, indications, and surgical technique. *Head Neck* 1989;11:111–22.
27. Lindberg R. Distribution of cervical node metastasis from squamous cell carcinoma of the upper respiratory and digestive tracts. *Cancer* 1972;29:1446–9.
28. Ballantyne A. Significance of retropharyngeal nodes in cancer of the head and neck. *Am J Surg* 1964;108:500–3.
29. Kalnins IK, Leonard AG, Sako K, Razack MS, Shedd DP. Correlation between prognosis and degree of lymph node involvement in carcinoma of the oral cavity. *Am J Surg* 1977;134:450–4.
30. Tytor M, Olofsson J. Prognostic factors in oral cavity carcinomas. *Acta Otolaryngol Suppl* 1992;492:75–8.
31. Johnson JT, Myers EN, Bedetti CD, Barnes EL, Schramm VL Jr, Thearle PB. Cervical lymph node metastases. Incidence and implications of extracapsular carcinoma. *Arch Otolaryngol* 1985;111:534–7.
32. Andersen PE, Cambronero E, Shaha AR, Shah JP. The extent of neck disease after regional failure during observation of the N0 neck. *Am J Surg* 1996;172:689–91.

33. Alvi A, Johnson JT. Extracapsular spread in the clinically negative neck (N0): implications and outcome. *Otolaryngol Head Neck Surg* 1996; 114:65–70.
34. Zelefsky MJ, Harrison LB, Fass DE et al. Postoperative radiotherapy for oral cavity cancers: impact of anatomic subsite on treatment outcome. *Head Neck* 1990;12:470–5.
35. Carter RL, Barr LC, O'Brien CJ, Soo KC, Shaw HJ. Transcapsular spread of metastatic squamous cell carcinoma from cervical lymph nodes. *Am J Surg* 1985;150:495–9.
36. Byers RM, El-Naggar AK, Lee YY et al. Can we detect or predict the presence of occult nodal metastases in patients with squamous carcinoma of the oral tongue? *Head Neck* 1998;20: 138–44.
37. Spiro RH, Huvos AG, Wong GY, Spiro JD, Gnecco CA, Strong EW. Predictive value of tumor thickness in squamous carcinoma confined to the tongue and floor of the mouth. *Am J Surg* 1986;152:345–50.
38. Candela FC, Kothari K, Shah JP. Patterns of cervical node metastases from squamous carcinoma of the oropharynx and hypopharynx. *Head Neck* 1990;12:197–203.
39. Cummings C, Goepfert H, Myers E. Squamous cell carcinoma of the base of the tongue. *Head Neck Surg* 1986;9:56–9.
40. Leemans CR, Engelbrecht WJ, Tiwari R et al. Carcinoma of the soft palate and anterior tonsillar pillar. *Laryngoscope* 1994;104:1477–81.
41. Byers RM, Weber RS, Andrews T, McGill D, Kare R, Wolf P. Frequency and therapeutic implications of "skip metastases" in the neck from squamous carcinoma of the oral tongue [see comments]. *Head Neck* 1997;19:14–9.
42. Davidson BJ, Kulkarny V, Delacure MD, Shah JP. Posterior triangle metastases of squamous cell carcinoma of the upper aerodigestive tract. *Am J Surg* 1993;166:395–8.
43. van den Brekel MW, Castelijns JA Stel HV et al. Occult metastatic neck disease: detection with US and US-guided fine-needle aspiration. *Radiology* 1991;180:457–61.
44. Shaha A, Webber C, Marti J. Fine-needle aspiration in the diagnosis of cervical lymphadenopathy. *Am J Surg* 1986;152:420–3.
45. van den Brekel MW, Stel HV, Castelijns JA et al. Cervical lymph node metastasis: assessment of radiologic criteria. *Radiology* 1990;177:379–84.
46. van den Brekel MW, Castelijns JA, Stel HV et al. Detection and characterization of metastatic cervical adenopathy by MR imaging: comparison of different MR techniques. *J Comput Assist Tomogr* 1990;14:581–9.
47. van den Brekel MW, Stel HV, Castelijns JA, Croll GJ, Snow GB. Lymph node staging in patients with clinically negative neck examinations by ultrasound and ultrasound-guided aspiration cytology. *Am J Surg* 1991;162:362–6.
48. van den Brekel MW, Castelijns JA, Croll GA et al. Magnetic resonance imaging vs palpation of cervical lymph node metastasis. *Arch Otolaryngol Head Neck Surg* 1991;117:663–73.
49. van den Brekel MW, Snow GB. Assessment of lymph node metastases in the neck. *Eur J Cancer B Oral Oncol* 1994;30:88–92.
50. Kang CJ, Lin CY, Yang LY et al. Positive clinical impact of an additional PET/CT scan before adjuvant radiotherapy or concurrent chemoradiotherapy in patients with advanced oral cavity squamous cell carcinoma. *J Nucl Med* 2015;56:22–30.
51. Schechter NR, Gillenwater AM, Byers RM et al. Can positron emission tomography improve the quality of care for head-and-neck cancer patients? *Int J Radiat Oncol Biol Phys* 2001;51:4–9.
52. Yao M, Smith RB, Graham MM et al. The role of FDG PET in management of neck metastasis from head-and-neck cancer after definitive radiation treatment. *Int J Radiat Oncol Biol Phys* 2005;63:991–9.
53. Yao M, Luo P, Hoffman H et al. Pathology and FDG PET correlation of residual lymph nodes in head and neck cancer after radiation treatment. *Am J Clin Oncol* 2007;30:264–70.
54. Shah J, Kraus D. Radical neck dissection and its modifications. In: Donohue J, Heerden JV, Monson J. (eds). *Atlas of Surgical Oncology*. Cambridge: Blackwell Science, 1994, 75–82.
55. Martin H. The case for prophylactic neck dissection. *CA Cancer J Clin* 1951;4:92–7.
56. Hughes CJ, Gallo O, Spiro RH, Shah JP. Management of occult neck metastases in oral cavity squamous carcinoma. *Am J Surg* 1993;166:380–3.
57. Ho CM, Lam KH, Wei WI, Lau SK, Lam LK. Occult lymph node metastasis in small oral tongue cancers. *Head Neck* 1992;14:359–63.
58. Kurita H, Kurashina K, Minemura T, Kotani A. Pitfalls in the treatment of delayed lymph-node metastases after control of small tongue carcinomas. *Int J Oral Maxillofac Surg* 1995;24:356–60.
59. van den Brekel MW, van der Waal I, Meijer CJ, Freeman JL, Castelijns JA, Snow GB. The incidence of micro-metastases in neck dissection specimens obtained from elective neck dissections. *Laryngoscope* 1996;106:987–91.
60. McGuirt WF Jr, Johnson JT, Myers EN, Rothfield R, Wagner R. Floor of mouth carcinoma. The management of the clinically negative neck. *Arch Otolaryngol Head Neck Surg* 1995;121:278–82.
61. Yuen AP, Wei W, Wong YM, Tang KG. Elective neck dissection versus observation in the treatment

of early oral tongue carcinoma. *Head Neck* 1997;19:583–8.
62. Vandenbrouck C, Sancho-Garnier H, Chassagne D, Saravane D, Cachin Y, Micheau C. Elective versus therapeutic radical neck dissection in epidermoid carcinoma of the oral cavity: results of a randomized clinical trial. *Cancer* 1980; 46:386–90.
63. Shrime MG, Bachar G, Lea J et al. Nodal ratio as an independent predictor of survival in squamous cell carcinoma of the oral cavity. *Head Neck* 2009;31:1482–8.
64. Gil Z, Carlson DL, Boyle JO et al. Lymph node density is a significant predictor of outcome in patients with oral cancer. *Cancer* 2009;115:5700–10.
65. Kraus DH, Rosenberg DB, Davidson BJ et al. Supraspinal accessory lymph node metastases in supraomohyoid neck dissection. *Am J Surg* 1996;172:646–9.
66. Remmler D, Byers R, Scheetz J et al. A prospective study of shoulder disability resulting from radical and modified neck dissections. *Head Neck Surg* 1986;8:280–6.
67. Soboi S, Jensen C, Sawyer WD, Costiloe P, Thong N. Objective comparison of physical dysfunction after neck dissection. *Am J Surg* 1985;150:503–9.
68. Leipzig B, Suen JY, English JL, Barnes J, Hooper M. Functional evaluation of the spinal accessory nerve after neck dissection. *Am J Surg* 1983;146:526–30.
69. DeSanto LW, Beahrs OH. Modified and complete neck dissection in the treatment of squamous cell carcinoma of the head and neck. *Surg Gynecol Obstet* 1988:167:259–69.
70. Spiro RH, Gallo O, Shah JP. Selective jugular node dissection in patients with squamous carcinoma of the larynx or pharynx. *Am J Surg* 1993;166:399–402.
71. Lingeman RE, Helmus C, Stephens R, Ulm J. Neck dissection: radical or conservative. *Ann Otol Rhinol Laryngol* 1977;86:737–44.
72. Byers RM. Modified neck dissection. A study of 967 cases from 1970 to 1980. *Am J Surg* 1985;150:414–21.
73. Byers RM, Wolf PF, Ballantyne AJ. Rationale for elective modified neck dissection. *Head Neck Surg* 1988;10:160–7.
74. Spiro JD, Spiro RH, Shah JP, Sessions RB, Strong EW. Critical assessment of supraomohyoid neck dissection. *Am J Surg* 1988;156:286–9.
75. Spiro RH, Strong EW, Shah JP. Classification of neck dissection: variations on a new theme. *Am J Surg* 1994;168:415–8.
76. Spiro RH, Morgan GJ, Strong EW, Shah JP. Supraomohyoid neck dissection. *Am J Surg* 1996;172:650–3.
77. Den Toom IJ, Heuveling DA, Flach GB et al. Sentinel node biopsy for early-stage oral cavity cancer: the VU University Medical Center experience. *Head Neck* 2015;37:573–8.
78. Ross G, Shoaib T, Soutar DS et al. The use of sentinel node biopsy to upstage the clinically N0 neck in head and neck cancer. *Arch Otolaryngol Head Neck Surg* 2002;128:1287–91.
79. Stoeckli SJ, Alkureishi LW, Ross GL. Sentinel node biopsy for early oral and oropharyngeal squamous cell carcinoma. *Eur Arch Otorhinolaryngol* 2009;266:787–93.
80. Suen JY, Goepfert H. Standardization of neck dissection nomenclature. *Head Neck Surg* 1987;10:75–7.
81. Bernier J, Domenge C, Ozsahin M et al. European Organization for Research and Treatment of Cancer Trial 22931. Postoperative irradiation with or without concomitant chemotherapy for locally advanced head and neck cancer. *N Engl J Med* 2004;350:1945–52.
82. Vikram B. Adjuvant therapy in head and neck cancer. *CA Cancer J Clin* 1998;48:199–209.
83. Bartelink H, Breur K, Hart G, Annyas B, van Slooten E, Snow G. The value of postoperative radiotherapy as an adjuvant to radical neck dissection. *Cancer* 1983;52:1008–13.
84. Peters LJ, Goepfert H, Ang KK et al. Evaluation of the dose for postoperative radiation therapy of head and neck cancer: first report of a prospective randomized trial. *Int J Radiat Oncol Biol Phys* 1993;26:3–11.
85. Cooper JS, Pajak TF, Forastiere AA et al. Radiation Therapy Oncology Group 9501/Intergroup. Postoperative concurrent radiotherapy and chemotherapy for high-risk squamous-cell carcinoma of the head and neck. *N Engl J Med* 2004;350:1937–44.
86. Bernier J, Cooper JS, Pajak TF et al. Defining risk levels in locally advanced head and neck cancers: a comparative analysis of concurrent postoperative radiation plus chemotherapy trials of the EORTC (#22931) and RTOG (# 9501). *Head Neck* 2005;27:843–50.
87. Chaturvedi AK, Engels EA, Pfeiffer RM et al. Human papillomavirus and rising oropharyngeal cancer incidence in the United States. *J Clin Oncol* 2011;29:4294–301.
88. Garden AS, Gunn GB, Hessel A et al. Management of the lymph node-positive neck in the patient with human papillomavirus-associated oropharyngeal cancer. *Cancer* 2014;120:3082–8.
89. Vikram B, Strong EW, Shah JP, Spiro R. Failure in the neck following multimodality treatment for advanced head and neck cancer. *Head Neck Surg* 1984;6:724–9.
90. Lore JM Jr. Early diagnosis and treatment of head and neck cancer [editorial]. *CA Cancer J Clin* 1995;45:325–7.
91. Whitehurst JO, Droulias CA. Surgical treatment of squamous cell carcinoma of the oral tongue: factors influencing survival. *Arch Otolaryngol* 1977;103:212–5.

92. Centers for Disease Control. Current trends: deaths from oral cavity and pharyngeal cancer—United States, 1987. *JAMA* 1990;264:678.
93. Sankaranarayanan R. Oral cancer in India: an epidemiologic and clinical review. *Oral Surg Oral Med Oral Pathol* 1990;69:325–30.
94. Hindle I, Downer MC, Speight PM. The epidemiology of oral cancer. *Br J Oral Maxillofac Surg* 1996;34:471–6.
95. Hoffman HT, Karnell LH, Funk GF, Robinson RA, Menck HR. The national cancer data base report on cancer of the head and neck. *Arch Otolaryngol Head Neck Surg* 1998;124:951–62.
96. Boyle P, Macfarlane GJ, Zheng T, Maisonneuve P, Evstifeeva T, Scully C. Recent advances in epidemiology of head and neck cancer. *Curr Opin Oncol* 1992;4:471–7.
97. Plesko I, Obsitnikova A, Vlasak V. Increasing occurrence of oropharyngeal cancers among males in Slovakia. *Neoplasma* 1997;44:77–83.
98. Swango PA. Cancers of the oral cavity and pharynx in the United States: an epidemiologic overview. *J Public Health Dent* 1996;56:309–18.
99. Ong SC, Schöder H, Lee NY et al. Clinical utility of ^{18}F-FDG PET/CT in assessing the neck after concurrent chemoradiotherapy for locoregional advanced head and neck cancer. *J Nucl Med* 2008;49:532–40.
100. Amit M, Yen TC, Liao CT et al. The origin of regional failure in oral cavity squamous cell carcinoma with pathologically negative neck metastases. *JAMA Otolaryngol Head Neck Surg* 2014;140:1130–7.

11

Surgical approaches to oral cavity and oropharynx

PABLO H. MONTERO AND JATIN P. SHAH

SURGICAL APPROACHES TO THE ORAL CAVITY

Surgery remains the mainstay for nearly all tumors of the oral cavity. On the other hand, non-surgical approaches have shown equally effective tumor control and better functional outcomes in selected patients with tumors of the oropharynx. This is particularly true for human papillomavirus (HPV)-positive tumors. However, significant short-term toxicities and long-term functional sequelae result from definitive radiotherapy with chemotherapy for oropharyngeal carcinomas. Therefore, currently there are several clinical trials accruing patients for considering "de-intensification" of treatment for HPV-positive oropharynx cancers, with a resurgence of interest in surgical extirpation in selected patients. Until the results of these trials are available, surgery should be considered only in very selected patients with low-volume (T1, T2) primary tumors and low-volume (N0, N1, without extranodal extension [ENE]) nodal disease to avoid the addition of chemotherapy to postoperative radiation and thus reduce long-term functional sequelae of treatment.

Multiple surgical approaches have been described for resection of primary oral cavity tumors, including peroral, mandibulotomy, lower cheek flap, visor flap and upper cheek flap approaches, as shown in Figure 11.1. The selection of a particular approach depends on several factors, including the tumor size and site, depth of infiltration and proximity to the mandible or maxilla (1–20). The principles of an adequate oncological resection should not be compromised by efforts to minimize the extent of the procedure.

GENERAL CONSIDERATIONS

Excision of small primary lesions located in the anterior aspect of the oral cavity and easily accessible through the open mouth can be accomplished even under local anesthesia. However, resection of most oral cavity tumors requires general endotracheal anesthesia and adequate muscle relaxation. Nasotracheal intubation is preferable in this setting, since it facilitates surgical access, exposure and instrumentation of the oral cavity during surgery. Peroral intubation and endotracheal tube fixation with tape can distort facial skin lines, resulting in misplaced incisions. Accordingly, surgical incisions are marked out prior to endotracheal intubation. In patients with bulky, potentially obstructive oropharyngeal tumors, a preliminary tracheostomy is performed under local anesthesia prior to the induction of general anesthesia.

Ideally, the patient is placed on the operating table in the supine position with the upper half of the body elevated at 30° (Figure 11.2). Careful assessment of the primary tumor with examination under anesthesia at this juncture is crucial to facilitate thorough understanding of the three-dimensional extent of the tumor, as well as invasion or the proximity of adjacent structures. The head and neck region

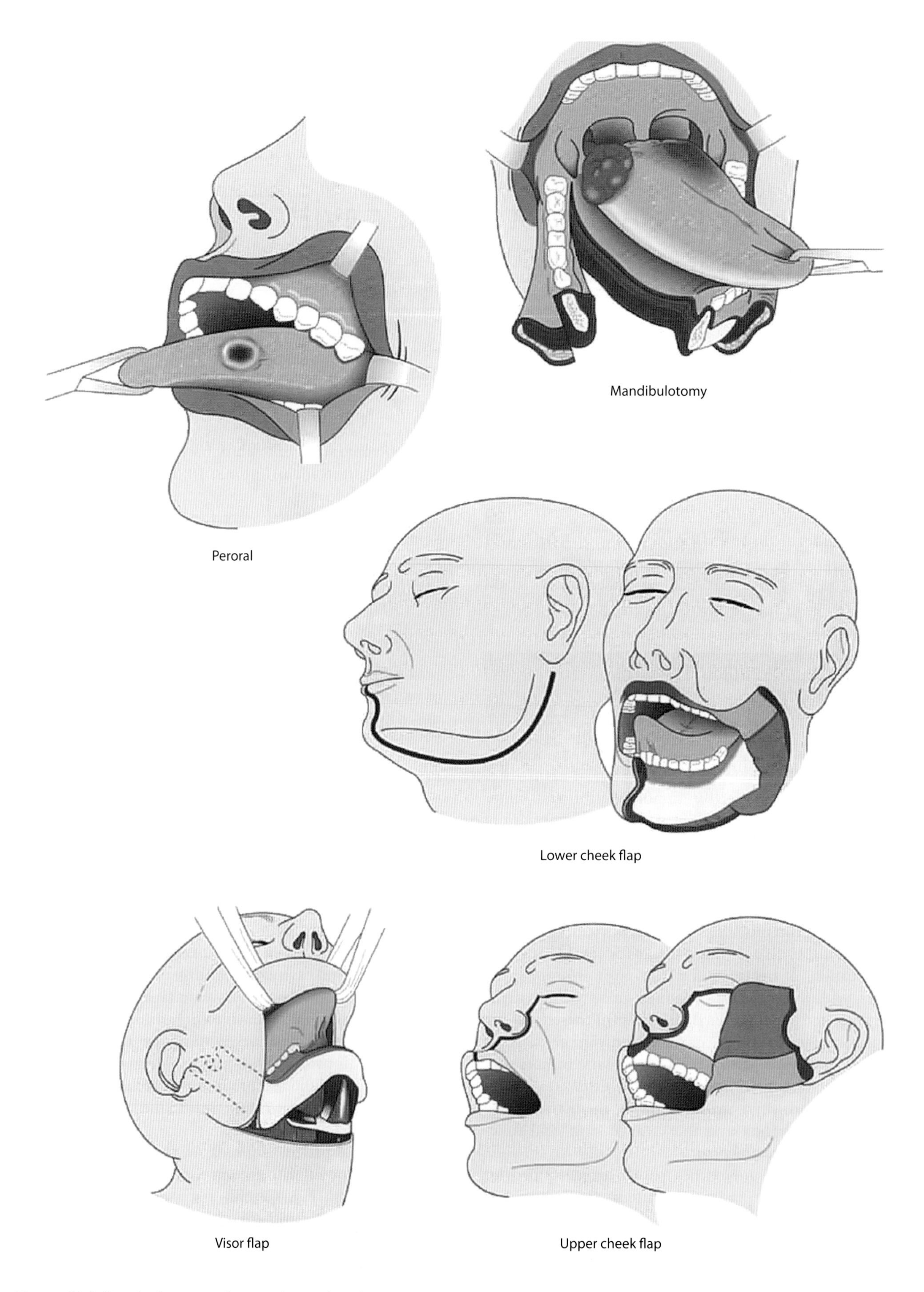

Figure 11.1 Surgical approaches to the oral cavity.

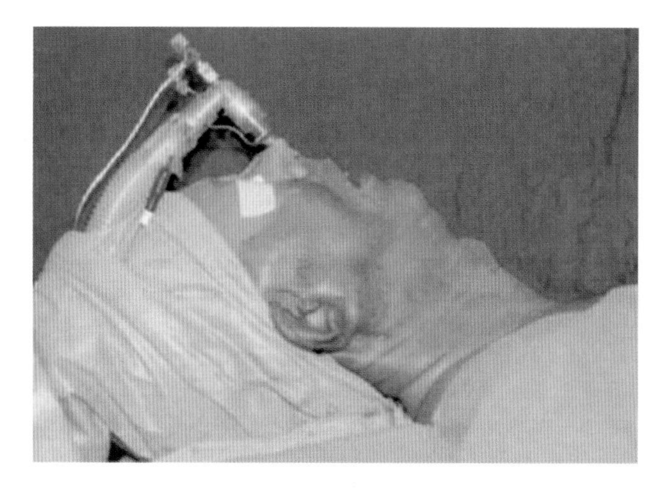

Figure 11.2 Position of the patient on the operating table.

is then prepared with antiseptic solution (Betadine; Purdue Frederick, Stamford, CT, U.S.A.) and draped according to whether the planned operative approach is solely intraoral or will require external incision either on the face or the neck. A transparent plastic drape is used to isolate the anesthetic tubing, with care taken to ensure that the patient's eyes, nose and endotracheal tube are clearly visible to both the surgeon and the anesthesiologist (Figure 11.3).

PERORAL SURGICAL APPROACH

Small tumors in easily accessible locations of the oral cavity are safely excised *via* an open mouth approach (Figure 11.4). Thus, small primary tumors of the oral tongue, floor of the mouth, gum, cheek mucosa and hard or soft palate are suitable for peroral excision. However, in patients with trismus or restricted oral apertures to provide access to the tumor, alternative approaches are required to allow for satisfactory resection.

Peroral partial glossectomy

All T1 and most T2 lesions of the oral tongue—that is, the anterior two-thirds of the tongue—are suitable for a partial

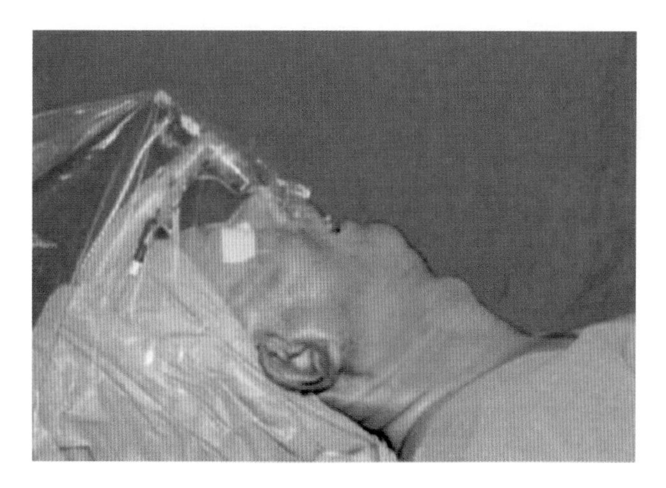

Figure 11.3 A transparent plastic drape provides a view of the anesthetic tubing and eyes.

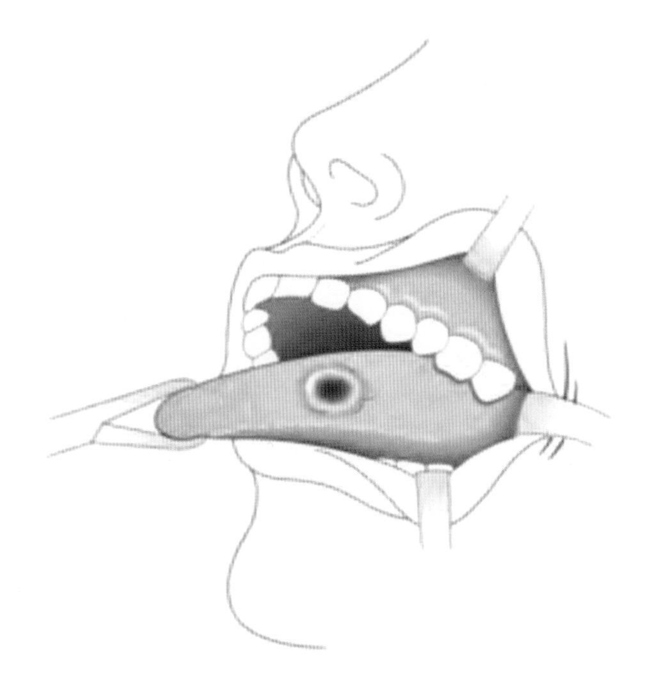

Figure 11.4 Peroral approach.

glossectomy through the open mouth. Tumors involving the lateral aspect of the oral tongue are amenable to a wedge excision oriented in a transverse fashion. Longitudinally oriented excision of a large tumor results in an elongated narrow tongue that often impairs speech and interferes with mastication. In contrast, transversely oriented wedge resections foreshorten the tongue, resulting in functionally and cosmetically superior results.

The procedure is best performed by electrocautery. First, the cutting current is used to incise the mucosa of the tongue on both its superior and inferior aspects. Following the mucosal incision, the coagulating current is used for resection of the underlying musculature of the tongue. Minor bleeding points in the musculature of the tongue are electrocoagulated while major branches of the lingual artery are ligated with chromic catgut. The excision should include a generous margin of the mucosa around the tumor and a full complement of the (third-dimension) thickness of the musculature of the tongue surrounding the palpable tumor. Frozen sections are taken from the mucosal margins, as well as from the depth of the surgical defect, to ensure adequate excision of the primary tumor. Repair of the surgical defect follows confirmation of negative margins by frozen section and attainment of complete hemostasis. A skin hook is used to retract the apex of the wedge-shaped surgical defect for transverse orientation of the closure. A two-layered closure is performed using interrupted 000 chromic catgut or 000 Vicryl sutures to approximate the musculature and the superior and inferior mucosal aspects of the tongue. Blood loss during the procedure is negligible. The patient can take clear liquids by mouth within 24–48 hours and is allowed a pureed diet on the third postoperative day. Most patients will be able to tolerate a soft diet by the end of the week.

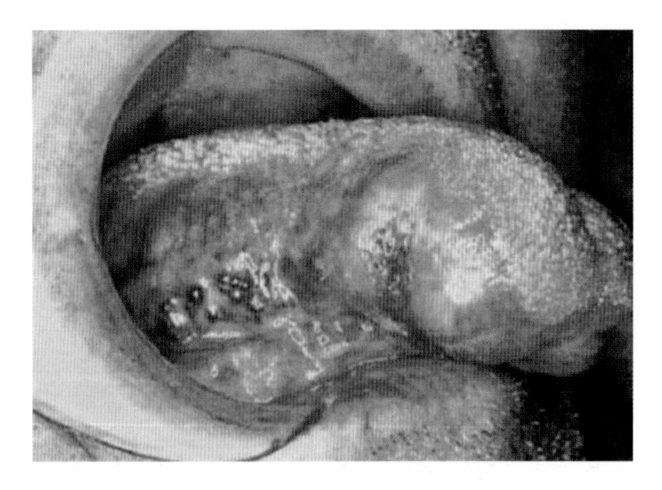

Figure 11.5 Squamous carcinoma of the lateral border of the oral tongue.

Initially, there is some degree of speech impairment, which improves as healing progresses and mobility of the tongue improve.

The lesion shown in Figure 11.5 is an ulcerated, endophytic, 2.5-cm carcinoma involving the right lateral border of the anterior and middle third of the tongue. The tumor does not extend across the midline, nor does it involve the adjacent floor of the mouth. Mobility of the tongue is not restricted. The steps of the operation are shown schematically in Figure 11.6.

The procedure is performed under general anesthesia with nasotracheal intubation. The oral cavity is isolated and cleaned with Betadine solution. A wedge-shaped incision is illustrated in Figure 11.7. The surgical specimen demonstrates full-thickness, three-dimensional resection of the tumor of the oral tongue with adequate mucosal and soft tissue margins (Figure 11.8). The surgical defect demonstrates satisfactory excision of the primary tumor (Figure 11.9). A two-layered closure is performed with interrupted catgut sutures. The postoperative appearance of the tongue approximately 3 months after partial glossectomy is shown in Figure 11.10. Note the transverse scar at the suture line, giving a normal configuration of the oral tongue. The patient now has practically no speech impairment and is able to tolerate all types of food by mouth.

Excision of the floor of the mouth and skin graft

Peroral excision can be performed for superficial lesions of the floor of the mouth, cheek mucosa or soft palate, leaving the surgical defect open to granulate and heal by secondary intention. However, when such an excision is in critical areas where mobility is essential or when the depth of excision extends to the underlying musculature, then healing by secondary intention leads to fibrosis and contracture, causing impairment of function. In these cases, it is desirable to cover such surgical defects with a full-thickness skin graft.

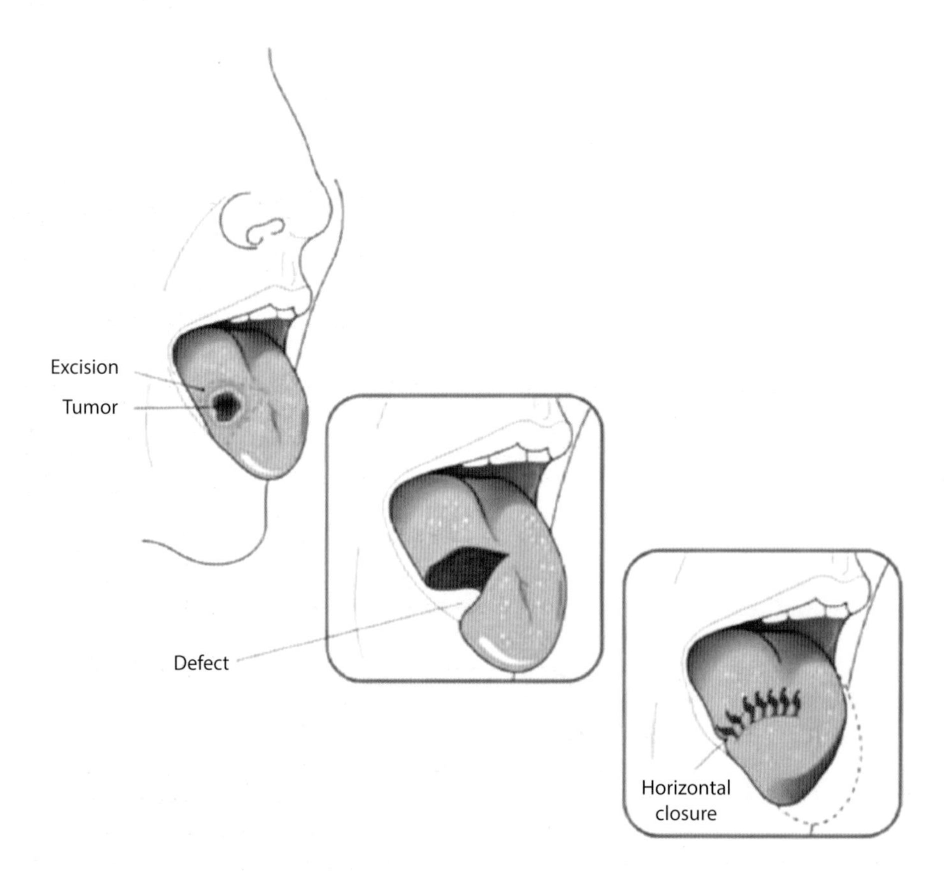

Figure 11.6 Transversely oriented wedge resection of tongue tumor.

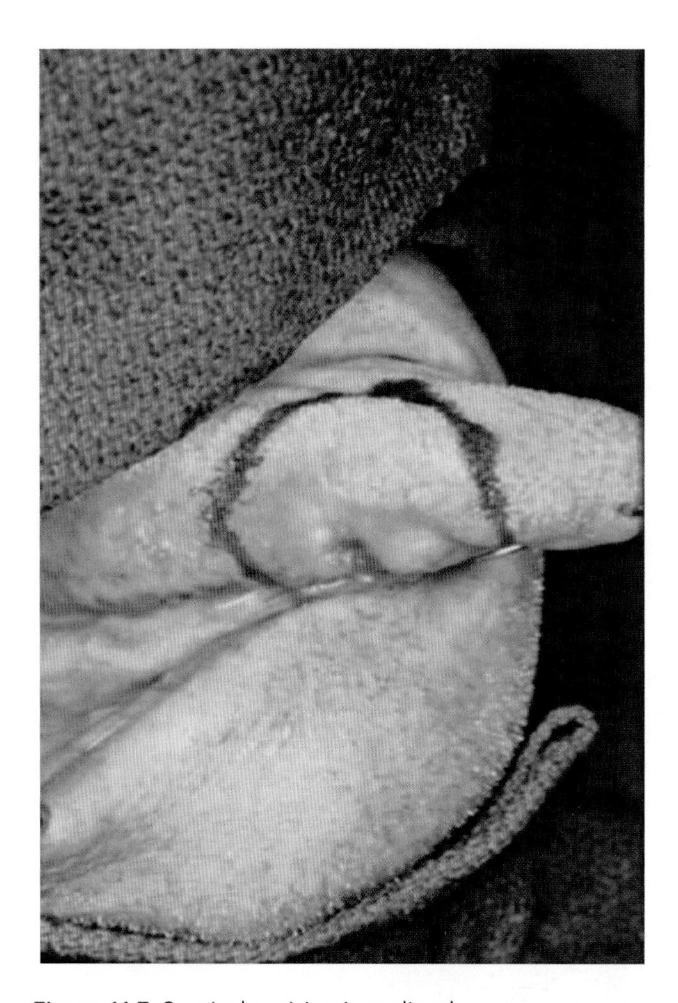

Figure 11.7 Surgical excision is outlined.

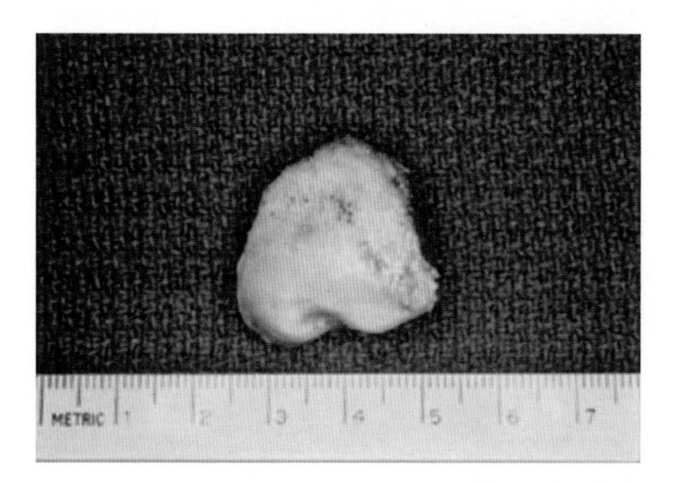

Figure 11.8 Wedge-shaped surgical specimen.

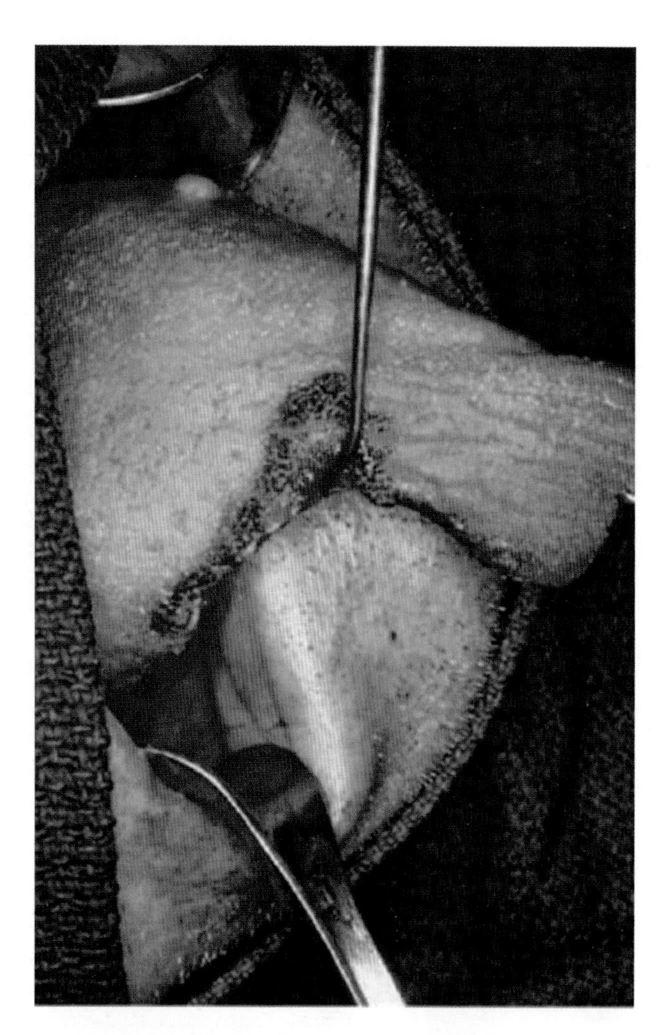

Figure 11.9 Wedge-shaped surgical defect.

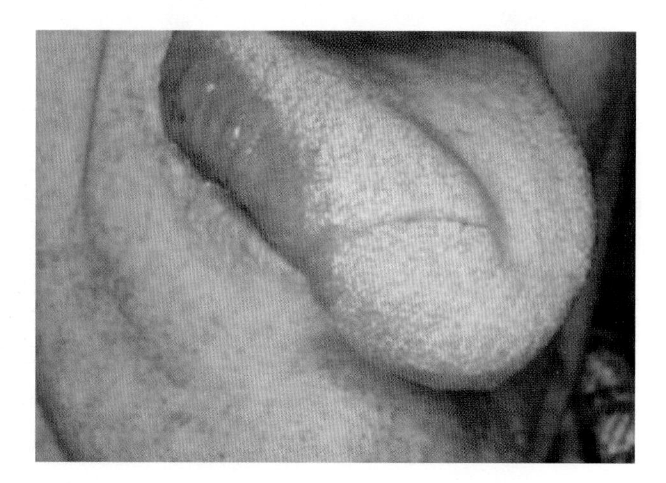

Figure 11.10 Postoperative appearance of the tongue at 3 months.

The patient shown in Figure 11.11 has squamous carcinoma of the anterior floor of the mouth invading the openings of Wharton's ducts on both sides. A generous margin around the tumor is obtained by the incision outlined with electrocautery (Figure 11.12). Excision of the lesion, including the underlying sublingual glands, is performed in a three-dimensional fashion (Figure 11.13). Note that Wharton's ducts are isolated bilaterally. The ducts are transected and tagged with a suture and the specimen is delivered. The surgical defect shows the underlying genioglossus muscle (Figure 11.14). The stumps of Wharton's ducts are transposed and sutured to the posterior edge of the mucosal defect and the skin graft.

The full-thickness skin graft is harvested from one of several areas, including the supraclavicular area of the neck. The skin graft is appropriately trimmed and sutured to the mucosal edges of the surgical defect using 000 chromic catgut interrupted sutures (Figure 11.15). Several stab incisions are made in the skin graft after it is sutured in place to permit drainage of blood and/or serum that may accumulate beneath the graft. A xeroform gauze bolster is made to fit the area of the skin graft and is anchored in position with 00 silk tie-over sutures (Figure 11.16). The patient is not allowed to take anything by mouth until the bolster

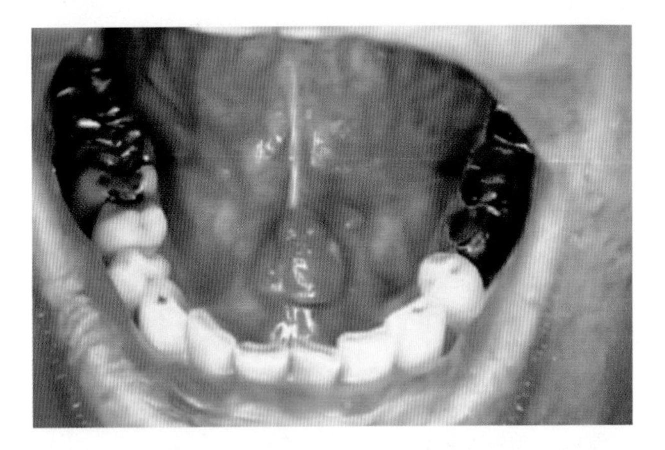

Figure 11.11 Squamous carcinoma of the anterior floor of the mouth.

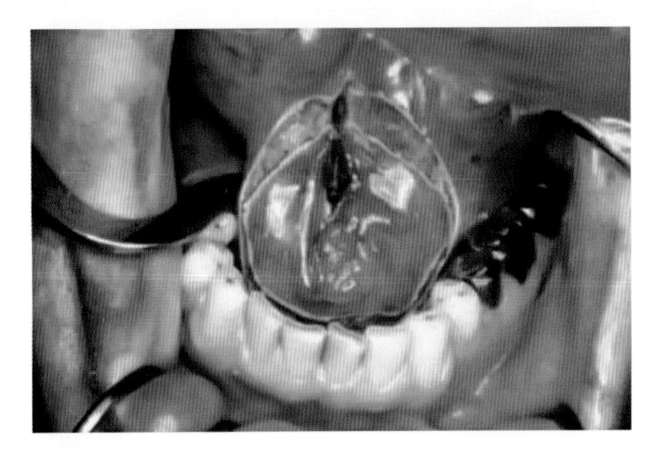

Figure 11.12 A circumferential mucosal incision is placed.

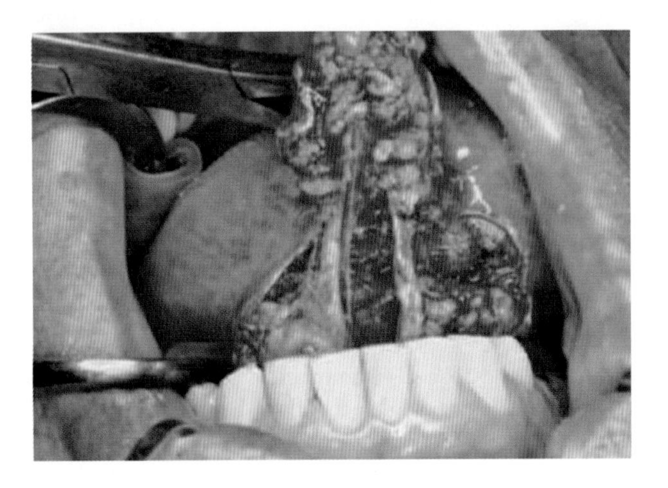

Figure 11.13 Wharton's ducts are dissected.

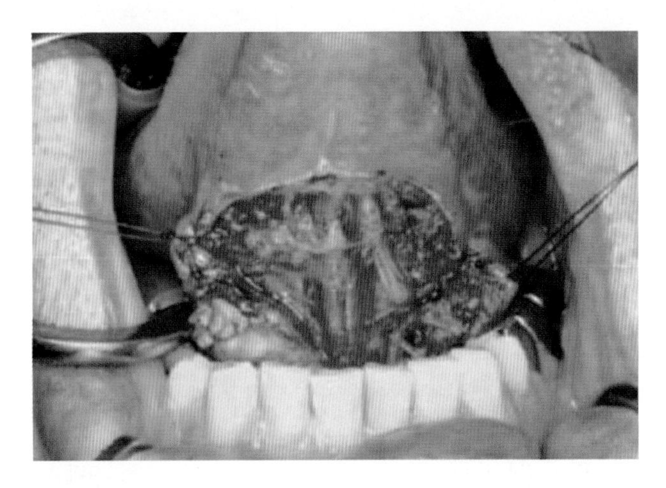

Figure 11.14 Wharton's ducts are resected and transposed.

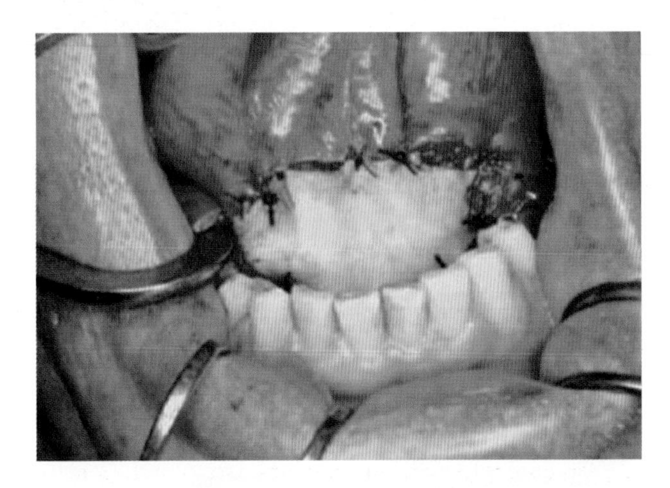

Figure 11.15 A skin graft is applied to the defect.

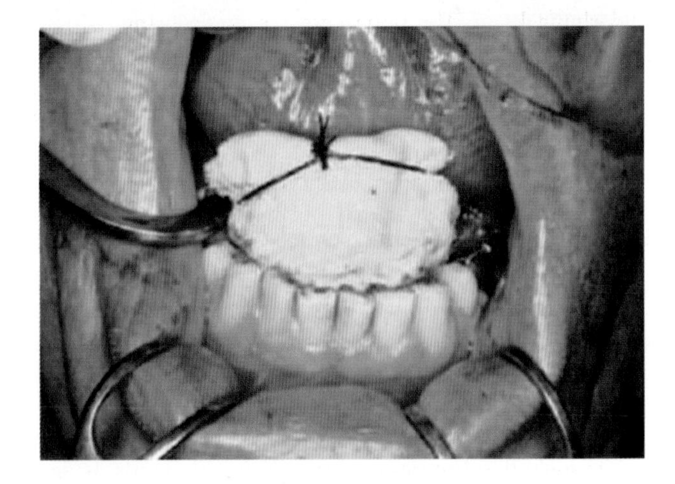

Figure 11.16 Bolus dressing holds the skin graft in position.

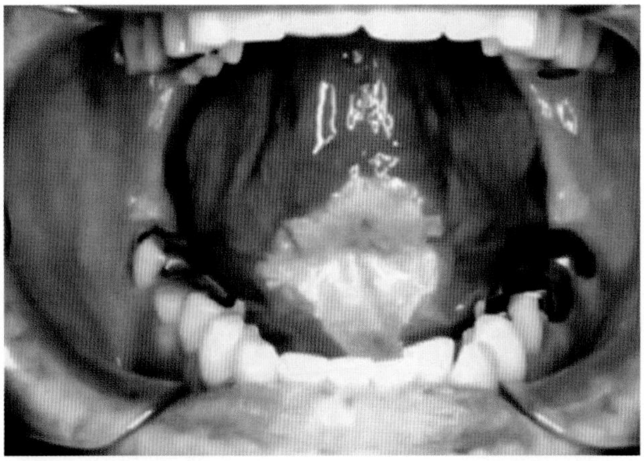

Figure 11.17 Healed skin graft at 8 weeks following surgery.

dressing is removed at approximately 1 week. Optimal oral hygiene is maintained with oral irrigation until the graft has satisfactorily healed. The patient can then take clear liquids and pureed foods by mouth. The postoperative appearance of the skin graft at approximately 8 weeks following surgery shows complete healing with normal mobility of the tongue, with no deficit in mastication or clarity of speech (Figure 11.17).

Peroral partial maxillectomy

Consideration for peroral tumor excision can also be extended to small tumors of dentoalveolar or mucosal origin of the upper alveolus *via* peroral alveolectomy or partial maxillectomy. However, it is important to remember that adequate radiographic assessment of the extent of bone invasion by the tumor is mandatory prior to embarking on this surgical procedure.

For anterior maxillary lesions, the first stage in the surgical procedure is to outline a circular incision in the mucosa around the visible tumor by electrocautery. The mucosal incision is then deepened through the soft tissue up to the underlying bone. The bone cuts are made using a high-speed saw and the specimen is fractured by the use of osteotomes. Every effort is made to achieve a monobloc removal and to avoid fragmentation of the specimen. The interior of the maxillary antrum is inspected for any pathology after completion of the tumor excision. If the mucosa of the antrum appears edematous, then it is curetted out as far as possible. If the mucosa appears normal and there is no other pathology within the maxillary antrum, then it is best left undisturbed.

Resection of posterior alveolar and maxillary tubercle lesions can also be accomplished in a similar manner. However, the pterygoid muscles will be exposed in the surgical defect, requiring skin grafting to avoid fibrosis and resultant trismus. A split-thickness skin graft is harvested from a suitable donor site and sutured to the edges of the mucosal defect with absorbable sutures. The graft is held in position with xeroform gauze packing and a dental obturator. If grafting is not required, then the maxillary antrum is packed with xeroform gauze and a temporary dental obturator is wired to the remaining teeth. The packing is left in position for approximately 1 week, but the patient can take liquids and pureed food by mouth from the first postoperative day. While the packing is in place, optimal oral hygiene is maintained by frequent oral irrigations and sprays in the oral cavity with half-strength hydrogen peroxide solution. The surgical dental obturator and the packing are removed after 1 week and an interim dental obturator with a soft liner is fabricated, which is used until soft tissue healing is complete.

The patient shown in Figure 11.18 has a squamous carcinoma arising on the buccal surface of the upper gum. The tumor is adherent to the underlying alveolar process of the maxilla. A computed tomography (CT) scan shows minimal bone invasion (Figure 11.19). The surgical specimen shows the canine and premolar teeth with a generous margin of mucosa, soft tissue and bone around the resected tumor (Figure 11.20). The postoperative view of the oral cavity approximately 3 months after the surgical procedure shows a well-healed surgical defect leading to the maxillary antrum (Figure 11.21). The permanent dental obturator is

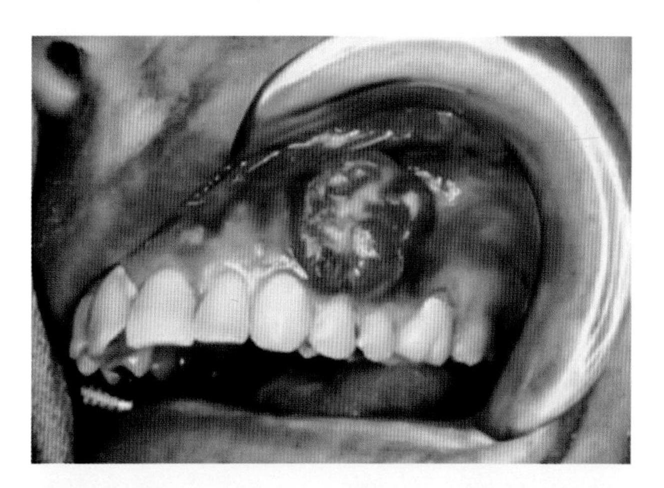

Figure 11.18 Squamous carcinoma of the left upper gum.

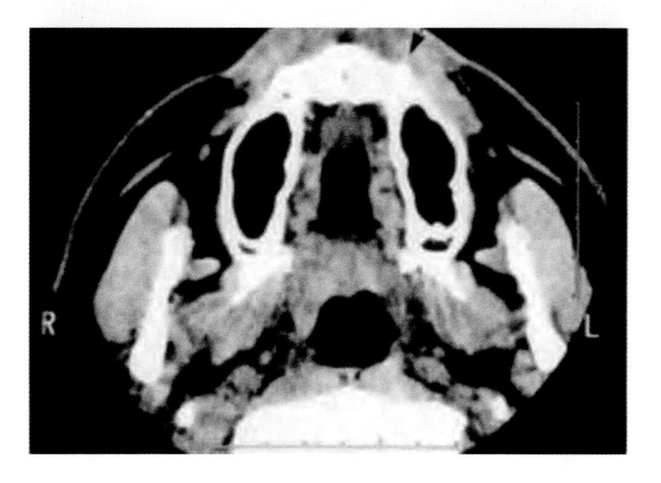

Figure 11.19 A CT scan showing minimal bone erosion.

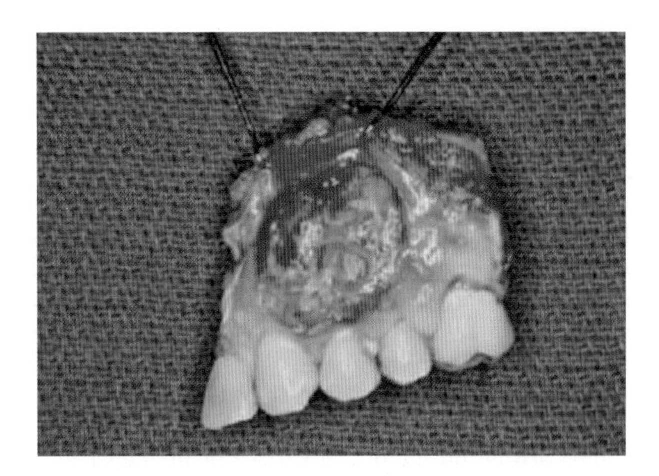

Figure 11.20 Surgical specimen showing adequate margins in all three dimensions.

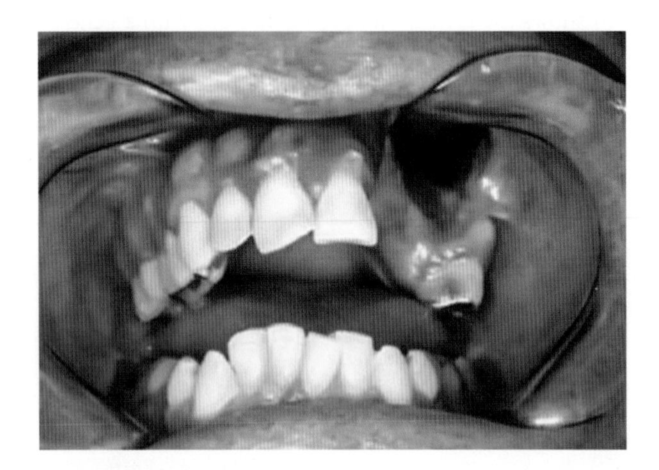

Figure 11.21 Healed surgical defect 3 months following surgery.

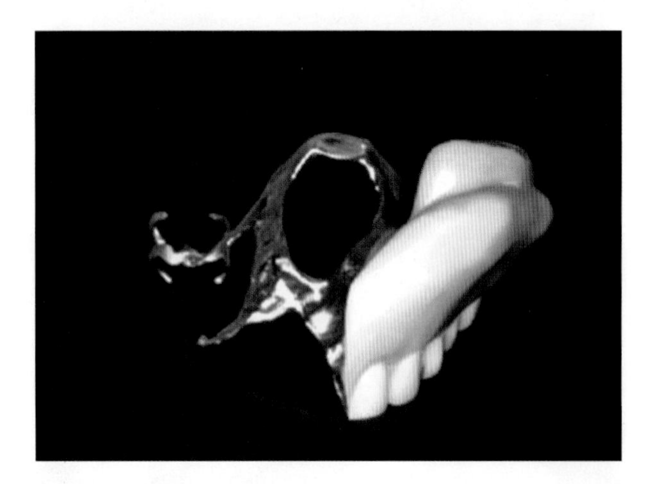

Figure 11.22 The dental obturator.

now made, which provides a plug to obliterate the opening of the maxillary antrum in the oral cavity and replaces the missing teeth (Figure 11.22). The patient is able to tolerate a regular diet by mouth and has no functional impairment with mastication or speech (Figure 11.23).

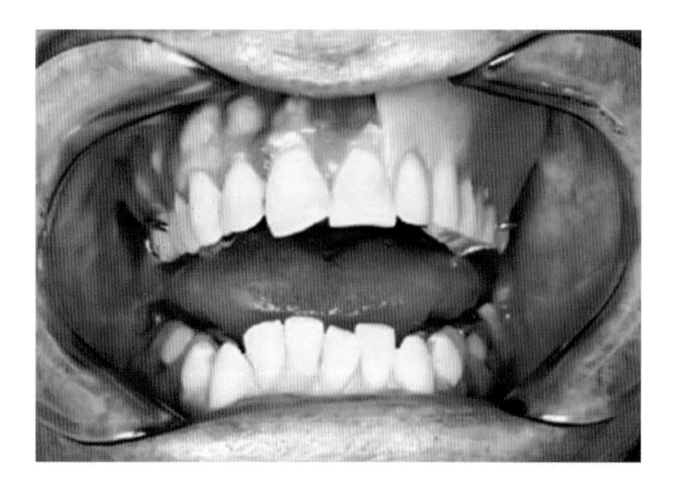

Figure 11.23 The dental obturator in place in the oral cavity.

MANAGEMENT OF THE MANDIBLE

Management of the mandible is an important consideration in oral cancer surgery for two reasons: (1) the proximity of the primary tumor to the mandible or invasion of the mandible by primary tumor requires resection of some part of the mandible; and (2) consideration of management of the mandible for resection of tumors not accessible thru the open mouth and where the mandible is not involved or in the vicinity of the tumor, but happens to be in the way to achieve complete resection of the tumor.

Thus, assessment of the mandible is essential for appropriate surgical planning and treatment. The mandible is considered at risk when the primary tumor overlies, is adherent to or lies in proximity to it. In order to establish the presence and extent of bone invasion, assessment of the mandible for invasion by tumor is performed by clinical and radiological examination. Careful examination under anesthesia by bimanual palpation is the most important aspect of mandibular assessment (5). Radiographic evaluation should be used to supplement findings of clinical evaluation (21–28). Thus, clinical assessment and radiographic findings are complementary to each other for thorough evaluation (29).

In addition to the risk of tumor involvement, management of the mandible also needs to be considered in large primary tumors of the oral cavity or oropharynx that are not accessible through the open mouth or even through a lower cheek flap approach due to anatomical restrictions posed by the intervening mandible. In the past, uninvolved mandible in such cases was routinely resected to gain access to the primary tumor in order to perform a composite resection ("commando" operation) so as to achieve a monobloc incontinuity resection of the primary tumor with neck dissection. However, sacrifice of uninvolved mandible to gain access to the oral cavity for facilitating resection of large intraoral tumors is no longer acceptable, since mandibulotomy provides the necessary exposure for resection without sacrifice of the intervening uninvolved mandible.

Tumor invasion of the mandible

In order to assess the need for and the extent of mandible resection required to encompass the primary tumor, it is essential to understand the process of invasion of the mandible by tumor (21,27,30–35). Primary carcinomas of the oral cavity extend along the surface mucosa and the submucosal soft tissues to approach the attached lingual, buccal and labial gingiva. From this point, tumors do not extend directly through intact periosteum and cortical bone toward the cancellous part of the mandible since the periosteum acts as a significant protective barrier (30,31,35). Instead, the tumor advances from the attached gingiva toward the alveolus. In patients with teeth, tumors invade the mandible by invading through the dental sockets and onto the cancellous part of the bone (Figure 11.24a). In edentulous patients, tumors extend up to the alveolar process then infiltrate the dental pores in the alveolar process to extend to the cancellous part of the mandible (Figure 11.24b). In patients who have been previously irradiated, however, the periosteal barrier is weak and direct invasion in the cancellous bone through the lingual cortex of the mandible may take place (30,31).

In non-irradiated, dentate patients with early invasion of the mandible, marginal mandibulectomy is feasible since the cortical part of the mandible inferior to the roots of the teeth remains uninvolved and can be spared safely (Figures 11.25 and 11.26) (36–38). In edentulous patients, however, the feasibility of marginal mandibulectomy depends on the vertical height of the body of the mandible. With aging, the alveolar process recedes and the mandibular canal comes closer and closer to the surface of the alveolar process. As shown in Figure 11.24, the resorption of the alveolar process eventually leads to a "pipestem" mandible. It is almost impossible to perform a satisfactory marginal mandibulectomy in such patients since the probability of iatrogenic fracture intraoperatively or postsurgical spontaneous fracture of the remaining portion of the mandible is very high (Figure 11.27). In general, marginal mandibulectomy in previously irradiated edentulous mandible is contraindicated; however, in select patients who have received previous radiotherapy, marginal mandibulectomy may be feasible if enough vertical height of the mandible is present, but it should be performed with extreme caution.

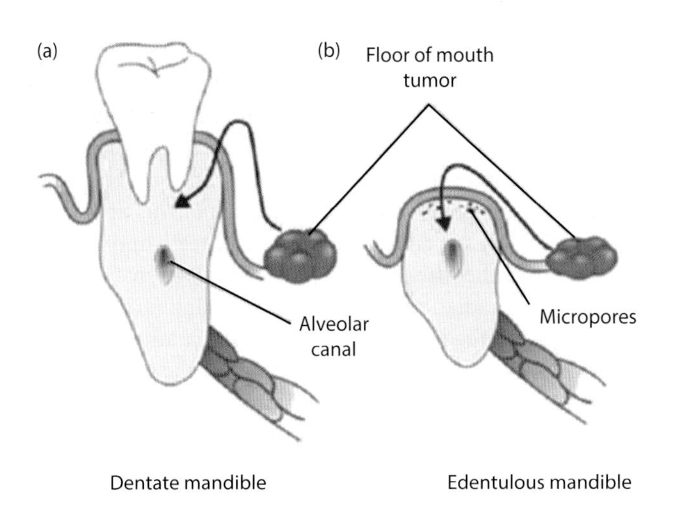

Figure 11.24 Mode of invasion of the mandible by cancer of the floor of the mouth. **(a)** Dentate mandible. **(b)** Edentulous mandible. Marginal mandibulectomy is feasible for minimal invasion of the alveolar process.

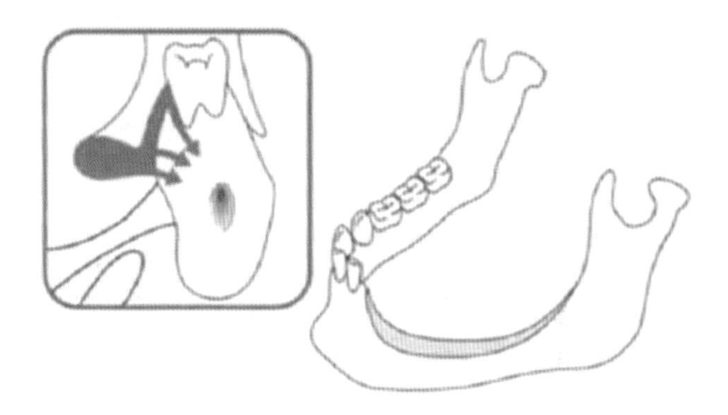

Figure 11.25 Feasibility of marginal mandibulectomy in dentate mandible.

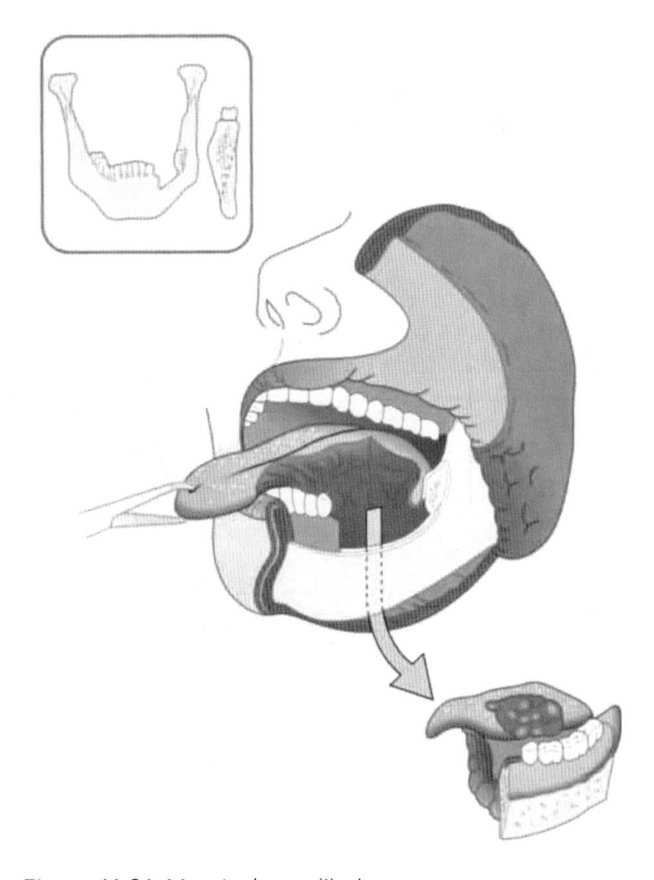

Figure 11.26 Marginal mandibulectomy.

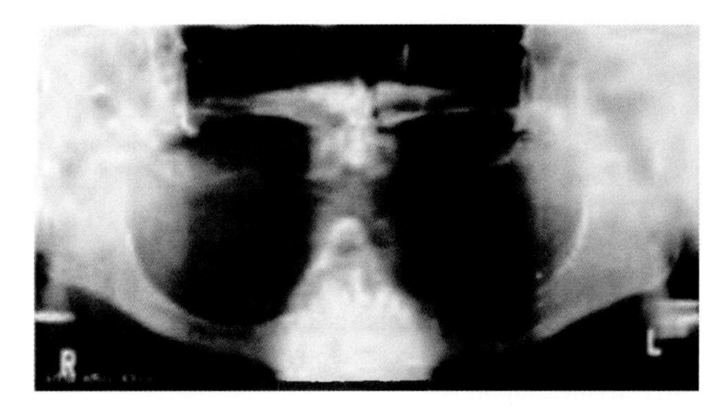

Figure 11.27 Pipestem mandible.

When the tumor extends to involve the cancellous part of the mandible, a segmental mandibulectomy must be performed (Figure 11.28). Generally, segmental mandibulectomy is also recommended in previously irradiated patients whose oral cancer is in close proximity to the mandible (5,39,40). Consideration of segmental resection should also extend to cases having significant soft tissue involvement adjacent to the mandible in association with a "massive primary tumor."

As mentioned earlier, segmental mandibulectomy should never be considered simply to gain access to primary cancers of the oral cavity or oropharynx not in the vicinity of the mandible (10,11,41). In addition, since there are no lymphatic channels passing through the mandible, there is no need for an incontinuity "composite resection (11,12,42)." Accordingly, the concept of the commando operation, with sacrifice of the normal uninvolved mandible to gain access to the primary tumors of the oral cavity or to accomplish an "in-continuity composite resection," cannot be justified.

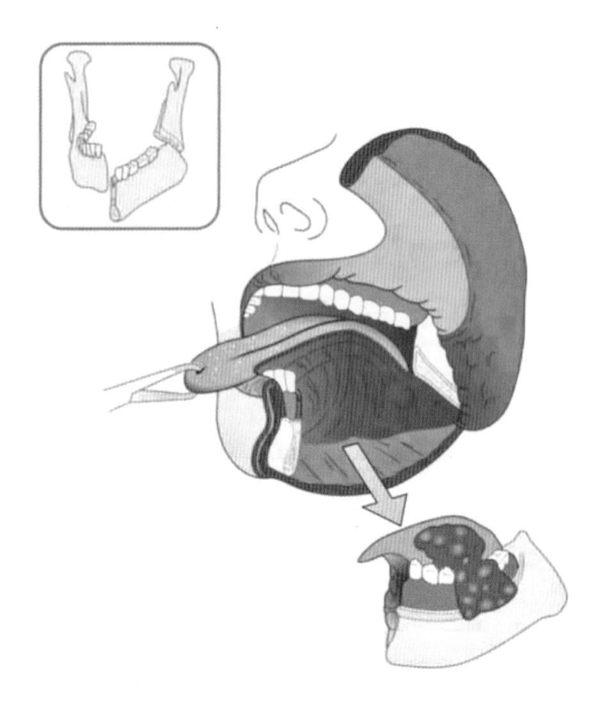

Figure 11.28 Segmental mandibulectomy.

The current indications for segmental mandibulectomy include:

1. Gross invasion by oral cancer
2. Proximity of oral cancer to the mandible in a previously irradiated patient
3. Primary bone tumor of the mandible
4. Metastatic tumor to the mandible
5. Invasion of the inferior alveolar nerve or canal by tumor
6. Massive soft tissue disease adjacent to the mandible (2)
7. Previously irradiated edentulous mandible

Understanding the process of tumor invasion of the mandible has enabled the development of mandible-sparing approaches. These include mandibulotomy for gaining access to large tumors of the oral cavity or posteriorly located tumors in the oropharynx and marginal mandibulectomy for minimal invasion of the alveolar process.

Mandibulotomy

Mandibulotomy or mandibular osteotomy is an excellent mandible-sparing surgical approach designed to gain access to the oral cavity or oropharynx for resection of primary tumors otherwise not accessible through the open mouth or by the lower cheek flap approach (Figure 11.29) (11,12,41). The mandibulotomy can be performed in one of three locations: (a) lateral (through the body or angle of the mandible), (b) midline or (c) paramedian.

Lateral mandibulotomy, however, has several disadvantages (43). First, the muscular pull on the two segments of the mandible is unequal due to the attachment of the pterygoid muscles to the ascending ramus of the mandible, putting the mandibulotomy site under significant stress. This results in delayed healing and may necessitate intermaxillary fixation. Second, the presence of intermaxillary fixation restricts access to the suture line in the oral cavity for cleaning, leading to poor oral hygiene and an increased risk of sepsis and wound breakdown. Furthermore, lateral mandibulotomy poses several anatomic disadvantages. Denervation of the teeth distal to the mandibulotomy site and the skin of the chin is a direct consequence of the procedure due to transection of the inferior alveolar nerve. Disruption of the endosteal blood supply is also a consequence of this approach, resulting in devascularization of the distal teeth and the distal segment of the mandible. In addition, in patients needing postoperative radiation therapy, the mandibulotomy site is directly within the lateral portal of the radiation field, leading to delayed healing and complications at the mandibulotomy site (44–46). For these reasons and the limited exposure afforded by the lateral mandibulotomy, this approach is not recommended.

By placing the site of mandibulotomy in the anterior midline, all of the disadvantages of lateral mandibulotomy are avoided (39–41). However, in order to avoid exposure of the roots of both central incisor teeth, putting them at the risk of extrusion, standard midline mandibulotomy

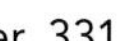

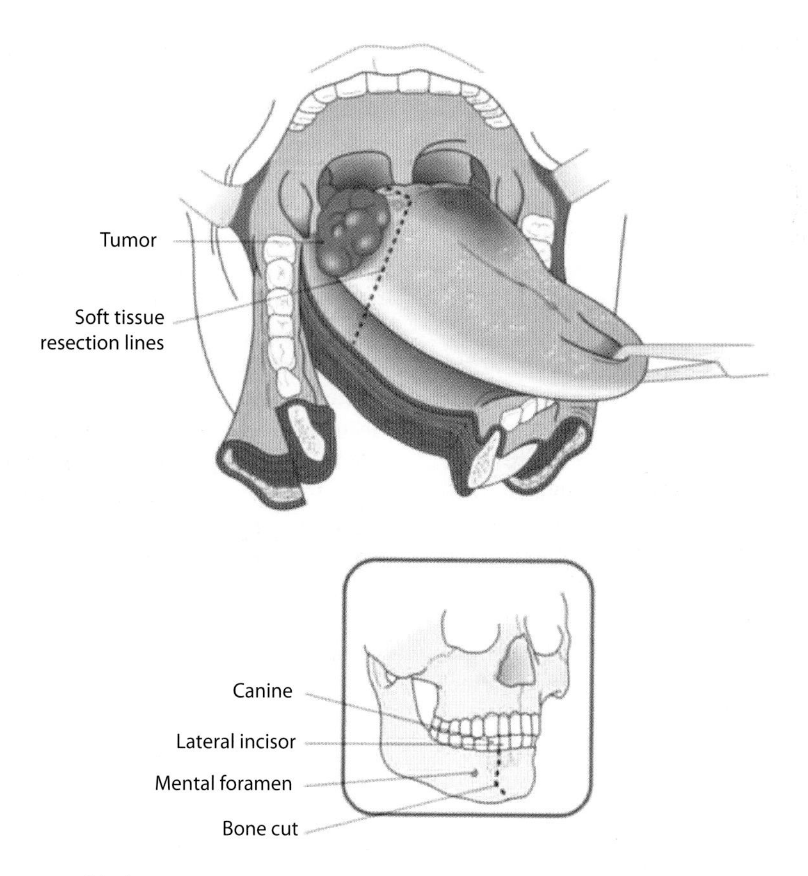

Figure 11.29 Paramedian mandibulotomy.

requires extraction of one central incisor tooth. This alters the esthetic appearance of the lower dentition. In addition, since midline mandibulotomy requires division of muscles arising from the genial tubercle—that is, the geniohyoid and genioglossus muscles—delayed recovery of the function of mastication and swallowing may occur. Therefore, a midline mandibulotomy is also not recommended for access to oral tumors.

Mandibulotomy performed in a paramedian position avoids the disadvantages of lateral mandibulotomy as well as midline mandibulotomy (45). The preferred site for paramedian mandibulotomy is between the lateral incisor and canine teeth. Since the roots of these two adjacent teeth diverge, a bone cut can be performed without risking tooth loss (2,39–41). Paramedian positioning of the mandibulotomy offers all the advantages of midline mandibulotomy, including wide exposure, and also allows preservation of the hyomandibular complex by avoiding division of the geniohyoid and genioglossus muscles. The mylohyoid is the only muscle that requires division, which results in minimal swallowing difficulties. Paramedian mandibulotomy does not cause denervation or devascularization of the skin of the chin or teeth and mandible. Fixation at the mandibulotomy site is easy and the mandibulotomy site does not fall within the lateral portal of radiation therapy. Thus, paramedian mandibulotomy is the optimal surgical approach for access to posteriorly located larger lesions of the oral cavity and tumors of the oropharynx.

Several non-tumor factors also impact on the selection of the mandibulotomy site, which need to be assessed in the preoperative setting. Mandibulotomy through an area of septic teeth should be avoided. If any other lesion such as a dental cyst is present at the proposed site of mandibulotomy, radiographic studies assist in the selection of an alternate site for mandibulotomy. Accordingly, in any patient requiring mandibulotomy, radiographic assessment of the mandible must be performed prior to surgery. A panoramic view of the mandible is usually satisfactory. If, however, facilities for a panoramic view are not available, then at least conventional radiographs of the mandible should be obtained prior to surgery.

MANDIBLE RESECTION FOR ORAL CANCER

Marginal mandibulectomy

The current indications for marginal mandibulectomy are:

1. For obtaining satisfactory three-dimensional margins around the primary tumor
2. When the primary tumor approximates the mandible
3. For minimal erosion of the alveolar process of the mandible (36–38,46–48)

Marginal mandibulectomy is contraindicated when there is gross invasion into the cancellous part of the mandible or when there is massive soft tissue disease. This procedure is also contraindicated in patients with previously irradiated edentulous mandibles or with significant atrophy of the alveolar process resulting in "pipestem mandible."

Marginal mandibulectomy can be performed to resect the alveolar process, the lingual plate or a combination of the alveolar process and lingual plate of the mandible for tumors of the anterior oral cavity. Marginal mandibulectomy can also be performed for lesions adjacent to the retromolar trigone, whereupon the anterior aspect of the ascending ramus of the mandible, including the coronoid process and the adjacent alveolar process of the body of the mandible, is resected. Reverse marginal mandibulectomy is indicated in patients who have tumors of the buccal mucosa or soft tissue disease such as fixation or prevascular facial lymph nodes to the lower cortex of the mandible.

When performing a marginal mandibulectomy, right-angled cuts should be avoided, since the angles create points of excessive stress, leading to the risk of spontaneous fracture. The marginal mandibulectomy should be performed in a smooth curve to evenly distribute the stress at the site of resection (Figure 11.30). Following marginal mandibulectomy, the exposed bone may be covered by primary closure of the mucosa of the tongue or floor of the mouth to the buccal mucosa. However, primary closure eliminates the lingual or the buccal sulcus and therefore fabrication and retention of a removable denture becomes exceedingly difficult. Alternatively, a skin graft can be applied directly over the exposed cancellous part of the mandible, which retains the sulci and the ability to wear a removable partial denture, which can be clasped to the remaining teeth. In edentulous patients, the ability to wear a denture over a marginally resected mandible is simply not possible. When there is significant soft tissue and mucosal loss in addition to marginal mandibulectomy, a radial forearm free flap provides ideal lining and reconstruction of the soft tissue defect. Osseointegrated implants are generally not feasible in the marginally resected mandible along the body of the mandible due to the lack of enough bone height over the mandibular canal. On the other hand, dental implants may be considered if the marginal mandibulectomy is performed in the anterior part of the mandible near the symphysis (from canine #22 to canine #27). There is usually sufficient vertical height of the mandible in this area, even in the edentulous patient, and there is no mandibular canal to worry about.

If the ultimate goal in the patient planned to have marginal mandibulectomy is to have total dental rehabilitation with restoration of dentition with dental implants, then marginal mandibulectomy should not be performed. Instead, that patient should undergo segmental mandibulectomy with fibula free flap reconstruction and either immediate or delayed placement of dental implants.

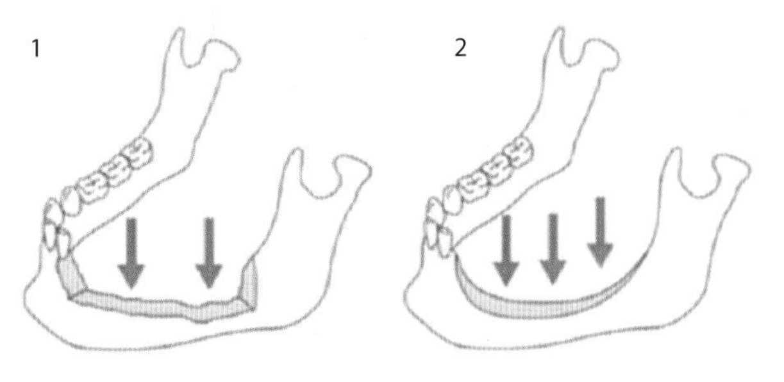

Figure 11.30 Technique of marginal mandibulectomy. It is essential to avoid sharp edges and to perform a smooth, rounded resection.

Segmental mandibulectomy

Resection of a segment of the mandible is required when there is gross bone destruction, tumor invasion in the cancellous part of the mandible, invasion of the inferior alveolar canal, primary malignant tumors of the mandible or metastatic lesions involving the mandible (Figures 11.31 through 11.33) (2,4,39). Massive soft tissue involvement around the mandible also occasionally requires segmental mandibulectomy (Figure 11.34). In a segmental mandibulectomy, the location of the segment of the mandible to be resected plays an

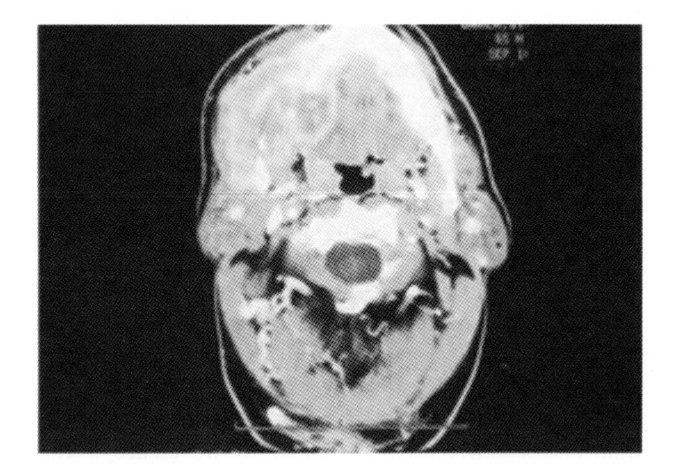

Figure 11.31 Gross destruction of the mandible by tumor.

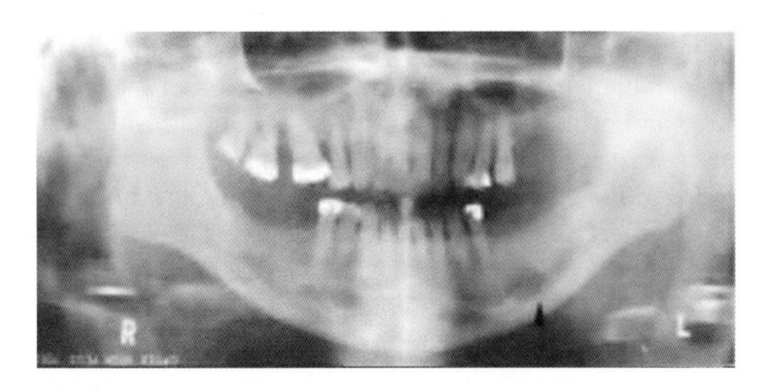

Figure 11.32 Invasion of the inferior alveolar canal by tumor.

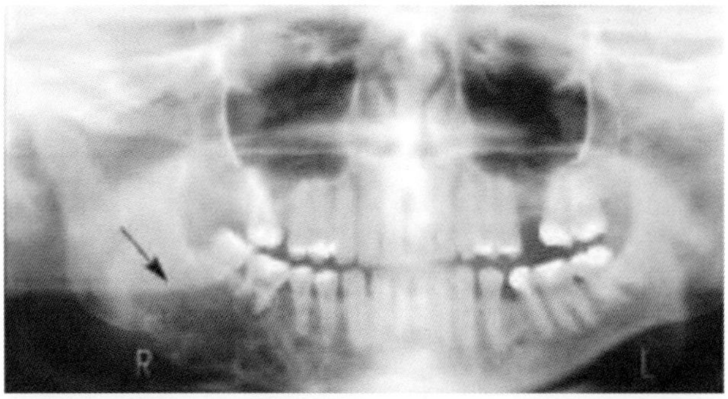

Figure 11.33 Panoramic X-ray showing gross invasion of mandible.

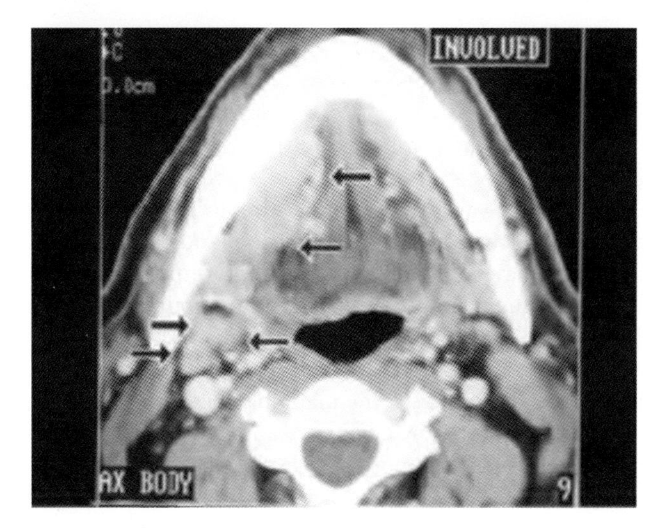

Figure 11.34 CT scan showing extensive soft tissue disease adjacent to the mandible.

important part in reconstruction and/or rehabilitation of the residual mandible. If any portion of the body of the mandible is resected and the remaining two stumps of the mandible are to be retained for secondary reconstruction, then fixation of the two segments of the mandible with a reconstruction plate (A–O plate) is required. Alternatively, primary reconstruction of the missing segment of the mandible can be undertaken with an appropriate microvascular free flap. If segmental mandibulectomy is performed on the posterior aspect of the body of the mandible and extending into the ascending ramus, then the residual portion of the ascending ramus is not useful, unless it is sufficient to permit immediate reconstruction with a vascularized free bone flap. The remaining portion of the ascending ramus should be sufficient in length to permit placement of plates and screws to anchor the free bone flap. If that much length of the remnant mandible is not available, then it is best to disarticulate the remnant stump from the temporomandibular joint and consider using the condyle to be placed on the free bone flap and snap back into the temporo-mandibular (TM) joint.

On the other hand, if mandible reconstruction is not planned and a primary closure of the surgical defect after segmental mandibulectomy is contemplated, then it is best to remove the remaining stump of the ascending ramus as it is not functional and is indeed a hindrance to adequate closure of the mouth. The unequal pull on the short stump of the ascending ramus of the mandible from the unopposed pterygoid muscles causes medial and cephalad deviation of the remnant ascending ramus toward the soft palate. With passage of time, this shift of the residual stump of the mandible causes pain and produces significant impairment in oral function. Therefore, if segmental mandibulectomy is performed on the posterior part of the body of the mandible beyond the angle into the ascending ramus and if reconstruction is not planned, then the residual ascending ramus should be resected.

It is imperative that immediate reconstruction of the mandible is undertaken when segmental resection of the anterior arch of the mandible is performed. Reconstruction plates are not a satisfactory solution for replacement of the anterior arch of the mandible, as they are esthetically and functionally unacceptable and are invariably exposed in a majority of patients, requiring their subsequent removal. Therefore, whenever a resection of a segment of the anterior arch of the mandible is performed, immediate bone reconstruction is necessary and should be factored in surgical treatment planning.

Paramedian to mandibulotomy for resection of cancer of the posterior third of the tongue

This procedure is best suited for resection of tumors of the oropharynx and particularly the base of the tongue not accessible through the oral cavity and where the mandible is not at risk. The patient shown in Figure 11.35 has a squamous carcinoma of the posterior third of the tongue. The patient is placed under general anesthesia with nasotracheal intubation on the operating table and adequate relaxation is obtained. An incision is planned, splitting the lower lip in the midline with extension of the incision up to the hyoid bone, at which point the incision extends laterally on the side of neck dissection along an upper neck skin crease

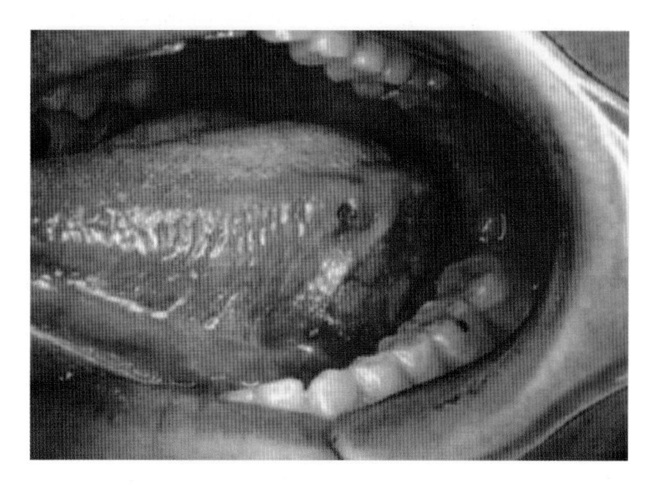

Figure 11.35 Squamous carcinoma of the posterior third of the tongue.

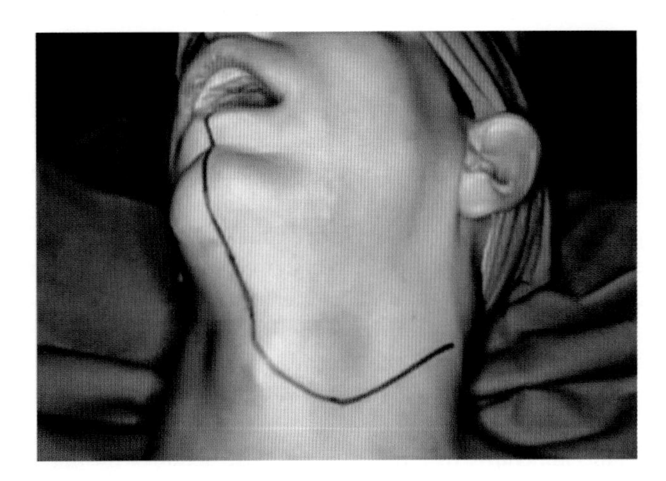

Figure 11.36 Lower lip-splitting incision with lateral extension.

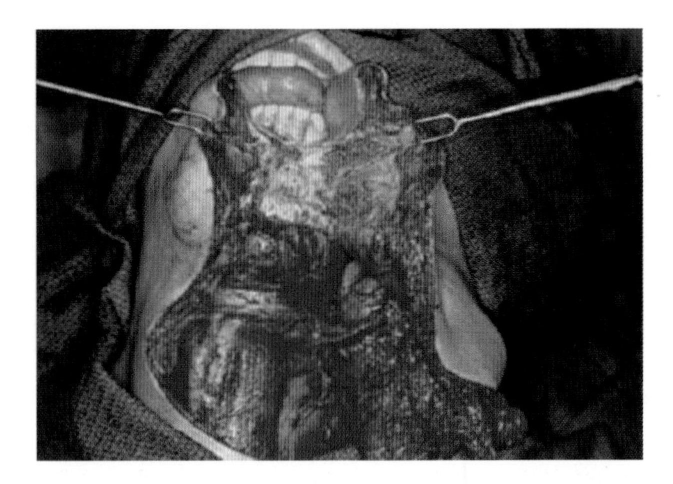

Figure 11.38 A short cheek flap is elevated to expose the mandible.

(Figure 11.36). Extension of the incision to the lateral aspect of the upper neck provides adequate exposure for an appropriate neck dissection as required.

Initially, only the transverse part of the neck incision is made and in this patient a supraomohyoid neck dissection is completed (Figure 11.37). The skin incision is then extended in the midline, dividing the chin and the lower lip through its full thickness up to the reflection of the mucosa at the gingivolabial sulcus. Approximately 5 mm of labial mucosa at the gingivolabial sulcus is left attached to the gum to facilitate closure. At that point, an incision is made in the labial mucosa on the left-hand side of the midline for a distance of approximately 2 cm and a short cheek flap is elevated (Figure 11.38). All the soft tissue attachments of the chin are elevated from the anterior aspect of the mandible to a distance of approximately 3 cm from the midline on the left-hand side, exposing the mandibulotomy site. Elevation of the cheek flap, however, should not extend up to the mental foramen; otherwise, the mental nerve is exposed to injury, resulting in loss of sensation of the skin of the chin. Elevation of the left-sided short cheek flap exposes the outer

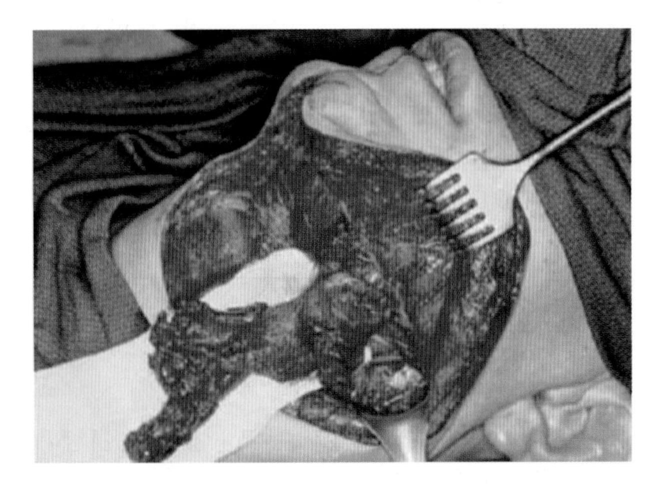

Figure 11.37 Supraomohyoid neck dissection is completed.

cortex and the inferior border of the mandible at the mandibulotomy site.

There are a variety of different ways in which an osteotomy may be performed to accomplish mandibulotomy. The mandible may be divided with a straight-line vertical cut. However, this is not desirable since immobilization of the mandible is difficult due to the possibility of sliding motion at the site of the mandibulotomy, causing delayed union or malunion. Alternatively, the mandible may be divided in a stepladder fashion to avoid upward and downward displacement. However, anteroposterior displacement would still be a problem with that approach. In addition, the transverse cut of a stepladder osteotomy may amputate or injure the roots of teeth at that site and devitalize them. Therefore, the preferred approach is an angular osteotomy performed in a zig-zag fashion, dividing the alveolar process between the lateral incisor and canine tooth in a vertical plane for a distance of approximately 10 mm, at which point the mandibular osteotomy is angled medially. The angulation in the osteotomy is approximately at a 45° angle, below the level of the roots of adjacent teeth. The angled cut provides a more stable osteotomy for fixation. We prefer to use a high-speed power saw with an ultra-thin blade to make the mandibular cuts. However, prior to division of the bone, appropriate drill holes are placed for fixation of the mandibulotomy site using titanium miniplates. Two-plane fixation is necessary. A four-hole miniplate is placed on the outer cortex of the mandible over the mandibulotomy site below the level of the roots of adjacent teeth. With the use of benders, the plate is appropriately bent and shaped to fit snugly over the mandibular surface. Four drill holes are now made through the plate holes in the mandible (Figure 11.39). Another similar plate is shaped to fit over the lower border of the mandible and four drill holes are made in a vertical plane through the holes in the plate, but avoiding entry into adjacent tooth sockets. These plates are saved for use later in the operation for repair of the osteotomy site. The drill holes are placed before the osteotomy is performed to allow accurate re-approximation of the two segments of the mandible during

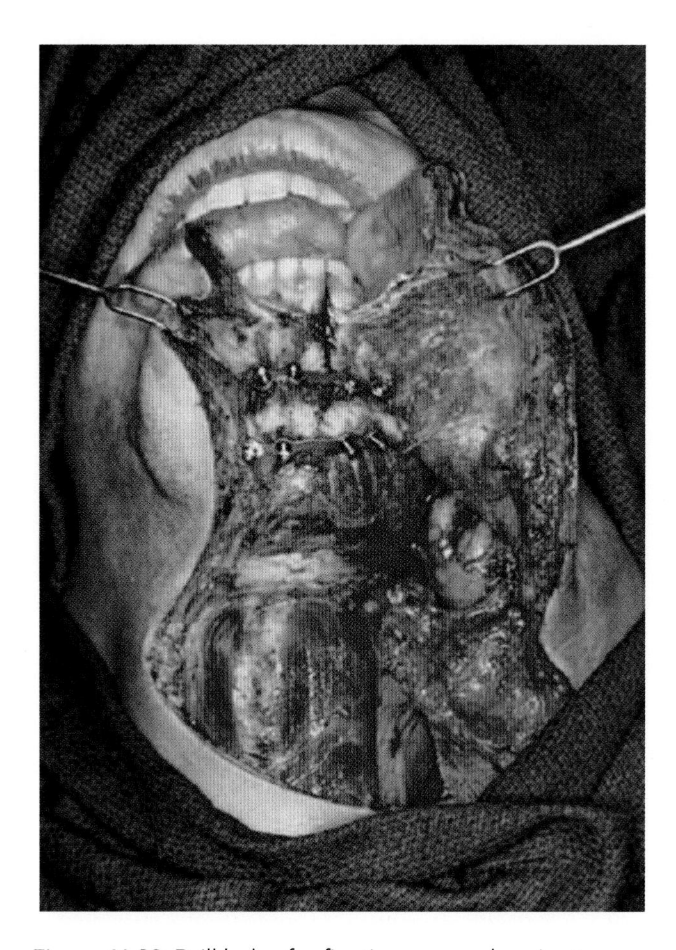

Figure 11.39 Drill holes for fixation are made prior to bone division.

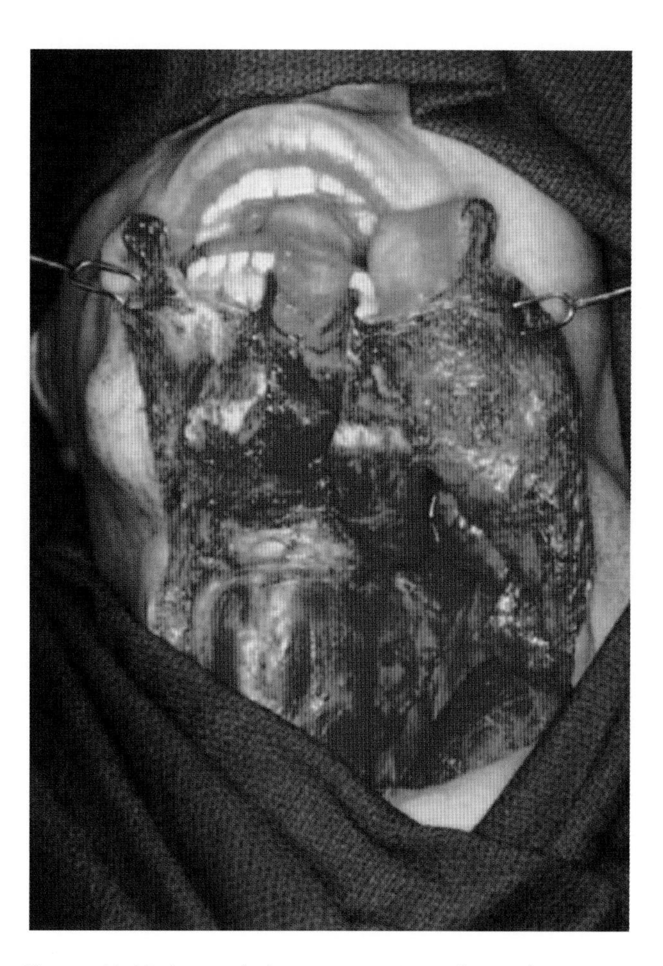

Figure 11.40 An angled osteotomy is performed.

closure, preserving the occlusal surfaces of the upper and lower dentition in perfect alignment. Accurate placement of both miniplates is vitally important to avoid injury to the roots of adjacent teeth. The mandible is divided exactly as planned using a high-speed power saw. Overriding of the bone cuts at the angulation should be avoided to prevent iatrogenic fracture at the mandibulotomy site.

Once the mandible is divided, its two segments are retracted laterally with sharp retractors (Figure 11.40). Brisk hemorrhage from each stump of the mandible is to be expected; however, this can be easily controlled with electrocautery or bone wax. Electrocautery is now used to divide the soft tissue and muscular attachments on the two sides of the mandible. As the two sides of the mandible are retracted, a mucosal incision is made in the floor of the mouth, leaving a curf of approximately 1 cm of mucosa at the gingiva. This is essential to facilitate closure of the floor of the mouth (Figure 11.41).

The mucosal incision in the floor of the mouth extends from the mandibulotomy site all the way up to the anterior pillar of the soft palate. If the incision has to be extended further posteriorly, it will require division of the lingual nerve that crosses the surgical field between the mandible and the lateral aspect of the tongue. The tongue is retracted medially in the oral cavity as the mandibular segment is retracted laterally, providing the necessary exposure.

The soft tissue attachments on the medial aspect of the mandible are divided and the two halves of the mandible are retracted (Figure 11.42). The sublingual salivary gland, if to be preserved, is swept medially to remain attached to the tongue. On the other hand, if it is planned to excise the sublingual gland along with the mylohyoid muscle and the submandibular gland in an en bloc fashion to remain in continuity with the neck dissection specimen, the sublingual gland needs to be retracted laterally. Note that the mucosal incision in the floor of the mouth should retain a curf of mucosa along the gingiva to facilitate closure. The mylohyoid muscle attached to the mandible is now exposed. It will have to be divided to permit mandibular "swing" and further exposure. It is divided in its center by electrocautery, leaving its lateral half attached to the mandible. Complete division of the mylohyoid muscle permits sufficient swing of the mandible to provide exposure of the tumor in the surgical field (Figure 11.43). On the other hand, if the plan is to do a monobloc incontinuity resection of a large primary tumor along with the sublingual gland, mylohyoid muscle, submandibular gland and neck dissection, then the mylohyoid muscle is detached from the mandible and divided at its medial end in the midline. In this setting, there will be a through-and-through defect between the mouth and the neck. Therefore, a free flap, such as a radial forearm flap, or a regional flap, such as a

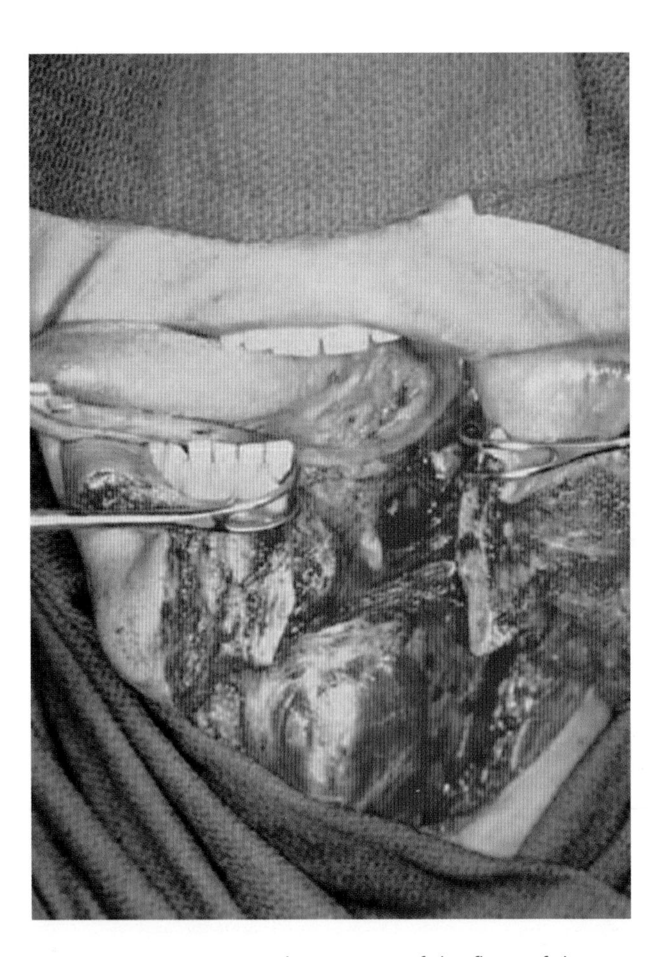

Figure 11.41 Incision in the mucosa of the floor of the mouth extends up to the soft palate.

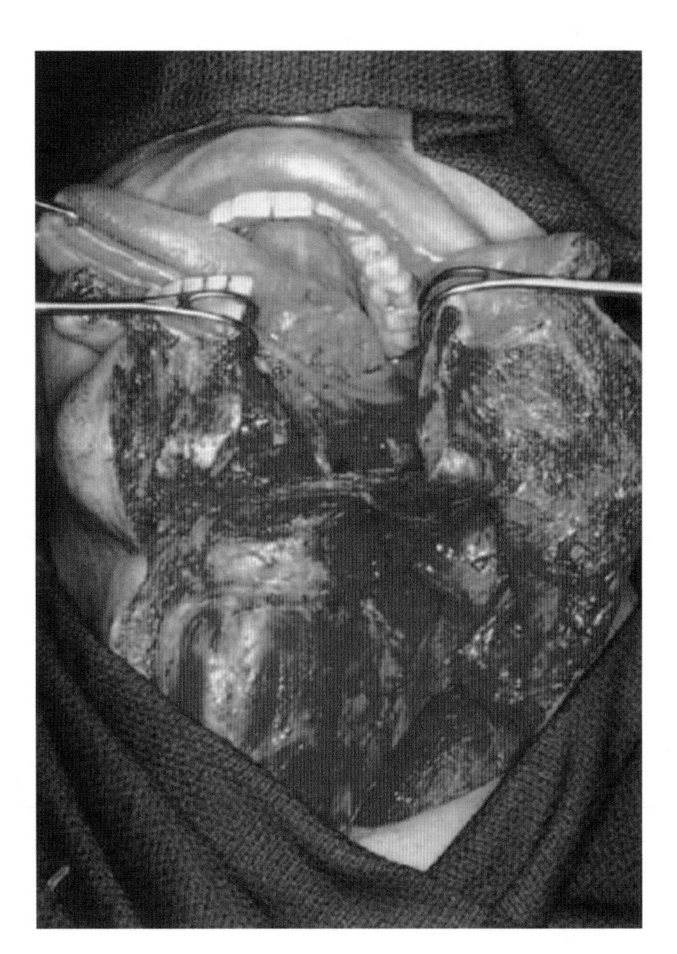

Figure 11.42 The mylohyoid muscle is exposed.

submental flap, will be required to close the surgical defect. The palpable extent of the tumor is examined and the proposed site of resection is marked out. A full-thickness, through-and-through, three-dimensional resection of the tumor is now performed using electrocautery with coagulating current. Note that the wedge-shaped resection is oriented transversely to permit re-approximation of the surgical defect by primary closure (Figure 11.44). Brisk hemorrhage from the lingual artery and/or its branches is to be expected during resection of the tongue; however, this is easily controlled with appropriate measures.

Upon completion of the surgical resection, frozen sections are obtained from the lateral mucosal margins and the deep soft tissue margin of the surgical defect (tongue musculature) to ensure adequacy of resection (Figure 11.45). A nasogastric feeding tube is inserted prior to beginning the closure. It is important to introduce the feeding tube at this point because if there is difficulty in the insertion of the tube after the wound is closed, then any digital manipulation may disrupt the suture line. A skin hook is placed at the apex of the wedge-shaped surgical defect on the dorsum of the tongue and traction is applied toward the right-hand side. This allows the front of the tongue to draw posteriorly, providing easy approximation of the raw areas. Closure is performed in two layers using interrupted 00 chromic catgut or Vicryl sutures for the muscular layer as well as the mucosa.

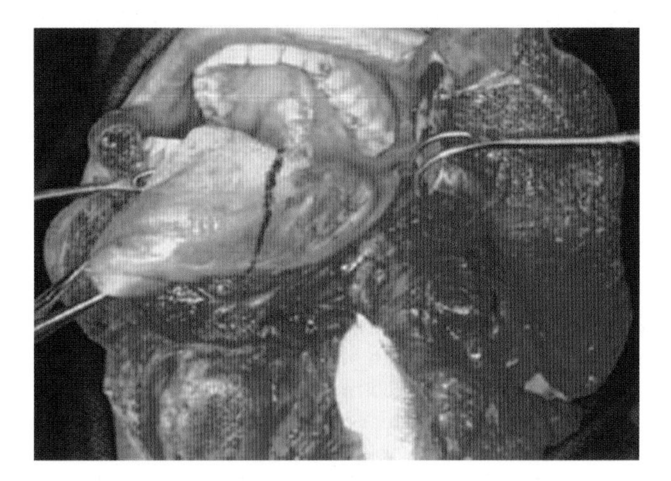

Figure 11.43 The tumor is exposed.

Following repair of the tongue, the retracted left half of the mandible is brought back into its normal position. Closure of the mucosa of the lateral aspect of the tongue to the mucosa of the floor of the mouth on the gingiva is completed with interrupted chromic catgut sutures. As the closure proceeds anteriorly, the mandible draws closer and closer to the mandibulotomy site until complete mucosal closure of the floor of the mouth is accomplished. At this point, the mandibulotomy site is repaired with

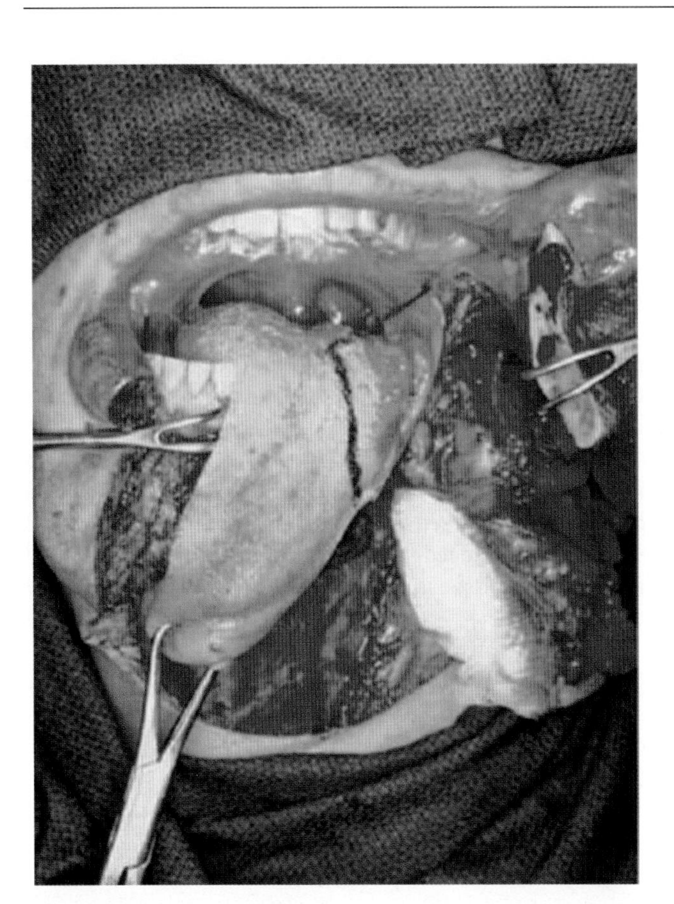

Figure 11.44 A transversely oriented wedge resection is outlined.

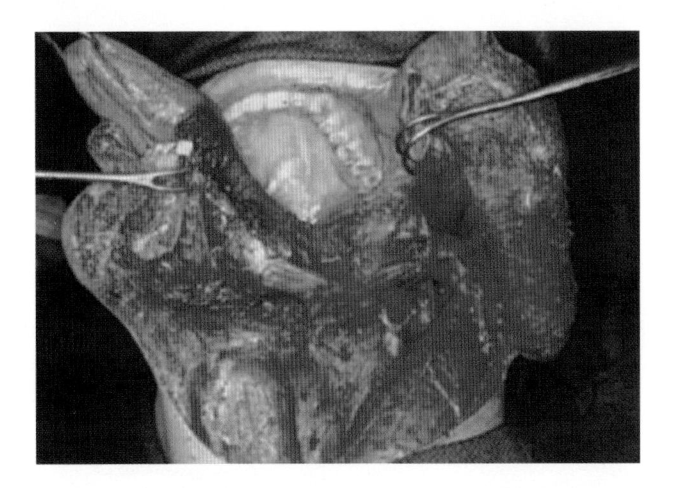

Figure 11.45 The surgical defect following resection.

fixation using the previously shaped miniplates and screws (Figure 11.46).

A depth gauge is used to select the length of the screws for the miniplates. We prefer to use screws long enough to enter the lingual cortex of the mandible for the lateral plate. On the other hand, the miniplate on the lower border of the mandible is fixed with relatively short screws to avoid injury to the roots of the adjacent teeth. Generally, 7-mm screws are appropriate for mandible fixation. Every attempt is made to secure perfect alignment of the two segments of

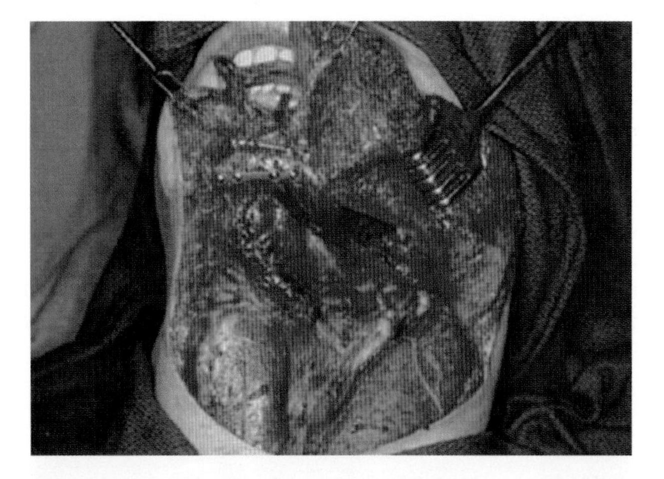

Figure 11.46 The mandibulotomy is reconstructed with miniplates.

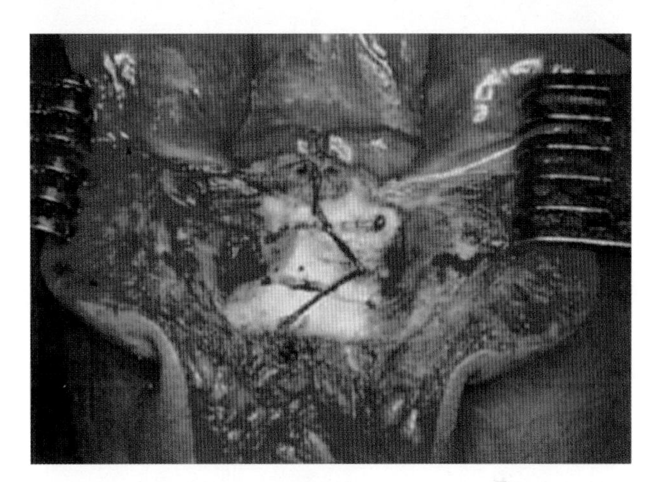

Figure 11.47 Mandibulotomy site and curfs for wire fixation.

the mandible to restore normal occlusion. The screws are tightened snug but not too tight, otherwise the heads of the titanium screws will break.

If titanium miniplates and screws are not available, fixation of the mandible can be accomplished reasonably well using No. 24 gauge stainless steel wire (49). In that case, four drill holes are made prior to mandibulotomy (Figure 11.47). Two horizontal wires and one oblique wire are used to stabilize the mandible. The wires are twist-tied and the stumps are bent and buried to avoid exposure through soft tissues (Figure 11.48). In the experience of the authors, miniplate fixation and wire fixation following mandibulotomy work equally well. The rigidity of immobilization and postoperative complications are comparable with these two techniques (49).

Mucosal closure now begins by re-approximating the cut edge of the labial mucosa to the curf of the mucosa at the gingivolabial sulcus on the alveolar process. This closure is accomplished using 000 chromic catgut interrupted sutures. Chromic catgut sutures are used for both the muscular layer and the mucosal layer of the lip, while nylon sutures are used for the skin and vermilion border. For perfect closure of the midline lip-splitting incision, a fine nylon suture is first placed accurately, aligning the mucocutaneous junction of the vermilion border. This suture is held as a retractor and closure of the labial mucosa progresses backward (retrograde) from the vermilion border up to the gingivolabial sulcus. Interrupted sutures are placed in order to approximate the muscular layer in a similar fashion. Finally, accurate re-approximation of the skin of the lip and chin is essential to obtaining an esthetically acceptable scar. The stumps of the divided mylohyoid muscle are re-approximated using interrupted chromic catgut sutures. Although this re-approximation is seldom accurate, it does permit reduction of the dead space in the submandibular region and provides support to the mucosal suture line in the floor of the mouth. A suction drain is placed in the wound and brought out through a separate stab incision. The neck incision is closed in two layers. The surgical specimen shows incontinuity resection of the primary tumor with the lymph nodes of levels I, II and III from the supraomohyoid triangle and the intervening submandibular salivary gland (Figure 11.49).

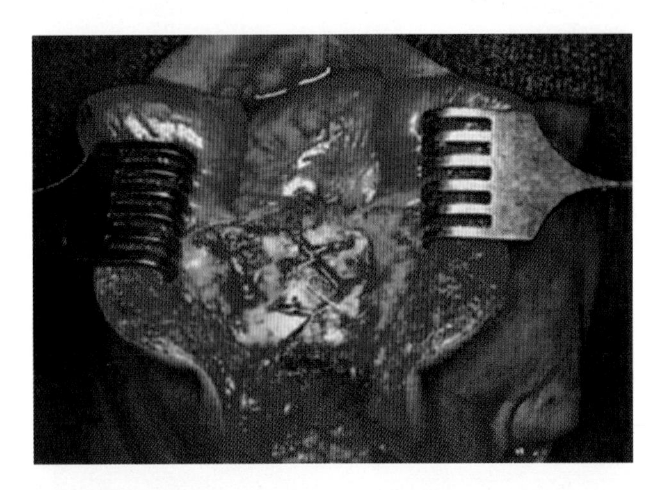

Figure 11.48 Mandibulotomy repair with wire fixation.

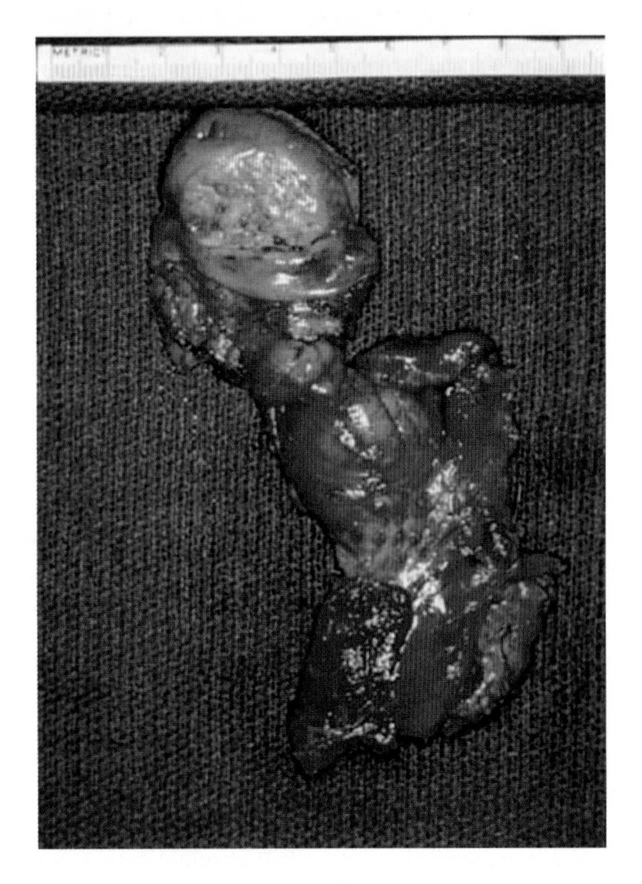

Figure 11.49 Surgical specimen showing primary tumor removed in continuity with regional lymph nodes.

In the postoperative period, the patient is maintained on nasogastric tube feeding for approximately 1 week, followed by a trial with pureed food to assess whether swallowing is successful. If, indeed, the patient is able to tolerate pureed food, then he or she is gradually advanced to a soft diet over the next few days.

A postoperative view of the patient 3 months after surgery shows a well-healed midline scar and esthetically acceptable external appearance (Figure 11.50). The intraoral view shows excellent shape and mobility of the tongue (Figure 11.51).

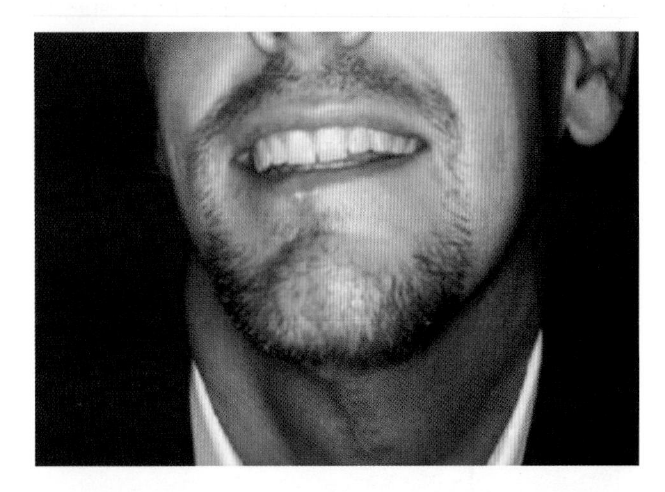

Figure 11.50 Postoperative view showing healed incision.

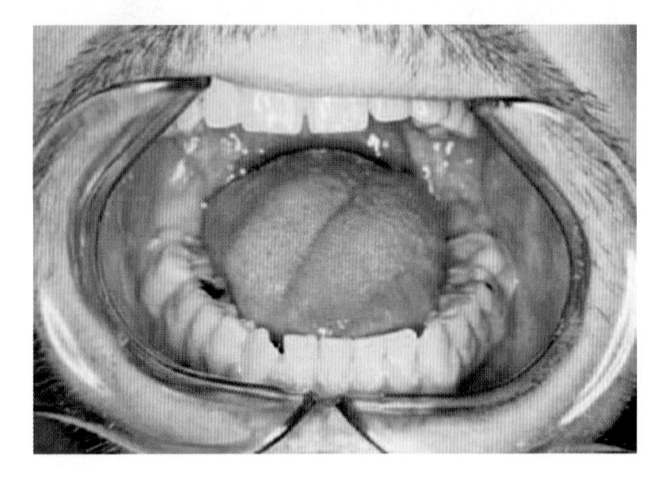

Figure 11.51 Postoperative intraoral view.

Mandibulotomy approach for hemiglossectomy in continuity with comprehensive neck dissection

Locally advanced primary tumors of the oral tongue can be resected in continuity with the regional lymph nodes in a monobloc fashion without the intervening mandible if it is not involved or at risk. For this to be accomplished, the primary tumor must not be adherent to the mandible. The extirpation is achieved by first completing a comprehensive neck dissection, followed by a paramedian mandibulotomy to facilitate resection. Then the mandible is swung laterally on the side of the tumor to expose the primary tumor of the oral tongue. The hemiglossectomy is carried out with electrocautery. The primary tumor remains attached to the specimen of the right neck dissection through the soft tissues and musculature of the floor of the mouth and the right submandibular and sublingual salivary glands as well as adjacent lymph nodes. A monobloc incontinuity resection can thus be performed without sacrificing the intervening mandible not involved by the tumor. The resulting surgical defect usually requires reconstruction by bringing soft tissue from elsewhere into the region in the form of either a pedicled regional flap or a free flap. Following reconstruction of the surgical defect, closure of the mucosal suture line is completed. The mandibulotomy site is repaired with miniplates and screws and the neck incision is closed in the usual fashion.

The patient shown in Figure 11.52 has a T3 carcinoma of the lateral border of the oral tongue with clinically palpable lymph node metastases in the right-hand side of the neck. The tumor did not involve the floor of the mouth or the gingiva and therefore the mandible could be safely spared. A comprehensive right neck dissection sparing the accessory nerve is completed and a paramedian mandibulotomy is performed. The mandible is swung laterally, exposing the primary tumor of the tongue (Figure 11.53). Due to the extent of the tumor, the patient requires a hemiglossectomy, extending from the tip up to and including a portion of the posterior third of the tongue on the right-hand side (Figure 11.54).

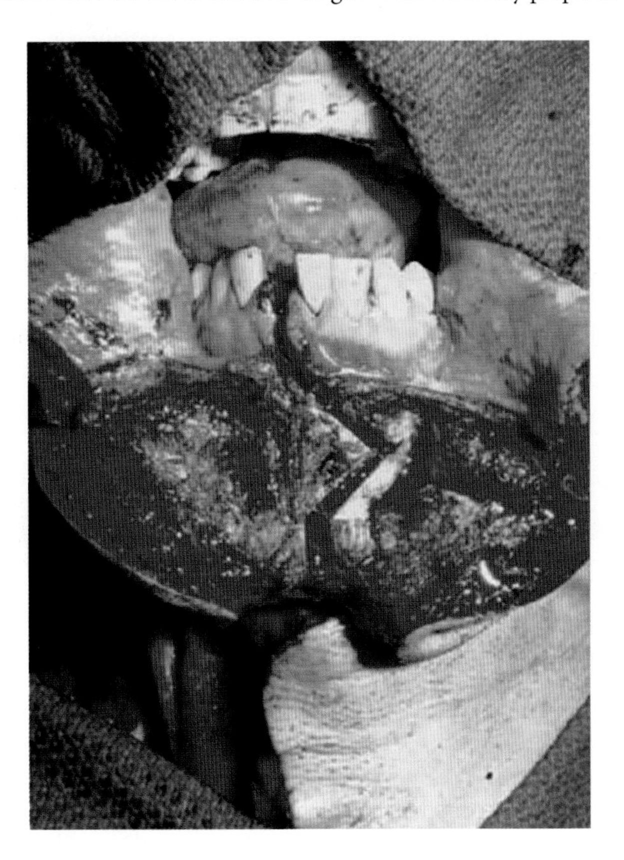

Figure 11.52 Paramedian mandibulotomy.

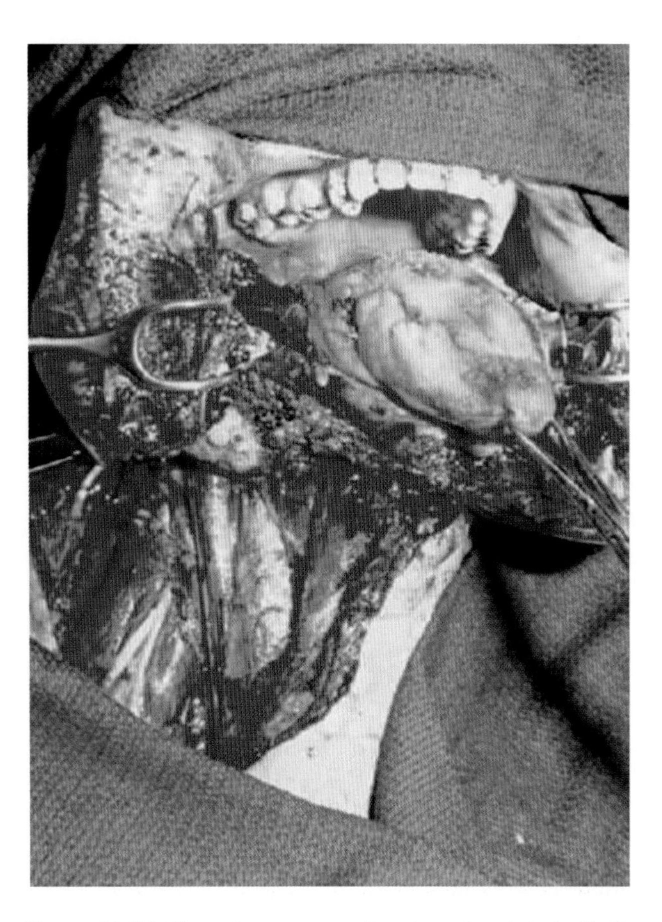

Figure 11.53 The primary tumor involves the right half of the tongue.

The surgical defect at the site of resection of the primary tumor shows the cut surface of the left half of the tongue from a lateral view (Figure 11.55). The anterior view shows excision of the right half of the tongue (Figure 11.56). The surgical specimen shows the primary tumor of the tongue resected in continuity with a right comprehensive neck dissection, including the intervening soft tissues of the floor of the mouth and the submandibular triangle (Figure 11.57).

The postoperative appearance of the oral cavity shows perfect alignment of the two segments of the mandible and satisfactory reconstruction of the tongue, maintaining acceptable mobility for speech, mastication and swallowing (Figure 11.58). The external appearance of the patient is shown in Figure 11.59. Note that the external contour of the face is essentially unchanged.

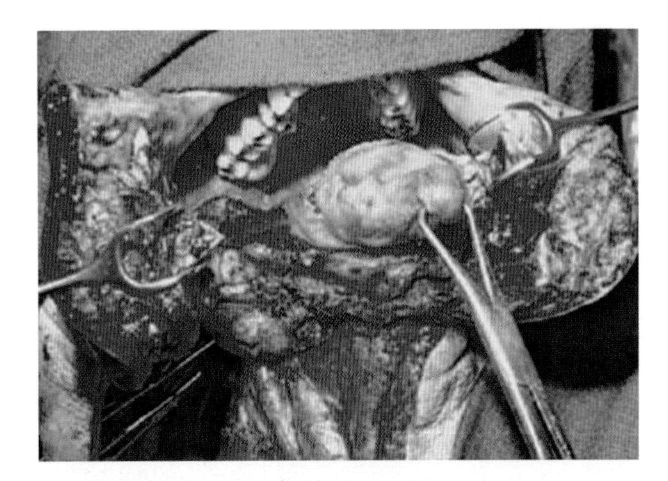

Figure 11.54 A right hemiglossectomy is performed.

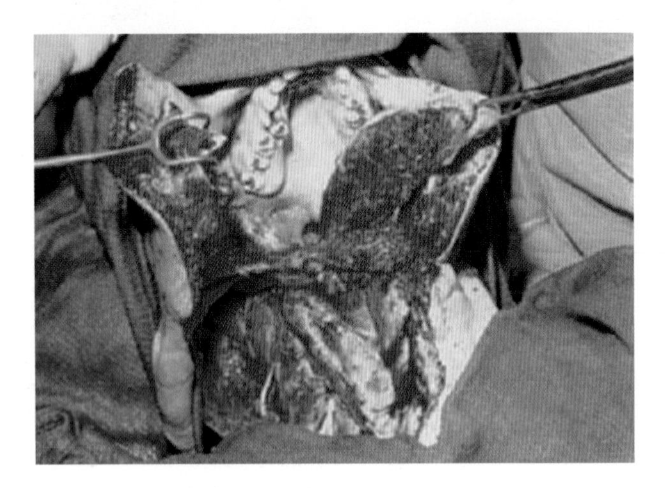

Figure 11.55 The surgical defect after tumor resection.

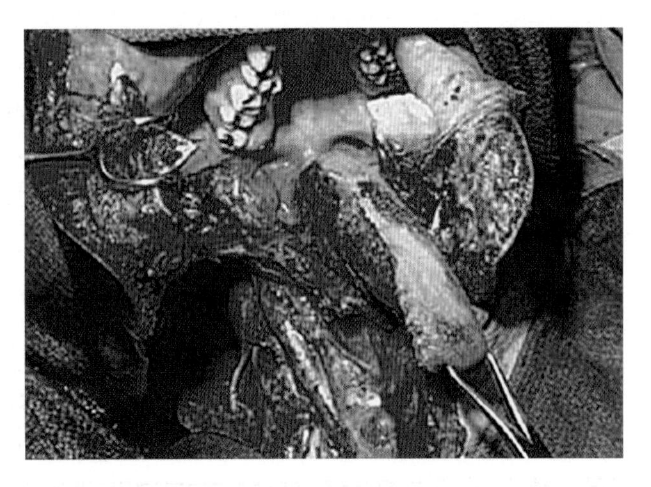

Figure 11.56 Right hemiglossectomy defect showing the remaining tongue.

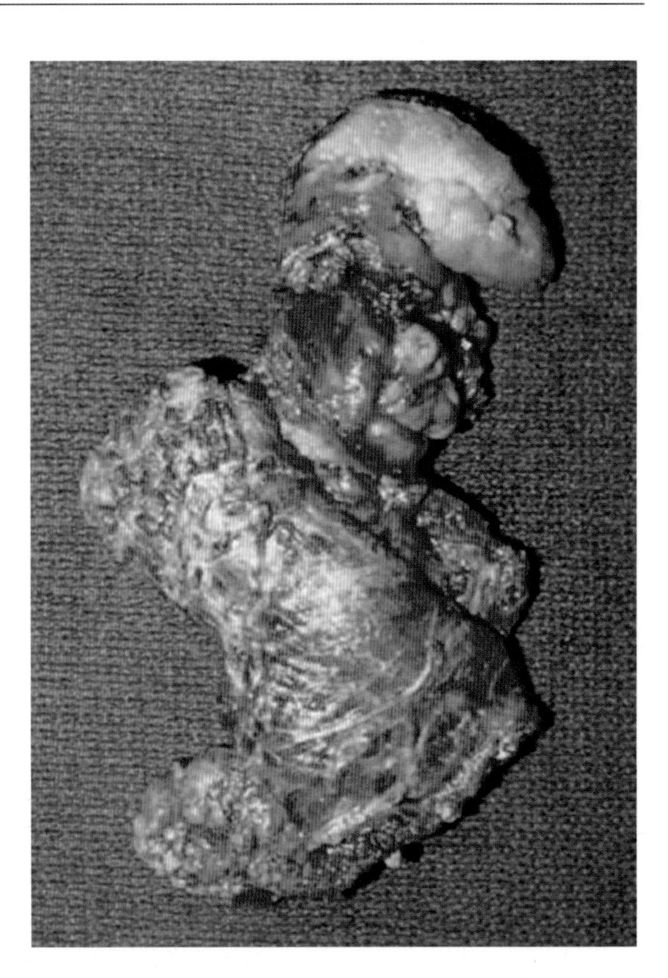

Figure 11.57 The surgical specimen of right hemiglossectomy and radical neck dissection done in continuity in a monobloc fashion.

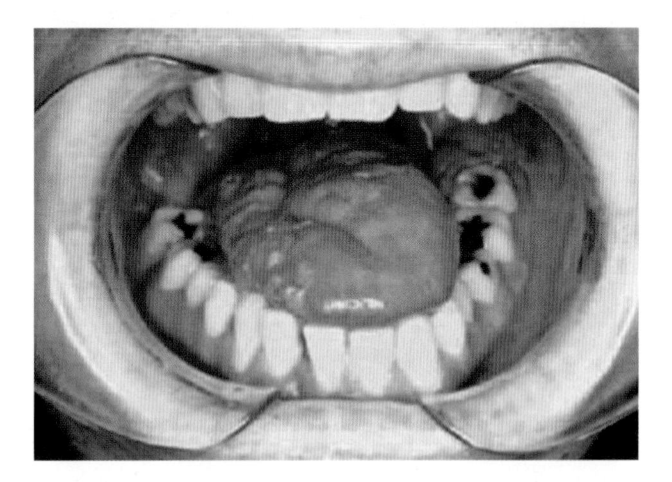

Figure 11.58 Postoperative intraoral view showing the reconstructed tongue.

Mandible resection in the management of intraoral cancer

Surgical resection of the mandible becomes necessary when a primary malignant tumor of the oral cavity extends to the gingiva over the alveolar process or directly infiltrates into the mandible. If there is direct extension of the tumor from the alveolar process to the cancellous part of the mandible or if contiguous tumor infiltration to the lingual or lateral cortex of the mandible is present, then a segmental mandibulectomy becomes necessary (Figure 11.60). However, if a primary

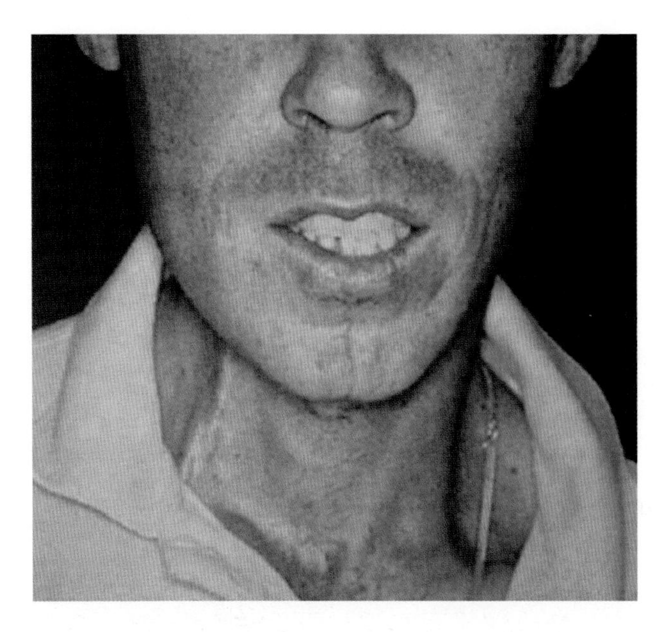

Figure 11.59 Postoperative picture of the patient showing well-healed incisions.

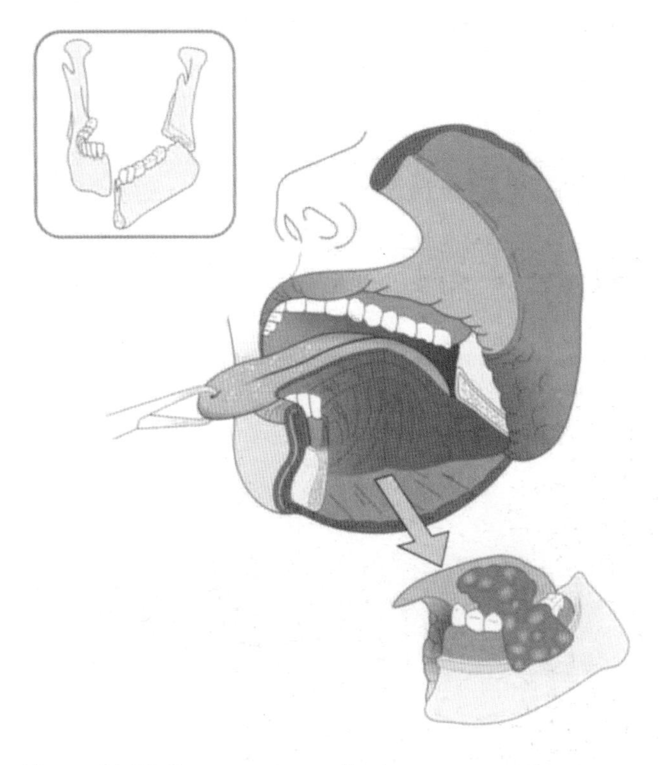

Figure 11.60 Segmental mandibulectomy.

tumor of the oral cavity approximates the alveolar process or the lingual plate of the mandible, then resection of a part of the mandible, preserving its arch, is adequate to obtain satisfactory margins around the primary tumor. In this clinical setting, segmental mandibulectomy is not indicated, but a marginal mandibulectomy proves to be satisfactory (Figure 11.61).

A marginal mandibulectomy may include resection of the lingual plate or the alveolar process, or both, but still retains the continuity of the arch of the mandible by preserving its

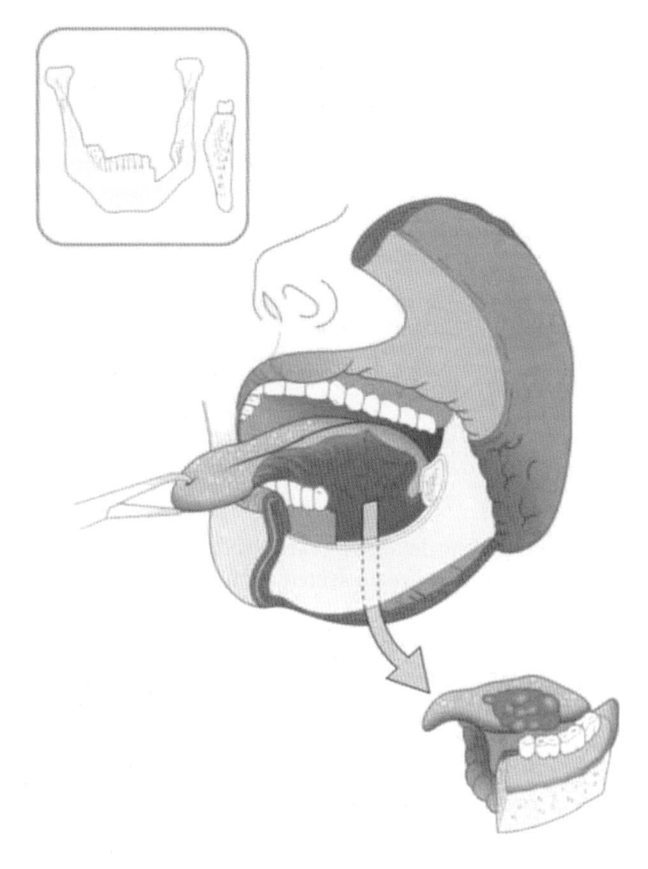

Figure 11.61 Marginal mandibulectomy.

lower border and/or the lateral cortex. The routes of spread of intraoral tumors in proximity to the mandible are such that marginal resection is feasible in either dentate or edentulous mandible (30,31). This procedure produces minimal, if any, esthetic and functional deformity. Marginal mandibulectomy can be performed on any part of the mandible; that is, the symphysis, body or retromolar trigone.

Marginal mandibulectomy provides an oncologically sound three-dimensional resection of tumors of the oral cavity that approach, approximate or superficially involve the mandible. The operative procedure leaves minimal esthetic and functional deformity, avoids the need for mandible reconstruction and offers local control of cancer in properly selected patients, comparable to that achieved by segmental mandibulectomy (39). However, dental rehabilitation with implants is not feasible in the remaining mandible after marginal mandibulectomy due to the lack of sufficient vertical height above the mandibular canal.

Marginal mandibulectomy can be performed safely through the open mouth for small lesions, particularly in the anterior aspect of the oral cavity. For larger lesions, a wider exposure is necessary for access to the primary tumor and its satisfactory resection. Either a lower cheek flap approach or a visor flap approach may be employed. In most instances, the lower cheek flap approach is desirable since it provides satisfactory exposure and permits resection of the primary tumor and ipsilateral cervical lymph nodes

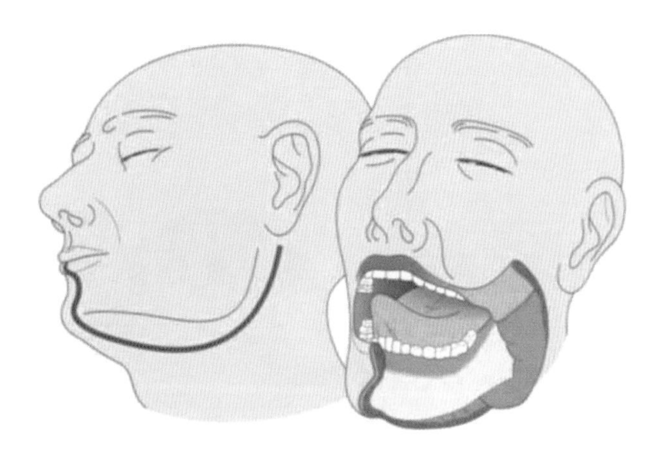

Figure 11.62 Lower cheek flap approach.

(Figure 11.62). The details of a variety of marginal mandibulectomy procedures are presented here.

PERORAL MARGINAL MANDIBULECTOMY

Small primary tumors of the anterior aspect of the lower gum are suitable for excision through the open mouth, including the alveolar process, regardless of the presence or absence of teeth. This operation is also indicated for lesions of the floor of the mouth or cheek mucosa approaching the lower alveolus.

In the long term, the patient shown in the example below may need dental implants for restoration of dentition or a secondary vestibuloplasty to create sulci to facilitate wearing a denture. Dental implants in this setting are satisfactory, since the vertical height at the symphysis is satisfactory and there is no mandibular canal in the remaining bone at this site to worry about. Alternatively, a split-thickness skin graft may be used primarily to cover the marginally resected mandible and thus restore the sulci. A vestibuloplasty and fabrication of a removable denture are not required if the patient is a suitable candidate for osseointegrated implants and a permanent fixed denture. Dental implants can be inserted either at the time of marginal mandibulectomy or later on if adequate vertical height of the remaining body of the mandible following marginal mandibulectomy is available. If the osseointegrated implants are inserted primarily, satisfactory coverage over the mandible should be secured to avoid exposure and loss of the implants.

The patient shown in Figure 11.63 has a 1-cm, ulcerated, superficial carcinoma involving the alveolus of the edentulous mandible adjacent to her central incisor tooth. A panoramic radiograph of the mandible did not show any evidence of bone destruction beneath this lesion. This tumor is therefore suitable for a marginal mandibulectomy. The surgical specimen of marginal mandibulectomy accomplished through the open mouth is shown in Figure 11.64. Note that satisfactory mucosal and soft tissue margins are secured, as seen on the surface view of the specimen. On the side view, the height of the surgical specimen is shown with ample deep bone margins for this superficial ulcerated

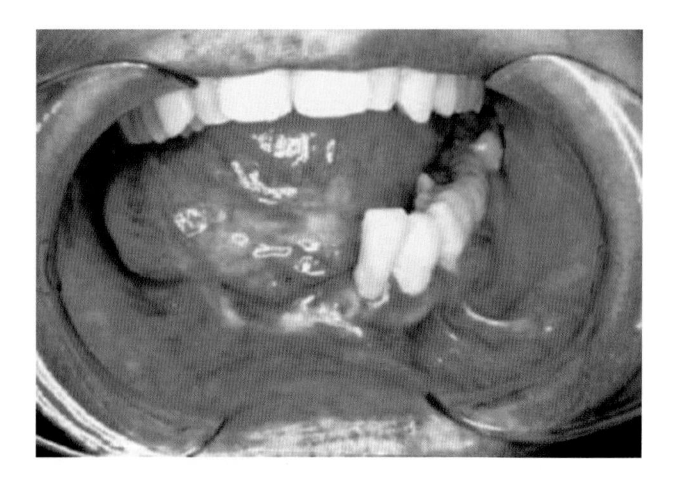

Figure 11.63 Superficial squamous carcinoma of the lower gum.

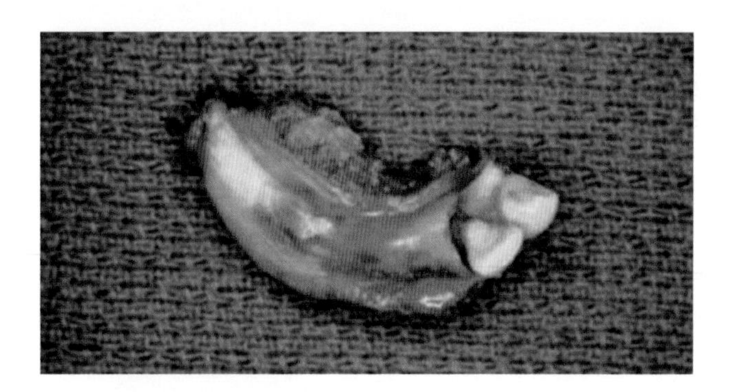

Figure 11.64 Specimen showing adequate mucosal margins.

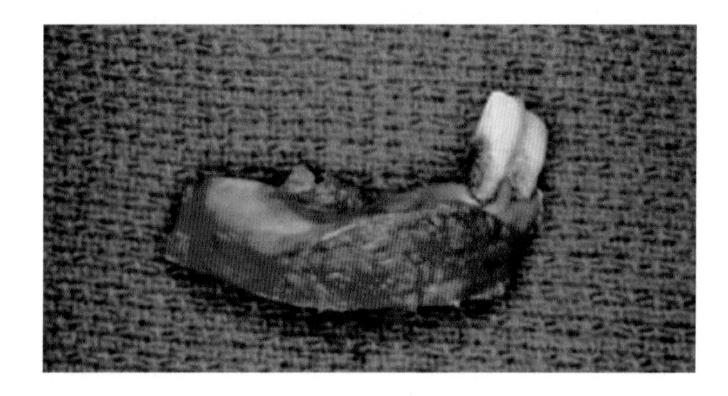

Figure 11.65 Specimen showing a satisfactory deep margin.

carcinoma (Figure 11.65). The surgical defect is repaired by primary closure of the mucosa of the floor of the mouth to the mucosa of the lower lip. Although the sulci at the site of the resected mandible in the floor of the mouth and the gingivolabial region are eliminated, the functional impairment in the immediate postoperative period is minimal. The postoperative appearance of the mouth at approximately 1 year shows a well-healed suture line (Figure 11.66). Note the absence of gingivolabial sulcus, as well as flattening of the mucosa of the floor of the mouth. At this time, she would be

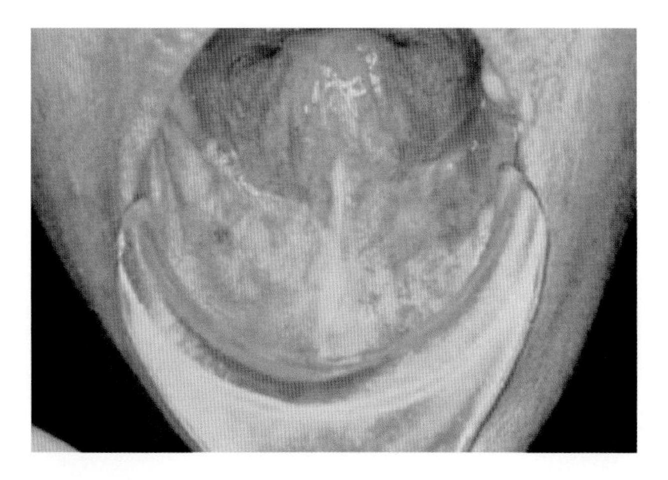

Figure 11.66 Postoperative intraoral view.

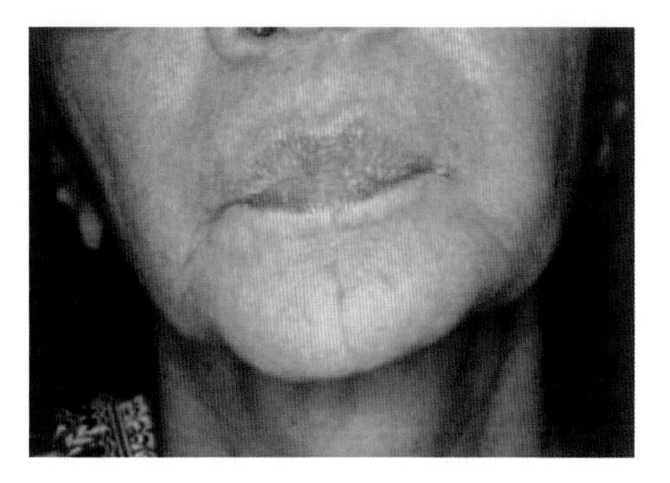

Figure 11.67 Postoperative external appearance.

an ideal candidate to consider dental implants. The external appearance of the patient, however, remains unchanged (Figure 11.67).

MARGINAL MANDIBULECTOMY AND REPAIR WITH SKIN GRAFT

The intraoral photograph of a patient with carcinoma of the lower alveolus adjacent to her remaining teeth is shown in Figure 11.68. The primary lesion is exophytic and relatively superficial, involving the alveolar process and attached gingiva of the adjacent teeth. A panoramic radiograph of the mandible fails to show any evidence of bone destruction (Figure 11.69). The extent of the tumor and the planned extent of marginal mandibulectomy are shown on the panoramic X-ray. Marginal mandibulectomy in this patient was performed using a lower cheek flap approach, splitting the lip in the midline to gain exposure of the lesion. A high-speed sagittal power saw is used to accomplish a marginal mandibulectomy in a smooth, curved fashion to evenly distribute the stress at the site of bone resection. The surgical specimen shows a satisfactory three-dimensional resection of the primary tumor (Figure 11.70). The surgical defect demonstrates a smooth, curved, marginal resection of the

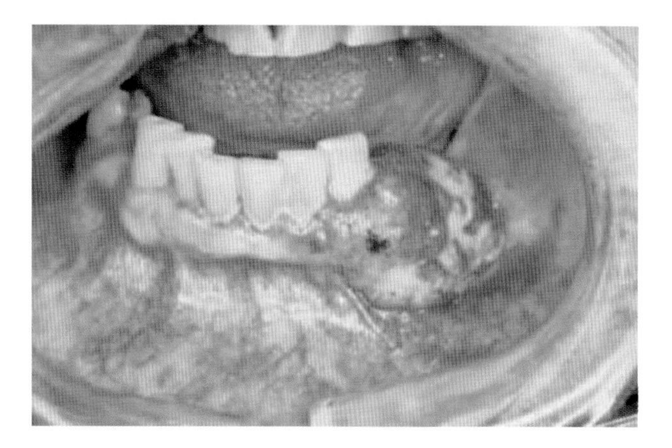

Figure 11.68 Squamous carcinoma of the lower alveolus.

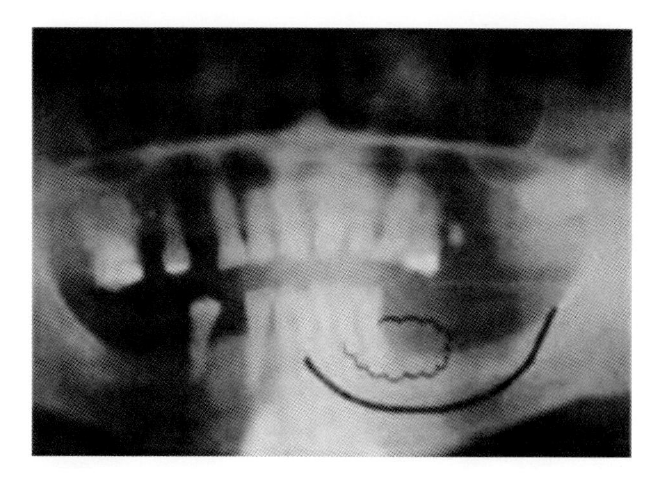

Figure 11.69 Panoramic X-ray of the mandible showing the location of the tumor and proposed marginal mandibulectomy.

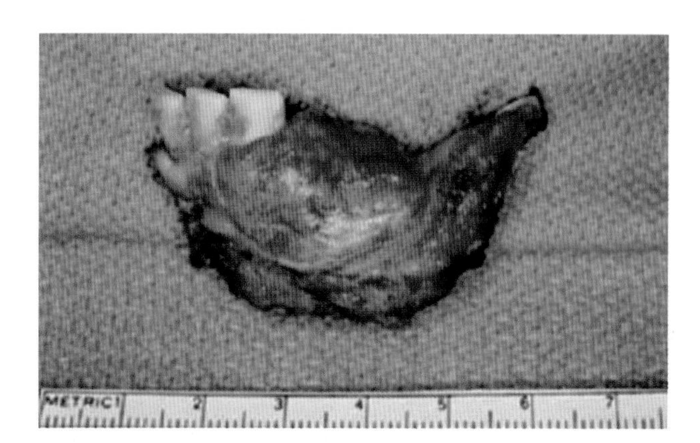

Figure 11.70 Surgical specimen of marginal mandibulectomy.

mandible with sufficient cortical bone remaining to provide stability to the mandible and to preserve the continuity of the arch of the mandible (Figure 11.71). The surgical defect in this patient was repaired using a split-thickness skin graft. The skin graft usually heals satisfactorily and provides excellent coverage of the exposed bone (Figure 11.72).

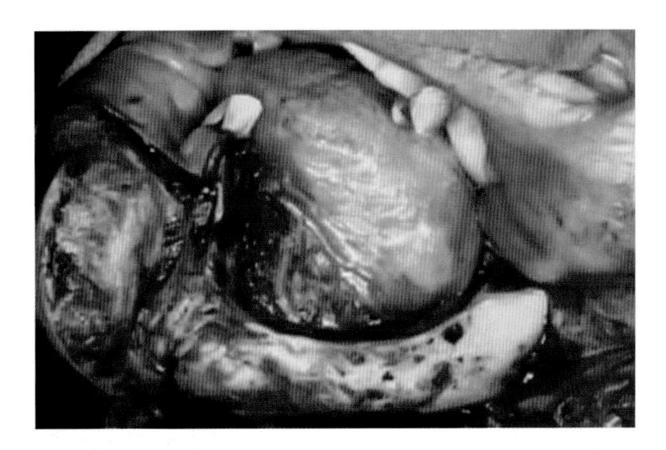

Figure 11.71 Surgical defect following marginal mandibulectomy.

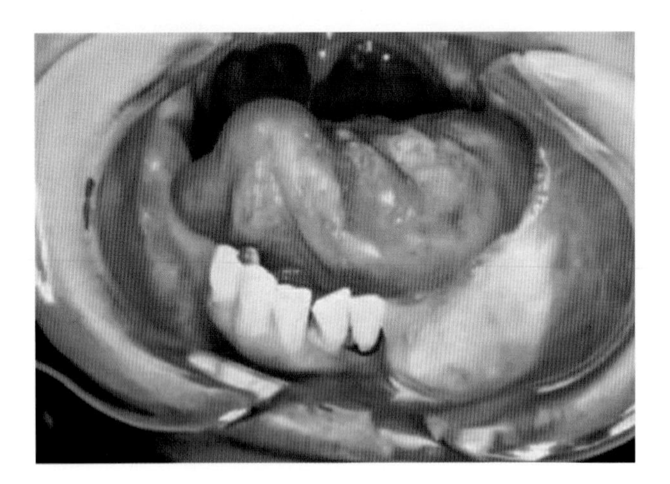

Figure 11.72 Healed skin graft over the marginally resected mandible.

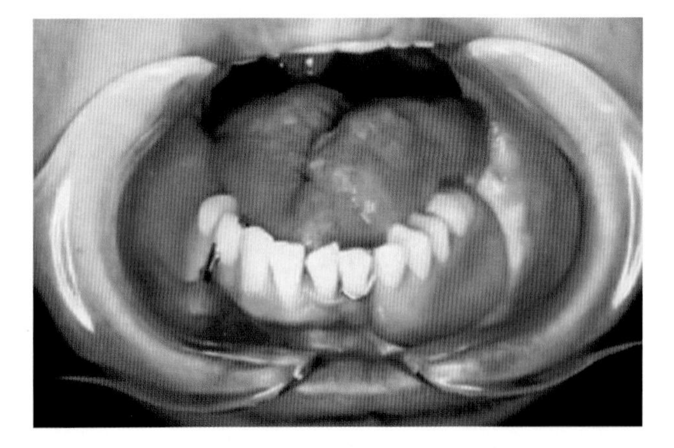

Figure 11.73 Partial denture at the site of marginal mandibulectomy.

Since the patient has remaining teeth in the lower dentition, a removable denture was fabricated that can be clasped to the teeth to restore lower dentition (Figure 11.73). Another patient who had undergone marginal mandibulectomy in a similar anterior location is shown in Figure 11.74, with the osseointegrated implants placed at the site of marginal mandibulectomy with a permanent fixed denture in place. Her panoramic radiograph shown in Figure 11.75 demonstrates satisfactory position of the implants anterior to the mental foramen in the mandible where marginal mandibulectomy was performed. The permanent dental implants restoring lower dentition with a fixed denture are shown in Figure 11.76. Thus, when feasible, osseointegrated implants should be considered for complete dental rehabilitation following marginal mandibulectomy.

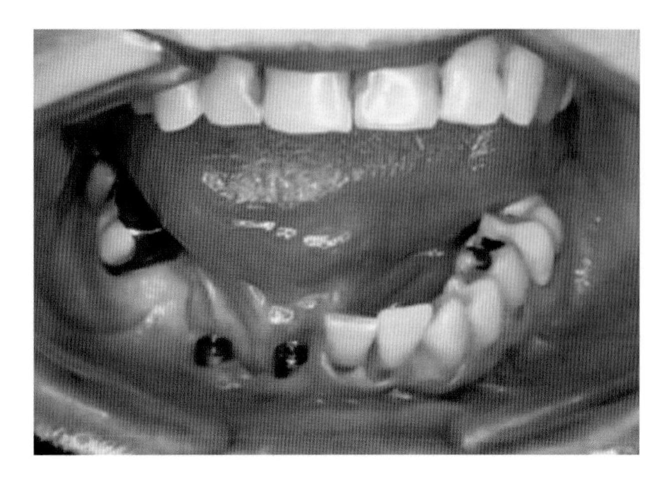

Figure 11.74 Osseointegrated implants at the site of marginal mandibulectomy.

MARGINAL MANDIBULECTOMY IN AN EDENTULOUS PATIENT

In general, marginal mandibulectomy is not advisable in an edentulous patient due to the lack of adequate vertical height of the mandible on the lateral aspect. However, in selected patients it may be feasible. Thus, if marginal mandibulectomy is performed in an edentulous patient, extreme caution must be exercised with regard to viability of the remaining mandible (30,32); otherwise, a pathological fracture is possible at that site. If such is feared to be the case, then the remaining mandible should be supported using a metallic plate as a buttress to prevent iatrogenic fracture.

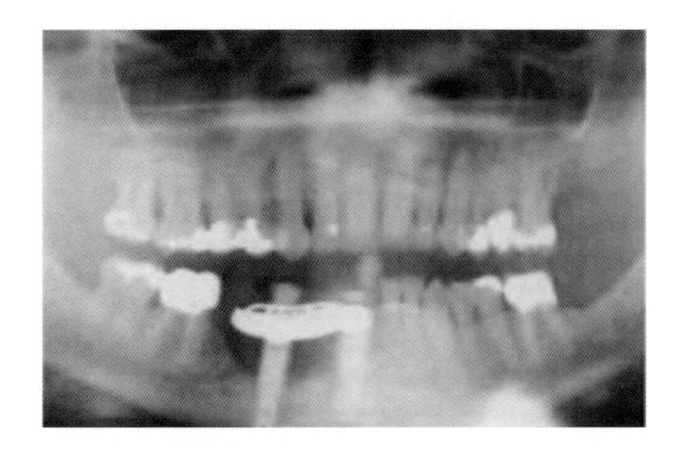

Figure 11.75 Panoramic X-ray showing the osseointegrated implants.

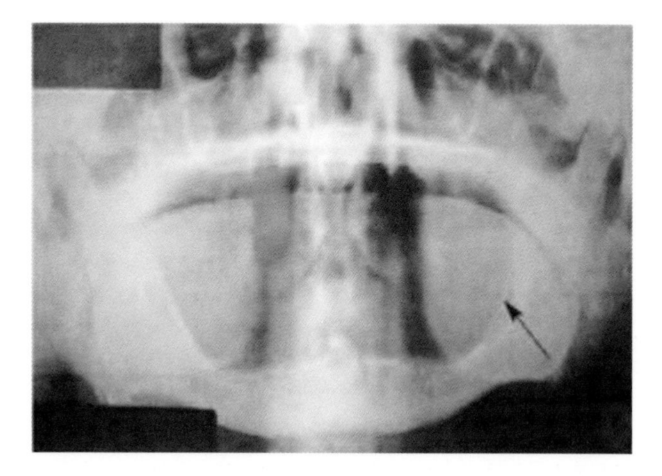

Figure 11.76 Permanent, fixed denture at the site of marginal mandibulectomy.

Figure 11.78 Panoramic X-ray showing minimal cortical erosion at the left retromolar region.

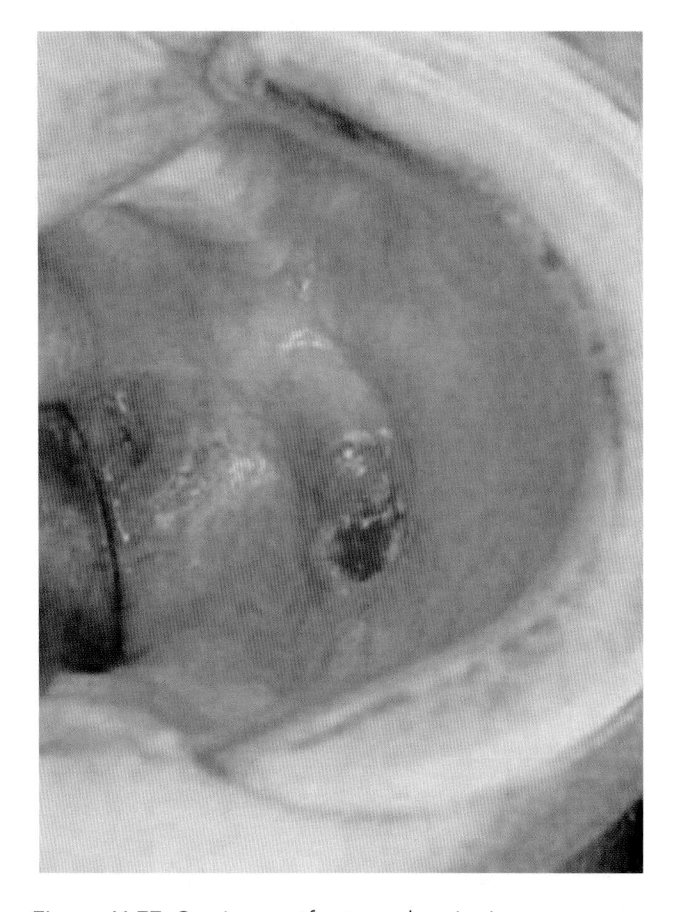

Figure 11.77 Carcinoma of retromolar gingiva.

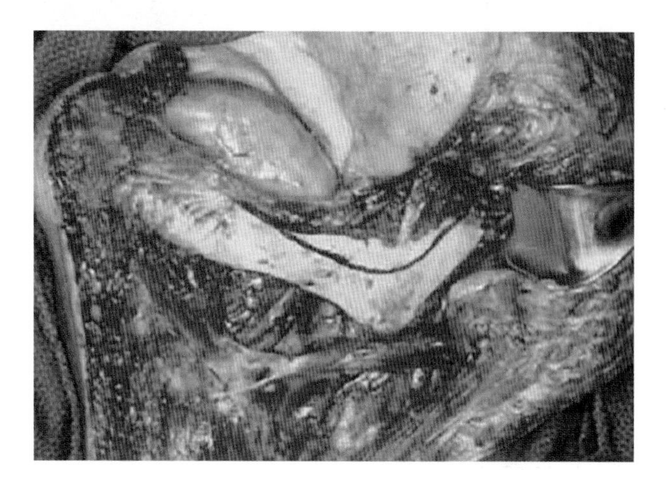

Figure 11.79 The proposed marginal mandibulectomy is outlined.

The patient shown in Figure 11.77 has carcinoma of the retromolar trigone and the adjacent lower gingiva on the left-hand side with invasion of the underlying cortical bone in an edentulous mandible. Panoramic radiograph of the mandible shows cortical erosion at the retromolar trigone, requiring at least a marginal mandibulectomy (Figure 11.78). A supraomohyoid neck dissection as a staging procedure is done and the lower cheek flap is elevated in the usual fashion so that it remains lateral to the outer cortex of the mandible from the symphysis at the anterior midline up to the mandibular notch posteriorly. The extent of bone resection to be undertaken at the site of the primary tumor is marked on the ascending ramus and the posterior aspect of the body of the mandible (Figure 11.79). Appropriate three-dimensional resection is then performed using a high-speed power saw with an ultra-thin blade. The surgical specimen viewed from the lateral aspect is shown in Figure 11.80. Note that a three-dimensional resection has been accomplished with a satisfactorily deep margin to excise the alveolar surface of the mandible in a monobloc fashion. The surface view of the surgical specimen shows adequate mucosal margins around the primary tumor (Figure 11.81). The sharp edges of the marginally resected mandible are smoothed out. Note that the remaining mandible is very thin, has a very limited height and is at risk for spontaneous fracture (Figure 11.82). Therefore, a long miniplate is used to support the remaining mandible in order to prevent spontaneous fracture. The miniplate is appropriately shaped to fit the lateral cortex of the mandible extending from the ascending

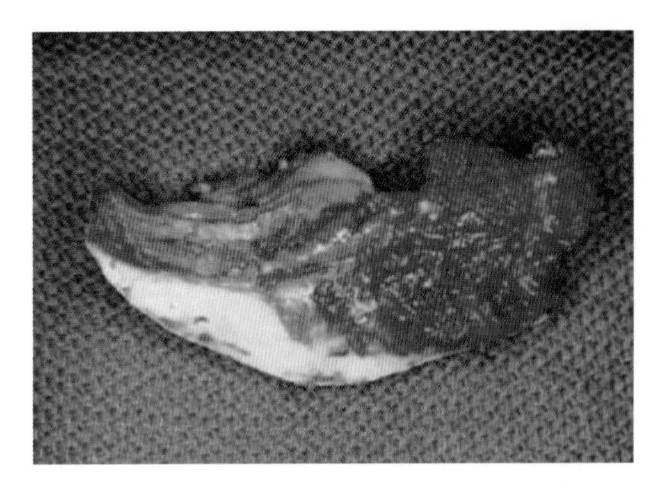

Figure 11.80 Specimen showing adequate deep margins.

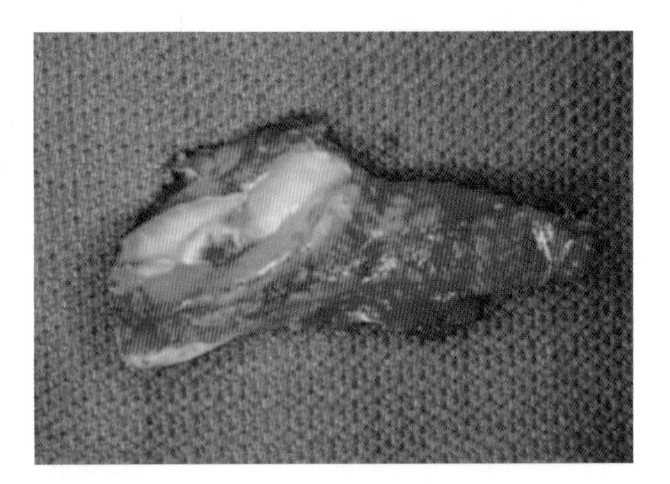

Figure 11.81 Specimen showing adequate mucosal margins.

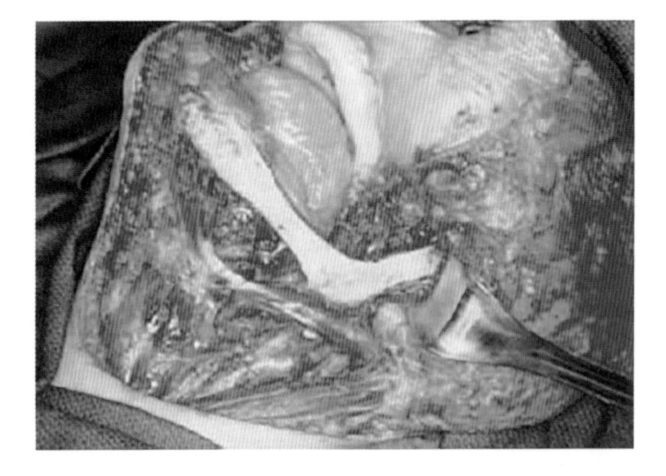

Figure 11.82 Surgical defect showing remaining edentulous mandible.

ramus up to the anterior aspect of the body of the mandible (Figure 11.83). Several screws are used to hold the miniplate in position. Primary closure of the mucosa of the floor of the mouth and cheek is performed and the wound is closed in the usual fashion.

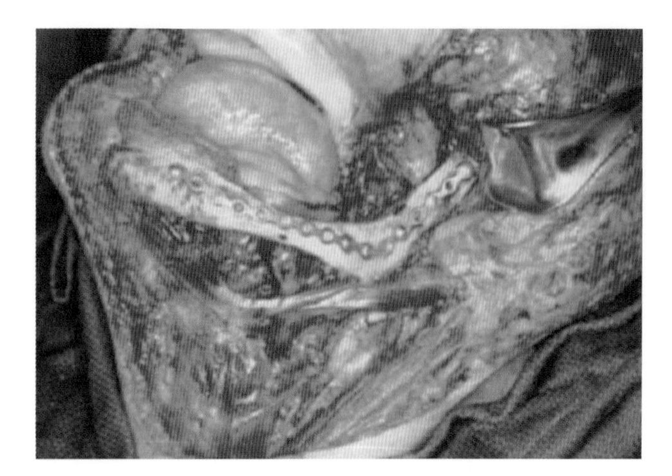

Figure 11.83 A long miniplate support is applied to the remaining mandible to prevent fracture.

AGGRESSIVE MARGINAL MANDIBULECTOMY AND RECONSTRUCTION WITH AN A–O PLATE AND RADIAL FOREARM FREE FLAP

When a large area of mucosa of the lower gum is involved by primary tumor, then clearly a secondary effort at reconstruction to provide surface lining in the oral cavity is essential. However, if the underlying bone is not involved, then a marginal mandibulectomy is technically feasible.

A primary verrucous carcinoma of the lower gum extending from the region of the first molar tooth to the retromolar trigone is shown in Figure 11.84. Panoramic radiograph of the mandible shows cortical erosion of the retromolar trigone region. The extent of bone resection is indicated on radiograph (Figure 11.85). A midline lower lip-splitting incision extended to the lateral aspect of the upper part of the neck is used to facilitate a supraomohyoid neck dissection (Figure 11.86). A supraomohyoid neck dissection is completed and a marginal mandibulectomy is performed through the lower cheek flap approach. A monobloc resection is accomplished (Figure 11.87). The medial surface view of the surgical specimen shows a large area of the mucosa of

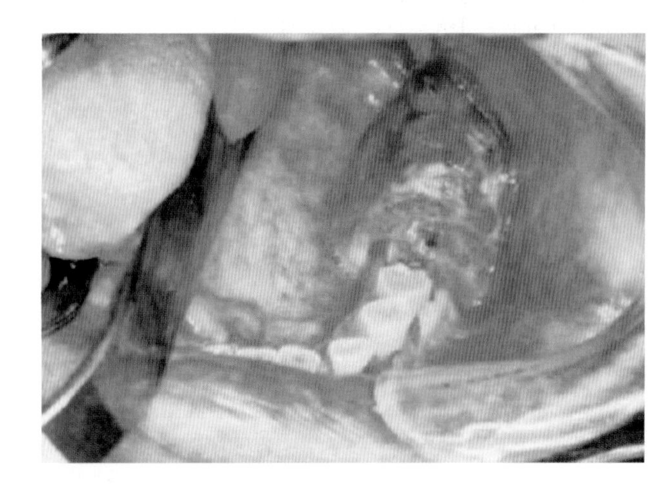

Figure 11.84 Verrucous carcinoma of the lower gum extending up to the retromolar trigone.

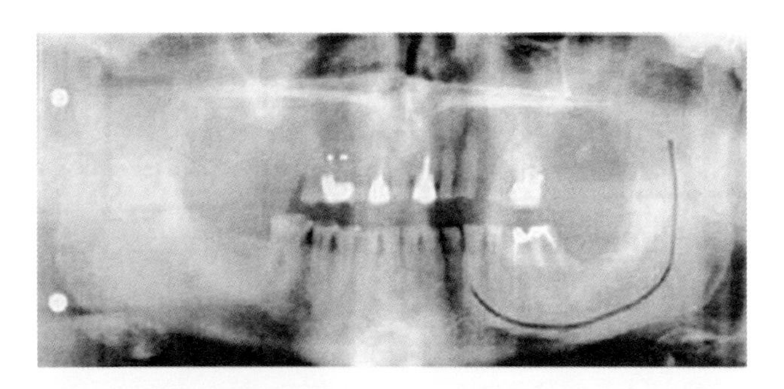

Figure 11.85 Proposed marginal mandibulectomy outlined on a panoramic X-ray.

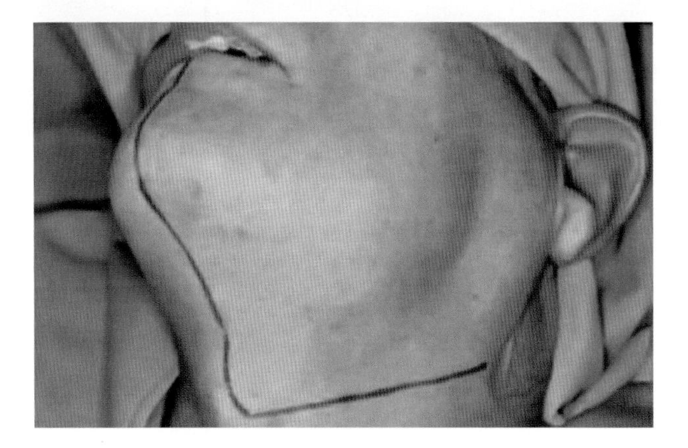

Figure 11.86 The skin incision is outlined for marginal mandibulectomy and modified neck dissection.

the lower gum and floor of the mouth as well as the cheek excised in a monobloc fashion, with the underlying mandible in continuity with the contents of the supraomohyoid neck dissection (Figure 11.88). The surgical field shows the bony defect in the body and the ascending ramus of the mandible (Figure 11.89). The remaining mandible is at significant risk of spontaneous fracture unless it is supported by a metallic buttress. An A–O plate is used to support the residual mandible (Figure 11.90).

A fascio-cutaneous radial forearm free flap is elevated from the patient's left arm (Figure 11.91). The free flap is used to resurface the lining of the oral cavity over the remaining portion of the mandible supported by the A–O plate. A postoperative intraoral view of the patient shows primary healing of the radial forearm free flap providing excellent coverage of the lining in the oral cavity (Figure 11.92).

A postoperative panoramic view of the mandible shows adequate placement of the A–O plate (Figure 11.93).

COMPOSITE RESECTION WITH SEGMENTAL MANDIBULECTOMY (COMMANDO OPERATION)

A composite resection with segmental mandibulectomy (commando operation) is indicated for primary tumors of the oral cavity or oropharynx that extend to involve the mandible (Figure 11.94). On occasion, a composite resection may be indicated for patients with primary tumors having extensive soft tissue disease around the mandible that necessitates the sacrifice of an intervening segment of mandible to accomplish an incontinuity monobloc resection of the primary tumor in conjunction with neck dissection. Thus, a commando operation or a composite resection entails excision of the intraoral primary tumor along with a segment of the mandible performed in conjunction with ipsilateral neck dissection in a monobloc fashion.

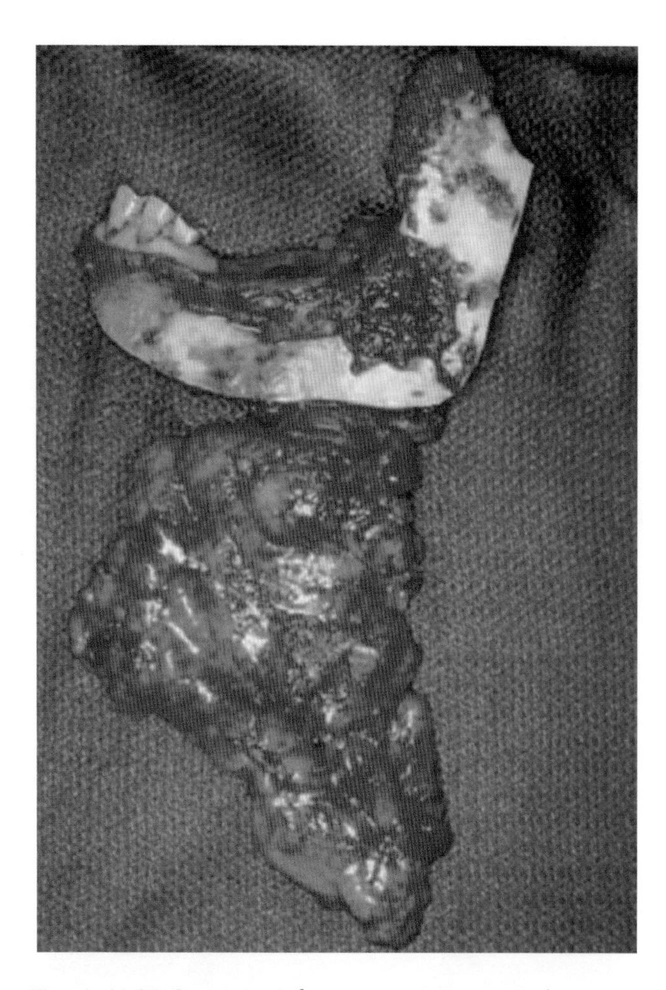

Figure 11.87 Specimen of an aggressive marginal mandibulectomy and supraomohyoid neck dissection.

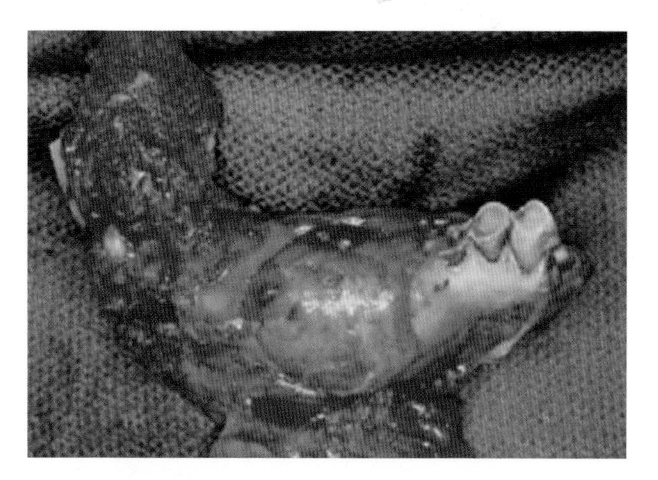

Figure 11.88 Specimen showing excision of a large mucosal surface.

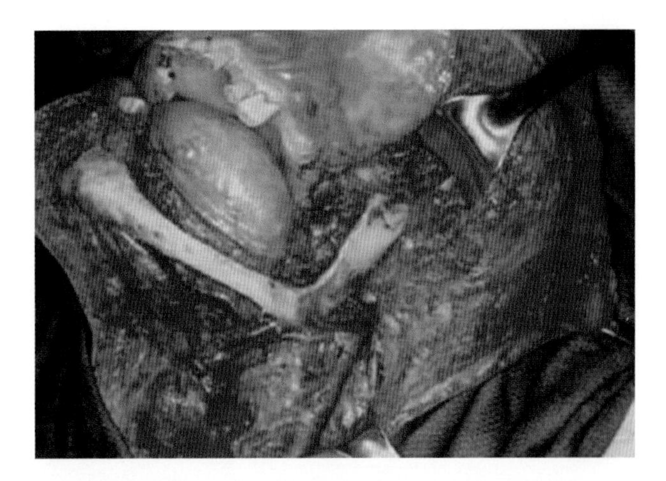

Figure 11.89 Surgical field showing residual mandible.

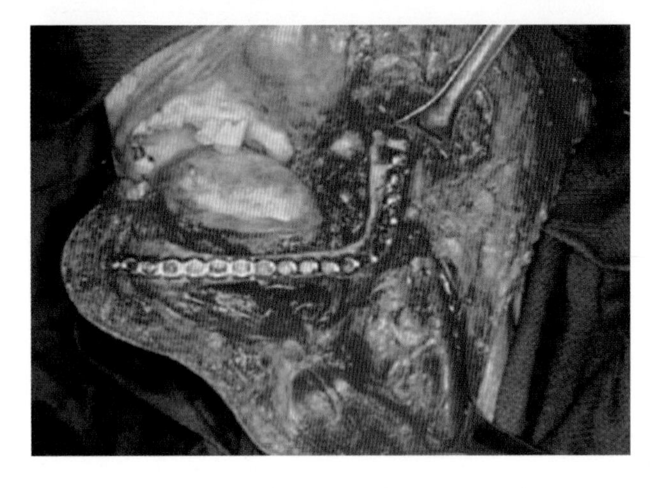

Figure 11.90 An A–O plate is used to support the remaining mandible.

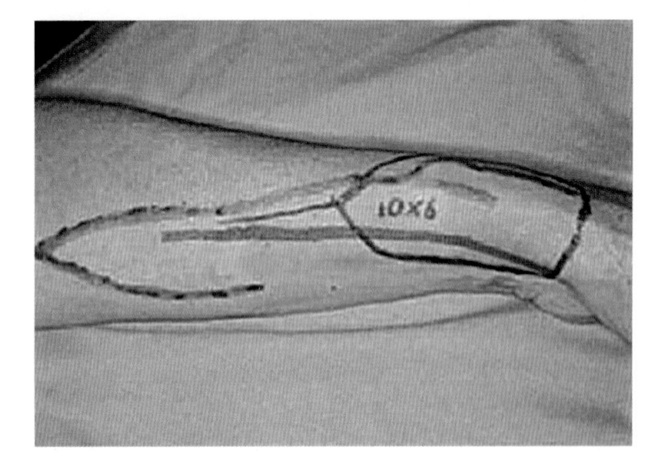

Figure 11.91 A radial forearm flap is used to reconstruct the mucosal defect.

The patient shown in Figure 11.95 has primary carcinoma of the lower gum with extension to the retromolar trigone and adjacent gingivobuccal sulcus. He had received previous radiotherapy with a curative intent, but the tumor persisted and hence the surgical procedure of composite

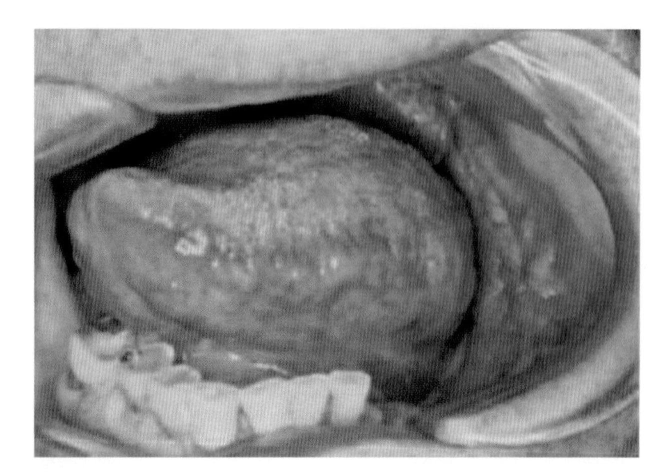

Figure 11.92 Postoperative intraoral view showing the radial forearm flap.

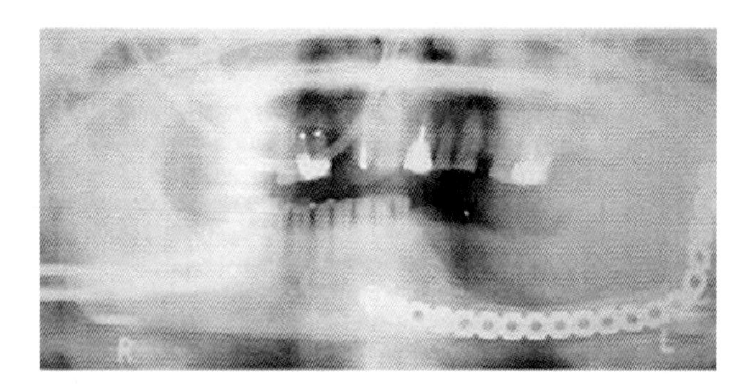

Figure 11.93 Postoperative panoramic X-ray showing the A–O plate.

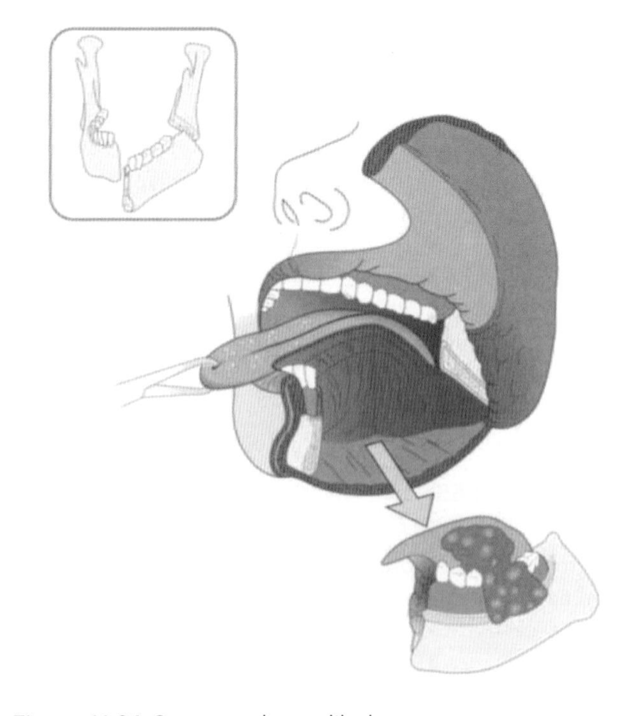

Figure 11.94 Segmental mandibulectomy.

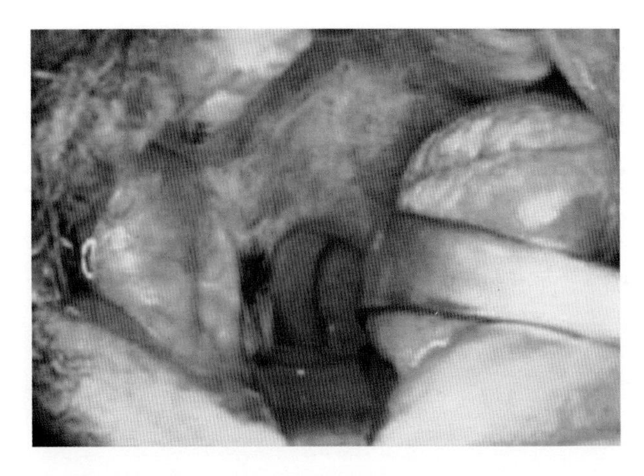

Figure 11.95 Previously irradiated squamous carcinoma of the lower gum.

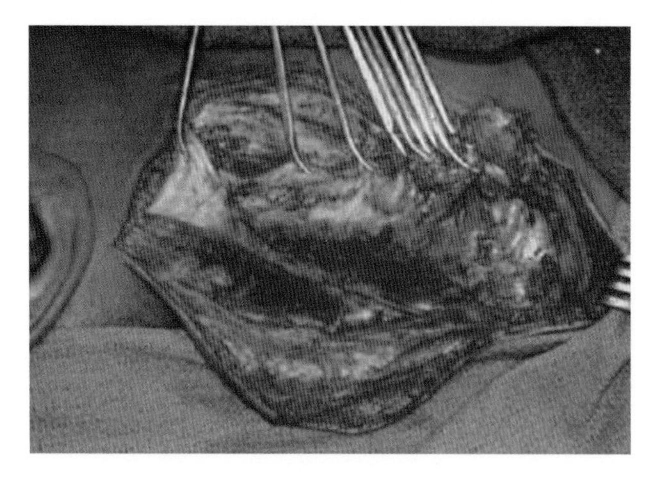

Figure 11.97 Neck dissection begins in the posterior triangle.

resection was indicated. He has clinically palpable cervical lymph node metastasis. The incision for the operation is a standard transverse cervical incision for neck dissection beginning at the tip of the mastoid process and curving anteriorly, remaining approximately two fingerbreadths below the body of the mandible up to the midline of the neck at the level of the hyoid bone (Figure 11.96). At that point, the incision turns cephalad, dividing the skin and soft tissues of the chin and the lower lip in the midline. If this transverse incision is made in a natural skin crease in the mid-cervical region, then a vertical component of the incision is not required. On the other hand, if the transverse incision is high in the neck, then a vertical incision will be necessary for exposure of the lower neck in order to accomplish the neck dissection clearing lymph nodes at levels IV and V. Due to the presence of clinically palpable cervical lymph nodes, this patient requires a comprehensive neck dissection clearing all five levels. In this patient, the vertical curvaceous component of the incision begins at the region of the posterior border of the sternocleidomastoid muscle on the transverse incision and extends down to the clavicle at the midclavicular point. The sequential steps of various types of neck dissections are described in Chapter 10 on the management of the neck. Dissection of the posterior triangle and lower neck is completed in the usual fashion, preserving the accessory nerve if it is not directly involved by metastatic disease (Figure 11.97). The phrenic nerve is preserved and the cutaneous roots of the cervical plexus are divided (Figure 11.98). The lower anterior skin flap is now elevated and the insertion of the sternomastoid muscle is detached from the sternum and the clavicle (Figure 11.99). After ligation of the internal jugular vein at the lower end, dissection proceeds cephalad along the carotid sheath toward level I (Figure 11.100). No attempt is made to dissect the contents of the submandibular triangle, which remain attached through the floor of the mouth and the soft tissues medial to the mandible and the primary site (Figure 11.101).

At this point, the neck incision is extended cephalad in the midline, dividing the skin of the chin and the lower lip through its full thickness (Figure 11.102). The upper skin

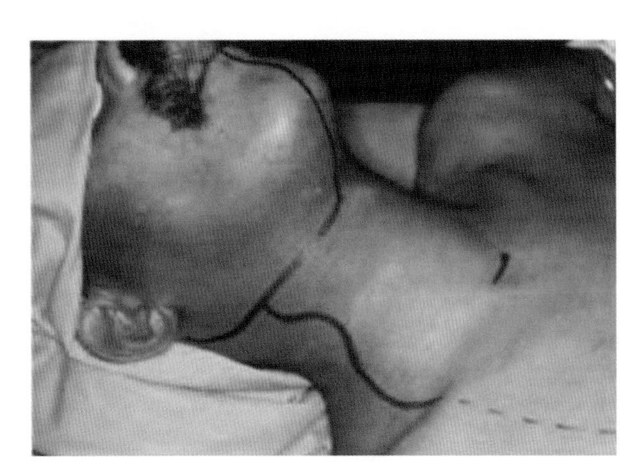

Figure 11.96 Skin incision outlined for composite resection of the lower gum with neck dissection.

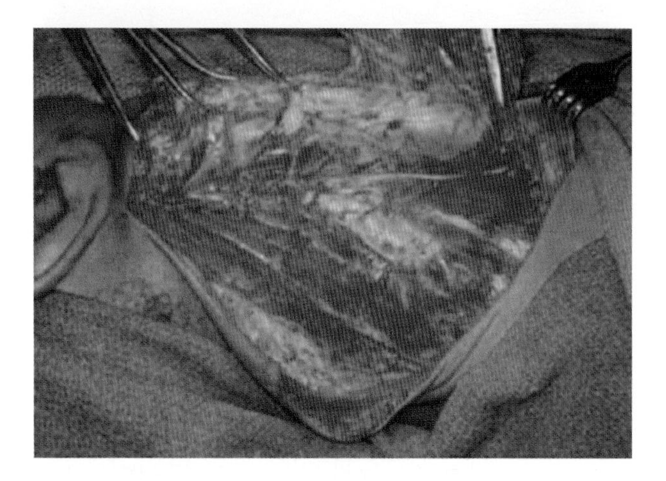

Figure 11.98 The accessory and phrenic nerves are preserved, but the cutaneous cervical roots are divided.

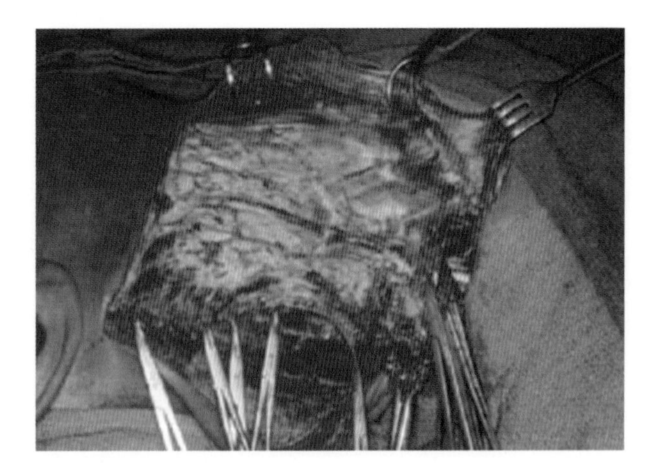

Figure 11.99 The anterior skin flap is elevated to expose the lower end of the sternomastoid muscle.

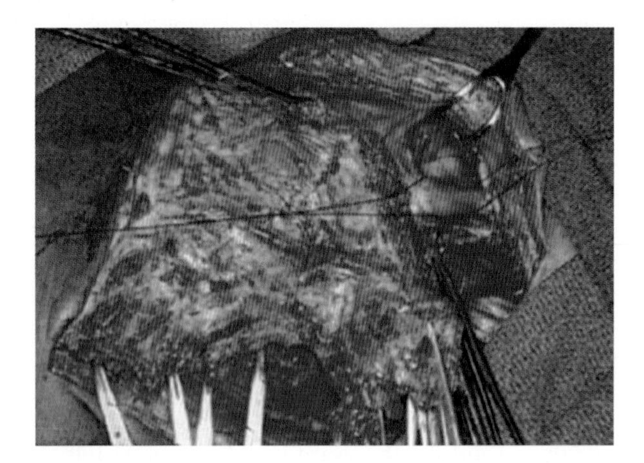

Figure 11.100 The internal jugular vein is doubly ligated and divided.

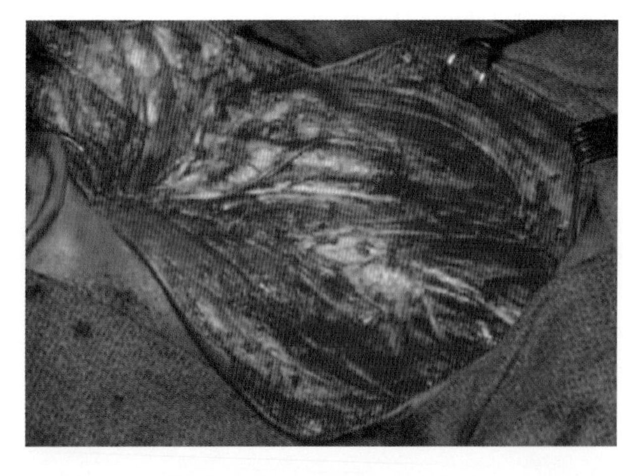

Figure 11.101 Dissection proceeds along the carotid sheath up to the hypoglossal nerve.

flap of the neck dissection is now elevated, remaining deep to the platysma, which is retained on the flap. Meticulous attention should be paid to identification and careful preservation of the marginal branch of the facial nerve to maintain the function of the lower lip and competency of the

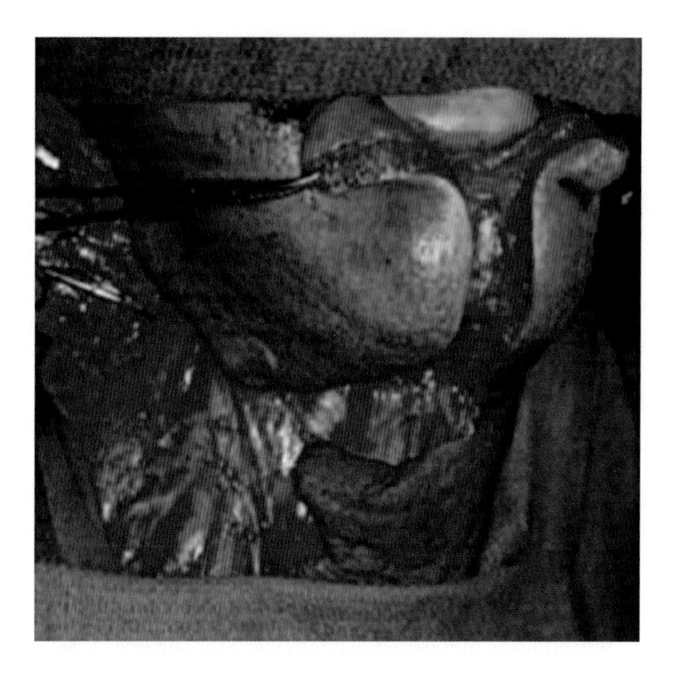

Figure 11.102 The lower lip is split in the midline and the outer cortex of the mandible is exposed.

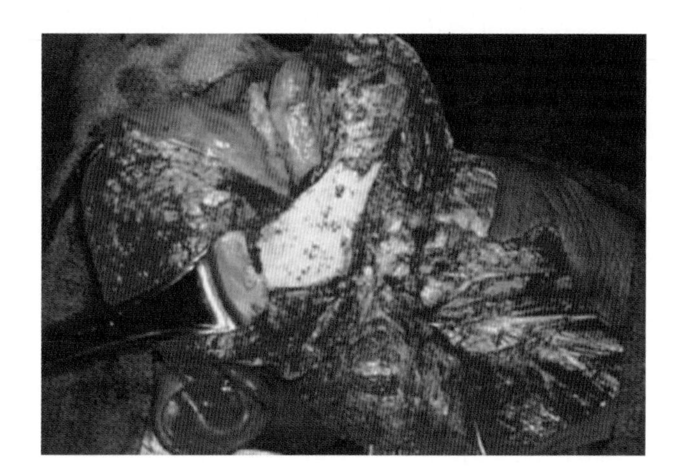

Figure 11.103 The lower cheek flap is elevated.

oral cavity. The upper skin flap is elevated up to the lower border of the mandible, extending from the angle of the mandible all the way up to the midline of the chin. Division of the lower lip in the midline through its full thickness is now completed up to the anterior cortex of the mandible at the symphysis.

A mucosal incision is placed in the gingivolabial and gingivobuccal sulcus, leaving adequate mucosal and soft tissue margins around the primary tumor (Figure 11.103). In this patient, the cheek flap is elevated, leaving all soft tissues, including prevascular facial nodes, attached to the mandible. The lateral surface of the masseter is exposed and the masseter is detached from the ascending ramus of the mandible up to the mandibular notch. This maneuver provides exposure of the entire lateral cortex of the mandible from the mandibular notch up to the midline at the symphysis menti. An appropriate site on the mandible for division is marked (Figure 11.104).

The muscular attachments of the temporalis muscle over the coronoid process of the mandible are detached. A sagittal power saw is now used to divide the mandible through the ascending ramus. Brisk hemorrhage ensues from the two cut ends of the mandible following division of the condyloid process. Bone wax is used to control bleeding from the cut ends of the bone. Extreme caution should be exercised to prevent the power saw from cutting through the soft tissues medial to the mandible, otherwise excessive hemorrhage will result from laceration of the pterygoid muscles and the rich network of terminal branches of the internal maxillary artery. In order to avoid laceration of the soft tissues medial to the mandible, it is desirable to introduce a small, malleable retractor medial to the condyloid process of the mandible before dividing the bone. Alternatively, a Mixter clamp may be introduced to support the condyloid process of the mandible and prevent the blade of the sagittal saw from lacerating the soft tissues situated medially. Attention is now focused on dividing the mandible distally at an appropriate place depending upon the site, size and surface extent of the tumor, as well as the extent of the soft tissue disease contiguous to the mandible. A straight cut through the body of the mandible is performed at the appropriate site. Bone wax is used again to control hemorrhage from the cut ends of the mandible. The mandible, having been divided at two places, permits its lateral retraction and exposure of the intraoral tumor.

Using electrocautery, a mucosal incision is placed around the primary tumor with a generous curf of normal mucosa to secure satisfactory margins. A three-dimensional resection of the primary tumor along with the adjacent floor of the mouth, underlying soft tissues and musculature of the tongue is performed with the use of electrocautery, remaining in continuity with the mandible and the contents of the dissected neck. Hemostasis is secured as the procedure proceeds by ligation or electrocoagulation of the bleeding points as they are encountered. The final part of the procedure requires division of the medial and lateral pterygoid muscles from the pterygoid plates. Again, brisk bleeding occurs at this time; however, it is easily controllable with electrocautery and using an absorbable over and over, figure-of-eight suture through the stumps of the pterygoid muscles. The extent of mucosa and soft tissue resection clearly depends on the extent and invasive nature of the primary tumor and the involvement of the underlying musculature, soft tissues and neurovascular bundles.

After removal of the specimen, the surgical field shows a satisfactory monobloc resection of the primary tumor in conjunction with the contents of the dissected neck and the intervening soft tissues and lymphatics (Figure 11.105). Frozen sections are obtained from appropriate areas according to the extent of the primary tumor and the judgment of the surgeon regarding the proximity of the tumor to the surgical margins, as seen in a close-up view (Figure 11.106).

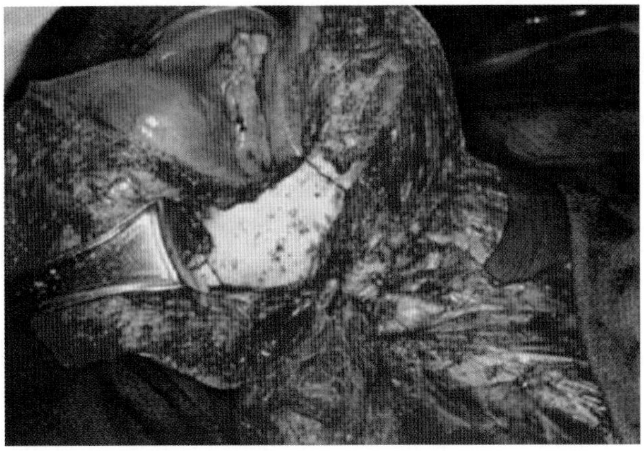

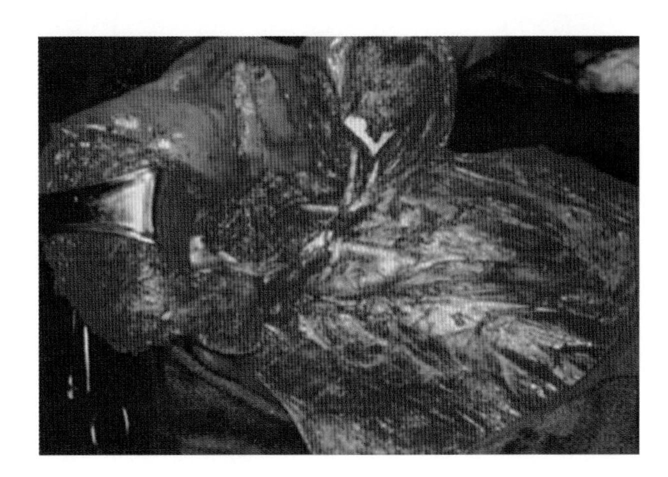

Figure 11.105 The surgical defect following composite resection.

Figure 11.104 Mucosal incisions are placed around the tumor and the extent of bone resection is outlined.

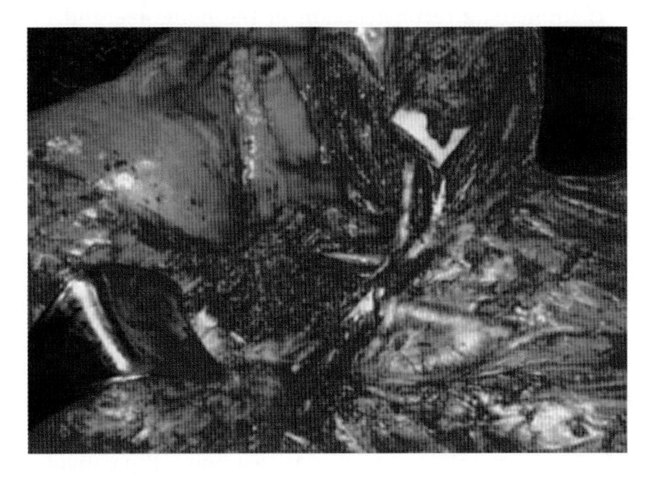

Figure 11.106 Close-up view of the surgical defect at the primary site.

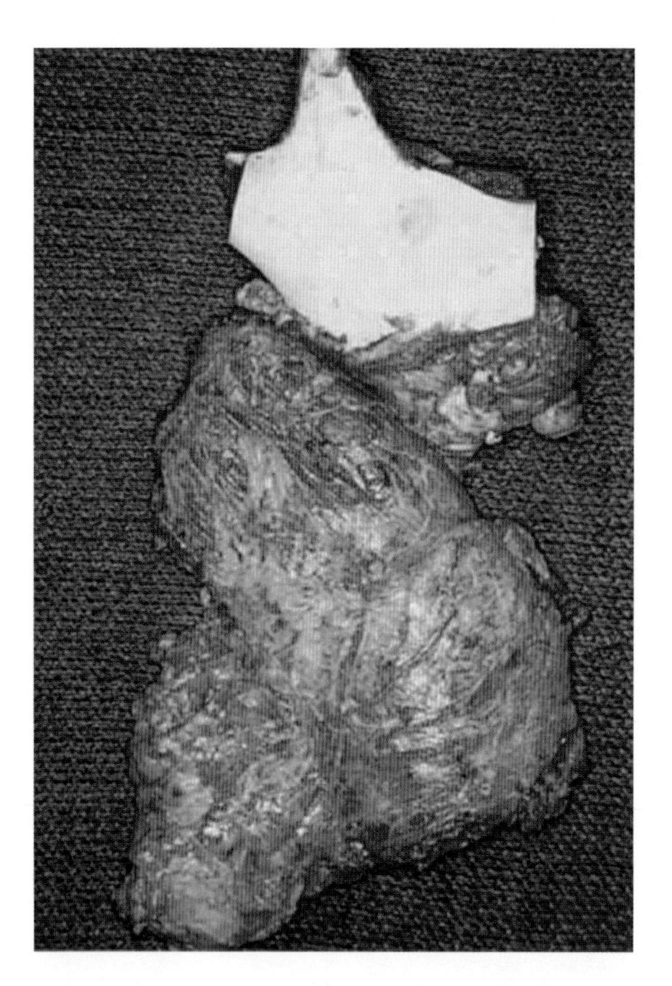

Figure 11.107 Lateral view of the surgical specimen.

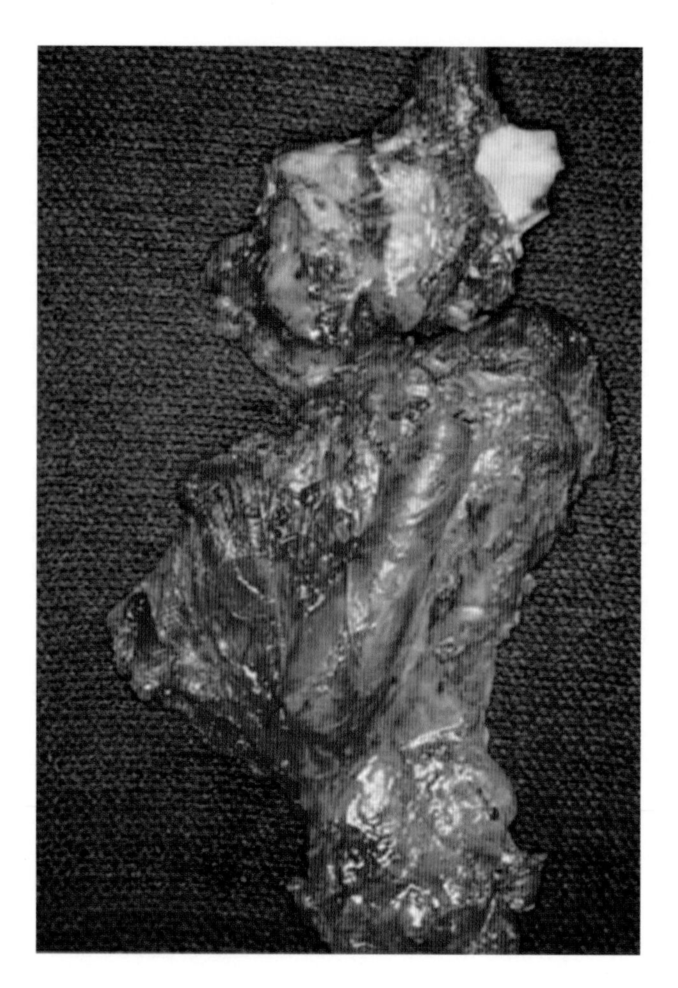

Figure 11.108 Medial view of the surgical specimen.

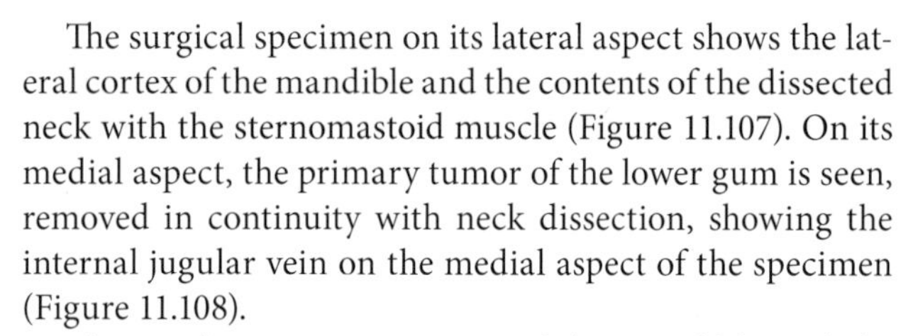

The surgical specimen on its lateral aspect shows the lateral cortex of the mandible and the contents of the dissected neck with the sternomastoid muscle (Figure 11.107). On its medial aspect, the primary tumor of the lower gum is seen, removed in continuity with neck dissection, showing the internal jugular vein on the medial aspect of the specimen (Figure 11.108).

If immediate reconstruction of the mandible and the mucosal lining is planned with a composite microvascular free flap, then the appropriate reconstructive procedure begins at this point. On the other hand, if no specific effort at reconstruction of the surgical defect is planned, then primary closure of the surgical defect should be performed.

A tracheostomy is done at the conclusion of the operation to facilitate clearance of pulmonary secretions postoperatively and for provision of a satisfactory airway to facilitate smooth postoperative recovery. Blood loss during this operative procedure is minimal. Blood transfusion is seldom necessary. If there is no tension on the suture line of the mucosa in the oral cavity, then primary healing should be expected within 1–2 weeks. At that point, the patient is started on pureed foods by mouth and gradually advanced to soft diet.

Dental rehabilitation following mandible reconstruction

Complete anatomic and functional rehabilitation of the oral cavity following cancer ablative surgery and reconstruction of the mandible requires either a satisfactorily removable lower denture clasped to the remaining teeth or the use of osseointegrated implants to facilitate a permanent fixed denture (50–53). The choice of dental rehabilitation with implants is based on several factors, including the status of the oral cavity after tumor resection, the need for adjuvant postoperative radiotherapy (PORT) with or without chemotherapy, available resources and patient preferences.

If osseointegrated dental implants are to be placed, we prefer that they be placed secondarily after satisfactory healing of the bone has occurred, rather than primarily at the time of free flap reconstruction of the mandible. A minimum of 12 months is allowed to elapse before osseointegrated implants are considered. A panoramic radiograph of the reconstructed mandible should show satisfactory bony union between the graft and the mandible and satisfactory bony healing of the osteotomized segments in the graft. Ideally, the placement of the implants should be performed by an appropriately trained oral surgeon with expertise in implantology. The first step is to assess the site for positioning of the implants. If metallic titanium plates and screws used for reconstruction of the mandible are impeding implant placement, then they are removed first to clear that area to receive the implants.

The location and number of implants to be placed are best assessed by the oral surgeon, who will assume the responsibility of placement of the implants and their subsequent exposure, as well as the eventual fabrication and placement of the permanent fixed denture. Satisfactorily integrated implants are exposed at between 4 and 6 months following placement. For details on the technical aspects of the placement of osseointegrated implants, their subsequent exposure and fabrication and fixation of a permanent fixed denture, the reader is referred to appropriate textbooks of oral surgery and dental implantology.

The patient shown in Figure 11.109 had a central salivary carcinoma of the lower gum on the left-hand side. His preoperative CT scan shows expansion of the involved segment of the mandible by tumor (Figure 11.110). He underwent segmental mandibulectomy. The specimen is shown in Figure 11.111. A radiograph of the specimen shows the extent of bone invasion (Figure 11.112). The mandible was reconstructed with a free flap of fibula. The postoperative intraoral picture shows satisfactory mucosal healing (Figure 11.113). Osseointegrated implants were placed after satisfactory bone healing of the fibula free flap. Serial panoramic views of the mandible show the immediate postoperative appearance of the reconstructed mandible after removal of plates and screws and after insertion of implants (Figure 11.114). The finished permanent, fixed

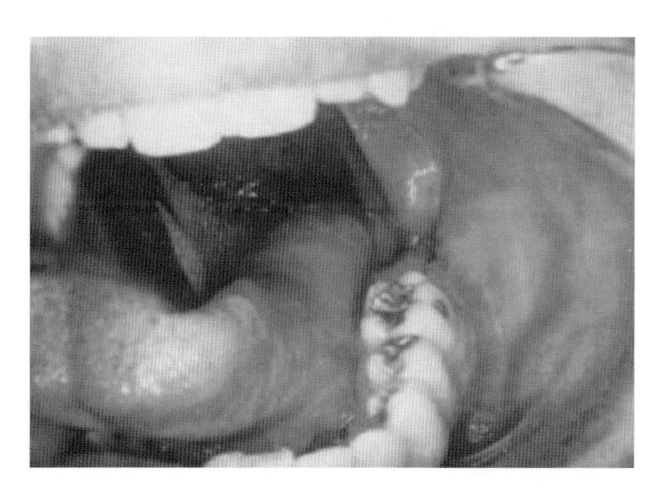

Figure 11.109 Intraoral view of left lower gum lesion.

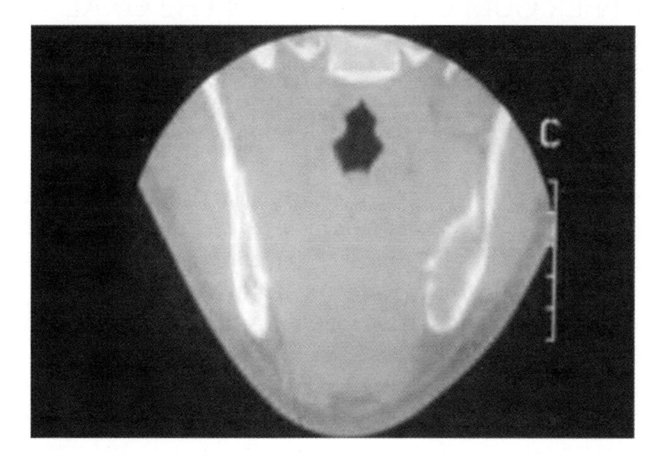

Figure 11.110 Coronal view of a CT scan of the mandible showing an expansive lesion.

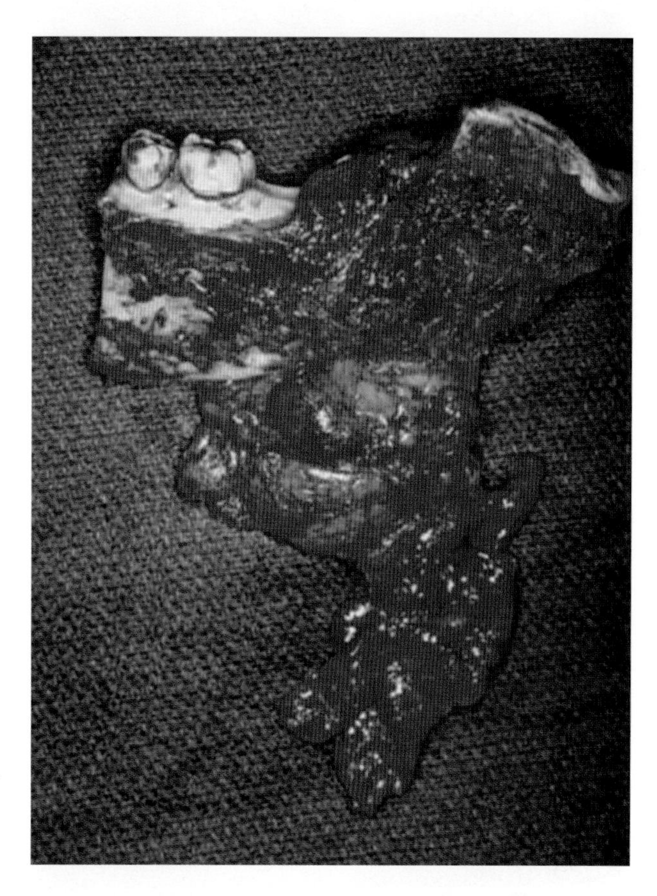

Figure 11.111 Surgical specimen of segmental mandibulectomy and supraomohyoid neck dissection.

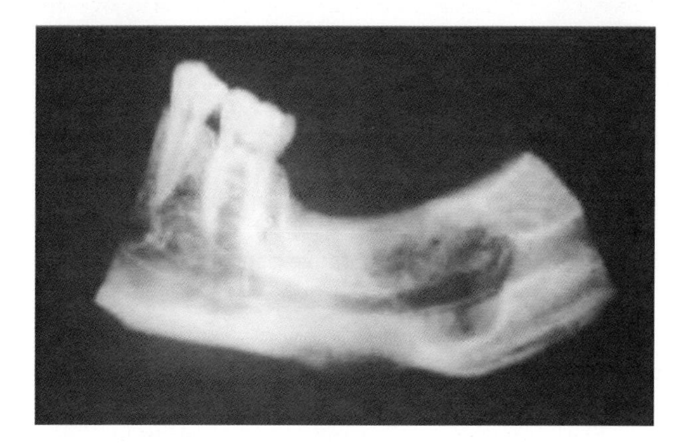

Figure 11.112 Plain radiograph of the specimen showing the lytic lesion.

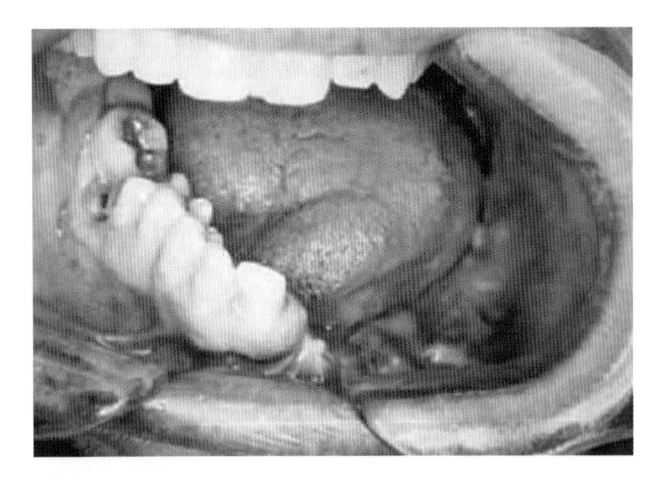

Figure 11.113 Postoperative intraoral view showing primary healing.

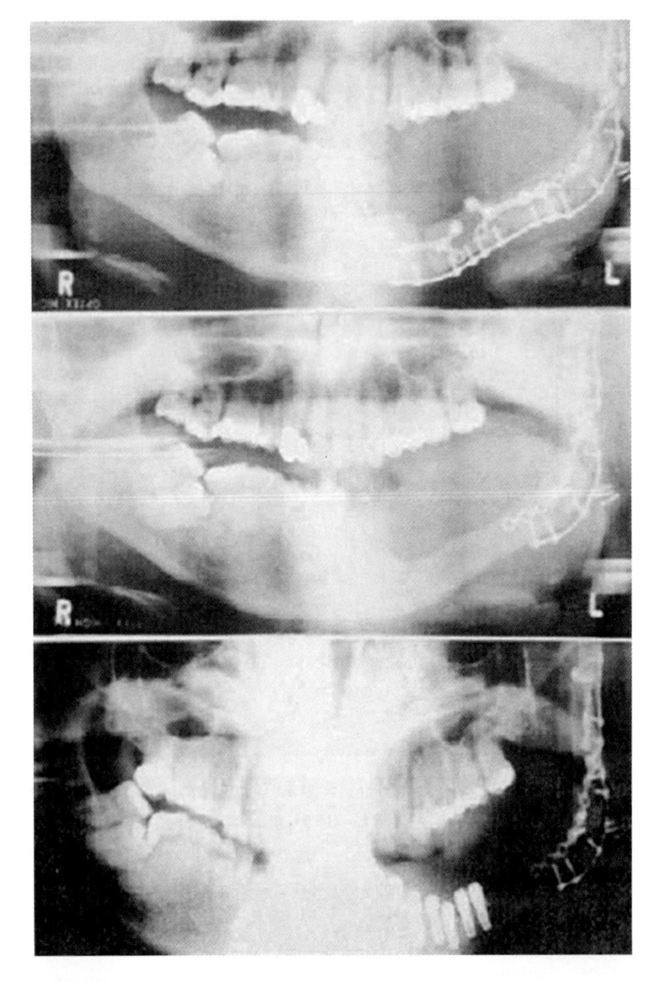

Figure 11.114 Serial postoperative panoramic X-rays of the mandible.

denture in the oral cavity is shown in Figure 11.115. At this time, the patient is considered fully rehabilitated following ablative cancer surgery and reconstruction to restore form and function. His external appearance is seen in Figure 11.116.

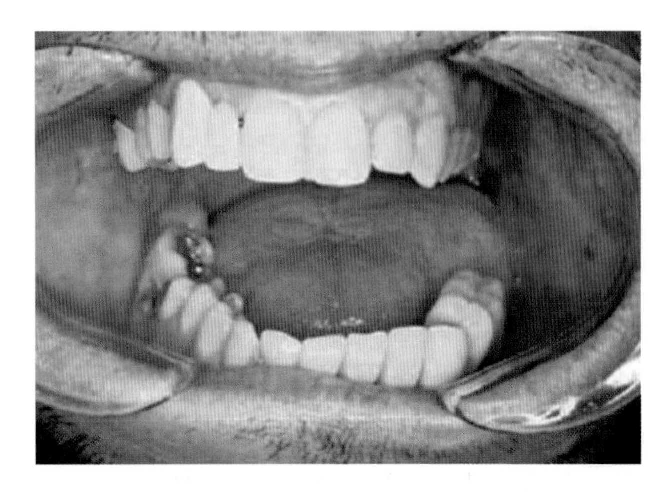

Figure 11.115 Intraoral view showing permanent fixed denture.

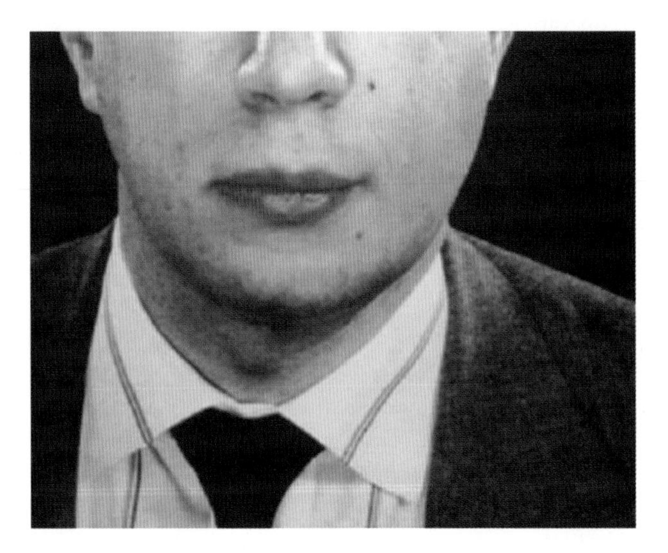

Figure 11.116 Postoperative appearance of the patient.

RESECTION OF THE MAXILLA FOR PRIMARY TUMORS OF THE PALATE, UPPER GUM OR MAXILLA IN THE ORAL CAVITY

Resection of a part of the maxilla is required in some patients undergoing surgical resection of primary epithelial tumors of the oral cavity arising on the hard palate, upper gum, upper gingivobuccal sulcus and anterior aspect of the soft palate. If the primary tumor involves the underlying hard palate or the upper gum, then resection of the maxilla is mandatory. Maxillary resection should be considered even when a tumor is only adherent to or in direct contiguity with the maxilla. Maxillary resections range from simple alveolectomy, to palatal fenestration and partial maxillectomy of the infrastructure (Figure 11.117) (54). However, the extent of maxillary resection is dictated by the location and extent of the tumor. A maxillectomy is also indicated in patients with primary neoplasms of the maxilla of either epithelial

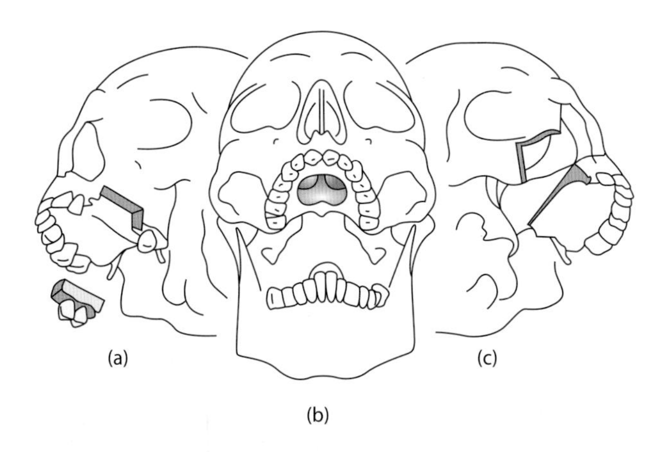

Figure 11.117 Maxilla resection. **(a)** Alveolectomy, **(b)** palatal fenestration and **(c)** partial maxillectomy.

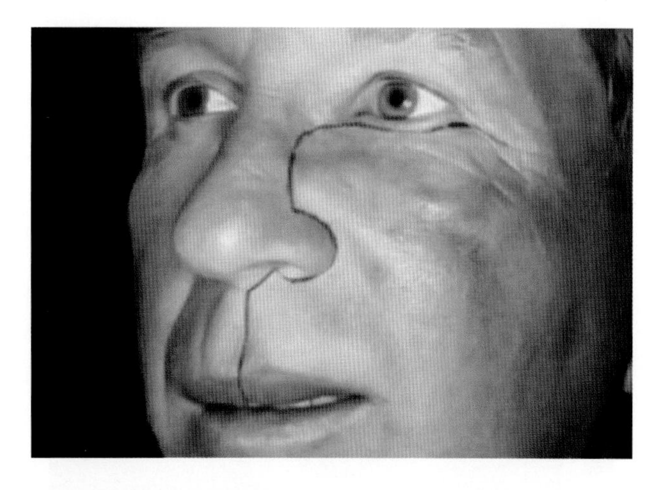

Figure 11.118 Modified Weber–Ferguson incision.

origin or mesenchymal origin, such as osteosarcoma, chondrosarcoma, fibrosarcoma, etc. Radiographic evaluation is essential to supplement clinical evaluation for assessment of bone invasion, but it must be remembered that early invasion is often not demonstrated on radiographic studies. Satisfactory evaluation of the hard palate requires CT scans in the coronal and sagittal planes, with soft tissue and bone windows.

Assessment of the status of dentition in the vicinity of the primary tumor is vitally important and is performed in the preoperative setting. If any dental care is necessary, it is completed either preoperatively or intraoperatively, with appropriate assistance from a dental surgeon. Impressions of the upper alveolus and hard palate are obtained preoperatively if any part of the upper gum or hard palate is to be resected with resultant communication between the oral cavity and the nasal cavity or the maxillary sinus. The impressions are used to make dental cast models, which facilitate fabrication of an immediate surgical obturator to be used intraoperatively for restoration of the palatal defect.

The final dental prosthesis with teeth is fabricated approximately 3 months after surgery. This dental prosthesis effectively plugs the surgical defect and also incorporates the remaining denture. When inserted in the oral cavity, the prosthesis provides satisfactory restoration of speech and mastication. It is important to re-emphasize that in any type of surgery for primary tumors of the oral cavity where removal of the alveolar process or hard palate is indicated, continuous communication between the surgeon and the prosthodontist is essential for satisfactory outcome of function and esthetics (55).

Small lesions that are easily accessible through the open mouth can be resected in conjunction with a limited partial maxillectomy *via* a peroral approach. However, when access is difficult or the primary tumor is large, then an upper cheek flap approach is necessary. This requires a modified Weber–Ferguson incision respecting the nasal subunits, with either a Lynch or a (Diffenbach) subciliary extension depending on the location of the primary tumor and the exposure necessary. In most instances, if only the hard palate or the upper gum is to be resected, then neither of these extensions is necessary.

The modified Weber–Ferguson incision is very important for cosmetic reasons. Esthetic improvement in the appearance of the healed Weber–Ferguson incision is clearly superior if modifications in the incisions are made respecting the nasal subunits (Figure 11.118). The incision begins exactly in the midline of the upper lip, dividing the philtrum, and extends up to the lower end of columella, where it turns lateral and into the floor of the nasal cavity. The incision then exits the nasal cavity, leaving a 60° notch in the floor of the nasal cavity where the triangular portion of the skin of the upper lip is inserted back into this defect during closure. The incision then follows the crease of the nasal ala all the way up to its superomedial end on the lateral aspect of the nose. A sharp 90° turn of the incision then extends as a straight line on the lateral aspect of the nose overlying the nasal bone up to a point about 6–8 mm medial to the medial canthus. At this point, it may be extended up to the inferomedial end of the eyebrow (Lynch extension) or extended laterally along a natural skin crease on the lower eyelid. This line is often demarcated by the junction of the slightly pigmented skin of the lower eyelid with the lighter skin of the cheek. All the angles and corners of the incision are accurately aligned at the time of closure to achieve a superior cosmetic result.

The patient shown in Figure 11.119 presented to her local otolaryngologist with complaints of nasal congestion. Imaging studies done at that time consisted of a CT scan and magnetic resonance imaging (MRI) of the sinuses. The CT scan shown in Figure 11.120 in a coronal view with bone windows shows a mass lesion occupying the maxillary sinus, with extension into the left nasal cavity. The lesion breaks through the lateral wall of the maxillary sinus (arrow). In an axial view of the CT scan, inflamed mucosal thickening is seen throughout the maxillary sinus (Figure 11.121). Both the medial and lateral walls are involved by the tumor and are thinned out. The MRI scan in a T2-weighted coronal view shows a bright white shadow in the lower half of the left maxillary antrum (Figure 11.122). It is difficult to differentiate between the tumor and the overlying inflamed mucosa of the maxillary sinus. With the presumed diagnosis of inflammatory polyps, she underwent an attempt at endoscopic sinus

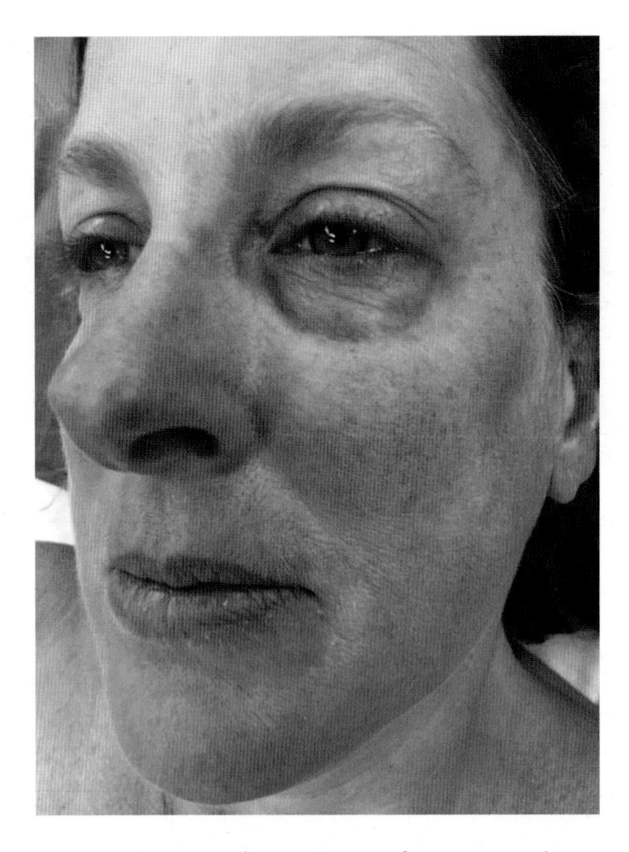

Figure 11.119 External appearance of a patient with a fibrosarcoma of the maxilla.

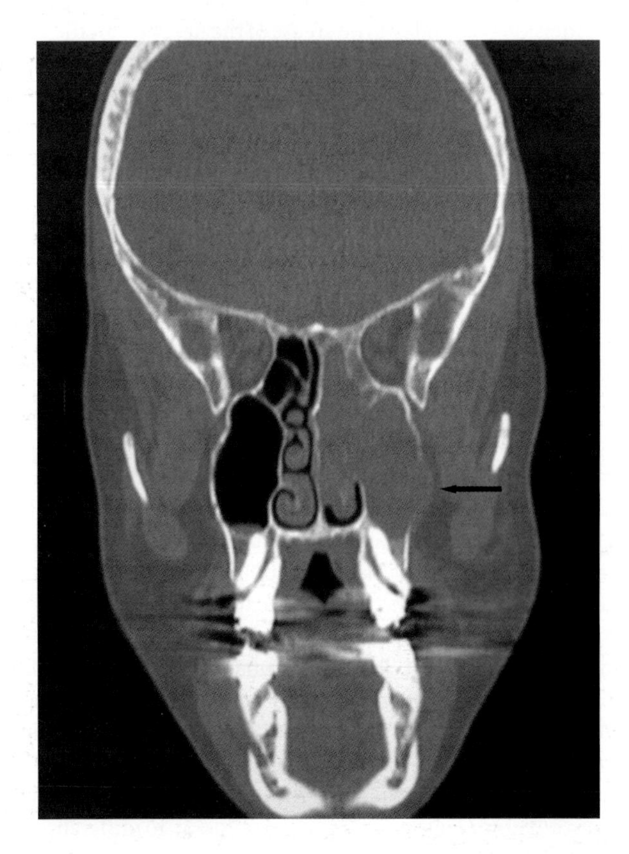

Figure 11.120 CT scan of the sinuses in the coronal plane and bone windows showing tumor occupying the maxillary sinus and breaking through the lateral wall (arrow).

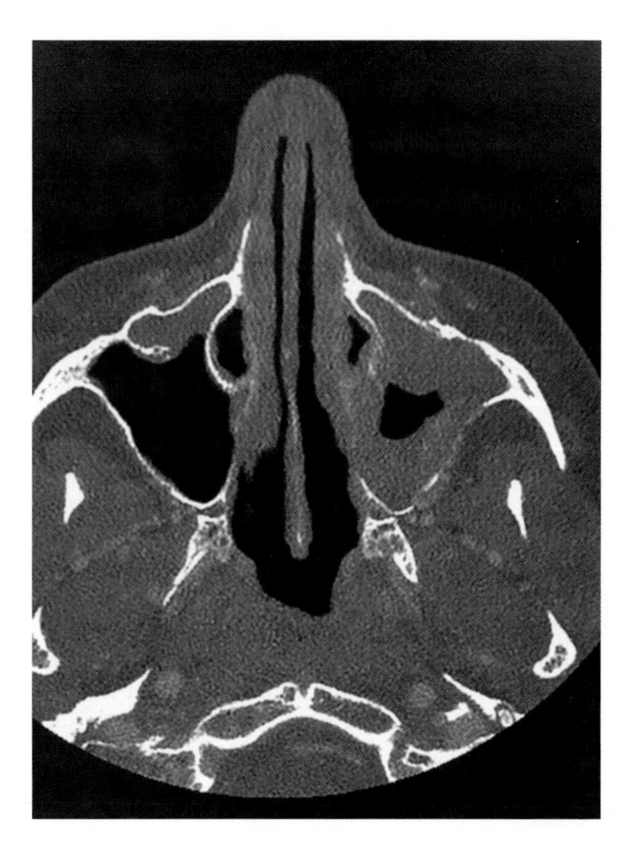

Figure 11.121 CT scan of the sinuses in an axial view shows tumor and inflamed and thickened mucosa of the antrum.

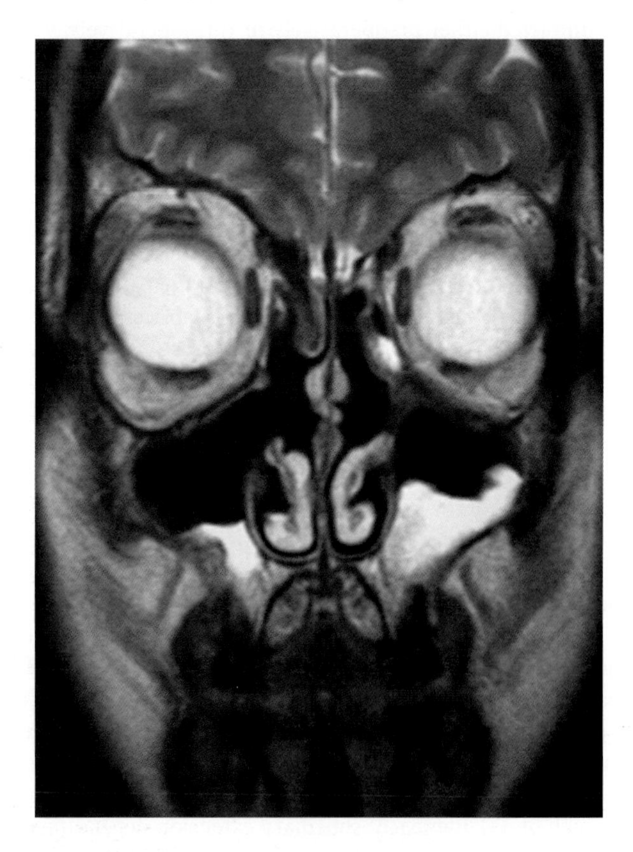

Figure 11.122 Coronal view of the sinuses on a T2-weighted MRI scan showing the tumor occupying the floor of the maxillary sinus.

surgery. The tissue biopsy, however, showed this lesion to be a fibrosarcoma. She now presents for definitive treatment.

Detailed review of the scans showed that the tumor is localized to the "infrastructure" of the left maxilla, but extends through its lateral wall into the masticator space. The patient therefore requires a partial maxillectomy of the infrastructure, preserving the floor of the orbit and the zygomatic process of maxilla. A modified Weber–Ferguson incision is marked out on the patient's face (Figure 11.123). Note that the Weber–Ferguson incision is modified respecting the nasal subunits. The incision begins in the midline of the vermilion border of the upper lip and is extended up to the columella. At that point, it follows the curve of the columella into the floor of the nasal cavity. It then exits the nasal cavity at a 60° angle following the ala of the nostril. It then curves around in the alar groove up to the upper end of the alar cartilage. At that point, it is extended straight up on the lateral wall of the nose up to the level of the medial canthus. The incision is then extended laterally in a skin crease of the lower eyelid at the junction of the slightly pigmented skin of the lower eyelid and the lighter skin of the cheek. The incision ends at about the lateral edge of the orbit in the region of the lateral canthus. The skin incision is made with a scalpel, but thereafter, all dissection is carried out with a needle point electrocautery to elevate the upper cheek flap.

The cheek flap is elevated in full thickness right up to the bony anterior wall of the maxilla in its lower half. This part of the flap contains skin, underlying fat and facial muscles up to the bony anterior wall of maxilla. However, the upper part of the cheek flap consists of only the skin overlying the orbicularis oculi muscle. This is very thin skin and extreme care should be exercised in not perforating the skin in this region (Figure 11.124). The cheek flap is then retracted laterally, exposing the orbicularis oculi muscle. The muscle is then elevated from the underlying bone as a separate layer up to the orbital rim. This maneuver preserves the "ring" of the orbicularis muscle with its nerve supply intact, preventing ectropion in the postoperative period. The entire anterior and lateral surface of the maxilla is now exposed, permitting the required bone cuts (Figure 11.125). The proposed bone cuts are marked out in Figure 11.126 with a purple marking pen. The canine tooth is extracted and a bone cut is marked out through its socket and into the nasal cavity. A thin rim of bone is preserved at the orbital rim to support the orbit. This bone

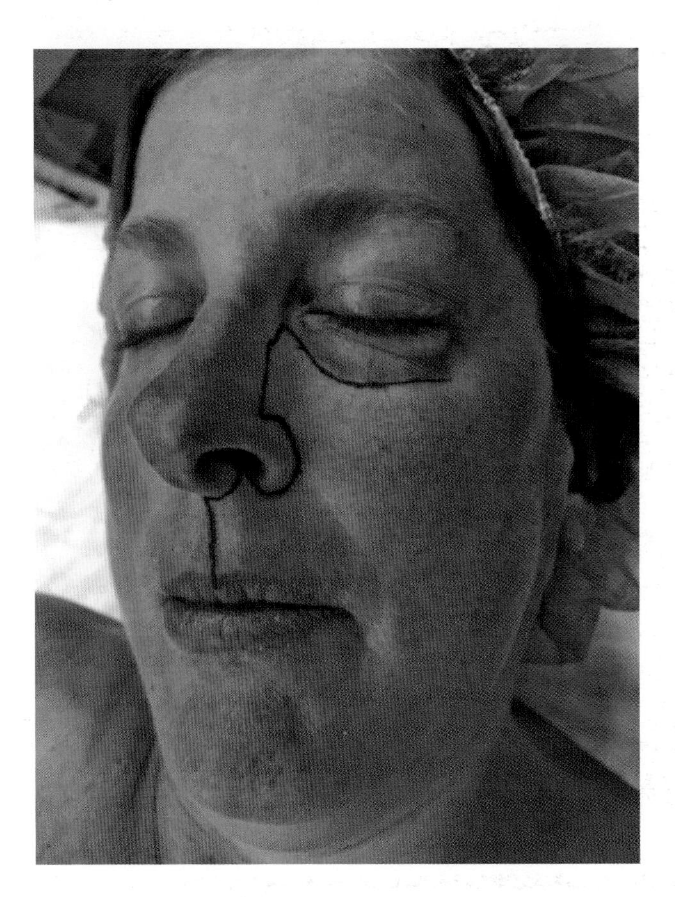

Figure 11.123 Modified Weber–Ferguson incision.

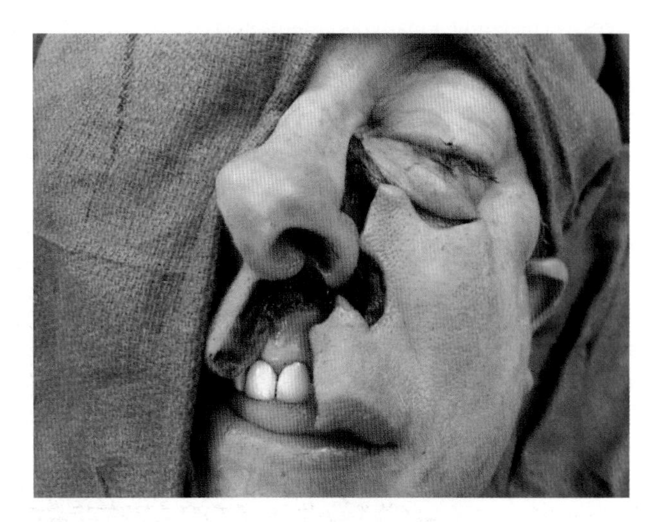

Figure 11.124 The upper cheek flap is elevated over the anterior wall of the maxilla and superficial to the orbicularis oculi muscle.

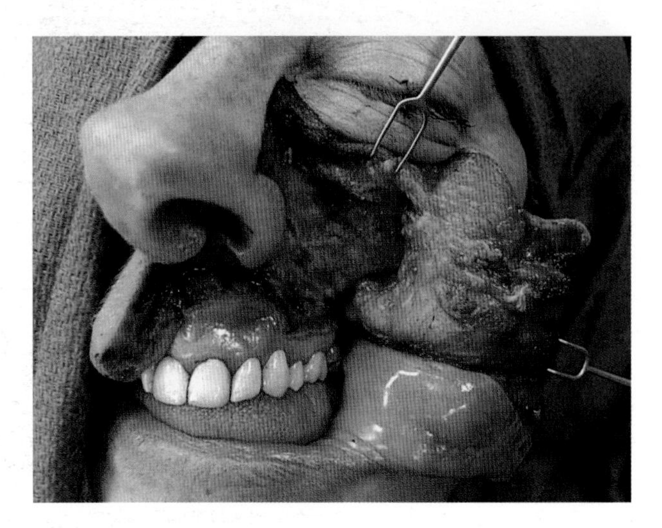

Figure 11.125 The orbicularis oculi muscle is exposed and retracted cephalad up to the orbital rim.

cut connects with the bone cut at the zygomatic process of maxilla.

An incision is now made in the mucosa of the hard palate extending from the socket of the canine tooth up to the midline. It then extends along the midline up to the junction of the hard and soft palate. At that point, it turns lateral, up to the maxillary tubercle, where it meets the mucosal incision in the gingivobuccal sulcus, thus completing circumferential incision on the mucosal surface of the specimen, containing the upper alveolus and hard palate. The incision in the palatal mucosa is made with electrocautery and is deepened up to the underlying bone. Deeper soft tissue and muscular attachments to the maxilla on its posterior surface are now divided with the electrocautery.

A sagittal power saw with an ultra-thin blade is now used to make the bone cuts on the anterior wall of the maxilla, as well as through the hard palate. These bone cuts are made only through the bone, carefully avoiding laceration of the underlying soft tissues or muscular attachments to avoid excessive bleeding. Finally, an osteotome is used to "fracture" the specimen through these bone cuts from the remaining bony attachments to remove the specimen in a monobloc fashion. Care should be exercised to not fragment the specimen. After all bony attachments are divided, Mayo scissors are used to divide the remaining muscular attachments in the pterygoid fossa and the specimen is delivered. Brisk bleeding from the branches of the internal maxillary artery is expected, but it is easily controlled with sutures and electrocautery. The surgical defect is carefully examined to ensure that the entire tumor has been resected (Figure 11.127).

The surgical specimen viewed from the lateral aspect shows en bloc resection of the lower half of the maxilla with the tumor contained within (Figure 11.128). The medial view of the specimen shows tumor (pale) in the floor of the maxillary antrum and edematous mucosa of the lateral wall of the maxilla (Figure 11.129). Depending on the extent of the exposed raw area, a decision is made at this point as to whether a skin graft is required to line the inner defect. In general, it is preferable to avoid a skin graft for relatively small raw areas. The eventual defect healed by secondary intention has a smooth and moist mucosa, which is much

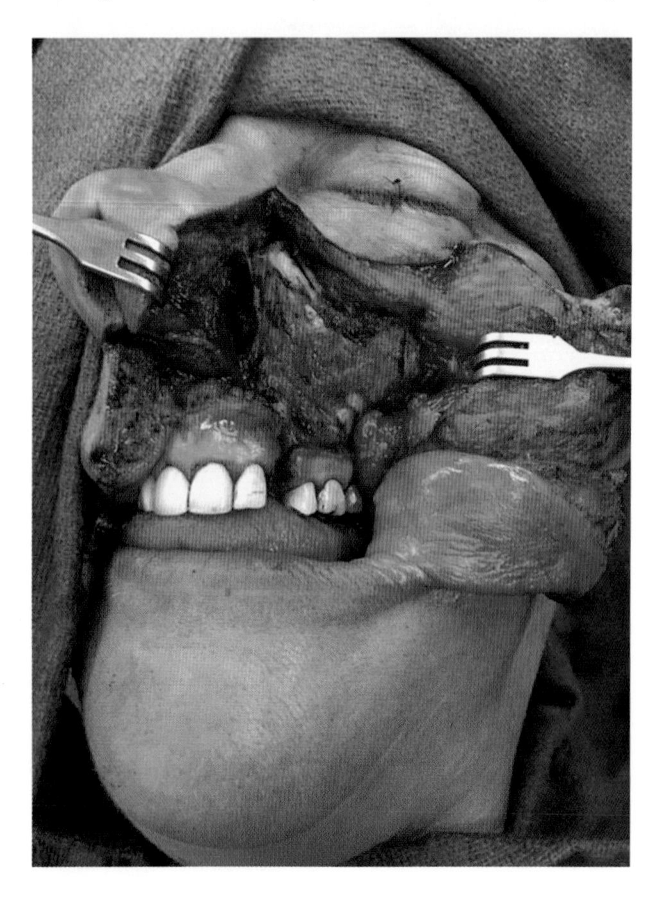

Figure 11.126 Bone cuts are marked on the anterior surface of the maxilla.

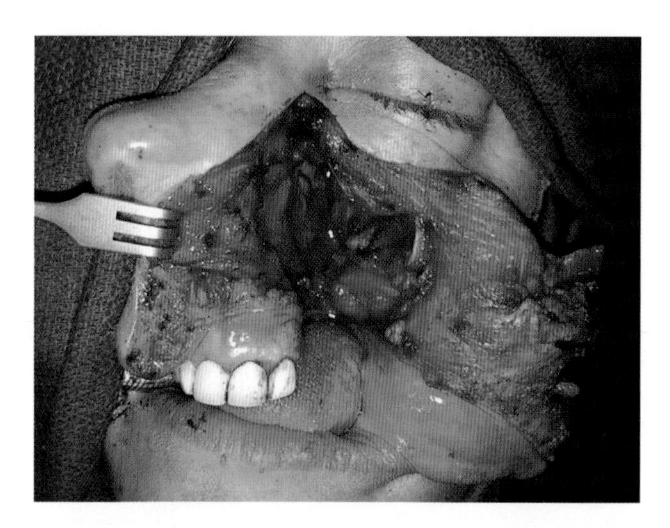

Figure 11.127 Surgical defect of maxillectomy after removal of the tumor.

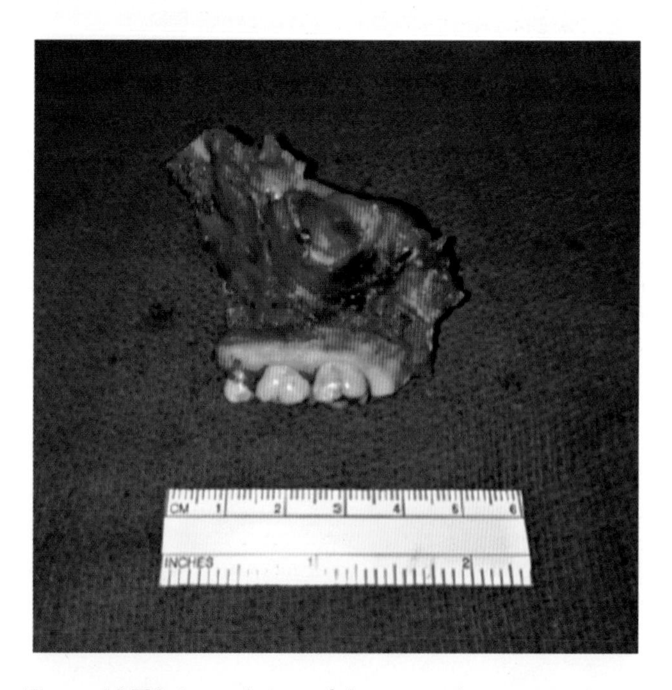

Figure 11.128 Lateral view of the surgical specimen showing clear superior margins with the tumor located in the floor of the maxillary sinus.

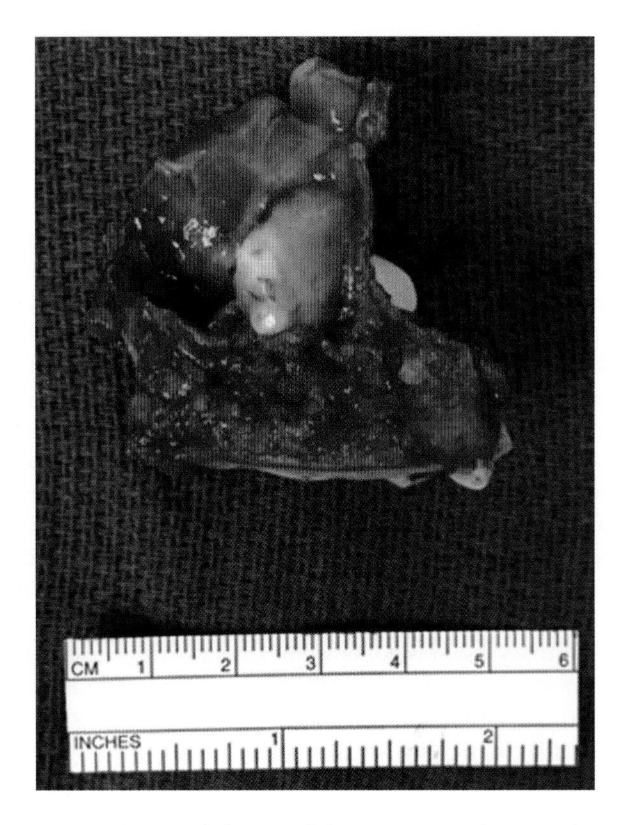

Figure 11.129 Medial view of the specimen showing the tumor (pale) and edematous mucosa of the lateral wall of the maxilla.

better for keeping the defect clean and moist. However, if the raw area is too large, particularly in the masticator space, then a skin graft will be necessary. While the skin graft provides nice coverage of the defect and early healing, it does have some drawbacks in the long term. Secretions from the skin get dried up and produce crusting with odor. It requires regular irrigations to prevent dry crusting and the odor from dry secretions is unpleasant.

A xeroform gauze packing if now placed in the surgical defect to support the skin graft if used or to prevent bleeding and oozing from the raw area in the postoperative period. A prefabricated dental prosthesis is now placed to replace the resected hard palate and to retain the packing. The obturator prosthesis is wired to the remaining teeth. The packing remains in place for at least 7 days. The wound is closed in two layers using absorbable sutures for muscles and subcutaneous soft tissues and 5-0 nylon for skin. Meticulous attention should be paid to match every corner of the incision accurately in order to get an esthetically good result (Figure 11.130).

The patient is able to tolerate liquids by mouth within 24 hours and is started on a soft diet on the third postoperative day. The obturator prosthesis used to support the packing is removed on the eighth postoperative day. The packing is also removed and an interim obturator prosthesis is fabricated to separate the oral cavity from the surgical defect in the maxilla and nasal cavity. This prosthesis is made of soft resin material to avoid friction and bleeding and for

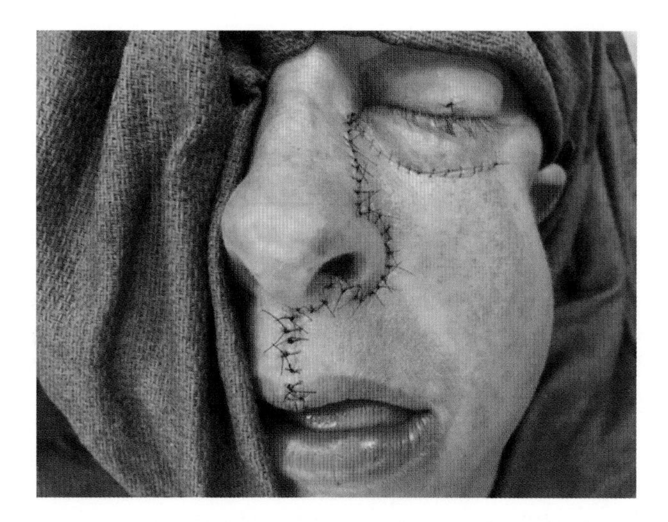

Figure 11.130 Closure of the incision with accurate alignment of all angulations of the incision.

comfort to the patient. In addition, the prosthesis needs to be revised regularly every few days while the defect is healing. The final obturator is made at approximately 3 months after surgery and after complete healing of the defect. The postoperative appearance of the patient approximately 1 year after surgery shows a nicely healed incision with very little esthetic deformity (Figure 11.131).

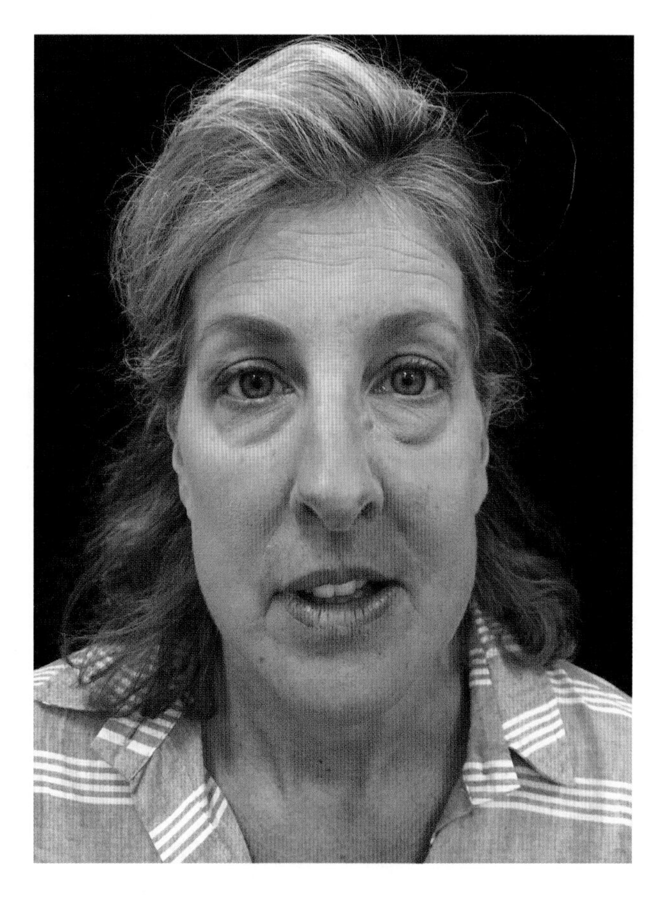

Figure 11.131 Postoperative appearance of the patient 1 year after surgery.

SURGICAL APPROACHES TO THE OROPHARYNX

GENERAL CONSIDERATIONS

The treatment of oropharyngeal cancer has been a subject of extensive controversy in the last few years. The usual treatment approaches include definitive surgery or radiotherapy alone for very-early-stage disease and either radical surgery with PORT or chemoradiotherapy (CRT). Alternatively, advanced-stage tumors are treated without surgery with concurrent CRT, keeping salvage surgery in reserve. Due to the significant morbidity of surgery with PORT or CRT and due to the excellent response rates to CRT alone, particularly in HPV-positive tumors, the pendulum swung toward nonsurgical treatment of nearly all oropharyngeal cancers. However, with increasing experience and long-term follow-up of surviving patients, the significant functional morbidity with CRT has raised concern and rejuvenated interest in initial surgical treatment for early-stage disease, with the goal to avoid CRT and even PORT in the very-early-stage patients. This surgical enthusiasm is also fueled by the introduction of new technologies of minimally invasive surgery, including transoral laser microsurgery (TOLM) and transoral robotic surgery (TORS). Furthermore, there has been a steep rise in the incidence of HPV-positive oropharyngeal cancers, usually occurring in young, healthy, non-smoking males, who have an excellent prognosis and prolonged longevity. Therefore, they would suffer the functional morbidity of CRT for their whole life if treated non-surgically. The current debate, therefore, in the management of oropharyngeal cancer revolves around de-intensification of treatment in patients with HPV-positive tumors to reduce functional morbidity while maintaining equally good oncologic efficacy (56,57). Several clinical trials are currently underway in the United States and abroad to define the optimal treatment for these patients (58). At present, primary surgery is considered in patients with T1–2 N0 or T1–2 N1 tumors of the tonsil or base of the tongue, with or without PORT. These are patients in whom there is a high probability to resect the primary tumor with negative margins and in whom there is limited, low-volume nodal metastasis without any clinical or radiologic evidence of ENE of disease. The goal is to avoid postoperative CRT. On the other hand, if preoperative assessment warrants the need for postoperative CRT by virtue of a large, invasive or ill-defined primary or clinical or radiologic evidence of ENE, then surgery is not undertaken and primary CRT is employed, with salvage surgery kept in reserve. This applies to all advanced-stage tumors (i.e. T3–4 or N2–3). The goal is to avoid using three modalities of treatment (i.e. surgery, radiotherapy and chemotherapy). Primary surgery for oropharyngeal squamous cell carcinomas thus is currently restricted to tumors that are suitable for transoral resection. This may be performed with electrocautery, laser or the robot. All other tumors such as minor salivary gland tumors and other non-epithelial tumors are treated using the conventional surgical approaches described earlier in the chapter.

Preoperative evaluation of these tumors requires careful clinical examination and flexible fiber-optic nasolaryngoscopy as well as palpation of the lesion to assess its third dimension. In addition, imaging studies, including contrast-enhanced CT, MRI and positron emission tomography (PET), are recommended in all patients. CT scanning has a high sensitivity for identifying nodal disease, while MRI is valuable in assessing the third dimension of tumors of the base of the tongue and tonsils. PET scanning can often identify nodal disease in unusual locations such as the retropharyngeal lymph nodes and occult, clinically not obvious primary tumors. Tissue diagnosis can often be obtained from a biopsy of the obvious primary tumor under local anesthesia in the office setting. A fine needle aspiration cytology is usually accurate in confirming the presence of metastatic disease in neck nodes. Examination under anesthesia and biopsy of the primary tumor is required sometimes when the primary lesion is not obvious. In that setting, ipsilateral diagnostic (and therapeutic) tonsillectomy is recommended, securing clear margins around the tonsil. Guided biopsy of suspicious areas from the base of the tongue is necessary in patients where there is no obvious lesion in the base of the tongue. The role of routine lingual tonsillectomy as a diagnostic procedure remains to be defined. All tissue harvested must be submitted for p16 staining as well as determination of HPV status by *in situ* hybridization.

Accurate preoperative staging is crucial in order to define the surgical resectability of oropharyngeal cancer. In addition to imaging and biopsies, accurate assessment of the primary lesion with reference to extension to the nasopharynx, soft palate, parapharyngeal soft tissues for tonsil tumors and the larynx and pyriform sinus and extrinsic muscles of the tongue for base of the tongue tumors is essential to assess resectability. The goal is to accomplish surgical resection with negative margins in all directions.

Cervical lymph node metastases occur often in patients with oropharyngeal primary tumors. The presence of large lymph node metastasis, matted nodes and any evidence of ENE might change the treatment plan to a non-surgical approach, even in a scenario with a small primary tumor (T1/T2). In HPV-positive patients, it is not uncommon to see a small primary tumor with bulky lymph node metastases. Sometimes, the primary is not even clinically evident and might be found through imaging studies such a CT scan or a PET/CT scan (59,60).

The ultimate goal of the decision-making process is to avoid three modalities of treatment (i.e. surgery and PORT with chemotherapy). The goal is either a single-modality treatment or at most two modalities of treatment.

TREATMENT OPTIONS

Small and superficial lesions of the oropharynx can be excised through the oral cavity with use of electrocautery, TOLM or TORS. Patients with larger lesions or those not

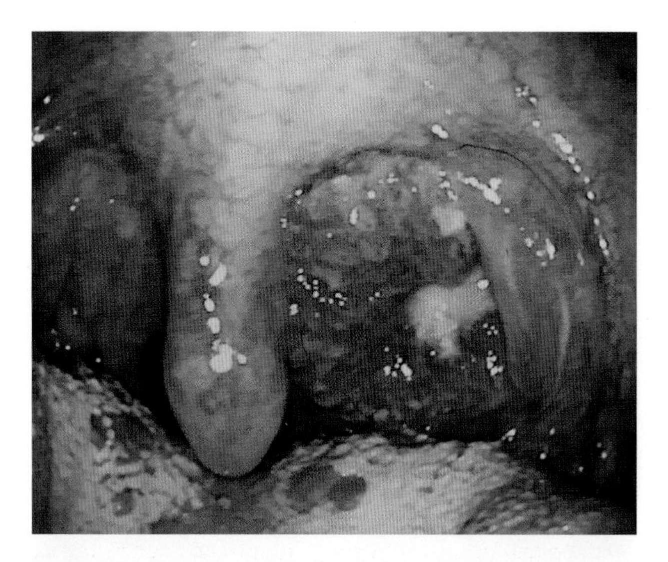

Figure 11.132 HPV-associated large carcinoma of the left palatine tonsil.

quite suitable for electrocautery or laser due to inadequate exposure and those typically who would have required a mandibulotomy for resection are considered for TORS (Figure 11.132). In the last decade, TORS has been extensively explored for resection of even larger lesions of the tonsils and base of the tongue. While postoperative morbidity is minimized, long-term tumor control rates are not reported in any comparative clinical trial. In addition, up to 30% of patients in reported series require postoperative CRT due to positive margins or ENE of disease. Thus, at this time, the role of TORS remains limited to early-stage tumors of the oropharynx. On the other hand, TORS is generally not recommended for tumors that are persistent or recurrent after initial CRT. These patients require conventional open surgery to get an oncologically complete and safe operation.

SURGICAL APPROACH TO THE OROPHARYNX

Small, superficial and well-circumscribed tumors of the tonsils, soft palate and pharyngeal wall are suitable for a peroral approach using conventional means, such as an electrocautery or CO_2 laser. For larger lesions of the tonsil, pharyngeal wall and base of the tongue, consideration should be given to TORS if such equipment and expertise is available. Alternatively, TOLM has been shown to be equally effective in selected cases.

The classical surgical approach for larger tumors of the base of the tongue not involving the mandible is resection through a mandibulotomy approach. A transhyoid or lateral pharyngotomy is rarely used because it provides limited exposure and incurs significant postoperative functional morbidity. For very advanced tumors with invasion of the mandible, a composite resection with segmental mandibulectomy is required. Similarly advanced tumors of the base of the tongue with invasion of the larynx may require a laryngectomy with appropriate reconstruction.

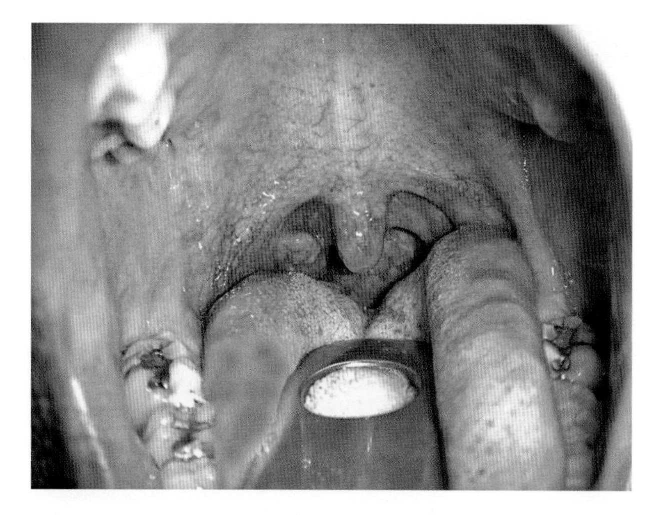

Figure 11.133 T1 carcinoma of the right tonsil suitable for peroral excision.

Peroral resection for carcinoma of the tonsils

Small, superficial (T1) lesions confined to the tonsils can be managed safely by a peroral tonsillectomy, simply with adequate exposure and electrocautery, securing adequate margins in all three dimensions (Figure 11.133). On the other hand, larger lesions (T2) are selected for TORS or TOLM. Caution needs to be exercised, however, before selecting the patient for a transoral resection by any method; that is, the surgeon must be reasonably sure that he or she will be able to perform the transoral resection with negative margins. Resection with positive margins defeats the very purpose of the "de-intensification" of treatment, since that patient will now need postoperative CRT, increasing the functional morbidity with the use of three modalities of treatment. Thus, stringent selection criteria must be employed for choosing patients for TORS or TOLM.

TORS of the tonsils

Resection of primary malignant tumors of the tonsils (T1 or T2) entails a monobloc resection with generous mucosal margins and resection of the underlying constrictor muscle of the pharyngeal wall as well as adjacent base of the tongue. This is accomplished either with TOLM or TORS.

The patient shown here has a HPV-positive squamous cell carcinoma of the right tonsil, staged T2N1M0. Flexible fiber-optic laryngoscopy clearly shows the exophytic component of the tumor in the right tonsil (Figure 11.134). A contrast-enhanced CT scan shows the tumor of the right tonsil as well as a metastatic lymph node at level II (Figure 11.135). Note that there is a fat plane at the deep margin of the primary tumor in the parapharyngeal space, ensuring a negative deep margin. Similarly, the metastatic node does not show any radiological features of ENE. An ^{18}F-fluorodeoxyglucose (FDG) PET scan shows intense FDG uptake in the primary tumor as well as the neck node,

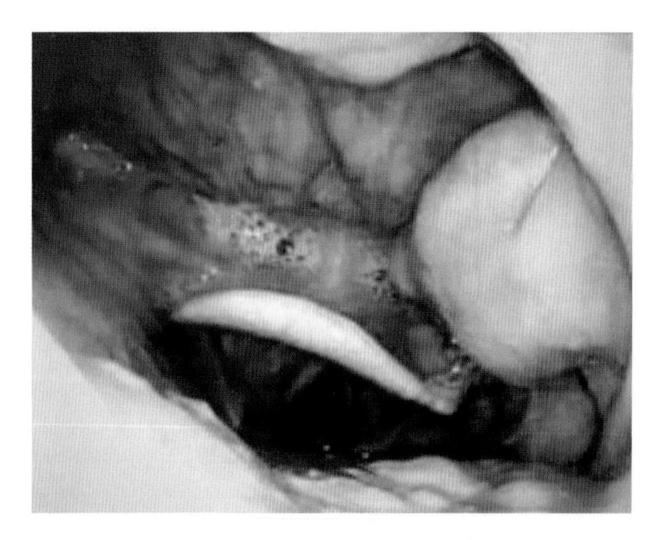

Figure 11.134 Flexible fiber-optic laryngoscopy showing exophytic tumor of the right tonsil.

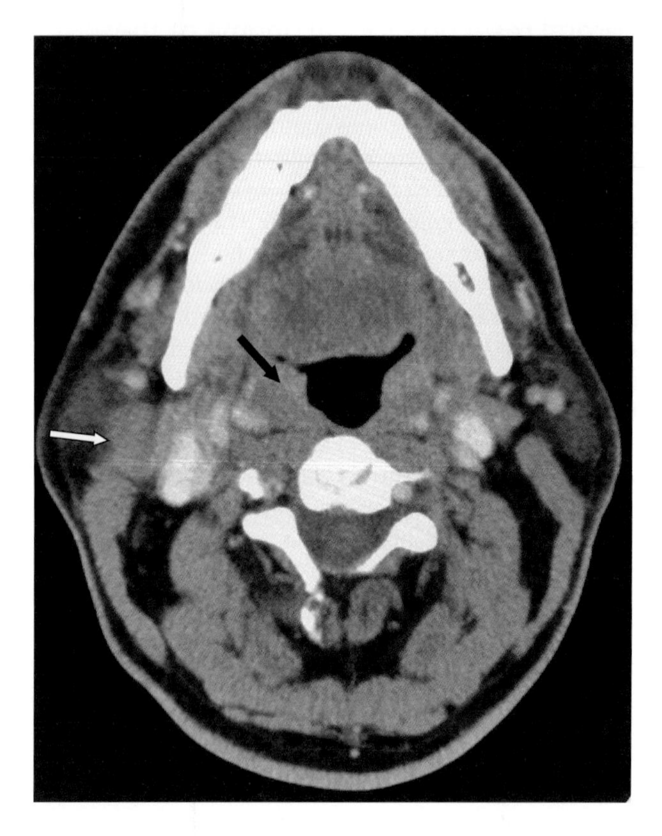

Figure 11.135 Contrast-enhanced CT scan showing primary tumor of the tonsil (black arrow) and a metastatic lymph node (white arrow).

without any other activity (Figure 11.136). Thus, this tumor is suitable for TORS. The surgical procedure is performed in an operating room equipped with the robotic platform.

The patient is placed under general anesthesia with nasotracheal intubation and good muscle relaxation is obtained. The neck dissection is completed first and the incision in the neck is closed. The patient is placed in the supine position to allow for appropriate setting for the robotic arms. The

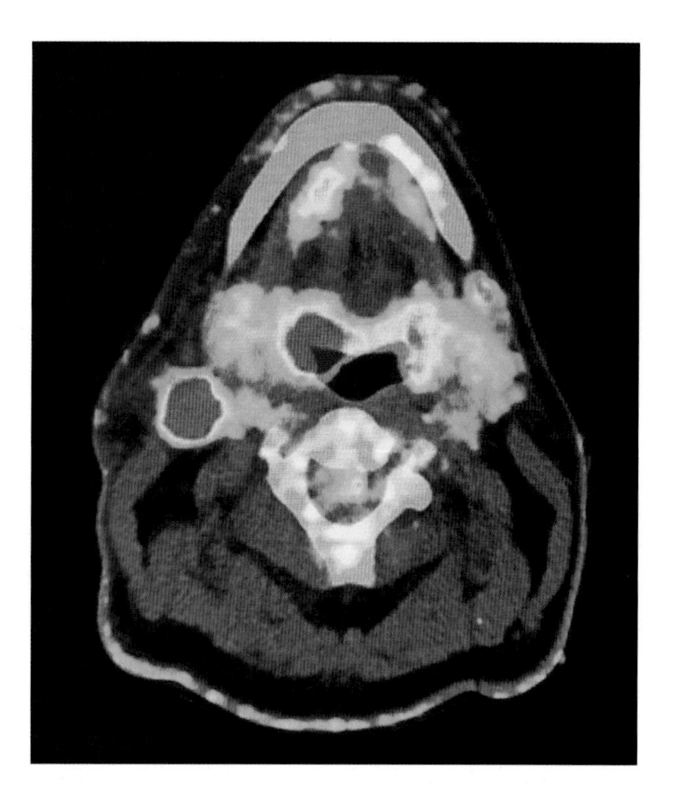

Figure 11.136 FDG-PET scan showing intense uptake in the primary tumor and neck node metastasis.

patient's eyes are protected with the use of safety goggles. Teeth are protected with the use of a mouth guard. The procedure usually starts with a direct laryngoscopy to accurately assess the tumor prior to resection. After this, a silk suture is placed in the anterior tongue in order to facilitate tongue retraction and manipulation. The oropharynx is exposed with the use of a Dingman self-retaining retractor. This is locked in position as soon as appropriate exposure is obtained, encompassing the entire surface of the tonsil, the lateral base of the tongue medially and the soft palate superiorly. Alternatively, a Feyh–Kastenbauer (FK) retractor may be used, particularly if the lesion extends to the base of the tongue (Figure 11.137).

Once the oropharyngeal exposure has been satisfactorily accomplished, the robotic arms are positioned in the patient's mouth at an approximately 45° angle with respect to the plane of the operating table. While many robotic systems are available around the world, the patient shown here is undergoing TORS with a da Vinci S Surgical System (Intuitive Surgical, Inc., Sunnyvale, CA, U.S.A.). For TORS, three out of the four arms available in the robot are actually used for surgery, one central arm for the camera and two lateral arms for an instrument and electrocautery. Further instrumentation (i.e. suction, suction-cautery and endoclips) is not attached to the robot and is provided free-handed by an assistant sitting at the head of the operating table assisted by a scrub nurse. The camera usually has a 0° lens, but a 30° lens may be necessary in certain steps of the procedure to ensure optimal visualization of the distal portion of the tonsil or the base of the

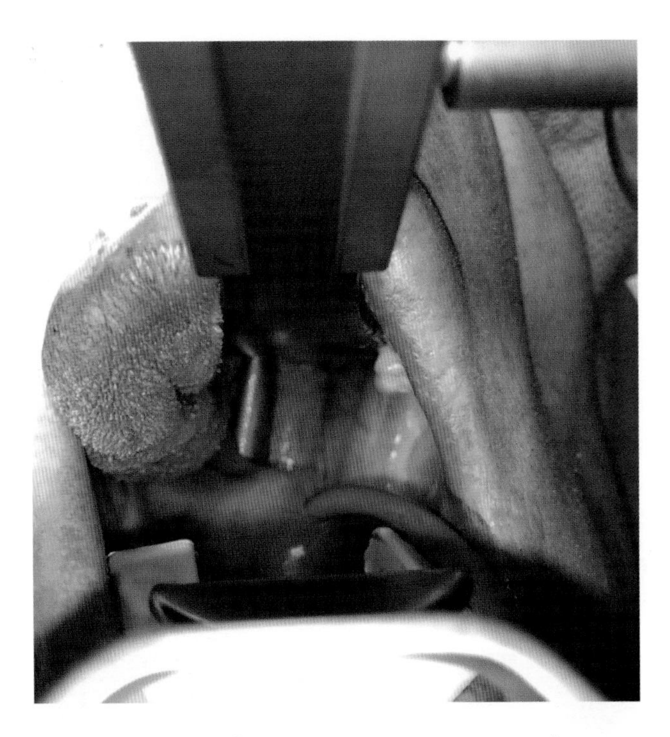

Figure 11.137 A self-retaining FK retractor is used to provide exposure of the right tonsil.

tongue. Proper positioning of the robot improves surgical performance and reduces risk to the patient. The surgeon seated on the robotic console personalizes the settings for their appropriate use (Figure 11.138). The surgeon and the assistant are continuously in communication throughout all aspects of the procedure in order to know if the positioning of the instruments in the oral cavity is safe and the procedure is being conducted smoothly and safely for the patient.

The dissection begins with the lateral pharyngotomy. The initial mucosal incision is placed on the lateral portion of the tonsil at the anterior tonsillar pillar (Figure 11.139). An adequate margin of normal mucosa is included in the specimen. The mucosal cuts are extended superiorly to the soft palate and inferiorly to the inferior portion of the tonsil. In the same fashion, the posterior pharyngeal wall is incised. Dissection continues through the submucosal plane. In the superior–lateral portion of dissection, the palatoglossus, palatopharyngeous and superior constrictor of the pharynx are all identified and sectioned, providing a safe lateral margin (Figure 11.140). It is important to emphasize that the plane of dissection is lateral to the pharyngeal musculature, unlike a standard tonsillectomy where it is medial to these muscles. Once deeper dissection is accomplished, the buccopharyngeal fascia is opened, allowing access to the parapharyngeal space (Figure 11.141). Dissection of this space should be performed carefully in order to avoid potential life-threatening hemorrhage from the carotid artery. Appropriate hemostasis of the pharyngeal and palatine branches of the external carotid artery should be secured at this point with electrocautery or vascular clips. Once this is completed,

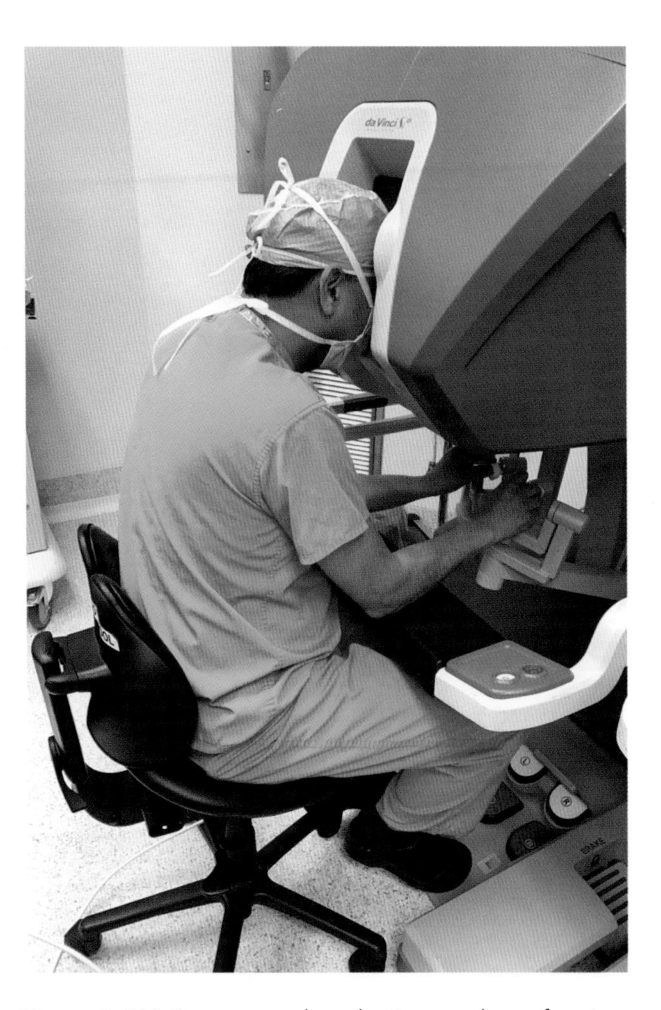

Figure 11.138 Surgeon at the robotic console performing TORS.

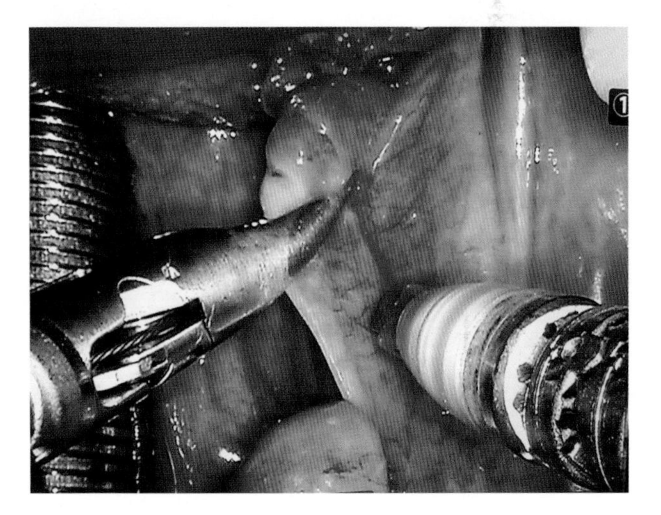

Figure 11.139 Initial incision is made on the lateral aspect of anterior pillar of the tonsil.

the dissection continues from lateral to medial. The inferior portions of the palatoglossus, palatopharyngeous and superior constrictor muscles are divided and the dissection continues to the inferior portion of the tonsil. The mucosal cuts are circumferentially completed at this point. The

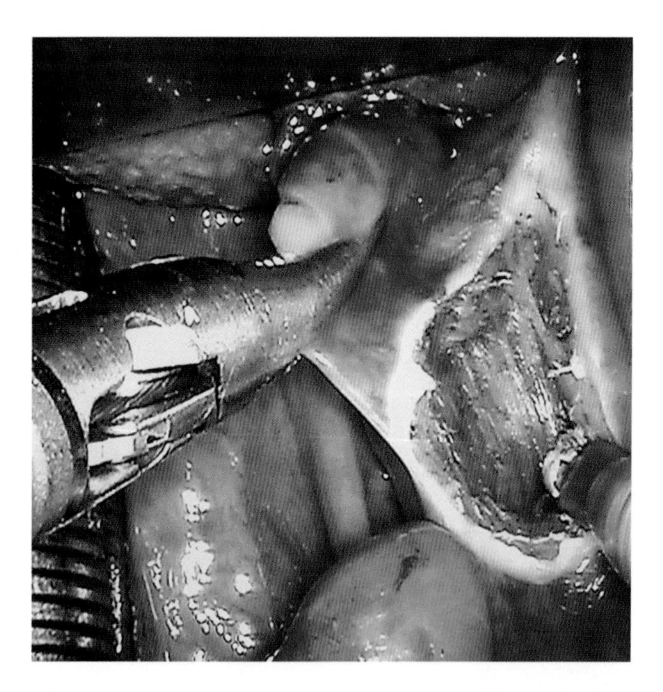

Figure 11.140 Muscles of the soft palette and lateral pharyngeal wall are incised.

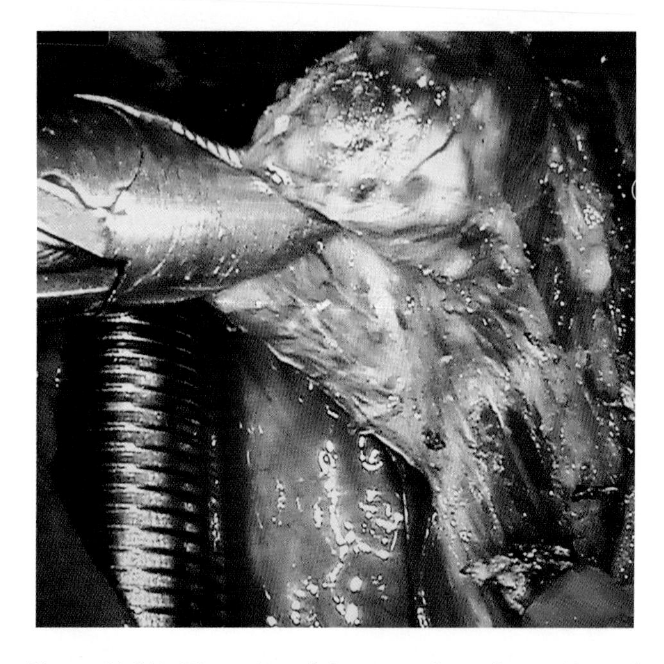

Figure 11.141 Dissection of the tumor is performed lateral to the pharyngeal constrictor muscle.

specimen remains attached to the prevertebral fascia and the posterior pharyngeal wall. The specimen is dissected from the prevertebral fascia and the medial portion of the superior constrictor of the pharynx, which is divided, allowing delivery of the specimen. Representative intra-operative margins are taken from the tumor bed and the specimen is sent to pathology, appropriately oriented and marked, for definitive pathology report. Additional remnants of the constrictor muscle in the bed of the surgical

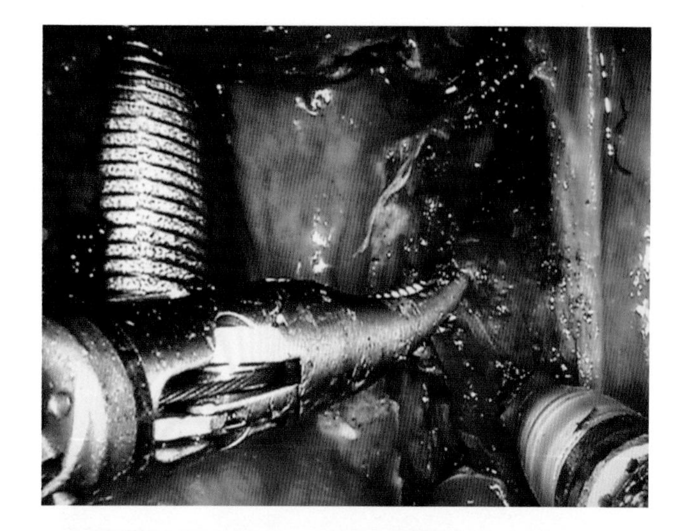

Figure 11.142 Additional deep margin is obtained from tissue in the parapharyngeal space.

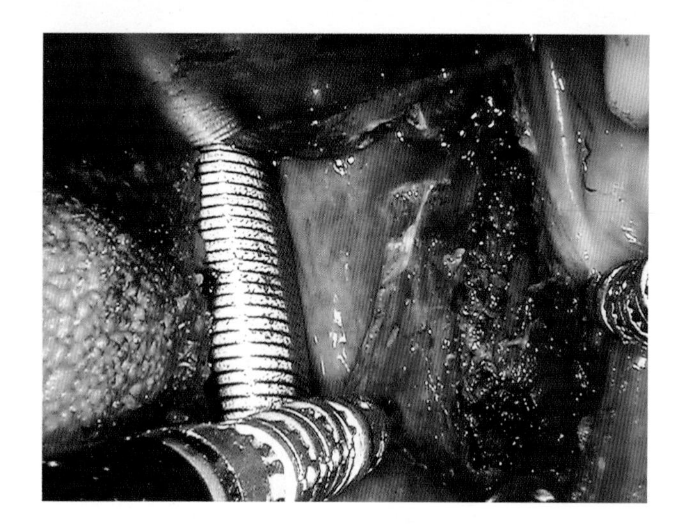

Figure 11.143 Surgical defect after three-dimensional resection of carcinoma of the right tonsil.

defect are removed as a separate specimen for deep margin analysis (Figure 11.142).

No attempt is made to close this surgical defect, which will be allowed to heal by secondary intention. Complete hemostasis is ascertained. The surgical defect is carefully reassessed for bleeding after removing the self-retaining retractor (Figure 11.143). A nasogastric feeding tube is inserted under direct visualization. Some patients remain intubated overnight depending on the surgeons' preference after assessment of the complexity of the surgery. The patient is permitted to drink clear liquids on the next day and progression to a full liquid diet occurs in the next 2 days according to the patient's oral tolerance. The nasogastric tube is removed on the third day if oral intake is adequate and there are no other complications. The patient is maintained with frequent oral irrigations, rinses and power sprays of the surgical defect, using half-strength hydrogen peroxide solution to provide mechanical cleaning of the defect.

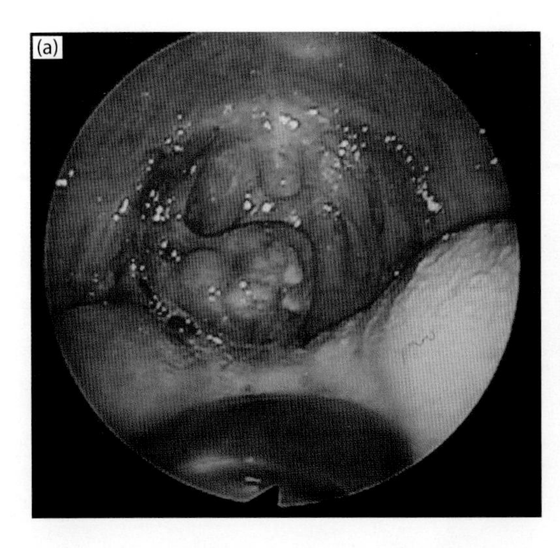

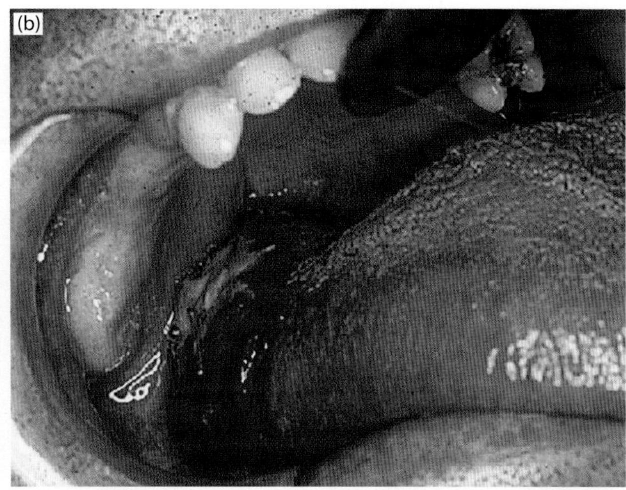

Figure 11.144 **(a)** Exophytic polypoid tumor of the base of the tongue. **(b)** Exophytic sessile tumor of the base of the tongue.

Transoral robotic resection of the base of the tongue

Primary neoplasms of the base of the tongue are difficult to access through the oral cavity, particularly if they have a significant infiltrative component into the musculature of the tongue base. Small, superficial lesions are amenable to transoral resection with a laser. When it is available, robotic surgery may be considered for resection of such tumors. Examples of tumors of the base of the tongue are shown in Figure 11.144a and b.

TORS for base of the tongue tumors has basically the same settings described before. For exposure of the base of the tongue, an FK retractor is preferred (Figure 11.145).

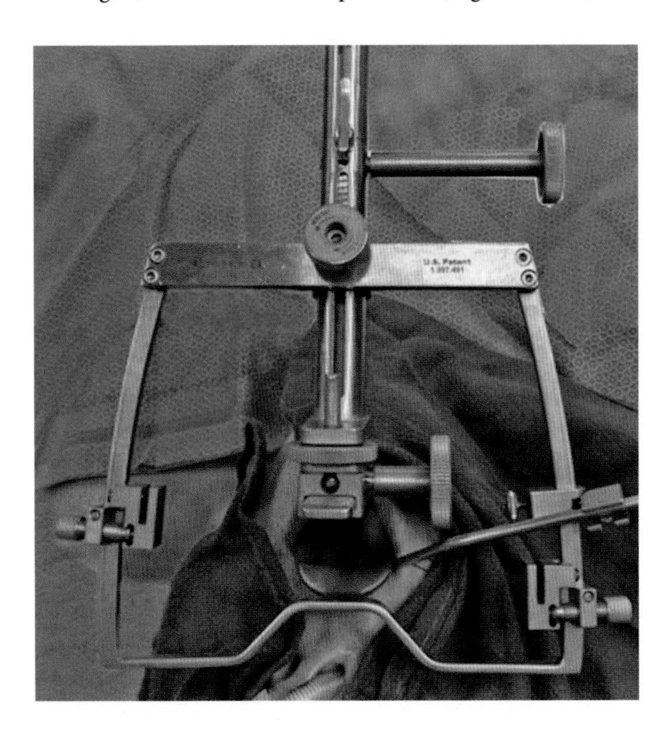

Figure 11.145 FK retractor used for exposure of base of the tongue lesion for peroral resection.

Robot positioning and settings are the same, but the camera is usually a 30° version that allows better visualization of the base of the tongue. The dissection might include the tonsil fossa as described in the previous section. During the resection of the base of the tongue, the lingual artery is usually identified and appropriately controlled. The tumor is usually resected in monobloc fashion, taking care to not violate the tumor or enter into it in its third dimension.

Resection of the base of the tongue *via* mandibulotomy

In the absence of the transoral options mentioned above, tumors of the base of the tongue can be approached *via* a mandibulotomy. The selection of the site of mandibulotomy has been discussed earlier in this chapter. A paramedian mandibulotomy is the less disruptive approach and thus leads to minimal postoperative morbidity regarding swallowing and speech. In patients with intact lower dentition, the mandibulotomy site is preferred between the lateral incisor and canine tooth. Details of the steps of the operation are described earlier in this chapter (Figures 11.35 through 11.51).

Salvage surgery for oropharynx cancer

The technical details for composite resection with marginal mandibulectomy and segmental mandibulectomy for recurrent carcinoma of the tonsils and retromolar region following previous radiation therapy have been discussed previously (Figures 11.86 through 11.92 and 11.95 through 11.108). The patient shown here had undergone a composite resection of the tonsillar fossa, adjacent soft palate, base of the tongue and floor of the mouth for squamous cell carcinoma of the tonsil that had failed to respond to radiation therapy. The monobloc three-dimensional resection of the tonsil tumor warranted the need for a marginal mandibulectomy, which entailed excising the coronoid process of the mandible along with the anterior half of the

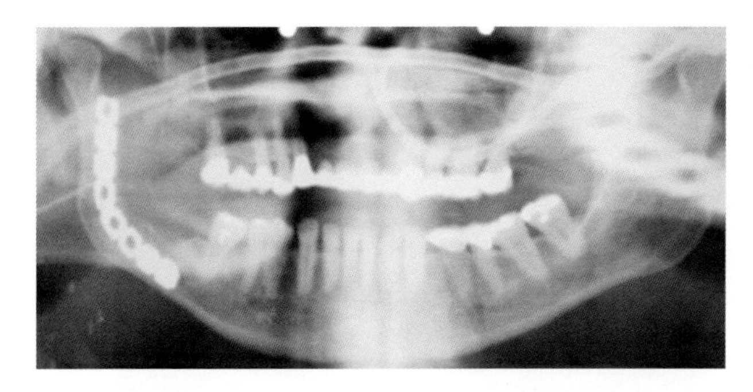

Figure 11.146 A–O plate supporting the angle of the mandible after marginal mandibulectomy.

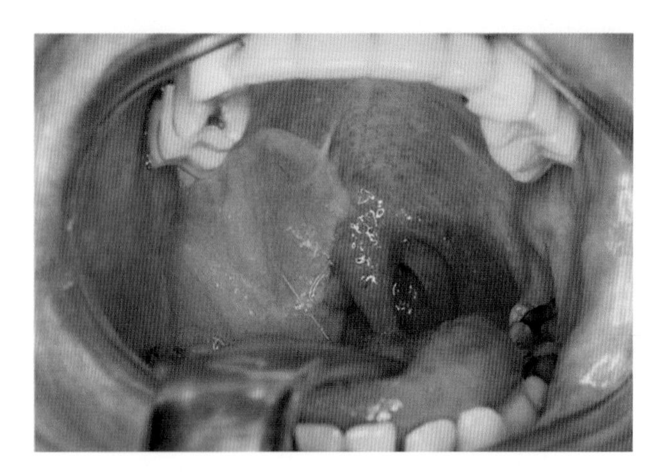

Figure 11.147 Radial forearm free flap reconstruction of the oropharyngeal defect after composite resection.

ascending ramus of the mandible and the alveolar process of the posterior part of the body of the mandible. However, the posterior and inferior cortex of the mandible could be preserved along with an intact temporomandibular joint. Due to the very high risk for spontaneous fracture of the previously irradiated remaining mandible, an A–O plate is used to support the angle of the mandible (Figure 11.146). The surgical defect in this patient was repaired with a radial forearm free flap to provide replacement of the soft tissue defect and mucosal lining. The postoperative intraoral photograph shows a well-healed radial forearm free flap replacing the soft palate, tonsillar fossa, posterior pharyngeal wall, retromolar region and adjacent base of the tongue (Figure 11.147).

Achieving a complete watertight closure of the mucosal defect is crucial in this situation to avoid sepsis and exposure of the A–O plate. Infection and exposure mandate removal of the plate and pose the risk of spontaneous fracture of the previously irradiated and now infected residual weakened mandible. Alternatively, in a setting such as this, consideration may be given to proceed with a segmental resection of the mandible and reconstruction with a fibula free flap. The postoperative external appearance of the patient shows excellent retention of the contour of the face with maintenance of the continuity of the arch of the

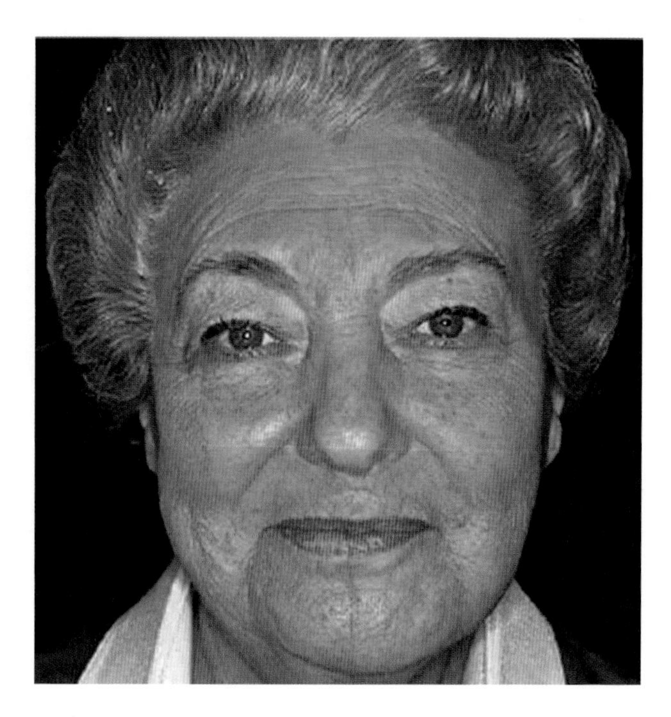

Figure 11.148 Postoperative appearance of the patient 1 year after surgery.

mandible and thus a very desirable functional and esthetic result (Figure 11.148).

REFERENCES

1. Shah JP, Candela FC, Poddar AK. The patterns of cervical lymph node metastases from squamous carcinoma of the oral cavity. *Cancer* 1990;66(1):109–13.
2. Shah JP. Surgical treatment of tumors of the oral cavity. In: Thawley S, Panje W (eds). *Comprehensive management of head and neck tumors.* Philadelphia: Saunders, 1987, 686–694.
3. Shah JP, Cendon RA, Farr HW, Strong EW. Carcinoma of the oral cavity. factors affecting treatment failure at the primary site and neck. *Am J Surg* 1976;132(4):504–7.
4. Shaha AR, Spiro RH, Shah JP, Strong EW. Squamous carcinoma of the floor of the mouth. *Am J Surg* 1984;148(4):455–9.
5. Shaha AR. Preoperative evaluation of the mandible in patients with carcinoma of the floor of mouth. *Head Neck* 1991;13(5):398–402.
6. Spiro RH, Strong EW. Epidermoid carcinoma of the mobile tongue. *Treatment by Partial Glossectomy Alone A J Surg* 1971;122(6):707–11.
7. Spiro RH, Strong EW. Epidermoid carcinoma of the oral cavity and oropharynx. *Elective vs Therapeutic Radical Neck Dissection as Treatment Archives of Surgery* 1973;107(3):382–4.
8. Spiro RH, Strong EW. Discontinuous partial glossectomy and radical neck dissection in selected patients with epidermoid carcinoma of the mobile tongue. *Am J Surg* 1973;126(4):544–6.

9. Spiro RH, Alfonso AE, Farr HW, Strong EW. Cervical node metastasis from epidermoid carcinoma of the oral cavity and oropharynx. *A Critical Assessment of Current Staging AJ Surg* 1974;128(4):562–7.
10. Spiro RH, Strong EW. Surgical treatment of cancer of the tongue. *Surg Clin North Am* 1974;54(4):759–65.
11. Spiro RH, Gerold FP, Strong EW. Mandibular "swing" approach for oral and oropharyngeal tumors. *Head Neck Surg* 1981;3(5):371–8.
12. Spiro RH, Gerold FP, Shah JP, Sessions RB, Strong EW. Mandibulotomy approach to oropharyngeal tumors. *Am J Surg* 1985;150(4):466–9.
13. Spiro RH. Squamous cancer of the tongue. *CA Cancer J Clin* 1985;35(4):252–6.
14. Spiro RH, Huvos AG, Wong GY, Spiro JD, Gnecco CA, Strong EW. Predictive value of tumor thickness in squamous carcinoma confined to the tongue and floor of the mouth. *Am J Surg* 1986;152(4):345–50.
15. Leemans CR, Tiwari R, Nauta JJ, Snow GB. Discontinuous vs in-continuity neck dissection in carcinoma of the oral cavity. *Arch Otolaryngol—Head Neck Surg* 1991;117(9):1003–6.
16. Leemans CR, Tiwari R, Nauta JJ, van der Waal I, Snow GB. Regional lymph node involvement and its significance in the development of distant metastases in head and neck carcinoma. *Cancer* 1993;71(2):452–6.
17. Leemans CR, Engelbrecht WJ, Tiwari R et al. Carcinoma of the soft palate and anterior tonsillar pillar. *Laryngoscope* 1994;104(12):1477–81.
18. Leemans CR, Tiwari R, Nauta JJ, van der Waal I, Snow GB. Recurrence at the primary site in head and neck cancer and the significance of neck lymph node metastases as a prognostic factor. *Cancer* 1994;73(1):187–90.
19. Guillamondegui OM, Oliver B, Hayden R. Cancer of the anterior floor of the mouth. *Selective Choice of Treatment and Analysis of Failures A J Surg*1980;140(4):560–2.
20. Byers RM, White D, Yue A. Squamous carcinoma of the oral cavity: choice of therapy. *Curr Probl Cancer* 1981;6(5):1–27.
21. Brown JS, Browne RM. Factors influencing the patterns of invasion of the mandible by oral squamous cell carcinoma. *Int J Oral Maxillofac Surg* 1995;24(6):417–26.
22. Campbell RS, Baker E, Chippindale AJ et al. MRI t staging of squamous cell carcinoma of the oral cavity: radiological–pathological correlation. *Clin Radiol* 1995;50(8):533–40.
23. Chan KW, Merrick MV, Mitchell R. Bone SPECT to assess mandibular invasion by intraoral squamous-cell carcinomas. *J Nucl Med* 1996;37(1):42–5.
24. Close LG, Merkel M, Burns DK, Schaefer SD. Computed tomography in the assessment of mandibular invasion by intraoral carcinoma. *Ann Otol Rhinol Laryngol* 1986;95(4 Pt 1):383–8.
25. Curran AJ, Toner M, Quinn A, Wilson G, Timon C. Mandibular invasion diagnosed by SPECT. *Clin Otolaryngol Allied Sci* 1996;21(6):542–5.
26. Muller H, Slootweg PJ. Mandibular invasion by oral squamous cell carcinoma. clinical aspects. *J Craniomaxillofac Surg* 1990;18(2):80–4.
27. Smyth DA, O'Dwyer TP, Keane CO, Stack J. Predicting mandibular invasion in mouth cancer. *Clin Otolaryngol Allied Sci* 1996;21(3):265–8.
28. Ator GA, Abemayor E, Lufkin RB, Hanafee WN, Ward PH. Evaluation of mandibular tumor invasion with magnetic resonance imaging. *Arch Otolaryngol—Head Neck Surg* 1990;116(4):454–9.
29. Werning JW, Byers RM, Novas MA, Roberts D. Preoperative assessment for and outcomes of mandibular conservation surgery. *Head Neck* 2001;23(12):1024–30.
30. McGregor AD, MacDonald DG. Patterns of spread of squamous cell carcinoma to the ramus of the mandible. *Head Neck* 1993;15(5):440–4.
31. McGregor AD, MacDonald DG. Routes of entry of squamous cell carcinoma to the mandible. *Head Neck Surg* 1988;10(5):294–301.
32. Haribhakti VV. The dentate adult human mandible: an anatomic basis for surgical decision making. *Plast Reconstr Surg* 1996;97(3):536–41. discussion 542–543.
33. Jones AS, England J, Hamilton J et al. Mandibular invasion in patients with oral and oropharyngeal squamous carcinoma. *Clin Otolaryngol Allied Sci* 1997;22(3):239–45.
34. Slootweg PJ, Muller H. Mandibular invasion by oral squamous cell carcinoma. *J Craniomaxillofac Surg* 1989;17(2):69–74.
35. Marchetta FC, Sako K, Murphy JB. The periosteum of the mandible and intraoral carcinoma. *Am J Surg* 1971;122(6):711–3.
36. Shaha AR. Marginal mandibulectomy for carcinoma of the floor of the mouth. *J Surg Oncol* 1992;49(2):116–9.
37. Barttelbort SW, Bahn SL, Ariyan SA. Rim mandibulectomy for cancer of the oral cavity. *Am J Surg* 1987;154(4):423–8.
38. Barttelbort SW, Ariyan S. Mandible preservation with oral cavity carcinoma: rim mandibulectomy versus sagittal mandibulectomy. *Am J Surg* 1993;166(4):411–5.
39. Dubner S, Heller KS. Local control of squamous cell carcinoma following marginal and segmental mandibulectomy. *Head Neck* 1993;15(1):29–32.
40. Dubner S, Spiro RH. Median mandibulotomy: a critical assessment. *Head Neck* 1991;13(5):389–93.
41. Shaha AR. Mandibulotomy and mandibulectomy in difficult tumors of the base of the tongue and oropharynx. *Semin Surg Oncol* 1991;7(1):25–30.
42. Spiro RH, Spiro JD, Strong EW. Surgical approach to squamous carcinoma confined to the tongue and the floor of the mouth. *Head Neck Surg* 1986;9(1):27–31.
43. Marunick M, Mahmassani O, Siddoway J, Klein B. Prospective analysis of masticatory function following lateral mandibulotomy. *J Surg Oncol* 1991;47(2):92–7.

44. Altman K, Bailey BM. Non-union of mandibulotomy sites following irradiation for squamous cell carcinoma of the oral cavity. *Br J Oral Maxillofac Surg* 1996;34(1):62–5.
45. Sullivan PK, Fabian R, Driscoll D. Mandibular osteotomies for tumor extirpation: the advantages of rigid fixation. *Laryngoscope* 1992;102(1):73–80.
46. Beecroft WA, Sako K, Razack MS, Shedd DP. Mandible preservation in the treatment of cancer of the floor of the mouth. *J Surg Oncol* 1982;19(3):171–5.
47. Fleming WB. Marginal resection of the mandible in treatment of cancer of the floor of the mouth. *Aust N Z J Surg* 1987;57(8):521–5.
48. Randall CJ, Eyre J, Davies D, Walsh-Waring GP. Marginal mandibulectomy for malignant disease: indications, rationale, and results. *J Laryngol Otol* 1987;101(7):676–84.
49. Shah JP, Kumaraswamy SV, Kulkarni V. Comparative evaluation of fixation methods after mandibulotomy for oropharyngeal tumors. *Am J Surg* 1993;166(4):431–4.
50. Zlotolow IM, Huryn JM, Piro JD, Lenchewski E, Hidalgo DA. Osseointegrated implants and functional prosthetic rehabilitation in microvascular fibula free flap reconstructed mandibles. *Am J Surg* 1992;164(6):677–81.
51. Mounsey RA, Boyd JB. Mandibular reconstruction with osseointegrated implants into the free vascularized radius. *Plast Reconstr Surg* 1994;94(3):457–64.
52. Butow KW, Duvenage JG. Implanto-orthognathic reconstructive surgery. A preliminary report. *J Craniomaxillofac Surg* 1993;21(8):326–34. discussion 335.
53. Urken ML, Moscoso JF, Lawson W, Biller HF. A systematic approach to functional reconstruction of the oral cavity following partial and total glossectomy. *Arch Otolaryngol—Head Neck Surg* 1994;120(6):589–601.
54. Spiro RH, Strong EW, Shah JP. Maxillectomy and its classification. *Head Neck* 1997;19(4):309–14.
55. Kornblith AB, Zlotolow IM, Gooen J et al. Quality of life of maxillectomy patients using an obturator prosthesis. *Head Neck* 1996;18(4):323–34.
56. Rutter CE, Husain ZA, Burtness B. Treatment de-intensification for locally advanced HPV-associated oropharyngeal cancer. *Am J Hematol Oncol* 2015;11:13–7.
57. An Y, Holsinger C, Husain ZA. De-intensification of adjuvant therapy in human papillomavirus-associated oropharyngeal cancer. *Cancer Head Neck* 2016;1:18.
58. Robert L, Ferris PI. Phase II randomized trial of transoral surgical resection followed by low-dose or standard-dose IMRT in resectable p16 locally advanced oropharynx cancer (ECOG-E3311). https://clinicaltrials.gov/ct2/show/NCT01898494.
59. Gődény M, Lengyel Z, Polony G, Nagy ZT, Léránt G, Zámbó O, Remenár É, Tamás L, Kásler M. Impact of 3T multiparametric MRI and FDG-PET-CT in the evaluation of occult primary cancer with cervical node metastasis. *Cancer Imaging* 2016;16(1):38.
60. Cheol Park G, Roh JL, Cho KJ, Seung Kim J, Hyeon Jin M, Choi SH, Yuhl Nam S, Yoon Kim S. F-FDG PET/CT vs. human papillomavirus, p16 and epstein–barr virus detection in cervical metastatic lymph nodes for identifying primary tumors. *Int J Cancer* 2017;140(6):1405–12.

12

Radiotherapy

SEAN McBRIDE

Since the discovery of radium and with the progressive availability of newer sources of ionizing radiation, radiotherapy has become an integral part of the treatment of cancers of the oral cavity and oropharynx. Radiation may be employed as a single modality or in combination with chemotherapy, either as a definitive treatment or as an adjuvant treatment following surgery. The goal of radiotherapy is to achieve maximal cell death with minimum tissue damage to normal structures and hence minimal acute toxicity and long-term sequelae.

MECHANISM OF ACTION OF RADIOTHERAPY AND RATIONALE FOR FRACTIONATION

The principle mechanism by which radiotherapy results in tumor cell death is *via* the induction of DNA damage in cancer cells. Broadly speaking, X-ray radiotherapy (as compared to charged particle radiotherapy) is indirectly ionizing; DNA damage is not directly produced by the X-rays, but is rather the result of the production of electrons when the X-rays interact with tissue. The secondary electrons produced by photon radiotherapy go on to ionize DNA either directly *via* interactions with the nuclei of the DNA molecule or indirectly *via* the creation of free radicals. With the energy used in modern linear accelerators, the predominant mechanism of DNA ionization is *via* the production of free radicals by these secondary electrons.

The ionization of DNA results in base damage, single-strand breaks, double-strand breaks and DNA protein cross-links. Double-strand breaks are thought to be the most critical to the initiation of mitotic cell death following radiation therapy. Mitotic cell death occurs when cells attempt to divide with heavily damaged chromosomes and is the most common type of cell death following irradiation. A second common mechanism of cell death following irradiation is apoptosis. Apoptotic cell death is a highly controlled, stepwise mechanism of cellular demise that involves chromatin condensation and fragmentation and the eventual creation of apoptotic cell bodies.

Most radiotherapy regimens in the upfront treatment of head and neck malignancies involve the delivery of relatively small doses of daily radiotherapy over multiple weeks. Canonical radiobiology suggests that, compared to a single large dose of radiation, spreading out the dose over multiple weeks allows for both decreased rates of late toxicities and an increased probability of local tumor control. The reduction in late toxicity comes from the potential repair of sub-lethal damage between the smaller doses of daily radiation. The improvement in local control is thought to stem from two factors: (1) in the time between daily fractions of radiation, a proportion of the tumor cells may enter more radiosensitive phases of the cell cycles; and (2) fluctuations in tumor oxygenation may place a portion of the tumor in a higher-oxygen and thus more radiosensitive environment.

TREATMENT STRATEGIES

For oral cavity and oropharynx squamous cell malignancies, the two most common treatment strategies involve either the use of radical (i.e. definitive) radiotherapy without the need for upfront surgery or the utilization of upfront surgery followed by postoperative radiotherapy (PORT), assuming certain risk factors are present. More recently, with the publication of a series of cooperative group trials, chemoradiotherapy (CRT), both in the definitive and postoperative settings, has been shown to improve survival for subsets of patients with oral cavity and oropharynx malignancies.

For oral cavity malignancies, with advances in free flap reconstructive techniques, the standard of care is upfront surgical resection, if feasible, followed by observation, adjuvant radiotherapy or adjuvant CRT depending upon the pathologic factors present at resection; definitive radiotherapy options are likely inferior to upfront surgical strategies (1). If surgery is not feasible, combined concurrent chemotherapy and external beam radiotherapy are often utilized; in centers with the requisite experience, interstitial brachytherapy may also be an option.

In the oropharynx subsite, the epidemic of human papillomavirus (HPV)-related malignancies, their responsiveness to CRT and the morbidity associated with traditional surgical techniques led to a shift in the standard of care toward concurrent CRT over the last decade. However, recent advances in transoral surgical techniques have led to a push for treatment de-intensification strategies that involve upfront resection (2).

RADICAL (DEFINITIVE) RADIOTHERAPY

DIFFERENT FRACTIONATION REGIMENS IN HEAD AND NECK RADICAL RADIOTHERAPY

For head and neck squamous cell malignancies, because of their putatively rapid doubling time, there is a relatively robust literature on alternative fractionation regimens designed to improve the probability of local control with radical radiotherapy. For these tumors with rapid doubling times, local control is impacted by total radiation dose delivered to the tumor and by total treatment time. Acute toxicities increase with a reduction in treatment time or an increase in dose per fraction; late toxicities increase with an increase in total dose or dose per fraction and are relatively insensitive to total treatment time. Balancing the benefit of improved local control with the clear detriments of increased acute and late toxicities is a critical component of optimizing the therapeutic ratio in head and neck radiotherapy.

Hyperfractionation is an attempt to increase tumor control by increasing total dose delivered and holding steady the rates of late effects by decreasing the dose per fraction. Accelerated fractionation, purely defined, involves no change in dose per fraction or total dose, but using twice a day (BID) treatment delivery in order to condense the overall treatment time, with the aim of improving local control by reducing the effects of tumor cell repopulation between fractions. An obvious downside of accelerated fractionation is a concomitant increase in acute toxicity. These two strategies were extensively examined in a series of clinical trials conducted in the 1980s and 1990s. While not specific to oral cavity and oropharynx cancer, the majority of patients in most of these trials had tumors arising from the oropharynx. Again, for operable oral cavity primary lesions, resection is the preferred initial therapeutic strategy. The results of several altered fractionation trials are summarized here.

EORTC 22791 compared two radiotherapy regimens in patients with locally advanced oropharyngeal carcinoma: 80.5 Gy in 1.15-Gy fractions delivered twice daily versus 70 Gy in 2-Gy fractions delivered daily. Local tumor control at 5 years increased from 40% to 59% with the hyperfractionated regimen. There was no comparative difference in acute or late toxicities.

EORTC 22851 looked at accelerated fractionation, comparing 72 Gy in 45 fractions (1.6 Gy three times a day [TID]) over 5 weeks with a 2-week mid-treatment break compared to 70 Gy in 2-Gy fractions delivered daily in patients with non-oropharyngeal, head and neck squamous cell carcinoma (SCC). While there was a 15% improvement in locoregional control (LRC), there was a significant increase in acute toxicities and an unexpected increase in late effects, including some lethal complications (3).

In the United Kingdom, the Continuous, Hyperfractionated, Accelerated Radiotherapy Trial (CHART) was designed to dramatically reduce overall treatment time and therefore increase local control but also, by reducing total dose and dose per fraction, reduce the late adverse effects of radiation. The investigators compared 54 Gy at 1.5 Gy per fraction delivered TID over 12 consecutive days versus 66 Gy at 2 Gy per fraction delivered 5 days per week over a period of 6.5 weeks. While there was no difference in locoregional relapse-free survival, disease-free survival, disease-specific survival or overall survival, there were statistically significant reductions in late dysphagia, xerostomia, laryngeal edema and mucosal necrosis (4).

Finally, RTOG 90-01 compared four different fractionation regimens: (1) 70 Gy in 35 fractions delivered over 7 weeks; (2) 81.6 Gy delivered in 1.2-Gy fractions twice daily over 7 weeks; (3) 67.2 Gy delivered in 1.6 Gy per fraction BID over 6 weeks with a 2-week break; and (4) 72 Gy delivered in 1.8-Gy fractions over 6 weeks with a 1.5-Gy boost field given BID for the final 12 days of treatment. Only the hyperfractionated regimen (regimen 2) significantly improved LRC and overall survival at 5 years compared to the standard fractionation arm. There were no significant differences in the prevalence of grade ≥3 toxicity when comparing the groups. However, when comparing the 6-week to the 7-week treatment arms, there did appear to be an increase in grade ≥3 toxicity at 5 years (5).

Perhaps the most significant contribution to the long debate about altered fractionation was the publication of a meta-analysis in 2006. Evaluating the two potential altered strategies in head and neck SCC, the authors concluded that, compared to standard fractionation, the hyperfractionated regimens had the greatest benefit in both locoregional and overall survival, although the accelerated options did provide for improved LRC as well (6).

More recently, the intensity of the once raging debate over fractionation schemes has been dampened by the findings that altered fractionation is likely not commensurate with standard fraction CRT and that, compared to conventionally fractionated CRT, chemotherapy combined with altered fractionation offers no additional benefit (7,8).

CONCURRENT CHEMOTHERAPY WITH RADICAL RADIOTHERAPY

The majority of patients in clinical trials that demonstrated efficacy of combined concurrent chemotherapy with definitive radiotherapy compared to radical radiotherapy alone had oropharynx primary lesions. Again, this enrollment pattern reflects the differences in the current standard of care between the treatments for these two primary sites.

GORTEC 94-01 specifically enrolled patients younger than 75 with stage III/IV oropharynx cancer, randomizing them to radical, conventionally fractionated radiotherapy or the same radiotherapy dose with concurrent administration of carboplatin and 5-fluorouracil at weeks 1, 4 and 7. The addition of carboplatin/5-fluorouracil resulted in statistically significant improvements in overall survival, disease-specific survival and LRC. Stage IV disease and hemoglobin levels <125 g/L were predictive of worse outcome. Grade 3 or 4 complications were more common in patients receiving concurrent chemotherapy (56% versus 30%).

The Head and Neck Intergroup trial randomized patients with unresesctable head and neck squamous cell carcinoma (HNSCC) to one of three arms: (1) radical radiotherapy alone to 70 Gy in 35 fractions; (2) radical radiotherapy with concurrent cisplatin; and (3) split course radiotherapy with cisplatin and 5-FU. If, after the first half of radiotherapy, disease became resectable, patients went for surgery; otherwise, the second half of the radiotherapy regimen was delivered. More than 50% of the patients on this trial had oropharynx SCC. Comparing arms 1 and 2, the addition of concurrent cisplatin improved overall survival at 3 years (37% versus 23%). The split-course arm (arm 3) was no better than conventional fractionated radiotherapy.

POSTOPERATIVE RADIOTHERAPY

For cancers of the oral cavity, upfront surgical resection remains the standard of care (9). In oropharynx cancer, with the proliferation of minimally invasive, transoral surgical techniques and the recognition that the extraordinarily high cure rates with CRT may allow for treatment de-intensification, upfront transoral robotic-assisted resection and transoral laser resection have become more popular. Surgery in this setting may allow for moderate reductions in radiotherapy dose and for the elimination of concurrent chemotherapy (10).

PORT is considered for patients with extranodal extension (ENE), positive margins, pT3 or T4 disease, pN2 or pN3 disease, nodal disease in levels IV or V, perineural invasion (PNI) or vascular emboli. For patients with ENE, concurrent chemotherapy is typically added to the radiotherapy regimen. In the case of positive margins, where re-resection is not feasible, concurrent chemotherapy is also recommended. These recommendations, based on National Comprehensive Cancer Network (NCCN) guidelines, hold for malignancies of both the oral cavity and oropharynx.

RTOG 73-03 randomized 320 patients with T2-4N any supraglottic larynx and hypopharynx SCC to 50 Gy preoperatively versus 60 Gy postoperatively. There was a significant improvement in LRC at 10 years (58% versus 70%). By logical deduction, if PORT is superior to lower-dose preoperative RT, it is very likely the case that PORT compared to observation in the aforementioned subgroup of patients could potentially confer an even greater benefit. Although it did not include patients with oral cavity and oropharynx SCC, there is no prima facie reason to believe that results for these primary sites would differ (11).

An MD Anderson Cancer Center (MDACC)-led prospective trial attempted to answer the question of which postoperative subgroups might benefit from PORT (12). The authors stratified patients into risk categories based on the presence of the following risk factors: ≥2 positive nodes, ≥2 nodal groups involved, PNI, margin status, oral cavity subsite, largest node >3 cm and ENE. The low-risk group had none of these risk factors, the intermediate-risk group had one of these factors (excluding ENE) and the high-risk group had ≥2 factors or ENE. The low-risk group was observed, the intermediate-risk group received 57.6 Gy in 6.5 weeks and the high-risk group was randomized to 63 Gy in 5 weeks or 63 Gy in 7 weeks. The majority of patients in this study had oropharynx or oral cavity primaries.

The low-risk group had excellent LRC with surgery alone (5-year LRC was 90%). The intermediate-risk group had similarly excellent outcomes with moderate-dose postoperative RT (LRC of 94%). In the high-risk group, the patients who underwent accelerated fraction had a trend toward a higher LRC (p = .11).

Data from the Memorial Sloan Kettering Cancer Center (MSKCC) specifically evaluating PORT in oral cavity cancer demonstrated that those who tend to benefit from PORT are patients with positive margins, higher N stages, higher T stages, younger age and female sex (13).

Surveillance, Epidemiology and End Results (SEER) database analyses have also provided data to show the benefit of PORT in oral cavity and oropharynx SCC. Shrime et al. evaluated the use of adjuvant radiation in patients with T1–2N1 oral cavity SCCs and found significant improvements in 5-year overall survival (41.4% versus 54.2%). These benefits were predominantly limited to patients with T2N1 disease and those with oral cavity and floor of the mouth primary lesions (14).

Kao et al. used SEER data to evaluate the benefits of PORT in HNSCC patients with node-positive disease. They found improvements in overall survival for patients with oropharynx, hypopharynx, larynx and oral cavity primaries. The benefit was seen regardless of nodal stage (15).

Although the MDACC study did suggest a benefit to altered fractionation in the postoperative setting, this was not confirmed in a subsequent study by Sanguineti et al. With a median follow-up of 30.6 months, there was no difference in LRC or overall survival comparing once-a-day treatment to a biphasic boost schedule with the beginning and end of treatment involving BID sessions (16).

POSTOPERATIVE CONCURRENT CRT

Two seminal studies evaluated the benefit of concurrent chemotherapy added to PORT in certain high-risk subgroups. RTOG 95-01 and EROTC 22931 had different eligibility criteria. Both trials included patients with ENE and positive margins, although with slightly different definitions of marginal positivity. The RTOG trial included patients with multiple positive nodes. The EORTC study did not strictly define eligibility based on multiple pathologically enlarged nodes; however, it did include patients with T3–4 primaries, those with PNI or LVI (lymphovascular invasion) and oral cavity patients with level IV or V nodal metastasis. RTOG had a primary endpoint of LRC; EORTC evaluated progression-free survival.

The 5-year update of the RTOG study showed a trend toward an improvement in LRC (79.5% versus 71.3%) and disease-free survival (37.4% versus 29.1%; both p = .10) (17). The EORTC study, with a median follow-up of 5 years, actually showed statistically significant improvements in progression-free survival, overall survival and LRC (18). As was expected, in both trials, the rates of acute mucosal toxicity were higher with the addition of cisplatin. Somewhat surprisingly, the addition of cisplatin did not influence the rate of distant failure.

RADIATION TECHNIQUES

INTENSITY-MODULATED RADIATION THERAPY

Traditional radiotherapy for head and neck SCC, whether definitive or postoperative, involved the use of parallel opposed radiation beams (almost always using photons of 6 MV energy) to treat the upper neck nodes and the primary site, with a matched low anterior neck (LAN) field to treat the more inferior nodal basins. Beyond the placement of blocks in order to spare the spinal cord and brainstem, little in the way of normal tissue dose reduction was possible.

Dramatic advances in computer and imaging technologies allowed for the introduction of intensity-modulated radiotherapy (IMRT) in the 1990s. IMRT allowed for exquisitely conformal radiotherapy plans. Because of the tight anatomical spaces and the proximity of tumor to critical normal tissues (parotid gland, carotid artery, spinal cord and pharyngeal constrictor muscles), IMRT was ideally suited for the treatment of patients with head and neck malignancies.

Briefly, IMRT involves the treatment of the patient from multiple (e.g., five to nine) different, typically co-planar directions (occasionally with continuous arcs) with photon beams of non-uniform fluences. The beams (or arcs) undergo an optimization process using a cost function that directs the dynamic movement of multi-leaf collimators in order to deliver high doses to prespecified targets (planning target volumes [PTVs]) and minimize doses to normal structures. The process of optimization utilizes a method known as "inverse planning." In inverse planning, beamlet weights or intensities are adjusted in order to achieve a specific desired dose to a certain volume of a target structure. In addition, normal tissue limits are specified (e.g., mean dose to the left parotid gland of <26 Gy). Because of the steep dose gradients involved in IMRT, knowledge of computed tomography (CT)-based axial anatomy has become a critical component for proper delivery of radiotherapy.

The data supporting the use of the more costly IMRT (as opposed to conventional radiotherapy) are most robust in head and neck SCC. As such, its use is widespread and should be considered the standard of care for patients with oral cavity and oropharynx SCC.

Nutting et al. reported the parotid-sparing intensity-modulated versus conventional radiotherapy in head and neck cancer (PARSPORT) phase III trial (49). The vast majority of the patients enrolled in the trial were undergoing radical radiotherapy for oropharynx SCC, although postoperative and hypopharynx patients were also allowed.

At 12 months, grade 2 or greater xerostomia was present in 74% of the patients treated with conventional radiotherapy versus 38% of those treated with IMRT. At 24 months, this dramatic difference remained. Furthermore, at both 12 and 24 months, significant benefits were seen in recovery of saliva secretion with IMRT compared to conventional radiotherapy. There were no reported differences in LRC or overall survival.

BRACHYTHERAPY

Since the advent and proliferation of IMRT, the use of brachytherapy for head and neck cancers has decreased. Its employment is very much institution dependent. When it is employed, interstitial brachytherapy can be used either alone or in combination with external beam radiation therapy (EBRT) and most often for select lesions of the oral tongue, lip and floor of the mouth (19). Iridium-192 is often employed in temporary, high-dose rate brachytherapy, whereas in permanent, low-dose rate brachytherapy, the radionuclide of choice is iodine-125.

Tumor thickness dictates whether the brachytherapy implant is to be single plane or double plane; for tumors of thickness <1 cm, generally a single-plane implant is sufficient. For larger tumors, the double-plane implant is preferred.

At the MSKCC, fractionated high dose rate (HDR) brachytherapy using iridium-192 sources is preferred. It remains unclear as to the optimal dose per fraction with HDR therapy, but generally twice daily fractions of between 3 and 4 Gy are thought to minimize the risk of late toxicity. Brachytherapy can be used in combination with EBRT postoperatively or as a single-modality treatment. It is generally recommended that the concurrent administration of brachytherapy and chemotherapy be avoided. Intraoperative planning should be done using 3D CT or magnetic resonance imaging (MRI)-based images. Gross tumor volume (GTV) and clinical tumor volume (CTV) should be delineated and the organs at risk contoured.

In early-stage (T1–2N0) oral tongue and floor of the mouth SCC treated definitively with radiation, the 5-year local control with HDR brachytherapy (60 Gy in ten fractions delivered BID) is approximately 87% with no significant increase in late effects compared to low dose rate (LDR) methods. For locally advanced oral tongue SCC not amenable to resection, EBRT is often combined with HDR brachytherapy (20,21).

Although not performed frequently at many institutions, surface mold brachytherapy can also be used for select primary superficial (<1 cm depth of invasion) lesions of the hard palate, lower gingiva and floor of the mouth. This involves an impression of the target surface with the subsequent creation of a mold in the form of a partial dental plaster plate. HDR remote afterloading is feasible with surface molds.

SIMULATION

Simulation often involves multiple imaging modalities, but at the very least a CT of the head and neck with intravenous contrast, with the patient immobilized in the precise position in which he/she will be for all subsequent treatments. Radiotherapy plans are then devised based on the CT images obtained at simulation after the proper delineation of target structures and normal tissues.

The patient is placed in the supine position with relevant anatomic detail (surgical incisions) outlined using radio-opaque markers. For oral cavity or oropharynx lesions, the supine position is most frequently used. A bite block is used for oral tongue, floor of the mouth or hard palate primary lesions in order to spare structures inferior or superior to the intended primary target. For buccal mucosal lesions, an intraoral stent should be used to shift the tongue to the contralateral side of the cavity.

Immobilization involves the use of a five-point mask that limits motion of the head, neck, shoulders and upper arms (Figure 12.1). Many institutions use an open-mask device that still effectively restricts patient motion but is more tolerable, avoiding feeling of claustrophobia.

If available, all head and neck patients should undergo positron emission tomography (PET)-CT simulation with intravenous contrast in order to improve target delineation for both primary and nodal disease. Even more ideal is the concurrent use of an MRI simulator. In our experience, magnetic resonance simulation may improve soft tissue delineation, allowing for a more precise determination of gross disease and for a more effective sparing of normal tissues, most especially the constrictor muscles. If magnetic resonance or PET technology is not available within the simulation suite, previously obtained diagnostic magnetic resonance and PET scans should fused to the planning CT scan. The use of maximum amperage for CT scanning can also improve resolution.

The determination of bolus need is also a critical component of head and neck radiotherapy simulation. Typically, the soft tissues within the oral cavity and oropharynx provide for enough secondary electron buildup to minimize the need for bolus placement. However, with buccal mucosa and lip primary lesions, this oftentimes becomes necessary. The bolus is placed either at the time of simulation or is created during the planning process as a result of dosimetric considerations.

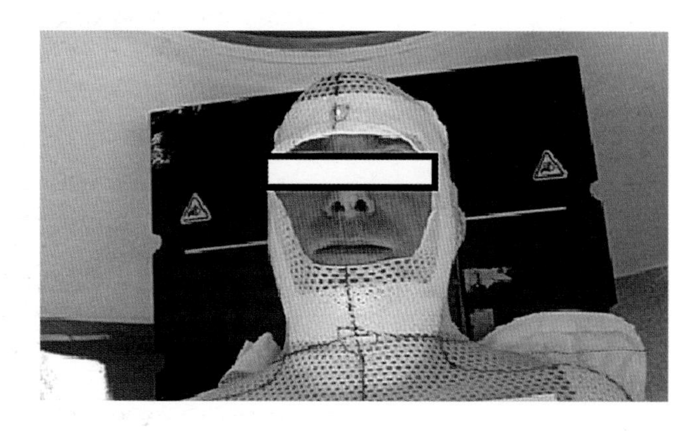

Figure 12.1 Five-point open face mask.

PLANNING TECHNIQUES AND ON-TREATMENT IMAGING

For almost all oral cavity and oropharynx lesions we prefer IMRT techniques because of improved conformality. However, for lip lesions, it is still feasible, and may be preferable from a dosimetric standpoint, to use three dimensional radiation therapy (3DRT) with an appositional electron field treating the primary and parallel opposed lateral photon fields treating the upper neck nodes (when necessary).

The question of whole-field IMRT versus an IMRT plan matched to a LAN field is one that is hotly debated. Broadly speaking, assuming no low-level neck disease, we tend to prefer IMRT for the primary lesion and upper neck nodes matched to a LAN field (22). Dosimetric studies have suggested that, compared to whole-field IMRT, a LAN field dynamically matched to an IMRT plan results in statistically significant reductions in larynx and constrictor dose (23). Although no study has shown clear differences in dysphagia between the two techniques, if feasible, based on the dosimetric studies alone, a LAN matched to an IMRT plan is preferred. The match line is placed just above the arytenoids.

We will discuss subsite-specific target dose recommendations below. However, coverage of the target and dose restrictions to organs at risk is the same regardless of oral subsite (Figure 12.2). It should be noted that with ipsilateral-only nodal treatment, we anticipate contralateral mean parotid and submandibular doses far below those listed. In addition, in the treated but radiographic node-negative neck, ipsilateral mean parotid doses should be kept below 15–16 Gy. This can be easily achieved.

Finally, because of the steep dose gradients associated with IMRT plans, on-treatment imaging becomes critical to the successful delivery of the prescribed dose. As such, daily 2DKV (two dimensional kilovoltage) imaging that includes both an AP film and a lateral film is recommended. Moreover, a weekly cone-beam CT image as an additional assurance of appropriate coverage is desirable.

PRETREATMENT NUTRITIONAL CONSIDERATIONS

Over 50% of patients undergoing concurrent CRT develop severe, acute odynophagia, taste alterations and thickened

	Target Criteria	
H&N	Coverage for each volume	D95 ≥ Prescription Dose
	Dose Homogeneity	D05 of Highest Dose Volume ≤ 108% of prescription for that PTV
		D05 of other targets ≤ Prescription of next higher dose volume
	Review a 3D isodose surface display to ensure that the hot spots are inside the PTV	

	Normal Tissue Criteria			
	Structures	Todal Dose* ≤	To:	Comments
H&N	Cord	45Gy(50Gy)	Max Point Dose	
	Brainstem	50Gy(60Gy)	Max Point Dose	
	Chiasm	54Gy(60Gy)	Max Point Dose	
	Optic Nerve	54Gy	Max Point Dose	
	Retina	45Gy	Max Point Dose	
	Lens	5Gy(10Gy)	Max Point Dose	
	Parotid	26Gy	Mean Dose	Each gland
	Cochlea	50Gy	Max Point Dose	
		55Gy	$D_{05\%}$	If Max dose constaint not possible
	Oral Cavity	35-40Gy	Mean Dose	
	Larynx	105% of Rx or 70Gy, whichever is lower	Max Point Dose	
		40-45Gy	Mean Dose	
	Mandible	No Hot Spots	Max Point Dose	
	Mandible_*not*_PTV	70Gy	Max Point Dose	
	Brachial Plexus	65Gy	Max Point Dose	The criteria for Brachial Plexus should take precedence over PTV coverage near the brachial plexus for any PTV with a prescription dose of ≥ 59.4Gy
	Submandibular Gland	39Gy	Mean Dose	Each gland. PTV coverage should take precedence over Submandibular Gland guideline
	Constrictor Muscle	58Gy	Mean Dose	
	Ipsilateral Medial Pterygoid	68Gy	Mean Dose	
	Ipsilateral Masseter	42Gy	Mean Dose	

Figure 12.2 Target coverage goals and dose restrictions to normal tissue. *The doses listed in parentheses are only used with the express approval of the attending physician.

saliva. This combination can significantly compromise oral intake. As a result, we routinely involve speech/swallow therapy and nutrition early on in the course of CRT.

The routine use of prophylactic feeding tubes should be discouraged. Prophylactic percutaneous endoscopic gastrostomy (pPEG) placement may compromise long-term swallowing outcomes. Reports from the MSKCC have demonstrated that placement of pPEG in patients with oropharyngeal head and neck cancer (HNC) undergoing definitive CRT failed to significantly improve mortality or albumin levels, decrease acute toxicity rates (dysphagia, mucositis and xerostomia), decrease chronic dysphagia and affect treatment duration as compared to patients who refused pPEG placement (24). Given these data, PEG tube placement should be reserved for patients who are at high risk of weight loss and dehydration that would likely require interventions that could potentially delay treatment.

OROPHARYNX

The anatomic delineations of the oropharynx include: anteriorly, the base of the tongue, the anterior tonsillar pillars and the boundary line of the hard and soft palate; posteriorly, the posterior pharyngeal wall mucosa; superiorly, the soft palate; and inferiorly, the oropharynx is demarcated by the hyoid bone. Amongst the oropharyngeal subsites, the vast majority of primary lesions arise in the palatine tonsils and base of the tongue (lingual tonsils).

Although traditionally related to tobacco exposure, the vast majority of oropharynx cancers now result from high-risk HPV infection, predominantly the HPV-16 subtype. HPV carcinogenesis arises from the overexpression of the viral oncoproteins Eg and E7 (25). Consequently, there has been a demographic shift in the patient population toward younger, male never-smokers (26).

TREATMENT STRATEGY

Multidisciplinary collaboration in the treatment of patients with oropharynx cancer is critical. Early stage (T1–2N0) oropharyngeal cancer is amenable to treatment with either radical radiotherapy or surgical extirpation alone without the need for any adjuvant therapy. The decision as to which modality is most appropriate depends in part on the surgeon's estimation of the functional detriments that might result from surgical intervention and the probability of achieving negative margins. A positive margin that is not amenable to re-resection may consign the patient to adjuvant therapy with either radiotherapy or CRT. In such cases, radical radiotherapy is preferred. In cases where the lesion is exophytic with radiographically negative neck nodes, a strong case can be made for surgery alone, especially in younger patients in whom the late effects of RT can be avoided.

Patients with T1–2N1 disease are somewhat more controversial. The first pertinent question is whether to pursue a radiotherapy or surgery-based regimen. If physical examination demonstrates a mobile node and imaging suggests encapsulated nodal disease, upfront surgery is preferred. If there is any question of ENE, in order to avoid tri-modal therapy and the consequent toxicities, radical radiotherapy is preferred. Although CT is not particularly sensitive for assessment of ENE, it is fairly specific (27); thus, when called by the head and neck radiologist, ENE is quite likely to be present on subsequent dissection.

Whether patients with radiographic and clinical N1 disease with small primaries benefit from the addition of concurrent chemotherapy to radiation is a question that remains controversial. The vast majority of the patients in the GORTEC oropharynx trial had T3–4 disease (87%); there were very few T1–2N1 patients, so application of the results of that trial to this setting is questionable. O'Sullivan et al. reported no difference in local, regional or distant control in patients with T1–2N1–2a oropharyngeal cancer treated with RT versus CRT (28). In T1–2N1 HPV-positive patients with a <10 pack-year smoking history, radical radiotherapy alone is likely sufficient. Evidence suggests that tobacco smoking increases the risk of distant failure, even in those with p16 (HPV) positivity (29). The MACH meta-analysis shows a small but significant benefit in distant control with concurrent chemotherapy (30). Therefore, in those with a more substantial tobacco history, if the decision is made to pursue radical radiotherapy, one might be more inclined to treat with CRT in these patients. The ECOG surgical trial in HPV-positive oropharynx patients consigns T1–N2N1 patients who achieve negative margins to observation alone, but does stratify by tobacco history (>10 pack-year history being the cut-off).

In patients with more locally advanced disease (T1–4N2–3), what is the most appropriate treatment regimen? For patients with bulky primary lesions, because of the morbidity that would be associated with surgical resection, concurrent CRT is preferred. In T1–2N2–3 patients, there exists continued controversy. Again, the benefit of upfront surgical resection is that, assuming negative margins and contained nodal disease, chemotherapy can often be omitted. However, in embarking on a surgery-first approach, it is often difficult to precisely quantify the risk, particularly of ENE; therefore, the chance for the need of tri-modal therapy is often uncertain. This presents issues when counseling patients. Furthermore, because of concurrent chemotherapy's benefits in reduction in distant failure, chemotherapy may positively impact groups of patients at high risk for metastasis.

Given that the ECOG trial in p16-positive patients has just begun to accrue, the current strategy is largely influenced by prior retrospective data, namely the report from O'Sullivan et al. (28). The Princess Margaret group argues that distant metastatic risk is substantial in N2c disease and tobacco-positive (>10 pack-years) patients with N2b disease (28). In these patients, therefore, concurrent CRT is recommended. For T1–2N2a–b HPV-positive never-smokers, if operative risk is acceptable and imaging affirms nodal encapsulation, surgery with the hopes of consequent chemotherapy omission is typically preferred.

A still outstanding question is when to pursue salvage neck dissection in HPV-positive oropharynx cancer treated with definitive radiation or chemoradiation. In the hopes of providing clinical guidance, the Princess Margaret Hospital (PMH) group investigated temporal nodal regression in their N2–N3 patients stratified by HPV status (50). In HPV-positive patients who did not have a complete response (lymph node <1 cm) by 8–12 weeks and who did not undergo salvage neck dissection, only six of 69 had a subsequent regional failure. The tempo of nodal regression in HPV-positive oropharynx cancer is prolonged. Within the HPV-positive cohort, complete response (CR) did not predict for subsequent regional recurrence; however, initial N3 disease did. Therefore, at the PMH, HPV-positive N2 patients often undergo continued imaging surveillance. As long as the nodes either continue to regress or are stable in size, no neck dissection is planned. For N3 disease without CR at 8–12 weeks, neck dissection is recommended.

VOLUMES

A thorough physical examination and appropriate imaging are critical to the proper delineation of primary and nodal contours. Specifically, nasopharyngoscopy must be performed in order to determine the extent of the primary lesion. MRI, CT and PET are crucial to defining primary disease contours and to determining the presence or absence of grossly involved lymph nodes. If not available in simulation, diagnostic images should be fused to the planning CT.

More specifically, the clinical target volume (CTV) for a tonsil primary should include the ipsilateral soft palate to midline, the anterior glossotonsillar sulcus, a portion of the retromolar trigone (RMT), a portion of the ipsilateral base of the tongue and the ipsilateral parapharyngeal space. It is desirable to cover superiorly the pharyngeal mucosa/parapharyngeal space up to the most inferior extent of the pterygoid plates.

For a base of the tongue primary, the entire lingual tonsil should be encompassed in the CTV primary volume. As one moves superolaterally, the glosso-tonsillar (G-T) sulcus should be included, as should the inferior pole of the palatine tonsil. Anteriorly, especially for bulky lesions, a portion of the muscles comprising the floor of the mouth should also be included on the ipsilateral side. Inferiorly, the field should extend to cover several slices into the pre-epiglottic space. A portion of the posterior pharyngeal wall should also be included.

In the postoperative setting, the CTV primary should be outlined based on initial imaging of gross disease, the intraoperative report and the postoperative examination. In general, any flaps should be covered in their entirety. Margins to account for intraoperative seeding may also be important.

For CTV nodal contours, one must first determine whether it is necessary to treat unilateral nodal basins or bilateral nodal basins. For primaries of the base of the tongue and soft palate, we routinely utilize bilateral nodal irradiation because of the proximity of the primaries to the midline. More uncertainty surrounds primary lesions of the tonsils. If there is extension into the base of the tongue or soft palate, again, we will recommend bilateral irradiation. For well-lateralized tonsil primaries, the American College of Radiology is comfortable with unilateral nodal irradiation in T1–2N1–2a disease. For N2b disease, they recommend bilateral irradiation (31). However, other groups are comfortable omitting the contralateral nodes even in the N2b setting. Still more confusingly, recent data from the Royal Marsden Hospital suggests that not only N2b disease, but ENE and a >10 pack-year history should be viewed as contraindications to unilateral radiation with tonsil primaries (32).

In the postoperative or definitive node-positive neck, we will routinely cover levels II, III, IV, VA, VB, retrostyloid and retropharyngeal nodal basins as defined by RTOG/DAHANCA/EORTC/NCIC/TROG guidelines in the nodal CTV (33). If the primary lesion extends into the oral tongue or floor of the mouth or positive nodes are found at the time of dissection, we will include ipsilateral levels IA/B. Otherwise, we do not routinely cover level I in the node-positive neck unless it is positive at initial dissection. The same holds true for level V.

In the radiographically or pathologically node-negative neck, we will cover level II to where the posterior belly of the digastric crosses the internal jugular vein, level III and level VA. In the postoperative setting, the entirety of the sternocleidomastoid should be contoured in areas where ENE was present.

The isotropic PTV expansions for the GTV primary and CTV primary, volumes should generally be 4–5 mm and expansions for CTV nodes generally 2–3 mm.

DOSE

For HPV-positive oropharyngeal cancer, the PTVs associated with gross disease are treated to 70 Gy in 35 fractions (2 Gy per fraction). The PTVs associated with the CTVs surrounding the primary lesion are treated to 54 Gy in 30 fractions (1.8 Gy per fraction). High-risk nodal CTVs are treated to 54 Gy in 30 fractions. Low-risk nodal CTVs are treated to 50.1 Gy in 1.67-Gy fractions (30 fractions). Finally, if a lymph node is indeterminate, in the HPV-positive setting, the node is treated to 60 Gy in 30 fractions. Given the exquisite radiosensitivity of HPV-positive disease, this relative de-escalation is considered justifiable and safe.

For the rare instances of HPV-negative oropharyngeal SCC, the gross disease is treated to 70 Gy. However, the CTV surrounding the primary and high-risk nodal basins is treated to 60 Gy. Low-risk nodal basins are treated to 54 Gy.

OUTCOMES

Outcomes with radical radiotherapy alone in early-stage oropharyngeal cancers are excellent, in part because of the inherent radiosensitivity of HPV-related malignancies. Selek et al. reported outcomes in 208 patients treated at the MDACC with early-stage (stage I or II) oropharyngeal cancer treated with radiotherapy alone. Although most were treated in the pre-HPV era, outcomes were excellent, with 5-year rates of LRC of approximately 81%. There was no apparent difference when comparing conventional fractionation with concomitant boost radiotherapy (34). RTOG 02-22 was a prospective phase II trial evaluating IMRT radiotherapy alone in 68 patients with T1–2N0–1 oropharyngeal cancer (39% were N positive) treated with an accelerated hypofractionation regimen (gross disease received 66 Gy in 2.2-Gy fractions). The 2-year rate of locoregional failure was 9%; the 2-year overall survival rate was 95.5% and the disease-free survival rate was 82.0%.

In locally advanced disease, both the MDACC and the MSKCC have reported their outcomes in large cohorts of oropharynx patients treated with concurrent CRT (35,36). LRC is excellent with the use of CRT. In the MSKCC series, the 3-year cumulative incidence rates of local and regional failure were 5.4% and 5.6%, respectively. In the MDACC series, the 5-year rate of LRC was 90%.

ORAL CAVITY

The oral cavity contains several distinct subsites including the lip, anterior two-thirds of the tongue (oral tongue), floor of the mouth, buccal mucosa, gingiva, hard palate and RMT. The floor of the mouth is bounded by the lower alveolar ridge in the anterolateral dimension and the ventral tongue surface and anterior tonsillar pillar posteriorly. The oral tongue is the portion of the tongue anterior to the circumvallate papillae. The buccal mucosa overlies the buccinator muscle and is bound by the gingiva in the superior and inferior dimensions and by the RMT in the posterior direction.

Approximately 65% of oral cavity cancers are attributed to tobacco exposure (37). Heavy alcohol intake also increases one's odds of developing oral cavity SCC (38). There is also a multiplicative interaction between tobacco and alcohol consumption in the causation of oral cavity SCC.

As is in keeping with other head and neck subsites, approximately 95% of cancers of the oral cavity are SCCs, with the majority arising in the oral tongue or floor of the mouth in the Western world. In other parts of the world where tobacco chewing habits are prevalent, the buccal mucosa, gum and RMT are the most common sites.

TREATMENT STRATEGY

In general, surgery followed by postoperative radiation or chemoradiation is the standard of care in the treatment of oral cavity cancer. However, there are some variations by subsite.

For T1–2N0 lesions of the lip, surgical resection is the preferred option, assuming an acceptable cosmetic outcome. Optimal surgical margins are ≥5 mm. Postoperative radiation is offered in the case of positive margins not amenable to re-resection, PNI, vascular invasion (VI) or lymphatic vessel invasion. In most instances, elective nodal dissection or elective nodal irradiation are unnecessary. However, patients with lip cancers with a depth of invasion of greater than 5 mm may benefit from elective nodal irradiation after surgical resection.

For patients with T3–4a or node-positive SCC of the lip, surgery is also preferred with ipsilateral or bilateral neck dissection depending upon the extent of nodal disease. In patients with N0 disease, observation may be considered. For those with one positive node without adverse features (namely ENE, positive margins, multiple positive nodes or PNI/LVI/VI), radiation should be considered and directed to the primary site and at-risk nodal basins. For patients with ENE or positive margins, adjuvant chemoradiation is recommended. For those with adverse features exclusive of ENE or positive margins, radiation alone is generally sufficient, although chemoradiation can be considered.

For patients with oral tongue, buccal mucosa, RMT, gingiva and hard palate primary lesions, surgical resection is the mainstay for T1–2N0 lesions, typically without the need for any major reconstructive effort. For patients with T1–2N0 lesions and a depth of invasion >5 mm, elective, selective neck dissection is generally recommended with extirpation of lymph nodes at levels I–III; bilateral neck dissection should be reserved for lesions near or crossing the midline. Elective neck dissection may be considered in patients with depth of invasion of <5 mm.

Assuming no adverse risk features (pT3 or T4 disease, pN2 or N3 nodal disease, nodal disease in levels IV or V, PNI, vascular embolism, ENE or positive margins), adjuvant therapy can be avoided in T1–2N0 patients. However, in oral tongue SCC, in lesions with >4 mm depth of invasion, the regional recurrence rate is quite high despite elective neck dissection. In these patients, postoperative irradiation should be considered. In patients with a single positive node without adverse risk features, postoperative radiation therapy may be considered. On the other hand, in patients with adverse risk features exclusive of ENE and positive margins, radiation should be offered. With ENE and positive margins, adjuvant CRT is required.

For patients with locally advanced disease (T3N0, T1–3N1–3 or T4a), upfront surgery with ipsilateral or bilateral neck dissection depending upon lesion location is the standard of care. Adjuvant radiation should be considered in all instances of locally advanced disease, with the addition of chemotherapy in cases of ENE or positive margins.

VOLUMES

A postoperative MRI or PET scan is desirable in order to determine whether any remnant gross disease is present. This is especially important in the setting of large primary lesions or extracapsular spread where, in the interval between surgery and the initiation of adjuvant therapy, the risk for interval locoregional recurrence or even distant metastasis is high (39,40).

Obviously, any gross disease should be outlined and treated to a therapeutic dose. The CTV primary in the postoperative setting should include the area of gross disease as determined by preoperative imaging and operative note, as well as the entire postoperative bed, including any regional or free flaps. It may be beneficial, if feasible, to fuse preoperative imaging to the simulation CT. A high-risk CTV primary should be contoured to include areas of soft tissue/bone invasion or microscopically positive margins. For deeply invasive oral tongue lesions, the CTV primary should encompass a large portion of the floor of the mouth as a possible location at risk for local recurrence. For buccal mucosa primaries, the CTV primary should extend cranially to the gingivobuccal sulcus and infratemporal fossa, caudally to the gingivobuccal sulcus and submandibular gland, anteriorly at least to the commissure of the lips and posteriorly to the RMT (Figure 12.3). The buccal fat pad is also clearly at risk for microscopic infiltration and should be included in the CTV primary. For larger RMT primary lesions that invade the pterygoid muscles, the CTV primary should include the pterygopalatine fossa.

For nodal contours, any areas of extracapsular spread (ECS) should be contoured out as a high-risk CTV node; ideally, the tissue overlying areas of ENE should be bolused to ensure adequate dose coverage. For all primary subsites except for buccal mucosa primaries, bilateral nodal basins should be covered. In the node-negative neck, CTV nodes should include levels IA, IB, II, III and IV. Coverage of level IV is critical in the oral tongue, even if levels II and III are uninvolved, since clinically occult skip metastases are possible (41). Level V is almost never involved in the clinically negative neck. For the pathologically or radiographically positive neck, levels IA, IB, II, III and IV should be covered. We would omit level V and the retropharyngeal nodes unless they were obviously involved. Including level V electively may be considered in the node-positive neck with oral tongue primaries, although the risk for involvement is still slight (42). In the positive neck, we would include the retrostyloid nodes.

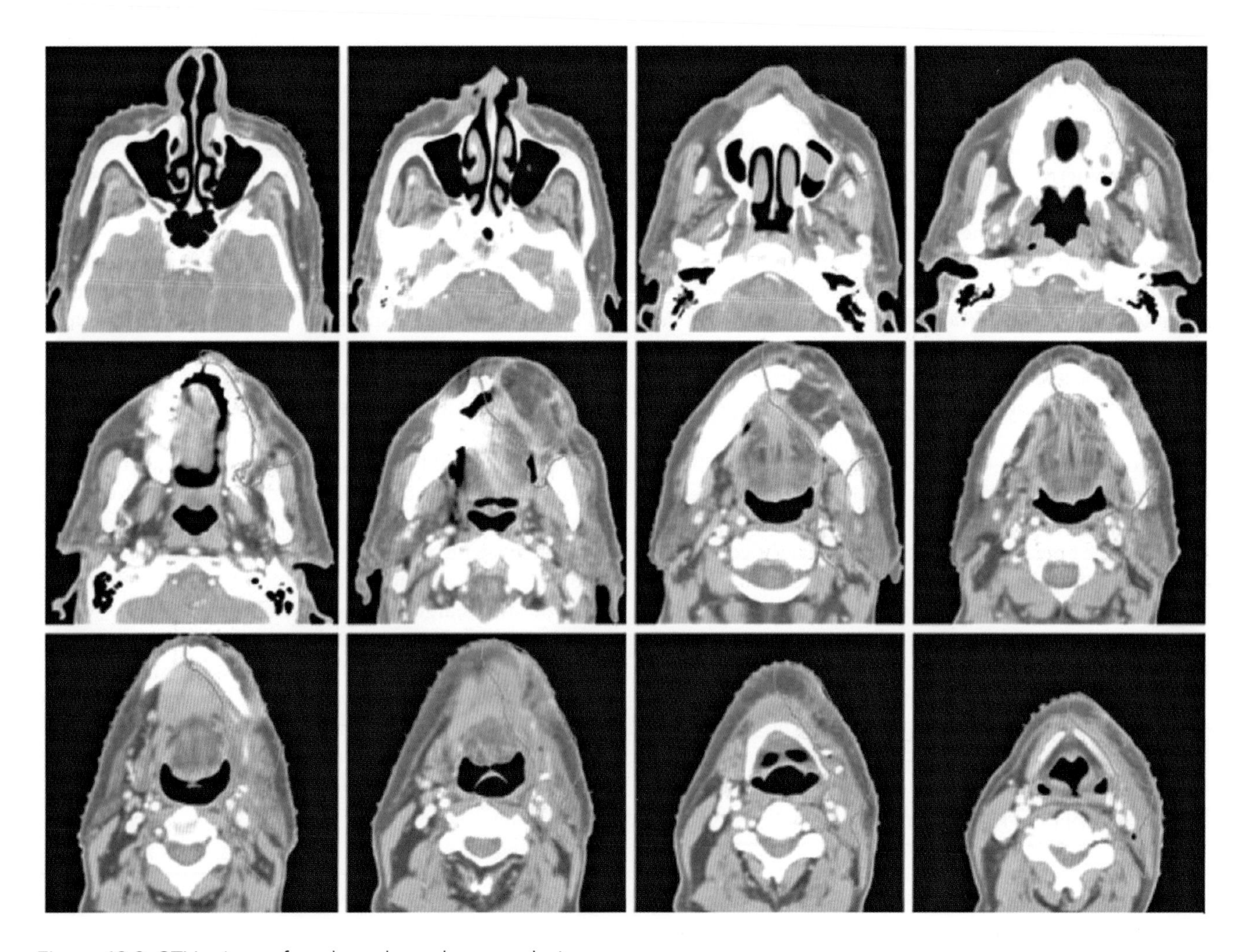

Figure 12.3 CTV primary for a large buccal mucosa lesion.

DOSE

The PTV for gross disease should be taken to 70 Gy. The PTV for the high-risk CTV primary and CTV nodes (e.g. those areas of positive margin or ENE) should be taken to 66 Gy in 2-Gy fractions. The remainder of the CTV postoperative primary should be treated to 60 Gy in 2-Gy fractions. The positive postoperative CTV nodal basins should be treated to 60 Gy in 2-Gy fractions. Finally, the CTV for nodal basins in the electively treated, node-negative neck should be up to 54 Gy in 1.8-Gy fractions.

OUTCOMES

The largest series on outcomes of postoperative radiation following primary surgery for oral cavity SCC was recently reported by Chan et al. (43). The vast majority of the 180 patients included in the study had oral tongue (46%) or floor of the mouth (23%) primary lesions. The majority of patients received bilateral neck irradiation. In the ipsilateral neck, levels IA, IB, II, III, IV and V were covered; in the contralateral neck, level V was omitted 46% of the time. Concurrent bolus cisplatin was given in instances of ENE or positive margins. The dosing used was similar to that previously outlined in the "Dose" section. The 2-year rates of overall survival, local control, regional control, LRC and distant control were 65%, 87%, 83%, 78% and 83%, respectively. For the oral tongue specifically, the LRC was 72%; for the floor of the mouth, the LRC was 84%. The bulk of locoregional failures were in-field, with seven marginal and five out-of-field failures (approximately a third of the total). The buccal mucosa, RMT, hard palate and gingival primary lesions were under-represented in this study, however.

A recent report from the University of Florida looking at RMT SCC treated with surgery followed by adjuvant radiotherapy showed a 5-year rate of LRC of 89% for stage I–III disease and 58% for stage IV disease; 5-year cause-specific survival was 82% for stage I–III disease and 43% for stage IV disease (44).

Bachar et al. reported on outcomes of 70 patients with buccal mucosa primary lesions (45). The majority of patients (n = 40) had early-stage, T1–2N0 disease. Sixty-one patients had upfront surgery, 23 of whom later underwent postoperative radiation. The most significant predictor of outcome was nodal status (N+ versus N−) and ENE. The 5-year overall survival was 87.3% for node-negative patients and 50.8% for node-positive patients.

Eskander et al. reported on outcomes in 97 patients with maxillary alveolus and hard palate SCC treated between 1994 and 2008 (46). Approximately 30% of patients received postoperative radiation. The indication for postoperative radiation in this cohort was multiple positive nodes. In the overall cohort, the 3-year disease-free survival rate was 70%. Hard palate site, advanced pathologic T stage and poorly differentiated tumors were predictive of failure; nodal involvement trended toward an association with disease-free survival.

TOXICITY

The most common acute toxicity in oral cavity and oropharyngeal radiotherapy is mucositis. By week 3 of treatment, most patients will develop a patchy (grade 2) mucositis; by the end of treatment, the vast majority will experience a confluent (grade 3) mucositis that causes significant odynophagia requiring opiate pain medication. At the MSKCC, gabapentin is used in an attempt to reduce the need for opiate pain medications and their attendant side effects (47). Management of pain secondary to mucositis involves initiation with liquid oxycodone by week 3 and, based on breakthrough requirements, a fentanyl patch for long-acting pain control. It is critical to have patients concurrently initiate Senna and Colace in order to reduce the risk of constipation.

Diligent oral hygiene promotes mucosal healing. The signs of oral *Candida* infection are critical to recognize and should be promptly treated with either nystatin or, in the event of resistance, systemic anti-fungal agents such as fluconazole (Figure 12.4).

The odynophagia along with the dysgeusia that patients experience by the second week of treatment can lead to decreased per oral (PO) intake. However, upfront placement of a pPEG tube is not recommended because of the risks of late swallowing dysfunction (48). PEG placement should be considered during treatment in patients who have lost more than 10% of their baseline body mass or in patients who are taking minimal PO despite a maximally tolerated outpatient pain regimen.

Patients often experience thickened saliva during radiotherapy. This can further contribute to both treatment-related weight loss and nausea. The upfront treatment recommended for increased salivary secretions is either guaifenesin or, failing that, glycopyrrolate.

Radiation dermatitis is also a common acute side effect of treatment. Low-grade dermatitis is traditionally treated with over-the-counter skin moisturizers such as Aquaphor and Eucerin. For higher-grade dermatitis, re-epithelialization is

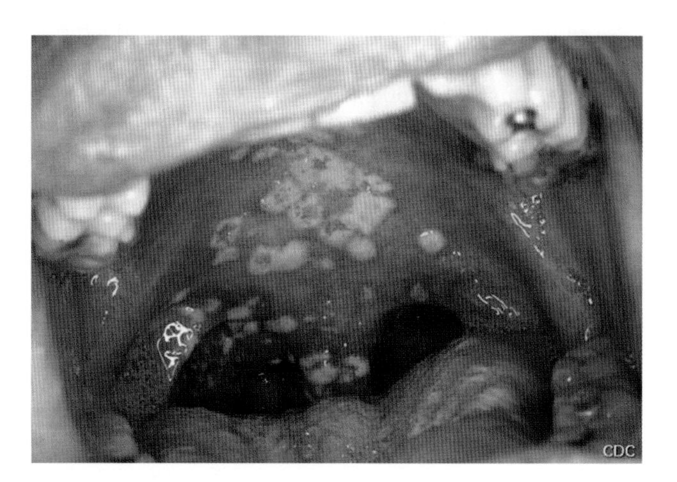

Figure 12.4 Oral candidiasis.

important and is promoted by use of Domeboro's solution to cleanse the wound site. Topical antibacterials may also help to desiccate a wet wound. Along with steroid creams such as mometasone, these are crucial in the treatment of dermatitis toward the end of therapy.

Late side effects must also be evaluated. The most common late complication of radiotherapy for oral cavity or oropharyngeal lesions is xerostomia. Although its incidence can be reduced with IMRT, a significant proportion of patients will still experience permanent decreases in salivary function. Several over-the-counter salivary stimulants may be used to manage xerostomia. Dry mouth tends to be most bothersome at night and the use of a bedside humidifier may be helpful. Furthermore, pharmacologic intervention with pilocarpine may help to increase salivary flow, although at the risk of headaches, hypertension, flushing, bowel and bladder motility and tachycardia.

Because of xerostomia and the risk for subsequent dental caries, diligent attention to oral hygiene is critical. This includes visits every 3–4 months to the dentist for teeth cleaning. Topical fluoride applications are also important, as well as fluoride-containing dentifrice.

A more serious late complication of radiotherapy is osteonecrosis, most commonly of the mandible. Its initial management is typically conservative with the use of systemic antibiotics and analgesis. Good oral hygiene is once again critical to prompt resolution. Healing can take place over several months, although surgical resection of the necrotic bone and reconstruction may be necessary in patients with an exposed and sequestered segment of the mandible.

REFERENCES

1. Sher DJ, Thotakura V, Balboni TA et al. Treatment of oral cavity squamous cell carcinoma with adjuvant or definitive intensity-modulated radiation therapy. *Int J Radiat Oncol Biol Phys* 2011;81(4):e215–22.
2. Kelly K, Johnson-Obaseki S, Lumingu J et al. Oncologic, functional and surgical outcomes of primary transoral robotic surgery for early squamous cell cancer of the oropharynx: a systematic review. *Oral Oncol* 2014;50(8):696–703.
3. Bernier J, Horiot JC. Altered-fractionated radiotherapy in locally advanced head and neck cancer. *Curr Opin Oncol* 2012;24(3):223–8.
4. Saunders MI, Rojas AM, Parmar MKB et al. Mature results of a randomized trial of accelerated hyperfractionated versus conventional radiotherapy in head-and-neck cancer. *Int J Radiat Oncol Biol Phys* 2010;77(1):3–8.
5. Beitler JJ, Zhang Q, Fu KK et al. Final results of local-regional control and late toxicity of RTOG 9003: a randomized trial of altered fractionation radiation for locally advanced head and neck cancer. *Int J Radiat Oncol Biol Phys* 2014;89(1):13–20.
6. Bourhis J, Overgaard J, Audry H et al. Hyperfractionated or accelerated radiotherapy in head and neck cancer: a meta-analysis. *Lancet* 2006;368(9538):843–54.
7. Bourhis, J, Sire C, Graff P et al. Concomitant chemoradiotherapy versus acceleration of radiotherapy with or without concomitant chemotherapy in locally advanced head and neck carcinoma (GORTEC 99-02): an open-label phase 3 randomised trial. *Lancet Oncol* 2012;13(2):145–53.
8. Nguyen-Tan PF, Zhang Q, Ang KK et al. Randomized phase III trial to test accelerated versus standard fractionation in combination with concurrent cisplatin for head and neck carcinomas in the Radiation Therapy Oncology Group 0129 trial: long-term report of efficacy and toxicity. *J Clin Oncol* 2014;32(34):3858–67.
9. Pfister DG, Spencer S, Brizel DM et al. Head and neck cancers, Version 2.2014. Clinical practice guidelines in oncology. *J Natl Compr Canc Netw* 2014;12(10):1454–87.
10. Morisod B, Simon C. A meta-analysis on survival of patients treated with trans-oral surgery (TOS) versus radiotherapy (RT) for early stage squamous cell carcinoma of the oropharynx (OPSCC). *Head Neck* 2016;38(Suppl 1):E2143–50. doi: 10.1002/hed.23995.
11. Tupchong L, Phil D, Scott CB et al. Randomized study of preoperative versus postoperative radiation therapy in advanced head and neck carcinoma: long-term follow-up of RTOG study 73-03. *Int J Radiat Oncol Biol Phys* 1991;20(1):21–8.
12. Peters LJ, Goepfert H, Ang KK et al. Evaluation of the dose for postoperative radiation therapy of head and neck cancer: first report of a prospective randomized trial. *Int J Radiat Oncol Biol Phys* 1993;26(1):3–11.
13. Wang SJ. Patel SG, Shah JP et al. An oral cavity carcinoma nomogram to predict benefit of adjuvant radiotherapy. *JAMA Otolaryngol Head Neck Surg* 2013;139(6):554–9.
14. Shrime MG, Gullane PJ, Dawson L et al. The impact of adjuvant radiotherapy on survival in T1–2N1 squamous cell carcinoma of the oral cavity. *Arch Otolaryngol Head Neck Surg* 2010;136(3):225–8.
15. Kao J, Lavaf A, Teng MS et al. Adjuvant radiotherapy and survival for patients with node-positive head and neck cancer: an analysis by primary site and nodal stage. *Int J Radiat Oncol Biol Phys* 2008;71(2):362–70.
16. Sanguineti G, Richetti A, Bignardi M et al. Accelerated versus conventional fractionated postoperative radiotherapy for advanced head and neck cancer: results of a multicenter phase III study. *Int J Radiat Oncol Biol Phys* 2005;61(3):762–71.
17. Cooper JS, Pajak TF, Forastiere AA et al. Postoperative concurrent radiotherapy and chemotherapy for high-risk squamous-cell carcinoma of the head and neck. *N Engl J Med* 2004;350(19):1937–44.

18. Bernier J, Domenge C, Ozsahin M et al. Postoperative irradiation with or without concomitant chemotherapy for locally advanced head and neck cancer. *N Engl J Med* 2004;350(19):1945–52.
19. Nag S, Cano ER, Demanes DJ et al. The American Brachytherapy Society recommendations for high-dose-rate brachytherapy for head-and-neck carcinoma. *Int J Radiat Oncol Biol Phys* 2001;50(5):1190–8.
20. Inoue T, Inoue T, Yoshida K et al. Phase III trial of high- vs. low-dose-rate interstitial radiotherapy for early mobile tongue cancer. *Int J Radiat Oncol Biol Phys* 2001;51(1):171–5.
21. Nicholas Lukens J, Gamez M, Hu K et al. Modern brachytherapy. *Semin Oncol* 2014;41(6):831–47.
22. Lee N, Mechalakos J, Puri DR et al. Choosing an intensity-modulated radiation therapy technique in the treatment of head-and-neck cancer. *Int J Radiat Oncol Biol Phys* 2007;68(5):1299–309.
23. Caudell JJ, Burnett OL, Schaner PE et al. Comparison of methods to reduce dose to swallowing-related structures in head and neck cancer. *Int J Radiat Oncol Biol Phys* 2010;77(2):462–7.
24. Romesser PB, Romanyshyn JC, Schupak KD et al. Percutaneous endoscopic gastrostomy in oropharyngeal cancer patients treated with intensity-modulated radiotherapy with concurrent chemotherapy. *Cancer* 2012;118(24):6072–8.
25. Steinau M, Saraiya M, Goodman MT et al. Human papillomavirus prevalence in oropharyngeal cancer before vaccine introduction, United States. *Emerg Infect Dis* 2014;20(5):822–8.
26. Chaturvedi AK. Epidemiology and clinical aspects of HPV in head and neck cancers. *Head Neck Pathol* 2012;6(Suppl 1):S16–24.
27. Prabhu RS, Magliocca KR, Hanasoge S et al. Accuracy of computed tomography for predicting pathologic nodal extracapsular extension in patients with head-and-neck cancer undergoing initial surgical resection. *Int J Radiat Oncol Biol Phys* 2014;88(1):122–9.
28. O'Sullivan B, Huang SH, Siu LL et al. Deintensification candidate subgroups in human papillomavirus-related oropharyngeal cancer according to minimal risk of distant metastasis. *J Clin Oncol* 2013;31(5):543–50. doi: 10.1200/JCO.2012.44.0164.
29. Gillison ML, Zhang Q, Jordan R et al. Tobacco smoking and increased risk of death and progression for patients with p16-positive and p16-negative oropharyngeal cancer. *J Clin Oncol* 2012;30(17):2102–11.
30. Pignon JP, Maître A, Maillard E et al. Meta-analysis of chemotherapy in head and neck cancer (MACH-NC): an update on 93 randomised trials and 17,346 patients. *Radiother Oncol* 2009;92(1):4–14.
31. Expert Panel on Radiation Oncology—Head and Neck Cancer et al. ACR Appropriateness Criteria® ipsilateral radiation for squamous cell carcinoma of the tonsil. *Head Neck* 2012;34(5):613–6.
32. Lynch J, Lal P, Schick U et al. Multiple cervical lymph node involvement and extra-capsular extension predict for contralateral nodal recurrence after ipsilateral radiotherapy for squamous cell carcinoma of the tonsil. *Oral Oncol* 2014;50(9):901–6.
33. Gregoire V, Ang K, Budach W et al. Delineation of the neck node levels for head and neck tumors: a 2013 update. DAHANCA, EORTC, HKNPCSG, NCIC CTG, NCRI, RTOG, TROG consensus guidelines. *Radiother Oncol* 2014;110(1):172–81.
34. Selek U, Garden AS, Morrison WH et al. Radiation therapy for early-stage carcinoma of the oropharynx. *Int J Radiat Oncol Biol Phys* 2004;59(3):743–51.
35. Setton J, Caria N, Romanyshyn J et al. Intensity-modulated radiotherapy in the treatment of oropharyngeal cancer: an update of the Memorial Sloan-Kettering Cancer Center experience. *Int J Radiat Oncol Biol Phys* 2012;82(1):291–8.
36. Garden AS, Dong L, Morrison WH et al. Patterns of disease recurrence following treatment of oropharyngeal cancer with intensity modulated radiation therapy. *Int J Radiat Oncol Biol Phys* 2013;85(4):941–7.
37. Lubin JH, Muscat J, Gaudet MM et al. An examination of male and female odds ratios by BMI, cigarette smoking, and alcohol consumption for cancers of the oral cavity, pharynx, and larynx in pooled data from 15 case–control studies. *Cancer Causes Control* 2011;22(9):1217–31.
38. Scoccianti C, Straif K, Romieu I. Recent evidence on alcohol and cancer epidemiology. *Future Oncol* 2013;9(9):1315–22.
39. Liao CT, Fan K-H, Lin C-Y et al. Impact of a second FDG PET scan before adjuvant therapy for the early detection of residual/relapsing tumours in high-risk patients with oral cavity cancer and pathological extracapsular spread. *Eur J Nucl Med Mol Imaging* 2012;39(6):944–55.
40. Kang CJ, Lin C-Y, Yang LY et al. Positive clinical impact of an additional PET/CT scan before adjuvant radiotherapy or concurrent chemoradiotherapy in patients with advanced oral cavity squamous cell carcinoma. *J Nucl Med* 2015;56(1):22–30.
41. De Zinis LO, Bolzoni A, Piazza C et al. Prevalence and localization of nodal metastases in squamous cell carcinoma of the oral cavity: role and extension of neck dissection. *Eur Arch Otorhinolaryngol* 2006;263(12):1131–5.
42. Parikh DG, Chheda YP, Shah SV et al. Significance of level V lymph node dissection in clinically node positive oral cavity squamous cell carcinoma and evaluation of potential risk factors for level V lymph node metastasis. *Indian J Surg Oncol* 2013;4(3):275–9.
43. Chan AK, Huang SH, Le LW et al. Postoperative intensity-modulated radiotherapy following surgery for oral cavity squamous cell carcinoma: patterns of failure. *Oral Oncol* 2013;49(3):255–260.

44. Hitchcock KE, Amdur RJ, Morris CG et al. Retromolar trigone squamous cell carcinoma treated with radiotherapy alone or combined with surgery: a 10-year update. *Am J Otolaryngol* 2015;36(2):140–5. doi: 10.1016/j.amjoto.2014.10.005.
45. Bachar G, Goldstein DP, Barker E et al. Squamous cell carcinoma of the buccal mucosa: outcomes of treatment in the modern era. *Laryngoscope* 2012;122(7):1552–7.
46. Eskander A, Givi B, Gullane PJ et al. Outcome predictors in squamous cell carcinoma of the maxillary alveolus and hard palate. *Laryngoscope* 2013;123(10):2453–8.
47. Bar Ad V, Weinstein G, Dutta PR et al. Gabapentin for the treatment of pain syndrome related to radiation-induced mucositis in patients with head and neck cancer treated with concurrent chemoradiotherapy. *Cancer* 2010;116(17):4206–13.
48. Langmore S, Krisciunas GP, Miloro KV et al. Does PEG use cause dysphagia in head and neck cancer patients? *Dysphagia* 2012;27(2):251–9.
49. Nutting CM, Morden JP, Harrington KJ et al. Parotid-sparing intensity modulated versus conventional radiotherapy in head and neck cancer (PARSPORT): a phase 3 multicentre randomised controlled trial. *Lancet Oncol* 2011;12(2):127–36. doi: 10.1016/S1470-2045(10)70290-4. https://www.ncbi.nlm.nih.gov/pubmed/21236730.
50. Huang SH, O'Sullivan B, Xu W et al. Temporal nodal regression and regional control after primary radiation therapy for N2-N3 head-and-neck cancer stratified by HPV status. *Int J Radiat Oncol Biol Phys* 2013;87(5):1078–85. doi: 10.1016/j.ijrobp.2013.08.049.

13

Chemotherapy

ANDRES LOPEZ-ALBAITERO AND MATTHEW G. FURY

INTRODUCTION

The management of patients with locally and/or regionally advanced head and neck squamous cell carcinoma (HNSCC) has evolved from purely surgical to a multidisciplinary effort that includes radiation and chemotherapy. Randomized trials and meta-analyses have led to widespread acceptance of organ preservation strategies with the combination of cytotoxic chemotherapy and radiation therapy (1–3). Single-modality or multimodality treatments are typically employed for early-stage and locoregionally advanced disease, respectively. For patients with unresectable, recurrent or metastatic disease, systemic therapy has shown efficacy in numerous well-designed clinical trials.

The choice of modality for the treatment of locally and/or regionally advanced HNSCC not only depends on subsite and stage, but also on the general medical condition and the functional status of each patient. Contemporarily, there are four scenarios in which chemotherapy is used in combined-modality treatment programs:

1. The first uses surgery as a primary treatment followed by concurrent chemoradiation. Surgical extirpation allows accurate staging of the disease and determines the need for adjuvant treatment by precisely identifying high-risk features (extranodal spread or positive margins).
2. Chemoradiation is used with curative intent, keeping surgery in reserve for salvage treatment of persistent or recurrent disease. This is the preferred approach when organ preservation is the goal, when surgery is not feasible or when the anticipated functional outcome of surgical resection is deemed to be unacceptable.
3. Chemotherapy can be used in neoadjuvant (induction) schemes. Induction regimens are usually followed by definitive local treatment: surgery or radiation therapy. This approach, mostly used for the treatment of advanced laryngeal cancer, is based on the findings from the landmark 1991 VA trial in which response to induction chemotherapy was associated with subsequent response to radiation treatment, leading to laryngeal preservation (4).
4. Chemotherapy is used either in combination with radiation or by itself for palliation of recurrent, unresectable or metastatic disease. In this setting, the patients are best entered into ongoing clinical trials if such are available at the institution where the patient is being treated.

In this chapter, evidence for the use of systemic therapy in the treatment of HNSCC is discussed in brief. Given the great progress seen in the treatment of other solid tumors, current advances in immunotherapy are also presented. Finally, because of its singular clinical characteristics, human papillomavirus (HPV)-related oropharynx SCC is discussed as a distinct entity.

AGENTS AVAILABLE FOR THE TREATMENT OF HNSCC

CYTOTOXIC CHEMOTHERAPY

The cytotoxic agents most commonly administered in the treatment of HNSCC include platinum-based anti-neoplastics (cisplatin and carboplatin), taxanes (paclitaxel and docetaxel) and antimetabolites (methotrexate and 5-fluorouracil [5FU]).

Platinum agents cross-link DNA, preventing cell replication. Although they share some side effects, cisplatin and carboplatin have slightly different toxicity profiles. Cisplatin is generally viewed as more emetogenic, but patients respond well to serotonin receptor antagonists like ondansetron. Cisplatin has more potent neurotoxic and nephrotoxic properties and this latter dose-limiting toxicity is prevented by aggressive hydration. Cisplatin can also cause high-frequency hearing loss and it is often prudent to obtain pre- and post-treatment audiograms for patients who receive cisplatin as part of essential workup for considering combined-modality regimen. For oropharynx SCC patients who are not deemed suitable candidates for cisplatin in the context of combined-modality therapy, the regimen of carboplatin plus 5FU may be considered (5).

Taxanes interfere with cell replication by interfering with microtubule function during mitosis. Docetaxel and paclitaxel are similarly efficacious clinically against HNSCC (6,7). Characteristic toxicities are neutropenia, neuropathy and alopecia. They can also induce hepatotoxicity and should not be used in patients with significant baseline hepatic dysfunction.

The antimetabolites with well-described clinical activity against HNSCC are methotrexate and 5FU (8,9). Methotrexate inhibits an enzyme involved in the synthesis of thymidine necessary for DNA synthesis. 5FU is a pyrimidine analogue with the same inhibitory mechanism of action. Methotrexate is mostly used for palliation in low doses, while 5FU is used in combination with other drugs, mainly in induction regimens. They both can produce diarrhea, myelosuppression and mucositis.

TARGETED THERAPY: SMALL MOLECULES AND BIOLOGICS

Targeted therapy uses a small molecule or biologic agent (antibody) to target a gene that is mutated or preferentially expressed in cancer cells. The overexpression or mutation of this gene may lead to aberrant activation of a specific pathway that not only is important for the tumor's malignant phenotype, but also is indispensable for tumor survival. Thus, targeted therapy is largely dependent on how much a tumor relies on the targeted pathway/gene being targeted. The dependency of the tumor on a specific gene is known as oncogene addiction. Tumors can, however, present resistance to this approach. Resistance can be present prior to the initiation of therapy (primary resistance) or develop as a consequence of it (acquired resistance). The concept of targeted therapy is enticing and has been largely effective in treating solid and non-solid tumors, but has not been clearly established in the clinical management of HNSCC.

Targeted therapy against HNSCC has focused on the epidermal growth factor receptor (EGFR or HER1). Over 90% of HNSCC tumors overexpress this receptor. There are several antibodies that are specific for EGFR, but cetuximab (C225) is the only one approved by the Food and Drug Administration of the United States for the treatment of HNSCC. Cetuximab is an IgG1 antibody that binds to the extracellular domain of EGFR and blocks activation of this receptor by preventing ligand binding. Cetuximab is also thought to induce an immune reaction against cancer cells (10).

EGFR has also been targeted using small molecules that block the tyrosine kinase domain. However, published randomized clinical trials of small-molecule EGFR inhibitors against advanced HNSCC have been negative (11,12). In view of oncogenic alterations in the *PIK3CA* gene in many HNSCCs (13–15), a current focus of intense research is the use of small-molecule inhibitors of phosphatidylinositol 3-kinase (PI3K).

IMMUNOTHERAPY

The goal of immunotherapy is to redirect the immune system against cancer cells. The concept of an immune response against cancer has a long history in oncology research, but convincing clinical validation of this approach has been obtained only in recent years.

The immune system has evolved to recognize cells that harbor mutations, including tumor cells. The mechanisms through which these immune responses occur are complex and in some cases only partially understood. The most active form of defense in the immune system is mediated by cytotoxic T-cells. Activation of T-cells is carefully controlled through a complex mechanism of checks and balances. Activation only occurs when the sum of the signals presented to the T-cell surpasses a certain threshold. Tumor cells exploit the mechanisms used to control T-cell activation, preventing T-cell activation and inducing tolerance.

Several approaches have been designed that attempt to redirect T-cells against tumor cells. CAR T-cells are T-cells that have been engineered to express a receptor that is able to recognize an antigen within a tumor cell, leading to T-cell activation and tumor killing. After these T-cells have been engineered, they are reinfused into patients and are able to mediate anti-tumor cellular responses. This technology is evolving and has not yet been reported for the treatment of solid tumors. The first trials to determine their effectiveness in this setting are underway.

Research efforts have also focused on blocking the inhibitory signals that prevent T-cell activation. One method to achieve this is by using antibodies that block these inhibitory receptors, so-called immune checkpoint inhibitors. The rationale behind the use of these antibodies is that T-cells can be activated against tumors by blocking the inhibitory signals on the surface of immune or tumor cells. The first positive randomized clinical trial results with this approach were obtained in patients with advanced melanoma, but more recently activity with checkpoint inhibition has been described in a growing list of solid tumor types.

The latest evidence suggests that patients with a higher rate of mutations may be more likely to benefit the most from these immune checkpoint inhibitors, although data are still evolving regarding which patients are most likely to benefit from this class of drug. HNSCCs arising in individuals with a smoking history may elicit a T-cell response due to the mutational burden created by carcinogens in tobacco, and HPV-related HNSCC may elicit a T-cell response due the presence of viral proteins. Numerous clinical trials to evaluate the efficacy of immune checkpoint inhibition in HNSCC are ongoing.

CURRENT SCHEMES USED IN THE TREATMENT OF HNSCC

CONCURRENT CHEMOTHERAPY AND RADIATION

There are three theoretical principles that support the use of concurrent chemotherapy and radiation in the treatment of HNSCC: first, chemotherapy can have an additive effect by sensitizing cancer cells to radiation, improving the rates of local control. Second, although it has long-term toxicity for some patients, concurrent chemoradiation can achieve organ preservation without the debilitating and life-changing consequences of surgical extirpation. Third, the administration of chemotherapy is the only systemic treatment for HNSCC and has the potential to eliminate minimally distant metastatic disease, although evidence for the latter has not been robust in clinical trials.

The Meta-Analysis for Chemotherapy in Head and Neck (MACH-HN) published in 2000 by Pignon et al. established that the use of concurrent chemoradiation in the treatment of advanced HNSCC provided an overall 8% survival advantage (3). The update on this meta-analysis, including the individual patient analyses of 17,436 patients, confirmed this finding with an absolute survival benefit of 6.5%. This paper consolidated the role of cytotoxic chemotherapy in the treatment of HNSCC.

The current dose used for the treatment of locally advanced HNSCC was described in the Intergroup phase III trial published by Adelstein et al. in 2003 (1). This trial was carried out to determine the benefit of adding chemotherapy to radiation in the treatment of unresectable HNSCC. This trial established the advantage of high-dose platinum (100 mg/m^2) on days 1, 22 and 43 of radiation treatment. Acute and long-term toxicities have been consistently shown in this and other trials.

In laryngeal cancer, concurrent chemotherapy was popularized as a regimen for laryngeal preservation based on the initial and subsequent reports of the RTOG 91-11 trial (2). This trial was designed to determine the utility of concurrent chemoradiation in the setting of advanced laryngeal cancer by comparing it to an induction regimen (cisplatin/5FU) or radiotherapy alone. The utility of concurrent chemoradiation was clearly established: the 10-year follow-up demonstrated that locoregional control and laryngeal preservation were superior with this approach.

In 2006, Bonner et al. showed that the combination of radiotherapy with cetuximab was superior to radiotherapy alone in the treatment of locoregionally advanced HNSCC (16). Patients treated with a combination of cetuximab and radiation had better progression-free survival without an increase in toxicity, one of the most feared complications seen with concurrent chemoradiation using cytotoxic agents. Prospective clinical trial data are needed because it is currently not known if locoregional control and overall survival with this regimen are better or worse than that which can be obtained with concurrent chemoradiation with cisplatin. Cetuximab has failed to provide an advantage even when added to concurrent chemoradiation using cisplatin (17). Because of these findings, the initial enthusiasm in the use of cetuximab in the treatment of HNSCC has been tempered by a realization of the limitations imposed by the lack of a validated predictive biomarker to guide the clinical use of this agent in HNSCC patients. Current research is focusing on the biologic markers that predict response as well as the mechanisms of resistance to cetuximab and ways to circumvent them.

INDUCTION CHEMOTHERAPY

Induction (or neoadjuvant) regimens are always followed by a definitive local treatment: radiation therapy or surgery. The optimal regimen for induction chemotherapy in locally advanced head and neck cancer is TPF (docetaxel, cisplatin and 5FU), but the role of sequential therapy in the treatment of locally/regionally advanced HNSCC has not been clearly established.

Induction chemotherapy usually includes multiple agents, most commonly cisplatin and 5FU. The combination of cisplatin/5FU in induction regimens can induce responses in a majority of patients, but evidence has shown that patients benefit from the addition of docetaxel. As such, TPF is the comparator for any new induction therapy regimens in HNSCC (18,19).

Induction regimens have been used for all HNSCC subsites, but principles were established in early studies of laryngeal cancer. This effort was encouraged by the results of the VA study from 1991. In this study, treatment groups were established based on the patient's initial response to induction chemotherapy with cisplatin and 5FU combined. Those patients who failed to respond received surgery versus chemoradiation for the initial responders. This study established that survival for induction chemotherapy followed by radiation therapy was comparable with the standard of treatment at the time—surgery followed by radiation. However, preservation of the larynx was feasible in 64% of patients who received radiation after response to induction chemotherapy. The RTOG 91-11 trial compared concurrent cisplatin and radiation with induction (again with cisplatin and 5FU) followed by radiotherapy (2). However, as discussed in the previous section, concurrent chemotherapy was found to be superior in this setting.

An update of the MACH-NH further analyzed these patients by subsite (20,21). The survival advantage of concurrent chemoradiation was statistically significant in patients with oropharyngeal and laryngeal tumors, with a trend of significance for oropharyngeal and oral cavity tumors. Interestingly, induction regimens appeared to be superior in the control of distant metastases.

However, there is no published randomized clinical trial to support widespread use of the sequential approach of TPF followed by radiation therapy (RT-based) treatment instead of primary chemoradiation. In fact, there are now three negative randomized published clinical trials that looked at this question (22–24). The negative results in the PARADIGM (22) and DeCIDE (23) trials have been attributed to poor accrual and unexpectedly favorable outcomes in the control arms. In the TTCC study (24), a central factor underlying the negative results appears to have been difficulty with deliverability of Induction Chemotherapy (ICT). Although the explanations for failure to achieve a positive primary endpoint vary among these three studies, there has been an accumulation of negative phase III trial data against the widespread adoption of TPF-based sequential therapy.

SPECIAL CONSIDERATIONS FOR HPV-RELATED OROPHARYNX SCC

HNSCC has been traditionally associated with carcinogen exposure, with a higher incidence of this disease in smokers and drinkers. On the other hand, the high-risk strains of the HPV are causative agents for anogenital SCCs. In 2000, Gillison et al. described an association between high-risk HPV infection and HNSCC (25). HPV-associated tumors were more frequently found in the oropharynx and were not associated with tobacco or alcohol consumption. Importantly, patients who had tumors that were HPV-related had a 59% reduction in risk of death from cancer compared to those who had HPV-negative tumors.

Kian Ang et al. published in 2010 an analysis of the association between HPV status and survival in patients receiving concurrent chemoradiation with cisplatin and different radiation therapy regimens in the context of a prospective clinical trial, RTOG 0129 (26). This study found a similar 58% reduction in the risk of death (hazard ratio: 0.42) among all patients with HPV-related oropharynx SCC compared to patients with HPV-negative tumors after adjustment for other variables. Three prognostic risk groups were defined based on HPV status, tobacco history and T and N stage.

HPV-related oropharynx SCC affects a younger patient population who may endure decades of impediments to quality of life due to the long-term toxicities of combined-modality therapy. The following question has been posed: can long-term toxicities be avoided by de-escalation of treatment in HPV-related oropharynx cancer with the same therapeutic effect?

One concept under study is the use of the monoclonal antibody cetuximab instead of cisplatin. In the cetuximab trial by Bonner et al., where patients were not stratified by HPV status, there was a suggestion that patients with oropharyngeal cancer benefited the most from this targeted therapy (16). This generated great interest in the use of cetuximab in HPV-positive patients. The RTOG-1016 and De-ESCALATE trials were designed to investigate this question, but have different primary endpoints. Both studies randomize patients with HPV-related oropharynx SCC to receive concurrent chemoradiation with cisplatin or cetuximab. Accrual for RTOG-1016 has been completed, but results have not yet reached maturity for reporting purposes. Accrual for the De-ESCALATE trial is ongoing. It is hoped that the results of these studies will help clarify the current dilemma regarding the role of cetuximab in the management of patients with newly diagnosed, locoregionally advanced, HPV-associated OPSCC. In contrast to the Bonner et al. data, subgroup analyses in the RTOG-0522 study did not demonstrate improved progression-free survival or overall survival with the addition of cetuximab to cisplatin, compared to cisplatin alone, for oropharynx cancer patients, regardless of p16 status, when given concurrently with radiation therapy (27). It is anticipated that the results of the RTOG-1016 and De-ESCALATE trials will better define the utility of cetuximab in this patient population.

Trials to determine the optimal dose of radiation and also the potential role of surgery for these patients are also underway. Available evidence to date does not support any changes from the current treatment protocols for patients with HPV-related disease. Modifications of treatment protocol for these patients should only occur in the setting of a clinical trial.

CONCLUSION

HNSCC is a complex and diverse disease in which therapeutic advantages with systemic therapy have been demonstrated in various contexts. As with other tumor systems, the current advances in genomics, molecular medicine, immunology and tumor biology will continue to guide clinical researchers on the path toward more efficacious and less toxic therapy. In this era of burgeoning incidence of HPV-related oropharynx SCC, results of ongoing trials are eagerly awaited to help define the optimal way to reduce toxicities without compromising survival.

REFERENCES

1. Adelstein DJ, Li Y, Adams GL et al. An intergroup phase III comparison of standard radiation therapy and two schedules of concurrent chemoradiotherapy in patients with unresectable squamous cell head and neck cancer. *J Clin Oncol* 2003;21:92–8.
2. Forastiere AA, Goepfert H, Maor M et al. Concurrent chemotherapy and radiotherapy for organ preservation in advanced larynx cancer. *New Engl J Med* 2003;349:2091–8.

3. Pignon J, Bourhis J, Domenge D, Designe L. Chemotherapy added to locoregional treatment for head and neck squamous cell carcinoma: three meta-analyses of updated individual data. *Lancet* 2000;355:949–55.
4. The Department of Veterans Affairs Laryngeal Cancer Study Group. Induction chemotherapy plus radiation compared with surgery plus radiation in patients with advanced laryngeal cancer. *N Engl J Med* 1991;324:1685–90.
5. Denis F, Garaud P, Bardet E et al. Final results of the 94-01 French Head and Neck Oncology and Radiotherapy Group randomized trial comparing radiotherapy alone with concomitant radiochemotherapy in advanced stage oropharynx carcinoma. *J Clin Oncol* 2004;22:69–76.
6. Forastiere A, Shank D, Neuberg D et al. Final report of a phase II evaluation of paclitaxel in patients with advanced squamous cell carcinoma of the head and neck: an Eastern Cooperative Oncology Group Trial (PA390). *Cancer* 1998;82:2270–4.
7. Dreyfuss AI, Clark JR, Norris CM et al. Docetaxel: an active drug for squamous cell carcinoma of the head and neck. *J Clin Oncol* 1996;14:1672–78.
8. Forastiere AA, Metch B, Schuller DE et al. Randomized comparison of cisplatin plus fluorouracil and carboplatin plus fluorouracil versus methotrexate in advanced squamous-cell carcinoma of the head and neck: a Southwest Oncology Group study. *J Clin Oncol* 1992;10:1245–51.
9. Taylor SG, McGuire WP, Hauck WW et al. A randomized comparison of high dose infusion methotrexate versus standard weekly therapy in head and neck squamous cancer. *J Clin Oncol* 1984;2:1006–11.
10. Srivastava RM, Lee SC, Andrade Filho P et al. Cetuximab-activated natural killer cells and dendritic cells collaborate to trigger tumor antigen-specific T-cell immunity in head and neck cancer patients. *Clin Cancer Res* 2013;19:1858–72.
11. Argiris A, Ghebremichael M, Gillbert J et al. Phase III randomized, placebo-controlled trial of docetaxel with or without gefitinib in recurrent or metastatic head and neck cancer: an eastern cooperative group oncology trial. *J Clin Oncol* 2013;31:1405–14.
12. Stewart JWS, Cohen EEW, Licitra L et al. Phase III study of gefitinib compared with intravenous methotrexate for recurrent squamous cell carcinoma of the head and neck. *J Clin Oncol* 2009;27:1864–71.
13. Stransky N, Egloff AM, Tward AD et al. The mutational landscape of head and neck squamous cell carcinoma. *Science* 2011;333:1157–60.
14. Agrawal A, Frederick MJ, Pickering CR et al. Exome sequencing of head and neck squamous cell carcinoma reveals inactivating mutations in NOTCH1. *Science* 2011;333:1154–56.
15. Nichols AC, Palma DA, Chow W et al. High frequency of activating *PIK3CA* mutations in human papillomavirus-positive oropharyngeal cancer. *JAMA Otolaryngol Head Neck Surg* 2013;139:617–22.
16. Bonner JA, Harari PM, Giralt J et al. Radiotherapy plus cetuximab for squamous cell carcinoma of the head and neck. *N Engl J Med* 2006;354:567–78.
17. Kian Ang K, Zhang Q, Rosenthal DI et al. Randomized phase III trial of concurrent accelerated radiation plus cisplatin with or without cetuximab for stage III and IV head and neck carcinoma: RTOG 0522. *J Clin Oncol* 2014;32:2940–50.
18. Vermorken JB, Remenar E, Van Herpen C et al. Cisplatin, fluorouracil, and docetaxel in unresectable head and neck cancer. *N Engl J Med* 2007;357:1695–704.
19. Posner M, Hershok DM, Blajman CR et al. Cisplatin and fluorouracil alone or with docetaxel in head and neck cancer. *N Engl J Med* 2007;357:1705–15.
20. DeVita VT, Lawrence TS, Rosenberg SA (eds). *Cancer: Principles and Practice of Oncology* (8th Edition). New York: Lippincott, Williams, and Wilkins, 2008.
21. Blanchard P, Baujat B, Holostenco V et al. Meta-analysis of chemotherapy in head and neck cancer (MACH-NC): a comprehensive analysis by tumour site. *Radiother Oncol* 2011;100:33–40.
22. Haddad RI, O'Neill A, Rabinowits G et al. Induction chemotherapy followed by concurrent chemoradiotherapy (sequential chemoradiotherapy) versus concurrent chemoradiotherapy alone in locally advanced head and neck cancer (PARADIGM): a randomised phase 3 trial. *Lancet Oncol* 2013;14:257–64.
23. Cohen EE, Karrison TG, Kocherginsky M et al. Phase III randomized trial of induction chemotherapy in patients with N2 or N3 locally advanced head and neck cancer. *J Clin Oncol* 2014;32:2735–43.
24. Hitt R, Grau JJ, Lopez-Pousa A et al. A randomized phase III trial comparing induction chemotherapy followed by chemoradiotherapy versus chemoradiotherapy alone as treatment of unresectable head and neck cancer. *Ann Oncol* 2014;25:216–25.
25. Gillison ML, Koch WM, Capone RB et al. Evidence for a causal association between human papillomavirus and a subset of head and neck cancers. *J Natl Cancer Inst* 2000;92:709–20.
26. Kian Ang K, Harris J, Wheeler R et al. Human papillomavirus and survival of patients with oropharyngeal cancer. *N Engl J Med* 2010;363:24–35.
27. Kian Ang K, Zhang QE, Rosenthal DI et al. A randomized phase III trial (RTOG 0522) of concurrent accelerated radiation plus cisplatin with or without cetuximab for stage III-IV head and neck squamous cell carcinomas. *J Clin Oncol* 2011;29S:5500.

14

Complications of surgical treatment and their management

PABLO H. MONTERO, JATIN P. SHAH, AND BHUVANESH SINGH

Post-surgical complications after oral and oropharyngeal cancer surgery are not rare occurrences. The combination of patient factors, such as a high prevalence of older patients, tobacco/alcohol abuse and comorbidities, in addition to surgery-related factors, such as extensive resections and the clean–contaminated nature of oral and oropharyngeal surgery, results in a significantly elevated risk for developing complications (1–4). The implications of surgical complications include functional and cosmetic morbidity, prolonged hospitalization, increased treatment cost, delay in starting postoperative adjuvant therapy and mortality (5,6).

Identification of factors that affect the incidence and severity of complications in head and neck cancer patients could be beneficial in preventing serious and life-threatening complications and reducing the burden of these events. The American Head and Neck Society (AHNS) through its Quality of Care Committee has identified specific quality measures for the management of oral cavity cancer (7). Another important step is the development of new tools for the quantification of risk in an individual patient, allowing surgeons to effectively identify patients at higher risk for complications and develop strategies to improve recognition and early management of these adverse events (8).

In general, complications in patients undergoing surgery for oral cancer can be divided into (1) local (those related to the surgical wound) and (2) systemic. In a recent analysis of a cohort of 9,365 oral cancer patients included in the United States National Inpatient Sample (NIS), the overall complication rate was 29%. Among them, 12% of the patients had a local complication and 21.5% had systemic complications (9). However, some series have reported a higher incidence of complication when a higher degree of scrutiny was employed. A recent review of the database on patients undergoing surgery for oral cancer at the Memorial Sloan Kettering Cancer Center (MSKCC) demonstrated a relatively high incidence (62%) of postoperative complications. The majority (47%) were systemic and 28% were local. Although there is no consensus about a grading system for oral cancer surgery complications, the use of the Clavien–Dindo classification (Table 14.1) (10) offers a standardized scale. This scale allows reproducible grading and results and allows comparison between institutions. Based on this classification, most of the complications in the MSKCC analysis were minor (grade I and II), the incidence of major complications (grade >II) was only 10% and the postoperative mortality rate was 0.8% (8). These observations demonstrate the high incidence of complications after oral cancer surgery due to accurate and detailed data recording and reporting, as well as the quality of the data source.

Table 14.2 shows the most common complications following surgery for oral cancer seen in a recent review at the MSKCC (1985–2012).

SYSTEMIC COMPLICATIONS

Systemic complications are the most common complications associated with oral cancer surgery, with the presence of baseline comorbid conditions being the most important predictor(12–14). Age by itself is not an important factor, but older patients tend to have more comorbid conditions and tend to develop more severe complications (4,15–17).

Systemic complications most commonly involve the pulmonary system and arise in about 15%–19% of cases (8,13,18,19). The co-existence of advanced medical disease,

Table 14.1 Clavien–Dindo classification of surgical complications

Grade	Definition
I	Any deviation from the normal postoperative course without the need for pharmacological treatment or surgical, endoscopic and radiological interventions. Allowed therapeutic regimens are drugs as antiemetics, antipyretics, analgetics, diuretics, electrolytes and physiotherapy. This grade also includes wound infections opened at the bedside
II	Requiring pharmacological treatment with drugs other than those allowed for grade I complications. Blood transfusions and total parenteral nutrition are also included
III	Requiring surgical, endoscopic or radiological intervention
IIIa	Intervention not under general anesthesia
IIIb	Intervention under general anesthesia
IV	Life-threatening complication (including CNS complications)[a] requiring IC/ICU management
IVa	Single-organ dysfunction (including dialysis)
IVb	Multiorgan dysfunction
V	Death of a patient

[a] Brain hemorrhage, ischemic stroke and subarachnoid bleeding, but excluding transient ischemic attacks.
CNS: central nervous system; IC: intermediate care; ICU: intensive care unit.

such as chronic obstructive pulmonary disease, combined with active tobacco use is the most important predictor for the development of a pulmonary complication (13,19). The risk can be reduced somewhat if the patient gives up tobacco use preoperatively or with optimization of pulmonary function by intensive respiratory therapy, rigorous postoperative pulmonary toilet and early ambulation (13,20).

Other systemic complications are less common. Cardiac complications occur in about 10% of patients with complications, usually as cardiac arrhythmias or congestive heart failure (8). Myocardial infarction occurs in less than 1% of patients undergoing head and neck surgery and is mainly related to pre-existing cardiac disease (12,21).

The most common neurologic complication is delirium. This was observed in 9% of patients in the MSKCC review. Postoperative delirium is directly associated with poor surgical outcomes including increased length of stay and even mortality (22). Other central nervous system complications, including cerebrovascular accidents (CVAs), meningitis and cerebrospinal fluid leaks, are rare unless skull base surgery or carotid artery manipulation or resection is performed (23–25). Resection of the carotid artery should be performed in highly selected patients with respect to both patient and tumor parameters. Angiographic balloon occlusion studies may help to identify patients at higher risk for CVA (26).

Table 14.2 Common complications after oral and oropharyngeal cancer surgery

Systemic complications

Pulmonary system
Pneumonia, COPD decompensation, etc.

Cardiac system
Arrhythmias, congestive heart failure, myocardial infarction, etc.

Neurologic system
Delirium, CVA, etc.

Vascular
Venous thromboembolism

Local complications

Intraoperative anesthesia complications
Anesthesia-related complications (volume overload, bradycardia and hypotension)

Intraoperative surgical complications
Nerve injury, neuropraxia and neurotmesis
Vascular injuries
Chyle fistulae
Mandible fractures
Tracheal injury

Immediate postoperative complications
Airway compromise
Hematoma
Seroma
Chyle leak
Skin flap necrosis
Free flap complications

Late postoperative complication
Wound infections
Salivary fistulae
Chyle fistulae
Skin necrosis

Delayed complications
Mandible and hardware exposure
Dysphagia
Altered speech
Trismus
Sensory and motor dysfunction
Xerostomia

COPD: chronic obstructive pulmonary disease; CVA: cerebrovascular accident.

In the MSKCC review, there was a venous thromboembolism (VTE) rate of 2%, including isolated deep venous thrombosis (four cases) and pulmonary embolism (three cases). The literature about the VTE in head and neck surgery is sparse. However, the incidence seems to be significantly higher for patients undergoing major head and neck surgery compared to those undergoing general otolaryngology procedures (27). This is likely associated with older age and the presence of malignancy in the head and neck surgery group. A recent review of the incidence of VTE events and the effectiveness of prophylaxis in otolaryngology and head and neck surgery found that the effectiveness and safety of VTE chemoprophylaxis differed between patients and procedures (28). Thus, a risk-based approach should be implemented in order to maximize the effectiveness of prophylaxis. The use of the Caprini risk score is recommended in selecting prophylactic measures (29). The effectiveness of VTE chemoprophylaxis significantly increases in patients with high Caprini risk scores and in cases of free flap reconstruction (28).

Identification of risk factors offers an opportunity for prevention of complications. Early identification of symptoms and signs and prompt institution of treatment are the pillars of effective management of these adverse events. Thus, the risk and morbidity of systemic complications can be satisfactorily controlled with collaborative multidisciplinary management to optimize care delivery before, during and after head and neck cancer surgery.

LOCAL (SURGICAL) COMPLICATIONS

Several factors are associated with an increased risk for the development of local complications, the most important of which is the type and extent of surgery, baseline medical status, presence of prior irradiation to the surgical bed and factors related to surgical technique (30–32). Surgical complications may be classified temporally into four groups: intraoperative, early postoperative, late postoperative and delayed complications. Careful preoperative assessment and meticulous surgical technique, combined with careful operative planning, can prevent many of the observed complications associated with surgery for oral cancer.

INTRAOPERATIVE ANESTHESIA-RELATED COMPLICATIONS

Anesthesia-related complications are rare with the use of modern anesthetic drugs and contemporary monitoring techniques. However, when they occur, they can be life-threatening if not identified and treated promptly (33–35). Intraoperative airway complications are of primary concern and are mainly due to shifting of the endotracheal tube. The use of clear plastic head and neck drapes to cordon off the endotracheal tube allowing its direct visualization throughout the operative procedure is desirable. If the tube is dislodged or disconnected during the procedure, it should be promptly repositioned or an emergency tracheostomy may be performed if necessary. Once in place, the endotracheal tube should be secured firmly with tape and tracheostomy tubes sutured to the skin to minimize the risk of dislodgement. When a tracheostomy tube has been placed in an emergency situation or if the procedure was complicated, a post-procedure chest radiograph should be performed to rule out the presence of pneumothorax (36,37).

Volume overload is the next most common intraoperative problem associated with anesthetic management and can lead to increased risks of pulmonary and wound complications (33–35). This risk can be minimized by limiting intravenous fluid to a volume sufficient to maintain an adequate urine output. Less common complications include intraoperative bradycardia and hypotension, which can result from manipulation of the carotid bifurcation during neck surgery. This can be counteracted by the injection of lidocaine into the adventitia in the region of the carotid bifurcation.

INTRAOPERATIVE SURGICAL COMPLICATIONS

Most intraoperative complications are associated with flaws in surgical technique, resulting in inadvertent injury to nerves and blood vessels. In the recent MSKCC review, 57 out of 247 patients (23%) who underwent neck dissection for oral cancer experienced some degree of nerve paresis (8). The accessory nerve is at greatest risk for iatrogenic injury, with 64% of cases experiencing some degree of nerve paresis in supraomohyoid and modified neck dissections. Some weakness in marginal mandibular nerve function was observed in 33%, which can result from direct physical trauma or from stretching associated with dissection and flap retraction. Injury to cervical plexus branches (2%), lower cranial nerves (2%) and the greater auricular nerve may also occur rarely during neck dissection. The lingual nerve may be injured in posterior floor of the mouth resections or during mandibulotomy. The mental nerve is sacrificed in cases that require a lower check flap approach. Careful identification and dissection around these verves allows preservation of nerve function. It should be remembered, however, that anatomic preservation of nerves does not necessarily ensure preservation of function. Most commonly, injury to nerves results from devascularization associated with circumferential dissection around the nerve and neuropraxia from stretching or by direct physical trauma to the nerve. Limiting the extent of circumferential dissection does not appear to reduce the risk for some functional loss. In fact, patient perceptions of shoulder dysfunction after supraomohyoid neck dissection or comprehensive modified radical neck dissection with accessory nerve preservation are similar in incidence and severity. In the MSKCC review, all postoperative nerve deficits proved to be transient and were managed conservatively with observation or physical therapy. Nearly all patients regained near-normal function within a year after surgery (8).

Vascular injury requiring repair or ligation of the injured vessel, including the internal jugular vein, common carotid artery or innominate artery, may also occur. However, inadvertent trauma can be minimized by meticulous attention to surgical technique and maintenance of a dry surgical field throughout the procedure. If significant bleeding is anticipated from a massive tumor, preliminary ligation of the feeding vessel or external carotid artery may be performed to minimize major blood loss.

Inadequate preoperative planning can also result in intraoperative complications. Skin or mucosal slough can be prevented by careful planning of incisions to avoid an acute angle, gentle handling of tissues and planned placement of sutures to avoid devitalization. If significant wound slough occurs in the postoperative period, it can be managed conservatively after debridement and packing. However, if the carotid artery is exposed, then regional or distant tissue transfer should be considered to close the defect and reduce the risk of carotid rupture.

Chyle fistulae can result from injury to the cervical portion of the thoracic duct. Typically, the duct is located in the lower portion of the left neck, lateral or posterior to the carotid sheath, but can extend as far as 5 cm superior to the clavicle and occur in the right neck in a small number of cases (2% in our series). If injury to the lymphatic duct is identified in the operating room, immediate attention should be paid to isolating the injury and suturing ligation of the duct. It is important to remember that the cervical thoracic duct is not always a single structure, but may have many tributaries, making several independent injuries possible. If injury to the duct is identified in the postoperative period, the dietary content should be modified and the volume of chyle drainage closely followed. If the chyle output is over 600 mL per day, re-exploration and ligation of the leaking duct is indicated. In cases with lower output, observation and conservative management will usually be sufficient for spontaneous closure of the fistula. The optimal time for re-exploration for a chyle fistula is within 48 hours postoperatively or after 2–3 weeks.

The management of the mandible might be complicated by an iatrogenic fracture during an overaggressive marginal mandibulectomy. This is usually secondary to an inadequate amount of bone stock remaining on the inferior border of the mandible, particularly in an edentulous mandible. Marginal mandibulectomy should be avoided in patients with "pipestem" mandibles and/or previously irradiated edentulous mandible (38). The risk of fracture can be minimized by planning resections to avoid sharp angles and maintaining the mandibular height of approximately 1 cm. In addition to this, the use of a sharp, well-controlled, high-speed saw allows for controlled and safe resection, avoiding fractures associated with the use of chisels to wedge and lever the specimen. If a fracture occurs, immediate repair should be performed using miniplates or wires.

IMMEDIATE POSTOPERATIVE COMPLICATIONS

The main complication in the immediate postoperative period is collection of blood or serum under the flap. Hematoma and seromas were observed in less than 2% of the patients undergoing neck dissection in the MSKCC series. This can result from non-functioning suction catheters or inadequate hemostasis. The placement of suction drains is not a substitute for the attainment of absolute hemostasis, as this will invariably result in the development of complications. The role of suction catheters is to evacuate fluid and keep the neck flaps in close apposition to the underlying soft tissue, thereby improving healing and decreasing the risk of infection. To minimize the risk of blockage, drains should be inserted during the final closure of the wound and immediately placed on high, continuous suction. The wound should be irrigated thoroughly to remove any clots and debris prior to drain placement. If a small collection of serum develops after removal of the drains, needle aspiration is performed. However, large accumulations of serum or re-accumulations require opening the wound, cleaning and leaving the wound open with a packing for secondary healing. Airway compromise in the immediate postoperative setting may be caused by many different factors. Traumatic laryngeal intubation may cause edema or hematoma, resulting in early postoperative stridor. Investigation should include fiber-optic examination to assess vocal cord function and to ascertain the extent of airway compromise. In severe cases, reintubation or tracheostomy should be performed. In less ominous cases, treatment with humidified oxygen and intravenous steroids may be attempted in a monitored setting. Other, less common causes of airway compromise include intraoral hemorrhage, tracheostomy tube plugging, pneumothorax and aspiration.

Although uncommon, the use of microvascular free tissue transfer introduces new scenarios for complication development (39–41). A pale appearance of the flap, combined with reduced temperature, delayed capillary refill and delayed or absent bleeding to pin prick in the early postoperative period, represents acute arterial obstruction. This usually results from complications at the anastomosis site. Management requires immediate return to the operating room for exploration of the anastomosis and appropriate intervention. Flap congestion with dark bleeding on pin prick typically occurring a few days after surgery represents problems with the venous anastomosis. Conservative management with the possible use of medical leeches may lead to resolution. However, in severe cases, re-exploration may be indicated. Early identification of ischemia of the flap is facilitated by the use of a Doppler monitor over the course of the flap pedicle, distal to the anastomostic site.

Another rare complication is nasal alar necrosis secondary to malpositioned nasogastric feeding tubes, which can result in significant cosmetic deformity. In addition, prolonged tube placement can also foster the development of ipsilateral sinusitis. Early nasogastric tube removal should be planned and proper positioning maintained while it is in place.

LATE POSTOPERATIVE COMPLICATIONS

Wound infections and fistulae are the most important complications in the late postoperative period, occurring in over 25%–50% of complex cases (42,43). Several risk factors have been associated with development of wound infection: age, American Society of Anesthesiologists (ASA) classification, poor nutritional status, recent dental extractions, tobacco history, large tumors, length of surgery, prior chemotherapy/radiotherapy, subsites such as the oral cavity or hypopharynx and reconstruction with local/regional flaps (44–50). The rate of wound infection associated with oral cancer surgery can be effectively reduced by the administration of preoperative antibiotics (51–58). The choice of antibiotic is not as important as the timing of its administration. Ideally, prophylactic antibiotics are started 1–2 hours prior to the skin incision (55). Antibiotic prophylaxis must cover a large bacterial spectrum made up of aerobes and anaerobes of oropharyngeal flora, Gram-negative bacteria and *Staphylococcus aureus*, likely the most important pathogen in wound infection after head and neck surgery (59). Cephalosporins (Ancef) and metronidazole (Flagyl) are usually given for clean–contaminated cases in the preoperative holding area. A second course of antibiotics is given in the operating room for cases lasting greater than 8 hours. In uncomplicated cases, prophylactic antibiotics only need be continued for 24–48 hours postoperatively (53). Although the duration of prophylactic therapy may need to be extended in high-risk cases, unrestricted use of antibiotics and for long periods might be associated with higher rates of multi-resistant pathogenic infections (60).

Once a mild wound infection develops, it can be treated by antibiotic therapy alone. However, it must be kept in mind that signs of mild or superficial local infection at the wound site may represent a more serious underlying infection in some cases. If suppuration is suspected, the wound should be opened widely, cleaned and appropriate cultures instigated. Empiric broad-spectrum antibiotic therapy directed against oral flora should be administered, since most infections associated with oral cancer surgery are polymicrobial. The choice of antibiotic should be modified according to the culture results, when available. The presence of a fistula should be suspected with all cases of wound suppuration, especially when there is a mucosal suture line in the depth of the wound. Other nonspecific manifestations of fistulization include fever, pain and leukocytosis. Fistula development occurs due to technical problems in closure of the mucosa under tension, advanced tumors with large defects and wound healing problems resulting from poor nutrition, diabetes mellitus or prior radiation exposure. The risk of fistulization can be reduced by minimizing technical errors, including performance of a tension-free closure, avoidance of devitalization of mucosal edges and adequate apposition with inversion of the mucosal edges (43,61). The use of free tissue transfer to close complex defects may further decrease the rate of fistulization. Preoperative nutritional optimization should also be considered in selected cases, as it improves wound healing (31,32,62–64). The role of previous radiation therapy in the development of wound breakdown and salivary fistulae may be debated. However, there is a consensus that fistulae in irradiated patients heal at a significantly slower rate and often require secondary surgical intervention for closure (65,66). The use of a muscle flap such as the pectoralis major to support a "high-risk" suture line reduces the risk of development of fistula and helps spontaneous closure if one develops in the postoperative period. Initial management of salivary fistulae consists of wide opening, debridement, cleaning and packing of the wound, along with the correction of the aggravating factors, when identified. Carotid coverage is performed in cases where it is exposed in the wound. For unresolving or large fistulae, regional or distant tissue transfer should be considered.

Exposure of the mandible may develop consequent to wound dehiscence or fistulization. Management is based on the severity of the problem. If minimal exposure is present, without hardware exposure, it can be managed with local wound care to promote secondary healing. In cases of extensive exposure, hardware removal, wound debridement and mandibular stabilization may be required through an open approach. Non-union can also result from infection and improper immobilization. If left untreated, non-union can be the nidus for more severe infections, including osteomyelitis. Treatment consists of open debridement and re-stabilization of the mandibular fragments.

DELAYED COMPLICATIONS

Long-standing sequelae after oral cancer surgery include dysphagia, trismus, shoulder dysfunction and sensory loss. Other complications are results of the combination of surgery and adjuvant treatments with radiation or chemoradiation, causing xerostomia, dental infections and osteoradionecrosis (67).

Dysphagia can result from neurological injuries to cranial nerves V, IX, X, and XII or from direct anatomical insults, as in glossectomy or partial laryngeal and pharyngeal surgery. The addition of postoperative radiation therapy amplifies the magnitude of dysphagia (67). Little can be done to avert these surgical sequelae, but anticipation and aggressive management are warranted if problems develop. Intensive postoperative rehabilitation with support from a speech/swallowing pathologist is crucial in functional recovery. If significant anatomical resections are planned, consideration should be given to early placement of a gastrostomy tube to maintain adequate nutrition (68).

Dysphagia assessment should be performed in collaboration with a speech and swallowing therapist (69–71). It must be kept in mind that swallowing is accomplished through a complex series of interrelated reflex mechanisms, which can be disrupted by sensory, qualitative and anatomical changes (71–73). A thorough examination analyzing the impact and extent of anatomic deficits and cranial nerve dysfunctions is performed, supplemented by functional fiber-optic examination of swallowing where possible. Modified barium swallow is used to identify the location and severity of the swallowing deficit and facilitate its treatment.

Anatomic resections resulting in significant loss in oral and pharyngeal soft tissue volume can cause problems with bolus formation and propulsion beyond the oral phase of swallowing (69–71). Tongue resection and denervation is a particularly difficult problem, resulting in significant deficits in both speech and swallowing rehabilitation. A palatal drop prosthesis can be used to compensate for soft tissue volume loss of the tongue to improve swallowing (74). Dental rehabilitation with dentures or osseointegrated implants also plays a significant role in improving deglutition. Conversely, neurological deficits are difficult to treat and require intensive swallowing therapy, with modifications in swallowing techniques to allow for partial restoration of swallowing function.

Trismus can be a significant dilemma in this population, causing problems with deglutition and oral hygiene, as well as limitations in oral and pharyngeal examinations (75–79). Once trismus develops, it is difficult to reverse; therefore, preventive management is best. The use of skin grafts and flaps can limit fibrosis in cases with exposure of pterygoid muscles. This results in significant reduction of trismus development. Aggressive jaw exercises, beginning in the immediate postoperative period and continued for several months, are of significant benefit. Oral rehabilitation exercises should also be initiated in patients receiving radiation to the pterygoid region to prevent fibrosis of the muscles of mastication (80).

Shoulder weakness and deformity are predictable sequelae in all patients undergoing radical neck dissection, consequent to sacrifice of the accessory nerve (81–89). The severity of shoulder dysfunction, however, is intensified with denervation of the nerve supply to the other supporting musculature, including the rhomboids and levator scapulae (72). The nerve supply to the latter is at greatest risk as it is derived from the cervical plexus in the neck. Functional deficit results from both pain on movement of the scapulohumeral joint and an inability to fully abduct the arm due to loss of muscular action. Treatment involves a combination of intensive physical therapy and pain control (81).

Sensory loss following neck dissections can be particularly troublesome. This results from injury to the branches of the greater auricular nerve and the cervical plexus (90). The resultant deficit extends from the temporal region to the chest. Gradual resolution of much of the deficit can be anticipated with time, but patients should initially avoid exposure to extremes of temperature in the region. Many other long-term complications can occur, including scar contractures, neuroma formation, Frey's syndrome, reflex sympathetic dystrophy and dysgeusia, but are relatively rare (91–93).

Xerostomia is a consequence of radiation therapy that can have several significant long-term sequelae, including tooth decay and perigingival caries. Regular and lifelong use of fluoride gel is necessary to reduce the risk of dental caries. Dental sepsis can lead to progression of infection into the mandible or maxilla, resulting in the development of osteoradionecrosis (75). Although it can involve the maxilla, the highest risk of osteoradionecrosis is in the mandible (75–78,94). Osteoradionecrosis is a delayed complication caused by the failure of bone healing as a result of poor blood supply (95). It may occur in approximately 5% of patients and, in its severe forms, can affect quality of life and functional prognosis. Lesions involving cortical bone may progress to pathologic fracture and fistula formation. Risk factors include the size and location of the primary lesion, time between dental extraction and radiotherapy, volume of the mandible within the radiation field, high radiation dose (more than 65 Gy), presence dental or periodontal disease, alcohol and tobacco abuse, diabetes and poor nutrition (96). The risk can be effectively reduced by the maintenance of optimal oral hygiene, combined with avoidance of dental manipulation and procedures. Ideally, dental interventions and procedures in irradiated mandibles should be provided by dentists and oral surgeons experienced in the management of head and neck cancer patients. In general, the treatment of osteoradionecrosis is conservative, with significant attention given to oral hygiene, wound debridement and removal of sequestrum. This is especially recommended for early and limited areas of osteoradionecrosis. The use of systemic antibiotics in these patients remains controversial. Patients with severe osteoradionecrosis unresponsive to conservative management benefit from aggressive surgical intervention to resect the necrotic segment and immediate microvascular reconstruction (97). Although it appears promising, the benefit from the use of hyperbaric oxygen therapy (11). both for prevention and treatment, remains controversial.

REFERENCES

1. Singh B, Bhaya M, Stern J et al. Validation of the Charlson comorbidity index in patients with head and neck cancer: a multi-institutional study. *Laryngoscope* 1997;107(11 Pt 1):1469–75.
2. Singh B, Bhaya M, Zimbler M et al. Impact of comorbidity on outcome of young patients with head and neck squamous cell carcinoma. *Head Neck* 1998;20(1):1–7.
3. Funk GF, Hoffman HT, Karnell LH et al. Cost-identification analysis in oral cavity cancer management. *Otolaryngol Head Neck Surg* 1998;118(2):211–20.
4. Shaari CM, Buchbinder D, Costantino PD, Lawson W, Biller HF, Urken ML. Complications of microvascular head and neck surgery in the elderly. *Arch Otolaryngol Head Neck Surg* 1998;124(4):407–11.
5. Bhattacharyya N, Fried MP. Benchmarks for mortality, morbidity, and length of stay for head and neck surgical procedures. *Arch Otolaryngol Head Neck Surg* 2001;127(2):127–32.
6. Ch'ng S, Choi V, Elliott M, Clark JR. Relationship between postoperative complications and survival after free flap reconstruction for oral cavity squamous cell carcinoma. *Head Neck* 2014;36(1):55–9.
7. AHNS Committee on quality care. The development of quality of care measures for oral cavity cancer. *Arch Otolaryngol Head Neck Surg.* 2008;134(6):672.

8. Awad MI, Shuman AG, Montero PH, Palmer FL, Shah JP, Patel SG. Accuracy of administrative and clinical registry data in reporting postoperative complications after surgery for oral cavity squamous cell carcinoma. *Head Neck* 2015;37(6):851–61. doi: 10.1002/hed.23682. Epub June 27, 2014.
9. Montero PH, Albornoz CR, Shuman AG et al. Incidence and risk factors of surgical complications in oral cavity cancer. *Abstracts of the American Head and Neck Society Annual Meeting 2013*, Orlando, Florida, 2013.
10. Dindo D, Demartines N, Clavien PA. Classification of surgical complications: a new proposal with evaluation in a cohort of 6,336 patients and results of a survey. *Ann Surg* 2004;240(2):205–13.
11. Epstein J, van der Meij E, McKenzie M, Wong F, Stevenson-Moore P. Hyperbaric oxygen therapy. *Oral Surg Oral Med Oral Pathol Oral Radiol Endod* 1996;81(3):265–6.
12. Papac RJ. Medical aspects of head and neck cancer. *Cancer Invest* 1985;3(5):435–44.
13. McCulloch TM, Jensen NF, Girod DA, Tsue TT, Weymuller EA Jr. Risk factors for pulmonary complications in the postoperative head and neck surgery patient. *Head Neck* 1997;19(5):372–77.
14. Piccirillo JF. Importance of comorbidity in head and neck cancer. *Laryngoscope* 2000;110(4):593–602.
15. Singh B, Cordeiro PG, Santamaria E, Shaha AR, Pfister DG, Shah JP. Factors associated with complications in microvascular reconstruction of head and neck defects. *Plast Reconstr Surg* 1999;103 (2):403–11.
16. Hosking MP, Warner MA, Lobdell CM, Offord KP, Melton LJ 3rd. Outcomes of surgery in patients 90 years of age and older. *Jama* 1989;261(13): 1909–15.
17. Hosking MP, Lobdell CM, Warner MA, Offord KP, Melton LJ 3rd. Anaesthesia for patients over 90 years of age. outcomes after regional and general anaesthetic techniques for two common surgical procedures. *Anaesthesia* 1989;44(2):142–7.
18. Weber RS, Hankins P, Rosenbaum B, Raad I. Nonwound infections following head and neck oncologic surgery. *Laryngoscope* 1993;103(1 Pt 1):22–7.
19. Rao MK, Reilley TE, Schuller DE, Young DC. Analysis of risk factors for postoperative pulmonary complications in head and neck surgery. *Laryngoscope* 1992;102(1):45–7.
20. Warner MA, Offord KP, Warner ME, Lennon RL, Conover MA, Jansson-Schumacher U. Role of preoperative cessation of smoking and other factors in postoperative pulmonary complications: a blinded prospective study of coronary artery bypass patients. *Mayo Clin Proc* 1989;64(6):609–16.
21. Jacobs C. The internist in the management of head and neck cancer. *Ann Intern Med* 1990;113(10):771–8.
22. Shuman AG, Patel SG, Shah JP, Korc-Grodzicki B. Optimizing perioperative management of geriatric patients with head and neck cancer. *Head Neck* 2014;36(5):743–9.
23. Snyderman CH, D'Amico F. Outcome of carotid artery resection for neoplastic disease: a meta-analysis. *Am J Otolaryngol* 1992;13(6):373–80.
24. Bilsky MH, Kraus DH, Strong EW, Harrison LB, Gutin PH, Shah JP. Extended anterior craniofacial resection for intracranial extension of malignant tumors. *Am J Surg* 1997;174(5):565–8.
25. Shah JP, Kraus DH, Bilsky MH, Gutin PH, Harrison LH, Strong EW. Craniofacial resection for malignant tumors involving the anterior skull base. *Arch Otolaryngol Head Neck Surg* 1997;123(12):1312–7.
26. Chung EJ, Kwon KH, Yoon DY, Cho SW, Kim EJ, Rho YS. Clinical outcome analysis of 47 patients for advanced H&N cancer with preoperative suspicion of carotid artery invasion. *Head Neck* 2016;38 (Suppl 1): E287–92. doi: 10.1002/hed.23987. Epub June 26, 2015.
27. Moreano EH, Hutchison JL, McCulloch TM, Graham SM, Funk GF, Hoffman HT. Incidence of deep venous thrombosis and pulmonary embolism in otolaryngology-head and neck surgery. *Otolaryngol Head Neck Surg* 1998;118(6):777–84.
28. Bahl V, Shuman AG, Hu HM et al. Chemoprophylaxis for venous thromboembolism in otolaryngology. *JAMA Otolaryngol Head Neck Surg* 2014;140(11):999–1005.
29. Caprini JA. Risk assessment as a guide for the prevention of the many faces of venous thromboembolism. *Am J Surg* 2010;199(1 Suppl):S3–10.
30. Johnson JT, Bloomer WD. Effect of prior radiotherapy on postsurgical wound infection. *Head Neck* 1989;11(2):132–6.
31. Copeland EM 3rd, Daly JM, Dudrick SJ. Nutritional concepts in the treatment of head and neck malignancies. *Head Neck Surg* 1979;1(4):350–65.
32. Copeland EM 3rd, Daly JM, Ota DM, Dudrick SJ. Nutrition, cancer, and intravenous hyperalimentation. *Cancer* 1979;43(5 Suppl):2108–16.
33. Cox RG. The anesthetic management of patients undergoing free flap reconstructive surgery following resection of head and neck neoplasms: a review of 64 patients. *Ann R Coll Surg Engl* 1989;71(2):143–4.
34. Inglis MS, Robbie DS, Edwards JM, Breach NM. The anaesthetic management of patients undergoing free flap reconstructive surgery following resection of head and neck neoplasms: a review of 64 patients. *Ann R Coll Surg Engl* 1988;70(4):235–8.
35. Manson PN, Saunders JR Jr. Anesthesia in head and neck surgery. Head and neck cancer surgery and maxillofacial trauma. *Clin Plast Surg* 1985;12(1):115–22.

36. Beahrs OH. Complications of surgery of the head and neck. *Surg Clin North Am* 1977;57(4):823–9.
37. Barlow DW, Weymuller EA Jr, Wood DE. Tracheotomy and the role of postoperative chest radiography in adult patients. *Ann Otol Rhinol Laryngol* 1994;103(9):665–8.
38. Song CS, Har-El G. Marginal mandibulectomy: oncologic and nononcologic outcome. *Am J Otolaryngol* 2003;24(1):61–3.
39. Hidalgo DA, Disa JJ, Cordeiro PG, Hu QY. A review of 716 consecutive free flaps for oncologic surgical defects: refinement in donor-site selection and technique. *Plast Reconstr Surg* 1998;102(3):722–32; discussion 733–4.
40. Khouri RK, Cooley BC, Kunselman AR et al. A prospective study of microvascular free-flap surgery and outcome. *Plast Reconstr Surg* 1998;102(3):711–21.
41. al Qattan MM, Boyd JB. Complications in head and neck microsurgery. *Microsurgery* 1993;14(3):187–95.
42. Cohen M, Marschall MA, Greager J 3rd, Early, aggressive management of postoperative oropharyngocutaneous fistulas. *Plast Reconstr Surg* 1992;89(1):56–61; discussion 62–3.
43. Friess CC, Fontaine DJ, Kornblut AD. Complications of therapy for oral malignant disease. *Otolaryngol Clin North Am* 1979;12(1):175–81.
44. Clayman GL, Raad II, Hankins PD, Weber RS. Bacteriological profile of surgical infection after antibiotic-prophylaxis. *Head Neck* 1993;15(6):526–31.
45. Cole RR, Robbins KT, Cohen JI, Wolf PF. A predictive model for wound sepsis in oncologic surgery of the head and neck. *Otolaryngol Head Neck Surg* 1987;96(2):165–71.
46. Doerr TD, Marunick MT. Timing of edentulation and extraction in the management of oral cavity and oropharyngeal malignancies. *Head Neck* 1997;19(5):426–30.
47. Penel N, Fournier C, Lefebvre D, Lefebvre JL. Multivariate analysis of risk factors for wound infection in head and neck squamous cell carcinoma surgery with opening of mucosa. study of 260 surgical procedures. *Oral Oncol* 2005;41(3):294–303.
48. Penel N, Fournier C, Lefebvre D et al. Previous chemotherapy as a predictor of wound infections in nonmajor head and neck surgery: results of a prospective study. *Head Neck* 2004;26(6):513–7.
49. Robbins KT, Favrot S, Hanna D, Cole R. Risk of wound-infection in patients with head and neck-cancer. *Head Neck* 1990;12(2):143–8.
50. Weber RS, Callender DL. Antibiotic-prophylaxis in clean–contaminated head and neck oncologic surgery. *Annals of Otology Rhinology and Laryngology* 1992;101(1):16–20.
51. Johnson JT, Schuller DE, Silver F et al. Antibiotic prophylaxis in high-risk head and neck surgery: one-day vs. five-day therapy. *Otolaryngol Head Neck Surg* 1986;95(5):554–7.
52. Girod DA, McCulloch TM, Tsue TT, Weymuller EA Jr. Risk factors for complications in clean–contaminated head and neck surgical procedures. *Head Neck* 1995;17(1):7–13.
53. Fee WE Jr, Glenn M, Handen C, Hopp ML. One day vs. two days of prophylactic antibiotics in patients undergoing major head and neck surgery. *Laryngoscope* 1984;94(5 Pt 1):612–4.
54. Clayman GL, Raad II, Hankins PD, Weber RS. Bacteriologic profile of surgical infection after antibiotic prophylaxis. *Head Neck* 1993;15(6):526–31.
55. Classen DC, Evans RS, Pestotnik SL, Horn SD, Menlove RL, Burke JP. The timing of prophylactic administration of antibiotics and the risk of surgical-wound infection. *N Engl J Med* 1992;326(5):281–6.
56. Brown BM, Johnson JT, Wagner RL. Etiologic factors in head and neck wound infections. *Laryngoscope* 1987;97(5):587–90.
57. Blair EA, Johnson JT, Wagner RL, Carrau RL, Bizakis JG. Cost analysis of antibiotic prophylaxis in clean head and neck surgery. *Arch Otolaryngol Head Neck Surg* 1995;121(3):269–71.
58. Becker GD. Identification and management of the patient at high risk for wound infection. *Head Neck Surg* 1986;8(3):205–10.
59. Penel N, Fournier C, Lefebvre D, Lefebvre JL. Multivariate analysis of risk factors for wound infection in head and neck squamous cell carcinoma surgery with opening of mucosa. study of 260 surgical procedures. *Oral Oncol* 2005;41(3):294–303.
60. Morimoto Y, Sugiura T, Tatebayashi S, Kirita T. Reduction in incidence of methicillin-resistant *staphylococcus aureus* (MRSA) after radical surgery for head and neck cancer. *Spec Care Dentist* 2006;26(5):209–13.
61. Krause CJ, Smits RG, McCabe BF. Complications associated with combined therapy of oral and pharyngeal neoplasms. *Ann Otol Rhinol Laryngol* 1972;81(4):496–500.
62. Dudrick SJ, Copeland EM 3rd, Daly JM et al. A clinical review of nutritional support of the patient. *JPEN J Parenter Enteral Nutr* 1979;3(6):444–51.
63. Daly JM, Reynolds HM, Dudrick SJ, Copeland EM 3rd. Effects of nutritional repletion on host and tumor response to chemotherapy. *Curr Surg* 1979;36(2):138–43.
64. Daly JM, Dudrick SJ, Copeland EM 3rd. Evaluation of nutritional indices as prognostic indicators in the cancer patient. *Cancer* 1979;43(3):925–31.
65. Shemen LJ, Spiro RH. Complications following laryngectomy. *Head Neck Surg* 1986;8(3):185–91.
66. Weingrad DN, Spiro RH. Complications after laryngectomy. *Am J Surg* 1983;146(4):517–20.
67. Hutcheson KA, Lewin JS, Barringer DA et al. Late dysphagia after radiotherapy-based treatment of head and neck cancer. *Cancer* 2012;118(23):5793–99.

68. Rosenthal DI, Lewin JS, Eisbruch A. Prevention and treatment of dysphagia and aspiration after chemoradiation for head and neck cancer. *J Clin Oncol* 2006;24(17):2636–43.
69. Poertner LC, Coleman RF. Swallowing therapy in adults. *Otolaryngol Clin North Am* 1998;31(3):561–79.
70. Machin J, Shaw C. A multidisciplinary approach to head and neck cancer. *Eur J Cancer Care (Engl)* 1998;7(2):93–6.
71. Kronenberger MB, Meyers AD. Dysphagia following head and neck cancer surgery. *Dysphagia* 1994;9(4):236–44.
72. Bigliani LU, Compito CA, Duralde XA, Wolfe IN. Transfer of the levator scapulae, rhomboid major, and rhomboid minor for paralysis of the trapezius. *J Bone Joint Surg Am* 1996;78(10):1534–40.
73. Valdez IH, Fox PC. Interactions of the salivary and gastrointestinal systems. II. Effects of salivary gland dysfunction on the gastrointestinal tract. *Dig Dis* 1991;9(4):210–8.
74. Johnson JT, Aramany MA, Myers EN. Palatal neoplasms: reconstruction considerations. *Otolaryngol Clin North Am* 1983;16(2):441–56.
75. Whitmyer CC, Waskowski JC, Iffland HA. Radiotherapy and oral sequelae: preventive and management protocols. *J Dent Hyg* 1997;71(1):23–29.
76. Jansma J, Vissink A, Spijkervet FK et al. Protocol for the prevention and treatment of oral sequelae resulting from head and neck radiation therapy. *Cancer* 1992;70(8):2171–80.
77. Dreizen S. Oral complications of cancer therapies. Description and incidence of oral complications. *NCI Monogr* 1990;(9):11–5.
78. Maxymiw WG, Wood RE. The role of dentistry in head and neck radiation therapy. *J Can Dent Assoc* 1989;55(3):193–8.
79. Cohen SG, Quinn PD. Facial trismus and myofascial pain associated with infections and malignant-disease. Report of Five Cases. *Oral Surg Oral Med Oral Pathol* 1988;65(5):538–44.
80. Bensadoun RJ, Riesenbeck D, Lockhart PB et al. A systematic review of trismus induced by cancer therapies in head and neck cancer patients. *Support Care Cancer* 2010;18(8):1033–38.
81. Saunders WH, Johnson EW. Rehabilitation of the shoulder after radical neck dissection. *Ann Otol Rhinol Laryngol* 1975;84(6):812–6.
82. Sobol S, Jensen C, Sawyer W 2nd, Costiloe P, Thong N. Objective comparison of physical dysfunction after neck dissection. *Am J Surg* 1985;150(4):503–9.
83. Ariyan S. Functional radical neck dissection. *Plast Reconstr Surg* 1980;65(6):768–76.
84. Hill JH, Olson NR. The surgical anatomy of the spinal accessory nerve and the internal branch of the superior laryngeal nerve. *Laryngoscope* 1979;89(12):1935–42.
85. Wright TA. Accessory spinal nerve injury. *Clin Orthop Relat Res* 1975;(108):15–8.
86. Nori S, Soo KC, Green RF, Strong EW, Miodownik S. Utilization of intraoperative electroneurography to understand the innervation of the trapezius muscle. *Muscle Nerve* 1997;20(3):279–85.
87. Zibordi F, Baiocco F, Bascelli C, Bini A, Canepa A. Spinal accessory nerve function following neck dissection. *Ann Otol Rhinol Laryngol* 1988; 97(1):83–6.
88. Short SO, Kaplan JN, Laramore GE, Cummings CW. Shoulder pain and function after neck dissection with or without preservation of the spinal accessory nerve. *Am J Surg* 1984;148(4):478–82.
89. Leipzig B, Suen JY, English JL, Barnes J, Hooper M. Functional evaluation of the spinal accessory nerve after neck dissection. *Am J Surg* 1983;146(4):526–30.
90. Swift TR. Involvement of peripheral nerves in radical neck dissection. *Am J Surg* 1970;119(6):694–98.
91. Kiroglu MM, Sarpel T, Ozberk P, Soylu L, Cetik F, Aydogan LB. Reflex sympathetic dystrophy following neck dissections. *Am J Otolaryngol* 1997;18(2):103–6.
92. Teague A, Akhtar S, Phillips J. Frey's syndrome following submandibular gland excision: an unusual postoperative complication. *ORL J Otorhinolaryngol Relat Spec* 1998;60(6):346–8.
93. Hays LL. The Frey syndrome: a review and double blind evaluation of the topical use of a new anticholinergic agent. *Laryngoscope.* 1978;88(11):1796–824.
94. Marx RE. Osteoradionecrosis: a new concept of its pathophysiology. *J Oral Maxillofac Surg* 1983;41(5):283–88.
95. Epstein JB, Wong FLW, Stevenson-Moore P. Osteoradionecrosis: clinical experience and a proposal for classification. *J Oral Maxillofac Surg* 1987;45(2):104–10.
96. Glanzmann C, Gratz KW. Radionecrosis of the mandibula: a retrospective analysis of the incidence and risk factors. *Radiother Oncol* 1995;36(2):94–100.
97. Shaha AR, Cordeiro PG, Hidalgo DA et al. Resection and immediate microvascular reconstruction in the management of osteoradionecrosis of the mandible. *Head Neck* 1997;19(5):406–11.

15

Reconstructive surgery: Soft tissue

ADRIAN SJARIF AND EVAN MATROS

Reconstruction following tumor extirpation of the oral cavity must take into account both the functional and esthetic needs of the patient. The oral cavity serves as the entryway to the gastrointestinal tract where the process of digestion is initiated with mastication, salivation and propulsion of the food bolus into the pharynx. As mobile structures, the lips ensure oral competence by preventing spillage of contents. Their motion also ensures proper speech enunciation. The tongue is a mass of skeletal muscle used for grasping food, maneuvering it within the oral cavity and propelling it into the oropharynx in swallowing. The movements of the tongue also help to articulate laryngeal sounds into comprehensible speech. The tongue surface, in addition to having tactile sensation, contains specialized receptors for the specialized function of taste.

The oral cavity is bounded above by the hard palate and laterally by the buccal surface of the cheeks. It is lined by a mucosal layer that is adherent to underlying deeper structures such as the periosteum of the hard palate and the cheek musculature. The pliability of the cheek mucosa allows for food pocketing, preventing chewed food from spilling out of the oral cavity during deglutition.

In terms of esthetics, the aim of reconstruction should be to resurface/reconstitute the surgical defect so that external facial contour and symmetry are maintained to the greatest degree possible. Thoughtful reconstructive decision-making should reflect all of these needs.

Since oral cavity cancers are locally invasive they do not respect anatomical boundaries. As such, resections simultaneously involve multiple specialized tissue types (i.e., mucosa, muscle, bone and nerve) and/or anatomic areas. Due to the high functional requirements of the oral cavity, these specialized tissues should be restored individually as best as possible to preserve function. The traditional reconstructive mantra "replace like with like" holds true for oral cavity reconstruction, perhaps more than in any other region of the body. A subunit approach should also be considered wherever possible. For example, a combined buccal mucosa and tongue defect may be better reconstructed with a skin graft for the defect of the buccal mucosa and a free flap for the tongue rather than using a single flap for both. Reconstruction in such a way reflects the separate functional and anatomic roles of these two sites.

RECONSTRUCTIVE PLANNING

A proper preoperative assessment should be performed prior to any reconstructive surgery. The patient should undergo a complete medical and surgical history as well as a physical examination. There should be access to a multidisciplinary team composed of head and neck, plastic and reconstructive, dental, medical and radiation oncologists, radiologists, pathologists as well as allied health services such as speech therapy and dieticians so that treatment decisions can be made that simultaneously take into account all aspects of the patient's condition. Medical comorbidities also need to be factored in. For example, the advanced elderly may have conditions precluding lengthy surgery due to a higher incidence of postoperative medical complications. They may be better candidates for a pedicled rather than free flap reconstruction or even non-surgical management.

Routine imaging is not a necessary part of strictly soft tissue reconstructive planning in most cases; however, in some circumstances, it may be beneficial. Patients with prior neck dissection, radiotherapy or reconstruction may not have useable recipient vessels available. Computed tomography or magnetic resonance angiography suggest vessel patency in advance, while secondarily minimizing unnecessary dissection in the operating room. As virtual surgical planning for osseus mandible and maxillary reconstruction is gaining popularity, imaging of the fibula and other donor sites will become a more common part of the reconstructive workup.

Once the details of the extirpation and reconstruction plan are formulated, only then is the patient taken to the operating room. The ideal situation is one in which there are two surgical teams: one responsible for tumor extirpation and a second for reconstruction. Having a single surgeon perform both the tumor ablation and the reconstruction is an enormous and exhausting undertaking. It is often possible for both the ablative and reconstructive teams to operate concurrently, thereby speeding up the surgical procedures and minimizing the length of anesthesia time.

GRAFTS VERSUS FLAPS

GRAFTS

Reconstruction may be achieved through use of either non-vascularized tissue (i.e., grafts) or vascularized tissues (i.e., flaps). Grafts serve a valuable role in reconstruction because of their simplicity, but the ability to heal needs to be carefully scrutinized in patients who have had prior radiotherapy or will need postoperative radiotherapy. Adjuvant treatments are an integral part of the multimodal treatment plan, particularly for advanced-stage tumors, and that should be taken into consideration while planning reconstructive surgery. An open wound following a failed skin graft reconstruction may delay the timely delivery of radiotherapy with a negative impact on patient outcome. Expeditious healing should be a goal contemplated at the time of planning of reconstruction.

Non-vascularized grafts include skin, bone and nerve. Split- or full-thickness skin grafts are straightforward and popular means of resurfacing superficial defects of the hard palate, buccal mucosa, floor of the mouth or tongue. As long as the wound base is vascularized, a skin graft should take reasonably well. Depending upon the defect location, bolsters to minimize skin graft movement are necessary. However, securing the bolster may be difficult in some locations, since it may produce airway obstruction, making some areas more favorable than others. Compared to partial-thickness grafts, full-thickness grafts have less secondary contracture, but a higher metabolic requirement to ensure reliable healing. Both skin graft types are advantageous in that they are easy to harvest, readily available in abundance and can be used to resurface large defects. Disadvantages include a poor color and contour match, limited neovascularization on structures such as bone or radiated tissues and susceptibility to local trauma. Perhaps the most important aspect of skin grafts is that they are prone to contraction, with negative effects on tissue range of motion, pliability and compliance (1). Small and superficial mucosal defects of the oral cavity can be left open to granulate with spontaneous epithelialization, but with even greater contraction than a graft. Areas with rigid bony support to counteract contraction are most amenable to grafting or secondary healing, particularly the hard palate.

Acellular dermal matrices have also found a place in the reconstructive surgeons' armamentarium in recent years. They have been used to resurface intraoral defects of the tongue, maxillary oral vestibule, mandible, floor of the mouth and hard palate. Success rates up to 90% have been achieved, with complete epithelialization achieved by 4 weeks. The advantages of acellular dermal matrices over skin grafts include lower potential cost, absence of donor site morbidity, a natural-appearing mucosal surface and comparable functional status.

FLAPS

Vascularized tissue can be transferred into ablative defects in a number of ways. Local flaps are elevated from a donor site immediately adjacent to the area requiring reconstruction, whereas regional flaps are brought in from more remote sites.

The most common examples of local flaps are cutaneous flaps such as those used to resurface small defects following skin cancer removal. They are generally small, survive *via* a random blood supply and usually have length to width ratios no greater than 2:1. In contrast, axial flaps have an identifiable vessel supplying them. For this reason, axial flaps can be safely elevated with greater reliability and with length to width ratios of as much as 5:1.

Examples of local flaps in the oral cavity include mucosal advancement flaps such as those used for resurfacing of vermilion defects (random blood supply) versus axial mucoperiosteal flaps based on the greater palatine vessels for palatal reconstruction. Local flaps have limited use in the oral cavity since most small defects amenable to these reconstructions can often be closed primarily. Furthermore, small amounts of tension at either the flap donor or recipient site can have significant functional compromise on either speech or swallowing, so a careful balance must be achieved in local flap selection. For this reason, regional flaps are commonly preferred.

Like axial local flaps, regional flaps contain an intrinsic blood supply. Depending on the flap length, they reach a significant distance away from the donor site. Regional flaps used for oral cavity reconstruction can be harvested from other intraoral sites (i.e., facial artery myomucosal flap), cutaneous locations (i.e., nasolabial or submental flaps) or more distant sites (i.e., pectoralis major or supraclavicular flaps). Regional pedicle flaps have a number of disadvantages. Because they are entirely dependent on an intact blood supply, the flap reach is limited. There is also a paucity of available pedicle flaps that can reach the oral cavity for reconstruction. For example, flaps from the upper torso such as the pectoralis major and supraclavicular flaps lose much of their volume in the distance that is required to reach the oral cavity. The portion of the flap that ultimately provides the reconstruction is at the distal portion of the flap where blood supply is most tenuous. Pedicle flaps usually need to be tunneled into the recipient defect in the oral cavity, creating unwanted bulk in cosmetically sensitive areas such as the neck. Tunneling can also be a source of vascular pedicle constriction leading to flap ischemia. Finally, the direct communication between the intraoral inset and the donor site is an opportunity for donor site bacterial contamination or fistula development.

With the advent of the operating microscope and the development of vascular surgery techniques, specialized microsurgical instruments and suture materials were developed, leading to the field of microvascular surgery. Microvascular free tissue transfer, with the ability to repair small vessels accurately, has become a very powerful technique within the reconstructive armamentarium (2). Free flaps have their blood supply temporarily divided at a distant donor site and reconstituted at the recipient site. Such an ability does away with the inherent constraints of pedicled flaps, significantly changing the way in which oral cavity reconstruction is approached. As long as there are adequate recipient vessels, nearly any defect can be reconstructed using a free flap of specialized tissues from around the body.

RECONSTRUCTION BY ANATOMIC AREA

The choice of reconstruction is dependent on a number of factors relating to the nature of the defect, aspects of the potential donor site and surgeon preference. Careful measurements need to be taken, especially of the surface area, as well as the depth of the defect so that a volume assessment can be made.

Isolated defects of the buccal mucosa or floor of the mouth generally involve a large surface area, but are small in volume. Appropriate reconstructions use thin fasciocutaneous flaps such as the radial forearm, ulnar forearm, lateral arm and, in non-obese patients, the anterolateral thigh (ALT) flap. The facial artery musculo-mucosal (FAMM) or submental flap can also be considered in limited scenarios if the supplying vessel has been preserved. Fasciocutaneous flaps are also useful because they are pliable, allowing them to conform to contour changes from one part of the oral cavity to another.

Reconstruction of tongue defects is aimed at restoring the bulk that is lost following resection. Tongue convexity is necessary to contact the palate for speech articulation and to push the food bolus into the oropharynx (3). Small tongue defects can be closed primarily as long as there is no tethering or compromise to mobility. Resection involving greater than a third of the tongue is ideally reconstructed with free tissue transfer. For defects of up to two-thirds of the tongue volume, a thin, pliable flap such as the radial forearm should be utilized to preserve tongue mobility (Figure 15.1). Subtotal or total tongue defects require bulkier flaps. The three flaps most commonly used in this scenario are the rectus abdominis myocutaneous, the ALT and pectoralis flap (4). Free flaps can be made sensate by harvesting them with a cutaneous nerve for coaptation with the lingual nerve stump; however, it remains unclear if this has any proven benefit in speech or swallowing (5). Low-volume free flaps, such as a radial forearm, have some spontaneous sensation recovery even in the absence of nerve repair.

If the oral cavity defect includes bone in addition to soft tissue, then a decision needs to be made as to whether or not an osteocutaneous free flap is required. The workhorse flap for this type of reconstruction is the fibula (6). Other less widely used osseous flaps include the radial forearm, scapula and iliac crest. As mandible defects involve increasing amounts of soft tissue relative to bone, the balance may shift away from bone in favor of a musculocutaneous flap to obliterate surgical dead space and ensure reliable healing. The only area where bone is an absolute necessity is for the anterior mandible to avoid creation of the Andy Gump deformity. For large lateral and posterolateral mandible defects, an ALT or vertical rectus flap may function adequately,

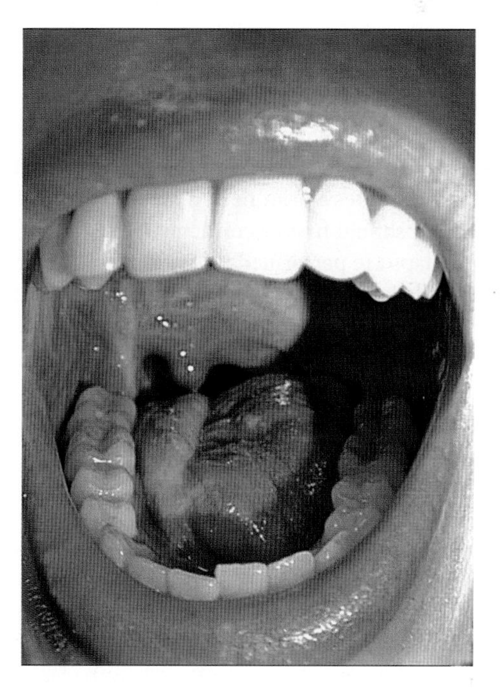

Figure 15.1 Radial forearm flap for reconstruction of right hemi glossectomy defect.

albeit without the opportunity for dental restoration (7). The alternative option is to combine a fibula with a second flap such as either a free radial forearm or pectoralis.

Composite defects of the oral cavity include the intraoral lining, intervening musculoskeletal tissues and external skin. Reconstruction can be performed with a folded multi-island free flap or two separate reconstructions for the internal and external portions. Depending upon the defect location and surface area to volume ratio required, either a thin or thick flap can be used. When more than one skin paddle is required, a flap with multiple perforators is favorable to allow maximal flexibility in the reconstruction. For this reason, the vertical rectus flap or radial forearm flap are preferred because of the ample number of supplying vessels to the skin islands emanating from the axial pedicle. Multiple skin paddles can be created with either an ALT or fibula flap; however, there is no way to ensure the presence of multiple perforators in a favorable reconstructive arrangement ahead of flap harvest. An alternative to creating two independent skin islands is to de-epithelialize an intervening section to create "pseudo-islands," although the degree of mobility is restricted.

INDIVIDUAL FLAP ANATOMY AND CONSIDERATIONS

TONGUE FLAP

The tongue is a structure made predominantly of skeletal muscle covered by mucosal epithelium. Because of its large size, it can be used as a donor source of tissue to resurface small defects of the palate, tonsils, alveolar ridge, floor of the mouth and lip vermillion. Tongue flaps can be based dorsally, laterally or from the ventral surface of the tongue.

The blood supply to these flaps is random, derived from either lingual artery. The tongue has a robust blood supply, so these flaps can be harvested safely and reliably. If the surgical history includes a prior neck dissection, patency of the lingual artery should first be confirmed (8).

Tongue flaps are performed in two stages. The first stage consists of flap elevation and partial inset into the area requiring resurfacing. Approximately 2–3 weeks thereafter, the second stage is performed with flap division and donor site closure. Dimensions of the tongue flap are limited with a base width no greater than 1.5–2 cm to allow for a primary donor site closure.

FAMM FLAP

The FAMM is a versatile flap used for resurfacing defects of the palate, alveolus, floor of the mouth and lip vermilion. The flap itself is composed of mucosa, submucosa and a portion of the buccinator muscle. Based on the facial artery, the FAMM flap is an intraoral, pedicled, locoregional flap that can be based either inferiorly or superiorly depending on the defect requiring reconstruction. As an axial pattern flap with an extended length to width ratio, the facial artery must be included along the entire length of the flap (9).

Flap dimensions are usually 2 cm wide by 8 cm long. Wider flaps can be problematic because of increased donor site complications at the buccal mucosa closure. Prior to flap elevation, the course of the facial artery is verified using a Doppler ultrasound. Inferiorly based flaps are vascularized by the facial artery, whereas the superiorly based flap is nourished retrograde *via* the angular vessel. If the surgical history includes a prior submandibular gland resection or neck dissection, the facial artery is likely ligated, precluding an inferiorly based flap. There is usually no obvious vein that travels with the artery, but instead a venous plexus that should be included with the flap to minimize the risk of venous insufficiency. For this reason, the artery should not be skeletonized, but a generous cuff of soft tissue is left around it.

Depending upon the defect location, the FAMM flap can be performed in one stage or may require a second stage for pedicle division in some instances.

The patient in Figure 15.2a developed osteonecrosis of her anterior mandible that required dental clearance and marginal mandibular resection. The resulting alveolar mucosal defect was unable to be closed primarily and not felt to be large enough to warrant a free flap reconstruction. Instead, an inferiorly based FAMM flap was designed as shown. The course of the facial artery was identified using a handheld Doppler machine.

In raising the flap, the mucosa is first incised. The facial artery is identified using a combination of needle tip cautery and blunt dissection, ensuring that the artery is included within the flap along its whole length. Figure 15.2b illustrates the length and breadth of flap that can be safely harvested. The flap is long enough to cover defects of the alveolus as illustrated in Figure 15.2c.

NASOLABIAL FLAP

More commonly used in reconstructing skin defects of the upper lip, cheek and nose, the nasolabial flap is occasionally employed to close small to moderate-sized defects of the floor of the mouth and buccal mucosa (10). Based on the facial/angular artery, a skin paddle 3 cm wide by 9 cm long can be elevated. It can be used as either a single- or two-stage reconstruction.

The flap is raised in a subcutaneous plane superficial to the facial muscles, with the medial aspect of the flap lying along the nasolabial crease. To transpose the flap from its donor site into the oral cavity, a transbuccal tunnel must be created posterior to the orbicularis oris muscle. The donor site is closed primarily after elevation of the adjacent cheek soft tissues.

SUBMENTAL FLAP

The submental flap is well suited for resurfacing skin defects of the external face, but can also be used for reconstruction

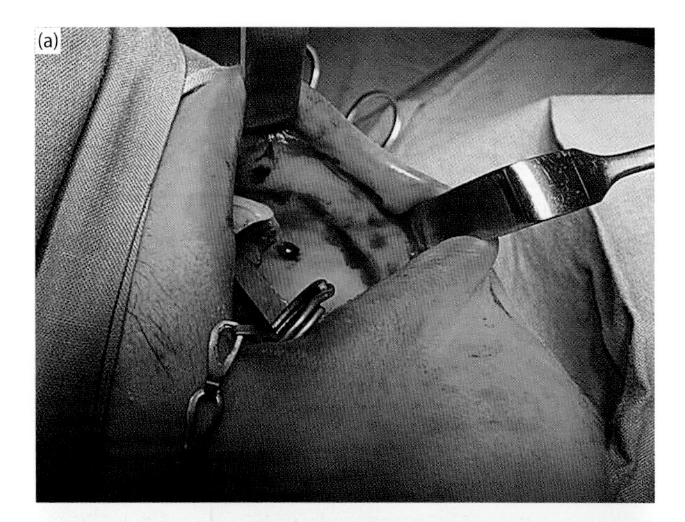

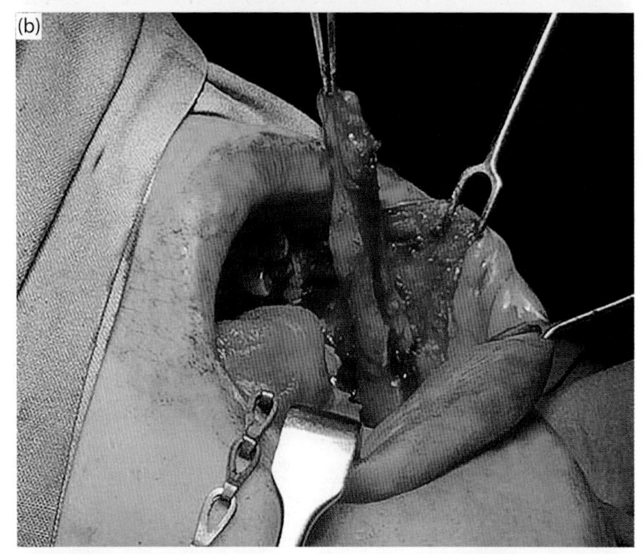

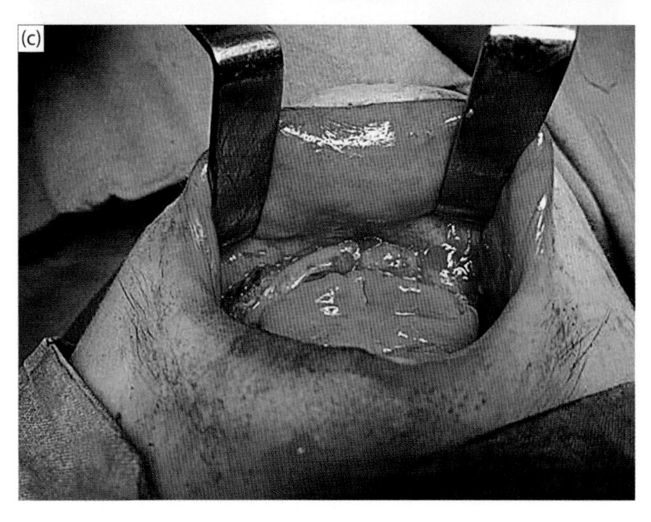

Figure 15.2 **(a)** FAMM outlined for reconstruction of a small lower alveolar defect. **(b)** The elevated FAMM flap showing the length and thickness that can be harvested. **(c)** FAMM flap used for closure of the lower alveolar defect.

of intraoral defects. It is primarily a fasciocutaneous flap composed of skin and soft tissue from the submental region raised with a portion of platysma muscle. The flap size is dependent on the amount of skin redundancy in the neck, commonly measuring 7 cm by 15 cm (11).

Dissection of the flap begins on the side opposite to its pedicle with elevation immediately deep to the platysma. Dissection proceeds across the midline until the anterior belly of the digastric is reached. The digastric muscle is divided here and included with the flap. The flap pedicle is then separated from the submandibular gland.

The arc of rotation allows the submental flap to reach defects of the buccal mucosa and floor of the mouth. If the operative defect does not provide a direct means for the flap to be introduced into the oral cavity, a tunnel needs to be created that is large enough to avoid compromising the pedicle.

The flap is based on the submental artery, a branch of the facial artery. Care needs to be taken when raising the flap in the setting of concurrent neck dissection. Removal of the submandibular gland is a risk for damage of the submental vessels. For this reason, some authors suggest raising the flap prior to the neck dissection. Similarly, in patients who have had prior neck dissection, flap reliability is questionable.

SUPRACLAVICULAR ARTERY PERFORATOR FLAP

The supraclavicular flap is used for reconstruction of oral cavity defects involving the floor of the mouth, lower dental alveolus and buccal mucosa. The supraclavicular artery flap is supplied by a perforating branch of the transverse cervical artery. The flap is based at the anatomic posterior triangle of the neck, bordered by the sternocleidomastoid muscle anteriorly, the trapezius muscle posteriorly and the clavicle inferiorly. Flap dimensions are approximately 7 cm wide by 35 cm long and can extend beyond the deltoid insertion. Flaps wider than 7 cm can be elevated, but require a skin graft to close the donor area. One disadvantage of the supraclavicular flap is that the perforator supplying the skin island is not uniformly present. Furthermore, due to its small size, the perforator cannot be reliably verified on preoperative imaging. Despite these limitations, large case series demonstrate few instances of flap loss, even in the setting of ipsilateral radiotherapy or neck dissection (12).

Figure 15.3 shows the flap design with the entry point of the supraclavicular perforator into the skin island. Flap dissection proceeds from distal to proximal in a subfascial plane. The initial dissection proceeds rapidly until the posterior triangle at the edge of the clavicle is reached. The investing fascia is incised to release the flap. The pedicle does not need to be skeletonized unless extensive reach is needed. Once the pedicle location is identified, the proximal aspect of the skin paddle is incised to create an island.

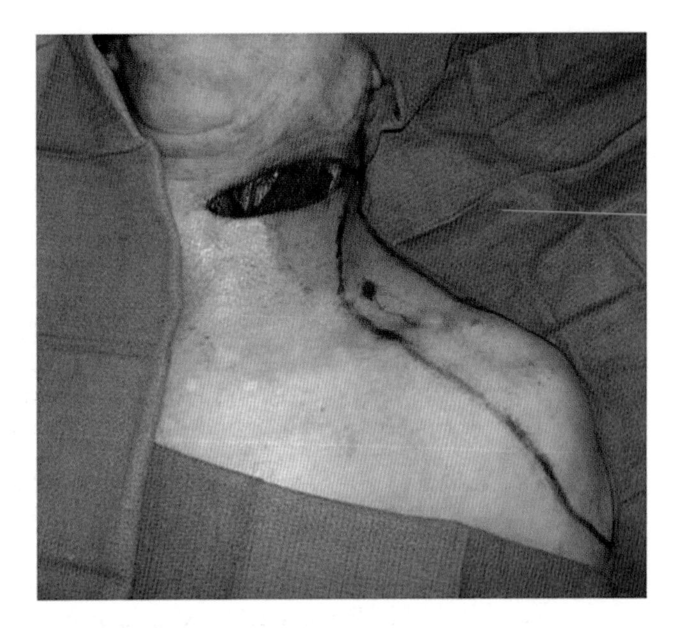

Figure 15.3 Supraclavicular artery perforator flap showing entry point of the supraclavicular perforator vessel.

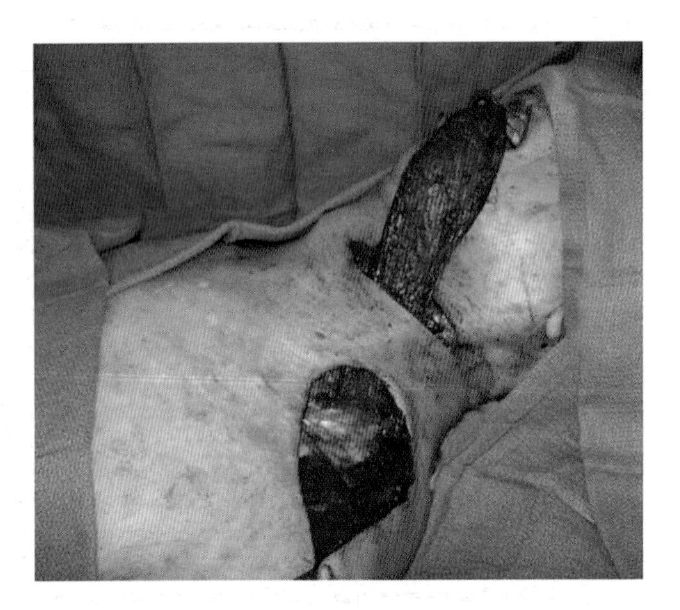

Figure 15.4 Arc of rotation of the FAMM flap.

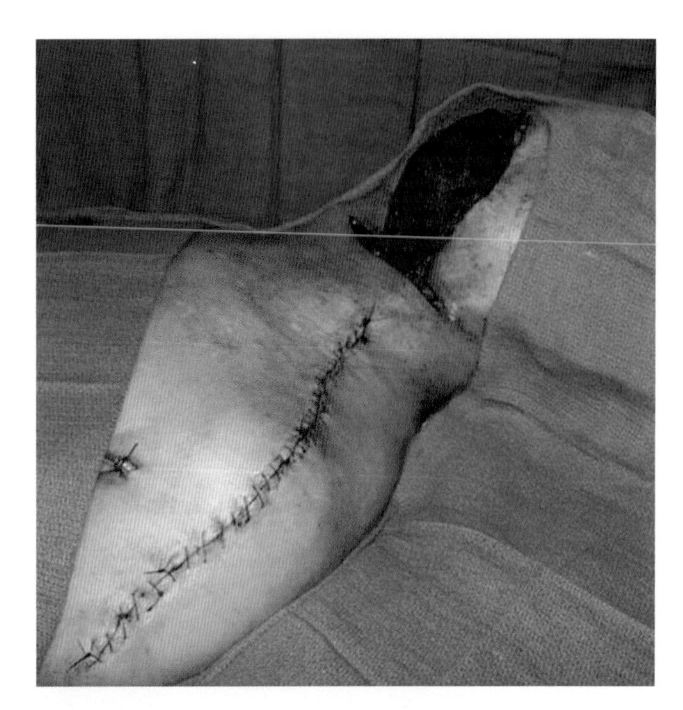

Figure 15.5 Closure of donor site by undermining skin flaps.

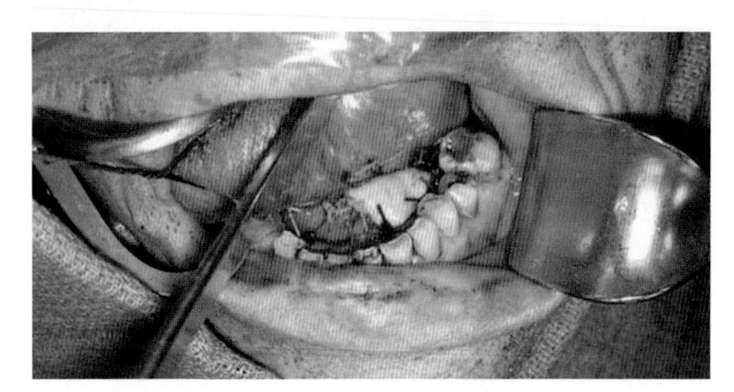

Figure 15.6 Skin island paddle of the FAMM flap for reconstruction of floor of the mouth.

The arc of rotation of the flap is shown in Figure 15.4. Primary closure of the donor site is achieved by undermining skin flaps over the pectoralis and trapezius muscles (Figure 15.5). The flap is tunneled into the oral cavity for insetting. Buried portions of the flap are de-epithelialized. The mucosal defect in the floor of the mouth is resurfaced with a small skin paddle (Figure 15.6).

PECTORALIS MAJOR FLAP

Long before the development of microvascular techniques, the pectoralis major myocutaneous flap was a workhorse for reconstruction of head and neck defects (13). Although it is no longer the first reconstructive choice for most oral cavity defects, it remains invaluable when there are relative contraindications to microvascular transfer.

The obvious benefits of the pectoralis major flap are its simplicity and reliability to close a variety of head and neck defects. The flap provides a generous amount of muscle, subcutaneous tissue and skin, which can be easily tailored. Its long arc of rotation is also a highly favorable feature. It can be raised as a muscle only to augment hypopharynx repairs in the neck, provide coverage for exposed vessels or seal orocutaneous fistulae. More commonly, however, the flap is raised with a skin paddle to resurface defects of the lower oral mucosa, gingiva and floor of the mouth. The skin island can seal the oral cavity; meanwhile, the muscle bulk is useful for replacing dead space following mandibulectomy (Figure 15.7a and b). The flap is also a useful option for closure of posterolateral mandible defects. If placement of the

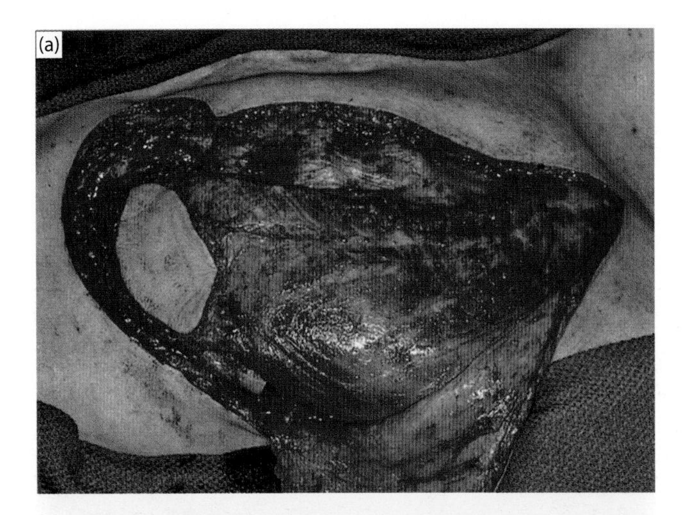

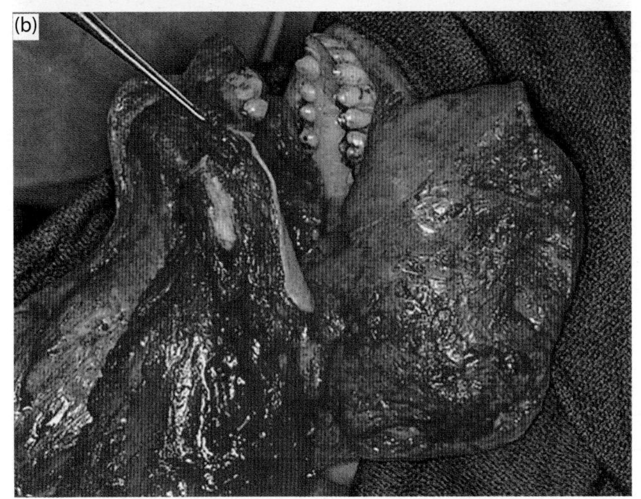

Figure 15.7 **(a)** Pectoralis major myocutaneous flap elevated with a skin island. **(b)** The skin island replaces the defect in the oral cavity and the muscle paddle replaces the dead space in the upper neck.

skin paddle on the upper oral cavity is attempted, such as following maxillectomy, it frequently dehisces in the postoperative period from the flap weight and force of gravity.

The blood supply to the pectoralis major muscle is *via* the pectoral branch of the thoracoacromial artery, which itself arises from the second part of the axillary artery. A robust and consistent blood supply from this vessel makes this flap highly dependable. The external surface markings of the vascular pedicle are determined by drawing a line from the shoulder to the xiphisternum and another line vertically from the midpoint of the clavicle to intersect the first line.

The skin paddle can be based anywhere over the muscle as long as a musculocutaneous perforator is present. Large skin paddles are safer because they maximize the chances of containing a perforator. Commonly, a large, vertically oriented ellipse, approximately 4–6 cm in width, is designed medial to the nipple–areola complex. The drawback of this skin paddle approach is the medialized position of the nipple–areola complex following donor site closure. In female patients, a crescentic skin paddle can be designed along the inframammary crease with minimal deformity to the breast. The trade-off of this design is that the skin paddle is positioned over the distal pectoralis muscle where there are fewer perforators. If the skin paddle is extended beyond the surface of the pectoralis muscle, the blood supply is more random, so it needs to be carefully evaluated intraoperatively.

RADIAL FOREARM FREE FLAP

The radial forearm flap is currently the mainstay for reconstruction of oral cavity defects involving a large surface area with a small volume (14). It is primarily used for resurfacing of buccal mucosa, partial/hemi-glossectomy and, less commonly, infrastructure maxillectomy defects. Its malleable nature and robust blood supply allow for the creation of multiple skin islands that can be folded for the reconstruction of composite oral cavity defects. The radial forearm flap can be harvested with the lateral antebrachial cutaneous nerve to restore sensation to the skin island. In cases of total lower lip reconstruction, the palmaris longus tendon can be harvested in continuity with the flap to reduce ptosis and oral incompetence (15). Although its donor scar is unfavorable, its many reconstructive advantages far outweigh this downside.

The skin of the volar forearm is generally very thin and pliable. A large skin paddle of up to 10 × 40 cm can be harvested based on the radial artery. When the skin paddle is designed distally on the forearm, a long pedicle up to 20 cm can be obtained. The pedicle can usually reach recipient vessels on either side of the neck, an important consideration in the setting of previous radiotherapy or neck dissection.

The vascular inflow of this flap is *via* the radial artery. Venous drainage can be based either on the paired venae comitantes or the cephalic vein. The flap is almost always wide enough to include the cephalic vein, so either system can be repaired for venous outflow. The cephalic vein is preferable because its large size allows a venous coupling device to be used for anastomosis.

Compared to other free flaps, the radial forearm has the advantage of a fairly easy dissection performed in under 1 hour. Prior to flap elevation, vascularization of the limb needs to be ensured with an Allen's test. A pulse oximeter placed on the thumb provides more valuable information than visual inspection alone following manual occlusion of the radial artery. The main disadvantage of the radial forearm flap is the unsightly donor site. Primary closure of the donor site is possible for flaps less than 4 cm in diameter. Any larger donor site defect needs to be reconstructed with a large bi-lobed flap based on ulnar artery perforators or resurfaced with a skin graft. Split-thickness skin grafts are generally used, but prelamination with Integra or a full-thickness graft can yield more cosmetically appealing results. A second disadvantage is that the flap skin paddle can be hairy in some patients. This problem can be circumvented by positioning the skin island more volar on the forearm or by using an ulnar forearm flap instead. Hair follicles are frequently destroyed by adjuvant radiotherapy as well.

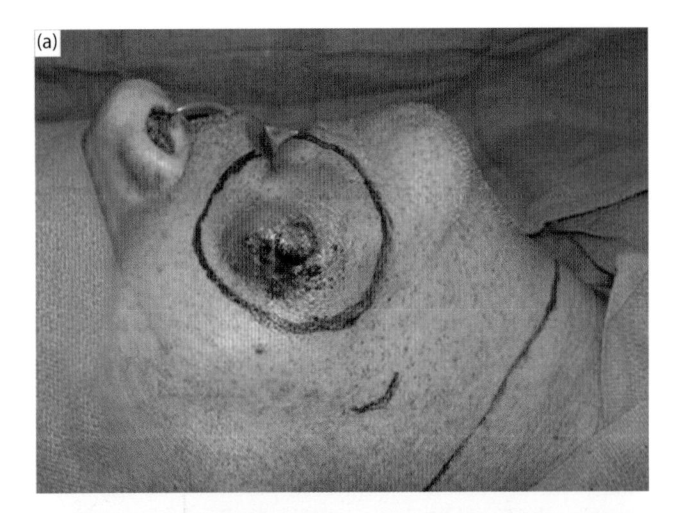

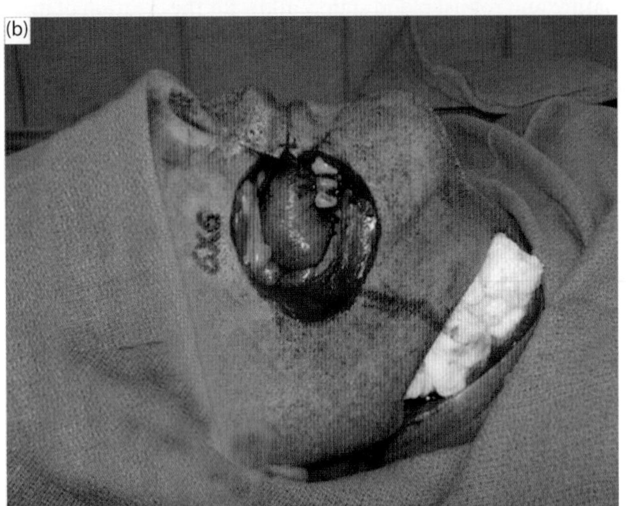

Figure 15.8 **(a)** Squamous cell carcinoma of the buccal mucosa perforating through the skin of the cheek. **(b)** Through and through defect of the right cheek after resection of buccal mucosa cancer.

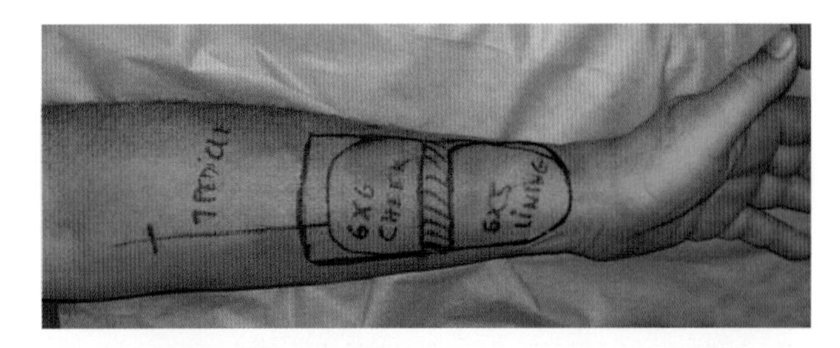

Figure 15.9 Radial forearm flap with two skin islands outlined for reconstruction of the buccal mucosa and skin of the cheek.

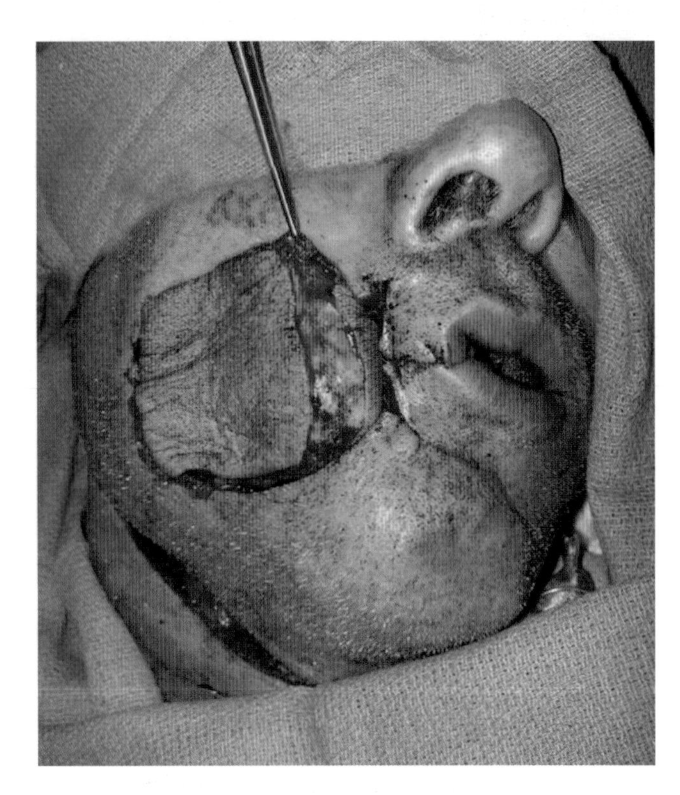

Figure 15.10 The double island radial forearm flap for closure of the through and through cheek defect showing inset of the inner island for replacement of mucosa and de-epithelization for separation of the second island to replace the skin of the cheek.

An example of a patient who presented with a neglected squamous cell carcinoma of the right buccal mucosa that had progressed to involve his external skin of the cheek is shown in Figure 15.8a. Once the tumor was removed, cut edges of the lip were approximated so the remaining defect size could be established in preparation for double island radial forearm free flap (Figure 15.8b). Accurate measurements are made of the intraoral and external skin defects. These dimensions are transferred to a paper template, adding a further 2 cm between the skin paddles for de-epithelialization and flap folding. Once the template is created, it is transposed onto the forearm skin. An assessment should also be made of the pedicle length required to reach the recipient vessels in the neck. The flap design is shown on the patient's non-dominant forearm. The flap is based on the radial aspect of the forearm to ensure that the cephalic vein can be included (Figure 15.9).

In general, flap inset is performed before the microvascular anastomosis. This establishes the pedicle length necessary for tension-free repair of the vessels and avoids inadvertent injury to the anastomosis that can occur during flap manipulation. Figure 15.10 shows the flap as it is inset into the intraoral defect followed by the buried portion of the flap, which is de-epithelialized. Finally, the skin paddle for external skin resurfacing is inset (Figure 15.11).

RECTUS ABDOMINUS FREE FLAP

The rectus abdominus myocutaneous flap is commonly utilized for reconstructing defects of the oral cavity where a large volume and surface area are required. For larger tumors of the tongue, when greater than 50% of the tongue has been resected, the vertical rectus abdominus muscle

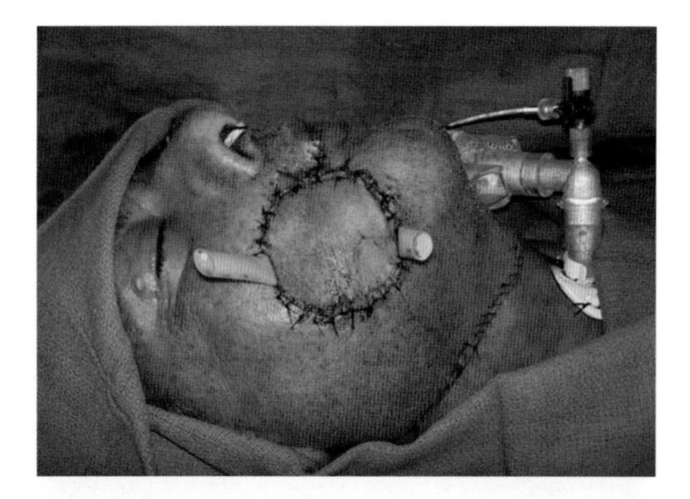

Figure 15.11 Second skin island of the radial forearm free flap achieving complete closure of the skin defect.

(VRAM) provides ample volume and skin for reconstruction. The VRAM flap is also useful in oral cavity reconstruction of large or composite defects involving multiple anatomic sites. It can simultaneously replace a significant number of missing intraoral structures such as the buccal mucosa, floor of the mouth, mandible, oropharynx and tongue, or it can be folded for composite defects involving intraoral structures and external skin (16).

The rectus abdominus is a vertically oriented muscle of the anterior abdominal wall extending between the costal margin and pubis. As opposed to breast reconstruction where a transversely oriented skin paddle is harvested Transverse Rectus Abdominis myocutaneous (TRAM), in head and neck reconstruction, a vertically oriented skin paddle is preferred. Although the design of the VRAM flap is less cosmetically favorable, the principle benefit of this arrangement is that the skin paddle overlies the rectus muscle along its entire length, capturing a maximal number of perforators. The flap harvest is straightforward with wide exposure and primary closure of the donor site, leaving a midline or paramedian scar.

The deep inferior epigastric artery, the dominant pedicle of the VRAM flap, gives off greater than 10–15 perforators to each hemi-abdominal wall. The length of the pedicle ranges between 8 and 10 cm and can be lengthened further by excising portions of the rectus muscle. The size of the skin paddle can be up to 45 × 15 cm, extending from the costal margin to just above the pubic skin crease. The width of the skin island is dependent on the laxity of the patient's abdominal wall that will allow for a primary skin closure.

The patient shown in Figure 15.12 underwent resection for a recurrent squamous cancer of the gingiva and mandible. A pervious marginal mandibulectomy was performed with primary closure of the defect using the floor of the mouth, causing tongue tethering. The current defect included external skin of the cheek and chin, a lateral segmental mandibulectomy, the buccal mucosa, the floor of the mouth and the retromolar trigone.

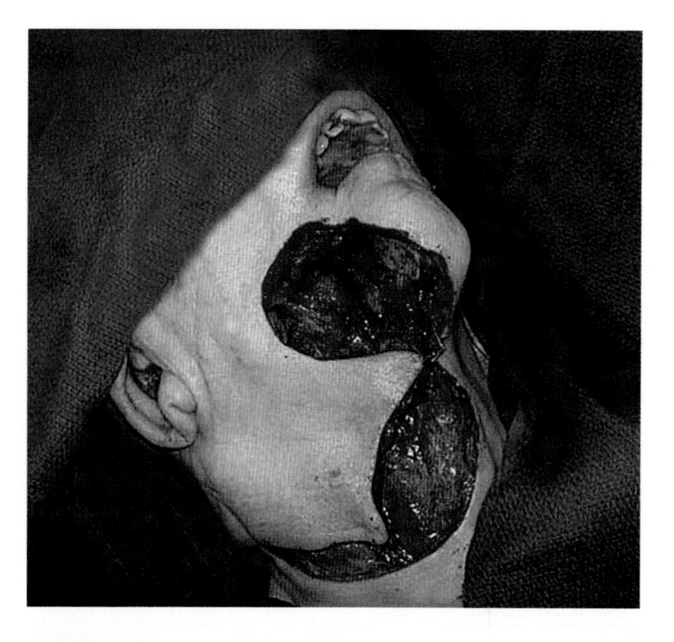

Figure 15.12 Composite defect following resection of the floor of the mouth, mandible and overlying skin for advanced recurrent carcinoma of the lower gum.

Because of the patient's advanced age and the large volume of the defect, a decision was made to use only soft tissue reconstruction instead of an osseus flap. A vertical rectus abdominus myocutaneous flap was designed with two separate skin islands (Figure 15.13). After measuring the external skin and intraoral defect, templates were created for transfer to the abdominal wall. The flap was raised after ensuring that the donor site could be closed primarily. As much anterior rectus sheath as possible is preserved to ensure that primary fascial closure is achieved without the use of a mesh.

Following division of the flap and transfer to the recipient site, the flap is first inset into the oral defect, beginning posteriorly at the retromolar trigone and working anteriorly, taking care to ensure that a watertight seal is obtained (Figure 15.14). The area for excision between the intraoral and external skin islands is established. Microsurgical anastomoses are then completed. Finally, attention is directed to resurfacing the external skin defect (Figure 15.15).

ALT FLAP

The ALT flap is ideal for reconstruction because of its minimal donor site morbidity and remote location away from the head and neck (17). It is commonly used for reconstruction of total glossectomy or buccal mucosal defects depending upon the thickness of the patient's thigh (4). For hemiglossectomy defects, the radial forearm flap is still preferred because the adipofascial tissues of the ALT are too rigid to allow for proper tongue motion.

The dominant pedicle of the flap is the descending branch of the lateral circumflex femoral artery, a branch off of the profunda femoris. After branching off the lateral circumflex femoral, the descending branch enters the vastus

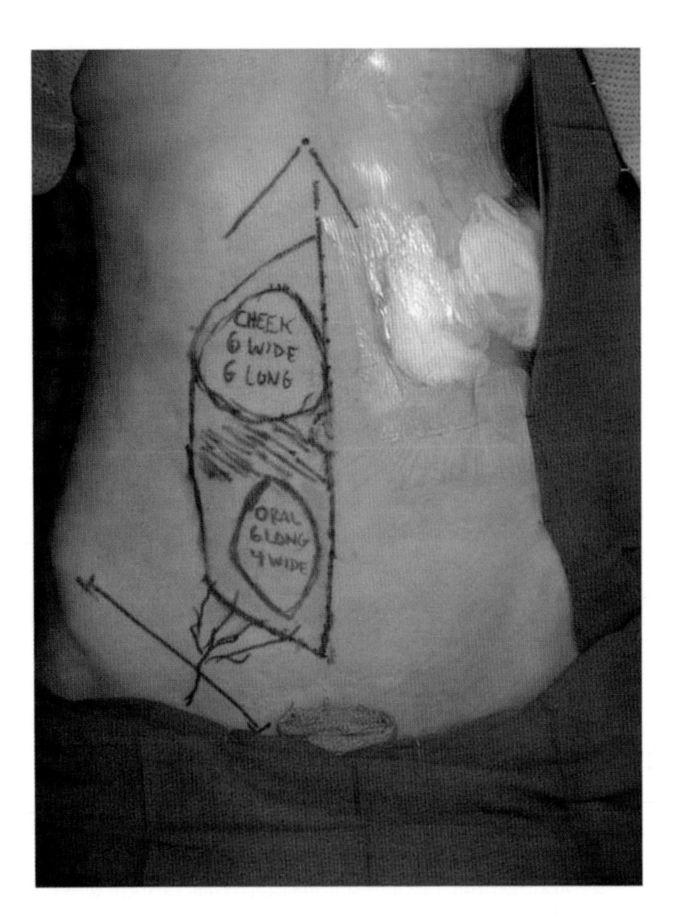

Figure 15.13 Double island vertical rectus abdominus myocutaneous flap for reconstruction of the composite through and through defect of the oral cavity.

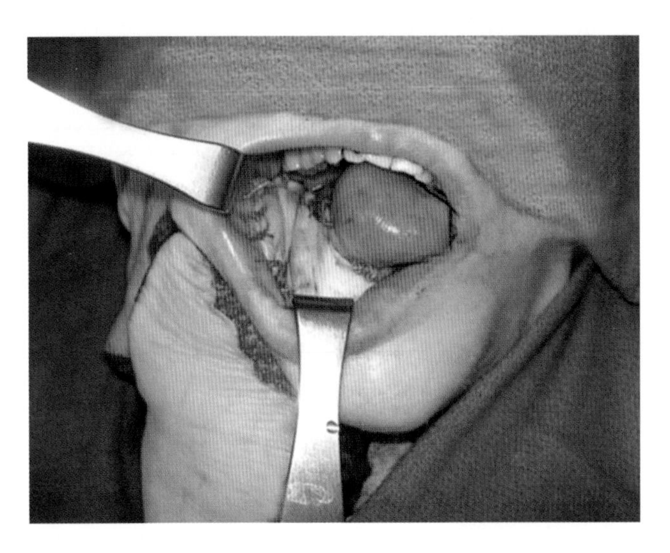

Figure 15.14 Distal island of the rectus abdominus myocutaneous flap for reconstruction of the intraoral defect.

lateralis muscle. It gives off a number of musculocutaneous perforating branches to the overlying skin. A skin paddle as large as 25 × 35 cm can be harvested. Flaps wider than about 7–9 cm require a skin graft for donor site closure.

To raise the flap, the patient is positioned supine with the thigh exposed. The surface marking is a line drawn from

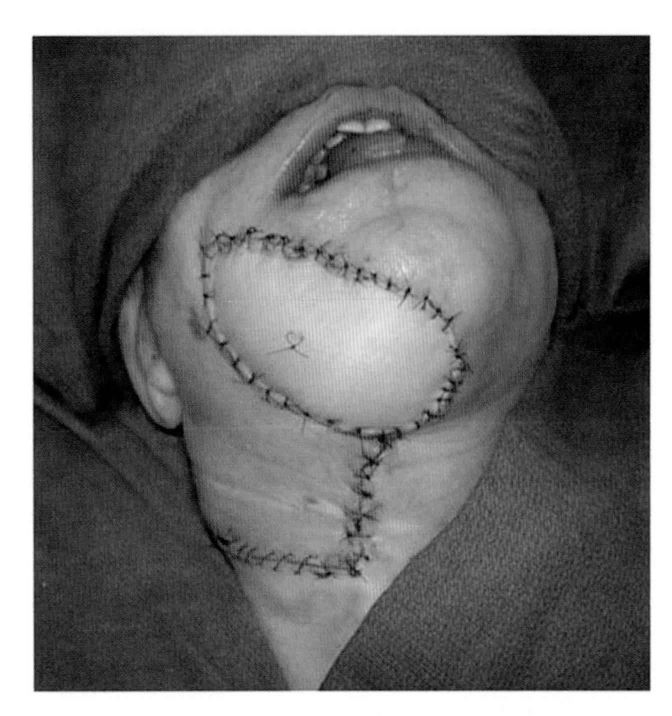

Figure 15.15 Proximal skin island of the rectus abdominus myocutaneous flap resurfacing external skin defect.

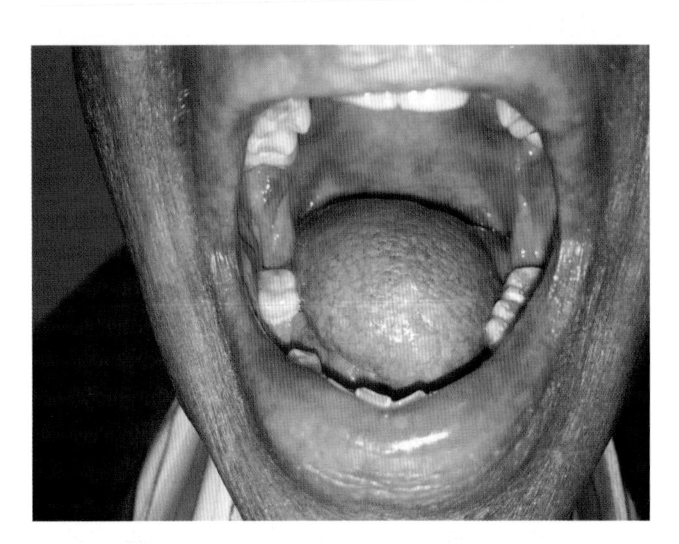

Figure 15.16 Anterolateral thigh flap for reconstruction after near-total glossectomy.

the anterior superior iliac spine to the superolateral border of the patella. A circle with a 3-cm radius is marked at the midpoint of this line where the main perforators can be located. In approximately two-thirds of patients, two usable perforators can be found. When more than one perforator exists, separate skin paddles can be created for use in composite defects.

In most situations, the ALT is harvested as a fasciocutaneous flap. Depending on the patient's subcutaneous tissues, the flap can be thick or thin. The flap can be thinned at the time of elevation, maintaining fascia of 5 cm in diameter around the perforator. In addition, variable amounts of vastus lateralis muscle can be included with the flap either directly below the skin island or in a chimeric fashion off the distal aspect of the lateral circumflex femoral system.

A subtotal glossectomy defect reconstructed with an ALT flap is shown in Figure 15.16. Flap inset demonstrates adequate bulk and convexity to reach the palate.

CONCLUSION

Oral cavity reconstruction requires thoughtful consideration of multiple aspects, including the nature of the surgically created defect and the patient's disease status and overall medical condition. Improved microsurgical techniques combined with the ability to harvest tissue from any part of the body have made free flaps the gold standard for reconstruction in the majority of cases.

REFERENCES

1. Chien CY, Hwang CF, Chuang HC, Jeng SF, Su CY. Comparison of radial forearm free flap, pedicled buccal fat pad flap and split-thickness skin graft in reconstruction of buccal mucosal defect. *Oral Oncol* 2005;41:694–7.
2. Panje WR, Bardach J, Krause CJ. Reconstruction of the oral cavity with a free flap. *Plast Reconstr Surg* 1976;58:415–8.
3. Engel H, Huang JJ, Lin CY, Lam W, Kao HK, Gazyakan E, Cheng MH. A strategic approach for tongue reconstruction to achieve predictable and improved functional and aesthetic outcomes. *Plast Reconstr Surg* 2010;126:1967–77.
4. Yu P. Reinnervated anterolateral thigh flap for tongue reconstruction. *Head Neck* 2004;26:1038–44.
5. Kimata Y, Uchiyama K, Ebihara S et al. Comparison of innervated and noninnervated free flaps in oral reconstruction. *Plast Reconstr Surg* 1999;104:1307–13.
6. Cordeiro PG, Disa JJ, Hidalgo DA, HU QY. Reconstruction of the mandible with osseous free flaps: a 10-year experience with 150 consecutive patients. *Plast Reconstr Surg* 1999;104:1314–20.
7. Hanasono MM, Zevallos JP, Skoracki RJ, Yu P. A prospective analysis of bony versus soft-tissue reconstruction for posterior mandibular defects. *Plast Reconstr Surg* 2010;125:1413–21.
8. Buchbinder D, St-Hilaire H. Tongue flaps in maxillofacial surgery. *Oral Maxillofac Surg Clin N Am* 2003;15:475–86.
9. Pribaz J, Stephens W, Crespo L, Gifford G. A new intraoral flap: facial artery musculomucosal (FAMM) flap. *Plast Reconstr Surg* 1992;90:421–9.
10. Lazaridis N, Tilaveridis I, Karakasis D. Superiorly or inferiorly based "islanded" nasolabial flap for buccal mucosa defects reconstruction. *J Oral Maxillofac Surg* 2008;66:7–15.
11. Martin D, Pascal JF, Baudet J, Mondie JM, Farhat JB, Athoum A, Le Gaillard P, Peri G. The submental island flap: a new donor site. Anatomy and clinical applications as a free or pedicled flap. *Plast Reconstr Surg* 1993;92:867–73.
12. Chiu ES, Liu PH, Friedlander PL. Supraclavicular artery island flap for head and neck oncologic reconstruction: indications, complications and outcomes. *Plast Reconstr Surg* 2009;124:115–23.
13. Ariyan S. The pectoralis major myocutaneous flap. A versatile flap for reconstruction in the head and neck. *Plast Reconstr Surg* 1979;63:73–81.
14. Yang GF, Chen BJ, Gao YZ. The free forearm flap. *Chin Med J* 1981;61:4.
15. Sadove RC, Luce EA, McGrath PC. Reconstruction of the lower lip and chin with the composite radial forearm–palmaris longus free flap. *Plast Reconstr Surg* 1991;88:209–14.
16. Patel NP, Matros E, Cordeiro PG. The use of the multi-island vertical rectus abdominis myocutaneous flap in head and neck reconstruction. *Ann Plast Surg* 2012;69:403–7.
17. Song YG, Chen GZ, Song YL. The free thigh flap: a new free flap concept based on the septocutaneous artery. *Br J Plast Surg* 1984;37:149–59.

16

Reconstructive surgery: Mandible

IVANA PETROVIC, COLLEEN McCARTHY, AND JATIN P. SHAH

INTRODUCTION

The mandible is a strategic structure in the craniofacial skeleton. Its complex three-dimensional structures are critical to facial form and function. More specifically, the mandible serves as a platform for the structures of the floor of the mouth, thereby playing a pivotal role in the maintenance of the airway. In addition to facilitating speech and swallowing, it also provides stability for the teeth that play a vital role in mastication and digestion. Finally, the mandibular bone largely determines the vertical height, transverse width and projection of the lower face. Any deviation from the normal contour of the lower border of the mandible will result in a very significant cosmetic deformity (1,2).

The vast majority of mandible defects result from excision of squamous cell cancer arising from oral mucosa. A small number of patients undergo mandibulectomy for osteogenic sarcomas or benign bone tumors. A smaller proportion of patients receiving head and neck radiotherapy develop complications such as osteoradionecrosis, which can result in bone sequestration and/or pathologic fracture that may necessitate segmental mandibulectomy with reconstruction.

The degree of functional and esthetic deficit after mandibulectomy depends upon the location and extent of mandible removed. Resection of the anterior mandibular arch results in loss of chin projection and lip support. In the absence of reconstruction, extensive soft tissue contracture may lead to loss of oral competence, known as the "Andy Gump" deformity. Resection of the lateral mandible does not result in a functional deficit of the same severity; however, without reconstruction, there will be a loss in lower lateral facial projection. Malocclusion in the patient with intact dentition commonly occurs as a result of the unimpeded action of the contralateral muscles of mastication. Patients with lateral segment resections can develop deviation of the mandible, which can subsequently lead to functional malocclusion, difficulty using dentures and an inability to masticate. Thus, in general, most mandibular defects should be reconstructed when technically possible and medically safe.

Reconstruction of a mandibular defect should aim to provide adequate wound closure, maintain oral competence, restore speech and mastication and maximize the contour of the lower third of the face (3).

HISTORY

The first reports of mandibular reconstruction described delayed reconstruction using external fixators on the remaining mobile bony segments (4). Subsequent advances involved internal wire fixation of non-vascularized bone grafts and the concomitant use of antibiotics (5,6). In the 1960s, more aggressive surgical resections were undertaken followed by postoperative radiation therapy, which led to problems with bone graft resorption, exposure and infection (7,8). The era of prosthetic and allograft mandible reconstruction followed. The use of metallic trays, Silastic, Dacron and Teflon implants allowed for good restoration of mandibular continuity, but long-term results were poor, with a high frequency of infection, exposure and fracture requiring removal of the prostheses (9–13). Mesh trays made of Dacron or metal were introduced in the 1970s as scaffold that were filled with bone graft chips, harvested from cancellous bone from the iliac crest and used for segmental bone defects. Long-term follow-up showed this method to be suboptimal and ineffective due to problems with bone graft dissolution and extrusion of the trays However, a very short segmental defect of up to 3 cm in the mandible without previous exposure to radiotherapy can be reconstructed with a non-vascularized bone graft, which usually is harvested from the iliac crest (3).

The use of pedicled flaps, including the pectoralis and trapezius myocutaneous flaps, then came into vogue. This reconstructive option was attractive in that given their location adjacent to the head and neck, rotation allowed for the importation of well-vascularized tissue into the defect. However, there were several important drawbacks. A significant portion of the flap volume is used up just to reach the recipient site. The portion of the flap that is used for the reconstruction is often the distal most part, has a marginal blood supply and is at risk for ischemic necrosis. The greatest limitation of these flaps, however, is that they do not provide enough tissue in the proper configuration to be useful. In addition, while they provide a large volume of soft tissue, the bone these flaps can bring in with them is of suboptimal quality. The bone available with the pectoralis major muscle (rib) and the trapezius (spine of the scapula) is limited compared to free flap alternatives. Although the pectoralis has been used to reconstruct the anterior mandible and the trapezius to reconstruct the lateral mandible, these flaps generally are not recommended as a preferred method of mandible reconstruction (3).

Metal reconstruction plates were developed as a result of advances in the development of hardware in the practice of orthopedics. Perceived advantages of this approach involved the ease with which the plate could be fixated as well as the avoidance of harvesting a bone graft from a distant site (Figures 16.1 and 16.2). Importantly, however, the use of a reconstruction plate without a reliable soft tissue flap had high rates of exposure, extrusion and fracture and even if complications could be avoided, the esthetic results were suboptimal (14–16).

In an attempt to ameliorate these problems, reconstruction plates were then covered with soft tissue flaps, most commonly the pectoralis myocutaneous flap. Unfortunately, despite the presence of well-vascularized soft tissue, extrusion was still seen with this method. This was particularly true with anterior reconstructions in which tension on the pectoralis flap tends to be excessive. Use of a free flap to cover a reconstruction plate has the lowest risk of plate exposure. The radial forearm donor site is an appropriate choice for this application (17). The anterolateral thigh flap is another alternative. Regardless of the donor tissue used to cover the reconstruction plate, however, this type of reconstruction is regarded as a "last resort" and is saved for situations in which a lack of suitable recipient vessels and/or appropriate donor tissue precludes use of a microvascular, osseous reconstruction.

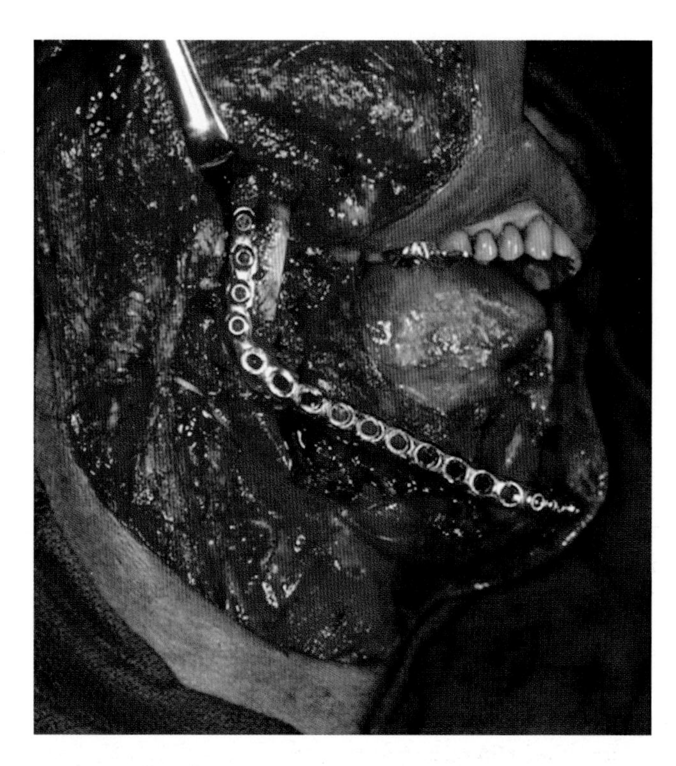

Figure 16.1 Intraoperative view of a reconstruction plate to replace a hemimandibulectomy defect.

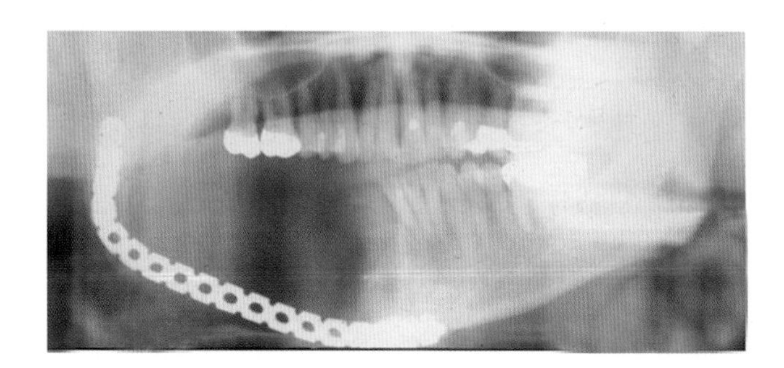

Figure 16.2 Postoperative panoramic view of the mandible showing the reconstruction plate used to replace the resected mandible.

STATE-OF-THE-ART RECONSTRUCTION

With the development of microvascular surgery, major advances took place in reconstructive surgery in the head

Table 16.1 Indications and contraindications for mandible reconstruction

Indications	Contraindications
1. Every patient with a segmental mandibular defect should be considered for reconstruction 2. The choice of reconstruction may be dictated by patient and disease factors 3. Central mandibular defect is an absolute indication for vascularized bony reconstruction	1. There are no contraindications to the concept of mandible reconstruction 2. Contraindications exist only to specific procedures 3. Contraindications may be mandated if a patient's comorbidities dictate

and neck. The indications for and timing of mandibular reconstruction are thus now well established (Table 16.1).

The vast majority of patients who undergo segmental mandibulectomy are candidates for primary reconstruction with vascularized bone flaps. It is the rare patient who is not reconstructed or is reconstructed with techniques such as non-vascularized bone grafts or reconstruction plates alone.

Since the transfer of large quantities of vascularized bone, soft tissue and skin with a single, composite flap is possible, almost any defect of the mandible can be reconstructed in a single stage. High bony union rates have made vascularized osseous free flaps the reconstructive option of choice. It has been demonstrated that vascularized bone will heal within a period of 2–3 months, even in the setting of preoperative or postoperative radiation (18). In addition, well-vascularized bone serves as an excellent bed for the placement of osseointegrated implants, which maximizes both functional and esthetic results.

Ideally, free flap mandible reconstruction should be done primarily at the time of surgical resection of the tumor, because the reconstruction is very precise and the goals of resection and reconstruction are accomplished in a single operation—unlike in secondary reconstruction, where the patient has to live for some time with a deformity (3). In addition, delayed reconstruction, has to be performed in an area of scarring and fibrosis of the remaining bone and soft tissues. Further, trismus may develop as a result of soft tissue contracture, which may not be correctable. Immediate reconstruction permits placement of well-vascularized tissue into the defect immediately in a single operation. Usually, one well-planned flap will be adequate to reconstruct most defects. Bone reconstruction should replace the missing segment of mandible while maintaining proper alignment of the remaining native mandible in order to minimize problems leading to trismus and malocclusion. Replacement of lining and intraoral soft tissue should be planned to maximize mobility of the tongue and buccal mucosa, restore an adequate buccal sulcus for dental rehabilitation and correct soft tissue contracture deformities. If external skin needs to be replaced, a second flap may be necessary (19).

Defects of the posterior aspect of the body of the mandible near its angle or of the ascending ramus may be left alone without consideration of any major reconstructive effort in elderly or poor-risk patients. The esthetic impact of this surgical defect in the early postoperative period is minimal. However, with the passage of time and soft tissue atrophy, the surgical defect becomes quite noticeable and unacceptable (Figures 16.3 and 16.4). In addition, resection of the ascending ramus of the mandible causes loss of function of the ipsilateral pterygoid muscles, leading to significant functional disability and malocclusion. Upward and medial pull by the unopposed contralateral masseter and medial pterygoid muscle produces rotation of the remaining mandible at the region of the molar teeth, leading to significant malocclusion and contracture. For these reasons, even for posterior defects of the mandible, reconstruction should be considered. On the other hand, resection of the anterior aspect of the body of the mandible and particularly the anterior arch of the mandible produces unacceptable functional and esthetic deformity that mandates an appropriate reconstructive effort to restore form and function (Figure 16.5).

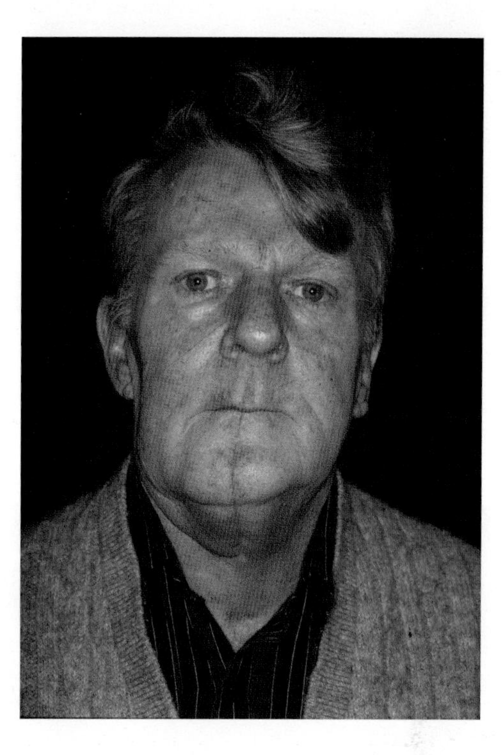

Figure 16.3 Postoperative appearance of a patient with resection of the ascending ramus of the mandible on the right-hand side.

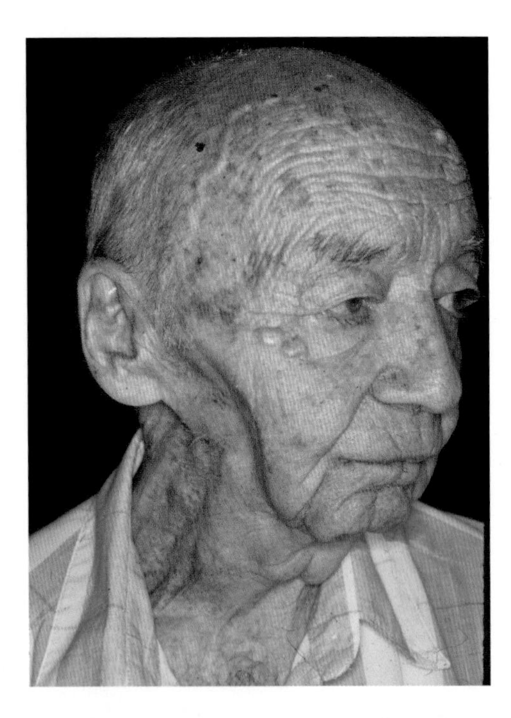

Figure 16.4 Postoperative appearance of a patient with resection of the body and ascending ramus of the mandible on the right-hand side.

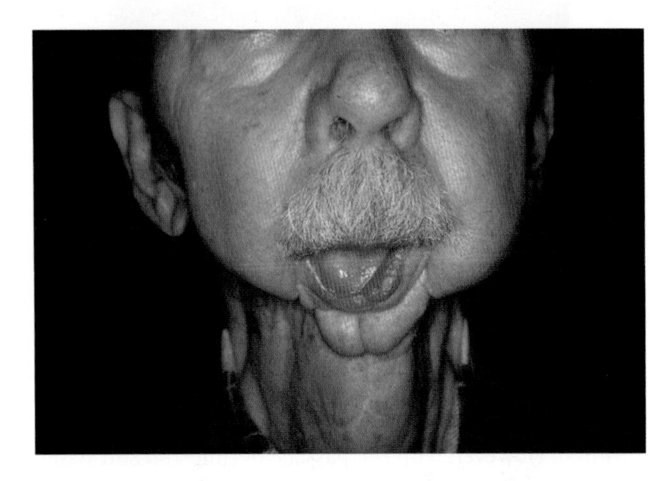

Figure 16.5 Postoperative appearance of a patient with resection of the anterior arch of the mandible.

ONCOLOGIC MANAGEMENT OF THE MANDIBLE

Primary squamous cell carcinomas in the oral cavity extend along the floor of the mouth or the buccal mucosa to approach the attached lingual or buccal gingiva. From here on the tumor does not extend directly through the intact periosteum and cortical bone toward the cancellous part of the mandible since the periosteum acts as a significant protective barrier. Instead, the tumor advances from the attached gingiva toward the alveolar process. In patients with teeth, the tumor extends through the dental sockets into the cancellous part of the bone and invades the mandible. In edentulous patients, the tumor extends up to the alveolar crest and then infiltrates through the dental pores in the alveolar process and extends to the cancellous part of the mandible. When there is extension of tumor to involve the cancellous part of the mandible, a segmental mandibulectomy must be performed. Segmental mandibulectomy should be considered only when there is gross invasion of the cancellous part of the bone by oral cancer, for primary bone tumors of the mandible, for metastatic tumors to the mandible, if there is invasion of the inferior alveolar nerve or canal by tumor and for massive soft tissue disease around the mandible (20).

PREOPERATIVE HISTORY AND CONSIDERATIONS

A multidisciplinary team approach is necessary and appropriate consultations should be sought prior to surgery to optimize the medical condition of the patient, particularly with reference to any existing comorbidities. History of prior treatment of the disease, such as prior radiation with or without chemotherapy, should be elucidated. A preoperative dental evaluation should also be performed in order to establish premorbid occlusion and manage any diseased dentition (1). The most serious postoperative problems in patients undergoing mandible reconstruction are cardiopulmonary in origin. Pneumonia, arrhythmias and myocardial infarction are life-threatening problems for which this patient population may be at risk. Therefore, thorough cardiopulmonary evaluation to assess the safety of a long operation and postoperative recovery should be performed in all patients.

Clinical assessment is performed to evaluate the appropriateness of the fibula and radial forearm donor sites; however, the routine use of preoperative angiography is not recommended. Patients are considered candidates for free fibula transfer if their peripheral vascular examination reveals normal posterior tibial and dorsalis pedis pulses and no signs of chronic arterial and/or venous insufficiency. In these patients, arteriography is unnecessary.

In patients with diminished pulses or a single absent pedal pulse, arteriography is indicated. Amongst these patients, those with evidence of a normal three-vessel run-off may still be considered candidates for flap harvest. Absolute contraindications to harvest of the fibula thus include congenital or acquired conditions in which harvest of the flap would result in an unusable flap or a compromised limb. The goal of preoperative arteriography is to identify such patients. For example, a vascular anomaly consisting of a dominant peroneal artery (peroneal arteria magna) exists, in which case harvesting of the fibula could lead to leg ischemia.

Similarly, in patients in whom the radial forearm flap is considered, neurovascular examination of the upper extremity should be performed. An Allen's test will confirm patency of the palmar arch. In cases where the clinical examination would suggest an incomplete arch such that harvest of the radial artery may compromise vascular supply to the hand, imaging is indicated (16).

CONCEPTUAL APPROACH TO RECONSTRUCTION

Segmental mandible resection often leads to composite defects of bone, mucosal lining in the oral cavity, the tongue and supporting structures, and occasionally external skin. As with any type of reconstruction, it is important to restore both form and function. Both the esthetic and functional objectives of reconstruction are best achieved by simultaneously addressing the bone, soft tissue and skin requirements of the defect. The use of osteocutaneous free flaps provides a source of composite tissue, including bone, muscle, fascia and/or skin. One well-planned flap will be adequate to reconstruct the majority of defects.

BONE REPLACEMENT

Bone reconstruction should replace the missing segment of mandible while maintaining proper alignment of the remaining native mandible. In doing so, this will minimize subsequent problems with trismus and malocclusion. Once the decision to reconstruct a segmental defect with vascularized bone has been made, the most important reconstructive choice is flap selection. There are several criteria that should dictate the selection of the donor site. The two most important decisions to be made are the quantity/quality of bone and the amount of skin/soft tissue that is needed. The combination of bone and soft tissue requirements will then establish the choice of flap.

Different segmental resections will require different amounts and qualities of bone for reconstruction. Anterior arch reconstructions, for example, require multiple osteotomies to duplicate the shape of the arch; the bone must be wide enough to take the placement of osseointegrated dental implants and strong enough to withstand the stresses of mastication. Lateral segment defects are less likely to require dental implants and, particularly in the ascending ramus, require smaller quantities of bone. Short segments may not require any osteotomies (3).

DONOR SITE SELECTION

The four osteocutaneous donor sites used most commonly for mandible reconstruction are the fibula, radial forearm, scapula and iliac crest. Each donor site differs with respect to the quality and quantity of available bone and soft tissue, the quality and length of the vascular pedicle and the potential for osseointegrated dental implants (21) (Figure 16.6).

The fibula donor site will be the first choice for a vast majority of patients, particularly those with large bony

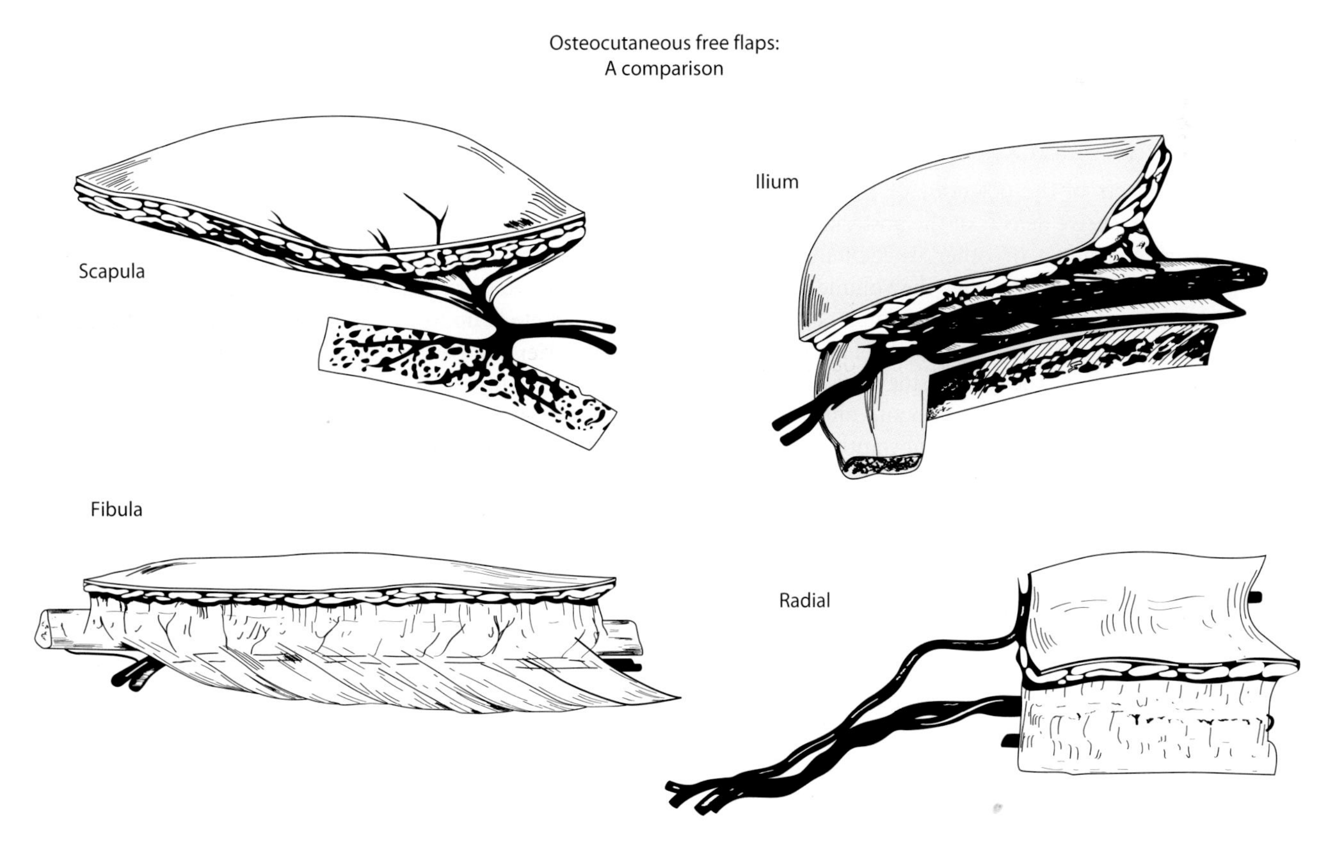

Figure 16.6 Osteocutaneous free flaps for mandible reconstruction.

defects requiring anterior reconstruction and multiple osteotomies. More specifically, the fibula flap is best suited for anterior, lateral or hemi-mandibular reconstructions with small to moderate-sized soft tissue defects of the external skin or intraoral lining.

The radius is sometimes a better alternative for the rare patient who requires a large quantity of thin, pliable skin for intraoral lining and/or who has a small, non-load-bearing lateral bony defect that does not require osteotomy. These defects are less likely to require dental implants and require smaller quantities of bone. An ideal example is a defect of the oropharynx after composite resection of cancer of the tonsil and lateral pharyngeal wall with resection of the ascending ramus of the mandible. By contrast, the radius is a poor choice for composite central defects. The relative lack of both bone and soft tissue bulk with this flap constitutes a strong contraindication for this particular application. Major anterior reconstructions performed with the radius typically have poor lower lip support, an accentuated edentulous appearance and a concavity of the anterior neck soft tissues (2,3).

Similarly, patients with extensive skin and soft tissue defects with minimal bone defects that do not require osteotomy tend to be the best candidates for the scapular osteocutaneous flap. For example, when an extensive soft tissue defect necessitates reconstruction of both the intraoral lining and external skin, the scapular flap may be the best option (2,3).

The iliac crest osteocutaneous flap provides a large amount of bone, with the shape of the crest resembling the hemimandible. However, the bone usually cannot be osteotomized without compromising the blood supply and therefore the shaping of anterior segment mandibular reconstructions becomes less precise. The iliac crest donor site can also be quite deforming and potentially morbid. This flap, therefore, is only indicated when the other options are unavailable (3).

Finally, in defects of the posterior or lateral mandible associated with extensive defects of the posterior and superior soft tissue, the fibula or other osteocutaneous flaps may not be adequate to meet either the volume or surface area requirements of the defect. For example, coverage of multiple zones including the soft palate, lateral inferior pharynx, tonsillar pillars and lateral sulcus of the cheek is often necessary. In addition to the skin and mucosal lining requirements, there are often very substantial soft tissue and volume/space-filling requirements. For example, the resection may include the soft tissue of the lateral pharynx with or without the masseter muscle, which can result in a very large-volume soft tissue defect. Resections extending superiorly into the glenoid fossa and/or all the way up to the temporal bone are also not uncommon. Furthermore, in addition to the mucosal lining, the ablative resection may result in a through-and-through defect extending to the skin, thereby requiring reconstruction of both the intraoral mucosa and external skin. In these circumstances, soft tissue flaps alone, such as the vertical rectus abdominus myocutaneous flap or anterolateral thigh flap, may be required. Composite soft tissue defects can also be closed with a single folded double island flap such as an anterolateral thigh or vertical rectus abdominus myocutaneous, rather than with a fibula skin island, which has a limited rotational degree of freedom around the intramuscular septum (2,21).

FIBULA OSTEOCUTANEOUS FREE FLAP

The fibula has become the flap of choice for reconstruction of most segmental mandibular defects. The exceptional attributes of the fibula flap make this the first choice in the majority of cases, particularly in anterior reconstruction and in patients requiring multiple osteotomies (3).

The fibula flap is based on the peroneal artery, one of three branches of the popliteal artery. In the proximal third of the lower leg, the peroneal artery descends beneath the flexor hallucis longus muscle to reach the medial aspect of the fibula. In the middle third of the fibula at its approximate midpoint, it gives rise to the nutrient artery, providing the major endosteal blood supply. In addition to the nutrient artery, there are usually vessels arising directly from the peroneal artery that supply the fibular diaphysis. Because the fibula has both an interosseous (nutrient artery) and segmental blood supply, multiple osteotomies can be made as close as 2 cm apart without concern for bone viability (22,23).

In fact, the fibula provides up to 26 cm of uniform, bicortical bone. The bone is available with enough length to reconstruct any mandible defect (24). The donor site morbidity is minimized by preserving 5–7 cm of distal fibula at the ankle and 4–6 cm at the knee (21).

The straight quality of the bone with adequate height and thickness makes it the ideal bone stock for precise shaping and receipt of osteointegrated implants. The flexor hallucis longus muscle can be harvested with the flap to provide extra soft tissue bulk. The flexor hallucis longus muscle, which can be harvested with the flap, can also be useful to fill soft tissue defects following neck dissection (2).

The peroneal vessels are of good quality and provide a long pedicle of up to 8 cm in length. The length of the pedicle can be effectively increased by stripping periosteum off the bone in the proximal portion of the flap.

The skin over the lateral aspect of the leg is supplied in part by septocutaneous perforators from the peroneal artery. These reach the skin by means of the posterior intermuscular septum that divides the lateral and posterior compartments. Although these vessels often appear tenuous, they are able to support a skin island raised with the fibular bone flap. We have found that incorporation of the flexor hallucis longus muscle with the flap results in greater reliability of the skin island. The skin island is based upon the perforating vessels, which travel within the posterior crural septum (21). Perforators entering the skin island are usually found at the junction of the middle and distal thirds of the fibula. The skin island component is reliable in approximately 91% of patients (23). When a large skin paddle is harvested, the donor site requires a skin graft for closure (Figures 16.7 through 16.9).

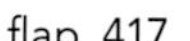

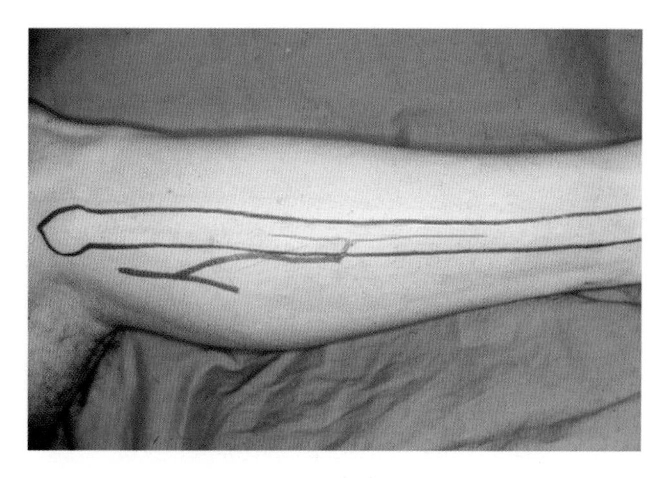

Figure 16.7 Outline of the fibula free flap showing the course of the peroneal artery, the primary blood supply to the fibula free flap.

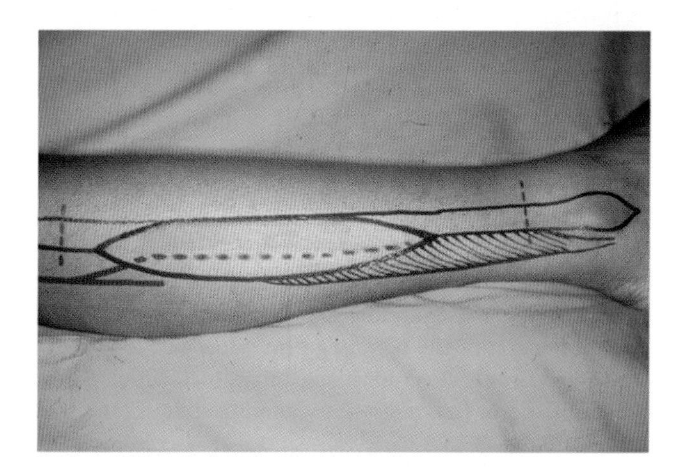

Figure 16.8 Outline of the fibula free flap showing the feasibility of including the flexor hallucis longus muscle and overlying skin in the free flap.

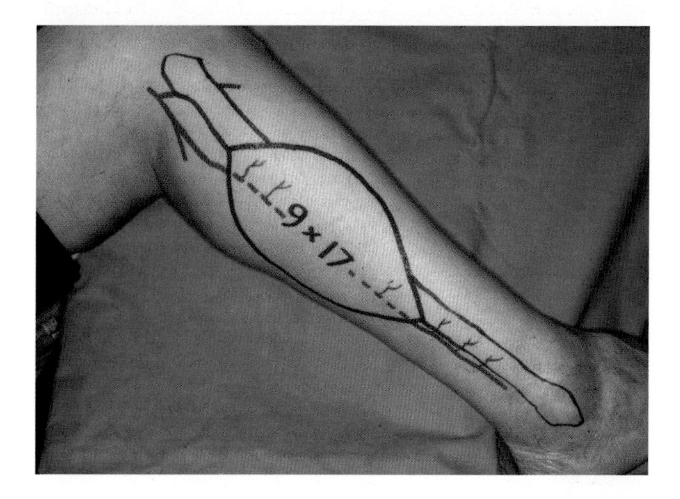

Figure 16.9 A large skin island can be harvested with the fibula free flap.

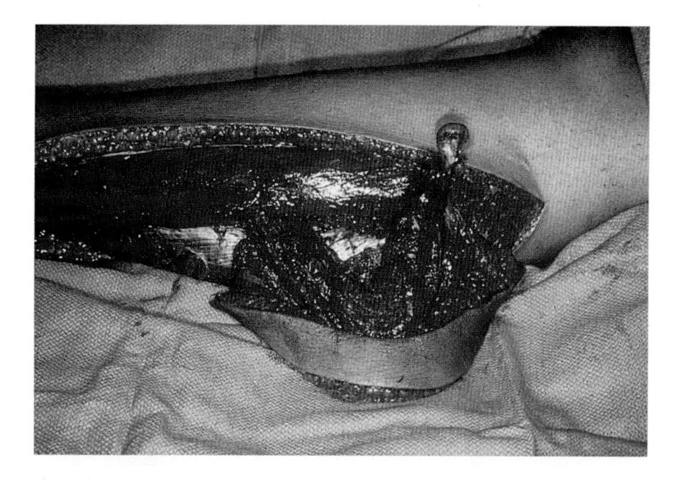

Figure 16.10 The fibula free flap is designed and fabricated at the donor site before transfer to the mandible to reduce ischemia time.

Fibular osteotomies and fixation are performed while the flap is still perfused at the donor site, thereby minimizing ischemia time. It is the ideal flap for simultaneous harvest during oncologic resections because it is located far from the head and neck. There is also minimal donor site morbidity (25) (Figure 16.10).

RADIAL FOREARM OSTEOCUTANEOUS FREE FLAP

The best indication for a radius free flap is a bone defect that is limited to the ascending ramus and the proximal body with a large associated intraoral soft tissue and lining defect. Dental rehabilitation is usually superfluous posteriorly and so the thin nature of the bone is not a factor. The radius is contraindicated for most anterior defects because adequate soft tissue and bone volume are essential in this area for the best functional and esthetic reconstruction.

The radial forearm osteocutaneous flap is based upon the radial artery, associated venae comitantes and cephalic vein (21). The cutaneous portion of the flap comprises the lateral half of the volar surface of the forearm, as well as a third of the posterior surface. It provides tissue that is thin, pliable and abundant. The vascular pedicle is also ideal, with long, large-diameter vessels capable of reaching the opposite side of the neck for difficult recipient vessel problems. The bone, in contrast, is not ideal compared to other choices (2) (Figure 16.11).

The length of bone available is limited and only half of the circumference of the cortex of the bone can be harvested as a graft. The blood supply to this segment of bone is non-segmental and somewhat precarious and therefore osteotomies are not feasible. This flap donor site has the potential for significant morbidity if a fracture of the donor site bone occurs (3).

There is insufficient soft tissue available with this flap to provide the necessary bulk to feel submandibular neck defects. The donor site appearance is often poor postoperatively

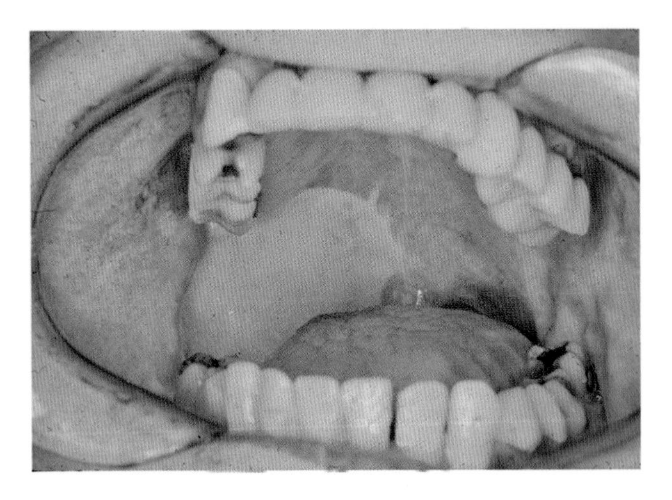

Figure 16.11 Postoperative intraoral view of a patient with reconstruction of a composite defect of resection of the tonsil, pharyngeal wall and ascending ramus of the mandible with a radial forearm osteocutaneous free flap.

owing to the need for a skin graft closure and an additional proximal forearm scar is necessary for obtaining adequate pedicle length.

SCAPULAR OSTEOCUTANEOUS FREE FLAP

The best indication for a scapular free flap in mandible reconstruction is for repair of a small bone gap associated with a large soft tissue defect (2). The major drawback is the marginal quality of the bone, which does not tolerate osteotomies or osseointegration reliably, and the location of the donor site, which prohibits simultaneous harvest of the flap and tumor resection.

The scapular free flap is based on the circumflex scapular artery and vein (21).

One of the advantages of the scapular osteocutaneous free flap is that the bone and the soft tissue components (skin and latissimus dorsi) are independent of each other in terms of their blood supply except for a common vascular pedicle (2) (Figure 16.12). A skin island as long as 30 cm that includes the entire latissimus dorsi muscle can be designed if needed. The blood vessels are reliable and there is minimal donor site morbidity. However, the bone characteristics of this flap are not ideal because the thickness is barely adequate for osteointegrated implants and the maximum length that can be harvested is limited to 14 cm from the lateral scapula. The bone does not have a segmental blood supply and therefore multiple osteotomies can be hazardous for the viability of some portion of the graft (3).

The skin island is somewhat thick compared to the forearm donor site. In addition, the color match is poor for replacement of the external facial skin. Finally, given the donor site location, resection of the tumor and reconstruction of the defect cannot be started simultaneously.

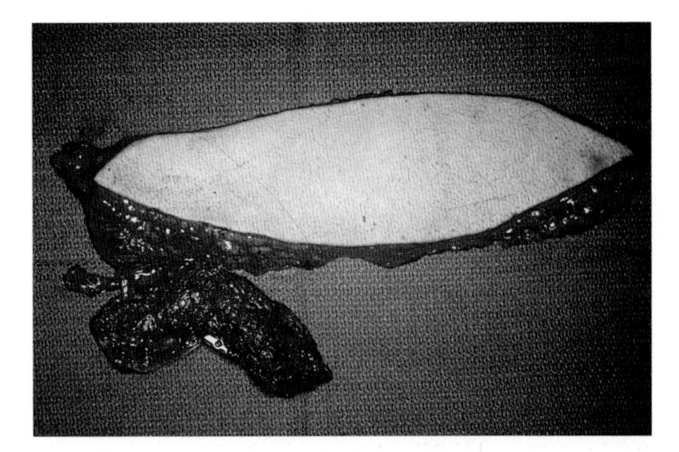

Figure 16.12 A scapula free flap showing an independent bone flap and skin paddle on the same vascular pedicle.

ILIAC CREST OSTEOCUTANEOUS FREE FLAP

A composite flap of ilium with the overlying skin is of limited value in mandible reconstruction. The ilium has abundant bone, but has a predetermined shape that makes graft shaping inherently less precise than in other donor site options (3) (Figure 16.13). The ilium is claimed to have a segmental blood supply from the deep circumflex iliac artery. This type of vascular anatomy is desirable when it is present because it allows segmental osteotomies to be performed with survival of each portion of the bone segment. However, long ilium grafts tend to have less robust, even marginal, circulation at the distal end of the multiply osteotomized graft. The skin

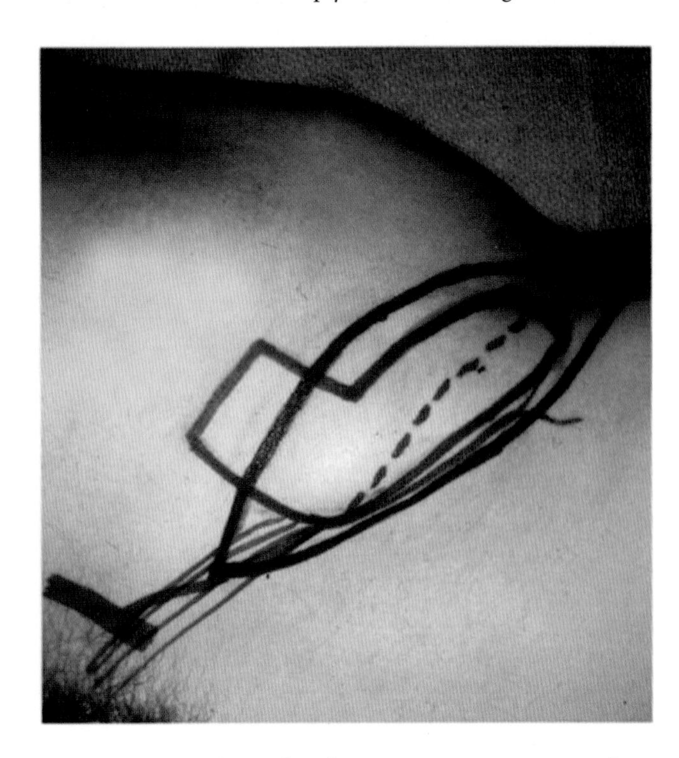

Figure 16.13 Outline of an iliac crest osteocutaneous flap.

island harvested with the ilium does not have a reliable circulation in many patients. In addition, the soft tissue components of the flap are often bulky and lack mobility with respect to the bone. The disadvantages of this flap include a short vascular pedicle and a lack of segmental perforators, which limit the ability to perform osteotomies for graft shaping. The skin island is thick, relatively non-mobile and unreliable. This limits its utility for intraoral reconstruction. In addition, the quantity of bone available is often not sufficient for osseointegration of dental implants (26). Significant morbidity occurs at the donor site because of a difficult closure with associated pain, leading to delayed ambulation. In some patients, a hernia develops at the donor site. Therefore, although abundant bone is available in the ilium free graft, its utility in mandible reconstruction is limited (3).

COMPUTER-ASSISTED MANDIBLE RECONSTRUCTION

Sculpting and designing of any vascularized bone reconstruction to exactly match the resected part of the mandible is a critical step in mandible reconstruction. The development of new technology has introduced approaches to virtual surgical planning by preparation of three-dimensional models of the fibula prior to surgery. Stereolithographic models of both the mandible *in situ* and the fibula can be obtained from computed tomography scan data preoperatively (27). In addition, it is possible to accurately estimate the length of the potential donor bone and the length of the vascular pedicle. These models assist in each step of the operation, including the osteotomies on the mandible for resection and on the fibula for planning reconstruction. Surgical cutting guides are then fabricated and reconstruction plates can be bent according to the model to increase the accuracy and reduce the length of the operation (28,29) (Figures 16.14 through 16.16). When the tumor has destroyed the contour of the lateral cortex of the mandible, a reconstructive plate can be designed by mirroring the contour of the healthy cortical bone on the contralateral hemimandible. If both hemimandibular cortical bones are involved with the tumor, it is possible to use a mandible from a library database that can then be adapted to the upper maxillary dental occlusion of the patient to obtain satisfactory esthetic and functional outcomes.

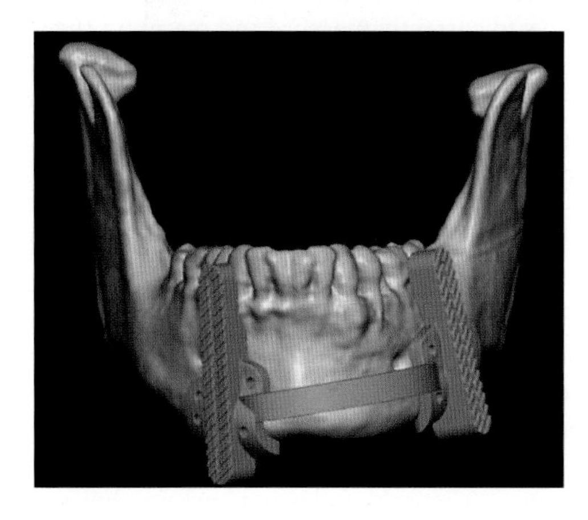

Figure 16.14 CAD-CAM fabricated cutting guides for resection of the mandible. (Courtesy of Evan Matros, MD.)

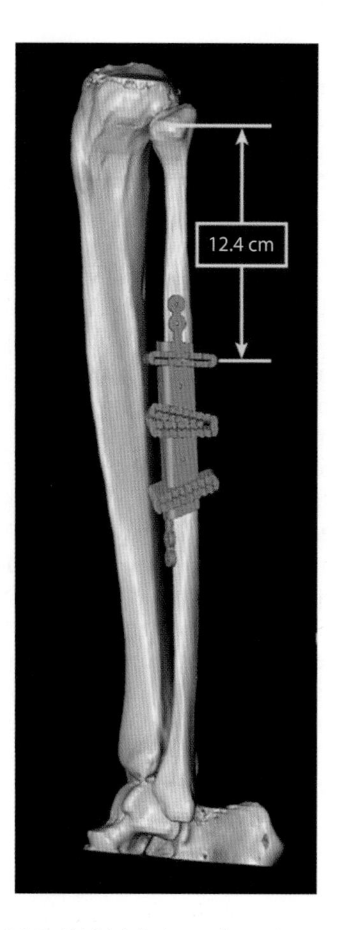

Figure 16.15 CAD-CAM fabricated cutting guides for the fibula free flap. (Courtesy of Evan Matros, MD.)

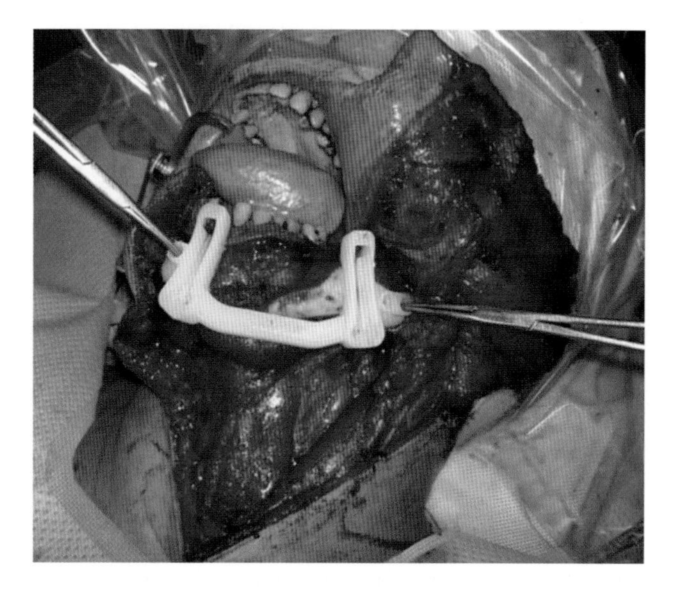

Figure 16.16 Cutting guides applied to the mandible for resection. (Courtesy of Evan Matros, MD.)

Thus, computer-assisted mandible reconstruction requires significant preoperative planning time for accuracy, resulting in greater surgical precision and a reduction in the duration of surgery (30). However, these models are expensive, require an accurate extent of the planned resection and are not easily adaptable to an uncertain surgical approach (31).

There are, however, some potential disadvantages of this technique, which include the cost of designing and prototyping the device, the increased time in preoperative planning and the difficulty in adapting to situations in which the intraoperative surgical plan changes due to unexpected findings during surgery, with either additional or lesser resection (e.g., positive margins on frozen section or reduced extent of bone resection based on intraoperative findings). To better adapt the computer-aided design and computer-aided manufacturing (CAD-CAM) process to intraoperative variations in resection, additional holes are designed, along with a small prolongation of the bone plate, to accommodate for such contingencies.

The postoperative outcomes of conventional methods of mandible reconstruction using templates from radiographs of the native mandible and individual surgeon's judgment versus using the CAD-CAM technology have been compared in both retrospective and prospective studies in small series (32,33). The results of these studies conclude that the esthetic and functional outcomes of both methods are comparable and that there is no particular advantage to the CAD-CAM technology, except a reduction in anesthesia and operating time, with a potential reduction in postoperative morbidity. There is also a possible reduction in cost due to shorter utilization of operating room facilities. Clearly, this has to be balanced against the increased cost of using this technology and the increased time in preoperative planning.

RECONSTRUCTION OF THE CONDYLE

There is one area in mandible reconstruction that deserves special attention and that is the hemimandibulectomy defect, which includes resection of the head of the condyle. If the condyle is not involved with the tumor (as judged by frozen section pathology confirmation of the marrow space and the clinical and radiological impression of the oncologic surgeon), its proximal 2.0–2.5 cm can be transplanted back onto the reconstructed mandible using rigid fixation (Figure 16.17). If it is necessary to resect more than 2 cm above the angle of the mandible, it is often easier to disarticulate the condyle with the specimen and transplant the condyle onto the fibula of the reconstructed mandible. Surgical exposure of the condyle *in situ* in the temporomandibular joint or high ascending ramus risks injury to the facial nerve and limits exposure for rigid fixation. If condyle transplantation is oncologically unsafe, the proximal end of the reconstructed mandible can be rounded to mimic the condyle. It can then be covered with fascia or left alone and inset into the glenoid fossa. A space of 1 cm should be left between the roof of the glenoid fossa and the end of the reconstructed mandible to reduce the risk of ankylosis. Patients generally function well with only one intact temporomandibular joint. There is a greater potential for trismus and malocclusion in this setting compared to condyle transplantation (34).

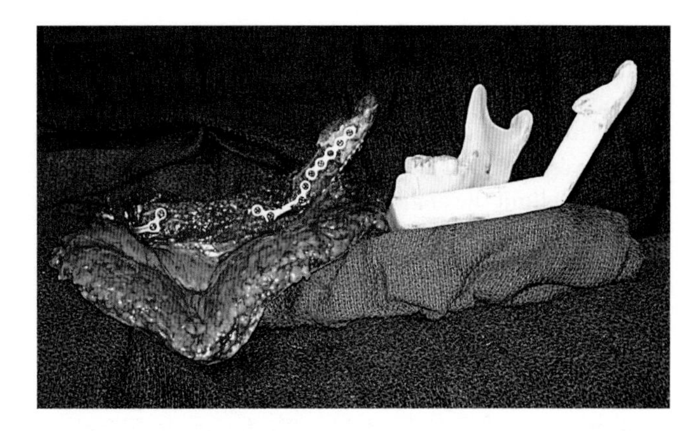

Figure 16.17 Native condylar head transplanted on the fibula free flap. (Courtesy of Evan Matros, MD.)

Several solutions have been recommended ranging from the use of a reconstruction plate incorporating a condylar head to the use of the resected condylar head reapplied as a non-vascularized graft (35). Our approach is to use either transplantation of the native condylar head on the fibula free flap or a modification of the fibula flap where vascularized periosteum is used as an interface between the fibula and the glenoid fossa. The periosteum of the fibula is incised in such a way that there is redundancy when the bone cut is made. The end of the fibula is then drilled down to replicate the size of the resected mandible. It is erroneous to believe that a temporomandibular joint is being reconstructed, but rather the bone is being reduced to the size of the mandibular condyle. The excess periosteum, which is retracted to facilitate the shaping of the fibula, is now pulled over the end of the bone and sutured to itself to provide a soft tissue interface between the bone and the glenoid fossa. It is imperative to correctly measure and maintain the mandibular width and height. Failure to do so not only will result in a deformity of the temporomandibular joint and mandible on the affected side, but also will negatively impact the temporomandibular joint dynamics on the unaffected side (1). The esthetic outcome with fibula free flap reconstruction clearly is superior to any other available free flap today. The patient shown in Figure 16.18 had a fibro-osseous lesion of the body and ascending ramus of the mandible. The surgical specimen of hemimandibulectomy is shown in Figure 16.19. Postoperative panoramic X-ray shows reconstruction of the resected mandible with a fibula free flap requiring multiple osteotomies (Figure 16.20). Postoperative appearance of the patient at 3 months following surgery shows excellent appearance and contour of the face (Figure 16.21).

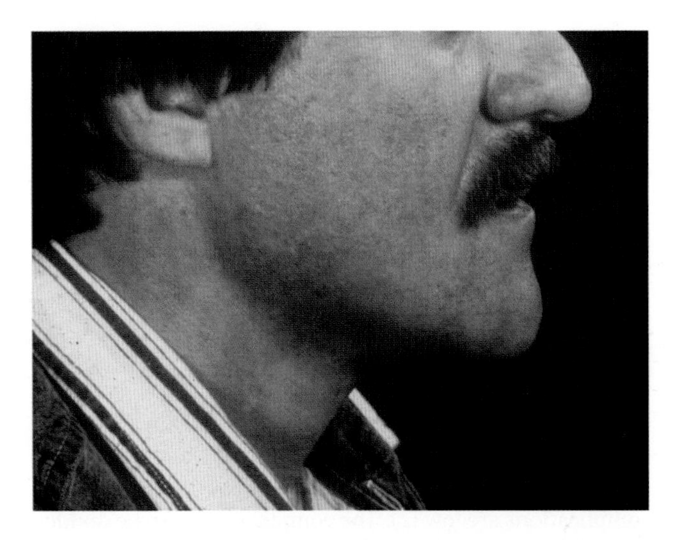

Figure 16.18 Preoperative lateral view of a patient with a fibro-osseous lesion of the right-hand side of the mandible.

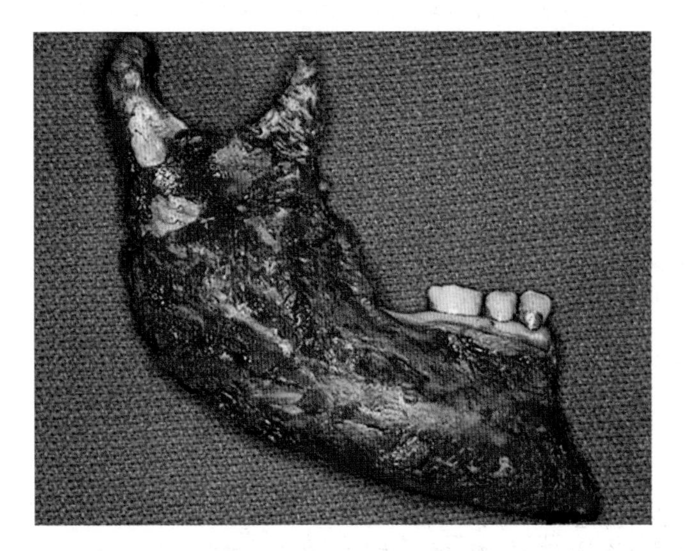

Figure 16.19 Surgical specimen of right hemimandibulectomy.

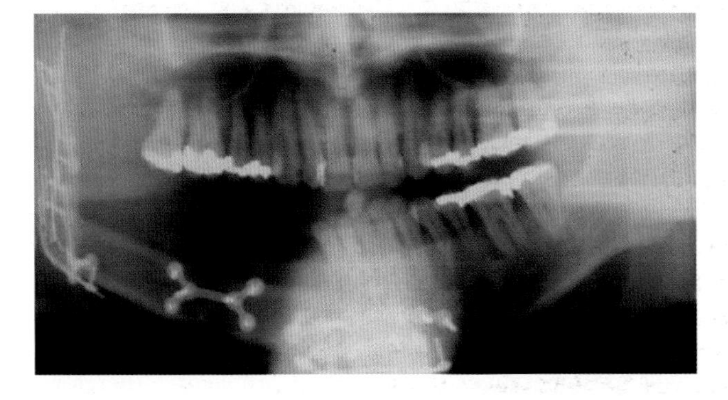

Figure 16.20 Postoperative orthopantomogram showing fibula free flap reconstruction of the right hemimandible with multiple osteotomies.

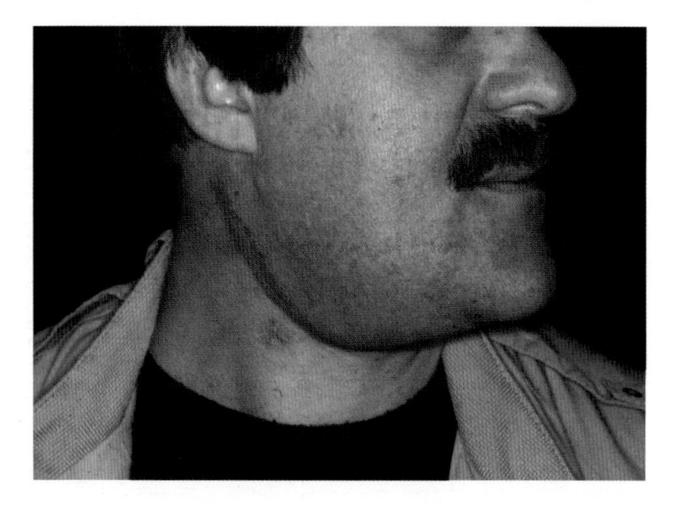

Figure 16.21 Postoperative lateral view of the patient shown in Figure 16.18 at 3 months following surgery.

DENTAL REHABILITATION

Consultation with and involvement of the dental surgeons is valuable in the management of mandible reconstruction patients. Intermaxillary fixation, intraoperative tooth extraction, custom splint fabrication and other ancillary procedures are best performed with the help of dental colleagues. Involvement of the dentist also sets the stage for postoperative dental rehabilitation with either conventional dentures or osseointegrated implants. These implants serve as a permanent foundation on which a dental prosthesis is mounted (21,36).

The obvious advantages of proceeding with osseointegrated implants for dental restoration in the reconstructed mandible are improvement in the esthetic appearance of the patient, restoration of the clarity of speech and restoration of oral competence and mastication. The requirement for successful osseointegration for the implants is the availability of adequate soft tissue coverage over the bone. The vertical height of the bone should be at least 1 cm and the width of the bone should be approximately 5–6 mm. Clearly, the best candidates are patients who are free of the disease and who have accurate reconstruction of the resected mandible. Patients with defects of the anterior arch of the mandible and those in whom no skin island is required for lining in the oral cavity are ideal candidates. Although immediate implants in the fibula at the time of mandible reconstruction have been advocated by some, we recommend that the implants be placed later for the following reasons. Immediate placement of implants has distinct disadvantages, such as: (a) occlusion alignment may not be ideal; (b) the implants may shift during healing of the bone; (c) the presence of the implants adds additional burden to the healing bony flap; and (d) postoperative radiation therapy will create "hot spots" around metallic implants with potential risk of extrusion of the implants. Therefore, secondary replacement of dental implants after complete healing of the fibula free flap is generally preferred. In addition, the miniplates and screws in the region of the site of the implant must be removed before the implants are placed. Thus, it may take up to 2 years before osseointegrated implants are completed with placement of teeth to achieve total mandibular reconstruction and rehabilitation (2,3). On the other hand secondary implants take an inordinate amount of time and expense of multiple procedures, and hospitalizations. Therefore, with the availability of CAD-CAM technology, now a days, primary dental implants are preferred, since they can be accurately placed at the desired locations, and it significantly reduces the time to total dental rehabilitation and cost. For more details, see Chapter 22. For more details, see Chapter 22.

POSTOPERATIVE CARE

Due to the prolonged nature of surgery for free flap mandible reconstruction and its consequent swelling of the upper aerodigestive tract, most patients will require a prophylactic tracheostomy as well as a nasogastric feeding tube. In addition, due to the need for fluid balance management, these patients need a central venous catheter and often an arterial line for monitoring oxygenation. Furthermore, monitoring of the perfusion of the flap is vital to ensure the viability of the flap. A surface Doppler along the course of the vascular pedicle is employed. Also, visual check for skin color (if a skin paddle is used) is employed on an hourly basis.

For optimal pulmonary clearance of secretions, frequent suctioning through the tracheostomy tube is required in the first 24 hours. The patient is taken off ventilatory support as soon as possible (within 24 hours) and is encouraged to do deep breathing exercises. A respiratory therapist attends to the patient for pulmonary support. Fluid balance is maintained for optimal urine output. If fluid overload is present, then fluid restriction and diuresis may be required. Intraoperatively, patients wear dynamic compression boots for prevention of venous thrombosis in the lower extremity. In many surgical units, routine administration of low-dose heparin or heparin analogues is also employed. The patient is encouraged to ambulate out of bed with support as early as possible, generally in 6–8 days. The compression boots are discontinued and patient is encouraged to do foot and leg exercises in bed within 24–48 hours. Anticoagulants are tapered off in 10 days. Nutrition is initiated through the nasogastric feeding tube as soon as the patient is awake and taken off the ventilatory support. Tube feedings are maintained until complete healing of the intraoral suture line and the patient is able to swallow his/her saliva. Constipation is a common complication in the postoperative period due to feeding with liquid formula. Therefore, stool softeners are recommended, beginning on the third day following surgery. Most patients are able to ambulate by the end of 1 week with the assistance of a walker. The tracheostomy tube is removed once the patient is ambulatory, the facial and oral swelling has reduced and the patient is able to breathe comfortably with a plug on the tracheostomy tube. In most patients, the nasogastric feeding tube and the tracheostomy tube are removed by the end of 1 week. A majority of patients are able to be discharged from the hospital by between 8 and 10 days following surgery.

COMPLICATIONS AND SIDE EFFECTS

In general, surgical complications following mandible reconstruction are few. In spite of the length and complexity of these surgical procedures, the frequency and severity of complications are low (2). The complications can be divided into: (a) locoregional at the site of surgery; or (b) systemic.

The local complications are largely related to flap viability due to compromised perfusion of the flap. This may lead to partial or complete flap failure. It may also cause significant wound healing problems including wound breakdown, necrosis, fistula formation and delayed healing, occasionally requiring secondary surgical intervention. Fortunately, the incidence of flap failure in most reported series is less than 5%. Similarly, wound healing problems can also occur at the donor site. In patients with compromised venous circulation in the lower extremity, delayed wound healing can lead to the need for prolonged wound care. Similarly, in the case of an ilial flap, abdominal wall hernia is a complication that may need secondary repair. The large field of muscular dissection in the scapula free flap occasionally leads to the formation of a seroma. In the case of the radial forearm free flap, exposure of tendons in spite of using a skin graft can be a tenacious problem, leading to contracture. Wound infection and cellulitis can occur at any site and will require appropriate treatment with antibiotics (2).

Late complications of free flap mandible reconstruction are largely related to tissue atrophy in the bone and soft tissues. These sequelae often produce esthetic and functional debility. Rarely, however, secondary efforts at further reconstruction are warranted. Occasionally, the fibula free flap may produce over-projection or recession of the chin, which produces significant esthetic morbidity. This is very difficult to correct. Similarly, alignment of the fibula accurately to the lower border of the native mandible to restore the contour of the jaw line is crucial, otherwise this may lead to contour discrepancy and its negative impact on esthetics (2).

Systemic complications are related to the patient's age, general medical condition, nutrition and cardiopulmonary status. In addition, the prolonged anesthesia and fluid overload commonly seen in long operations add to the immediate postoperative management problems. Therefore, optimization of patient cardiopulmonary status preoperatively and restricting fluid overload intraoperatively are crucial in preventing systemic complications. Management of systemic complications requires the involvement of a multidisciplinary team in an intensive care setup for close monitoring and appropriate interventions.

CONCLUSION

Microvascular free flap reconstruction is currently the best method of mandible reconstruction, with very high success rates with good to excellent esthetic and functional results in the majority of patients (21). Lateral and anterior defects constitute two distinct types of reconstructive problems. Mandible reconstruction has reached such a level of sophistication that we can predictably offer our patients good results with minimal donor site morbidity. The fibula osteocutaneous flap is currently the most popular and arguably the most effective reconstructive option and has become the gold standard for this challenging surgical defect (1).

The exceptional attributes of the fibula donor site make this the first choice in the majority of cases, particularly in anterior reconstruction and in patients requiring multiple osteotomies. The radius can be a better alternative for patients requiring a large quantity of thin, pliable skin for oral cavity lining, with a small lateral bone defect not requiring osteotomy. Patients with extensive skin and soft tissue defects with minimal bone defects tend to be the best candidates for the scapula flap. The ilium is recommended only when no other options are available. Osseointegration is recommended in cases in which bone is not irradiated, particularly in anterior defects (21).

REFERENCES

1. Neligan PC, Novak CB, Gullane PJ. Mandibular reconstruction. In: Guyuron B (ed). *Plastic Surgery: Indications and Practise,* Saunders, Philadelphia: Expert Consult Premium Edition, 2010, 1111.
2. Disa JJ, Hidalgo DA. Mandible reconstruction. In: Thorne CH, Chung KC, Gosain AK et al (eds). *Grabb and Smith's Plastic Surgery* (7th edition). Philadelphia: Wolters Kluwer Health/Lippincott Williams & Wilkins, 2014, 1311–2.
3. Shah JP, Patel SG, Singh B. (eds). Reconstructive surgery. In: *Jatin Shah's Head and Neck Surgery and Oncology* (4th Edition). Philadelphia: Elsevier/Mosby, 2012, 712–51.
4. Ivy R, Epes BM. Bone grafting for defects of the mandible. *Milit Surg* 1927;60:286–300.
5. Blocker TC, Stout RA. Mandibular reconstruction, World War II. *Plast Reconstr Surg* 1949;4:153–7.
6. Millard DR Jr, Deane M, Garst WP. Bending an iliac bone graft for anterior mandibular arch repair. *Plast Reconstr Surg* 1971;48:600–2.
7. Phillips CM. Primary and secondary reconstruction of the mandible after ablative surgery. *Am J Surg* 1967;114:601–4.
8. Kudo K, Fujioka Y. Review of bone grafting for reconstruction of discontinuity defects of the mandible. *J Oral Surg* 1978;36:791–3.
9. Obwegeser HL. Simultaneous resection and reconstruction of parts of the mandible *via* the intraoral route in patients without gross infections. *Oral Surg Oral Med Oral Pathol* 1966;21:693–705.
10. Lawson W, Loscalzo LJ, Baek SM et al. Experience with immediate and delayed mandibular reconstruction. *Laryngoscope* 1982;92:5–10.
11. Brown JB, Fryer MP, Kollias P et al. Silicon and Teflon prosthesis, including full jaw substitution: laboratory and clinical studies of etheron. *Ann Surg* 1963;157:932–43.
12. Leake DL, Rappoport M. Mandibular reconstruction: bone induction in an alloplastic tray. *Surgery* 1972;72:332–6.
13. Terz JJ, Bear SE, Brown PW et al. An evaluation of the wire meshes prosthesis in primary reconstruction of the mandible. *Am J Surg* 1978;135:825–7.
14. Chow JM, Hill JH. Primary mandibular reconstruction using the AO reconstruction plate. *Laryngoscope* 1986;96:768–73.
15. Snyder CC, Bateman JM, Davis CW, Warden GD. Mandibulo-facial restoration with live osteocutaneous flaps. *Plast Reconstr Surg* 1970;45:14–9.
16. Disa JJ, Cordeiro PG. The current role of preoperative arteriography in free fibula flaps. *Plast Reconstr Surg* 1998;102:1083–8.
17. Davidson J, Boyd B, Gullane P et al. A comparison of the results following oromandibular reconstruction using a radial forearm flap with either radial bone or reconstructive plate. *Plast Reconstr Surg* 1991;88:201–8.
18. Payne WG, Naidu DK, Wheeler CK, Barkoe D, Mentis M, Salas RE, Smith DJ Jr, Robson MC. Wound healing in patients with cancer. *Eplasty* 2008;8:e9.
19. Disa C. Mandibular reconstruction with microvascular surgery. *Semin Surg Oncol* 2000;19:226–34.
20. Shah JP, Gil Z. Current concepts in management of oral cancer—surgery. *Oral Oncol* 2009;45:394–401.
21. Disa C. Mandibular reconstruction with microvascular surgery. *Semin Surg Oncol* 2000;19:226–34.
22. Hanasono MD. Important aspects of head and neck reconstruction. *Plast Reconstr Surg* 2014;134:968e–80e.
23. Hidalgo DA. Fibula free flap: a new method of mandible reconstruction. *Plast Reconstr Surg* 1989;84:71–9.
24. Hidalgo DA. Aesthetic improvements in free-flap mandible reconstruction. *Plast Reconstr Surg* 1991;88:574–85. discussion 586–7.
25. Cordeiro PG, Disa JJ, Hidalgo DA, Hu QY. Reconstruction of the mandible with osseous free flaps: a 10-year experience with 150 consecutive patients. *Plast Reconstr Surg* 1999;104:1314–20.

26. Shenaq SM, Klebuc MJ. The iliac crest microsurgical free flap in mandibular reconstruction. *Clin Plast Surg* 1994;21:37–44.
27. Pellini R, Mercante G, Spriano G. Step-by-step mandibular reconstruction with free fibula flap modelling. *Acta Otorhinolaryngol Ital* 2012;32:405–9.
28. Hirsch DL, Garfein ES, Christensen AM et al. Use of computer-aided design and computer-aided manufacturing to produce orthognathically ideal surgical outcomes: a paradigm shift in head and neck reconstruction. *J Oral Maxillofac Surg* 2009;67:2115–22.
29. Mazzoni S, Marchetti C, Sgarzani R, Cipriani R, Scotti R, Ciocca L. Prosthetically guided maxillofacial surgery: evaluation of the accuracy of a surgical guide and custom-made bone plate in oncology patients after mandibular reconstruction. *Plast Reconstr Surg* 2013;131:1376–85.
30. Succo G, Berrone M, Battiston B et al. Step-by-step surgical technique for mandibular reconstruction with fibular free flap: application of digital technology in virtual surgical planning. *Eur Arch Otorhinolaryngol* 2015;272:1491–501.
31. Moro A, Cannas R, Boniello R et al. Techniques on modeling the vascularized free fibula flap in mandibular reconstruction. *J Craniofac Surg* 2009;20:1571–3.
32. Ritschl LM, Mücke T, Fichter A, Güll FD, Schmid C, Duc JM, Kesting MR, Wolff KD, Loeffelbein DJ. Functional outcome of CAD/CAM-assisted versus conventional microvascular, fibular free flap reconstruction of the mandible: a retrospective study of 30 cases. *J Reconstr Microsurg* 2017;33(4):281–91. doi: 10.1055/s-0036-1597823. Epub January 18, 2017.
33. Ritschl LM, Mücke T, Fichter AM, Roth M, Kaltenhauser C, Pho Duc JM, Kesting MR, Wolff KD, Loeffelbein DJ. Axiographic results of CAD/CAM-assisted microvascular, fibular free flap reconstruction of the mandible: a prospective study of 21 consecutive cases. *J Craniomaxillofac Surg* 2017;45:113–9.
34. Hidalgo DA. Condyle transplantation in free flap mandible reconstruction. *Plast Reconstr Surg* 1994;93:770–83.
35. Tarsitano A, Battaglia S, Ramieri V, Cascone P, Ciocca L, Scotti R, Marchetti C. Short-term outcomes of mandibular reconstruction in oncological patients using a CAD-CAM prosthesis including a condyle supporting a fibular free flap. *J Craniomaxillofac Surg* 2017;45:330–7.
36. Frodel JL Jr, Funk GF, Capper DT et al. Osseointegrated implants: a comparative study of bone thickness in four vascularized bone flaps. *Plast Reconstr Surg* 1993;92:449–55.

17

Reconstructive surgery: Maxilla

RALPH W. GILBERT

BASIC CONCEPTS

The past 30 years have seen a remarkable transformation and development of options for reconstruction of the maxilla. The fundamental tenet that all defects of the maxilla should be reconstructed with a prosthetic device has been transformed into a selective approach based on remarkable innovation in the use of myo-osseous or osteocutaneous free tissue transfer and the use of osseointegrated implants for comprehensive and functional dental restoration. The current approach integrates therapeutic decision-making, selecting the right reconstruction for the right patient based on maxillary defect extent and patient-specific goals and objectives.

GOALS OF RECONSTRUCTION

The goals of reconstruction are to restore the oral cavity functions of speech, mastication and swallowing, while minimizing esthetic contour deformities and in some cases correcting facial deformity. In order to achieve these goals, the reconstructive technique must create functional closure of the palate defect and at the same time create the opportunity for functional dentition. When a maxillary obturator is used, these objectives are met with a retained prosthetic device or in some cases an implant retained prosthesis through the use of zygomatic osseointegrated implants (1). When a reconstructive approach is used, the reconstruction should ideally close the palate with a mucosally lined surface or an equivalent and contain bone that is appropriately placed to allow the use of osseointegrated implants for dental restoration. The reconstructions should also allow the recreation of the facial skeleton in order to maintain normal facial contour.

A number of options exist to achieve these goals, ranging from the use of obturators, to a combination of techniques including vascularized bone and soft tissue with implant retained dental restoration. Numerous authors have described the use of free non-osseous myocutaneous flaps such as the rectus abdominus or latissimus dorsi flap for extensive infrastructure defects of the maxilla (2). In the palliative setting, these non-osseous options may be suitable; however, in the majority of patients, this option eliminates the ability to prosthetically restore dentition and does not meet the fundamental goals of maxillary reconstruction. We prefer the use of myo-osseous or osseocutaneous flaps in the majority of maxillary defects in order to provide the opportunity for prosthetic reconstruction of dentition and recreation of the skeletal structure of the midface.

CLASSIFICATION OF MAXILLARY DEFECTS

In order to discuss and describe maxillary reconstruction, it is useful to have a classification system of defects that allows for appropriate description and the development of treatment algorithms based on defect and patient factors.

In North America, two classifications have been described: the Okay classification (3) and the Memorial classification (2). The Okay classification is a defect-based classification based on suitability for prosthetic reconstruction, while the Memorial classification described by Cordeiro and Santamaria is based on a surgical reconstructive paradigm. In Europe, a defect-based classification based on suitability for prosthetic reconstruction described by Brown and Shaw (4) is widely used. In our institution, we prefer the Brown classification, as in our view it provides an appropriate classification for defect description and allows the development of treatment-specific paradigms. The Brown classification is illustrated in Figure 17.1 and has two component classifications for maxillary defects: the vertical extent class I–IV and the horizontal component A–D. Class I defects do not created an oronasal fistula, class II defects involve the resection of the maxilla without involvement of the orbital floor, class III defects include the orbit with preservation of the orbital contents and class IV defects include an orbital exenteration. The horizontal definitions are as follows: type A defects—not involving the alveolus; type B defects—involving half or less unilaterally; type C defects—involving half or less bilaterally or anteromedially; and type D defects—involving more than half of the infrastructure of the maxilla.

CLASS I DEFECTS

Class I defects are relatively rare in surgical practice and do not result in oronasal fistulae. Numerous options exist to resurface the palate, including a mucosal graft, palatal island rotation flap, buccal fat flap and rotation flaps, including the facial artery myomucosal flap in non-dentate maxillae or posterior defects. Some authors have described the use of the forearm flap to resurface larger defects.

CLASS IIA

Class IIA refers to defects involving less than half of the horizontal component of the palate without involvement of the alveolus. These defects can be reconstructed with a key-style obturator or with soft tissue and rarely need bone reconstruction. If a tissue reconstruction is desired, the best local flap is the palatal island rotation flap, particularly for more posteriorly placed defects. Other options for posterior defects include the temporalis flap or temporoparietal fascial flap. In larger defects, the preferred option is usually the free forearm flap as the flexibility of pedicle positions makes it ideal for large central palate reconstructions.

Class IIA maxilla defect: palatal island rotation flap

The palatal island rotation flap as described by Gullane and Arena (5,6) has great utility in palatal reconstruction. The flap based on the greater palatine vessels is a local rotation flap based on one vascular pedicle. The flap is harvested in a subperiosteal plane and great care must be taken to avoid stretching or traumatizing the pedicle. The flap occasionally has issues with venous congestion and partial losses are common in larger flaps. The donor site defect re-mucosalizes quickly and is not a major issue in patient recovery (Figure 17.2).

Class IIA maxilla defect: forearm flap for central palate

In central palate defects extending into the pre-maxilla such as cleft patients, the forearm flap can be an excellent reconstructive option. The only issue in using this flap is the path of the vascular pedicle, which must traverse the medial and anterior maxillary walls through the maxillary sinus before extending through the buccal space to the facial vessels. This can be easily accomplished through a traditional sublabial Caldwell–Luc approach with the pedicle traversing the lateral wall of the nose, passing through the maxillary sinus and extending to the facial vessels in the soft tissue space between the facial musculature and the buccinator (Figure 17.3).

CLASS IIB

Class IIB defects involve the infrastructure of the maxilla and less than half of the palate. These defects can range from posterior alveolar defects to the standard

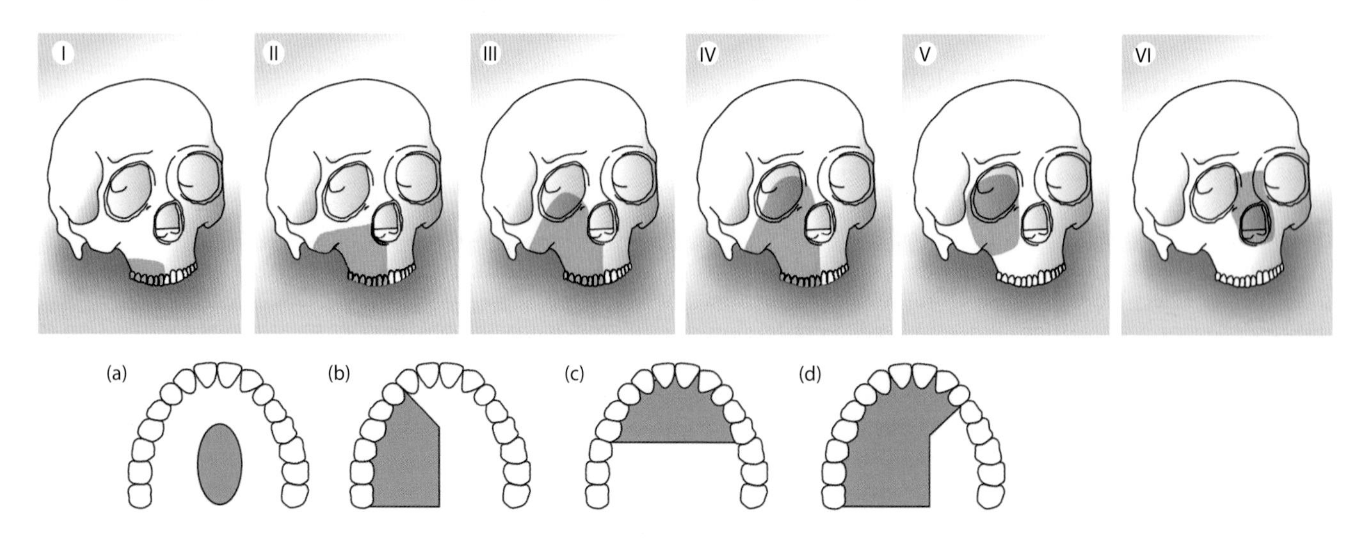

Figure 17.1 Brown classification of maxillary defects.

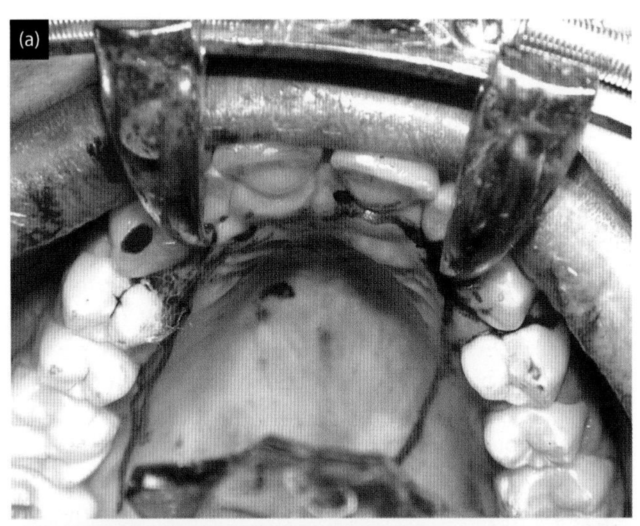

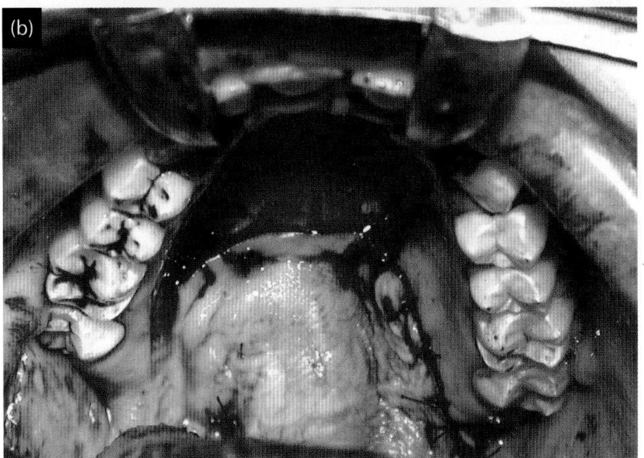

Figure 17.2 Palatal island rotation flap illustration.

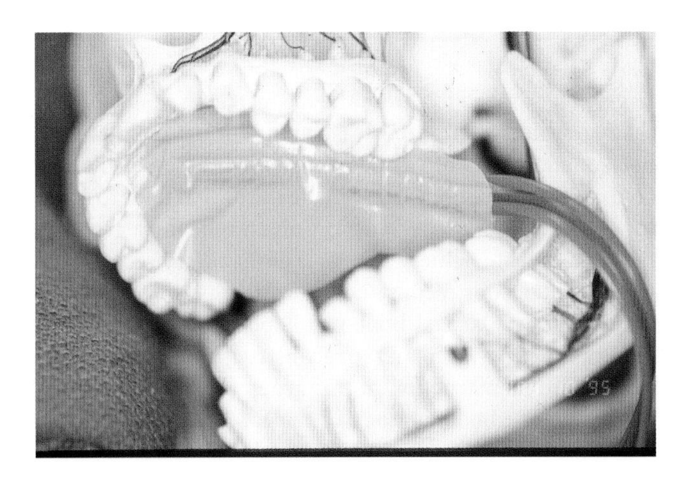

Figure 17.3 Forearm flap for class IIA, with extension through the maxillary sinus.

hemi-maxillectomy defects. Numerous options exist for these defects, including obturation, local flap reconstruction in posterior defects, free fasciocutaneous transfers and myo-osseous bone transfers. In patients with small posterior defects where prosthetic dental reconstruction is not required or would not be functional, we prefer the free

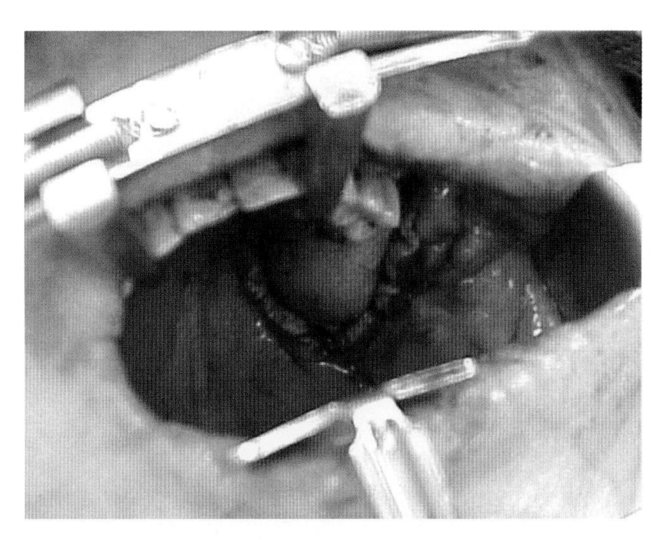

Figure 17.4 Maxillary tuberosity and alveolus reconstruction with forearm.

forearm flap or the anterolateral thigh flap (Figure 17.4). In patients with extensive defects, bone reconstruction is desired for optimal dental and esthetic reconstruction. In this case, three options exist: the horizontally positioned deep circumflex iliac artery (DCIA) myo-osseous flap (7,8); the osseocutaneous fibular flap (9,10); and the osseocutaneous thoracodorsal artery scapular tip (TDAST) (11,12).

Class IIB maxilla: horizontal myo-osseous DCIA

The DCIA flap has many unique advantages in infrastructure maxillary reconstruction. Two-team surgery including ablation and flap harvest is easily accomplished, the bone quality is ideal for osseointegrated implants and there is an ample bone supply for reconstruction. Disadvantages of this flap include the short vascular pedicle, a problem partially addressed by moving the harvested bone segment back from the anterior superior iliac spine. The major issue with this flap is donor site morbidity including late hernia formation and donor site pain. The hernia risk can be reduced by replacing the harvested internal oblique muscle with an appropriate alloplastic mesh; however, there may be long-term issues with mesh extrusion.

Class IIB maxilla defect: the osseocutaneous free fibular transfer

The osseocutaneous free fibular transfer has been widely used for maxillary reconstruction, particularly for complex defects of the maxilla. The advantages are the length of the vascular pedicle and available bone quality for osseointegrated implantation. In addition, because of the periosteal blood supply, the fibula can be osteotomized into unique shapes that closely approximate the resected structures. The disadvantages are the complexity of osteotomies in creating a three-dimensional maxilla and the risk of non-vascularized

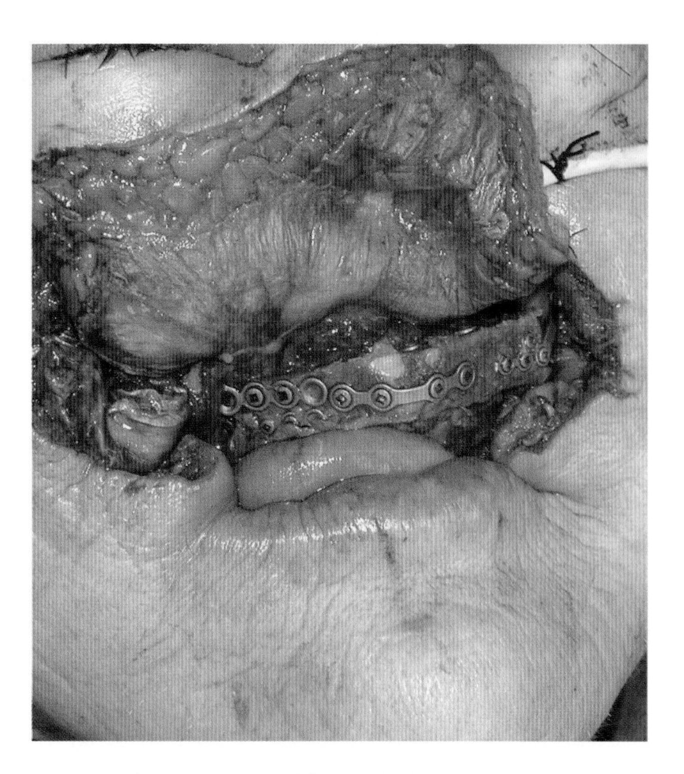

Figure 17.5 Illustration of fibular flap geometry for maxillary reconstruction.

segments (Figure 17.5). The skin island can be relatively mobile from the bone, which can create a problem for the implant interface. The donor site is well tolerated but in some older patients can be problematic in terms of gait disturbance. One unique feature of the fibular site is the ability to prefabricate an implanted maxilla in the leg. Through the use of virtual surgical planning, some groups have been able to plan the implant position and create implant retained maxillary reconstruction with dental restoration in a single procedure (13).

Class IIB maxilla defect: osseocutaneous TDAST

The osseocutaneous TDAST flap is an excellent option in infrastructure maxillary defects, particularly when placed horizontally. The pedicle can be up to 12 cm in length, making the selection of high-risk recipient vessels less of an issue. The scapula has a natural shape for maxilla reconstruction as it has been shown to almost uniformly match the native maxilla in contour. The major potential disadvantages of the flap are the bone quality for osseointegration, particularly in older female patients, and the inability to two-team the flap harvest. The flap can be harvested without repositioning the patient during the surgical procedure and the donor site morbidity appears to be limited, making it an excellent choice in older patients.

CLASS IIC

Classes IIC defects for the most part involve anterior defects of the maxilla and are often infrastructure defects that may also involve the central lip and nose. Obturation can be used in this site, but is problematic in patients without dentition. Most significantly, these defects require bone reconstruction for projection of the nose and midface in order to avoid a dramatic facial deformity. The options for reconstruction include the osseocutaneous radial forearm, the osseocutaneous fibula and the TDAST flap. Our preference is to avoid the osseocutaneous forearm flap for high-volume bone reconstruction given the poor quality of the available bone and the need to prophylactically plate the distal radius to avoid fracture. Of the other available flaps, the best choices are likely the TDAST and the osseocutaneous fibula. We prefer these largely because the midline location of the deformity requires a particularly long vascular pedicle and the bone available from these flaps is ideally suited to this defect.

CLASS IID

Class IID defects represent a group of patients with extensive infrastructure defects of the maxilla. In these patients, obturation is usually not an effective option as little normal bone and few dental elements remain to maintain a stable and functional prosthetic rehabilitation. The current reconstructive options include the DCIA, osseocutaneous fibula and TDAST flaps. Each of these flaps has advantages and disadvantages and flap selection should be based on patient and defect factors. We favor the use of the TDAST flap because of its limited donor site morbidity. As outlined earlier, in our opinion, this defect should never be reconstructed with a myocutaneous flap as this reconstructive option merely closes the palate defect and does not address any of the major functional issue with this defect.

CLASS IIIB, IIIC AND IIID

Class III defects are grouped together as they represent largely the same defect from the reconstructive perspective; that is, orbital floor and infrastructure of the maxilla with horizontal defects of various extents. In these defects, the goal of reconstruction is to recreate the orbital floor to allow for orbital prosthetic reconstruction and the infrastructure of the maxilla to achieve the goals of maxillary reconstruction. Orbital floor reconstruction can be performed either with non-vascularized bone or alloplasts provided this is accompanied by vascularized reconstruction of the maxilla. Maxillary reconstruction in this group of patients involves recreating the bone contour of the face of the maxilla to maintain the soft tissue contour of the infraorbital structures. In this defect, the options for reconstruction include the DCIA, osseocutaneous fibula and TDAST flaps.

Class IIIB, IIIC and IIID maxilla defect: vertically positioned DCIA with internal oblique

This reconstruction, originally described by Brown (8), is an excellent option for reconstructing this complex defect.

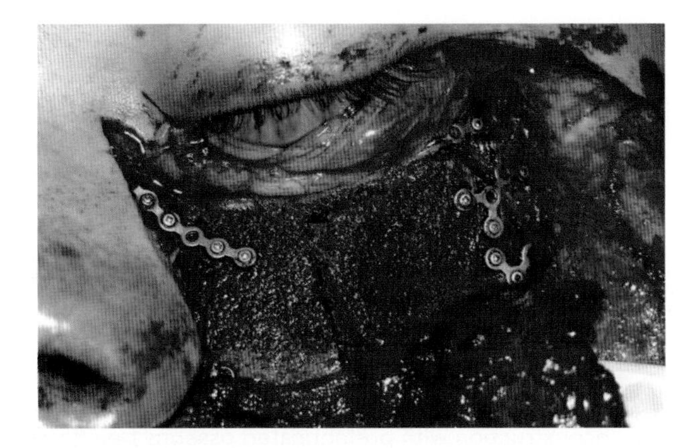

Figure 17.6 Illustration of iliac crest transfer for infrastructure reconstruction.

In this case, the DCIA is positioned vertically, with the internal oblique used to close the horizontal aspects of the infrastructure of the maxilla. It has the same limitations as when used in the horizontal defect, but provides outstanding bone quality for osseointegrated implants. The bone construct usually requires a single osteotomy and there is sufficient bone available to reconstruct the orbital floor with non-vascularized bone (Figure 17.6).

Class IIIB, IIIC and IIID maxilla defect: osseocutaneous fibular flap

The osseocutaneous fibular flap is an excellent option for this defect. The bone can be sectioned into a three-dimensional shape with three or four bone segments. The fibular flap is technically complicated, particularly the planning of the osteotomies, and requires significant preoperative planning facilitated by the use of virtual surgical planning.

Class IIIB, IIIC and IIID maxilla defect: osseocutaneous TDAST

The TDAST flap has significant advantages in this defect. The scapular can be positioned vertically, with the lateral edge of the scapula placed inferiorly and the tip placed anteriorly. The horizontal elements of the infrastructure of the maxilla are repaired with a large cuff of teres major muscle and the natural shape of the scapula usually mitigates the need for an osteotomy. There is available bone in the scapula to acquire a non-vascularized bone graft for the orbital floor, which often perfectly replaces the natural shape of the orbit. A significant advantage of this flap is the long vascular pedicle mitigating the risk of a short pedicle and issues with revascularization (Figure 17.7).

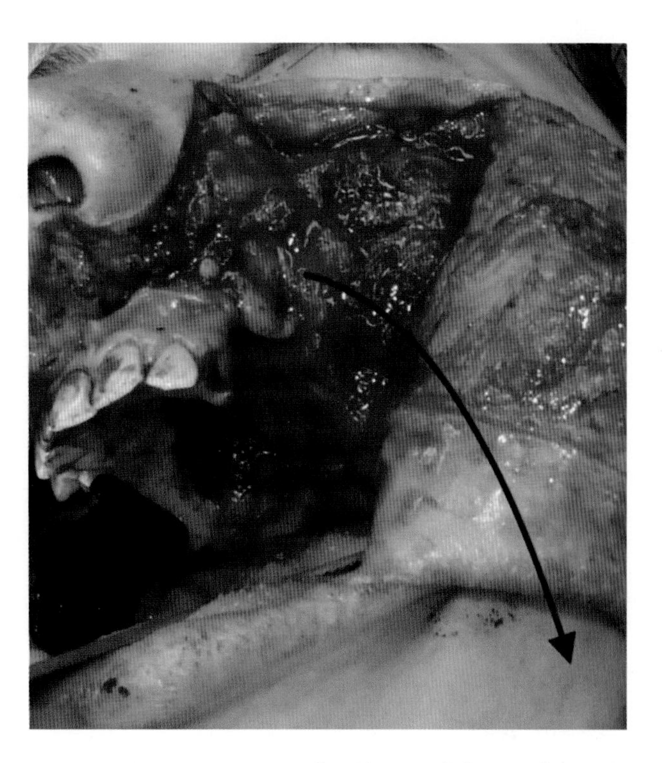

Figure 17.7 Reconstruction for Class III defect with TDAST flap (arrow is pedicle position).

CONCLUSION

Reconstruction of the maxilla has developed dramatically in the past three decades. Patients treated today have numerous options extending from the most simple—obturation—to the most complicated—two-stage, virtually planned, implant retained free tissue transfer with primary dental restoration. This defect site demands the most sophisticated and complex reconstructions currently performed in head and neck surgery. Patients with ablative maxillary defects are best managed by surgeons with a clear understanding of the principles of reconstruction of each of these unique defects. The reconstructive head and neck surgeon taking on these patients and defects must have a broad repertoire and experience with a wide variety of reconstructive options to optimally rehabilitate this complex group of patients. These patients are likely best served by being treated in centers that have a functional multidisciplinary team including head and neck oncology, reconstructive microsurgery and maxillofacial prosthetics.

REFERENCES

1. Schmidt BL, Pogrel M, Young CW, et al. Reconstruction of extensive v zygomaticus implants. *J Oral Maxillofac Surg* 2004;62:82–9.
2. Cordeiro PG, Santamaria E. A classification system and algorithm for reconstruction of maxillectomy and midfacial defects. *Plast Reconstr Surg* 2000;105:2331–46.
3. Okay DJ, Genden E, Buchbinder D, et al. Prosthodontic guidelines for surgical reconstruction of the maxilla: a classification system of defects. *J Prosthet Dent* 2001;86:352–63.

4. Brown JS, Shaw RJ. Reconstruction of the maxilla and midface: introducing a new classification. *Lancet Oncol* 2010;11:1001–8.
5. Gullane PJ, Arena S. Palatal island flap for reconstruction of oral defects. *Arch Otolaryngol* 1977;103:598–9.
6. Gullane PJ, Arena S. Extended palatal island mucoperiosteal flap. *Arch Otolaryngol* 1985;111:330–2.
7. Brown J, Jones D, Summerwill A, et al. Vascularized iliac crest with internal oblique muscle for immediate reconstruction after maxillectomy. *Brit J Oral Max Surg* 2002;40:183–90.
8. Brown JS. Deep circumflex iliac artery free flap with internal oblique muscle as a new method of immediate reconstruction of maxillectomy defect. *Head Neck* 1996;18:412–21.
9. Futran ND, Mendez E. Developments in reconstruction of midface and maxilla. *Lancet Oncol* 2006;7:249–58.
10. Futran ND, Wadsworth JT, Villaret D, et al. Midface reconstruction with the fibula free flap. *Arch Otolaryngol* 2002;128:161–6.
11. Clark JR, Vesely M, Gilbert R. Scapular angle osteomyogenous flap in postmaxillectomy reconstruction: defect, reconstruction, shoulder function, and harvest technique. *Head Neck* 2008;30:10–20.
12. Uglešić V, Virag M, Varga S, et al. Reconstruction following radical maxillectomy with flaps supplied by the subscapular artery. *J Cranio Maxill Surg* 2000;28:153–60.
13. Rohner D, Jaquiéry C, Kunz C, et al. Maxillofacial reconstruction with prefabricated osseous free flaps: a 3-year experience with 24 patients. *Plast Reconstr Surg* 2003;112:748–57.

18

Palliative care for head and neck cancer

CATRIONA R. MAYLAND AND SIMON N. ROGERS

INTRODUCTION

Despite the overall advances in terms of the accuracy of diagnosis and improvements in treatments, it is important to remember that some patients with head and neck cancer will die from their disease. In 2003, head and neck cancer accounted for around 7,000 cases per year in England and Wales (1). In 2012, however, a total of 11,725 head and neck cancers were diagnosed and this represented a year on year increase in the number of diagnoses, with "lip, tongue and oral cavity" cancer being the most common grouping (3,864 cases) (2). A recent report from England from 2012 presented an analysis of death certificates and indicated that 3,020 people died from a cancer of the head and neck (0.6% of all deaths) (2). Further, the report found that one in five men and one in six women died within a year of diagnosis and that deaths from head and neck cancer tended to occur at a younger age compared with deaths from "all cancers" and "all causes."

Patients with head and neck cancer represent a group with particular complexities, partly due to the unique properties of the disease itself and the profound impact the illness and treatments have on different organ systems essential for human functioning (e.g. communication, swallowing and breathing) (1,3). The resulting functional deficit and symptoms that arise can be challenging to treat (4) and can have an impact on the patients' psychological well-being due to resulting social isolation and depression (4). Additionally, there remains a traditional view that head and neck cancer only affects older men who have made particular lifestyle choices such as smoking and this results in a risk of stigma and an associated feeling of culpability (2).

The anti-cancer treatments themselves pose particular challenges. In those with advanced disease who are treated with curative intent, the actual treatment is radical in the form of major surgery and adjuvant radiotherapy or chemoradiotherapy. These treatments are associated with treatment burden and toxicity. Those who undergo potentially curative surgery for advanced or recurrent cancer can still have significant morbidity and a limited prognosis and may be considered by some to be palliative (5). Also, the health-related quality of life outcomes in patients with advanced cancer are relatively poor and are associated with many problems, perhaps most notably anxiety, depression, disfigurement, speech impairment, swallowing difficulties and loss of social interactions (6).

It is imperative, then, that early involvement of palliative care is considered by those initially making a diagnosis where the overall prognosis is poor.

In this chapter, we will look to examine the origins and development of palliative care, provide an overview of the medical and surgical management of common symptoms and discuss advance care planning (ACP) and the implications for care at the end of life.

ORIGINS OF THE MODERN HOSPICE DEVELOPMENT

By as early as the fifth century, there are recordings of hospices used as shelters for travelers and sick people (7). It is not until later in the 19th century, however, that the term "hospice" began to represent institutions primarily focusing on the care of dying patients (7). These institutions were often founded and run by religious organizations. The modern palliative care and hospice movement was founded by Cicely Saunders in the U.K. during the 1960s. She recognized that the care of dying patients could be improved through skilled nursing and medical care (8) and that combining clinical care, teaching and research was the essence to improving overall patient care at the end of life (9). Saunders worked to develop more effective ways of controlling pain and to ensure that the psychosocial and spiritual needs of both patients and their families were addressed (10). This model of holistic care became the hallmark of the contemporary hospice philosophy (10) and led to the opening of the first modern hospice, St. Christopher's, London, in 1967. The modern hospice movement was then subsequently established in the United States, Canada (11) and New Zealand during the 1970s before further international expansion. Since then, hospice care has emerged as the "humane alternative to the highly technical, depersonalized care" frequently found in the modern hospital (12). Unfortunately, even today, the traditional view of hospices as solely places for the care of the dying still holds sway with the general public and many healthcare professionals. Conversely, concerns have been expressed about the "medicalization" of hospices—that increasing medical presence and the ability to undertake more complex procedures and interventions has threatened the "essence" of hospice care; that is, the emotional and spiritual care of patients (13). Hospices should, however, be seen as specialist units that can integrate active and supportive treatment along with expert symptom control and psychosocial support.

WHAT IS PALLIATIVE CARE?

One of the key challenges is defining what palliative care entails, how it interlinks with specialist palliative care and how each should best be integrated into the care of patients with head and neck cancer.

In 2002, the definition initially put forward by the World Health Organization (WHO) was revised to clarify that palliative care is relevant to both malignant and non-malignant disease and that palliative care-focused interventions should be considered early, where appropriate, in patients' illness trajectories (Box 18.1). This care can generally be provided by health and social care professionals who are involved in and provide the day-to-day care at patients' homes and hospitals, but can also be provided by those who specifically specialize in palliative care. In essence, any individual who has an advanced, progressive and incurable illness should receive palliative care.

BOX 18.1: WHO's definition of palliative care

Palliative care is an approach that improves the quality of life of patients and their families facing the problems associated with life-threatening illness through the prevention and relief of suffering by means of early identification and impeccable assessment and treatment of pain and other problems that are physical, psychosocial and spiritual.[17]

Palliative care:

- Provides relief from pain and other distressing symptoms
- Affirms life and regards dying as a normal process
- Intends neither to hasten nor postpone death
- Integrates the psychological and spiritual aspects of patient care
- Offers a support system to help patients live as actively as possible until death
- Offers a support system to help the family cope during the patient's illness and in their own bereavement
- Uses a team approach to address the needs of patients and their families, including bereavement counselling, if indicated
- Will enhance quality of life and may also positively influence the course of illness
- Is applicable early in the course of illness, in conjunction with other therapies that are intended to prolong life, such as chemotherapy or radiation therapy, and includes those investigations needed to better understand and manage distressing clinical complications

SPECIALIST PALLIATIVE CARE

Specialist palliative care tends to be provided by specialist multidisciplinary palliative care teams that are composed of individuals who have undergone specific training in this area. They try to focus on the care of those patients who have particular needs (physical, psychosocial, social and spiritual) that cannot be met by the health and social care professionals who are involved in the day-to-day care of patients at home or in the hospital. In particular, this would include:

- Unresolved symptoms and complex psychosocial issues
- Complex end-of-life issues
- Complex bereavement and pre-bereavement issues

The specialist teams include palliative medicine consultants and palliative care nurse specialists together with a range of expertise provided by physiotherapists, occupational therapists, dieticians, pharmacists, social workers and those able to give spiritual and psychological support (14). Rather than solely existing within hospices, specialist palliative care teams are established within hospital and community settings to provide assessment and advice to all care settings. Often this involves the specialist palliative care team working alongside the patient's own doctor(s) and nurses and may include extended teams to provide support and care in the patient's home, often known as a "hospice at home" service.

One of the current issues relates to the fact that specialist palliative care involvement is often sporadic and late in the disease trajectory. This is not an isolated problem for head and neck cancer alone and it is recognized that oncologists can tend to refer later in the patient's illness or when pain is uncontrolled (15,16)

These delays are in part due to physicians' concerns that palliative care referral would induce anxiety in both patients and families, that patients prefer to focus on curative treatments and that patients do not want to discuss prognosis (16). This is despite the fact that there are many studies demonstrating the benefit of integrating specialist palliative care involvement. These benefits would include:

- Improved symptom control (18,19)
- Improved quality of life (20)
- Reduced depression (19)
- More efficient use of healthcare resources (21)
- Greater patient and family satisfaction with care (18)

Generally, when deciding whether to involve specialist palliative care teams, the decision for referral should be based on need rather than diagnosis, although clear explanations to both the patient and palliative colleagues may be required regarding roles and responsibilities. Certainly within the last decade, there has been recognition that specialist palliative care involvement needs to move "upstream" in the disease trajectory and integrate more with potentially curative and rehabilitative therapies rather than the more traditional involvement immediately prior to death (4,13).

MEDICAL AND SURGICAL OPTIONS TO AID SYMPTOM MANAGEMENT

Within this section, an overview will be provided on the medical and surgical management of common symptoms. The focus will be on the following: pain, hemorrhage, airway obstruction and nutritional support. This is not an exhaustive list, but describing all symptoms is beyond the scope of this chapter. For more specific details about other symptoms and specific medications, reference to specialist palliative care textbooks such as the *Oxford Textbook of Palliative Medicine* (22) and the *Palliative Care Formulary* (23) is advised.

PAIN

In advanced head and neck cancer patients, pain can be a common and complex symptom. In one study looking at the prevalence in the last 6 months of life, pain was reported by 62% of patients (24). In two further studies looking at the prevalence of pain during the last hospice admission, 77%–79% of patients reported pain (25,26).

Pain can be broadly subdivided into two main categories:

- *Nociceptive pain*: Arising due to ongoing activation of primary afferent nerves by noxious stimuli (nociceptors) (27)
- *Neuropathic pain*: Due to dysfunction or disease affecting the peripheral and/or central nervous system (28)

Within clinical practice, there can often be a mixture of both nociceptive and neuropathic pain, which can arise either due to the cancer itself (local compression or invasion) or related to previous treatments. Patients frequently have more than one pain and each pain should be appraised separately. As part of the assessment, the following factors should be considered: site, intensity, quality or nature of pain, onset, relieving and aggravating factors and associated factors (e.g., impact on activities of daily living, sleep and eating). By using this approach, the type and likely cause of the pain can be elicited. Pain charts offer a systematic way of collecting and monitoring this information. If possible, pain sites should be examined carefully, checking for tenderness, inflammation and altered sensation or allodynia (when light touch induces pain, suggesting a neuropathic component to the pain). Cicely Saunders developed the concept of "total pain" that, in addition to the traditional physical components of pain, encapsulates the psychological, spiritual, social and emotional elements (29). Hence, an exploration of these aspects is extremely important, focusing on fears about what the pain could mean, concerns about the future and the impact the pain has on the whole individual.

Most cancer pain can be managed effectively using the analgesic "stepladder" developed by the WHO (30). The logical, stepwise approach is illustrated in Figure 18.1. Although more recently this approach has been questioned, it has been validated through a number of studies (31,32). Simple analgesics such as paracetamol are used first, then supplemented with a weak opioid (such as codeine) and progressing to a strong opioid if pain is not relieved. Morphine is still the opioid of choice for moderate to severe pain (33). As pain relief does not differ between modified-release or immediate-release preparations, titration can be given *via* either method (34). There are an increasing array of different strong opioids including fentanyl, alfentanil, oxycodone, hydromorphone and methadone. These tend to be used second or third line if there are side effects due to opioid-induced neurotoxicity (35), with signs and symptoms such as myoclonus, peripheral shadows, hallucinations, confusion and drowsiness caused by the accumulation of opioid metabolites. Opioids such as alfentanil and fentanil are safer to use in renal impairment as their active metabolites are not excreted *via* the kidneys (36); methadone is also relatively safe in renal impairment but, due to its complex pharmacokinetic profile, should be used under the direct supervision of a specialist palliative care team.

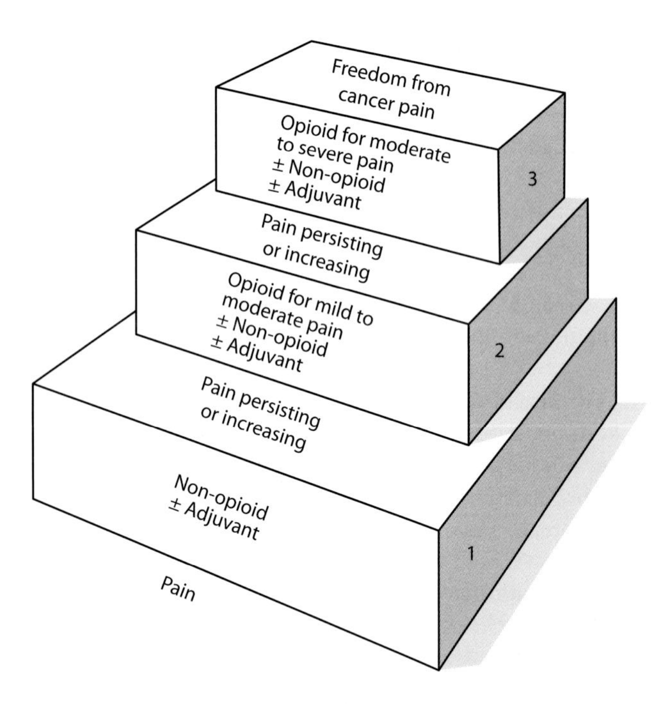

Figure 18.1 WHO's pain relief ladder. (Reproduced from World Health Organization. *Cancer Pain Relief and Palliative Care. Technical Report Series 804*. World Health Organization: Geneva, 1990.)

The transdermal method of delivery can be a useful way to deliver opioids (e.g. a fentanyl patch), but these should only be used in a clinical situation where pain control is relatively stable and controlled.

Using non-steroidal anti-inflammatory drugs (NSAIDs) has been widely accepted to help with cancer pain (37). Recent issues relating to their increased risk of cardiovascular and cerebrovascular events, however, led to the withdrawal of some specific medications and generally more cautious prescribing (38). With head and neck cancers, risk factors need to be closely examined (e.g. significant comorbidities, history of smoking and risk of bleeding) before using NSAIDs, and their use with these patients is probably more limited.

Adjuvant treatments are considered for specific pain problems. In terms of addressing neuropathic pain, in addition to using the WHO ladder, the first-line approach to treatment is either using an anti-convulsant (e.g. gabapentin or pregabalin) or an anti-depressant (amitriptyline) medication. If there is evidence of nerve compression, a trial of corticosteroids (dexamethasone) can be considered. Other therapeutic interventions would include the use of ketamine and topical preparations such as lidocaine transdermal patches, although specialist palliative care advice would be recommended.

The concept of "breakthrough pain" has been formally defined and further developed. Breakthrough pain is defined as "a transient exacerbation of pain that occurs either spontaneously, or in relation to a specific predictable or unpredictable trigger, despite relatively stable and adequately controlled background pain" (39). Traditionally, in this situation, an immediate-release form of morphine is given (e.g. Oramorph® or OxyNorm®). There have been a number of new formulations of strong opioids (fentanyl) that can be administered *via* sublingual, buccal and intranasal routes for this type of pain. They have been shown to have equal efficacy compared with traditional oral medications (40) and quicker onset of action, but are more expensive. Additionally, randomized controlled trials, particularly head-to-head trials, into the most effective way of managing breakthrough pain are relatively lacking (39). In practice, they tend to be reserved for pain related to a particular event (e.g. movement or pain that is sudden in onset and short-lived). It is noteworthy that prior to use of these strong, short acting opioids, patients should already be on a daily dose of 60 mg oral morphine or its equivalent.

The role of surgery in the palliation of pain in head and neck cancer is limited because of the anatomical configuration of nerves. Nerve blocks using alcohol or phenol and surgical nerve transection can be applied if pain is limited to a discrete neural distribution. It is relatively easy to block the maxillary (infra-orbital) and mandibular divisions (mental and inferior alveolar) of the trigeminal nerve, glossopharyngeal nerve and the cervical plexus (C3/4). Trigeminal ganglion ablation, percutaneous radiofrequency rhizotomy, stereotaxic thalamotomy or leucotomy, though described, are seldom indicated (40). Pain of dental cause needs to be treated by an experienced hospital-based practitioner. Dental extractions can invariably be performed using local anesthesia. Caution is necessary in situations where the jaws have been exposed to previous radiotherapy as extraction sites may fail to heal and osteoradionecrosis might ensue.

HEMORRHAGE

Minor bleeding is not uncommon from fungating head and neck cancers and may present as external hemorrhage, epistaxis, blood-stained saliva or hemoptysis depending on the site of the tumor.

The actual occurrence of a terminal hemorrhage (defined as "bleeding from an artery which is likely to result in death within a period of time that may be as short as minutes" (41)) is low, with rupture of the carotid artery system occurring in an estimated 3%–5% of patients who have undergone major head and neck resections (42).

The focus of care should be on minimizing the risk as much as possible. In terms of surgical options, ligation of the carotid artery and it branches has been superseded by endovascular stenting (43,44). This interventional radiological approach can have a significant risk of mortality and neurological morbidity, yet is usually a better option to open surgery. There should be exploration as to whether any definitive anti-cancer treatment (e.g. radiotherapy or laser treatment) should be considered. A review of the patient's current medication should be conducted. Any anti-coagulants (e.g. warfarin or heparin) should be discontinued and other medications that affect platelet function or the coagulation pathway should be reviewed and potentially discontinued (e.g. non-steroidal anti-inflammatory medications, aspirin and selective serotonin reuptake inhibitor anti-depressants). Whether anti-fibrinolytic agents are appropriate needs to be considered in the context of the patient's other comorbidities.

Sometimes there can be a herald or warning bleed that precedes the life-threatening hemorrhage or evidence of a ballooning or visible pulsation of arterial vasculature (45). Minor superficial bleeding may be reduced with topical adrenaline.

The key principles in terms of managing terminal hemorrhage are (46)

- Always have somebody staying with the patient (and family if present) to help reduce the anxiety and distress associated with the event.
- Use dark towels to help reduce the visibility of blood.
- Give an anxiolytic (e.g. 10 mg of midazolam given *via* deep intramuscular injection due to its rapid onset and short duration of action).

If there is a recognized risk of hemorrhage, midazolam should be pre-emptively prescribed. In practice, however, due to the potential rapidity of the event, it is often not needed and certainly it is better to stay with the patient than leaving them to get an injection. The aim of giving midazolam is to reduce the patient's awareness and hence distress regarding the event. Additionally, it provides retrograde amnesia so that if the patient did recover, they would not have recollection of the event. Generally, opioids are not needed unless the hemorrhage is more minor and the patient is reporting pain. Providing sufficient support to both the family and the healthcare professionals involved is a key factor after the event.

AIRWAY OBSTRUCTION

The most pertinent aspect of care for this issue is proactive decision-making about the appropriate level of treatment escalation so a structured care plan can be clearly executed. The decision to perform a tracheostomy for palliation is a difficult one. A tracheostomy may help with breathing difficulties but will limit communication. Additionally, a tracheostomy does not guarantee airway patency and, in the presence of uncontrolled disease in the laryngeal region, compromise of the airway can arise due to retention of secretions or by tumor encroachment into the stomal wall. Another indication for a tracheostomy is to secure the airway at the time of palliative surgery. Awake fiber-optic intubations might be appropriate if conventional intubation is hazardous and, if needs be, the procedure can be performed under local anesthesia. Although percutaneous dilatational tracheostomies under ultrasound guidance are successful (47), an open procedure by an experienced surgeon is favored because of the difficult airway with distorted anatomy due to previous surgery, radiation or tumor infiltration. In the event that surgical interventional is not appropriate, ensuring that pre-emptive prescribing of an anxiolytic, such as midazolam, is appropriate. Additionally, addressing the concerns of the patient and their family is important as this situation can cause considerable anxiety and distress (25). If there is clinical evidence of stridor, high-dose (8–16 mg) dexamethasone (48) given *via* a subcutaneous or intravenous injection may be beneficial.

NUTRITIONAL SUPPORT

The need for fluid and nutritional support in patients with head and neck cancer is widely appreciated and this would include those who are being treated with palliative intent (49). Percutaneous endoscopic gastrostomy (PEG) is an effective method for providing alimentation and is often inserted as part of their earlier treatment. In situations where the cancer prevents the passage of a gastroscope, a radiologically inserted gastrostomy (RIG) can be utilized. Generally, these methods are recommended on a more long-term basis compared with the use of a nasogastric tube, which can be easily displaced, can have particular challenges in the community setting necessitating recurrent hospital admission and can be uncomfortable for the patient. Unless prognosis is anticipated to be less than 2 months, PEG or RIG can be valuable in helping maintain hydration and nutrition, as well as providing an alternative route to administer medication if swallowing is difficult.

ROLE OF ACP

A key aspect of good care for all patients with incurable and progressive disease involves offering the opportunity to discuss and plan for the future. This is particularly of relevance to head and neck cancer patients because of the potential challenges that can occur in the last weeks and days of life due to the perceived risk of acute catastrophic events such as airway obstruction or acute hemorrhage (1,4). Not all patients will wish to do this or have these types of discussion, but all should be offered the opportunity.

ACP is a discussion between an individual and a professional (with or without the family) with the aim to identify:

- Wishes/preferences for care
- Concerns
- Understanding of illness and prognosis

Additionally, it can involve formal decision-making such as decisions regarding resuscitation and Advance Decisions to Refuse Treatment. The evidence of benefit demonstrates mixed results. In particular, a large study undertaken in North America showed that despite an intensive intervention using skilled nurses to elicit patient preferences and facilitate communication, there remained issues regarding unwanted interventions and doctor–patient communication (50). More recent studies have shown more favorable results, however, with the promotion of patient autonomy and increased patient and family satisfaction with care (51,52).

PREFERRED PLACE OF CARE AND PLACE OF DEATH

One area which relates to ACP and is especially noteworthy is that of preferred place of care and preferred place of death. Currently, there is a major mismatch between where patients wish to be cared for and where they actually die. The majority of individuals (up to 74%) express a preference to die at home, although many do not achieve this choice (53,54). Although a European study demonstrated national variation in the proportions of hospital deaths (55), a significant proportion of patients within many developed countries continue to die in hospitals (56–58). Recent end-of-life care policies have focused on enabling more people to die in their preferred place of care, which generally is at home (59,60). It is important to be mindful, however, that for some individuals, the hospital is the right place for people to die in, as the home can represent a "lonely and frightening place" (61). This issue is particularly pertinent for patients with head and neck cancer who may have breathing difficulties or a risk of hemorrhage. In view of the increased risk for acute events and the complexity of their symptoms, achievement of patients' preferences may be more challenging for head and neck cancer patients compared with other individuals. Patients who clearly express or record their wishes and preferences with healthcare professionals and family members, however, are more likely to have these wishes adhered to compared with those who do not.

In terms of head and neck cancer patients, there appears to be variation on place of death due to a number of factors. Within England, the following factors had a particular influence regarding place of death (2):

1. *Type of head and neck cancer*: Patients with thyroid and laryngeal cancer tend to die in hospital (50%) compared with those suffering from lip, tongue and oral cavity, salivary gland, nose, ear and sinus cancer, who tend to die at home (28%).
2. *Age*: The highest proportion of deaths at home (29%) or in a hospice (25%) occur in under 65-year-olds, whereas those over 85 years of age tend to die in care homes (27%).
3. *Socioeconomic deprivations*: In total, 44% of those from the most deprived areas of England will die in hospital compared with 38% from the least deprived; 21% from the most deprived areas die in hospices compared with 23% from the most affluent areas.

According to a recent national survey of bereaved people within the U.K., the quality of care for dying patients within hospital is not perceived to be as good compared with care provided within the home, hospice or care home setting (62). Recommendations to have more accessibility to specialist palliative care teams and mandatory training about care for dying patients for all healthcare professionals have followed (62). It is imperative that, no matter where the patient wishes to die, a focus on providing good quality of care and adequate support in all care settings is achieved.

CONCLUDING COMMENTS

Head and neck cancer patients pose unique challenges in terms of the individuals affected by the illness, the manner in which the cancer and its treatments impact on patients and families and the proactive planning for unexpected events. Close collaborative working between surgical, community and specialist palliative care is imperative if patient and family needs are to be adequately met. Early identification of those with poor prognosis and those likely to have complex symptoms may be challenging. Nevertheless, this identification is important so that specialist palliative care services can be linked in an integrated manner and potentially involved at an early stage of disease. ACP is of particular relevance for this group of patients if wishes and preferences are to be elicited and for patients to be cared for and to die in the place of their choosing.

REFERENCES

1. National Institute of Clinical Excellence. *Guidance on Cancer Services. Improving Outcomes in Head and Neck Cancer. The Manual.* London: NICE, 2004.
2. National End of Life Care Intelligence Network. *Head and Neck Cancers in England: Who Died from Them and Where Do They Die?* London: Public Health England, 2014.
3. Ferlito A, Rogers SN, Shaha AR et al. Quality of life in head and neck cancer. *Acta Otolaryngol* 2003;123:5–7.
4. Shuman AG, Yang Y, Taylor JMG et al. End-of-life care among head and neck cancer patients. *Otolaryng Head Neck* 2010;144:733–9.
5. Shaw HJ. Palliation in head and neck cancer. *J Laryngol Otol* 1985;99:1131–42.
6. Rogers SN, Ahad SA, Murphy AP. A structured review and theme analysis of papers published on "quality of life" in head and neck Cancer: 2000 to 2005. *Oral Oncol* 2007;43:843–68.
7. Clark D, Seymour J. History and development. In: Clark D, Seymour J (eds). *Reflections in Palliative Care.* Buckingham: Open University Press, 1999, 65–78.
8. Thoresen I. A reflection on Cicely Saunders' views on a good death through the philosophy of Charles Taylor. *Int J Pall Nurs* 2003;9:19–23.
9. Clark D. From margins to centre: a review of the history of palliative care in cancer. *Lancet Oncol* 2007;8:430–8.
10. Seale CF. What happens in hospices: a review of research evidence. *Soc Sci Med* 1989;28:551–9.

11. Ferris FD, Balfour HM, Bowen K et al. A model to guide patient and family care: based on the nationally accepted principles and norms of practice. *J Pain Symp Manage* 2002;24:106–23.
12. Dawson NJ. Need satisfaction in terminal care-settings. *Soc Sci Med* 1991;32:83–7.
13. Clark D. Between hope and acceptance: The medicalization of dying. *Br Med J* 2002;324:905–7.
14. National Council for Palliative Care. The Palliative Care explained. http://www.ncpc.org.uk/palliative-care-explained (accessed December 2014).
15. Wentlandt K, Krzyzanowska MK, Swami N et al. Referral practices of oncologists to specialized palliative care. *J Clin Oncol* 2012;30:4380–6.
16. Smith CB, Nelson JE, Berman AR et al. Lung cancer physicians' referral practices for palliative care consultation. *Ann Oncol* 2012;23:383–7.
17. World Health Organization. *National Cancer Control Programmes: Policies and Managerial Guidelines* (2nd Edition). Geneva: World Health Organization, 2002.
18. Ellershaw JE, Peat SJ, Boys LC. Assessing the effectiveness of a hospital palliative care team. *Palliat Med* 1995;9:145–1552.
19. Bandieri E, Sichetti D, Romero M et al. Impact of early access to a palliative/supportive care intervention on pain management in patients with cancer. *Ann Oncol* 2012;23:2016–20.
20. Temel JS, Greer JA, Muzikansky A et al. Early palliative care for patients with metastatic non-small cell lung cancer. *N Engl J Med* 2010;363;733-42.
21. Morrison RS, Penrod JD, Cassel JB et al. Cost savings associated with US hospital palliative care team. *Arch Intern Med* 2008;168:1783–90.
22. Hanks G, Cherny NI, Christakis NA et al. *Oxford Textbook of Palliative Medicine* (4th Edition). Oxford University Press, Oxford, 2011.
23. Twycross R, Wilcock A. *Palliative Care Formulary* (4th Edition). Palliativedrug.com Ltd, Nottingham, 2011.
24. Price KA, Moore EJ, Moynihan T et al. Symptoms and terminal course of patients who died of head and neck cancer. *J Pall Med* 2009;12:117–8.
25. Forbes K. Palliative care in patients with cancer of the head and neck. *Clin Otolaryngol* 1997;22:117–22.
26. Talmi YP, Roth YR, Waller A et al. Care of the terminal head and neck cancer patient in the hospice setting. *Laryngoscope* 1995;105:315–8.
27. Portenoy RK, Forbes K, Lussier D et al. Chapter 8.2.11. In: Doyle D, Hanks G, Cherny N, Calman K. (eds). Difficult Pain Problems: An Integrated Approach, in *Oxford Textbook of Palliative Medicine* (3rd Edition). Oxford: Oxford University Press, 2005, 438–58.
28. Saarto T, Wiffen PJ. Antidepressants for neuropathic pain. *Cochrane Database Syst Rev* 2007;4:CD005454.
29. Clark C. "Total pain," disciplinary power and the body in the work of Cicely Saunders, 1958–1967. *Soc Sci Med* 1999;49:727–36.
30. World Health Organization. *Cancer Pain Relief and Palliative Care. Technical Report Series 804*. Geneva: World Health Organization, 1990.
31. Ventafridda V, Tamburini M, Caraceni A et al. A validation study of the WHO method for cancer pain relief. *Cancer* 1987;59:850–6.
32. Zech DFJ, Grond S, Lynch J et al. Validation of world health organization guidelines for cancer pain relief: A 10 year prospective study. *Pain* 1995;63:65–76.
33. Hanks GW, de Conno F, Chery N et al. Morphine and alternative opioids in cancer pain: the EAPC recommendations. *B J Cancer* 2001;84:587–93.
34. Wiffen PJ, Wee B, Moore RA. Oral morphine for cancer pain (review). *The Cochrane Collaboration 2016*. http://onlinelibrary.wiley.com/doi/10.1002/14651858.CD003868.pub4/full (accessed January 2018).
35. Lawlor P, Lucey M, Creedon B. Opioid side effects and overdose. In: Walsh D. (ed). *Palliative Medicine*. Philadelphia: Saunders Elsevier, 2009, 1411–6.
36. Douglas C, Murtagh FE, Chambers EJ et al. Symptom management for the adult patient dying with advanced chronic kidney disease: a review of the literature and development of evidence-based guidelines by a United Kingdom Expert Consensus Group. *Palliat Med* 2009;23:103–10.
37. McNicol ED, Strassels S, Goudas L et al. NSAIDs or paracetamol, alone or combined with opioids, for cancer pain. 2011. The Cochrane Collaborative. http://www.thecochrancelibrary.com (accessed December 2014).
38. Antman EM, Bennett JS, Daugherty A. Use of nonsteroidal anti-inflammatory drugs. An update for clinicians. A scientific statement from the American Heart Association. *Circulation* 2007;1115:1634–42.
39. Davies AN, Dickman A, Reid C, Stevens AM, Zeppetella G. The management of cancer-related breakthrough pain: recommendations of a task group of the Science Committee of the Association for Palliative Medicine of Great Britain and Ireland. *Eur J Pain* 2009;13:331–8.
40. Davies A, Sitte T, Elsner F et al. Consistency of efficacy, patient acceptability and nasal tolerability of fentanyl pectin nasal spray compared with immediate-release morphine sulphate in breakthrough cancer pain. *J Pain Symptom Manage* 2011;41:358–66.
41. Harris DG, Noble SI. Management of terminal haemorrhage in patients with advanced cancer: a systematic literature review. *J Pain Symptom Manage* 2009;38:913–27.
42. Powitzky R, Vasan N, Krempl G et al. Carotid blowout in patients with head and neck cancer. *Ann Otol Rhinol Laryngol* 2010;119:476–84.
43. Tatar EC, Yildirim UM, Dündar Y et al. Self-expandable polytetrafluoro-ethylene stent for carotid blowout syndrome. *B-ENT* 2012;8:61–4

44. Upile T, Triaridis S, Kirkland P et al. The management of carotid artery rupture. *Eur Arch Otorhinolaryngol* 2005;262:555–60.
45. Rimmer J. Management of vascular complications of head and neck cancer. *J Laryngol Otol* 2012;126: 111–5.
46. Ubogagu E, Harris DG. Guideline for the management of terminal haemorrhage in palliative care patients with advanced cancer discharged home for end-of-life care. *BMJ Support Palliat Care* 2012;2:294–300.
47. Aadahl P, Nordgard S. Percutaneous dilatational tracheostomy in a patient with thyroid cancer and severe airway obstruction. *Acta Anaesthesiol Scand* 1999;43:483–5.
48. Davies C. ABC of palliative care. Breathlessness, cough, and other respiratory problems. *BMJ* 1997;315:931–4.
49. Roland NJ, Bradley PJ. The role of surgery in the palliation of head and neck cancer. *Curr Opin Otolaryngol Head Neck Surg* 2014;22:101–8.
50. The SUPPORT principle investigators. A controlled trial to improve care for seriously ill hospitalized patients. The study to understand prognosis and preferences for outcomes and risks of treatment (SUPPORT). *JAMA* 1995;274:1591–8.
51. Hayhoe B, Howe A. Advance care planning under the Mental Capacity Act 2005 in primary care. *Br J Gen Pract* 2011;61(589):e537–41. doi: https://doi-org.liverpool.idm.oclc.org/10.3399/bjgp11X588592.
52. Mullick A, Martin J, Sallnow L. An introduction to advance care planning in practice. *BMJ* 2013;347:f6064. doi: https://doi.org/10.1136/bmj.f6064.
53. National Audit Office. *End of Life Care*. London: The Stationary Office, 2008.
54. Higginson IJ, Sen-Gupta GJ. Place of care in advanced cancer: a qualitative systematic literature review of patient preferences. *J Palliat Med* 2000;3:287–300.
55. Cohen J, Houttekier D, Onwuteaka-Philipsen B et al. Which patients with cancer die at home? A study of six European countries using death certificate data. *J Clin Oncol* 2010;28:2267–73.
56. Costantini M, Balzib D, Garronecc E et al. Geographical variations in place of death among Italian communities suggest an inappropriate hospital use in the terminal phase of cancer disease. *Publ Health* 2000;114:15–20.
57. Yang L, Sakamoto N, Marui E. A study of home deaths from 1951 to 2002. *BMC Palliat Care* 2006;5:2.
58. Gomes B, Higginson IJ. Where people die (1974–2030): Past trends, future projections and implications for care. *Palliat Med* 2008;22:33–41.
59. Commonwealth of Australia. *Supporting Australians to Live Well at the End of Life. National Palliative Care Strategy 2010*. Commonwealth of Australia, 2010. https://www.health.gov.au/internet/main/publishing.nsf/Content/EF57056BDB047E2FCA257BF000206168/$File/NationalPalliativeCareStrategy.pdf (last accessed January 2018).
60. Department of Health. *End of Life Care Strategy. Promoting High Quality Care for all Adults at the End of Life*. London: Department of Health, 2008.
61. Johnston B. Is effective, person-centred, home based palliative care truly achievable? *Palliat Med* 2014;28:373–4.
62. Office of National Statistics. National survey of bereaved people (VOICES), 2013. http://www.ons.gov.uk/ons/dcp171778_370472.pdf (accessed December 2014).

PART III

Outcomes and follow-up

19

Oncologic outcomes

PABLO H. MONTERO, JOCELYN C. MIGLIACCI, AND SNEHAL G. PATEL

The oral cavity and oropharynx are two major subsites in the head and neck region for squamous cell carcinoma (HNSCC) as reported in a 15-year study of the National Cancer Database (NCDB) from 1990 to 2004. These two sites consistently represented roughly 25% of head and neck cancers throughout the 15-year study, but the proportion of oral cavity cancers declined slightly from 1990 to 2004, accounting for 13.5% and 11.3%, respectively. On the other hand, the percentage of oropharyngeal tumors increased slightly from 12.0% to 13.7% (1). Although the incidence of oral cancer is decreasing (2), unfortunately, there has only been a marginal improvement in survival (3).

HNSCC in general and oral/oropharyngeal cancer in particular have traditionally been etiologically associated with tobacco and alcohol use (4). However, human papillomavirus (HPV) has emerged as a predominant etiologic factor in oropharyngeal carcinoma over the last 15 years (5). This etiological shift to HPV-related tumors has not been shown for oral cancer (6).

The increase in the incidence of oropharyngeal cancer has been attributed mainly to the emergence of HPV infection (7). The prognosis of these HPV-related oropharyngeal cancers seems to be quite different from and superior to non-HPV-related tumors (5). Treatment paradigms for cancer of the oral cavity and oropharynx are substantially different. Oral cancer is primarily treated with surgery followed by appropriate adjuvant treatment, while primary radiation therapy with or without chemotherapy is equally effective as surgery in the treatment of oropharyngeal cancer.

In this chapter, we will show the contemporary outcomes of therapy for oral and oropharyngeal cancer patients treated at the Memorial Sloan Kettering Cancer Center (MSKCC). All patients were treated by a multidisciplinary "disease management team" with relatively uniform treatment philosophies. The data collection and statistical methods used for our analyses were similar for both sites (8).

Clinical, treatment and outcomes data were entered into a computerized database, and statistical analysis was carried out using commercially available computer software packages (9,10). The overall survival interval was calculated in months from the date of initial treatment to the date of last follow-up or death and the recurrence-free survival (RFS) was calculated from the date of initial treatment to the date of first recurrence. For cancer-specific survival, patients who died of non-oral/oropharyngeal cancer-related causes and those who were alive with disease at the last follow-up were censored. Patients who died with a secondary primary malignancy of the head and neck region were considered as having died of the disease. Overall, cancer-specific and relapse-free survival rates were calculated by the Kaplan–Meier method and univariate comparisons were performed using the log-rank test. A p-value of 0.05 or less was considered statistically significant and all significant factors were entered into a multivariate analysis using the Cox proportional hazard model.

For the purpose of this discussion, we have also included data from the NCDB of the Commission on Cancer of the American College of Surgeons and the Surveillance, Epidemiology and End Results (SEER) program. The NCDB is supported by the American Cancer Society and the National Tumor Registrars Association. Over 1,400 hospitals across the U.S.A. voluntarily contribute data each year to this national database. Data analysis is performed at the American College of Surgeons (11). This information offers national trends in therapeutic choices and outcomes data that reflect cross-sectional observations nationwide in the U.S.A. Similarly, the SEER database, which is supported by the National Cancer Institute, started data collection for cancer patients in 1974 from 20 different registries across the U.S.A.

ORAL CAVITY

We retrospectively analyzed patients treated at the MSKCC from 1985 to 2012. During this 28-year period, 1,866 previously untreated patients received surgery with or without postoperative radiotherapy for invasive squamous cell carcinoma of the oral cavity. The median age of the cohort was 62 years (range: 15–96), and 56.3% were males. The most common site of the primary tumor was the tongue (50.2%), followed by the floor of the mouth (15.1%), lower gum (13.8%), upper gum (6.4%), buccal mucosa (6.4%), retromolar trigone (5.8%), and hard palate (2.4%; Figure 19.1). Forty-three percent of patients with a clinically negative neck underwent elective neck dissection, and clinically occult nodal disease was reported in 248 (19.0%) of these patients. Five hundred and forty eight patients (29.4%) received a therapeutic neck dissection due to clinically positive nodes. Postoperative radiation therapy was used in 658 patients (35.3%) and postoperative chemoradiation therapy in 99 patients (5.3%).

CLINICAL PREDICTORS OF OUTCOME

Stage of the tumor is an important factor predicting survival in patients with oral cavity cancer (Figure 19.2). The presence of clinically positive lymph nodes is the single most important factor in determining outcome (Figure 19.3).

Aside from regional lymph node metastasis, there are several other ominous clinical signs related to the primary

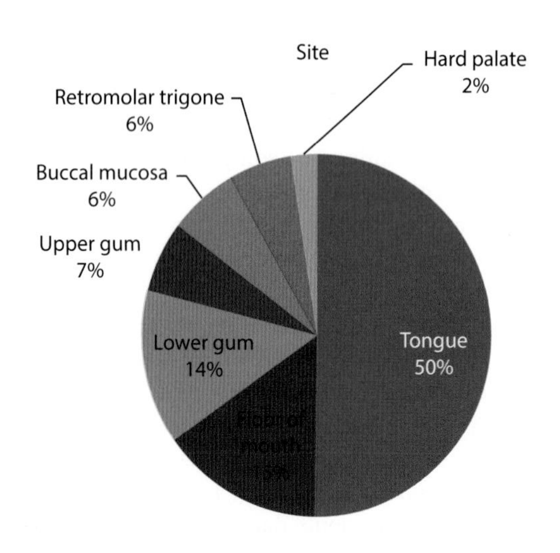

Figure 19.1 Distribution of patients by site of disease within the oral cavity.

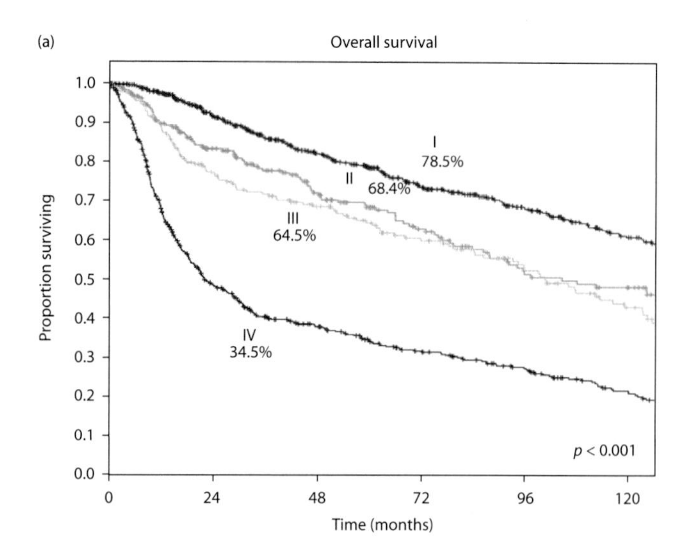

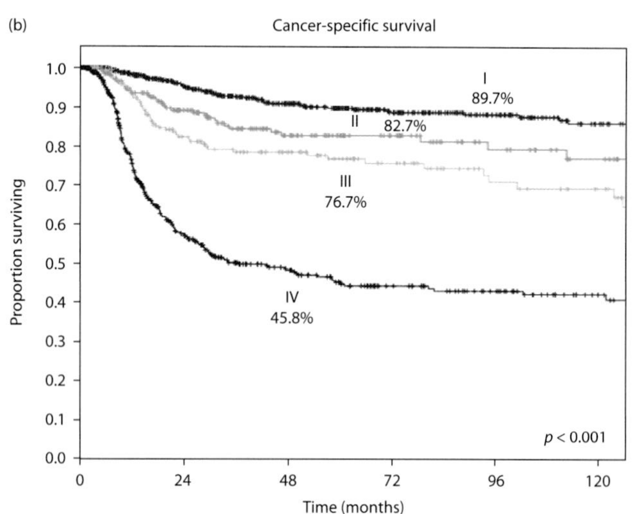

Figure 19.2 The clinical stage of the disease is a significant predictor of outcome **(a)** overall survival and **(b)** cancer-specific survival in squamous cell carcinoma of the oral cavity.

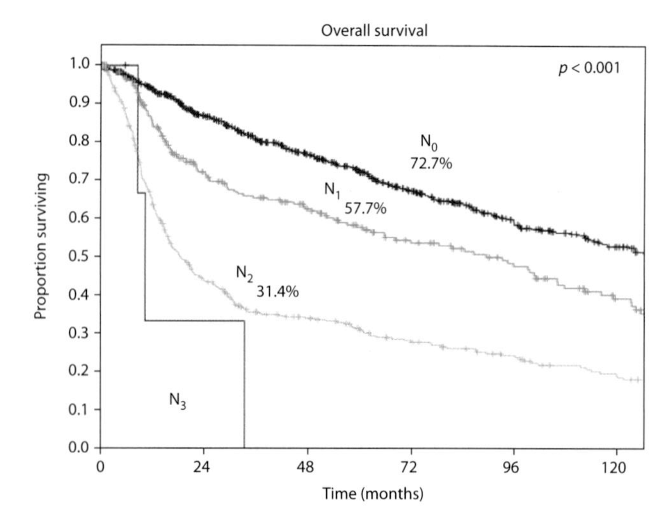

Figure 19.3 Impact of clinically palpable lymph node metastasis on overall survival in squamous cell carcinoma of the oral cavity.

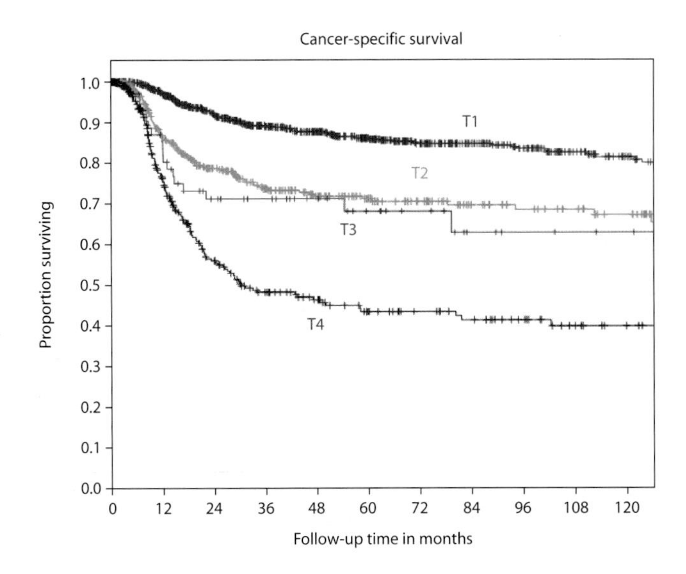

Figure 19.4 Cancer-specific survival by pathologic T stage.

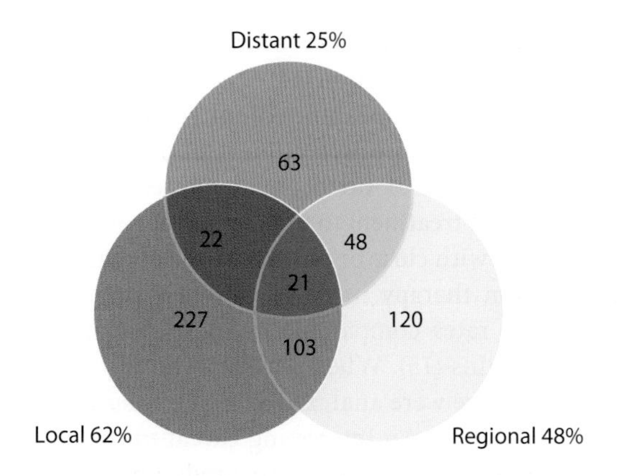

Figure 19.5 Patterns of failure in patients that failed treatment for cancer of the oral cavity. Treatment failure was noted in 171/595 patients (29%).

tumor that imply locally advanced disease (T4) (Figure 19.4). Similarly, when a tumor has grown to an extent where the skin is involved, the chance of cure is relatively low. Another ominous sign is bone invasion, particularly in gum tumors. The presence of trismus, which suggests invasion of the pterygoid, temporalis or masseter muscles, is also an adverse prognostic feature.

LOCOREGIONAL CONTROL

Approximately one-third of patients (32%) treated for oral cavity cancer fail treatment. Locoregional recurrence is the most common pattern of failure (Figure 19.5). The rate of local control after treatment of tumors of the oral cavity is influenced by several factors. The status of the surgical margins is probably the single most important factor determining local control (Figure 19.6). Following earlier reports (12), margin status was classified as positive if it met one of the following four criteria:

1. Close margin (tumor within 0.5 cm)
2. Premalignant change in the margin
3. *In situ* carcinoma in the margin
4. Invasive microscopic cancer at the margin

A significant aspect of margin assessment and reporting is that, after resection and processing, the average specimen has been shown to shrink by approximately 22% (13). A lesion resected with an appropriate margin *in vivo* might be reported to have a close or positive margin on final pathology. The implication of this observation is that, especially for certain sites in the oral cavity, the margin status should be interpreted in the context of adequacy of surgical resection. For tumors of the oral tongue, we have recently reported the tumor: specimen index as an indicator of adequacy of

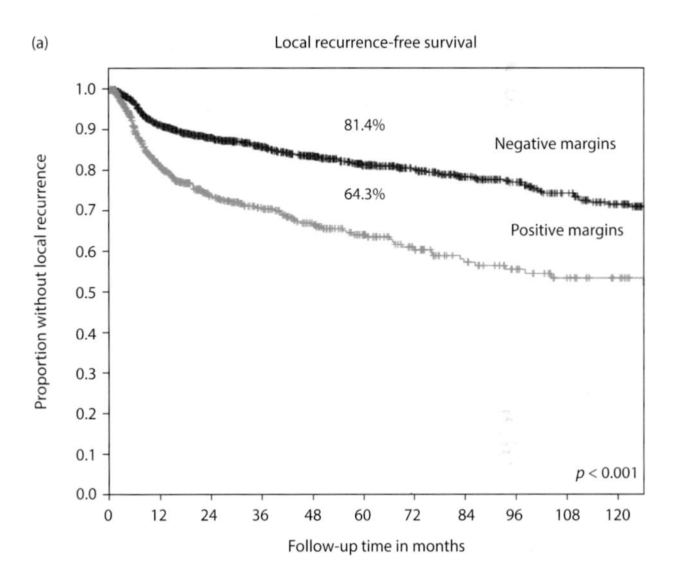

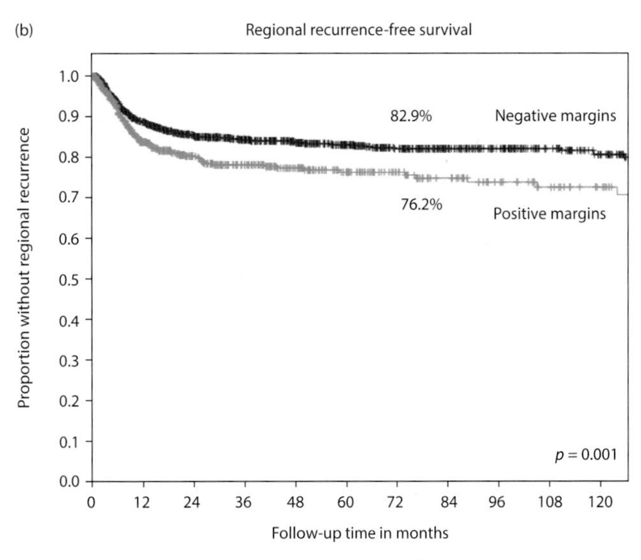

Figure 19.6 Local **(a)** and regional **(b)** control rates drop significantly in patients with positive surgical margins.

surgical resection and an aid to interpretation of close or positive margins of resection (14).

Nevertheless, the appearance of microscopic tumor cells at or near the margin of resection is of concern and warrants consideration of further wider resection if feasible and/or adjuvant treatment to improve local control.

In patients with close or positive surgical margins, adjuvant radiation therapy in doses of 60 Gy or more yields local control rates comparable to those in patients with negative margins (15). When patients who received a dose of 60 Gy or more were analyzed as a subgroup, the control rate exceeded 90%. An interesting caveat to this, however, is that the efficacy of postoperative radiation therapy was dependent on the site of the primary tumor; floor of the mouth tumors had a better 5-year local control rate compared to oral tongue tumors (89% versus 62%) (15). In spite of the option to use postoperative radiation therapy, it is crucial for the surgeon to strive for adequate total resection of the tumor with microscopically negative margins.

Another histopathological feature that has been correlated with local control is the presence of perineural invasion. Patients with histologic evidence of perineural invasion have a lower control rate (77%) compared to those without (91%) (16). When perineural invasion is seen in the specimen, consideration should be given to the use of adjuvant radiation therapy to enhance local control (17).

Other features of the primary lesion have been utilized to predict the risk of occult cervical lymph node metastasis that in turn directly relates to survival. The thickness of the primary tumor is one of the most predictive and reliable methods currently available to the clinician for estimating the risk of regional lymph node involvement (18). Thus, patients with deeply infiltrative tumors will have a higher rate of lymph node metastasis and thus a lower rate of survival (Figure 19.7). These findings have been duplicated by others (19–21). This parameter is now included in the 8th edition American Joint Committee on Cancer (AJCC)/International Union Against Cancer (UICC) T staging of primary tumors of the oral cavity and lips. Tumors are upstaged by one T stage with each 5-mm increase in tumor thickness for stages T1–T3. The three cutoff points are <5, 5–10 and >10 mm (22).

SURVIVAL AND PROGNOSTIC FACTORS

Surgery and radiation therapy are the mainstays of treatment of oral cavity cancer and "equivalent" results have been reported using either modality for early-stage tumors. However, it is important to note that most early-stage oral cancers can be easily resected surgically with minimal functional impact, whereas the morbidity associated with radiation therapy (e.g. xerostomia, loss of taste, life-long risk to dentition and the risk of radionecrosis of the mandible) can be considerable. For more advanced tumors, the two modalities are used in combination; our preference in tumors of the oral cavity is to employ radiation therapy in a postoperative adjuvant setting.

The overall 5-year survival for all comers in the current cohort of patients at the MSKCC was 63%. This represents a modest but appreciable improvement in treatment results over the years (Figure 19.8). Although a direct comparison of this nature is statistically irrelevant, it does provide some insight into trends. Factors that may have contributed to better results include: downstaging of the primary tumor due to earlier detection; an enhanced ability to resect large tumors and reconstruct large and complex defects, particularly with the availability of microvascular free flaps; an improved understanding of the patterns of regional lymphatic metastatic pathways; more aggressive regional therapy, including increasing use of elective selective neck dissections; and the use of postoperative radiation therapy with or without chemotherapy. On a nationwide basis in the U.S.A., however, the 5-year relative survival in almost 59,000 patients with oral cancer analyzed by the NCDB was reported to be 49.8% for squamous cell carcinoma (11). This may be a better reflection of contemporary outcomes of therapy, since it represents national data from all parts

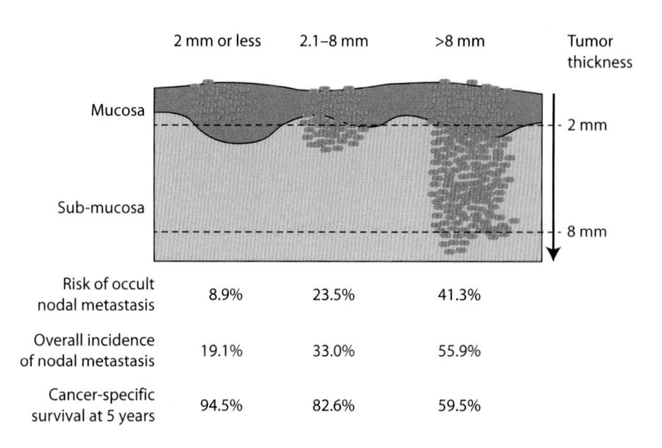

Figure 19.7 The depth of invasion of the primary tumor is a significant predictor of nodal metastasis and cancer-specific survival.

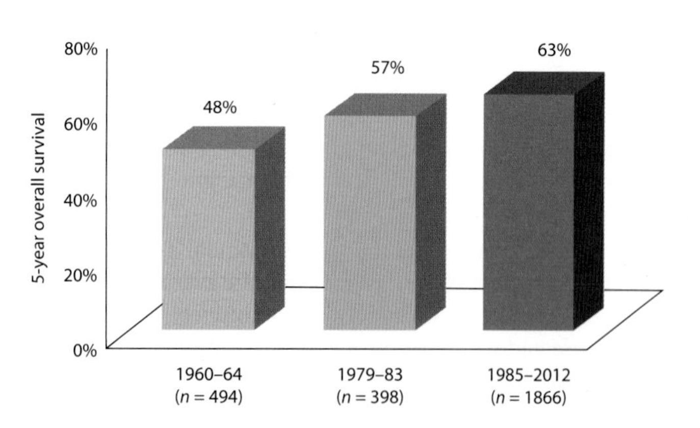

Figure 19.8 Improving outcomes in oral cavity cancer: Results of treatment in three cohorts treated during different time periods at the Memorial Sloan Kettering Cancer Center (1960–2012).

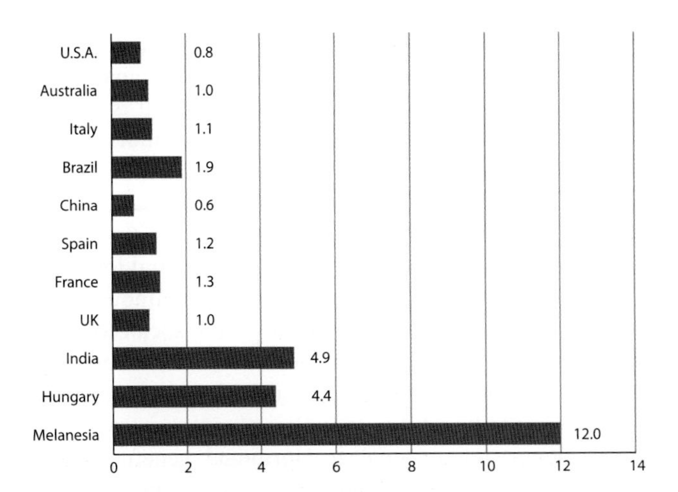

Figure 19.9 Estimated mortality rates for the year 2012 in patients treated for squamous carcinoma of the oral cavity (age-standardized [worldwide] death rates per 100,000 population). (Data from: Ferlay JSI et al. GLOBOCAN 2012 v1.0, cancer incidence and mortality worldwide: IARC cancer Base No. 11 [Internet]. *International Agency for Research on Cancer*, 2013. Available from: http://globocan.iarc.fr (23).)

of the U.S.A. and not institutional data from a leading tertiary care cancer center. Mortality rates from oral cancer also vary according to geographic location; certain high-incidence regions such as Melanesia, Eastern Europe and India have considerably higher death rates compared to the rest of the world (Figure 19.9) (23).

Oral carcinomas have mostly affected patients over the age of 45. Our dataset supports this observation as 79% of patients were ≥45 years of age and the median age of our cohort was 62 years. These patients are more likely to suffer from other comorbid conditions secondary to tobacco and alcohol abuse that may contribute to outcome. This is reflected in the fact that the 5-year cancer-specific survival (75%) is better than the corresponding overall survival (63%) (Figure 19.10). The proportion of patients dying from other causes has been reported to have increased from 14.1% at 5 years to approximately 50% at 10 years after treatment (11). There are reports speculating that oral cavity tumors in younger patients are more aggressive than similar tumors in older patients. When patients are stratified for age, however, survival is not statistically different between the older and younger groups. In our experience, cancer-specific survival was comparable while overall survival was poorer in older patients (Figure 19.11). Younger patients also had a significantly superior locoregional RFS ($p = .009$). A similar finding was reported in the NCDB study (11). These observations underscore the importance of comorbid conditions as determinants of outcome in patients with oral carcinoma.

Interestingly, the number of younger patients diagnosed with oral carcinomas has started to increase. A review of the literature done by a group in Poland reported conflicting evidence as to causes associated with this increase, resulting in uncertainty. Some groups have attributed it to smokeless

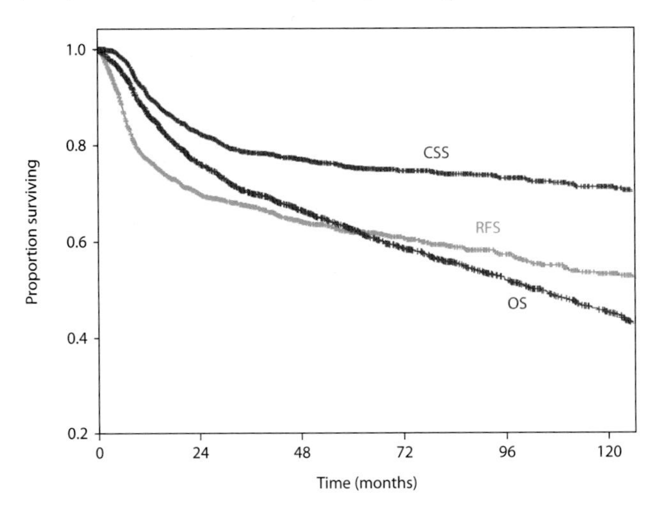

Figure 19.10 Five-year overall survival (OS) and cancer-specific survival (CSS) in a recent cohort of patients with oral cavity cancer treated at the Memorial Sloan Kettering Cancer Center.

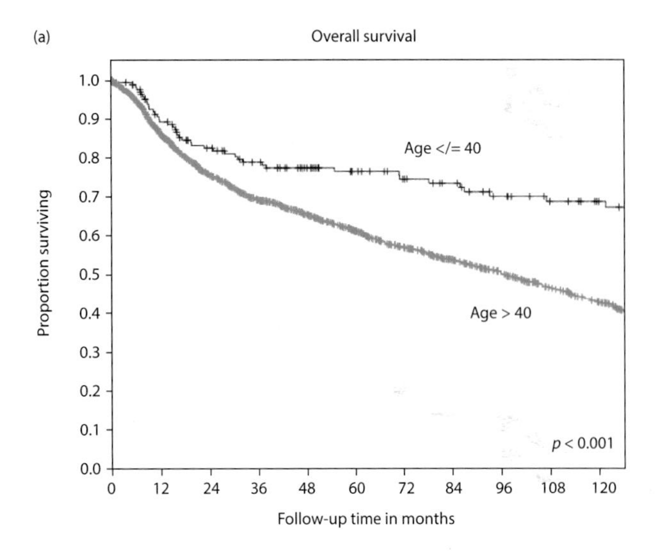

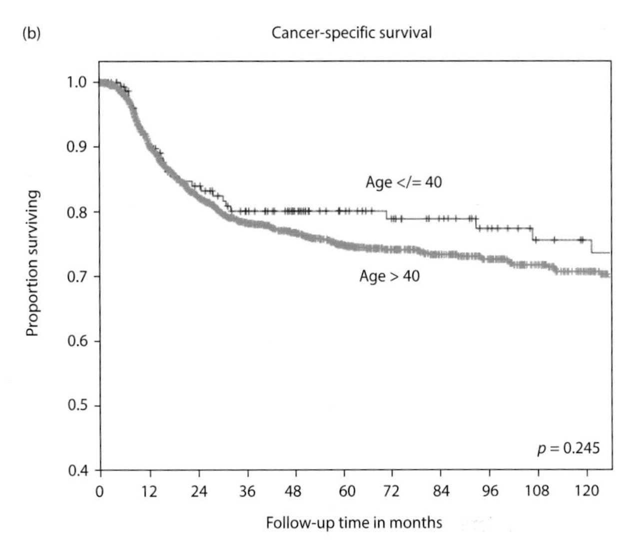

Figure 19.11 Overall survival **(a)** is poorer in older patients while cancer-specific survival **(b)** is comparable to younger patients.

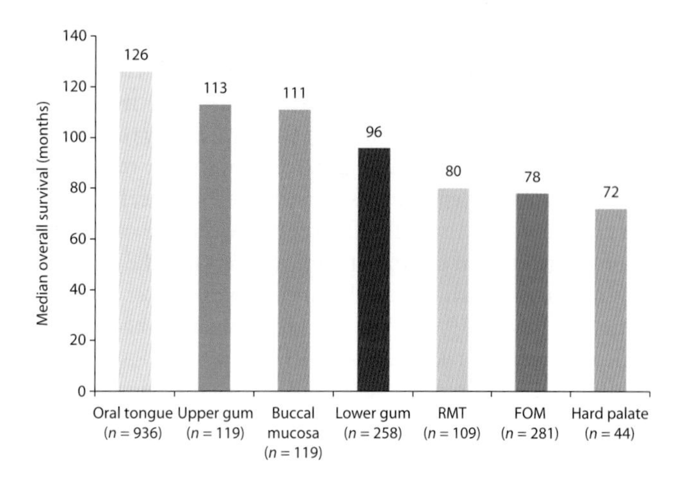

Figure 19.12 Overall survival is related to the site of the primary tumor within the oral cavity. FOM: floor of mouth; RMT: retromolar trigone.

tobacco products, but this has not been confirmed by subsequent studies (24). There is some suspicion that tumors in some younger patients who do not have the usual risk factors behave differently from the tobacco and/or alcohol-associated tumors in the older age group (25). These tumors may be related to HPV, and such tumors are reported to have a better prognosis than tobacco/alcohol-induced carcinomas (26). On the other hand, a subset of pathologically aggressive tumors that has a worse prognosis has been reported in patients younger than 35 years of age, especially females who do not have associated behavioral risk factors. It is unclear if these patients have biologically distinct tumors and/or if these differences are related to the host's immune status (27,28).

A significantly worse outcome has been reported for African–Americans compared to Caucasians and for males compared to females after treatment for squamous carcinoma of the oral cavity (11). Although the socioeconomic status of the host may contribute to ethnicity-related differences, the role of other factors such as aggressive tumor biology, host vulnerability, compliance with treatment and social support remain unclear. Hormonal, genetic, immunologic and behavioral and compliance issues may be related to the better survival reported in women (29).

The site of the tumor within the oral cavity can influence outcome (Figure 19.12). For example, patients with tumors arising in the tongue have better overall survival when compared with patients with tumors in other sites. On the other hand, patients with primary tumors in the buccal mucosa, retromolar trigone, floor of the mouth and hard palate had the poorest overall survival. This observation may be less related to the inherent biology of the tumor than to other factors such as proximity of the tumor to bone (retromolar trigone or alveolus) or the density of lymphatics (tongue). Tables 19.1 and 19.2 list some results of treatments in patients

Table 19.1 Overall 5-year survival (%) in patients with cancer of the floor of the mouth

Series	Total no. of patients	Stage I	Stage II	Stage III	Stage IV
Harrold, 1971 (57)	634	69	49	25	7
Panje et al., 1980 (58)	103	57	60	43	19
Nason et al., 1989 (59)	198	69	64	46	26
Shaha et al., 1984 (60)	320	88	80	66	32
Fu et al., 1976 (61)	153	83	71	45	10
Pernot et al., 1996 (62)	207	(T1)	(T1)	(T1)	—
		71	42	35	
MSKCC, 2017[a]	242	63	62	47	38

[a] Unpublished data.

Table 19.2 Overall 5-year survival (%) in patients with cancer of the tongue

Series	Total no. of patients	Stage I	Stage II	Stage III	Stage IV
Callery et al., 1984 (63)	252	75	60	40	20
Decroix et al., 1981 (64)	602	59	45	25	13
Wallner et al., 1986 (65)	424	68	50	33	20
Ildstad et al., 1983 (66)	122	48	48	18	26
O'Brien et al., 1986 (67)	97	73	62	—	—
Pernot et al., 1996 (62)	565	(T1)	(T1)	(T1)	—
		70	42	29	
MSKCC, 2017[a]	887	82	68	65	28

[a] Unpublished data.

treated for cancers of the floor of the mouth and oral tongue reported in the literature. Histologic variants of squamous cell carcinoma also have vastly different clinical behaviors and survival rates. Verrucous carcinoma of the oral cavity tends to have a more indolent course and carries a relatively low potential for regional lymph node metastasis. The survival of patients with verrucous carcinoma is more favorable than for patients with invasive squamous cell carcinoma and better survival rates have been reported using surgery compared to radiation therapy for oral verrucous tumors (30).

The clinical and pathological stages of the tumor are obviously important determinants of outcome, but the presence of nodal metastasis is the single most powerful predictor of survival (Figure 19.3). While the T stage measures the primary tumor in two dimensions, the depth of invasion represents the third dimension that relates to risk for lymph node metastasis (Figure 19.7). Deeply infiltrative tumors, measured by thickness of tumor, have significantly higher locoregional recurrence rates and poorer outcomes compared to more superficial tumors (Figure 19.13).

Complete surgical excision of the tumor, achieving negative surgical margins, is crucial to locoregional control and cancer-specific survival (Figure 19.14). Various other parameters such as perineural and vascular invasion and the grade of the primary tumor have been reported to be significant prognostic factors. However, positive surgical margins and lymph node metastasis are the only independent predictors on multivariate analysis of locoregional control and cancer-specific survival in patients with squamous carcinoma of the oral cavity. While the majority of oral cavity tumors are squamous cell carcinomas, a vast array of other tumor histologies may occur in this location. Minor salivary gland tumors, sarcomas, metastatic tumors, lymphomas, osseous tumors of the skeletal framework and mucosal melanomas represent a few of the possibilities. Although the principles of surgical treatment for

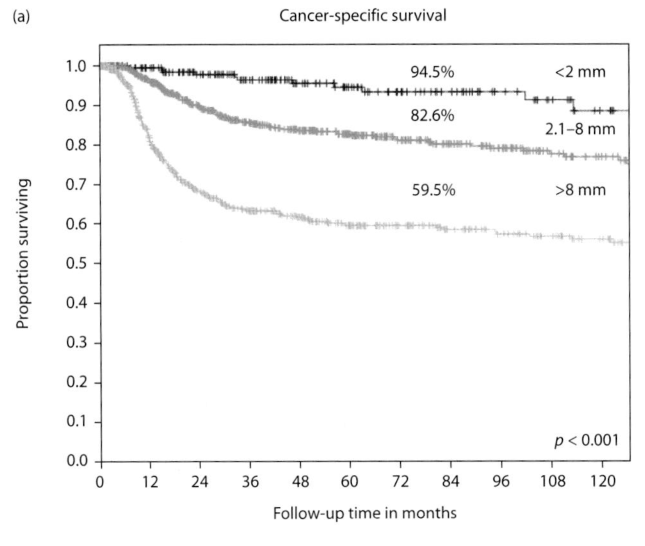

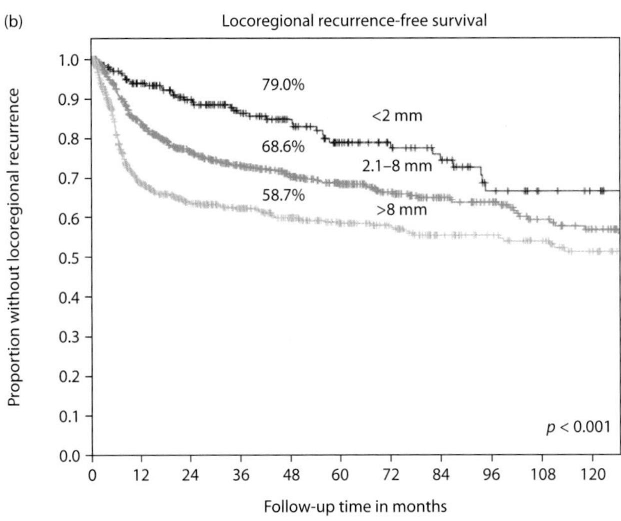

Figure 19.13 Deeply infiltrative tumors are more difficult to control locoregionally and have a poorer outcome compared to superficial tumors; **(a)** cancer-specific survival and **(b)** locoregional recurrence free survival.

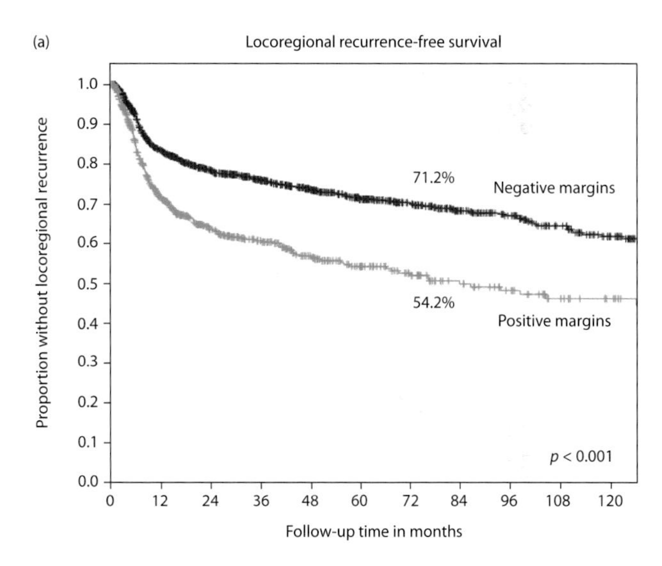

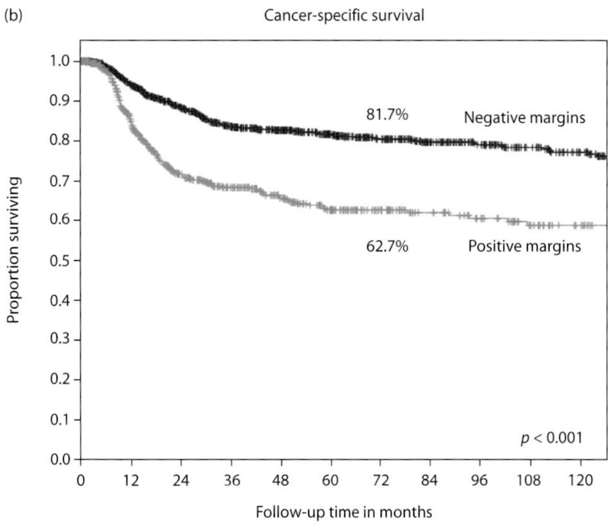

Figure 19.14 Positive surgical margins are significant predictors of locoregional failure **(a)** and cancer-specific survival **(b)**.

these tumors remain similar, the treatments and outcomes in all of these are widely divergent and beyond the scope of this chapter.

OROPHARYNX

The incidence of oropharynx carcinoma has risen during the last 20 years (31,32). This phenomenon has been called an "epidemic" and is attributed to changes in the etiological pattern of oropharyngeal carcinomas (33,34). The oropharynx is the most likely site to be HPV positive in head and neck and this accounts for the increasing incidence of HPV-related cancers. It has been estimated that 70% of oropharyngeal cancers are HPV related (35).

The treatment of oropharyngeal cancer has evolved over the last few decades. The standard treatment of oropharyngeal cancer 30 years ago was surgery followed by postoperative radiation therapy. Although acceptable oncologic outcomes were achieved with this approach (i.e. cancer-specific survival reported between 60% and 75%), the high burden of complications and functional sequelae of the surgery prompted a shift in therapy to an organ preservation approach. At that time, increasing availability of chemoradiation options propelled this paradigm shift. Currently, the most frequently employed primary treatment for early-stage oropharyngeal carcinoma is radiation therapy and for advanced-stage oropharyngeal carcinoma is chemoradiation therapy. However, there is renewed interest in less aggressive and intense therapies based on our understanding of HPV-related disease and there have been recent advances in minimally invasive surgery (robotic surgery and transoral laser microsurgery [TLM]) and a growing awareness of the short- and long-term sequelae of the concurrent chemoradiation therapy approach.

Our knowledge of survival in HPV-associated oropharyngeal cancer is based on information from large retrospective series and fewer prospective studies that strongly suggest that HPV-positive oropharyngeal cancers have a better prognosis (Table 19.3). Retrospective analyses by several authors have shown significantly better overall and disease-specific survival in patients with HPV-positive compared to HPV-negative tonsillar carcinoma treated with radiotherapy, even when adjusted for age, gender, tumor characteristics and treatment (36,37). These results are similar to the risk of local failure for HPV-positive patients after the analysis was adjusted by T stage and alcohol consumption (38). Authors have often attributed this benefit to being a favorable increase in sensitivity to radiotherapy. When clinical trials for locally advanced oropharyngeal cancer are reviewed, the results show similar trends in survival (Table 19.3). The first prospective analysis by Kumar et al. showed a better overall and disease-specific survival among HPV-positive tumor patients when compared with HPV-negative patients (39). Subsequently, Fakhry et al. in 2008 prospectively analyzed a cohort of patients treated with chemoradiation therapy. They demonstrated a 61% reduction in risk of death and a 62% lower risk of progression for patients with HPV-positive oropharyngeal carcinoma. Additionally, patients with HPV-positive disease had a significantly better response rate to chemoradiation when compared to HPV-negative patients (84% versus 57%, respectively) (40).

Results published by the Radiation Therapy Oncology Group (RTOG 0129) showed with a *post hoc* analysis that HPV status is an independent predictor of survival. HPV-positive patients with stage III and IV oropharyngeal carcinoma had a significantly better overall survival (3-year overall survival of 82.4% versus 57.1% for HPV-negative cancer). They developed a risk model for death from oropharyngeal squamous cell carcinoma on the basis of HPV status, pack-years of tobacco smoking, tumor stage and nodal stage that showed that the risk of death significantly increased with each additional pack-year of tobacco smoking (41).

Other clinical trials have shown similar favorable outcomes for HPV-positive oropharyngeal cancer patients. The Trans Tasman Radiation Oncology (TROG) phase III trial on 172 oropharynx cancer patients (59% of them HPV positive) also reported a better overall survival (91% versus 74%) and RFS for HPV-positive patients (87% versus 72%)

Table 19.3 Clinical trials analyzing on the effect of HPV status on survival

Authors	Patients (*n*)	Outcome HPV positive versus HPV negative		
		Endpoint	Hazard ratio or odds ratio (95% confidence interval)	*p*-value
Fakhry et al. (40)	96	Tumor progression	0.27 (0.10–0.75)	.01
Ang et al. (41)	323	Overall survival	0.42 (0.27–0.66)	<.001
		Progression-free survival	0.49 (0.33–0.74)	<.001
Rischin et al. (42)	185	Overall survival	0.36 (0.17–0.74)	.004
		Failure-free survival	0.39 (0.20–0.74)	<.001
Posner et al. (43)	111	Overall survival	0.20 (0.10–0.38	<.0001
Lassen et al. (68)	794	Overall survival	0.62 (0.49–0.78)	<.001
		Disease-specific survival	0.58 (0.41–0.81)	.001

Source: From Ang KK, Sturgis EM. *Semin Radiat Oncol* 2012;22(2):128–42 (69).

than HPV-negative patients (42). A subset analysis of oropharyngeal cancer patients in a prospectively randomized, international phase III trial (TAX 324) where 50% of the evaluable patients were HPV positive showed a significantly better survival for HPV-positive patients of 82% versus 35% for HPV-negative patients at 5 years (43).

The prognostic interaction of HPV infection and tobacco use has been addressed by Ang et al. in their analysis of the RTOG 0129 data. They found a deleterious effect of smoking history on the otherwise positive impact of HPV infection on survival in oropharyngeal cancer patients. Among HPV-positive patients, 82% were never-smokers versus 58% among HPV-negative patients. Smoking was an independent predictor of worse survival in both groups and was directly related to the pack per year history. Using HPV status, smoking history, lymph node categories and T status, they could stratify patients into three different risk groups. Although most of the patients with HPV-positive tumors fall into the low-risk category (3-year survival: 94%), patients with HPV-positive tumors but with smoking history of more than 10 pack-years were at an intermediate risk of survival (3-year survival: 67%) (41). This interaction of HPV disease and tobacco has also been reported by other authors (44).

The positive influence of HPV status on survival in oropharyngeal cancer is widely demonstrated by the information gathered in randomized clinical trials and case series. HPV-associated disease seems to be highly responsive to treatment. This information has fueled the basis for de-intensification of treatment based on risk stratification in oropharyngeal carcinoma. Changes in treatment schemes or less aggressive treatments for HPV-positive oropharyngeal carcinomas should be expected in the future if current expectations about favorable prognosis are fulfilled. However, any changes should be based on randomized clinical trials specifically designed to address the most effective treatment for HPV-positive and HPV-negative patients (45).

RADIOTHERAPY

In recent years, radiation therapy for oropharyngeal cancer has progressed from conventional radiation (parallel opposing ports) to intensity-modulated radiotherapy (IMRT). Several studies demonstrated that local control was directly related to the total dose and treatment length (46). After the RTOG 90-03 study (47), the use of hyperfractionation and concomitant boost demonstrated superiority over other schemes of fractionation and was rapidly adopted as the standard of care in the late 1990s. However, developments in IMRT at the end of the last century quickly resulted in wide acceptance of this new technology because of its improved accuracy and benefits of improved normal tissue sparing. These benefits were demonstrated in a UK multicenter phase II trial (PARSPORT) showing a significant improvement in quality of life and reduction in xerostomia among patients treated with IMRT compared to conventional radiotherapy (48).

Table 19.4 Results of treatment of oropharyngeal cancer with radiotherapy (IMRT)

Authors	Year	Patients (*n*)	Locoregional control
Chao et al. (70)	2004	74	87%
Yao et al. (71)	2006	66	99%
Garden et al. (72)	2007	51	93%
Huang et al. (73)	2008	71	94%
Daly et al. (74)	2009	107	92%
RTOG 00-22 (75)	2009	69	91%
MSKCC (53)	2010	442	LC: 94.6%; RC: 94.4%

LC: local control; RC: regional control.

Currently, IMRT has demonstrated very good locoregional control rates in patients with oropharyngeal cancer. Several reports showed over 90% control at up to 2 years with a low toxicity profile. This is summarized in Table 19.4.

CHEMORADIATION THERAPY

In a large meta-analysis of 63 previously published trials, Pignon et al. demonstrated that the concomitant use of chemotherapy and radiotherapy in advanced head and neck cancer offers an absolute survival benefit of 6.5% at 5 years (49). This benefit was superior to the use of neoadjuvant or adjuvant chemotherapy. The proportion of oropharyngeal cancer patients in this analysis was 37%. After this finding, a Groupe d'Oncologie Radiothérapie Tête Cou (GORTEC) study showed a statistically significant improvement in overall survival and locoregional control in patients treated with concomitant chemoradiation therapy versus radiation therapy alone (50). With this evidence, the use of concomitant chemoradiation was established in the last 10 years as the standard of care for advanced oropharyngeal carcinoma. However, this approach is associated with a higher incidence of short-term and long-term toxicities, like mucositis, dermatitis, fibrosis and chronic dysphagia. The incidence of late complications (grade 3 and 4, common terminology criteria for adverse events [CTCAE] v3.0) has been described to be high as 56% (50,51).

The role of new therapeutic approaches to oropharyngeal cancer is consistently being researched. One area gaining interest examines the use of de-intensifying chemoradiation treatment regimens for patients with HPV-positive oropharyngeal cancer. Other areas of investigation include the use of lower doses of radiation, smaller radiation fields or different chemotherapy agents, hypothesizing that these approaches may contribute to reducing the short- and long-term complications of chemoradiation therapy. The recently closed RTOG 1016 trial compared the efficacy of concurrent chemoradiation therapy with cisplatin versus cetuximab for the treatment of HPV-positive oropharyngeal cancer and its results are awaited (52).

THE MSKCC EXPERIENCE WITH CHEMORADIATION THERAPY IN OROPHARYNGEAL CANCER

Between 1998 and 2009, 472 oropharyngeal cancer patients were treated at the MSKCC with IMRT. The median dose of RT was 70 Gy in 2.12-Gy daily fractions over 33 days. In total, 88% of these patients received concurrent chemotherapy; 50% of patients had primary tumors of the tonsil, 46% of the base of the tongue and 5% of the pharyngeal wall and soft palate. The results of treatment are summarized in Figure 19.15. The reported 3-year overall survival was 84.9%. The most significant factors associated with poor survival were T stage (T3–4 versus T1–2) and N stage (N2–3 versus N0–1). The local failure rate at 3 years was 5.4%, with all local failures occurring within the first 2 years after treatment was completed. Advanced T stage was the only significant factor associated with local recurrence. The regional failure was 5.6% at 3 years. No significant predictors of regional failure were found. There were no significant differences in outcome by tumor subsite. With respect to acute toxicities, only three patients developed grade 4 mucositis and one patient developed grade 4 dermatitis. The most common grade 3 toxicities were mucositis (22%), dysphagia (16%) and dermatitis (7%). Late toxicities such as grade ≥2 xerostomia and grade ≥2 late dysphagia were noted in 29% and 11% of patients, respectively. The outcomes reported in this study were similar to those of other published series (53).

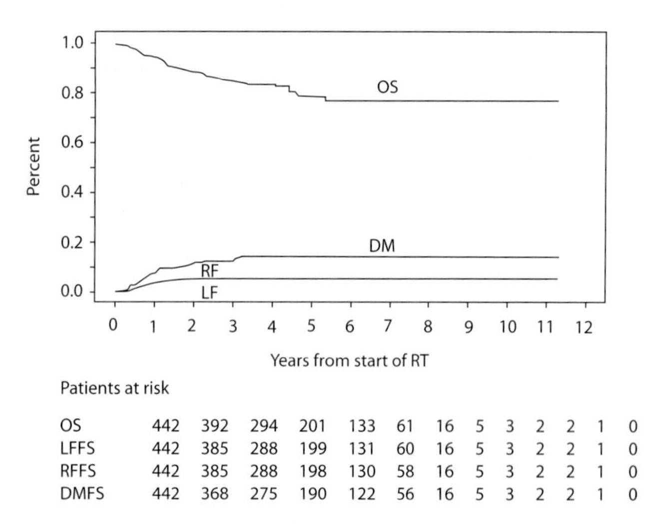

Figure 19.15 Results of treatment of oropharyngeal cancer at the Memorial Sloan Kettering Cancer Center using IMRT. Kaplan–Meier OS rate and cumulative incidence of LF, RF and DM. OS = overall survival; LF = local failure; RF = regional failure; DM = distant metastasis; LFFS = local failure-free survival; RFFS = regional failure-free survival; DMFS = distant metastasis-free survival. (Adapted from Setton J et al. *Int J Radiat Oncol Biol Phys* 2012;82(1):291–8 (53).)

SURGERY

Traditionally, the use of surgery in oropharyngeal cancer included the use of mandibulotomy to gain adequate access for resection and reconstruction. With the progressive use of radiation therapy and, more recently, chemoradiation therapy, surgery for oropharyngeal cancer was largely relegated to the salvage of persistent or recurrent disease. However, with the development of new minimally invasive technologies and new surgical techniques, there has been renewed interest in primary surgical treatment of oropharyngeal cancer.

The two techniques currently used are TLM and transoral robotic surgery (TORS). TLM is performed using an operating microscope with the usual instrumentation and the CO_2 laser used for laryngeal surgery. TORS requires the use of a surgical robot to facilitate the interaction between the surgeon and the patient. Since the first report by O'Malley et al. in 2006 (54), TORS has rapidly become the preferred technique for transoral surgical treatment of oropharyngeal cancer.

The published results have shown local control similar to chemoradiation therapy, with the caveat that these studies are small series with short follow-up periods. These results are summarized in Table 19.5. Locoregional control can be achieved for more than 90% of patients, at least in the first year of follow-up. Complications such as percutaneous endoscopic gastrostomy (PEG) dependency and aspiration are under 20% and comparable to other treatment approaches. A downside is the need for adjuvant treatment, specifically chemoradiation therapy in 20%–50% of patients.

THE MSKCC EXPERIENCE WITH SURGERY IN OROPHARYNGEAL CANCER

The results of surgical treatment of oropharyngeal cancer at the MSKCC have been recently published (55). These patients were treated with traditional surgical techniques prior to the era of TORS. A total of 213 patients with tonsillar squamous cell carcinoma treated between January 1985 and December 2005 were identified from an institutional database. Of these, 88 patients (41%) were treated exclusively with surgery and/or radiotherapy and were used in the analysis. No patients had postoperative chemoradiation. Patients were mainly cT1–2 (52%) and cN0–1 (52%). The HPV status was available in 75% of patients. The results of treatment are summarized in Figure 19.16. Overall survival, disease-specific survival and RFS at 5 years were 66%, 82%, and 80%, respectively. The 5-year local RFS, regional RFS and locoregional RFS rates were 89%, 98% and 88%, respectively. In this analysis, age >60 years, female sex, clinical and pathological T classification, margin status, lymphovascular invasion and p16 status were predictive of overall survival on univariate analysis. However, on multivariate analysis, only lymphovascular invasion remained a

Table 19.5 Results of treatment of oropharyngeal cancer with surgery

Authors	Year	Patients (*n*)	Site	5-year OS (%)	5-year DSS (%)	5-year RFS (%)	LVI	HPV
Moore et al. (76)	2009	102	Tonsil	85	94	—	—	—
Moncrieff et al. (77)	2009	92	OP	—	83	—	—	—
Yildirim et al. (78)	2010	120	Tonsil	86	—	92	—	—
Chuang et al. (79)	2011	86	Tonsil	—	—	—	NS	NS
Haughey et al. (56)	2011	204	OP	78	84	74	—	S
Haughey and Sinha (80)	2012	171	OP	91	94	—	S	S
MSKCC (55)	2012	88	Tonsil	66	82	80	S	S

OS: overall survival; DSS: disease-specific survival; RFS: recurrence-free survival; LVI: lympho-vascular invasion; OP: oropharynx; NS: not significant; S: significant.

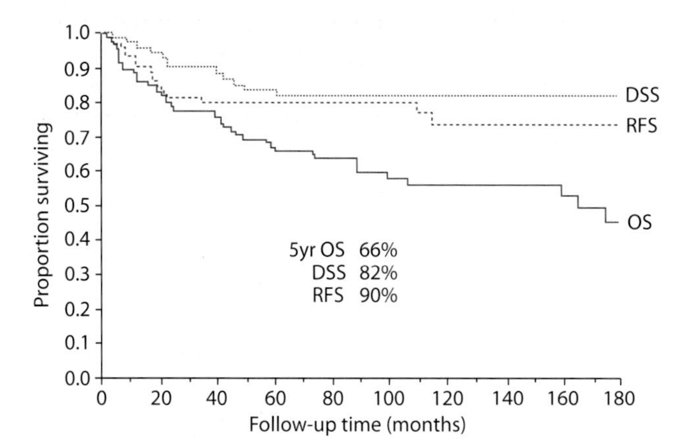

Figure 19.16 Overall, disease-specific and recurrence-free survival in patients with squamous cell carcinoma of the tonsil managed by surgery with postoperative radiotherapy. OS = overall survival; RFS = recurrence-free survival; DSS = disease-specific survival. (Adapted from Rahmati R et al. *Head Neck* 2015;37(6):800–7 (55).)

significant independent predictor (Figure 19.17). Similarly, lymphovascular invasion was the only independent predictor of disease-specific survival and recurrence. Also, on univariate analysis, HPV status was a significant predictor of overall survival and disease-specific survival (Figure 19.18). Finally, with respect to long-term sequelae of treatment at 1 year after surgery, only one patient (1.1%) was tracheostomy-dependent and 11 patients (12%) were still PEG-dependent.

Interestingly, some well-known prognostic factors were non-significant in this study: margin status, the presence of extensive lymph node disease and the presence of extracapsular extension were not independent predictors of recurrence. The lack of prognostic significance of ECS in HPV-positive oropharyngeal cancer was also recently reported by Haughey et al (56). Conversely, when extra capsular spread (ECS) was analyzed in the HPV-negative patients, it had a significant negative impact on survival. A similar finding was also observed when we assessed the impact of positive/close margins on disease specific survival (DSS) in patients who were p16 positive. These findings suggest that HPV-positive tumors have less aggressive behavior than HPV-negative tonsillar cancer.

In conclusion, the results of the analysis of tonsillar squamous cell carcinoma treated with conventional surgery and postoperative radiation therapy showed very promising results. Overall survival, disease-specific survival and recurrence rate are comparable to other studies published in the literature evaluating tonsillar squamous cell carcinoma

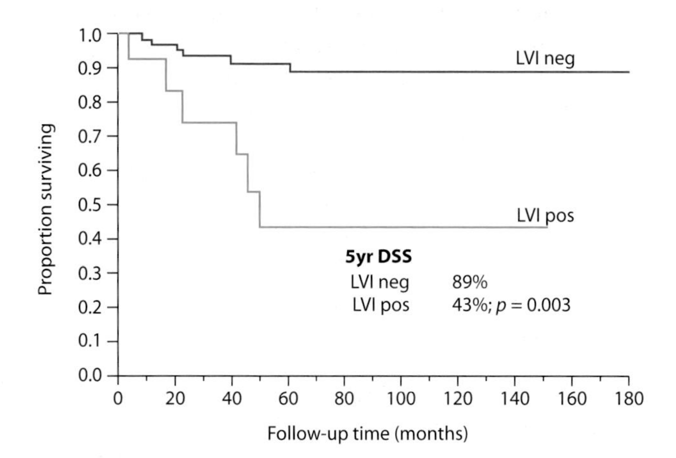

Figure 19.17 Disease-specific survival stratified by lymphovascular invasion.

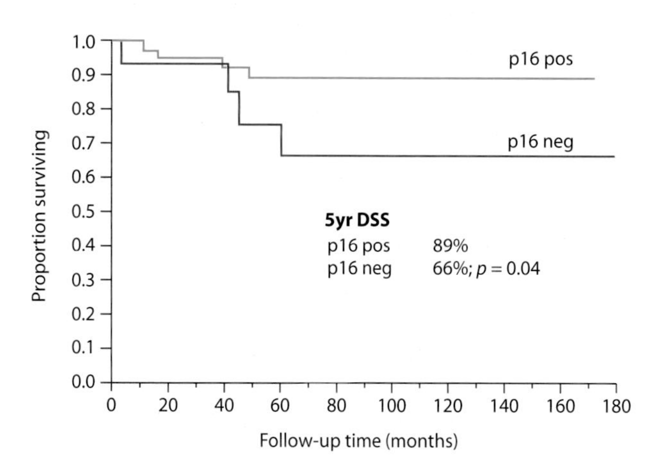

Figure 19.18 Disease-specific survival stratified by p16 status.

Table 19.6 Results of treatment of oropharyngeal cancer with TORS

Authors	Patients (n)	T1–2	N0–2b	Additional RT	Additional CTRT	PEG dependent	Aspiration	Locoregional control
Moore et al. (81)	45	73%	76%	18%	56%	18%	NA	90% at 1 year
Boudreaux et al. (82)	36	81%	19%	NA	NA	25%	3%	NA
Genden et al. (83)	20	100%	100%	44%	17%	0%	NA	100% at 5 months
Iseli et al. (84)	54	80%	NA	41%	20%	17%	6%	NA
Weinstein et al. (85)	31	100%	97%	40%	40%	NA	NA	93% at 2 years

RT: radiotherapy; CTRT: chemoradiotherapy.

managed by primary surgery, radiation or both (Table 19.6). A multicenter prospective study of 204 patients with oropharyngeal cancer treated with TLM reported comparable 3-year overall survival, DSS and disease-free survival (56). These outcomes also compare favorably with primary radiation and concomitant chemoradiation, for which treatment results range from 87% to 97% (Table 19.5), but with less long-term toxicity. Minimally invasive transoral surgical techniques in conjunction with adjuvant postoperative radiotherapy offers comparable treatment outcomes to radiotherapy alone and chemoradiation therapy. These outcomes make an argument for primary surgical therapy in a selected group of patients whose primary tumors are amenable to surgical resection by transoral endoscopic or robotic techniques. Surgery with radiotherapy is a reliable approach to de-intensifying treatment and might benefit selected patients.

FUTURE TRIALS

Currently, the appropriate treatment for early- and advanced-stage oropharyngeal cancer is controversial. Future directions of oropharyngeal cancer treatment are under study. Two major clinical trials have been designed to address the treatment of HPV-related and non-related tumors, with focus on modifying therapy and incorporating transoral surgery in treatment. The Eastern Cooperative Oncology Group has initiated a trial (ECOG 3311) that will evaluate de-intensified radiotherapy and chemotherapy against transoral surgical resection of HPV-positive oropharyngeal cancer. The RTOG 1221 trial was designed to compare outcomes of treatment of HPV-negative tumors with transoral surgery and adjuvant postoperative radiotherapy versus chemoradiation therapy, but was terminated due to a lack of accrual.

Other studies are addressing the de-intensification of therapy from a non-surgical point of view. The ECOG 1308 trial for stage III/IV HPV-associated cancer tested the use of induction chemotherapy (combination paclitaxel, cisplatin and cetuximab followed by concurrent cetuximab and radiotherapy) in order to reduce the dose to the primary site and involved neck nodes (from 69.3 to 54 Gy). This study is currently closed. A second study is the RTOG 1016 trial designed to test the use of a standard dose of radiotherapy with either concurrent cisplatin or concurrent cetuximab.

REFERENCES

1. Cooper JS, Porter K, Mallin K et al. National cancer database report on cancer of the head and neck: 10-year update. *Head Neck* 2009;31(6):748–58.
2. Howlader N, Noone AM, Krapcho M et al (eds). *SEER Cancer Statistics Review, 1975–2008*. Bethesda, MD: National Cancer Institute, 2011. https://seer.cancer.gov/archive/csr/1975_2008.
3. Pulte D, Brenner H. Changes in survival in head and neck cancers in the late 20th and early 21st century: a period analysis. *Oncologist* 2010;15(9): 994–1001.
4. Hashibe M, Brennan P, Chuang SC et al. Interaction between tobacco and alcohol use and the risk of head and neck cancer: pooled analysis in the international head and neck cancer epidemiology consortium. *Cancer Epidemiol Biomarkers Prev* 2009;18(2):541–50.
5. Gillison ML. Human papillomavirus-associated head and neck cancer is a distinct epidemiologic, clinical, and molecular entity. *Semin Oncol* 2004;31(6): 744–54.
6. Sturgis EM, Cinciripini PM. Trends in head and neck cancer incidence in relation to smoking prevalence: an emerging epidemic of human papillomavirus-associated cancers? *Cancer* 2007; 110(7):1429–35.
7. Chaturvedi AK, Engels EA, Anderson WF et al. Incidence trends for human papillomavirus-related and -unrelated oral squamous cell carcinomas in the United States. *J Clin Oncol* 2008;26(4):612–9.
8. Edge S, Byrd DR, Comtpon CC, Fritz AG, Greene FL, Trotti A (eds). *AJCC cancer Staging Manual* (7th Edition). Lyons, France: Springer, 2010.
9. SPSS Inc. IBM SPSS Statistics for Windows [computer program]. *Version 22*. Armonk, NY: IBM Corp., 2013.
10. R Development Core Team. *R: A Language and Environment for Statistical Computing [computer program]*. Vienna: The R Foundation for Statistical Computing, 2014.

11. Funk GF, Karnell LH, Robinson RA et al. Presentation, treatment, and outcome of oral cavity cancer: a national cancer data base report. *Head Neck* 2002;24(2):165–80.
12. Loree TR, Strong EW. Significance of positive margins in oral cavity squamous carcinoma. *Am J Surg* 1990;160(4):410–4.
13. Mistry RC, Qureshi SS, Kumaran C. Post-resection mucosal margin shrinkage in oral cancer: quantification and significance. *J Surg Oncol* 2005;91(2): 131–3.
14. Montero PH, Montero PH, Palmer FL et al. A novel tumor: specimen index for assessing adequacy of resection in early stage oral tongue cancer. *Oral Oncol* 2014;50(3):213–20.
15. Zelefsky MJ, Harrison LB, Fass DE, Armstrong JG, Shah JP, Strong EW. Postoperative radiation therapy for squamous cell carcinomas of the oral cavity and oropharynx: impact of therapy on patients with positive surgical margins. *Int J Radiat Oncol Biol Phys* 1993;25(1):17–21.
16. Fagan JJ, Collins B, Barnes L et al. Perineural invasion in squamous cell carcinoma of the head and neck. *Arch Otolaryngol* 1998;124(6):637–40.
17. Chinn SB, Spector ME, Bellile EL et al. Impact of perineural invasion in the pathologically N0 neck in oral cavity squamous cell carcinoma. *Otolaryngol Head Neck Surg* 2013;149(6):893–9.
18. Spiro RH, Huvos AG, Wong GY et al. Predictive value of tumor thickness in squamous carcinoma confined to the tongue and floor of the mouth. *Am J Surg* 1986;152(4):345–50.
19. Mohit-Tabatabai MA, Sobel HJ, Rush BF, Mashberg A. Relation of thickness of floor of mouth stage I and II cancers to regional metastasis. *Am J Surg* 1986;152(4):351–3.
20. Yuen AP, Lam KY, Wei WI et al. A comparison of the prognostic significance of tumor diameter, length, width, thickness, area, volume, and clinicopathological features of oral tongue carcinoma. *Am J Surg* 2000;180(2):139–43.
21. International Consortium for Outcome Research in Head and Neck Cancer, Ebrahimi A, Gil Z, Amit M et al. Primary tumor staging for oral cancer and a proposed modification incorporating depth of invasion: an international multicenter retrospective study. *JAMA Otolaryngol Head Neck Surg* 2014;140(12):1138–48.
22. Amin MB, Edge SB, Greene FL et al (eds). *AJCC Cancer Staging Manual* (8th Edition). Lyons, France: Springer, 2017.
23. Ferlay JSI, Ervik M, Dikshit R et al. GLOBOCAN 2012 v1.0, cancer incidence and mortality worldwide: IARC cancer Base No. 11 [Internet]. *International Agency for Research on Cancer*, 2013.
24. Majchrzak E, Szybiak B, Wegner A et al. Oral cavity and oropharyngeal squamous cell carcinoma in young adults: a review of the literature. *Radiol Oncol* 2014;48(1):1–10.
25. Koch WM, Lango M, Sewell D et al. Head and neck cancer in nonsmokers: a distinct clinical and molecular entity. *Laryngoscope* 1999;109(10): 1544–51.
26. Gillison ML, Koch WM, Capone RB et al. Evidence for a causal association between human papillomavirus and a subset of head and neck cancers. *J Natl Cancer Inst* 2000;92(9):709–20.
27. Byers RM. Squamous cell carcinoma of the oral tongue in patients less than thirty years of age. *Am J Surg* 1975;130(4):475–8.
28. Kuriakose M, Sankaranarayanan M, Nair MK et al. Comparison of oral squamous cell carcinoma in younger and older patients in India. *Eur J Cancer, B, Oral Oncol* 1992;28B(2):113–20.
29. Franco EL, Dib LL, Pinto DS et al. Race and gender influences on the survival of patients with mouth cancer. *J Clin Epidemiol* 1993;46(1):37–46.
30. Koch BB, Trask DK, Hoffman HT et al. National survey of head and neck verrucous carcinoma: patterns of presentation, care, and outcome. *Cancer* 2001;92(1):110–20.
31. Frisch M, Hjalgrim H, Jaeger AB et al. Changing patterns of tonsillar squamous cell carcinoma in the United States. *Cancer Causes Control* 2000; 11(6):489–95.
32. Shiboski CH, Schmidt BL, Jordan RC. Tongue and tonsil carcinoma: increasing trends in the U.S. population ages 20–44 years. *Cancer* 2005;103(9):1843–9.
33. Sturgis EM, Ang KK. The epidemic of HPV-associated oropharyngeal cancer is here: is it time to change our treatment paradigms? *J Natl Compr Canc Netw* 2011;9(6):665–73.
34. Gillison ML, D'Souza G, Westra W et al. Distinct risk factor profiles for human papillomavirus type 16-positive and human papillomavirus type 16-negative head and neck cancers. *J Natl Cancer Inst* 2008;100(6):407–20.
35. Kreimer AR, Clifford GM, Boyle P et al. Human papillomavirus types in head and neck squamous cell carcinomas worldwide: a systematic review. *Cancer Epidemiol Biomarkers Prev* 2005;14(2):467–75.
36. Li W, Thompson CH, O'Brien CJ et al. Human papillomavirus positivity predicts favourable outcome for squamous carcinoma of the tonsil. *Int J Cancer* 2003;106(4):553–8.
37. Mellin H, Friesland S, Lewensohn R, Dalianis T, Munck-Wikland E. Human papillomavirus (HPV) DNA in tonsillar cancer: clinical correlates, risk of relapse, and survival. *Int J Cancer* 2000;89(3):300–4.
38. Lindel K, Beer KT, Laissue J, Greiner RH, Aebersold DM. Human papillomavirus positive squamous cell carcinoma of the oropharynx: a radiosensitive subgroup of head and neck carcinoma. *Cancer* 2001;92(4):805–13.

39. Kumar B, Cordell KG, Lee JS et al. EGFR, p16, HPV Titer, Bcl-xL and p53, sex, and smoking as indicators of response to therapy and survival in oropharyngeal cancer. *J Clin Oncol* 2008;26(19):3128–37.
40. Fakhry C, Westra WH, Li S et al. Improved survival of patients with human papillomavirus-positive head and neck squamous cell carcinoma in a prospective clinical trial. *J Natl Cancer Inst* 2008;100(4): 261–9.
41. Ang KK, Harris J, Wheeler R et al. Human papillomavirus and survival of patients with oropharyngeal cancer. *N Engl J Med* 2010;363(1):24–35.
42. Rischin D, Young RJ, Fisher R et al. Prognostic significance of p16INK4A and human papillomavirus in patients with oropharyngeal cancer treated on TROG 02.02 phase III trial. *J Clin Oncol* 2010;28(27):4142–8.
43. Posner MR, Lorch JH, Goloubeva O et al. Survival and human papillomavirus in oropharynx cancer in TAX 324: a subset analysis from an international phase III trial. *Ann Oncol* 2011;22(5):1071–7.
44. Maxwell JH, Kumar B, Feng FY et al. Tobacco use in human papillomavirus-positive advanced oropharynx cancer patients related to increased risk of distant metastases and tumor recurrence. *Clin Cancer Res* 2010;16(4):1226–35.
45. Mehanna H, Olaleye O, Licitra L. Oropharyngeal cancer: is it time to change management according to human papilloma virus status? *Curr Opin Otolaryngol Head Neck Surg* 2012; 20:120–124.
46. Withers HR, Peters LJ, Taylor JM et al. Local control of carcinoma of the tonsil by radiation therapy: an analysis of patterns of fractionation in nine institutions. *Int J Radiat Oncol Biol Phys* 1995;33(3):549–62.
47. Fu KK, Pajak TF, Trotti A et al. A radiation therapy oncology group (RTOG) phase III randomized study to compare hyperfractionation and two variants of accelerated fractionation to standard fractionation radiotherapy for head and neck squamous cell carcinomas: first report of RTOG 9003. *Int J Radiat Oncol Biol Phys* 2000;48(1):7–16.
48. Nutting CM, Morden JP, Harrington KJ et al. Parotid-sparing intensity modulated versus conventional radiotherapy in head and neck cancer (PARSPORT): a phase 3 multicentre randomised controlled trial. *Lancet Oncol* 2011;12(2):127–36.
49. Pignon JP, Bourhis J, Domenge C et al. Chemotherapy added to locoregional treatment for head and neck squamous-cell carcinoma: three meta-analyses of updated individual data. MACH-NC collaborative group. meta-analysis of chemotherapy on head and neck cancer. *Lancet* 2000;355(9208): 949–55.
50. Denis F, Garaud P, Bardet E et al. Final results of the 94-01 French head and neck oncology and radiotherapy group randomized trial comparing radiotherapy alone with concomitant radiochemotherapy in advanced-stage oropharynx carcinoma. *J Clin Oncol* 2004;22(1):69–76.
51. Machtay M, Moughan J, Trotti A et al. Factors associated with severe late toxicity after concurrent chemoradiation for locally advanced head and neck cancer: an RTOG analysis. *J Clin Oncol* 2008;26(21):3582–9.
52. Trotti AG, Harari M, Sturgis P et al. RTOG 1016: Phase III Trial of Radiotherapy Plus Cetuximab Versus Chemoradiotherapy in HPV-Associated Ororpharynx Cancer. 2014, http://www.rtog.org/ClinicalTrials/ProtocolTable/StudyDetails.aspx?study=1016.
53. Setton J, Caria N, Romanyshyn J et al. Intensity-modulated radiotherapy in the treatment of oropharyngeal cancer: an update of the memorial sloan-kettering cancer center experience. *Int J Radiat Oncol Biol Phys* 2012;82(1):291–8.
54. O'Malley BW Jr, Weinstein GS, Snyder W et al. Transoral robotic surgery (TORS) for base of tongue neoplasms. *Laryngoscope* 2006;116(8):1465–72.
55. Rahmati R, Dogan S, Pyke O et al. Squamous cell carcinoma of the tonsil managed by conventional surgery and postoperative radiation. *Head Neck* 2015;37(6):800–7.
56. Haughey BH, Hinni ML, Salassa JR et al. Transoral laser microsurgery as primary treatment for advanced-stage oropharyngeal cancer: a United States multicenter study. *Head Neck* 2011;33(12):1683–94.
57. Harrold CC Jr. Management of cancer of the floor of the mouth. *Am J Surg* 1971;122(4):487–93.
58. Panje WR, Smith B, McCabe BF. Epidermoid carcinoma of the floor of the mouth: surgical therapy vs combined therapy vs radiation therapy. *Otolaryngol Head Neck Surg* 1980;88(6):714–20.
59. Nason RW, Sako K, Beecroft WA et al. Surgical management of squamous cell carcinoma of the floor of the mouth. *Am J Surg* 1989;158(4):292–6.
60. Shaha AR, Spiro RH, Shah JP et al. Squamous carcinoma of the floor of the mouth. *Am J Surg* 1984;148(4):455–9.
61. Fu KK, Lichter A, Galante M. Carcinoma of the floor of mouth: an analysis of treatment results and the sites and causes of failures. *Int J Radiat Oncol Biol Phys* 1976;1(9–10):829–37.
62. Pernot M, Hoffstetter S, Peiffert D et al. Role of interstitial brachytherapy in oral and oropharyngeal carcinoma: reflection of a series of 1344 patients treated at the time of initial presentation. *Otolaryngol Head Neck Surg* 1996;115(6):519–26.
63. Callery CD, Spiro RH, Strong EW. Changing trends in the management of squamous carcinoma of the tongue. *Am J Surg* 1984;148(4):449–54.
64. Decroix Y, Ghossein NA. Experience of the curie institute in treatment of cancer of the mobile

tongue: I. Treatment policies and result. *Cancer* 1981;47(3):496–502.

65. Wallner PE, Hanks GE, Kramer S, McLean CJ. Patterns of care study. Analysis of outcome survey data-anterior two-thirds of tongue and floor of mouth. *Am J Clin Oncol* 1986;9(1):50–7.
66. Ildstad ST, Bigelow ME, Remensnyder JP. Squamous cell carcinoma of the mobile tongue. Clinical behavior and results of current therapeutic modalities. *Am J Surg* 1983;145(4):443–9.
67. O'Brien CJ, Lahr CJ, Soong SJ et al. Surgical treatment of early-stage carcinoma of the oral tongue—wound adjuvant treatment be beneficial? *Head Neck Surg* 1986;8(6):401–8.
68. Lassen P, Eriksen JG, Krogdahl A et al. The influence of HPV-associated p16-expression on accelerated fractionated radiotherapy in head and neck cancer: evaluation of the randomised DAHANCA 6&7 trial. *Radiother Oncol* 2011;100(1):49–55.
69. Ang KK, Sturgis EM. Human papillomavirus as a marker of the natural history and response to therapy of head and neck squamous cell carcinoma. *Semin Radiat Oncol* 2012;22(2):128–42.
70. Chao KS, Ozyigit G, Blanco AI et al. Intensity-modulated radiation therapy for oropharyngeal carcinoma: impact of tumor volume. *Int J Radiat Oncol Biol Phys* 2004;59(1):43–50.
71. Yao M, Nguyen T, Buatti JM et al. Changing failure patterns in oropharyngeal squamous cell carcinoma treated with intensity modulated radiotherapy and implications for future research. *Am J Clin Oncol* 2006;29(6):606–12.
72. Garden AS, Morrison WH, Wong PF et al. Disease-control rates following intensity-modulated radiation therapy for small primary oropharyngeal carcinoma. *Int J Radiat Oncol Biol Phys* 2007;67(2):438–44.
73. Huang K, Xia P, Chuang C et al. Intensity-modulated chemoradiation for treatment of stage III and IV oropharyngeal carcinoma: the University of California-San Francisco experience. *Cancer* 2008;113(3):497–507.
74. Daly ME, Le QT, Maxim PG et al. Intensity-modulated radiotherapy in the treatment of oropharyngeal cancer: clinical outcomes and patterns of failure. *Int J Radiat Oncol Biol Phys* 2010;76(5): 1339–46.
75. Eisbruch A, Harris J, Garden AS et al. Multi-institutional trial of accelerated hypofractionated intensity-modulated radiation therapy for early-stage oropharyngeal cancer (RTOG 00-22). *Int J Radiat Oncol Biol Phys* 2010;76(5):1333–8.
76. Moore EJ, Henstrom DK, Olsen KD et al. Transoral resection of tonsillar squamous cell carcinoma. *Laryngoscope* 2009;119(3):508–15.
77. Moncrieff M, Sandilla J, Clark J et al. Outcomes of primary surgical treatment of T1 and T2 carcinomas of the oropharynx. *Laryngoscope* 2009;119(2):307–11.
78. Yildirim G, Morrison WH, Rosenthal DI et al. Outcomes of patients with tonsillar carcinoma treated with post-tonsillectomy radiation therapy. *Head Neck* 2010;32(4):473–80.
79. Chuang HC, Fang FM, Huang CC et al. Clinical and pathological determinants in tonsillar cancer. *Head Neck* 2011;33(12):1703–7.
80. Haughey BH, Sinha P. Prognostic factors and survival unique to surgically treated p16+ oropharyngeal cancer. *Laryngoscope* 2012;122(Suppl 2):S13–S33.
81. Moore EJ, Olsen KD, Kasperbauer JL. Transoral robotic surgery for oropharyngeal squamous cell carcinoma: a prospective study of feasibility and functional outcomes. *Laryngoscope.* 2009;119(11):2156–64.
82. Boudreaux BA, Rosenthal EL, Magnuson JS et al. Robot-assisted surgery for upper aerodigestive tract neoplasms. *Arch Otolaryngol Head Neck Surg* 2009;135(4):397–401.
83. Genden EM, Desai S, Sung CK. Transoral robotic surgery for the management of head and neck cancer: a preliminary experience. *Head Neck* 2009;31(3):283–9.
84. Iseli TA, Kulbersh BD, Iseli CE et al. Functional outcomes after transoral robotic surgery for head and neck cancer. *Otolaryngol Head Neck Surg* 2009;141(2):166–71.
85. Weinstein GS, Quon H, O'Malley BW Jr et al. Selective neck dissection and deintensified postoperative radiation and chemotherapy for oropharyngeal cancer: a subset analysis of the University of Pennsylvania transoral robotic surgery trial. *Laryngoscope* 2010;120(9):1749–55.

20

Functional outcomes and rehabilitation

JOCELYN C. MIGLIACCI, ALLISON J. KOBREN, AND SNEHAL G. PATEL

INTRODUCTION

The structures in the oral cavity and the oropharynx serve vital functions in mastication, deglutition and articulation of speech. Hence, patients with oral and oropharyngeal tumors often present with complaints of difficulty eating and speaking. While these tumors themselves can create functional deficits, treatment (including surgical resection and radiation with or without chemotherapy) often results in additional functional impairment. The magnitude of these post-treatment functional deficits is related to several factors, including (1–6):

1. Soft tissue volume loss
2. Sensory loss
3. Motor function loss
4. Post-treatment limitations in mobility of the tongue and pharyngeal musculature secondary to scar contracture and fibrosis
5. Alteration in the volume and viscosity of saliva

Speech and swallowing in patients with oral and oropharyngeal tumors may also be influenced by factors unrelated to the tumor or its extirpation or non-surgical treatment such as radiation therapy (7,8). All of these factors should be considered in the rehabilitation of a patient who has been treated for oral/oropharyngeal cancer.

NORMAL PHYSIOLOGY OF SPEECH AND SWALLOWING

In order to understand the functional outcomes of patients treated for tumors of the oral cavity and oropharynx, one must first understand the complex and intricate physiologic interplay of the pertinent structures as they relate to normal speech and swallowing. Swallowing has classically been divided into four phases (Table 20.1) (9). While this classification serves as a useful conceptual framework, it is rather artificial and oversimplifies this complex and dynamic process. Although oral and oropharyngeal cancers may affect all four phases, they most commonly and most profoundly impact the first three: the oral preparatory, oral transit and pharyngeal phases.

The oral preparatory phase involves the formation of a cohesive bolus. This is accomplished by rotary mastication and the mixing of the pulverized material with saliva. This mixture is ultimately compacted together into what is commonly referred to as a bolus. Although liquid boluses do not require chewing, the structures of the oral cavity must still work to place and contain the bolus between the tongue and hard palate.

The oral preparatory phase requires the coordinated use of the lips, labiobuccal musculature, jaws, teeth, muscles of mastication, tongue and hard and soft palate. A lesion involving any of these structures is likely to affect this phase of swallowing. For example, loss of a significant volume of the oral tongue will limit the ability to transport the food into position for grinding by the molars. Similarly, loss of a segment of the mandible and associated dentition may affect the process of mastication. The treatment of all but the earliest of oral cavity tumors is likely to affect this first phase of deglutition.

The second phase of swallowing is the oral phase. This phase begins with the initiation of the movement for posterior transport of bolus and ends with the initiation of the pharyngeal phase of swallowing. During this phase, the tongue plays a particularly integral role in moving the bolus backwards toward the oropharynx. The tongue establishes

Table 20.1 Phases of normal deglutition

I: Oral preparatory phase
II: Oral phase
III: Pharyngeal phase
IV: Esophageal phase

and maintains contact with the hard palate as it propels the bolus posteriorly. As this occurs, the velum (soft palate) elevates to seal off the nasopharynx, preventing nasal regurgitation of bolus material. Ultimately, the bolus reaches the base of the tongue, where the pharyngeal phase of swallowing is triggered by the activation of sensory receptors. The oral phase in its entirety is relatively brief, often lasting less than 1.0–1.5 seconds. Tumors in the oral cavity can result in difficulty during this phase, as a result of both the tumor and its treatment. Transit time might increase with increasing bolus viscosity (10), as is seen in patients who have xerostomia following radiation therapy. Surgery for lesions of the oral tongue can be particularly detrimental to this phase from restricted mobility and loss of volume of the tongue, as the tongue plays a crucial role in mastication and propulsion of the bolus posteriorly.

The next phase of swallowing, the pharyngeal phase, begins with the triggering of the pharyngeal swallow. The pharyngeal swallow refers to a series of simultaneous pharyngeal events that ultimately result in the arrival of the bolus at the upper esophageal sphincter (UES), situated atop the esophagus. In young, healthy individuals, the pharyngeal swallow is typically triggered when the bolus arrives at the level of the ramus of the mandible (as visualized via videofluoroscopy). Older adults, however, might trigger the swallow slightly beyond this region. Upon initiation of the pharyngeal swallow, the base of the tongue makes contact with the lateral and posterior pharyngeal walls, "squeezing" the bolus inferiorly through the pharynx. This "squeezing" movement is continued by the contraction of the pharyngeal constrictor muscles that line the pharynx. As these muscles contract, the bolus is pushed inferiorly, toward the UES. As all of this is occurring, the larynx moves superiorly and anteriorly and the epiglottis acts as a baffle to divide the bolus into two segments, which skirt the aryepiglottic (AE) folds and slide along the pyriform sinuses into the post-cricoid region. This movement prevents the bolus from entering the airway. At this time, triggered by the sensory response from the supraglottic larynx, the vocal folds, aryepiglottic folds and arytenoids adduct as additional means of airway protection. The upward and anterior movement of the larynx results in distention and opening of the UES (which remains closed during non-feeding activities). The bolus passes through the open UES and enters the esophagus, thus beginning the esophageal phase of swallowing.

The fourth and final phase of swallowing, the esophageal phase, consists of transmission of the bolus through the esophagus via involuntary muscle contractions known as peristalsis. Ultimately, the bolus enters the stomach through the lower esophageal sphincter.

Adequate rehabilitation of patients with oral and oropharyngeal cancer requires recognition of not only the site of the tumor, but also the effect that its location might have on any of the aforementioned physiological processes. Treatment must then address ways to minimize or counter these adverse effects.

Although a great deal of attention has been devoted to the motor aspects of swallowing, it is important to not neglect the role of sensory function in this process. Diminished sensation of oral and oropharyngeal structures can have several adverse effects, including decreased awareness of food entering or being placed in the oral cavity (10), consumption of non-food items (i.e., a piece of a wrapper stuck to a food item), excessive oral residue and difficulty triggering the pharyngeal swallow. When formulating a rehabilitation plan, potential sensory deficits must therefore be taken into consideration. Restoration of sensation following surgical excision of oral cavity tumors has become an area of interest with the increasing use of sensate microvascular free flaps. Microneural anastomosis between a sensory nerve supplying a fasciocutaneous flap (e.g. the lateral antebrachial nerve of the radial forearm flap) and a recipient nerve in the vicinity of the surgical defect (e.g. the lingual nerve) is relatively technically simple. However, the practical impact in terms of improved sensation and function after sensate flap reconstruction remains unclear (11–13). As a general rule, better recovery of sensation may be expected in patients whose lingual and/or inferior alveolar nerves are either intact or have been used for neurorrhaphy compared to other nerves (14). In addition, because of the innate differences in sensitivity of the oral mucosa and cutaneous surfaces, a considerable degree of sensory re-education may be necessary for useful sensation to return (15).

Speech is also a concern amongst this patient population, as the structures of the oral cavity play a crucial role in the articulation of speech. These structures alter the spectral quality of the sound produced by the vocal folds, creating distinctively different phonemes (speech sounds). Phonemes such as /p/ and /b/, for example, require a complete labial seal. Vowels and many consonants require precise lingual placement within the oral cavity. From a voice perspective, adequate velar function is necessary not only to produce nasal consonants such as /m/ and /n/, but also to prevent the escape of air into the nasal cavity, resulting in hypernasal speech (5–7,16–18). Treatment of oral/oropharyngeal tumors can significantly alter speech and patients must be appropriately counseled regarding the degree of rehabilitation that might be necessary and the expected outcomes.

FUNCTIONAL OUTCOMES

One of the major difficulties in reporting functional outcomes after treatment of oral and oropharyngeal tumors is the lack of adequate and standardized measures of function. The main problem in creating a comprehensive system that is universally applicable is the vast number of parameters that can be measured to quantify deficits in speech and swallowing. In addition, the interpretations of tests such as videofluoroscopy and some aspects of quality of life measurements are subjective and prone to variability. Notwithstanding these limitations, several tests have been reported that attempt to measure functional outcome with respect to speech and swallowing. These include videofluoroscopy, scintigraphy, speech tasks, articulation tests, water holding tests and evaluation of general health, food, intake, mastication and tongue mobility.

Assessment of function and quality of life can be either general or more specific to the disease of interest (e.g. head and neck or oral cancer). Disease-specific instruments are more relevant to the oral cancer population because they allow comparison of different treatment modalities in defined populations. Table 20.2 lists the salient features of some commonly used head and neck-specific instruments (19). As measurement of quality of life and function is largely indirect and subjective, no particular questionnaire can be expected to be globally useful. Notwithstanding their limitations, instruments that use summary scores (e.g. EORTC QLQ-C30/H&N35, HNQOL or QL-H&N) are practical and have therefore gained common usage. Instruments that are self-administered (e.g., EORTC QLQ), concise and quick to complete are also likely to be more commonly favored in clinical practice. There are several reports in the literature that have used these instruments to document the functional outcome after surgical treatment of tumors of the oral cavity. Not surprisingly, the postoperative functional deficit is directly proportional to the size and location of the primary tumor and hence the magnitude of the surgical defect (2,4,18). Additionally, the site of the tumor within the oral cavity affects functional outcome. There is a progressive worsening in swallowing function as the location of the index primary tumor changes from anterior to posterior (4,17). Additionally, resection of the mandible further impairs speech and swallowing postoperatively (18). From these observations, it can be concluded that the larger and more posterior the primary tumor, the greater the functional impairment postoperatively.

Another factor that has been shown to affect functional outcome is the method of reconstruction. In one study, patients were matched with regard to T stage and volume of tongue resected and then evaluated for functional outcome based on the method of reconstruction. Patients who had a primary closure of their surgical defect showed better function then similar-stage patients who had a free flap reconstruction (17). This observation is not entirely surprising because of the bias that would be expected in selecting patients for reconstruction; for instance, surgical defects in smaller T3 lesions are more likely to be closed primarily than those in larger T3 lesions, which would be reconstructed with a free flap. On a practical basis, free flaps have become standard of care following major resection and in this setting the use of free tissue transfer adds tremendously to the functional and esthetic outcome. While free flap reconstruction of the tongue does not add mobility to or sensation of the flap skin, it prevents tethering of the remnant tongue, fills up the soft tissue defect and retains mobility of the remnant tongue.

The use of adjuvant postoperative radiation therapy can also influence functional outcome. Although alterations in speech were reported in one study, patients who received postoperative radiation therapy showed poorer swallowing function than those who did not (7). Again, the selection bias inherent to such a retrospective study does not allow meaningful interpretation of the data since the patients who need postoperative radiation therapy are more likely to have had larger and more ominous primary tumors.

Finally, in one study, the benefit of rehabilitation treatment in the form of range of motion exercises was evaluated. It was demonstrated that a benefit in swallowing function was seen in those patients who performed range of motion exercises throughout their rehabilitative process (3). This certainly argues for the routine use of such exercises after treatment of oral cavity tumors.

REHABILITATION

Speech and swallowing rehabilitation of the patient can be considered in two broad categories: structural reconstruction of the surgical defect and rehabilitation of the functional deficit.

With regard to reconstruction of the surgical defect, several general principles can be applied. The reconstructive procedure of first choice should be the simplest option likely to provide maximal restoration of form and function. Small defects can be closed primarily without restriction of function. Likewise, if a small superficial defect can be adequately resurfaced with a split-thickness skin graft or allowed to heal by secondary re-epithelialization, then the use of free tissue transfer is unwarranted. The second principle in the reconstruction of surgical defects of the oral cavity is to replace like with like. With the evolution of free tissue transfer, this aim is much more readily achievable. The variety of donor sites with their unique composition of bone, muscle, skin and even neural innervation allows most defects to be reconstructed with a satisfactory restoration of form and even sensation (20,21). The challenges that remain in the oral cavity for the reconstructive surgeon include the restoration of intricate sensory and motor function of the resected structures as well as the complex three-dimensional tissues of critical regions such as the oral commissure.

It should be realized that the balance in achieving these two overriding principles is often at odds. Striking a balance between the principles of simplicity and sufficiency is governed by the surgical defect, its functional and esthetic implications and the resources available to the head and neck surgeon. Regardless of the clinical situation, a variety

Table 20.2 Head and neck quality of life instruments: Content analysis

Domains	General QOL									Voice	Dysphagia	Disfigure
	EORTC H&N35	FACT-H&N v4	HN QOLQ	HN Q	UWQOL v4	NDII	AQLQ	H&NS	FSS-SR	LASA for Voice quality	MDADI	DSHNC
Facial appearance												
Satisfaction with appearance	♦	♦	♦	♦			♦		♦			
Noticeable change in self-esteem				♦				♦				
Effects social contact/activities					♦			♦				
Type of H&N surgery												
Size of disfigurement												♦
Affects facial expression												♦
Distortion of face or neck												♦
Visibility of disfigured area												♦
Speech												
Voice quality/understand ability		♦	♦	♦	♦			♦	♦	♦		
Voice strength/volume			♦	♦				♦		♦		
Hoarseness	♦			♦						♦		
Communication/talking	♦	♦	♦	♦			♦			♦		
Voice fatigue/loss										♦		
Ability to sing/whistle										♦		
Satisfaction with voice				♦						♦		
Swallowing												
Saliva/dry mouth	♦	♦	♦	♦	♦		♦		♦	♦		
Bad breath												
Chewing			♦	♦	♦				♦			
Problems with teeth/dentures	♦			♦								
Swallowing	♦	♦	♦	♦	♦			♦	♦		♦	
Trismus	♦		♦									
Normalcy of diet quality		♦		♦			♦	♦			♦	
Normalcy of diet quantity	♦	♦		♦							♦	
Speed of eating				♦								
Appetite							♦					
Food enjoyment	♦											
Social eating	♦						♦	♦	♦		♦	
Taste	♦		♦		♦				♦			
Smell	♦											
Others												
Pain (head and neck)	♦	♦	♦	♦	♦		♦	♦	♦			
Respiratory sx (breathing/cough)	♦	♦					♦		♦			
Others												
Shoulder pain/function			♦		♦	♦	♦		♦			

(Continued)

Table 20.2 (*Continued*) Head and neck quality of life instruments: Content analysis

	General QOL									Voice	Dysphagia	Disfigure
Domains	EORTC H&N35	FACT-H&N v4	HN QOLQ	HN Q	UWQOL v4	NDII	AQLQ	H&NS	FSS-SR	LASA for Voice quality	MDADI	DSHNC
Hearing loss												
Loss of vision												
Skin symptoms												
Smoking and alcohol use		♦				♦						
General quality of life												
Physical/functional/sexual well-being	♦	♦	♦	♦	♦	♦	♦		♦		♦	
Social well-being	♦	♦		♦		♦	♦				♦	
Emotional well-being	♦	♦	♦				♦				♦	
Overall health-related quality of life			♦	♦	♦		♦		♦			
Satisfaction with treatment	♦											
Life satisfaction							♦					
Total	35	39	27	30	14	10	41	13	16	16	20	1

Source: Reproduced with permission from SAGE Publications. Pusic A et al. *Otolaryngology—Head & Neck Surgery*. 2007;136(4):525–35 (19).
Abbreviations: EORTC H&N35: European Organization for Research & Treatment of Cancer H&N 35; FACT-H&N: Functional Assessment of Cancer Therapy Scale—Head & Neck; HNQOLQ: University of Michigan H&N Quality of Life Questionnaire; HNCI: Head and Neck Cancer Inventory; UWQOL: University of Washington Quality of Life scale; NDII: Neck Dissection Impairment Index; AQLQ: Auckland Quality of Life Questionnaire; H&NS: head and neck surgery; FSS-SR: Functional Status Scale Impairment Index; LASA for Voice Quality: Linear Analog Self-Assessment Scale for Voice Quality; MDADI: MD Anderson Dysphagia Inventory; DSHNC: Disfigurement Scale for H&N Cancer; sx: symptoms; H&N: Head and Neck.

of reconstructive options exist for almost any surgical defect, as outlined in the section on reconstruction.

Once the surgical defect has been adequately reconstructed, rehabilitative efforts are directed toward maximizing the function of the residual and transposed tissue. The initial aspects of this rehabilitation process occur shortly after surgery as the operative bed heals and residual sensation and mobility return. Additionally, if innervated free tissue flaps have been utilized, sensation will often return to these tissues with time. During this early postoperative period, it is critical for the patient to maintain maximal mobility. Often progressive increase in the movements of the jaws and tongue over time will prevent fibrosis and longer-term restriction in movement.

A special note must be made with regard to the preservation of the ability to open the mouth widely and the prevention of trismus. The prevention of trismus is obviously critical to all aspects of the rehabilitation of speech and swallowing after treatment of tumors of the oral cavity. Any patient who undergoes treatment of a lesion in the oral cavity/oropharynx is at risk for the development of trismus. Trismus is much easier to prevent than it is to correct once it has set in. Performing exercises in which the mouth is opened as widely as possible several times a day can prevent trismus. An easy method of actively promoting jaw excursion is to instruct the patient to use fingers to pull the mandible and maxilla in opposite directions as frequently as possible during the post-treatment phase. A stack of wooden tongue depressors may also be used to progressively widen the interincisoral opening over time. A simple device called a "Cork Screw" fabricated by the dentist is easy to use and is effective in the prevention of trismus. Finally, various commercial devices, such as TheraBite® and the Jaw Dynasplint® System, are available to act as aids that facilitate active opening of the mouth. These devices, however, are often cumbersome and difficult to use in all but the most highly motivated patients and the rehabilitation plan must be designed to maximize compliance by taking into account the patient's ability to adhere to instructions.

If an anatomical defect persists following surgery and adequate healing, prosthetics can often be used to further restore form and function. One area where great success has been observed with this approach is the use of a palatal obturator in the rehabilitation of the post-maxillectomy defect. The obturator restores velopharyngeal competence, prevents nasal regurgitation and preserves the esthetic contour of the cheek. Similarly, a palatal drop prosthesis can be fabricated in those patients who do not have sufficient tongue volume to approximate to the hard palate during the bolus transport phase of swallowing.

While many of the aforementioned techniques are passive methods of rehabilitation, there are various active techniques that can be utilized. The speech–language pathologist is a critical player in these efforts. The sophisticated nature and scope of the speech and swallowing evaluation performed by the speech pathologist is beyond the scope of this text. In simple terms, however, an examination is conducted to investigate any structural or functional deficits. This may include radiographic examination of the swallowing process in the form of a modified barium swallow, flexible endoscopic evaluation of swallowing with sensory testing using a fiberoptic nasolaryngoscope or informal observation. A treatment plan is then formulated that addresses the patient's specific rehabilitation needs. This will likely include various exercises and treatment techniques to maximize the function of the remaining structures as well as to facilitate the adaptation of compensatory strategies (e.g., swallowing using certain techniques or postural adaptations). It is important for everyone involved in the patient's care to realize that speech and swallowing rehabilitation is typically a long and ongoing process. A considerable degree of patience, perseverance and compliance is necessary on the part of both the patient and the caregiver to achieve the goal of optimal rehabilitation.

Finally, it should be noted that the best postoperative rehabilitation will not overcome the deficits caused by poor surgical planning that does not respect the functional subunits of the oral cavity. A vivid illustration of this fact is the impact on function of the method of closure of the surgical defect after resection of early anterior tongue lesions. When a transverse wedge of tissue is resected that encompasses the tumor and is closed primarily, minimal functional or esthetic deficits result. In contrast, when the same lesion is resected in a longitudinal fashion resulting in a serpentine elongated tongue, significant effects on speech and swallowing are often seen.

The optimal rehabilitation of patients treated for tumors of the oral cavity therefore requires adequate preoperative planning, optimal reconstruction, postoperative assessment of deficits and limitations and rehabilitative methods that will allow the patient's quality of life to approximate or return to normal levels.

PSYCHOSOCIAL IMPAIRMENT

In addition to functional impairment, many patients treated for head and neck cancers experience some level of disfigurement from change in their appearance. These changes can cause patients to feel ashamed or uncomfortable in social situations, which may lead to psychological issues such as depression, anxiety or isolation (22). The inability to eat normally or speak correctly can cause patients embarrassment to the point where they prefer to eat alone and avoid social outings (23). These concerns are less, however, with older patients who have significantly better views of their esthetics and mental health (24). Sexuality issues were reported in a third of patients after treatment, especially in older patients (22). Sexuality changes happen over time and can often be related to radiotherapy (25). Radiation therapy and chemotherapy were also associated with significantly worse outcomes in eating and social disruptions (24). Patients without psychosocial issues mainly attributed their readjustment to the fact that they are grateful to be alive with the elimination of the disease (23,26).

There have been some discrepancies in the literature as to the severity or existence of psychosocial issues; some report patients getting worse over time, while others report patients getting better over time (23,27,28). Despite these discrepancies, recognition of the possibility of psychosocial issues following treatment for oral and oropharyngeal cancers is important. Therefore, the need for assessment and supportive care should be addressed. For many patients, poor coping techniques have been associated with worse quality of life. However, in most cases, these issues had potential for improvement with appropriate support (22). One study reports that two-thirds of outpatient referrals are young females and suggests that this might be a high-risk group (29). Establishing tools to identify these high-risk patients in a postoperative setting may be useful in order to help patients return to their preoperative mental status.

At the MSKCC, the head and neck surgery service in collaboration with the department of psychiatry and behavioral sciences has developed a scale to assess psychological impact of treatment in patients with oral cancer: the Shame and Stigma Scale (SSS) (30). This scale was created by prospectively studying a cohort of patients with squamous cell carcinoma of the oral cavity. The SSS consists of a 20-question survey that was given to patients at baseline and ≥3 months postoperatively. Factor analysis was used to relate questions and to develop four major categories: shame with appearance, sense of stigma, regret and social/speech concerns. These categories can be used to identify the specific type of intervention to be recommended. This internally validated scale shows promising reliability for patients.

Timely recognition of individuals who will be helped by psychological intervention is crucial to avoiding long-term social or mental effects and thereby achieving the goal of restoring overall health after treatment of oral and oropharyngeal cancer.

REFERENCES

1. Dejonckere PH, Hordijk GJ. Prognostic factors for swallowing after treatment of head and neck cancer. *Clin Otolaryngol Allied Sci* 1998;23(3):218–23.
2. Denk DM, Swoboda H, Schima W, Eibenberger K. Prognostic factors for swallowing rehabilitation following head and neck cancer surgery. *Acta Otolaryngol* 1997;117(5):769–74.
3. Logemann JA, Pauloski BR, Rademaker AW, Colangelo LA. Speech and swallowing rehabilitation for head and neck cancer patients. *Oncology* 1997;11(5):651–6, 659; discussion 9, 663–4.

4. McConnel FM, Logemann JA, Rademaker AW et al. Surgical variables affecting postoperative swallowing efficiency in oral cancer patients: a pilot study. *Laryngoscope* 1994;104(1 Pt 1):87–90.
5. Pauloski BR, Logemann JA, Rademaker AW et al. Speech and swallowing function after anterior tongue and floor of mouth resection with distal flap reconstruction. *J Speech Hear Res* 1993;36(2): 267–76.
6. Pauloski BR, Logemann JA, Rademaker AW et al. Speech and swallowing function after oral and oropharyngeal resections: one-year follow-up. *Head Neck* 1994;16(4):313–22.
7. Pauloski BR, Rademaker AW, Logemann JA, Colangelo LA. Speech and swallowing in irradiated and nonirradiated postsurgical oral cancer patients. *Otolaryngol Head Neck Surg* 1998;118(5):616–24.
8. Rademaker AW, Pauloski BR, Colangelo LA, Logemann JA. Age and volume effects on liquid swallowing function in normal women. *J Speech Lang Hear Res* 1998;41(2):275–84.
9. Ardran GM, Kemp FH. The mechanism of swallowing. *Proc R Soc Med* 1951;44(12):1038–40.
10. Logemann JA. *Evaluation and treatment of swallowing Disorders* (2nd edition). PRO-ED, Inc.: Austin, Texas 1998.
11. Vriens JP, Acosta R, Soutar DS, Webster MH. Recovery of sensation in the radial forearm free flap in oral reconstruction. *Plast Reconstr Surg* 1996;98(4): 649–56.
12. Lvoff G, O'Brien CJ, Cope C, Lee KK. Sensory recovery in noninnervated radial forearm free flaps in oral and oropharyngeal reconstruction. *Arch Otolaryngol* 1998;124(11):1206–8.
13. Netscher D, Armenta AH, Meade RA, Alford EL. Sensory recovery of innervated and non-innervated radial forearm free flaps: functional implications. *J Reconstr Microsurg* 2000;16(3):179–85.
14. Santamaria E, Wei FC, Chen IH, Chuang DC. Sensation recovery on innervated radial forearm flap for hemiglossectomy reconstruction by using different recipient nerves. *Plastic Reconstructive Surgery* 1999;103(2):450–7.
15. Cordeiro PG, Schwartz M, Neves RI, Tuma R. A comparison of donor and recipient site sensation in free tissue reconstruction of the oral cavity. *Ann Plast Surg* 1997;39(5):461–8.
16. Muz J, Mathog RH, Hamlet SL, Davis LP, Kling GA. Objective assessment of swallowing function in head and neck cancer patients. *Head Neck* 1991;13(1):33–9.
17. McConnel FM, Pauloski BR, Logemann JA et al. Functional results of primary closure vs flaps in oropharyngeal reconstruction: a prospective study of speech and swallowing. *Arch Otolaryngol* 1998;124(6):625–30.
18. Haribhakti VV, Kavarana NM, Tibrewala AN. Oral cavity reconstruction: an objective assessment of function. *Head Neck* 1993;15(2):119–24.
19. Pusic AA. A systematic review of patient-reported outcome measures in head and neck cancer surgery. *Otolaryngol Head Neck Surg* 2007;136(4):525–35.
20. Urken ML, Buchbinder D, Weinberg H et al. Functional evaluation following microvascular oromandibular reconstruction of the oral cancer patient: a comparative study of reconstructed and nonreconstructed patients. *Laryngoscope* 1991;101(9):935–50.
21. Urken ML. The restoration or preservation of sensation in the oral cavity following ablative surgery. *Arch Otolaryngol* 1995;121(6):607–12.
22. Moore KA, Ford PJ, Farah CS. Support needs and quality of life in oral cancer: a systematic review. *Int J Dent Hyg* 2014;12(1):36–47.
23. Argerakis GP. Psychosocial considerations of the post-treatment of head and neck cancer patients. *Dent Clin North Am* 1990;34(2):285–305.
24. Funk GF, Karnell LH, Christensen AJ. Long-term health-related quality of life in survivors of head and neck cancer. *Arch Otolaryngol* 2012;138(2):123–33.
25. Bjordal K, Kaasa S. Psychological distress in head and neck cancer patients 7–11 years after curative treatment. *Br J Cancer* 1995;71(3):592–97.
26. Bronheim H, Strain JJ, Biller HF. Psychiatric aspects of head and neck surgery. Part II: body image and psychiatric intervention. *Gen Hosp Psychiatry* 1991;13(4):225–32.
27. de Graeff A, de Leeuw JR, Ros WJ, Hordijk GJ, Blijham GH, Winnubst JA. A prospective study on quality of life of patients with cancer of the oral cavity or oropharynx treated with surgery with or without radiotherapy. *Oral Oncol* 1999;35(1):27–32.
28. Dropkin MJ. Anxiety: coping strategies, and coping behaviors in patients undergoing head and neck cancer surgery. *Cancer Nurs* 2001;24(2):143–8.
29. Espie CA, Freedlander E, Campsie LM, Soutar DS, Robertson AG. Psychological distress at follow-up after major surgery for intra-oral cancer. *J Psychosom Res* 1989;33(4):441–8.
30. Kissane DW, Patel SG, Baser RE et al. Preliminary evaluation of the reliability and validity of the shame and stigma scale in head and neck cancer. *Head Neck* 2013;35(2):172–83.

21

Prognostic nomograms

PABLO H. MONTERO, JOCELYN C. MIGLIACCI, AND SNEHAL G. PATEL

INTRODUCTION

The prediction of outcomes of oncologic treatment and prognosis is a fundamental need in the minds of patients and physicians alike. William Halsted, the father of surgical oncology, theorized that cancer progression follows an orderly, stepwise process beginning from primary tumor formation to distant theorized metastasis, passing through regional lymph nodes (1). In 1905, Steinthal in Germany first attempted to clinically stage breast cancer based on Halsted's theory (2). This simple concept of stepwise tumor progression was widely used in the first part of the 20th century and has essentially shaped the way we view and comprehend the behavior of a malignant tumor. It has also influenced the way we diagnose cancer, treat it and predict its course. The first systematic approach to stage cancer in a consistent way was done at Institut Gustave Roussy by Pierre Denoix. From 1942 to 1952, Denoix developed a system to stage solid malignancy based mainly on three anatomic characteristics: tumor (T), lymph node spread (N) and distant metastasis (M) (3). In 1953, a Special Committee on Clinical Stage Classification was established by the International Union Against Cancer (UICC) under the leadership of Denoix (4). In 1959, the American Joint Committee on Cancer (AJCC) was established to "formulate and publish systems of classification of cancer, including staging and end results reporting, which will be acceptable to and used by the medical profession for selecting the most effective treatment, determining prognosis, and continuing evaluation of cancer control measures" (5). After an initial course that was independent of each other and often contradictory, both organizations have worked in collaboration through the publication of the UICC/AJCC TNM Classification since 1987, and this has helped to standardize the way cancer is staged and results of treatment are reported around the world (6).

The TNM system offers a reliable method to estimate the prognosis of patients with cancer based on certain anatomic characteristics of the tumor. Over the last 60 years, the TNM has been widely used to plan treatment, summarize prognostic information, evaluate treatment results and compare outcomes between institutions around the world (7). Although the main T, N and M categories remain almost unchanged since their initial conception, the staging system has been periodically fine-tuned to incorporate newer anatomical prognostic factors. Examples include more detailed T4 categories for head and neck cancers; the introduction of sentinel lymph node and isolated tumor cells in the N categories of breast cancer (8,9); and the depth of invasion, ulceration and mitotic rate as major T determinants in malignant melanoma (10). Although the original TNM system was based solely on the anatomic extent of the tumor, other non-anatomic parameters related to both the tumor and the host have been included on a periodic basis. Examples of this trend include the incorporation of age and histology into thyroid cancer staging in 1983 (11); histological grade into soft tissue sarcoma and bone tumor staging in 1988 (12); and serum markers in testicular cancer, gestational trophoblastic tumors and prostate cancer in 1997 (13,14).

The TNM system is the most widely accepted prognostic system currently used in clinical practice around the world because of its relatively simple design and user-friendliness. Despite this popularity, criticism is common about the slow adoption of changes into the TNM staging system. It has been called anachronistic, and its use as the gold standard of cancer staging is accepted as "good enough" rather than optimal (15). Many disadvantages have been highlighted: lack of predictive power, lack of balance and differentiation between groups, failure to account for other tumors and host factors. The majority of this criticism is predicated by the enormous amount of new prognostic information now available to clinicians from radiographic imaging, histopathological examination, immunohistochemical studies and molecular analysis, in addition to patient factors such as comorbidity and lifestyle (tobacco, alcohol, human papillomavirus [HPV] status, HIV infection, Epstein–Barr virus [EBV] status, etc.). The design of the current system unfortunately does not allow for easy addition of further variables without compromising on its biggest advantage: simplicity and user-friendliness. The challenge facing us now is to find a solution that can strike the ideal balance between complexity and user-friendliness (16).

THE CURRENT TNM STAGING SYSTEM

The TNM system is based on the assumption that cancers grow first at the site of the primary tumor and then spread in a predictable, progressive fashion to regional lymph nodes and, finally, metastasize to distant sites in the body. Based on these three broad categories, patients with cancer are assigned into distinct categories. Thus, the TNM system uses compartments or "bins" to segregate patients into distinct categories that predict outcome. The T category (Tis, T1, T2, T3 and T4), N category (N0, N1, N2 and N3) and the M category (M0 and M1) are then combined into different "bins" (stage groupings). For most tumors, excluding the M1 category, this amounts to around 20 bins ($T = 5 \times N = 4$). Each of these bins is then assigned to one of four stage groups that reflect progressively advanced extent of disease and therefore worsening prognosis. In recognition of the distinct implications of locoregional advanced diseased versus distant metastases, recent iterations of the system have stratified the advanced stage IV grouping into stage IVA (advanced surgically resectable disease), stage IVB (very advanced surgically unresectable disease) and stage IVC (advanced distant metastatic disease) (17,18). Any individual patient can be slotted into a unique "bin" and stage and therefore every patient should have representation in the bin model (19).

ADVANTAGES OF THE TNM SYSTEM

The major advantage of the TNM system is its simple design, which requires only very basic information about the tumor and its spread. This information can generally be derived largely from clinical examination and radiographic imaging studies. The data points used for staging can be extracted from patient records even by personnel with minimal training and this user-friendliness has been pivotal in its worldwide popularity. Ironically, the simplicity of the system is at once its main advantage and also its greatest limitation.

LIMITATIONS OF THE TNM SYSTEM

The main drawback of the TNM system is its inability to adapt to advances in our understanding of cancer biology and incorporate new prognostic variables as they become available. The rigid "bin" configuration means that any attempts to include new variables or categories would exponentially increase the number of bins, multiply the stages and make the system unwieldy. This would detract from its very core advantage of simplicity and user-friendliness. Any increase in the number of bins would also require a sufficient number of patients in each bin in order to maintain the predictive value of the system. Addition of variables would generate changes in the previous system, causing upward or downward "stage migration," requiring a complete redefinition of the staging system itself (19,20). For these mechanistic reasons, changing the current TNM system has not been deemed advisable.

The main endpoint used by the TNM staging system is overall survival. However, the inclusion of other endpoints such as disease-specific survival, local control or regional control are more relevant to assessment of treatment results and differences among therapeutics options (16). Although the TNM system remains a very good tool for estimating prognosis at initial diagnosis and immediately after the initial treatment of cancer, one of its most important flaws is its inability to use subsequent events in the patient's course in recalibrating prognosis during follow-up. Thus, each patient has an initial TNM stage assigned to them at diagnosis and the system is unable to take into account the influence of recurrence-free interval on outcome. Thus, the TNM system is "static" and not "dynamic" reflecting the changes occurring in the patient during the natural history of the cancer.

Before we consider changing a system that has served us so well for several decades, it would be useful to examine the characteristics of an ideal staging system.

CHARACTERISTICS OF AN IDEAL STAGING SYSTEM

The characteristics of an efficient and effective staging system have been defined by Groome et al. (21) as: (1) hazard consistency, or the ability to have internal homogeneity within each group with similar survival for all individual patients included in the group; (2) hazard discrimination—groups should be different in composition and have distinct prognosis; (3) balance—each group and stage should have a similar number of patients; and (4) predictive power—the ability to predict an outcome of interest (overall survival, disease-specific survival, etc.). It is easy to see how the addition of prognostic factors to the current TNM system would make it increasingly difficult to maintain homogeneity within each group and at the same time maintain hazard discrimination across groups. The central challenge in improving the staging paradigm is to understand this basic interaction between hazard consistency and hazard discrimination that maintains balance between groups and yet has optimal predictive power.

Outcome prediction models in cancer patients have a similar overarching goal, but are more focused on the individual patient. The advantage of this approach is that it still provides the flexibility for grouping patients based on either certain basic characteristics or on distinctions in outcomes of any particular interest. Burke and Henson (19), in 1993, have described the ultimate goals of any system for cancer outcome prediction as:

1. It should be easy for physicians to use. Ideally, it should have input prompts. It should be available on programmable handheld calculators, iPhones, microcomputers and work stations.
2. It should provide predictions for all types of cancer.
3. It should provide the most accurate relapse and survival predictions at diagnosis and for every subsequent year lived for each patient.
4. It should provide group survival curves, where the grouping can be by any variable, including outcome and therapy.
5. It should accommodate missing data and censored patients and should be tolerant of noisy and biased data.
6. It should make no *a priori* assumptions regarding the type of data, the distribution of the variables or the relationships among the variables. It should efficiently capture nonmonotonic phenomena and complex interactions among variables.
7. It should be able to test putative prognostic factors for significance, independence and clinical relevance.
8. It should accommodate treatment information in the evaluation of prognostic factors.
9. It should accommodate new prognostic factors without changing the model.
10. It should accommodate emerging diagnostic techniques: not only molecular tests, but also new imaging modalities (e.g. endoscopy, computed tomography and magnetic resonance imaging).
11. It should provide information regarding the importance of each predictive variable.
12. It should be automatic; that is, the model's output should not depend on the operator.

With constant advances in our understanding of the mechanism and biologic behavior of cancer, many of these goals are suddenly becoming more achievable. The ongoing discovery of new information about cancer has fueled an increasing demand among caregivers and patients alike for customized treatment selection and outcome prediction. Commensurate with these trends in cancer discovery, there has also been a trend toward more accurate data collection and better follow-up of patients, as well as an explosion in statistical techniques for analysis and prediction of outcomes. Therefore, we now have a realistic ability to consider changing the conventional TNM staging paradigm.

DO WE NEED TO CHANGE THE STAGING SYSTEM?

Contrary to the relative stability in the structure and design of the TNM system, several new prognostic factors have come into common clinical use over the past several decades. The vast majority of these factors have not made their way into the staging system because of the limitations described above, but also because most of these variables do not predict outcome "independently" in multivariate models of prognostication. It is, however, very clear that cancer is a multidimensional disease. Many of the recognized descriptors of the disease that fail to independently predict prognosis in multivariate statistical analyses do actually work in tandem. Therefore, their exclusion from the staging system and prognostic models could potentially diminish accuracy. Advances in technology now allow consideration that a virtually limitless number of variables can be combined with the conventional TNM paradigm in order to improve the accuracy of the prognostic model (19,22). While more detailed conventional anatomic information about the tumor can be easily incorporated, better definitions of subclinical or clinical distant disease are also required (23). The potential prognostic categories that may be considered for inclusion in a revised staging system are summarized below.

HOST-RELATED FACTORS

Demographic factors such as age, sex, race, family history of cancer, socioeconomic status, lifestyles and habits (tobacco, alcohol and substance abuse) are only a few of the many factors that impact upon outcomes of treatment (24–27). Clinicians regularly use this information in the decision-making process for the treatment of patients with cancer. However, with the exception of the age of the patient, which is used in the TNM staging system for thyroid cancer, none of the other host characteristics have representation in the current staging paradigm. Medical comorbidity is also a significant determinant of outcome, especially overall survival. Patients with significant medical problems may not be capable of receiving treatment equivalent to the ideal situation in healthier patients. Comparing outcomes in patients with head and neck cancer without accounting for the influence of medical comorbidity therefore introduces significant bias in reporting. The behavior of squamous cell carcinoma in patients with genetic and familial syndromes is also different. An extreme example is the dismal prognosis of patients with Fanconi anemia. Another host-related characteristic that has come into prominence recently is the etiologic role of viruses in cancer pathogenesis (e.g. HPV for oropharyngeal cancer or EBV for nasopharyngeal cancer) (28,29). HPV-related oropharyngeal cancer is now recognized to behave differently from its more traditional tobacco- and alcohol-related counterparts. Moreover, viruses can also significantly impact the immune status of the host with resultant impact on outcome. The aggressive and explosive course of squamous cell carcinoma in immunosuppressed individuals who have had organ transplantation or HIV infection is a drastic example of the devastating influence of a host characteristic on outcomes and yet there is no way of accounting for such factors in the current staging system.

HISTOPATHOLOGICAL VARIABLES

Many features of the tumor such as gross characteristics of the tumor (exophytic, endophytic or ulcerative), tumor volume, depth of invasion or thickness, histological subtype (verrucous, basaloid, adenosquamous, etc.), microscopic pattern of invasion (invasive front, pushing border or invasive islands), presence of lymphovascular and/or perineural invasion and histologic differentiation grade are prognostic factors that have been extensively analyzed but have not been included in the TNM staging system (30–32). It is only in the most recent revision of the AJCC/UICC staging for oral cancer that the depth of invasion is included in the T staging of primary tumors. The impact of lymph node metastases on prognosis in patients with head and neck cancer is well recognized (33). The TNM system accounts for the metastatic burden in lymph nodes by stratifying N stage using the size, number and laterality of involved nodes. The influence of other features of metastatic lymph nodes such as extracapsular nodal spread was only introduced in 2017 the most recent revision of the nodal staging for head and neck cancer. The modalities for the detection of metastases in lymph nodes are also evolving and, as these methods become more accurate, we will need to account for the inclusion of micrometastatic nodal disease in the staging system. An example of this dilemma is the detection of submicroscopic melanoma using molecular methods in patients with malignant melanoma who now routinely undergo sentinel lymph node mapping and biopsy. Although our ability to identify nodal disease is improving with advances in radiographic imaging techniques, detailed histopathologic examination of the neck dissection specimen remains the best modality for the detection of metastatic disease. It is well recognized that the probability of detecting metastatic nodal disease depends on the level of scrutiny (extent of neck dissection, number of lymph nodes examined and modalities used to examine the nodes) and therefore the chances of detection of microscopic lymph node metastases are highest in patients who undergo elective neck dissection. The concept of lymph node density attempts to address the bias related to level of scrutiny by accounting for the number of metastatic nodes in the total number of nodes dissected at neck dissection. We have shown that lymph node density is superior to N stage in predicting survival in patients treated for oral cavity cancer (34).

BIOLOGICAL AND MOLECULAR MARKERS

With advances in understanding of cancer biology in general and head and neck cancer in particular, we are now faced with a deluge of information on molecular and genetic predictors of prognosis. Some molecular markers such as the epidermal growth factor receptor have been shown to have prognostic influence in certain situations such as laryngeal cancer (35,36). We now also have an improved understanding of the etiopathology of some cancers; HPV infection in oropharyngeal cancer and EBV infection in nasopharyngeal cancer are two prime examples. HPV infection is now considered the major etiologic determinant of oropharyngeal cancer and specific treatment paradigms are being considered based on the HPV status of oropharyngeal cancers (29), as patients who are HPV-positive have a significantly better prognosis than HPV-negative patients (37). Prognostic data of this nature will have to be incorporated into staging systems in order to maintain relevance of any staging system as our understanding of cancer continues to evolve.

NEWER TECHNOLOGY AND TOOLS

Several statistical tools such as artificial neural networks and nomograms have been reported widely in the prediction of outcomes (38).

Artificial neural networks have been used in computerized decision-making for a long time, but have only recently been introduced in clinical practice. This is a non-linear statistical data model that initially was inspired by biological neuronal networks, but now uses advanced statistics and signal processing to integrate massive amounts of data. It is a very flexible tool because of its property "to learn"; it uses a set of observations to determine which solution resolves a task optimally (39) and incorporates new information in the process. It has been tested in several tumors such as prostate, esophageal, gastric, colorectal and lung cancer, showing comparable or better results than traditional prognostic models. In head and neck cancer, its utility has been analyzed for the assessment of malignancy in thyroid nodules (40,41), to predict the likelihood of oral cancer based on risk factors and in laryngeal cancer (42,43). In laryngeal cancer, survival analysis based on neural networks demonstrated results similar to Cox's model in observed survival prediction (43).

Over the last 10 years, prognostic nomograms have become a competitive alternative to artificial neural networks, especially in regard to oncology, for predicting individualized patient risk.

NOMOGRAMS

A nomogram is a graphical representation of a statistical model that can be easily used by clinicians to predict a specified endpoint. The first use of nomograms dates back to the 1880s, when these tools were used mainly by mathematicians and engineers to offer a quick and accurate solution to complex calculations (44). Some have referred to nomography as a lost art; however, its use in cancer has been widely studied, with over 1,000 publications in the literature (45). The Memorial Sloan Kettering Cancer Center (MSKCC) alone has over 150 publications involving nomograms across multiple specialties. Most of these have been developed for use in prostate cancer and have focused on various applications such as predicting the probability of cancer in a biopsy, estimating prognosis before and after treatment or predicting the risk of locoregional recurrence (46). Nomograms have also been widely used for prognostic prediction in sarcoma, melanoma and pancreatic cancer.

In contrast to these cancers, nomograms have been used only sparingly for head and neck tumors. In 2008, we first reported a nomogram to predict the likelihood of local recurrence after treatment in patients with oral cancer and to assess the need for adjuvant treatment (47). We have also developed nomograms to predict other outcomes, such as the risk of cancer in thyroid nodules and the risk of hypocalcemia after thyroid surgery (48,49). Others have developed nomograms for selection of treatment in patients with advanced-stage head and neck carcinoma based on factors such as tumor volume and other host variables (50), as well as to predict overall survival and local failure in laryngeal patients (51).

The type of model to be utilized when creating a nomogram is determined by the outcome of interest. Frequently, this outcome is based on survival, but even within survival analyses, there are multiple endpoints that can be explored, such as overall survival, disease-free survival, recurrence-free survival, etc. For these types of analyses, multivariable Cox proportional hazard regression is the method most commonly used. Although the examples in this chapter will focus on survival analyses, nomograms can predict a variety of events. When predicting binary events at a fixed time point, such as hypocalcemia, logistic regression can be used. Nomograms will likely find widespread use in cancer prognostication, especially with the availability of good-quality data and increasing sophistication in computing software and technology.

DEVELOPMENT

Iasonos et al. have described the process of the creation and interpretation of a nomogram (52). Although the details are not within the scope of this review, this process could be summarized in the five following steps. (1) Identify a patient population: nomograms could be generated from single- or multi-institutional datasets, even from a population-based cohort, but the applicability of the nomogram will depend on the similitude between the source population and the subject or population to be analyzed. (2) Define the outcome: the event to be analyzed will define use of the nomogram; that is, overall survival, disease-specific survival, recurrence-free survival, etc. (3) Identify potential covariates: clinical evidence and data availability will define the prognostic factors that would be incorporated in the nomogram. (4) Construction of the nomogram: the nomogram is based on a formula obtained from a statistical model and correct selection of the predictors. The predictors are selected according to clinical and statistical significance, with special attention to detecting interaction between them or confounder effects. (5) Validation of the model: it is essential to assess how well the nomogram will perform when it is used in a new and independent cohort of patients. Validation is performed using different methods (cross-validation, external validation, etc.) and the predictive accuracy of the nomogram is expressed through a concordance index.

UNDERSTANDING A NOMOGRAM

Nomograms can take multiple forms when used for different objectives in science, but for our purposes, a nomogram is a series of horizontal lines that is used to obtain the probability of an event for a specific patient. Figure 21.1 shows a published nomogram utilizing preoperative details to predict 5-year disease-specific survival for oral cavity cancer (44). Each line is identified with a label directly to its left. The first line, labeled "Points," is the score given to an individual parameter. The next four lines represent the parameters included in the model: primary size dimension, clinical nodal status, subsite and bone invasion. The fifth line, labeled "Total Points," is the sum of the four individual parameter points. Finally, the last line in the nomogram shows the predicted 5-year disease-specific death probability.

To find the individual parameter score, one must identify a patient's result on the horizontal parameter line. From the parameter line at the patient's result, a perpendicular line is drawn up to the "Points" line and the individual parameter points should be recorded. This step is then repeated for each variable. Next, sum all four individual parameter points to obtain the total points for the patient's results. Find the sum on the horizontal "Total Points" line and draw

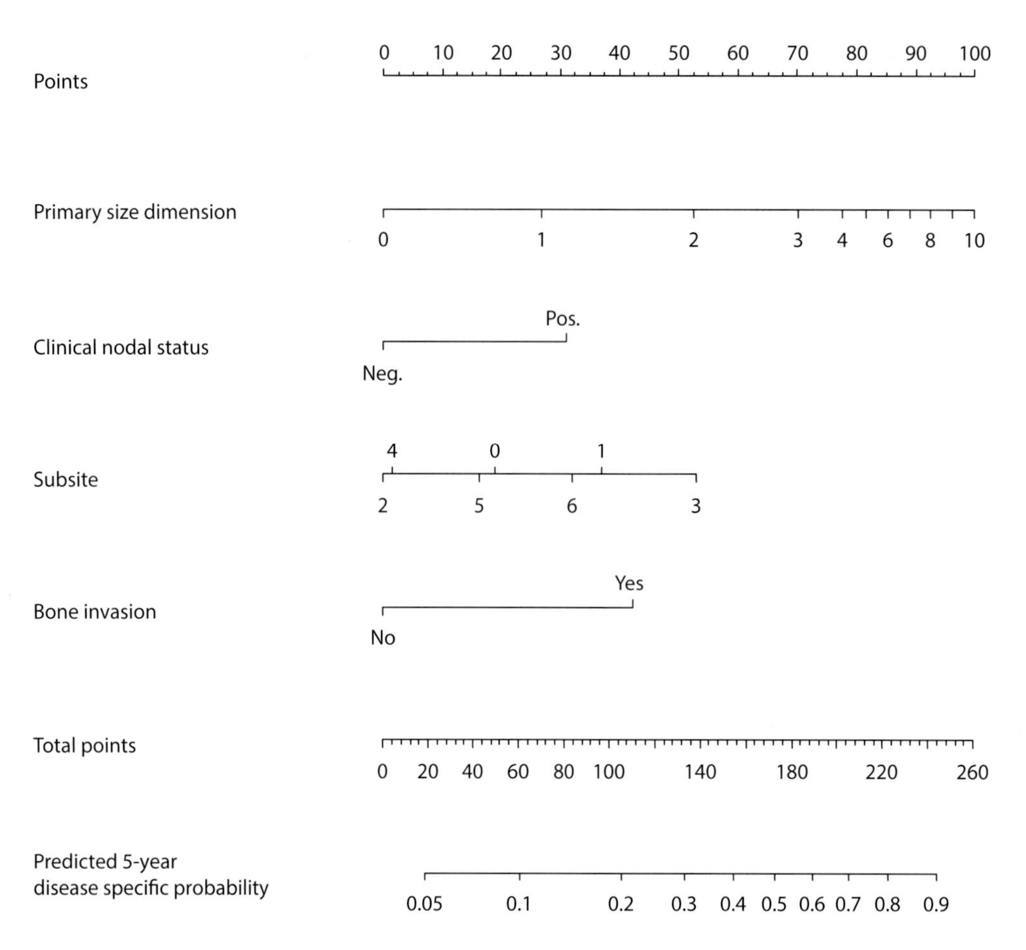

Figure 21.1 Preoperative prognostic nomogram for oral cavity cancer predicting 5-year disease-specific survival with Cox proportional hazard regression.

a perpendicular line down to the predicted 5-year disease-specific death probability. This indicates the patient's individualized risk of dying of the disease at 5 years post-surgery.

Figure 21.2 illustrates use of the nomogram with a sample patient. Patient A has a primary tongue tumor with clinically positive lymph nodes and no bone invasion. A 3-cm tumor, shown by the red line, corresponds to approximately 70 parameter points. Clinically positive nodal status, shown by the purple line, corresponds to approximately 32 parameter points. Tongue anatomic site, indicated with the yellow line, corresponds to approximately 37.5 parameter points. Finally, no bone invasion, indicated with the green line, corresponds to zero parameter points. Summing all parameter points determines the total points score for this patient is 139.5 points. The blue line in Figure 21.2 indicates the result of the total points and shows that Patient A has a 32.5% probability of dying of the disease by 5 years post-surgery.

In this chapter, we have illustrated the use of a nomogram in its literal form for educational purposes, but in practice, drawing physical lines on a paper copy of a nomogram would be cumbersome and far from ideal. Preferably, these nomograms will be used to create a dashboard-style computer interface where physicians can enter the required parameters. The computer will then calculate and report the risk for an individual patient. At the MSKCC, we have

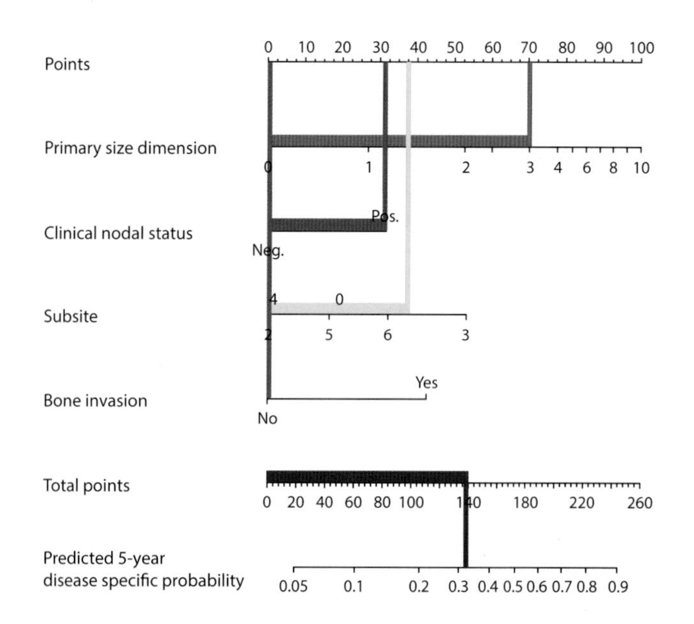

Figure 21.2 Patient A has a 3-cm tumor (red line), clinically positive nodes (purple line), tongue disease (yellow line), and no bone invasion (green line). The total sum of points (blue line) indicates that Patient A has a 32.5% chance of dying of the disease by 5 years post-surgery.

a website with this type of interface where our published nomograms can be used by outside physicians (http://www.mskcc.org/nomograms).

NOMOGRAMS FOR CANCER STAGING VERSUS CONVENTIONAL TNM STAGING

The rigid "bin" configuration of the TNM system limits any changes in its structure because addition of new variables would make the system very complicated, destroying its user-friendliness. Moreover, the addition of variables and increasing the number of "bins" would significantly affect the prognostic power of the system by altering the internal homogeneity of the groups and the hazard consistency of the stages (19). As shown in Chapter 19, staging groups are no longer producing clear distinctions in survival. This lack of distinction may be attributed to the TNM staging system's variable restrictions and/or the heterogeneity within staging groups. It is for this reason that any major changes in the way we stage cancer requires thinking "outside of the box" and is only achievable using novel technology and tools (16).

TNM staging uses limited information to compartmentalize patients into heterogeneous groups. Nomograms breakdown these groups and help disease management teams supply patients with important personalized information that will help them make the tough decisions they will face regarding cancer care. In this section, we consider two patients, Patient B and Patient C, who with traditional staging would be grouped together with similar outcomes, but by using a new postoperative nomogram recently created at the MSKCC (Figure 21.3), we show that these patients and their predicted outcomes are notably different.

Patient B, shown in Figure 21.4, is a 60-year-old white male who was a 20 pack-year smoker. He has diabetes and coronary artery disease and a maximum tumor dimension of 3.5 cm. His tongue tumor does not invade deep muscle, but has positive margins. Patient B also has vascular invasion, perineural invasion and positive level II lymph nodes.

Patient C, shown in Figure 21.5, is a 30-year-old white female non-smoker. She has a 2.5-cm tongue cancer but is otherwise healthy. Her tumor does not invade deep muscle and has negative margins. She does not have vascular invasion or perineural invasion, but she has positive level I lymph nodes.

By staging these patients using the traditional TNM staging system, both patients would be grouped as stage III (Table 21.1) with a predicted 5-year overall survival of 34.1%. However, by using the nomogram shown in Figure 21.5 to incorporate new prognostic variables, the 5-year overall survival predictions for Patient B and Patient C

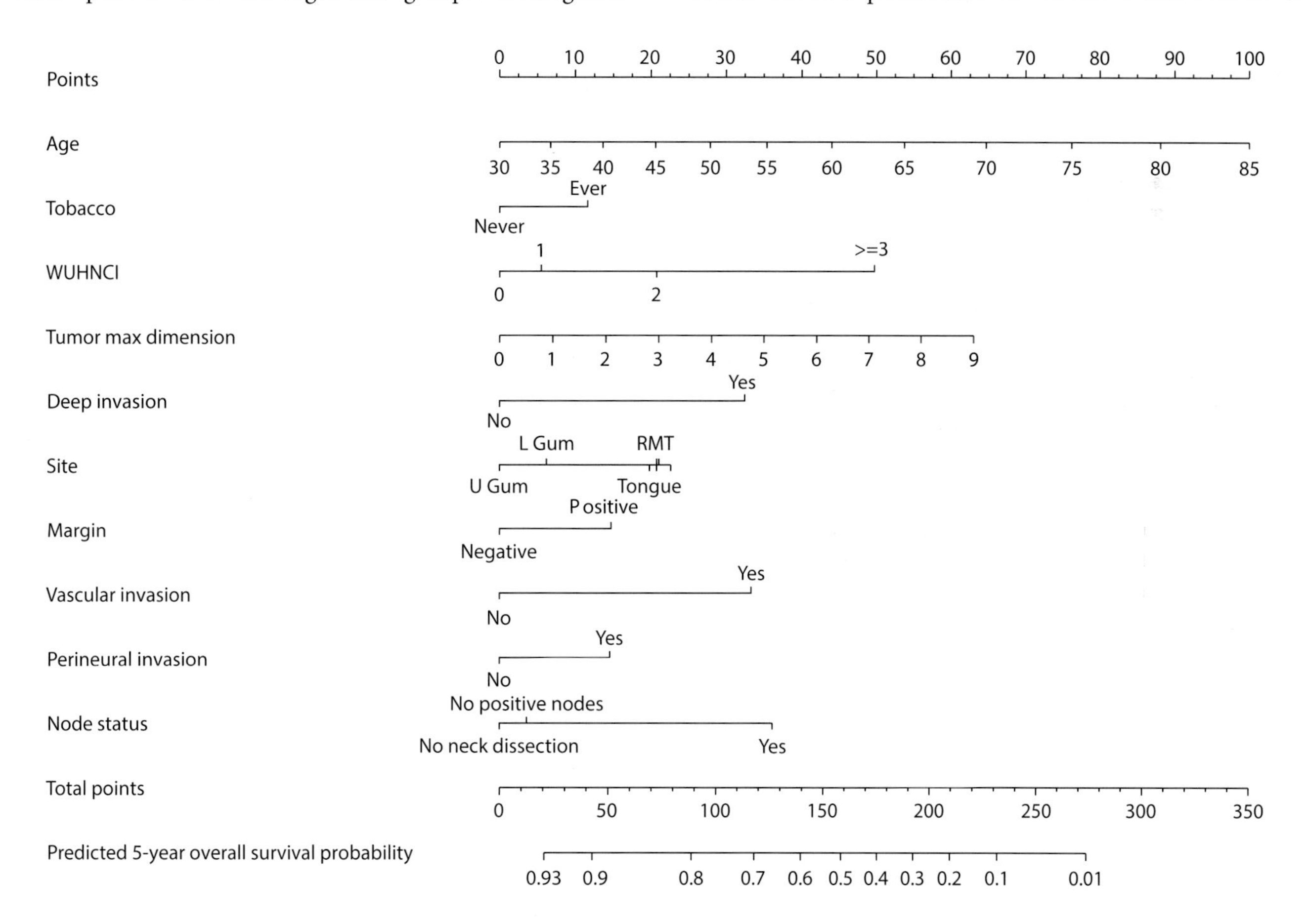

Figure 21.3 Postoperative nomogram developed at the MSKCC to predict 5-year overall survival.

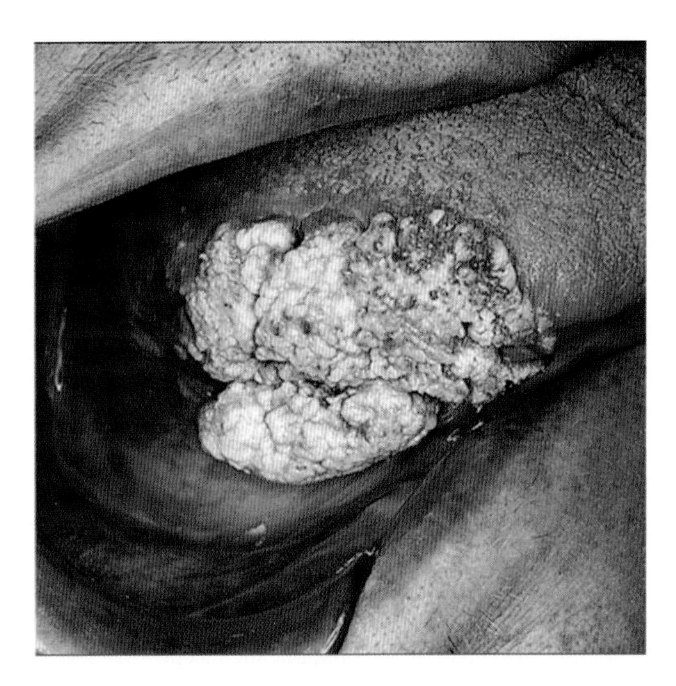

Figure 21.4 Photograph of Patient B's tumor. Patient B has a maximum tumor dimension of 3.5 cm.

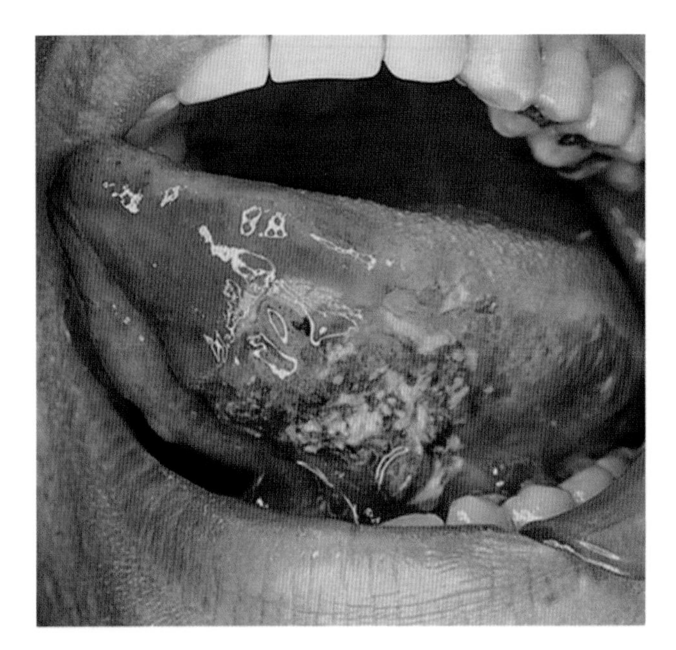

Figure 21.5 Photograph of Patient C's tumor. Patient C has a maximum tumor dimension of 2.5 cm.

are quite different. Figure 21.6 shows the nomogram with Patient B's results, indicating a 10% predicted 5-year overall survival. Figure 21.7 shows the nomogram with Patient C's results, indicating an 80% predicted 5-year overall survival.

This flexibility in the number of variables allows a modular design that would allow novel and advanced integration of predictive tools in a manner that was previously impossible. So, it would be possible to retain the currently accepted TNM staging variables as the very basic core around which a more complex, detail-oriented prognostication system could be constructed incorporating additional information on host characteristics, non-anatomic tumor parameters, treatment variables and even future advances in molecular biology and our understanding of the genetic characteristics of tumors (16). Unlike the current TNM system, such a modular system could be designed to predict not just survival, but any other oncologic or non-oncologic outcome of interest.

It is well recognized that the risk of some adverse tumor-related events such as locoregional relapse decreases with increasing time interval after treatment. Conversely, patients who survive their head and neck cancer may be at increasing risk for developing subsequent primary tumors. Thus, the risk of a particular outcome is not accurately represented by a static number, but actually changes dynamically based on many factors. Some of these may include lifestyle issues such as continued smoking or alcohol use. Our current staging paradigm is unable to account for these dynamic influences on probability of survival or disease control.

Table 21.1 Comparison of host and tumor characteristics, and outcomes in two patients who would be assigned stage III in the TNM system

Parameter	Patient B	Patient C
Age	60 years old	30 years old
Tobacco user	20 pack-year smoker	Non-smoker
WUHNCI	DM-2 and CAD	No comorbidities
Tumor maximum dimension (cm)	3.5	2.5
Deep muscle invasion	No	No
Site	Lateral tongue	Ventral tongue
Margin	Positive	Negative
Vascular invasion	Yes	No
Perineural invasion	Yes	No
Lymph node status	Positive level II LN	Positive level I LN
TNM stage	III	III
Staging prediction (5-year OS)	34.1%	34.1%
Nomogram prediction (5-year OS)	10%	80%

WUHNCI: Washington University Head and Neck Comorbidity Index; DM-2: Diabetes mellitus type 2; CAD: computer aided design; LN: lymph node; OS: overall survival.

PREDICTIVE VALUE

These multivariate models are created from large datasets of retrospectively reviewed patients, with the intent of predicting the endpoint as accurately as possible. Discrimination and calibration should be considered important measures of how a model performs.

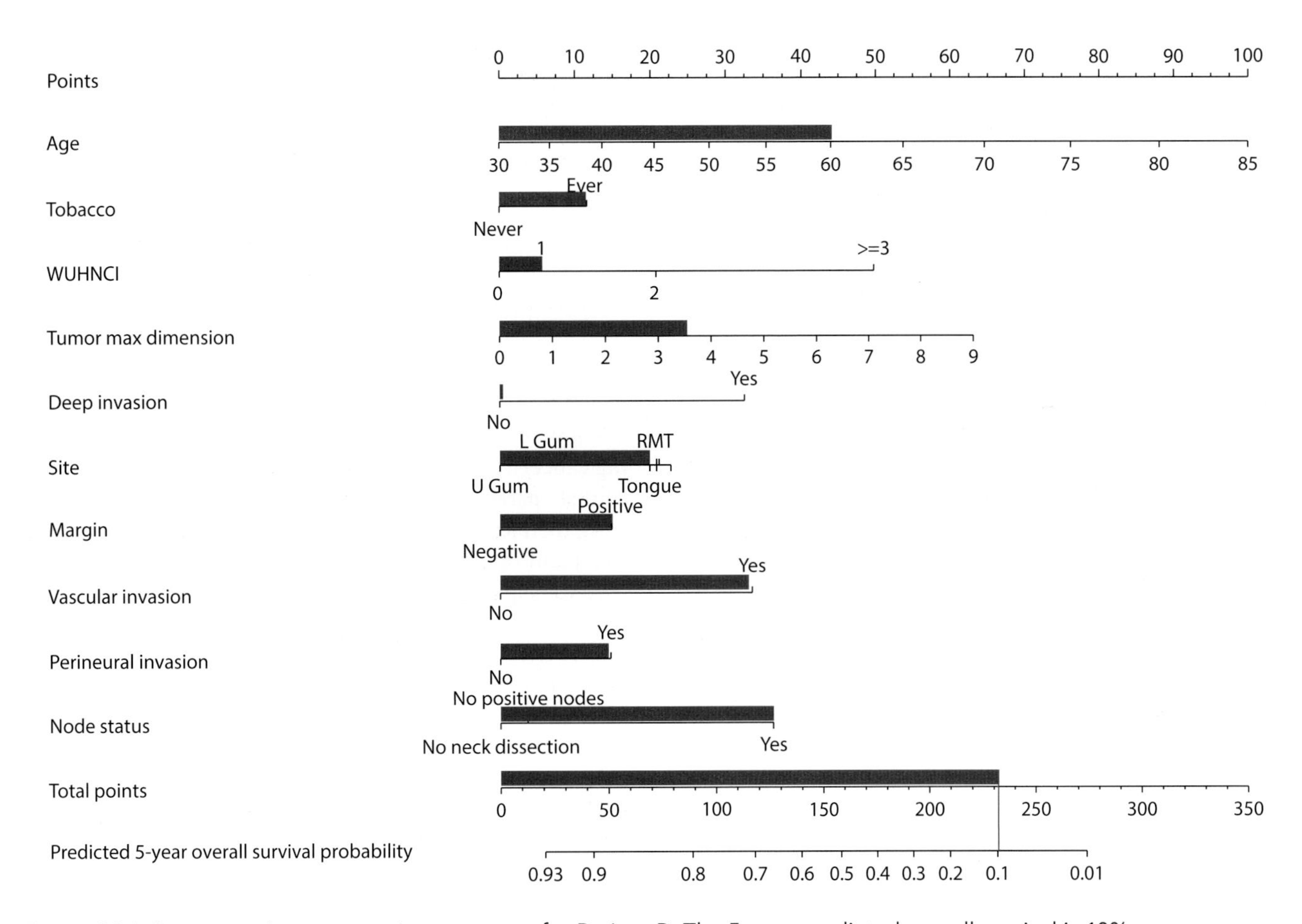

Figure 21.6 Postoperative prognostic nomogram for Patient B. The 5-year predicted overall survival is 10%.

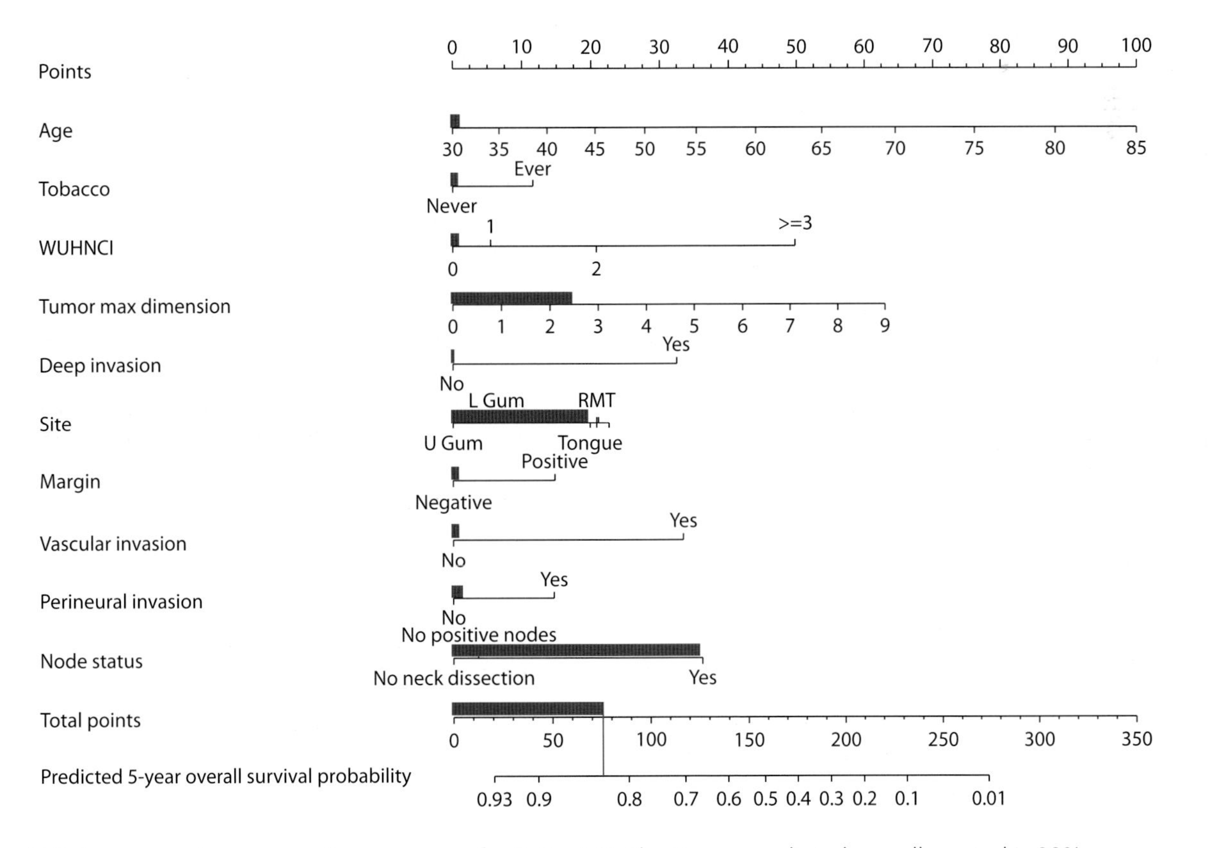

Figure 21.7 Postoperative prognostic nomogram for Patient C. The 5-year predicted overall survival is 80%.

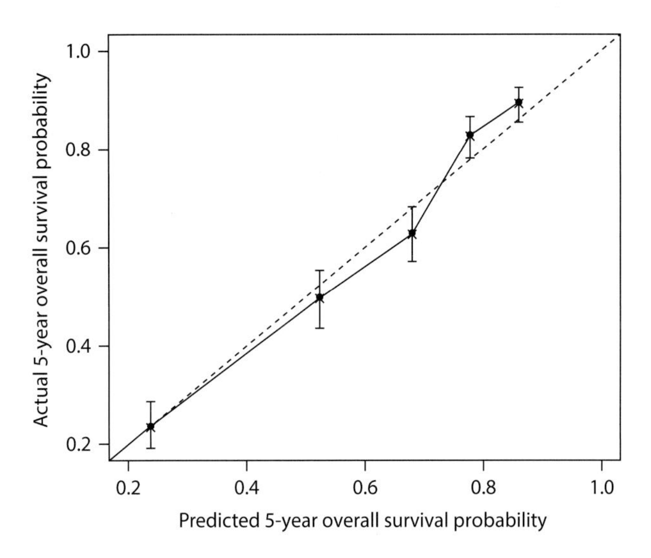

Figure 21.8 Calibration plot for postoperative predictive nomogram predicting 5-year overall survival from Figure 21.3. A perfect predictive model would produce a straight 45° line.

Discrimination examines how accurately a model will correctly quantify an outcome as an event or a non-event (53). The concordance index (c-index) is commonly used to assess discrimination. The c-index is comparable (and in the case of binary outcomes it is identical) to the area under the receiver operator curve (ROC), which plots true-positive rates against false-positive rates at all cutoffs for the probability of a specific outcome (54). Relatively recent statistical work has shown that the concept of area under the ROC can be extended and c-indices are now routinely used as measures of discrimination in survival analyses (53). The c-index is a measurement from 0.5 to 1, where 1 represents perfect discrimination (55).

Calibration is most often used as a graphical assessment of agreement between predicted and observed outcomes. The x-axis is the predicted probability determined by the model. The y-axis is the actual probability of the outcome specified by the model. A calibration plot for a perfectly predictive model will produce a 45° line on the plot (54).

Generally, all models are internally validated with bootstrapping, a technique from which a sample of patients is drawn with replacement from the original group of patients. The original model is then fit with the "new" sample patient cohort to see how well it predicts. Bootstrapping is done for a specified number of times, usually 100 to 1,000, and a new sample of patients is chosen each time (52). Ideally, the models are then validated on external datasets; however, large datasets with good-quality data are sometimes difficult to obtain.

The bootstrapped c-index for the model represented in Figure 21.3 is 0.73. This is a sufficient level of accuracy and is comparable to other published predictive nomograms (56–58). Figure 21.8 shows the calibration plot for the postoperative from nomogram represented in Figure 21.3.

CLINICAL UTILITY

Nomograms and the computerized interfaces created from them can be implemented in many ways. Individualized risk prediction is perhaps the most studied, and these tools are being used to predict a wide variety of outcomes of interest, such as diagnosis, cancer-related outcomes, treatment-related outcomes, etc. For instance, as a diagnostic tool, nomograms have been utilized to aid physicians in predicting malignancy in incidentally found thyroid nodules based on biological, clinical, ultrasonographic and cytologic features (48). After a diagnosis is made, predicting cancer-related outcomes can be useful for physicians to counsel patients when making tough decisions in dealing with their cancer care. As there are sometimes multiple treatment options for patients, these types of tools can be used to help decide between surgery, radiation, chemotherapy and combined-modality treatments. For example, in the oral cavity, we have validated a nomogram to predict the benefit of postoperative radiation therapy (59). Furthermore, nomograms could be useful in determining the intensity of surveillance or treatment-related outcomes. Individualized risk prediction using host, tumor and treatment variables and the event-free survival time after treatment can allow dynamic prediction of risk as the patient progresses along their post-treatment course. Such a tool could prove to be an invaluable resource in designing surveillance protocols for optimal utilization of healthcare expenditure as the cancer burden increases and more effective treatments widen the cancer survivor pool. At the MSKCC, we have also looked at treatment-related outcomes by creating a nomogram to predict the risk of developing a major complication following surgery for oral cancer. Predicting postoperative complications may be important because major complications can carry the possibility for serious morbidity. In thyroid cancer, we have also used individualized risk prediction to predict postoperative hypocalcemia, allowing our institution to predict patients prone to long-term postoperative hospitalization (49).

Nomograms are ideally suited to prediction of outcomes in individual patients based on their own unique characteristics. However, this information can be used for comparison of outcomes across "stage groups" of patients. By establishing a range of prognostic scores equivalent to stage grouping in the traditional TNM "bin" system, we can simplify the interpretation of individualized risk prediction by grouping patients with other patients that carry the same risk (16). Although it seems like we are returning to the compartmentalized groups that we have been trying to avoid, this stratification method will take into account multiple variables that traditional staging systems are not equipped to handle, making it superior.

Beyond physician utility, these types of predictive nomograms can be used by hospital administration to efficiently allocate hospital resources. If nomograms can be used to predict the duration of a patient's hospital stay or their probability of intensive care unit admission, high-demand departments could utilize nomograms to adjust the amount of required staff and supplies. Additionally, being able to predict that a patient will require more than the amount of time allowed for a short-stay surgery procedure could influence surgeons to perform those procedures on an inpatient basis. This would potentially eliminate unplanned return visits and hospital admissions, which use precious resources.

LIMITATIONS OF NOMOGRAMS

The most obvious limitation to the acceptance of nomograms in clinical use could be their perceived complexity. The use of a computerized interface in predicting outcomes is a shift in paradigm for clinicians who are accustomed to using a simple, non-graphical, tabular system for staging and estimating prognosis. The key to successful widespread acceptance will be to maintain or even increase user-friendliness when developing nomograms so that the statistical complexity and sophistication remain hidden behind the scenes. This will ensure that the user is presented with a very simple graphical interface that is readily accessible in the clinic on a computer screen or mobile device.

Another key issue with nomograms that utilize individualized patient information is that not all data points may be available to users in less sophisticated health systems. Therefore, a modular design that allows flexibility in usage depending on the quality of data available is desirable for widespread acceptance of such technology.

The sensitivity of a prediction tool in predicting outcomes depends on the number of individual prognostic variables that it is able to incorporate. Therefore, adequate validation is crucial to account for subtle variations in patient populations that may not be apparent on gross comparisons of established prognostic variables (52,60).

CONCLUSION

The TNM classification has been fundamental in staging, prognostication and outcomes reporting in oncology for more than half a century. It has been the standard and most widely accepted prognostic system. With improved understanding of the biologic behavior of cancer, the relevance of the traditional and static TNM system has been increasingly challenged. In spite of the realization that some newer prognostic variables merit inclusion in the staging paradigm, our ability to change the TNM system has been limited by its rigid "bin" configuration. Advances in statistical methodology and computer technology have converged so that we now have the ability to use tools such as nomograms to not only predict outcomes of interest in individual patients, but also compare groups of patients. This chapter provides a broad understanding of prognostic nomograms and the important role that they will likely play in the future of cancer care. These types of tools are extremely accessible and user-friendly. As we explore this newfound freedom, our challenge will be to preserve the fundamental user-friendliness that has been the hallmark of the TNM system and yet have a tool that accurately incorporates all factors that might influence a plethora of different outcomes of interest.

REFERENCES

1. Halsted WS. The results of operations for the cure of cancer of the breast performed at the Johns Hopkins Hospital from June, 1889, to January, 1894. *Ann Surg* 1894;20:497–555.
2. Steinhal C. Zur Dauerheilung des Brustkrebses. *Beitr Z Klin Chir* 1905;47:226.
3. Denoix PF. Tumor, node and metastasis (TNM). *Bull Inst Natl Hyg* 1944;1:1–69.
4. Denoix PF. [Note on the possible role of the International Union against Cancer in nomenclature, classification, analytical index, bibliography and documentation]. *Acta Union Int Contra Cancrum* 1952;8:92–6.
5. American joint committee for cancer staging and end results reporting. *Manual for staging of cancer.* 1977. American Joint Committee, 1977. Chicago, Illinois.
6. Beahrs O, Rubin P, Carr D. Toward a unified TNM staging system. *Int J Radiat Oncol Biol Phys* 1977;2:1185–89.
7. Sobin LH. TNM: evolution and relation to other prognostic factors. *Semin Surg Oncol* 2003;21:3–7.
8. Gusterson BA. The new TNM classification and micrometastases. *Breast* 2003;12:387–90.
9. Singletary SE, Greene FL, Sobin LH. Classification of isolated tumor cells: clarification of the 6th edition of the American Joint Committee on Cancer Staging Manual. *Cancer* 2003;98:2740–41.
10. Balch CM, Gershenwald JE, Soong SJ, Thompson JF. Update on the melanoma staging system: the importance of sentinel node staging and primary tumor mitotic rate. *J Surg Oncol* 2011;104:379–85.
11. Shaha AR. TNM classification of thyroid carcinoma. *World J Surg* 2007;31:879–87.
12. Peabody TD, Simon MA. Principles of staging of soft-tissue sarcomas. *Clin Orthop Relat Res* 1993: 19–31.
13. Lawton AJ, Mead GM. Staging and prognostic factors in testicular cancer. *Semin Surg Oncol* 1999;17:223–9.
14. UICC. *TNM History.* Evolution & Milestones. International Union Against Cancer, Geneva, Switzerland, 2010.
15. Eggener S. TNM staging for renal cell carcinoma: time for a new method. *Eur Urol* 2010;58:517–19; discussion 519–21

16. Patel SG, Lydiatt WM. Staging of head and neck cancers: is it time to change the balance between the ideal and the practical? *J Surg Oncol* 2008;97:653–7.
17. O'Sullivan B, Shah J. New TNM staging criteria for head and neck tumors. *Semin Surg Oncol* 2003;21:30–42.
18. *AJCC Cancer Staging Manual*. (8th ed). Amin M (ed). Springer, 2017.
19. Burke HB, Henson DE. The American Joint Committee on Cancer. Criteria for prognostic factors and for an enhanced prognostic system. *Cancer* 1993;72:3131–35.
20. Feinstein AR, Sosin DM, Wells CK. The Will Rogers phenomenon. Stage migration and new diagnostic techniques as a source of misleading statistics for survival in cancer. *N Engl J Med* 1985;312:1604–8.
21. Groome PA, Schulze K, Boysen M, Hall SF, Mackillop WJ. A comparison of published head and neck stage groupings in carcinomas of the oral cavity. *Head Neck* 2001;23:613–24.
22. Burke HB. Outcome prediction and the future of the TNM staging system. *J Natl Cancer Inst.* 2004;96: 1408–9.
23. Manikantan K, Sayed SI, Syrigos KN et al. Challenges for the future modifications of the TNM staging system for head and neck cancer: case for a new computational model? *Cancer Treat Rev* 2009;35:639–44.
24. Jones AS, Beasley N, Houghton D, Husband DJ. The effects of age on survival and other parameters in squamous cell carcinoma of the oral cavity, pharynx and larynx. *Clin Otolaryngol Allied Sci* 1998;23:51–6.
25. Arbes SJ, Jr., Olshan AF, Caplan DJ, Schoenbach VJ, Slade GD, Symons MJ. Factors contributing to the poorer survival of black Americans diagnosed with oral cancer (United States). *Cancer Causes Control* 1999;10:513–23.
26. Dikshit RP, Boffetta P, Bouchardy C et al. Lifestyle habits as prognostic factors in survival of laryngeal and hypopharyngeal cancer: a multicentric European study. *Int J Cancer* 2005;117:992–5.
27. Paleri V, Wight RG, Silver CE et al. Comorbidity in head and neck cancer: a critical appraisal and recommendations for practice. *Oral Oncol* 2010;46:712–9.
28. Ragin CC, Taioli E. Survival of squamous cell carcinoma of the head and neck in relation to human papillomavirus infection: review and meta-analysis. *Int J Cancer* 2007;121:1813–20.
29. Sturgis EM, Ang KK. The epidemic of HPV-associated oropharyngeal cancer is here: is it time to change our treatment paradigms? *J Natl Compr Canc Netw* 2011;9:665–73.
30. Spiro RH, Huvos AG, Wong GY, Spiro JD, Gnecco CA, Strong EW. Predictive value of tumor thickness in squamous carcinoma confined to the tongue and floor of the mouth. *Am J Surg* 1986;152:345–50.
31. Po Wing Yuen A, Lam KY, Lam LK et al. Prognostic factors of clinically stage I and II oral tongue carcinoma—a comparative study of stage, thickness, shape, growth pattern, invasive front malignancy grading, Martinez–Gimeno score, and pathologic features. *Head Neck* 2002;24:513–20.
32. Oc P, Pillai G, Patel S et al. Tumour thickness predicts cervical nodal metastases and survival in early oral tongue cancer. *Oral Oncol* 2003;39:386–90.
33. Shah JP. Cervical lymph node metastases—diagnostic, therapeutic, and prognostic implications. *Oncology* 1990;4: 61–69; discussion 72, 76.
34. Gil Z, Carlson DL, Boyle JO et al. Lymph node density is a significant predictor of outcome in patients with oral cancer. *Cancer* 2009;115: 5700–10.
35. Maurizi M, Almadori G, Ferrandina G et al. Prognostic significance of epidermal growth factor receptor in laryngeal squamous cell carcinoma. *Br J Cancer* 1996;74:1253–57.
36. Almadori G, Bussu F, Cadoni G, Galli J, Paludetti G, Maurizi M. Molecular markers in laryngeal squamous cell carcinoma: towards an integrated clinicobiological approach. *Eur J Cancer* 2005;41:683–93.
37. Chaturvedi AK, Engels EA, Pfeiffer RM et al. Human papillomavirus and rising oropharyngeal cancer incidence in the United States. *J Clin Oncol* 2011;29:4294–301.
38. Kates R, Schmitt M, Harbeck N. Advanced statistical methods for the definition of new staging models. *Recent Results Cancer Res* 2003;162:101–13.
39. Abbod MF, Catto JW, Linkens DA, Hamdy FC. Application of artificial intelligence to the management of urological cancer. *J Urol* 2007;178:1150–56.
40. Tsantis S, Dimitropoulos N, Cavouras D, Nikiforidis G. Morphological and wavelet features towards sonographic thyroid nodules evaluation. *Comput Med Imaging Graph* 2009;33: 91–9.
41. Lim KJ, Choi CS, Yoon DY et al. Computer-aided diagnosis for the differentiation of malignant from benign thyroid nodules on ultrasonography. *Acad Radiol* 2008;15:853–8.
42. Speight PM, Elliott AE, Jullien JA, Downer MC, Zakzrewska JM. The use of artificial intelligence to identify people at risk of oral cancer and precancer. *Br Dent J* 1995;179:382–7.
43. Jones AS, Taktak AG, Helliwell TR et al. An artificial neural network improves prediction of observed survival in patients with laryngeal squamous carcinoma. *Eur Arch Otorhinolaryngol* 2006;263:541–7.
44. Doerfler R. The lost art of nomography. *The UMAP Journal* 2009;30:457–93.
45. Montero PH, Yu C, Palmer FL et al. Nomograms for preoperative prediction of prognosis in patients with oral cavity squamous cell carcinoma. *Cancer* 2014;120:214–21.

46. Kattan MW. Nomograms are superior to staging and risk grouping systems for identifying high-risk patients: preoperative application in prostate cancer. *Curr Opin Urol* 2003;13:111–6.
47. Gross ND, Patel SG, Carvalho AL et al. Nomogram for deciding adjuvant treatment after surgery for oral cavity squamous cell carcinoma. *Head Neck* 2008;30:1352–60.
48. Nixon IJ, Ganly I, Hann LE et al. Nomogram for predicting malignancy in thyroid nodules using clinical, biochemical, ultrasonographic, and cytologic features. *Surgery* 2010;148:1120–27; discussion 1127–8.
49. Ali S, Yu C, Palmer FL et al. Nomogram to aid selection of patients for short-stay thyroidectomy based on risk of postoperative hypocalcemia. *Arch Otolaryngol Head Neck Surg* 2011;137:1154–60.
50. van den Broek GB, Rasch CR, Pameijer FA et al. Pretreatment probability model for predicting outcome after intraarterial chemoradiation for advanced head and neck carcinoma. *Cancer* 2004;101:1809–17.
51. Egelmeer AG, Velazquez ER, de Jong JM et al. Development and validation of a nomogram for prediction of survival and local control in laryngeal carcinoma patients treated with radiotherapy alone: a cohort study based on 994 patients. *Radiother Oncol* 2011;100:108–15.
52. Iasonos A, Schrag D, Raj GV, Panageas KS. How to build and interpret a nomogram for cancer prognosis. *J Clin Oncol* 2008;26:1364–70.
53. Pencina MDA, D'Agostino RB. Overall C as a measure of discrimination in survival analysis: model specific population value and confidence interval estimation. *Stat Med* 2004;23:2109–23.
54. Steyerberg EW, Vickers AJ, Cook NR et al. Assessing the performance of prediction models: a framework for traditional and novel measures. *Epidemiology* 2010;21:128–38.
55. Harrell FE. *Regression Modeling Strategies: With Applications to Linear Models, Logistic Regression, and Survival Analysis*. New York: Springer, 2001.
56. Gail MH, Brinton LA, Byar DP et al. Projecting individualized probabilities of developing breast cancer for white females who are being examined annually. *J Natl Cancer Inst* 1989;81:1879–86.
57. Kattan MW, Eastham JA, Stapleton AM, Wheeler TM, Scardino PT. A preoperative nomogram for disease recurrence following radical prostatectomy for prostate cancer. *J Natl Cancer Inst* 1998;90:766–71.
58. Kattan MW, Leung DH, Brennan MF. Postoperative nomogram for 12-year sarcoma-specific death. *J Clin Oncol* 2002;20:791–6.
59. Wang SJ, Patel SG, Shah JP et al. An oral cavity carcinoma nomogram to predict benefit of adjuvant radiotherapy. *JAMA Otolaryngol Head Neck Surg* 2013;139:554–9.
60. Vickers AJ, Cronin AM. Everything you always wanted to know about evaluating prediction models (but were too afraid to ask). *Urology* 2010;76:1298–301.

22

Prosthetic restoration and rehabilitation

IVANA PETROVIC, GEORGE BOHLE, AND JATIN P. SHAH

INTRODUCTION

The current management of the majority of head and neck cancers has evolved over the past several decades into a multidisciplinary specialty, with participation by head and neck surgeons, radiation oncologists, medical oncologists, maxillofacial surgeons, reconstructive surgeons, dentists and prosthodontists, rehabilitation specialists and supporting services. The goal of the multidisciplinary team is to maximize tumor control and minimize treatment-related sequelae, which impact upon the quality of life. Nowhere in the head and neck region is this more important than in the oral cavity and the oropharynx. The role of the dental surgeon and the prosthodontist is crucial from the day of initial diagnosis until after completion of treatment, rehabilitation and, thereafter, lifelong for management of the long-term sequela and complications of treatment. Thus, the involvement of the dental surgeon begins with pretreatment assessment of the patient's dentition, appropriate interventions and prophylactic treatments for effective and safe delivery of initial definitive treatment of the cancer. Intraoperative and perioperative dental management is crucial to the successful outcome of a surgical procedure. Similarly, pre-radiation assessment of dentition, fabrication of protective devices during radiation and post-radiation management of the radiated dentition are crucial to the successful outcome of treatment with radiation with none or minimal impact of radiation exposure on the teeth. Management of the dentition in patients receiving chemotherapy is equally important and complex. Avoidance of complications due to long-term bisphosphonate therapy is an integral part of the overall care of the patient. Finally, when reconstructive surgery has not or cannot restore a patient's appearance and function, the availability of external prosthetic devices should be considered. These personalized, individually fabricated devices significantly improve form and function and thus the quality of life after treatment of patients with head and neck cancers (1).

EVALUATION OF THE PATIENT AND DENTAL PROPHYLAXIS

Patients with oral and oropharyngeal cancers during their initial medical workup should be referred to an oncologic dentist to evaluate their oral and dental health. This should be done prior to any invasive intervention, during the treatment planning phase, either preoperatively or pre-radiation. The initial examination by the dentist involves assessment of the teeth clinically and by at least a screening orthopantomogram. Septic teeth that are not salvageable are extracted, unless they are in a tumor-bearing area. Septic but salvageable teeth are appropriately treated. If possible, restorative dentistry should be completed prior to radiation treatment. Preferably, dental caries and periodontal lesions and conditions should be treated before

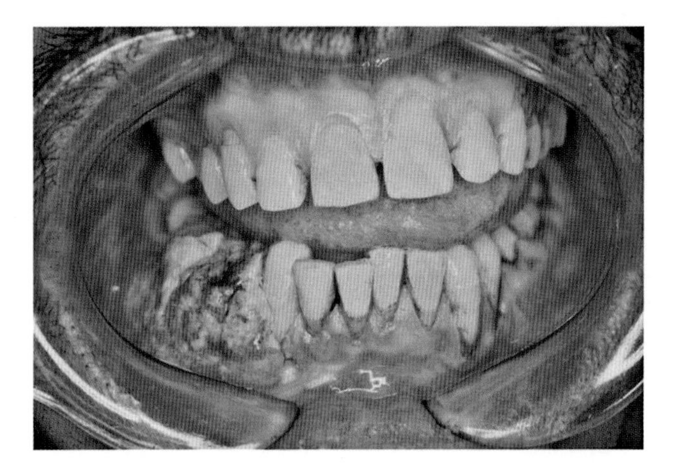

Figure 22.1 Squamous cell carcinoma of the lower gum.

the initiation of cytotoxic treatment or exposure to ionizing radiation. Ideally, a period of at least 2 weeks should be available to allow healing of soft tissue manipulations and dental extractions so that mucosal integrity is restored before treatment begins. It must be emphasized that dental extraction in the proximity of the tumor opens up a route for implantation of malignant cells through the alveolar process/dental socket and therefore it should be avoided. Two examples of these are shown in Figure 22.1, a squamous cell carcinoma of the lower gum, and in Figure 22.2, a sarcoma of the mandible. However, prolonged dental treatments should be delayed until after completion of cancer therapy because it is imperative that the cancer treatment takes priority over long-term elective dental treatment. The general practice dentist and hygienist can use the interval between initial screening appointment and commencement of external beam radiation therapy to complete all hygiene procedures such as scaling, polishing, soaking, root planning and curettage. Overhanging and faulty restoration can be removed and replaced appropriately and ill-fitting dentures should be corrected. Home care should include infective daily plaque removal and use of soft toothbrushes with application of high-potency fluoride. Fluoride trays are made for most patients and the need for daily topical fluoride is emphasized to reduce the risk of dental caries. This risk has not been eliminated by the use of intensity-modulated radiotherapy (IMRT). Factors such as the type of fluoride used or the modality of its application are less important to outcome than is daily compliance in using high-potential fluoride for the reminder of the patient's life. Patients are instructed to floss daily and brush their teeth after every meal, which includes liquid supplements, because they contain cariogenic carbohydrates. A toothpaste or gel that contains neutral 1% sodium fluoride is preferred over stenosed fluoride, which has an unpleasant taste and adverse effects such as sensitivity of the teeth and gingiva. The toothpaste can be used with a brush every night for 2 minutes. One may expectorate as much as desired, but patients should not rinse the mouth clean in the evening, leaving a thin film of fluoride on the teeth while sleeping (1).

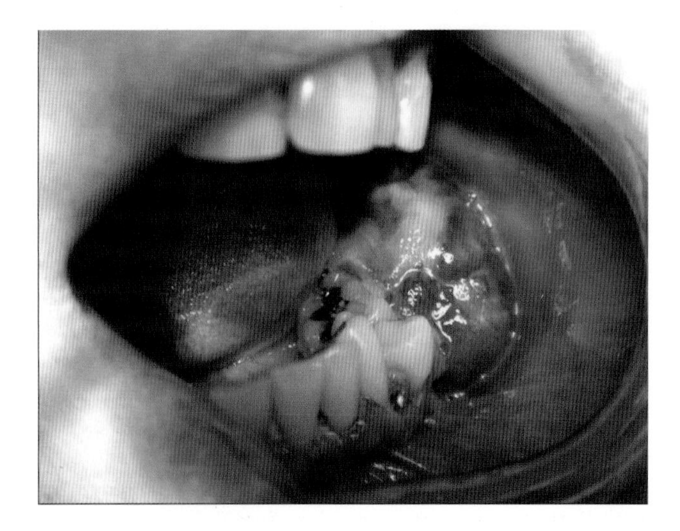

Figure 22.2 Sarcoma of the mandible.

Dental extractions should be done as soon as possible in those patients that require them (Table 22.1). Teeth may be extracted if they are decayed and unrestorable, lack opposing teeth, prosthetically useless and are likely to be lost during the course of treatment or in patients who are unwilling to carry out the rigorous oral care and hygiene regimen required. In addition, partly erupted third molar teeth and those with severe periodontal disease should be removed to prevent pericoronitis or other infections. Teeth with periodontal inflammatory disease or non-vital teeth may be kept if the patient is willing to undergo root canal treatment. As previously mentioned, all extractions should be completed in time for mucosal healing to occur prior to starting cancer treatment. It is important to avoid sharp ridges and bony spicules after dental extraction. These should be smoothed out by filing and, if possible, the mucosa of the gingiva at the extraction site should be closed with sutures (2). Upon extraction, it is imperative to consider alveoloplasty and primary mucoperiosteal flap closure to expedite healing. This is especially true in areas where the alveolus has been expanded to permit delivery of divergent root tips. Areas of thin, friable mucosa overlying bony prominences such as tori or exostosis can also be excised and the bone smoothed out to avoid problems secondary to delay in wound healing. Teeth with a poor prognosis should be extracted before irradiation

Table 22.1 Indications for dental extractions before radiation therapy.

- Poor oral hygiene and multiple missing or decayed teeth
- Dental caries non-amenable to restoration
- Extensive periodontal disease with mobility, bone loss and root furcation involvement
- Residual root tips
- Exposed, impacted or incompletely erupted teeth

or chemotherapy. Reducing sites of infection decreases the chance of osteoradionecrosis (ORN) in patients who undergo irradiation and infectious episodes in patients who receive chemotherapy (3).

ORAL CARE DURING RADIATION THERAPY

The mucosal surfaces of the oral cavity are exposed to significant doses of radiation during treatment. The indirect effect on these structures can also result from exposure of the parotid and submandibular glands to radiation with consequent alteration of the composition and quantity of saliva production. However, with increasing use of IMRT in radiation delivery, major salivary glands are often protected and thus normal saliva production is retained at least to a certain extent. Patients who have extensive metallic restorations require custom mouth guards to reduce scatter that causes increased mucositis. These guards should be fabricated in time for them to be delivered before the simulation appointment (1).

Patients should be seen by the dentist as necessary, but at least once during the course of their radiation treatment. During this visit, patients should be assessed for the presence of radiation-related side effects. Such visits also provide an opportunity to remove any immediate RT-related side effects on the teeth and to re-emphasize to the patient about the importance of continued dental care.

All patients will undoubtedly experience some degree of radiation mucositis. Mucositis generally occurs 5–7 days after initiation of external bean radiation therapy. The extent and intensity of mucosal changes depend on the fractionation, energy source, total dose of radiation and oral and dental status (4). Grade IV mucositis is infrequent and is usually seen toward the end of the treatment (Figure 22.3). Patients with metallic filings have an increased risk of severe mucositis as a result of "double-dose" radiation to the mucosa adjacent to the metallic filings due to the radiation

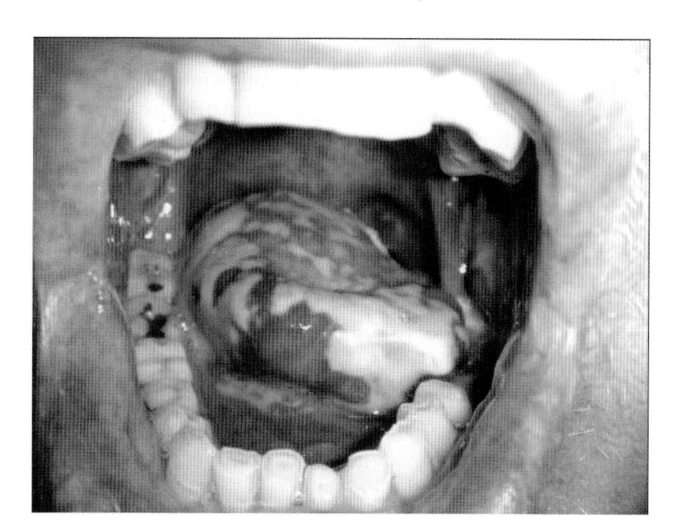

Figure 22.3 Extensive (grade IV) mucositis in a patient at 4 weeks during radiation for cancer of the oral tongue.

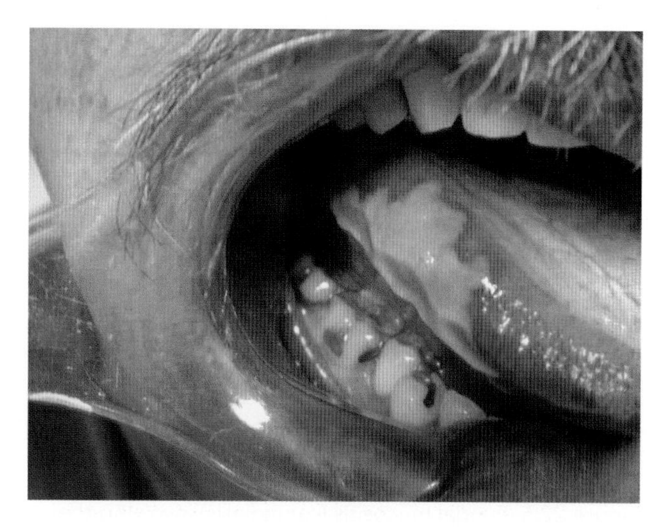

Figure 22.4 Severe mucositis of the tongue adjacent to metallic filings in the molar teeth.

beam bouncing off the metal (Figure 22.4). The mucosal reactions on the side of the entering beam may consist of patchy or confluent exudate, whereas the contralateral side may show only erythema. During the course of radiation therapy, the mucosa becomes thin as a result of direct cell death and the sloughing of radically replicating epithelial cells (5). Hot foods, smoking, alcohol or phenol-containing mouth rinses and sodium should be avoided (6). Treatment of mucositis typically consists of palliative pain reduction therapy. Good oral hygiene is essential to improving oral comfort and reducing the risk of oral contamination. This is easily maintained with frequent rinses and gargles with a solution of one quart of warm water with a teaspoonful of table salt and a teaspoonful of baking soda. Bacterial fungal and viral infections can occur as superinfections with mucositis, but are less likely to induce septicemia in patients undergoing radiation therapy than in patients receiving chemotherapy (7).

Candidiasis occurs in most patients receiving radiation therapy to the oral cavity, sometimes during the course of their treatment. It can manifest as pseudomembranous, hyperplastic or atrophic (erythematous or white) patchy lesions (8). The sites most frequently affected are the tongue, buccal mucosa, hard or soft palate or commissure labiorum oris (i.e. angular cheilitis) (Figure 22.5). Clinically, it can manifest as a whitish patch of the oral mucosa that may be removed with gentle pressure on wet gauze. Treatment consists of such topical antifungal agents as nystatin oral suspension or clotrimazole troches depending on the degree of xerostomia (8–10). Mastication and swallowing may be altered or hindered during radiation treatment. Patients should be encouraged to follow a soft diet and to receive an adequate caloric and nutrition intake. For patients in whom the tongue is involved, dysphagia may occur, lessening motivation to eat (2). In such patients, a nasogastric feeding tube or a percutaneous gastrostomy may be considered. The acute and long-term side effects of radiation therapy to the oral cavity are summarized in Table 22.2.

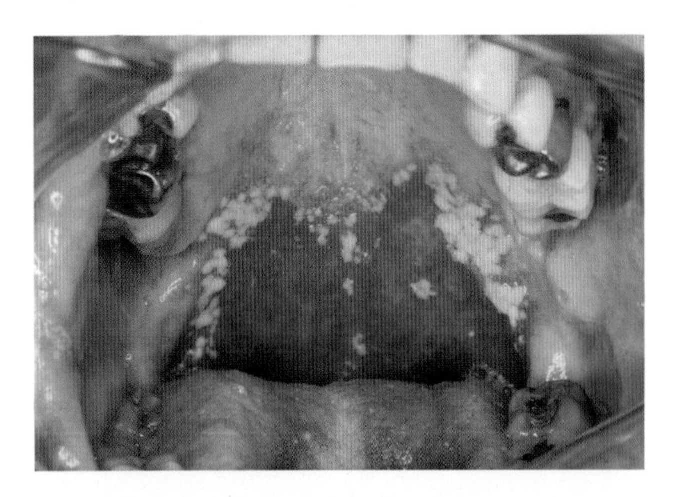

Figure 22.5 Fungal mucositis (candidiasis) involving the hard and soft palate.

Table 22.2 Acute and long-term effects of radiation on the oral cavity

Acute side effects	Long-term side effects
Mucositis	Xerostomia
Dysgeusia	Caries
Dysphagia	Periodontal diseases
Ropey saliva	Trismus
Risk of fungal infection	Osteoradionecrosis
	Fungal infections

LONG-TERM SEQUELAE OF RADIATION THERAPY TO THE ORAL CAVITY

Xerostomia is probably the most common long-term sequela of radiating the oral cavity. The severity of xerostomia depends on the total dose of radiation, the source, the fractionation and poor dose delivery. Radiation results in atrophy of salivary gland elements, causing cessation of normal saliva production. The problem is compounded when the patient receives chemotherapy concurrently with radiation. Apart from the impact on quality of life because of difficulty with eating, oral discomfort, fit of prosthesis and speech, xerostomia also increase the risk of caries, periodontal disease and, ultimately, ORN. Pharmacologic agents such as pilocarpine and amifostine have been investigated with mixed results for relief of xerostomia. However, most patients obtain symptomatic relief through frequent use of water (1). Prevention of dental caries and ORN of the mandible requires long-term prophylactic measures and daily dental care (Table 22.3).

Other long-term sequelae are related to effects on soft tissue, bone and blood vessels. Long-term effects on skin and subcutaneous soft tissues produce tissue atrophy and contractures with significant esthetic morbidity (Figure 22.6). Irradiation of the extrinsic muscles of mastication can produce fibrosis, which leads to trismus over time. Regular stretching exercises of the muscles can decrease or even prevent this dreadful complication. Patients may be instructed to use their thumb and fingers to forcefully open the mouth at the point of tolerance (Figure 22.7). It is crucial for the clinician to bring forth the importance of preventing trismus at every opportunity because difficulty in opening the mouth not only affects the quality of life, but also interferes with adequate post-treatment monitoring of the oral cavity and oropharynx for recurrence or new cancer. Patients should begin to perform this exercise before radiation therapy commences and if the exercises are stopped during treatment they must be resumed as soon as the acute side effects of radiation therapy have subsided. The exercises should be performed in multiple cycles throughout the day. If, however, trismus appears to be developing, then the use of special appliances such as an acrylic resin corkscrew, tongue depressors taped together or commercially available devices, such as Therabite or Dynasplint, is recommended (Figure 22.8) (1).

The risk for ORN increases if the bone is irradiated with more than 55 Gy. The mandible is more commonly affected

Table 22.3 Recommendations for dental prophylaxis in patients who have received radiation to the oral cavity

- Daily application of neutral sodium fluoride gel. This is done preferably with custom-made dental trays applied for at least 1 hour. The best time to do this is prior to retiring at night
- Floss daily
- Brush teeth after oral intake of any liquids or solids
- Gargle with salt and baking soda solution after every meal

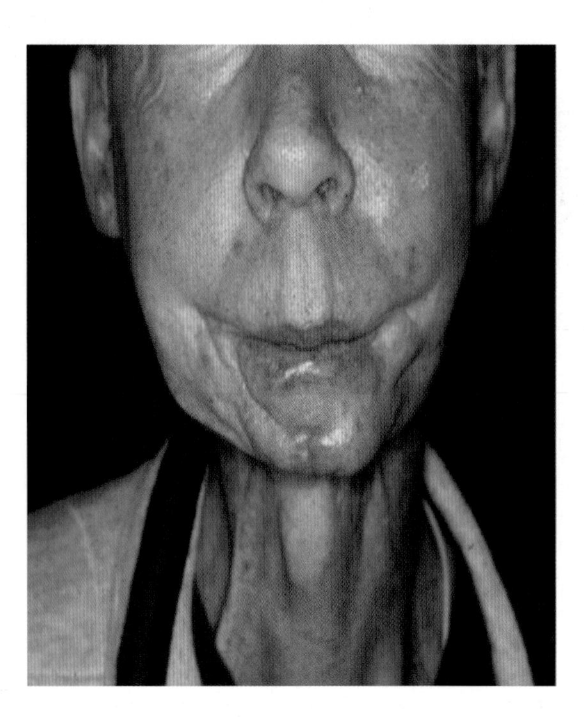

Figure 22.6 Skin and soft tissue atrophy following radiation therapy to the oral cavity.

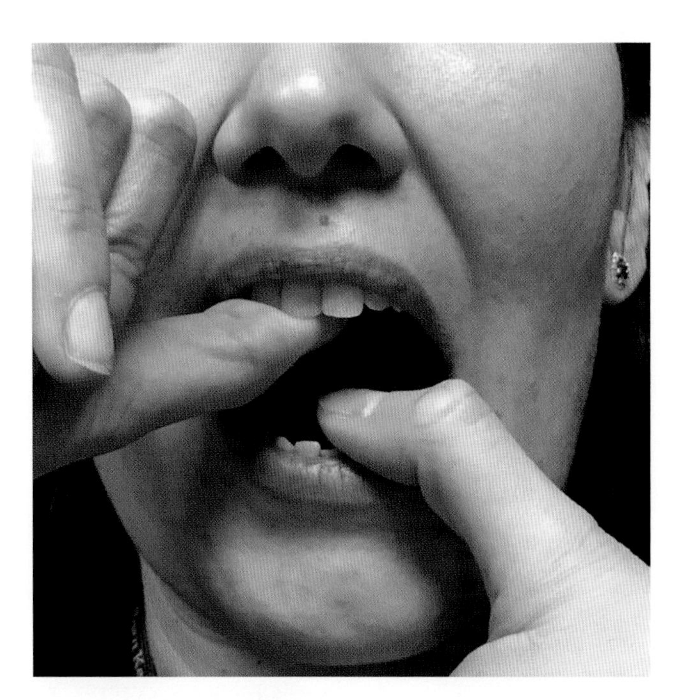

Figure 22.7 Jaw-stretching exercises for prevention of trismus.

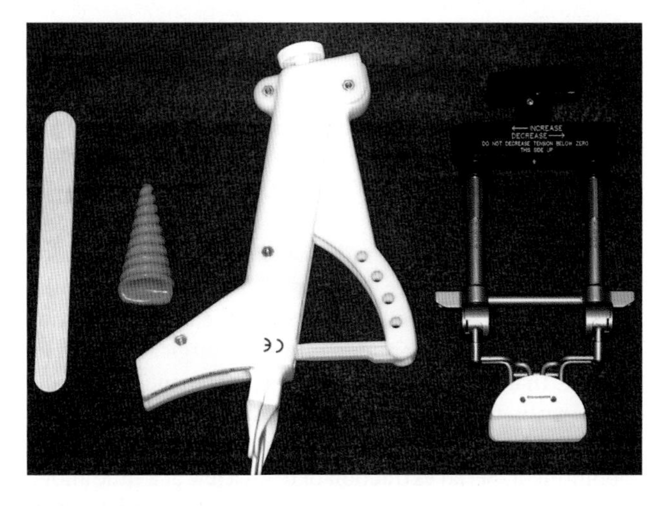

Figure 22.8 Appliances used for prevention of trismus. Tongue blades, acrylic cork screw, Therabite and Dynasplint.

because of endothelial damage to the relatively sparse intraosseous blood vessels. The maxilla has a profuse blood supply and therefore ORN of this bone is uncommon. The process can take many months or even years to develop and patients are at risk for the development of ORN for the remainder of their lives. Dental caries and periodontal disease leading to extractions are the most common precipitating factors. Prevention of this complication by rigorous oral hygiene is crucial because conservative measures such as antibiotics, debridement and curettage are effective only in the early stage of this disease process before bone necrosis takes place. Advanced ORN of the mandible with sequestrum formation and with exposed intraoral bone,

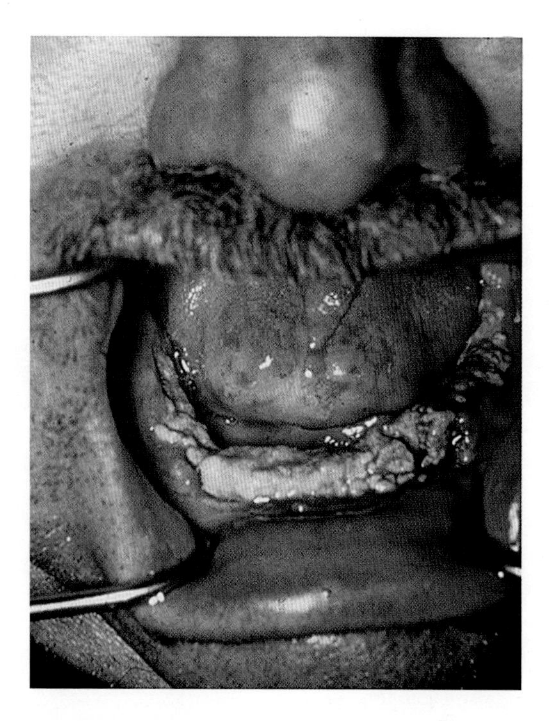

Figure 22.9 Osteoradionecrosis of the mandible with exposed sequestrum.

does not respond to conservative means of treatment and generally requires segmental resection and reconstruction (Figure 22.9) (1).

The role of hyperbaric oxygen (HBO) in the treatment of ORN has been debated over several decades and remains controversial. It is important for the clinician to realize that HBO cannot revitalize necrotic bone, for which the only effective treatment is sequestrectomy or mandible resection. However, HBO may be useful in the treatment of ORN if detected in its early stages. The sequential orthopantomograms of a patient with an exposed impacted tooth #17 requiring extraction and early onset of ORN treated with HBO are shown in Figure 22.10. On the other hand, ORN may develop in an unexposed mandible, which is treatable and is often controlled with HBO treatment (Figure 22.11). The major concern in using HBO for ORN revolves around whether replenishing oxygen in the affected tissue can lead to the activation of cancer cells that otherwise were dormant. However, no systematic study to address this question or other questions regarding the use of HBO in patients with ORN has been conducted. Sporadic reports appear in the literature about reactivation of a tumor in this setting. Therefore, HBO should be used with caution, especially if any doubt exists about the cancer status of the patient (1). Furthermore, the role of HBO in treating ORN was studied in a European multicenter, randomized, placebo-controlled trial. The trial was aborted at 1 year since the placebo group had better outcomes than the treatment group. Although many criticisms regarding the conduct of this trial have been reported, the fact remains that the role of HBO in established ORN remains controversial (11). Currently, HBO treatment is recommended in a prophylactic setting

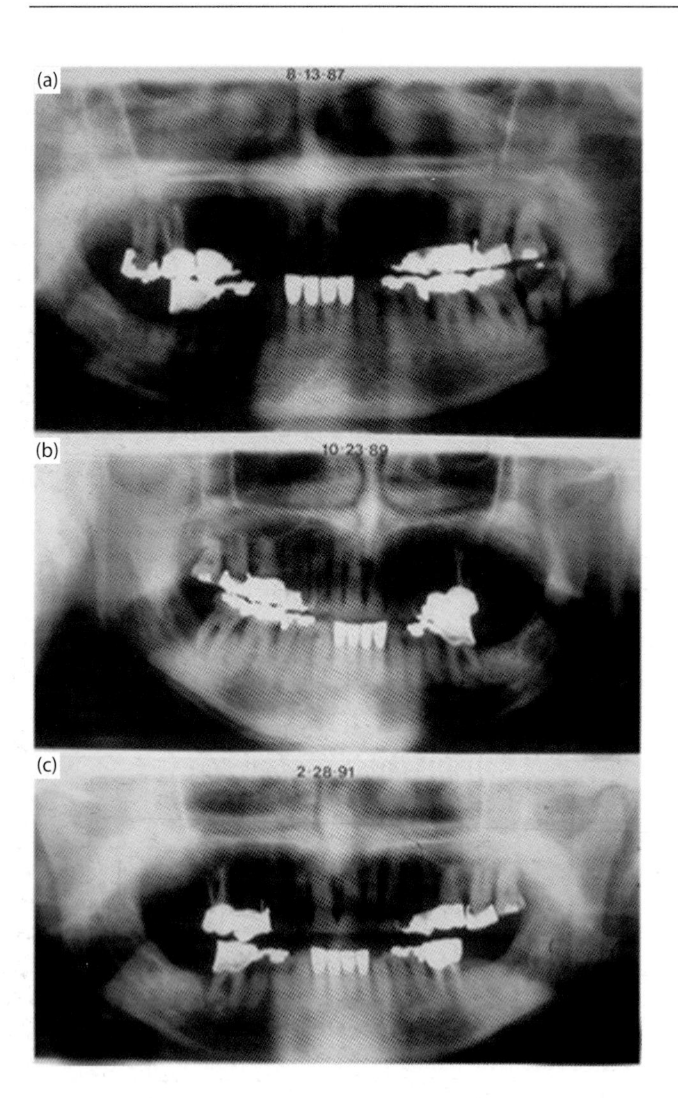

Figure 22.10 Orthopantomograms showing (a) an exposed impacted tooth #17 requiring extraction, (b) early onset of radionecrosis at the extraction site and (c) healed extraction site after HBO treatment.

when tooth extraction is required in a previously irradiated mandible. This is particularly important for extraction of molars since radiation exposure is usually the highest at the angle of the mandible. HBO treatment is delivered prior to extraction and postextraction to facilitate healing of the socket.

DENTAL CARE POST-RADIATION THERAPY

An oncologic dentist should see the post-radiated patient at least annually to determine that they are compliant with respect to their oral hygiene measures and to that they are free of post-radiation caries. Teeth affected by post-radiation caries are difficult to restore. Teeth that are unrestorable due to post-radiation caries may require extraction. Alternatively, they may be treated with root canal therapy and then allowed to exfoliate on their own. If extractions are required, it is important to discuss the location of the teeth with respect to the radiation field with the radiation oncologist. Teeth that are well outside the field do not require any special management. Teeth within the field of radiation should be extracted without raising a surgical flap when possible. In addition, the use of low epinephrine-containing local anesthetic and perioperative systemic antibiotics is recommended (12). It is better to not extract all teeth at one appointment. Serial extraction of teeth a few at a time allows the dentist to observe the progression of wound healing. Generally, in post-radiated patients, it is better to manage a small wound rather than many small wounds or several large ones. The role of HBO in the prevention of ORN in patients requiring extractions in a previously radiated mandible has been studied in a randomized trial and has shown benefit in reducing the risk of ORN following extractions (13).

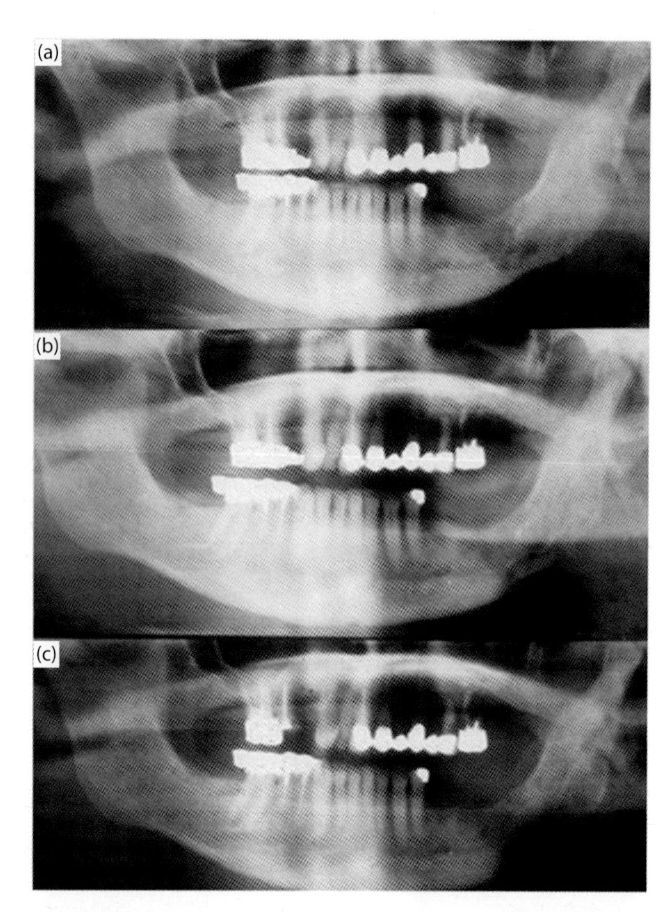

Figure 22.11 Orthopantomograms showing (a) early onset of ORN in unexposed mandible, (b) during HBO treatment and (c) complete healing at the site after HBO therapy.

Patients with very advanced cancer may be managed less aggressively from a dental standpoint, keeping their overall disease status and prognosis in mind. Asymptomatic teeth may be retained and managed conservatively even in the presence of caries, periodontal disease or periapical pathology. Abutment teeth for a removable prosthesis should be preserved if possible. Definitive restoration with crowns, fixed bridges and onlays for control of carious teeth may be delayed until completion of treatment with use of intermediate restorative materials (1).

Although commonly used chemotherapeutic agents such as cisplatin, 5-fluorouracil and methotrexate have the potential to cause acute mucositis on their own, their combination with each other and/or with radiation therapy can result in treatment-limiting stomatitis. Chemotherapy-related adverse effects can include mucositis and alteration of the milieu causing candidiasis and bacterial, other fungal or viral infections of the oral mucosa. In addition to their direct effect, these problems can cause a severe reduction in dietary intake, with other sequelae of malnutrition. As with patients scheduled to have radiation therapy, these patients also should be evaluated at least 3 weeks before chemotherapy is administered. The patient is carefully screened for potential sources of bacteria such as periodontal disease and appropriate therapy is undertaken if needed. Endodontic treatment or dental extraction is considered for symptomatic teeth with periapical lesions and third molar pathology is addressed. Oral hygiene during treatment should include frequent rinsing with a salt and baking soda solution, brushing of the teeth and washing the prosthesis (1).

MAXILLOFACIAL PROSTHETICS

Dental prosthetic support is required generally in all aspects of oral and oropharyngeal surgery where the function of speech, mastication, swallowing or external physical appearance is likely to be altered following surgery. Thus, it is crucial for the prosthodontist to see the patient preoperatively in order to get a baseline assessment of the basic problem and the anticipated functional/esthetic deformity that will result from surgery.

The need for prosthetic support can be divided into two major areas: bone and soft tissue. These are then related to: (a) palate (hard and soft) and upper gum; (b) mandible; and (c) tongue and floor of the mouth.

UPPER GUM AND HARD PALATE

Usually, there are three phases of prosthetic rehabilitation: surgical, (intraoperative), interim (postoperative) and definitive. Each phase may span from several days to several months or even up to a year depending on the size and location of the tumor, complexity and location of the defect, rate and quality of healing and post-radiation changes in the defect. Surgical and interim prosthesis may require frequent follow-up appointments and adjustments. The role of maxillofacial prosthodontist in the perioperative period is summarized in Table 22.4.

Maxillofacial prosthetic rehabilitation forms an integral component of a comprehensive treatment program for patients undergoing surgical resection of oral and oropharyngeal cancer. The common goals of rehabilitation are restoration of speech, mastication and swallowing, control of saliva and restoration of facial deficits. Prosthetic rehabilitation should begin prior to the cancer surgery. It is pivotal that the treating dentist or prosthodontist assesses the patient prior to surgery and devises the appropriate prosthesis to suit the individual patient and the surgeon's needs. Preoperative communication and discussion between the head and neck surgeon and the prosthodontist is crucial for optimum planning and achievement of a good functional and esthetic outcome at various stages of treatment. The head and neck surgeon should be aware of the functional sequelae from loss of the structures being resected so that the patient's rehabilitation is planned even before the extirpative surgical procedure is undertaken (1).

Table 22.4 The role of maxillofacial prosthodontist in dental/oral rehabilitation.

Preoperatively
- To obtain dental impression for surgical obturator
- Preoperative photographs
- Dental evaluation of patients undergoing segmental mandibulectomy and reconstruction
- Evaluation for external prosthesis
- Preparation of facial impressions and moulage

Intraoperatively
- Placement (wiring) of surgical obturator
- Intermaxillary fixation for free flap mandible reconstruction
- Placement of dental implants
- Dental extractions

Early postoperative period
- Adjustments of intermediate maxillary prosthesis
- Speech bulb prosthesis
- Partial augmentation prosthesis
- Partial dentures
- Lingual splints

Late postoperative period
- Definitive maxillary prosthesis
- Mandibular resection prosthesis
- Lingual splint for unstable mandibulotomy
- Palatal drop prosthesis
- Osseointegrated implants
- Fabrication of facial prosthesis (nasal, orbital, facial, auricular, complex)

MAXILLARY DEFECT AND OBTURATORS

The candidate for any type of maxillectomy or palatal, upper alveolar resection should be assessed by the prosthodontist preoperatively and the extent of surgery and structures to be removed and those that will remain discussed with the surgeon in detail. The prosthodontist should discuss with the surgeon three important principles that ultimately govern the success or failure of prosthetic rehabilitation: support, stability and retention. Support is the feature of the residual anatomy that will contribute to the resistance to intrusion of the denture, leaving horizontal bony areas on which the denture sits. If this does not compromise the surgical/oncologic resection, then it is desirable to maximize support. Stability is that feature of the denture base that makes the denture resistant to side-to-side and front-to-back movement. Teeth and vertical bony elements such as the alveolar prosthesis of the maxilla, which is protected by suitable mucosal coverage, contribute to the stability of the denture. Retention of denture is that property of the denture that keeps the denture affixed to the supporting structures. It is derived in the partially edentulous patient by placing clasp elements above residual teeth. In the partially and completely edentulous patients, the ability to mechanically adapt and learn to wear their prosthesis may be the biggest contributing factor to the denture's overall stability. Successful fabrication of a functional maxillary obturator is based on the principles of retention, stability and support (1).

The maxillofacial prosthodontist evaluates the patient before surgery to obtain impressions and participates in surgical planning of the resection and placement of the surgical obturator. An intraoperative photograph of a patient with carcinoma of the hard palate is shown in Figure 22.12. The prosthodontist takes impressions of the hard palate and produces a cast model. The head and neck surgeon marks the anticipated margins of resection on the dental cast model (Figure 22.13). The obturator usually is fabricated from polymethyl methacrylate acrylic resin and must be ready at the time of surgery. It is used in the operating room at the completion of the surgical resection. The prosthodontist is called into the operating room to affix the obturator prosthesis with wires to the remaining teeth or to the alveolar process in edentulous patients (Figure 22.14). In doing a maxillectomy, it is desirable to preserve as much of the adjacent/overlying mucosa/mucoperiosteum at the site of the bone cut to provide coverage on the excised bone margin. It is particularly important for resection of the hard palate where uninvolved mucoperiosteum of the palate is used to roll over the cut edge of the bone. A split-thickness skin graft after maxillectomy is employed under select circumstances. Simple infrastructure partial maxillectomy without any abnormality of the antral mucosa can be left alone to heal by secondary intention. This gives a much better mucosa-lined surgical defect in the long term. Use of skin grafts generally creates a skin-lined defect with dry sebaceous secretions and odor. However, a skin graft is necessary if the surgical defect extends into the masticator space with stumps of transacted pterygoid muscles. On some occasions, retention of the maxillary prosthesis is facilitated by excision of the inferior turbinate to create space for the prosthesis. In some patients with unopposed mandibular teeth at the site of maxillectomy, consideration should be given to extraction of these teeth, since they are dysfunctional and will cant medially, causing problems during mastication.

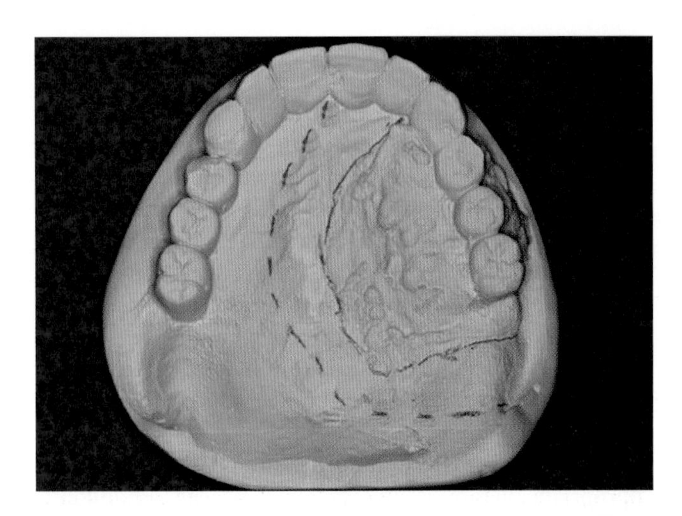

Figure 22.13 Dental cast model showing the extent of the tumor and the planned extent of resection.

Intraoperatively, when the dentist has positioned the prosthesis in its appropriate final position, the surgical obturator is ligated to the remaining teeth by twisting 24-gauge, pre-stretched, stainless steel wires between the teeth or, in the edentulous patient, through the alveolar ridge and palatal shelf. The surgical obturator prosthesis is placed over the surgical packing (14). If the patient is edentulous, implants could be placed at this time to allow for adequate healing before radiation if it is needed and to aid in retention and stability of the interim obturator.

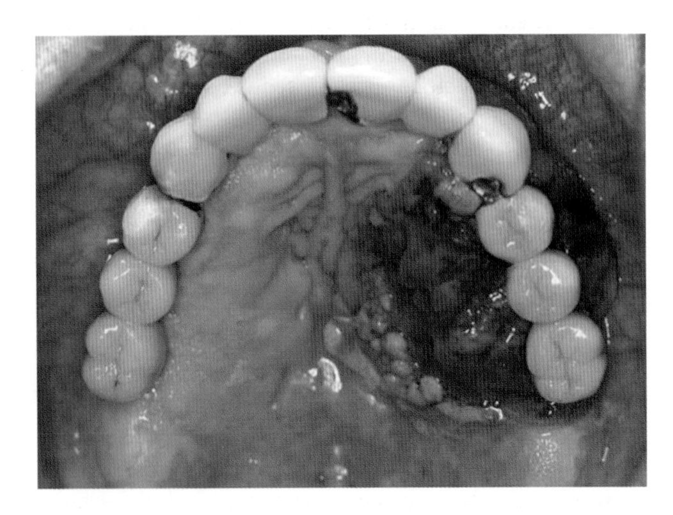

Figure 22.12 Intraoral view of squamous cell carcinoma of the hard palate.

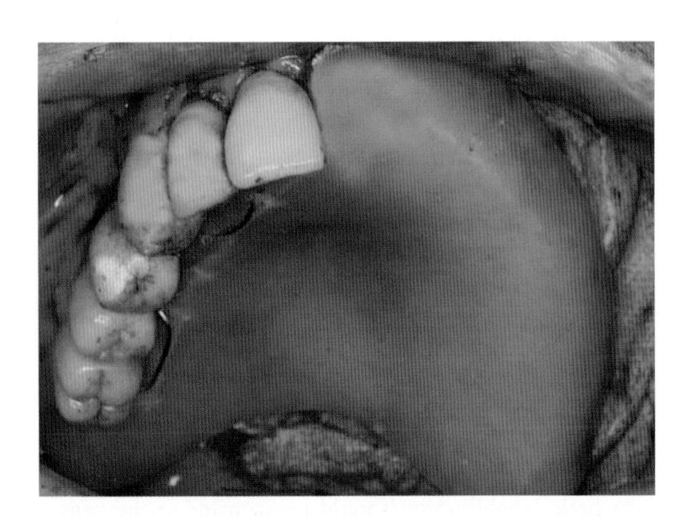

Figure 22.14 Surgical obturator placed in the oral cavity in the operating room following resection of the tumor.

The surgical obturator prosthesis may allow the patient to speak and swallow almost immediately after surgery and, in the interim, may alleviate the need for a nasogastric feeding tube. The prosthesis supports the packing used in the maxillectomy defect and maintains proper lip and cheek support during initial healing and thus increases resistance to the contracture and subsequent facial deformity due to scar tissue (15).

The surgical obturator is kept in place until the packing is ready to be removed in about 7–10 days after surgery and is replaced immediately with the interim obturator prosthesis (1). It is preferable to have the prosthodontist or the surgeon who placed the fixation device remove them as well as the packing. The prosthodontist and the patient are then both in the dental suit where the defect is debrided gently with moist gauze. It is very important to clean the defect and to keep the surgical site clean. The appliance and the cavity are cleaned thoroughly and then the appliance is adapted to the developing scar band using cold cure soft tissue conditioning material (2). The interim obturator prosthesis is modified as necessary to accommodate progressive change in the shape of the defect during the initial healing phase (Figure 22.15). A minimum of five to ten appointments may be needed to adjust and modify the prosthesis. The obturator portion of the prosthesis is fashioned with use of a soft lining material around the defect and as healing progresses and the configuration of the defect changes, the obturator is realigned every other week for the first 6–8 weeks after surgery (16).

Once healing is complete, usually about 4–6 months after surgery, a definitive obturator can be fabricated. Patients treated with postoperative radiation therapy may need to wait longer for the defect to stabilize. The definitive obturator should extend as high as possible along the lateral wall of the defect to provide maximal stability and retention. Routine care of the prosthesis requires that it be removed several times daily and cleaned with soap and water. In addition, excellent oral hygiene must be maintained for protection of the remaining teeth or implants (1).

In the partially dentate patient, the final appliance is frequently made of a combination of cast chrome–cobalt

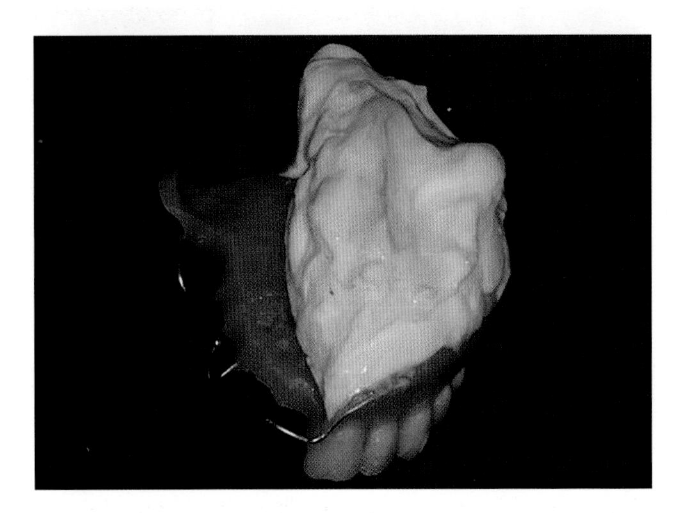

Figure 22.15 The interim obturator prosthesis.

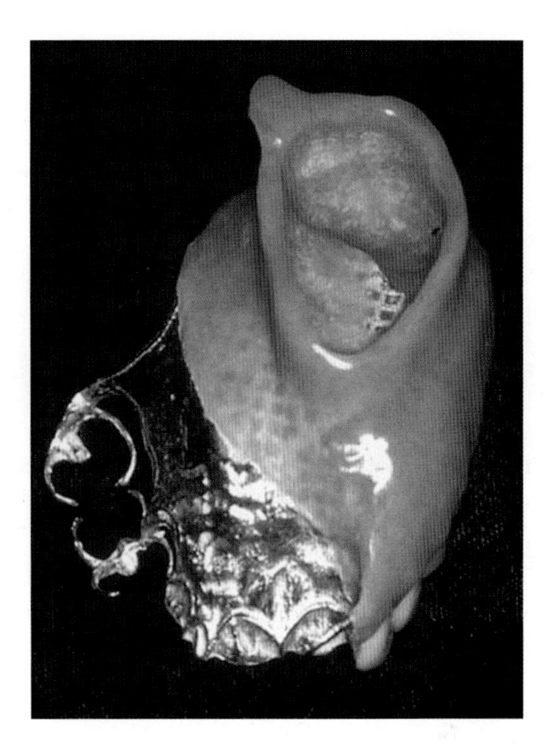

Figure 22.16 The permanent acrylic obturator prosthesis.

with cast wire clasps, rests, and an acrylic bulb with teeth of an appropriate shade and the soft tissue-colored denture acrylic base (Figure 22.16). The nasal aspect of the obturator bulb may be made hollow from above or be entirely hollow to lighten the weight of the appliance. If the entire nasal and sinus contents are removed at surgery, the bulb may be extended upwards to allow more normal-sounding speech. Occasionally, a two-part appliance may be fabricated with the upper portion fitted into the nasal sinus cavity and extended up to the orbital floor and the lower denture portion, which gets attached into this. The oral portion of the obturator should allow placement of the teeth in the prosthetic natural zone that is altered by surgery. Additionally, it should extend as far as possible for support, but should not cause alteration, nor interfere with normal occlusion or mastication. The oral surface should also be highly polished to allow the soft tissue to glide across them (2). This prosthesis maximizes esthetic appearance and function. The average lifespan of the definitive obturator prosthesis is 3–5 years and close follow-up is important to ensure an accurate fit (Figure 22.17) (17).

Soft palate

Restoration of function after resection of soft palate tumors resulting in velopharyngeal incompetence is one of the most challenging intraoral situations that confront maxillofacial prosthodontists (Figure 22.18). Surgical excision of a part or the entire soft palate alters normal palatopharyngeal closure, causing hyper-nasal speech and nasal regurgitation. A speech aid obturator allows palatopharyngeal closure in these patients by allowing the lateral and posterior walls of the nasopharynx to contract against the prosthesis (Figure

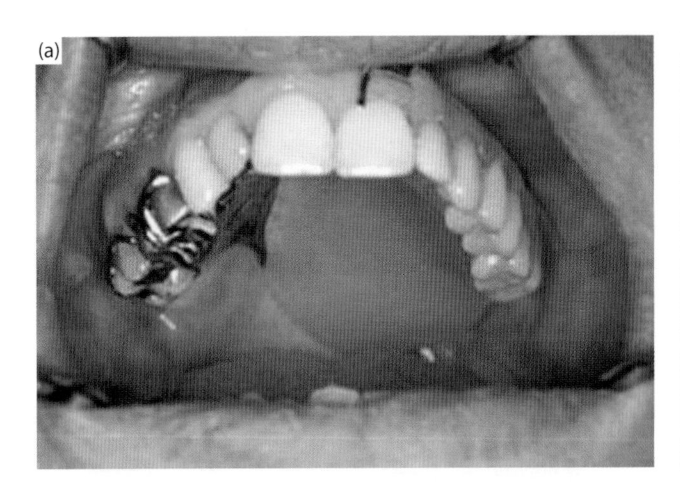

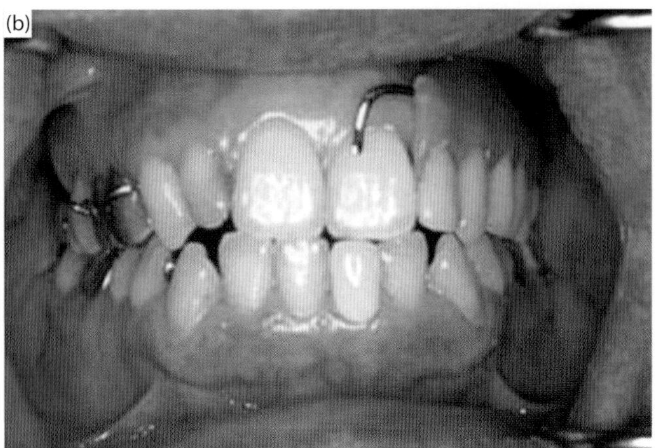

Figure 22.17 Permanent obturator prosthesis in a patient with partial maxillectomy showing (a) complete palatal closure and (b) excellent occlusion.

22.19). The obturator therefore must be sized appropriately to allow unimpeded nasal breathing and should not interfere with the tongue during swallowing and speech. The patient should be evaluated before surgery and an impression for a surgical obturator is obtained preoperatively (1). Removal of the soft palate allows easy access to the defect for fabrication of the prosthesis. Sometimes, preservation of a thin strip of soft palate becomes vitally important for prosthesis retention in patients with limited supporting tissue such as when a bilateral total maxillectomy has been done (18). However, when the remaining soft palate is non-functional, it should be completely removed. Primary radiation treatment of the soft palate may cause incompetency of the soft palate owing to fibrosis. In this situation, prosthetic rehabilitation may be impossible because of poor access to the oropharynx. In some cases, surgical removal of the soft palate may be required before prosthetic rehabilitation. Prosthetic rehabilitation may not restore the pretreatment function because of radiation-induced fibrosis in the muscles of the pharyngeal walls (19). Some soft palate defects are reconstructed laterally with a skin or myocutaneous flap. In such patients, the speech bulb must be placed posterior and superior to the flap in the nasopharynx. It is important to ensure that minimal contact occurs between the flap and the speech aid, which should be shaved and sized to allow the lateral and posterior pharyngeal musculature to contract around it (Figure 22.20) (1).

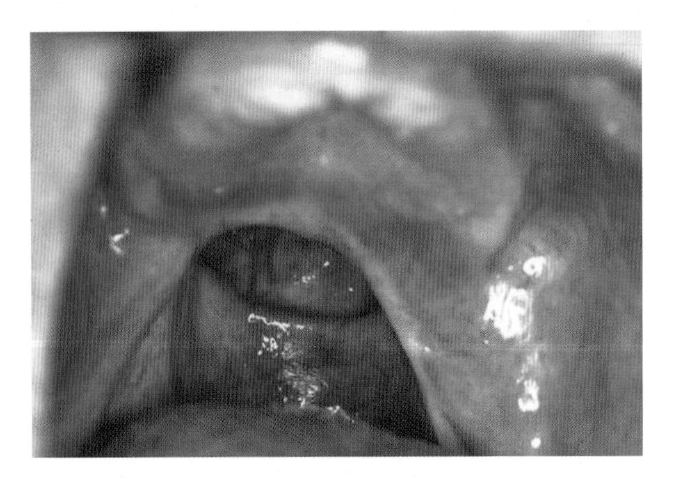

Figure 22.18 Intraoral view of the surgical defect following total resection of the soft palate in an edentulous patient.

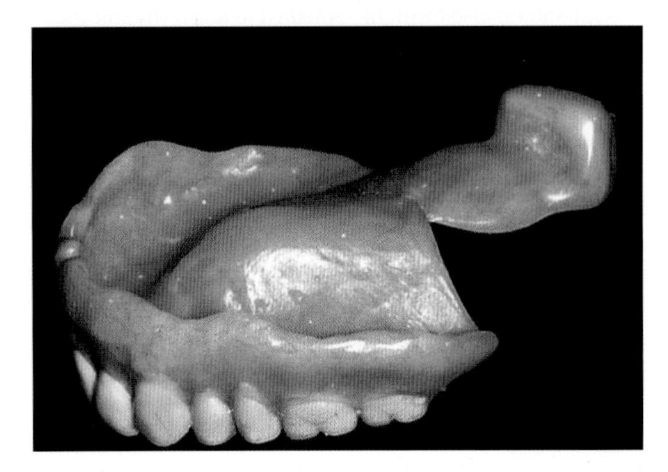

Figure 22.19 Speech bulb prosthesis attached to a full upper denture for rehabilitation of the soft palate defect.

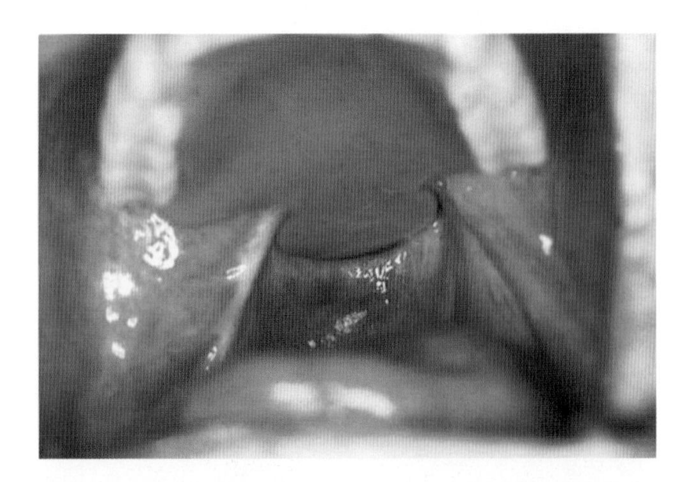

Figure 22.20 Upper dentures with speech bulb prosthesis in the oral cavity showing excellent apposition of the pharyngeal wall to the prosthesis.

Palatal augmentation prosthesis for defects of the tongue

Surgical resection of the tongue with significant loss of volume and/or mobility produces impairment of both speech and swallowing. With any loss of volume or limitation in range of motion, the tongue is unable to reach the hard palate to initiate the oral phase of deglutition. A palatal augmentation prosthesis is made to reduce the hollow of the arch of the hard palate to improve contact between the tongue and the palatal prosthesis during speech and swallowing (Figure 22.21) (20). A palatal augmentation prosthesis provides volume against which the dorsum of the remnant tongue can abut. An acrylic resin base is fabricated on the maxillary arch with an inferior extension that abuts against the dorsal surface of the tongue remnant or flap. The approximation of the remnant tongue against the surface of the prosthesis allows suction and provides improvement in and intelligibility of speech and better bolus transport and transit along with improvement in swallowing (Figure 22.22) (1).

The greatest improvement in function results when movement of the residual tongue remnant is retained. Replacing lost tissue bulk with a soft tissue flap may obliterate some of the space and allow retention of the mobility of the tongue. Patients with the greatest movement of the residual tongue benefit the most from the augmentation prosthesis and patients with a mobile tongue tip have the best speech function. The use of thin microvascular flaps for closure of the surgical site allows the residual innervated portion of the tongue to function with a minimal impairment of movement. Thus, the palatal augmentation prosthesis offers rehabilitation advantages to patients with impaired function of the tongue. The ultimate treatment goal is improvement in speech and swallowing, which may

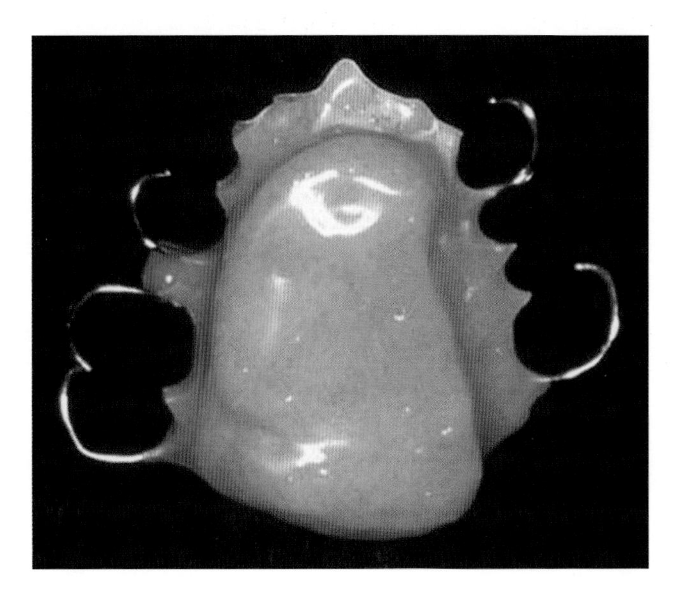

Figure 22.21 Palatal augmentation prosthesis.

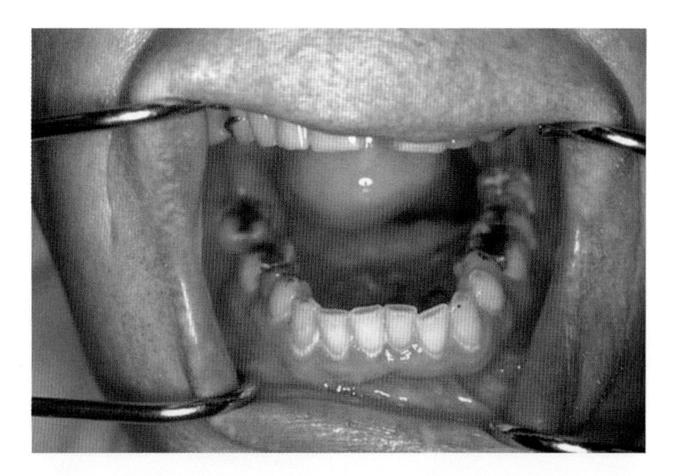

Figure 22.22 Palatal augmentation prosthesis in the oral cavity reducing the hollow of the palatal arch.

require the combination of soft tissue reconstruction and prosthetic support (20).

PROSTHETIC MANAGEMENT OF THE MANDIBLE

MANDIBULOTOMY

The mandibulotomy approach is used to gain access to the oral cavity and oropharynx for resection of large tumors not accessible through the open mouth and when the mandible is not involved by tumor. It is an alternative to a mandibular resection where there is no bony involvement or when excision of the primary tumor such as carcinoma of the base of the tongue requires excess not otherwise possible through the open mouth (21). During the course of the procedure, an osteotomy is made in the midline or in a paramedian location through either an edentulous area or an extraction socket. If a bone cut is made between two intact teeth, it is likely that both teeth may be lost in the postoperative period. If all teeth are present, then the osteotomy is made between the lateral incisor and canine tooth. The roots of these two teeth diverge, allowing for space to perform the mandibulotomy without injuring the sockets of these teeth. The distal ends of the right and left sides of the mandible are then retracted outwards, allowing a direct view of the posterior tongue and the oropharynx. During closure, the mandibulotomy site is realigned with miniplates and screws. Occasionally, in spite of such fixation, there is movement at the mandibulotomy site. In such instances, a mandibulotomy splint provides a buttress and offers rigid fixation. The splint is used to orient the teeth in three planes (coronal, axial and mediolateral) so that when the segments are realigned, the teeth and the temporomandibular joints are realigned in the same position they were prior to the splitting of the mandible. The preoperatively fabricated lingual splint may then be applied as an additional means of fixation and is removed at a later date (2). On occasion, sepsis develops around the screws and plates at the mandibulotomy site, requiring their removal, sometimes prior to satisfactory bone healing. In that setting, a lingual splint offers adequate immobilization at the mandibulotomy site until bony union is complete (Figures 22.23 through 22.25).

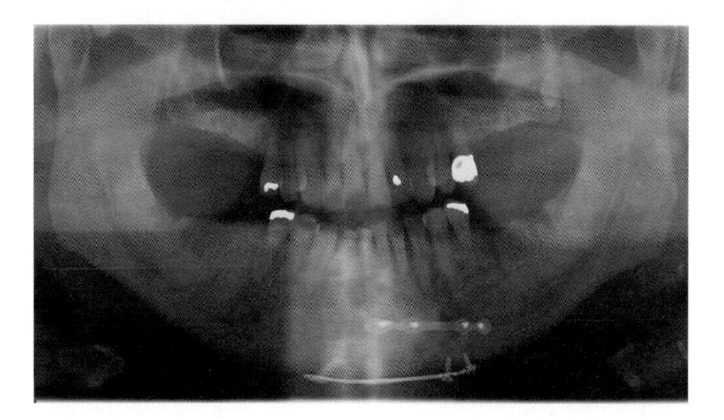

Figure 22.23 Orthopantomogram of a patient with sepsis at the mandibulotomy site showing bone loss and loose screws and plates.

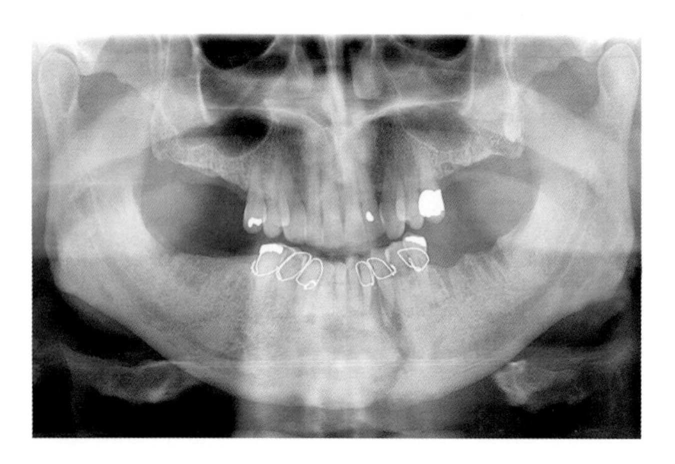

Figure 22.24 Orthopantomogram of the patient shown in Figure 22.23 showing a wired lingual splint at the site of mandibulotomy sepsis after removal of the screws and plates.

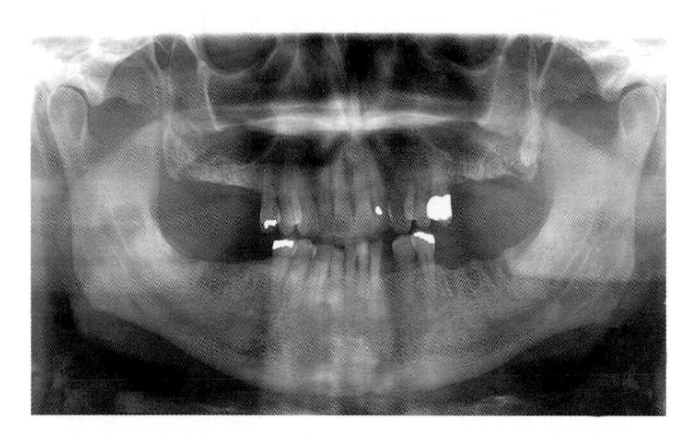

Figure 22.25 Orthopantomogram of the patient shown in Figure 22.24 after healing of the mandibulotomy site and removal of the lingual splint.

MANDIBLE RESECTION

Marginal mandibulectomy

Patients with uncomplicated marginal mandibulectomy may be treated using a variety of partial or complete lower dentures (Figure 22.26). Keeping in mind the triad of support, stability and retention, the surgeons should plan ahead to leave as much horizontal bony surface as possible for denture support. Stability can be improved by ensuring that the buccal and lingual sulci are not obliterated, but are kept as deep as possible. Obliteration of the buccal and lingual vestibular sulci is a prime cause for denying patients dental prosthetic rehabilitation. Retention is improved by ensuring that as many dental units are kept as possible and that they are well cared for (Figure 22.27). However, when marginal mandibulectomy is done followed by primary closure suturing the floor of the mouth mucosa to the buccal mucosa or a skin graft or a free flap, the lingual and buccal sulci are usually lost. Vestibuloplasty is a surgical

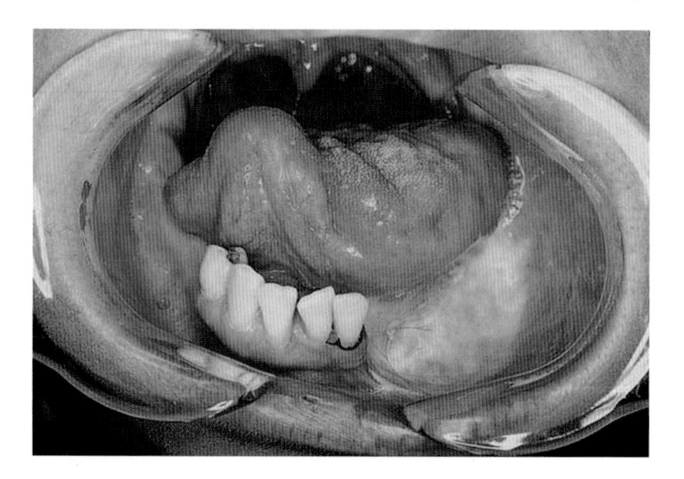

Figure 22.26 Intraoral view of a patient following marginal mandibulectomy and coverage with a skin graft.

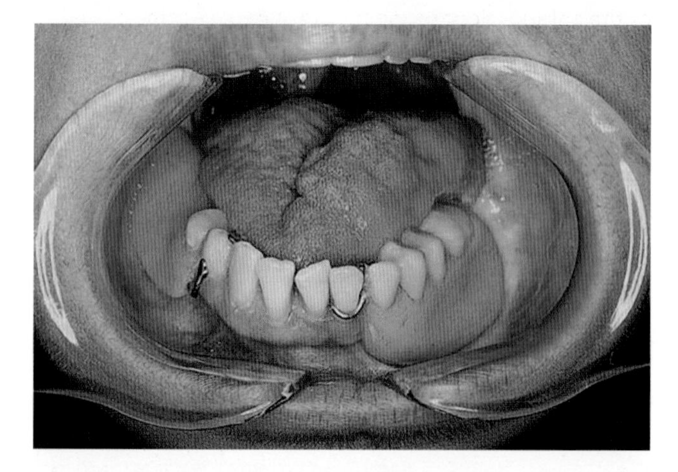

Figure 22.27 Intraoral view of the patient shown in Figure 22.26 with a removable partial denture clasped to the remaining teeth.

procedure designed to restore alveolar ridge support by reducing the attachment of muscles and soft tissues to the buccal, labial and lingual aspects of the jaw and trimming the existing tissues such as flaps used in the initial reconstruction. Split-thickness skin grafts are important because they provide a sound tissue base for the prosthesis and also can be used to separate the floor of the mouth from the buccal mucosa (22). When the tongue is sutured to the buccal or labial mucosa, prosthetic rehabilitation is limited if not impossible.

When a marginal mandibulectomy is performed in the body of the mandible, usually there is not sufficient vertical height to perform implants. However, if the marginal mandibulectomy is performed at the anterior aspect of the mandible (from canine to canine), then implants are possible (Figure 22.28). As stated before, a skin graft or mucosal lining coverage is ideal for implant placement. The implants are planned based on imaging studies of the mandible and a guided plane is fabricated (Figure 22.29). A computer model is developed for proper angulation of the implants for optimal occlusion (Figure 22.30). The implants are allowed to heal for several months. Following exposure of the implants, a fixed or removable denture can be fabricated (Figures 22.31 and 22.32).

Patients with partial mandibulectomy and rigid fixation with a plate may also be rehabilitated using variations of removable partial or full dentures if adequate support, stability and retention are present postoperatively (20).

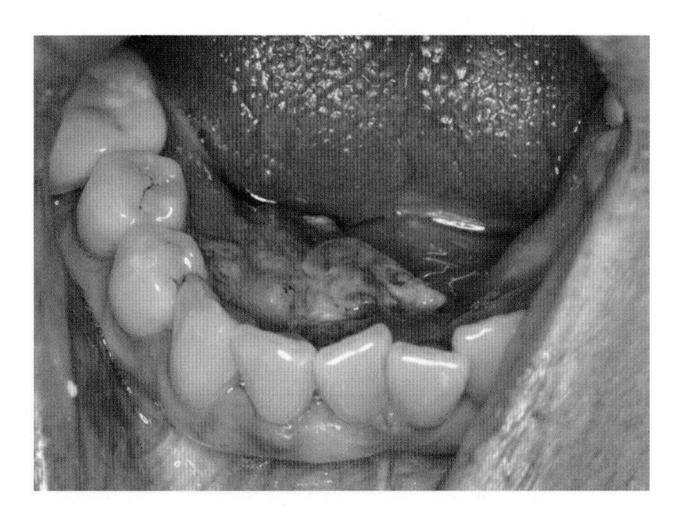

Figure 22.28 Intraoral view of a patient with carcinoma of the anterior floor of the mouth suitable for marginal mandibulectomy and subsequent dental implants for rehabilitation.

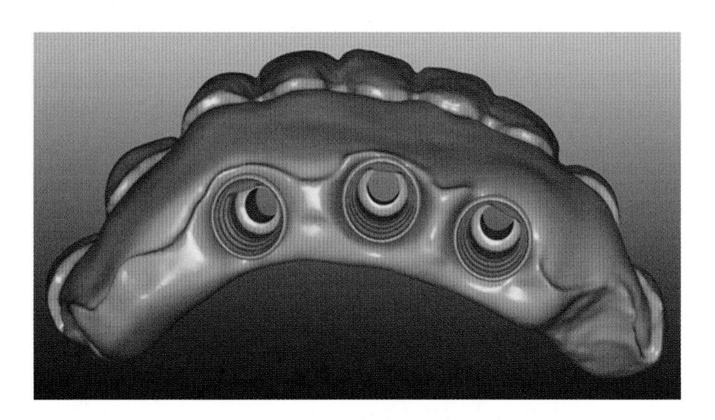

Figure 22.29 Guide plane for placement of implants.

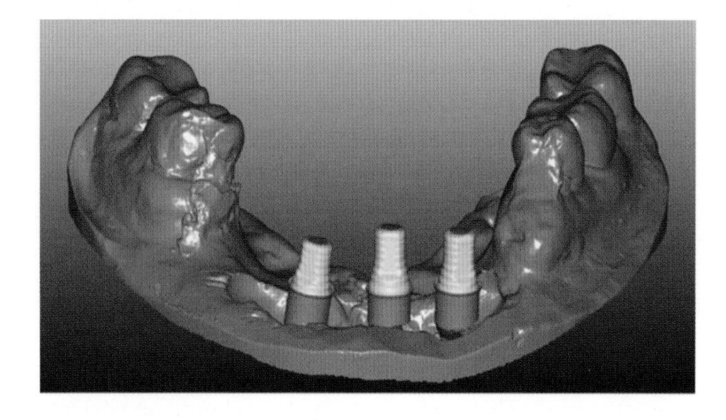

Figure 22.30 Computer model for placement and angulation of the implants.

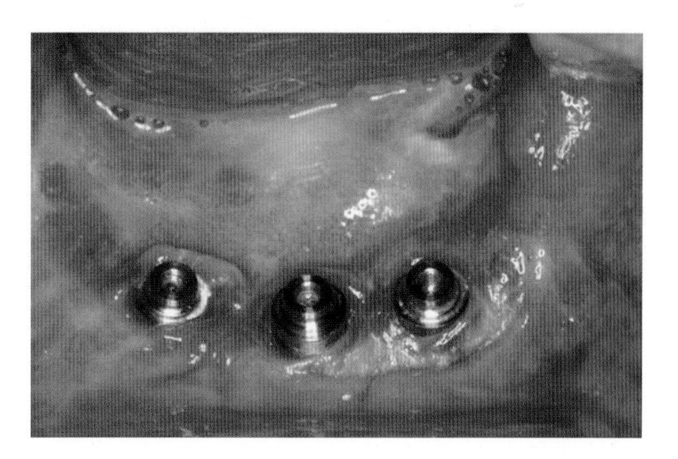

Figure 22.31 Exposed implants after satisfactory healing.

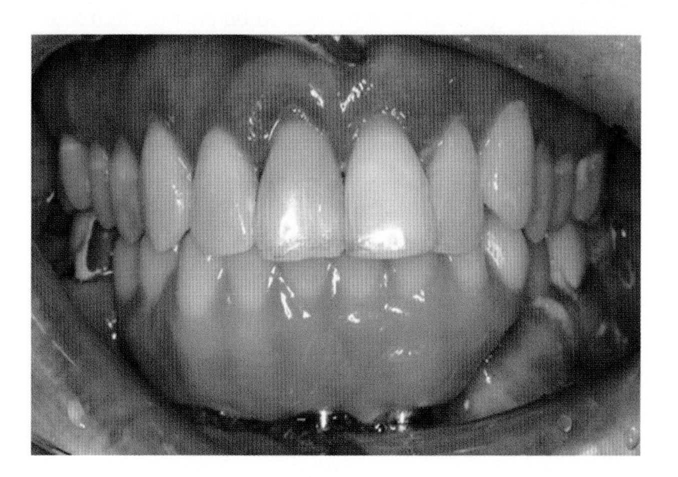

Figure 22.32 Implant-based removable denture in good occlusion.

Segmental mandibulectomy

After segmental resection, the non-reconstructed remnant mandible undergoes medial and upwards deviation and causes a deformity that can result in significant functional and cosmetic debility. This occurs due to unopposed traction by the contralateral pterygoid muscles, causing medial and posterior displacement. This deformity causes severe malocclusion and also esthetic deformity. Therefore, nearly all patients undergo some form of bone reconstruction after a segmental mandibulectomy. However, if for any reason the mandible continuity is not restored, then measures should be undertaken to reduce mandibular deviation to a minimum (1). In general, mandibular appliances are less well tolerated compared to maxillary prostheses. This is due to constant motion of the tongue and paramandibular muscular attachments, which makes prosthetic retention of the lower jaw a functional challenge.

A mandibular guide plane prosthesis may be used for patients who retain dentition in their remnant mandible and maxilla after segmental mandibulectomy and no reconstruction. This appliance can be used only on patients who have healthy dentition with adequate bony support to withstand diagonal forces. As the guide flanges engage, the mandible is directed to the appropriate intercuspal position during closure of the mouth. Definitive mandible guidance appliances are used when healing is complete and therefore the use may be delayed for several months for patients that undergo postoperative radiation therapy. In current practice, however, the rehabilitation of a patient undergoing segmental mandibulectomy is immediate reconstruction with an osseous or osteocutaneous free flap with dental reconstruction using osseointegrated implants (1).

IMPLANT REHABILITATION AFTER MANDIBLE RECONSTRUCTION

Microvascular free tissue transfer for surgical reconstruction has revolutionized repair of the deficits from ablative surgery of large tumors. If bone is to be part of the reconstructive effort, then a method of fixation to ensure the flap's stability is required until bony union occurs. Composite free flaps from the fibula, iliac crest and scapula are designed and harvested to address tissue volumetric loss, restore mandible continuity, separate oral from sinonasal cavities and provide a platform for fixture placement (23–26). Vascularized bone free flaps (VBFFs) from the fibula donor site provide excellent bone volume and the quality required by underlying bone for the application of osteointegration to prosthetic devices (27). Iliac crest free flaps can also support implants, but are not as good as the fibula. The VBFFs will either restore this continuity of the mandible or reproduce the stable base of the maxilla (28).

The decision to use fixed dental prosthesis versus removable dental prosthesis is dependent on clinical factors such as bone ability, the number of positions of implants, the need to assist or support restorations, hygiene maintenance and manual dexterity. Aside from these clinical factors, other considerations such as comfort and psychosocial implications affect prosthetic design. Fixed dental prosthetic restorations are associated with superior chewing performance and esthetics while causing less psychological discomfort and disability than removable counterparts. Fixed dental prosthetic restorations are usually screw retained and the prosthesis is retrievable. This design consideration is an important factor in cases in which direct revisualization of tissue is necessary. Implant surgery is performed once bony union of the vascular bone free flap osteotomies is established (29). Ideally, implant surgery should be performed with a transmucosal approach or within the incision to visualize the osteotomy site. Implant position favors abutment screw access either on the occlusal or lingual surface for esthetic conventional screw-retained fixed dental prosthesis. Incorporating an immediately loaded restoration at implant surgery is dependent on patient selection, prosthodontic design consideration and improvement in the implant position from computer design planning. Three-dimensional simulations/software provide the panoramic, axial and trans-sagittal plans to perform accurate implant placement with selected diameter and length according to bone availability. The implants are positioned to take advantage of the best bone stalk to avoid small structures and to ensure safety. The angulation of the fixtures is such that the screw access is confined to the occlusal surface rather than perforating a static facial surface, which is desirable for a screw-retained restoration (28).

Use of the fibula and the iliac crest can present a geometric challenge for prosthetic reconstruction. The fibula is usually positioned to reproduce the contour of the lower border of the mandible. This may lead to an intraoral height discrepancy with the native mandible. In addition, the dental arch lies on the lingual side above the reconstruction such that implants placed would be positioned on the facial side of the dental arch and the occlusal plane. There are surgical techniques to overcome the height discrepancy. One option is to position the fibula higher and use the construction plating system to reproduce the contour or the inferior border. The other option is the double-barrel technique in which the fibula is folded to increase the height of the fibula free flap (30). Thus, with fibula free flap mandible reconstruction, the orientation of the implant may be difficult owing to the height discrepancy of the native mandible and the lingual portion of the dental arch in relation to the inferior border of the mandible. However, resolving these factors does not solely rely on computer-assisted planning. The use of a supra-structure framework is necessary in time to overcome the severe height discrepancy of the mandible reconstruction with a fibula free flap.

When planning reconstruction of the complete dental arch with osseointegrated implants, a minimum of five or six implants is recommended. For unilateral defects, three to four implants are necessary. If the defect crosses the midline, more implants are necessary to support the replaced dental arch. Technical details and the process of selection of patients, as well as the technique of placement of implants and fabrication of removable or permanent implant-based dentition, are specialties in themselves and are beyond the scope of this book.

FACIAL PROSTHETICS

The defects of the face present special challenges for both the reconstructive surgeon and the maxillofacial prosthodontist. Reconstructive efforts for substantial facial defects are limited by the qualities of donor tissues such as texture, color and pliability. The efforts of the maxillofacial prosthodontist, on the other hand, are limited by the mobility of the tissue bed in the face, which causes problems with regard to the retention of prosthesis and the difficulty in matching the permanence and the feel and texture of replaced tissue (1). In general, a successful prosthesis is esthetically pleasing, retentive and tissue compatible. The prosthesis should be simple in design so that the patient can place and remove it easily. Material used in constructing facial prosthesis should be easy to clean, color stable, resistant to bacterial and fungal growth, durable and well tolerated by tissues (20). When prosthetic restoration of a facial defect is planned, pre-surgical photographs, digital images or laser scans are required. Irreversible hydrocolloid, vinyl polysiloxane or plaster is used to obtain an accurate impression of the patient's face or a medical model is produced from the digital data. The contours of the missing anatomy are then sculpted in a wax or clay model on the cast. Appropriate contouring, coloring and placement of margins are some of the many considerations that contribute to a successful outcome (1). Alternatively, the prosthesis can be designed using software and then "printed" in different materials, leading to fabrication of the prosthesis. This method then allows for rapid reproduction and alterations for future patient needs. The two materials that meet these criteria most are methyl methacrylate (plastic) and medical-grade silicones. An extraoral prosthesis may be combined with an intraoral prosthesis to enhance retention and esthetics (20).

An example of a composite defect following resection of the premaxilla, nose and upper lip, creating a complex three-dimensional defect, is shown in a patient in Figures 22.33 and 22.34. A two-component design for an intraoral obturator and external nasal prosthesis is created with magnets for retention (Figure 22.35). When used simultaneously, excellent dental and facial rehabilitation is accomplished (Figure 22.36).

Another factor that determines whether a prosthesis is utilized is its ease of placement and retention. A variety of retention techniques have been used. Lack of retention contributing to poor patient compliance or acceptance of a facial prosthesis and can be overcome with skin adhesive, design of the prosthesis into undercuts and mechanical means (attachments to glasses, straps and cranial facial implants with clips or magnets). Decisions regarding the selection of the type of retention technique are made on the basis of the complexity of the prosthesis, hygiene, type of skin, daily activity, dexterity of the patient and other handicaps such as blindness

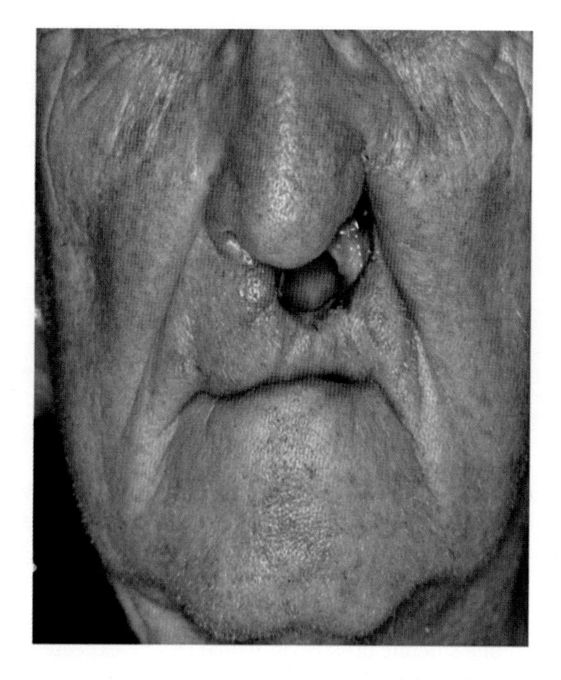

Figure 22.33 External appearance of a patient with a composite defect of the upper lip, nose and palate.

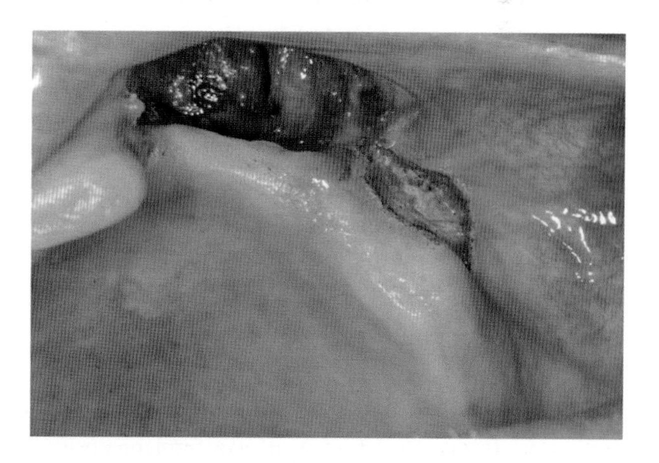

Figure 22.34 Intraoral view of the patient shown in Figure 22.33 demonstrating a through-and-through defect between the oral cavity and nose.

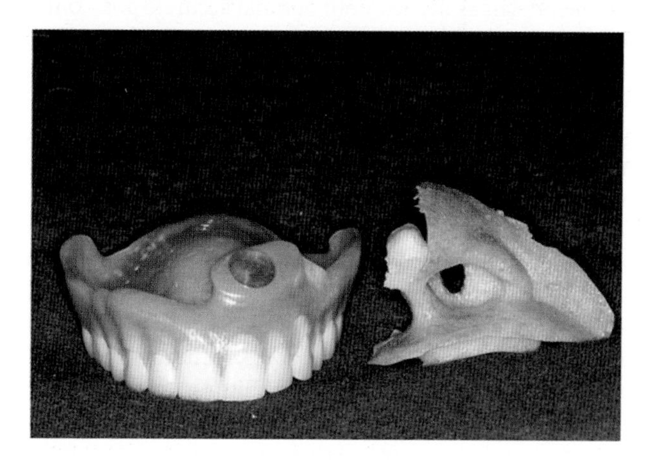

Figure 22.35 Dental obturator and nasal prosthesis with magnets for retention.

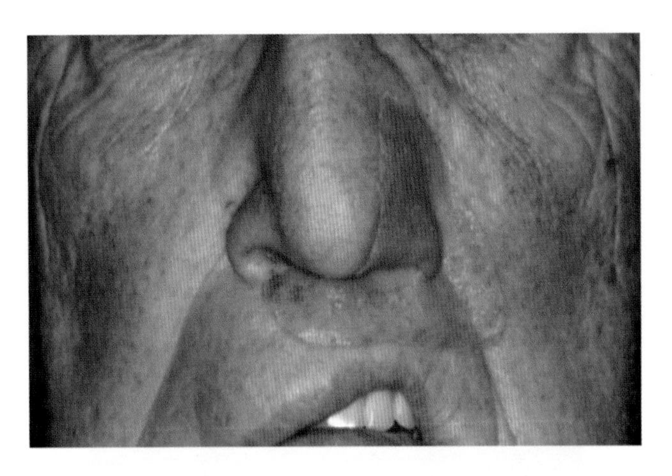

Figure 22.36 External appearance of the patient shown in Figure 22.33 with the intraoral and external prostheses in place.

or missing appendages. Prosthesis hygiene is crucial to the lifespan of a silicone prosthesis, which can be expected to be 12–24 months. Evaluation of these patients on a semi-annual basis ensures that instruction of prosthesis maintenance is re-enforced and adjustments such as additional tinting for continued color match are undertaken (1).

A stable and consistent prosthetic attachment is crucial to the successful rehabilitation of the patient who undergoes maxillofacial surgery. For the anaplastologist or practitioner who is designing and fabricating the prosthesis, implementing cranial implants can significantly help with meeting the needs of the patient (31).

The maxillofacial prosthodontist and the anaplastologist can assess the thickness of the soft tissue and guide the surgical team in locating implant abutments for the prosthetic framework. The surgical team can plan implant positions that best comply with surgical and the prosthetic principles. The team can preoperatively position implants, evaluate elongation of the trajectory, select final abutments and modify the treatment plan as needed until optimal accurate positioning for the support of the maxillofacial prosthesis is obtained.

There are several means of retention used in the maxillofacial prosthesis. Among the choices are adhesives, eyeglasses retention, magnet implants and combinations of these methods. The adhesives require patients to apply them to the prosthesis periphery at each time of usage. Some patients are uncomfortable with this and some develop an allergic reaction to the adhesive. Those patients who do not wear eyeglasses may not prefer the option of having to wear them. Although the implant is the newest option available, the availability of bone in the defect region is necessary (32). The magnet attachment is an attractive option that permits easy multiple prosthesis insertions and removals of its parts, making it more advantageous in cases such as a mid-face defect.

In addition, the lifespan of an implant-retained prosthesis is much longer than those requiring adhesives because of the wear and tear associated with the adhesive removal process. When the surgically placed, implant-retained prosthesis is chosen, the bar and cleft versus magnetic attachment options should be decided intraoperatively. This decision will determine how many exposed implants are needed. However, it has been shown that the gold bar arrangements prove to be more difficult for many patients to clean than the free-standing abutments for magnetic attachment. The magnetic attachment requires very little manual dexterity.

Implant-retained prosthesis offers several advantages over more traditional prosthetic techniques. Cranial implants provide secure attachment of the prosthesis that obviates the need for adhesives, double-sided tape, glasses or other more traditional fixation methods that give suboptimal prosthetic stability. Cranial implants enhance the patient's quality of life *via* improved self-image, greater activity level due to superior retention and ease of prosthetic management. Traditional adhesives have several disadvantages such as discoloration of the prosthesis, skin reactions (especially in irritated areas) and poor performance during movements of facial muscles or perspiration. Another significant advantage of cranial implantation is that the technique avoids distortion of tissues inherent in traditional surgical reconstruction, which allows for superior tumor surveillance. It has been suggested that, despite difficulty with osseointegration in irradiated bone, cranial implants may have an advantage in the irradiated patient who has poor-quality soft tissue available for reconstruction. Several disadvantages to prosthetic reconstruction exist, including the necessity of prosthetic or implant maintenance because of normal wear and tear, discoloration and, depending on the level of the patient's activity, the prosthesis may be dislodged at inopportune times, such as during social or athletic events. Some patients may have adverse psychological effects due to prosthesis-related problems.

EXTERNAL EAR DEFECT

Partial or total amputation of the pinna (external ear) is very difficult to accurately reconstruct surgically. On the other hand, it is an ideal situation for prosthetic replacement. The patient shown in Figure 22.37 has undergone complete amputation of the right external ear. Three implants in the mastoid process of the temporal bone have been placed and exposed. Magnets have been anchored to the implants. A full ear prosthesis is fabricated, with accurate color match (Figure 22.38). On the back of the prosthesis, magnets are embedded to align with the implants (Figure 22.39). The prosthesis is applied and retained with the magnets (Figure 22.40).

ORBITAL DEFECT

If the bone structures of the orbit are left intact, then a split-thickness skin graft can be placed in the orbital defect to allow a prosthesis contact with tissue at the depth of the defect (Figures 22.41 and 22.42). When the orbital contents

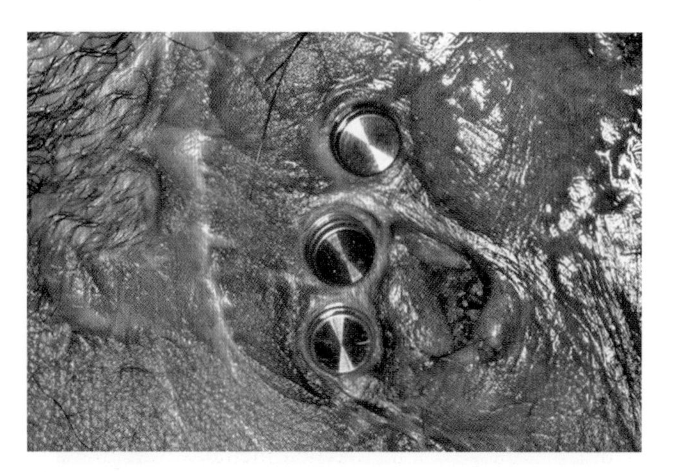

Figure 22.37 Implants in the mastoid process for retention of a total external ear prosthesis with anchored magnets.

are removed in conjunction with maxillary resection, reconstruction of the infraorbital rim improves the facial contour and enhances prosthetic rehabilitation. This reconstruction can be accomplished by using free tissue transfer with bone. Because of the osseous anatomy of the orbit, orbital implants must be placed radially within the orbital rim to provide adequate bone thickness for retention. Generally, implant placement within the lateral rim is recommended because of the increased thickness of the bone in this region. The medial orbit can be problematic in most cases secondary to a lack of adequate bone thickness and increased anatomic complexity due to the lacrimal fossa. Placement of two to three implants is generally adequate for support of the substructure and the orbital prosthesis. The preferred site is the lateral supraorbital rim if it has not been resected; however, implants may be placed in the residual periorbital bony rim as well. A special consideration for treatment planning of

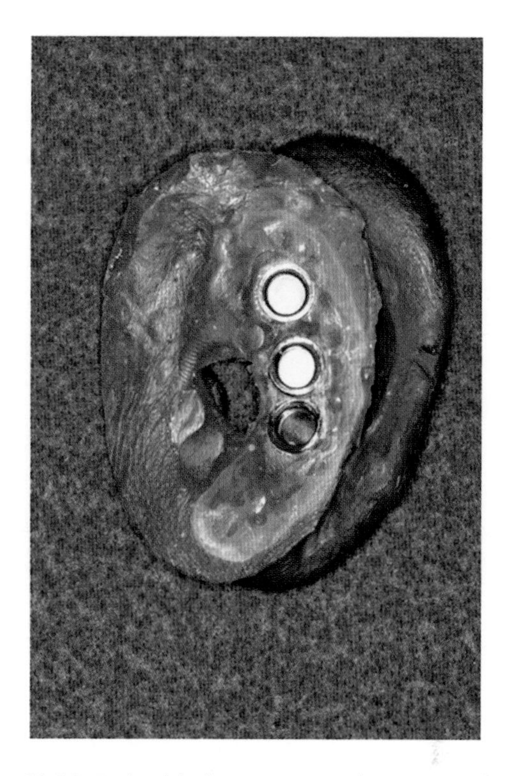

Figure 22.39 Embedded magnets on the inner surface of the prosthesis.

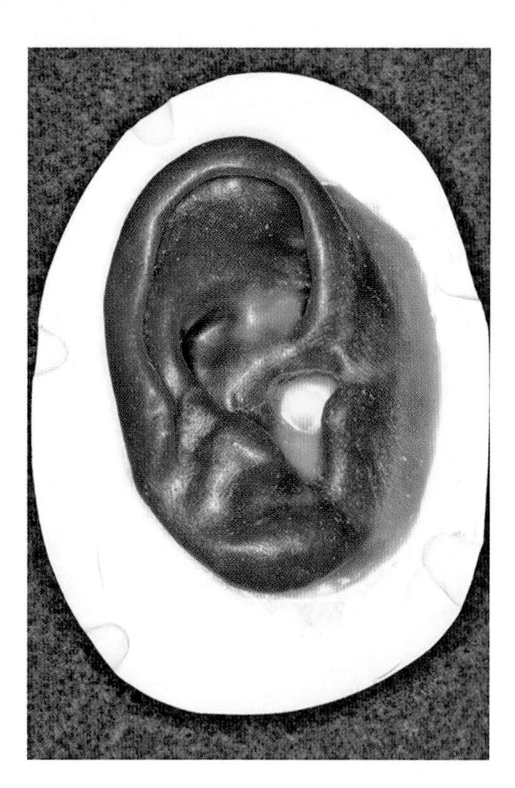

Figure 22.38 Surface view of a total external ear prosthesis.

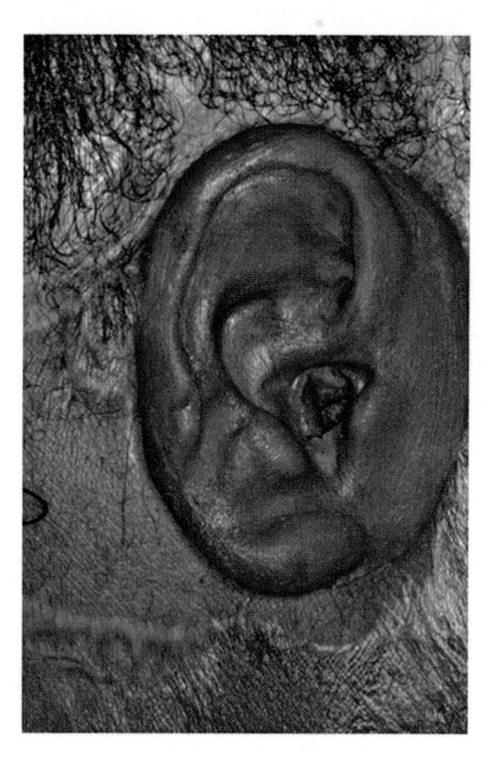

Figure 22.40 Total ear prosthesis in place, retained by magnets.

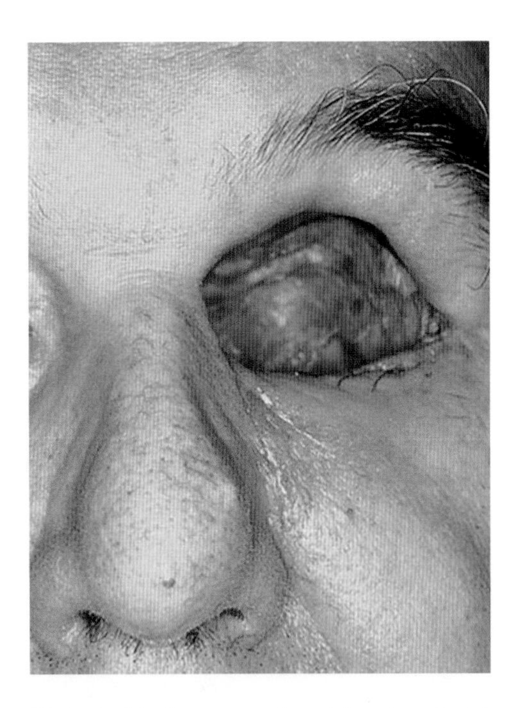

Figure 22.41 Orbital exenteration defect lined with a skin graft.

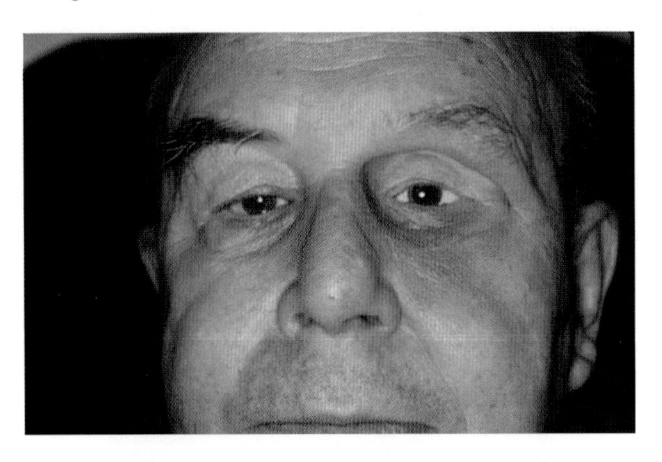

Figure 22.42 Orbital prosthesis retained in the orbital socket with glue in the patient shown in Figure 22.41.

the orbital prosthesis is the available depth of the orbital defect. Virtual planning of the implant is performed and the orbital depth is established intraoperatively by debulking the orbital contents. Computer-guided treatment planning allows positioning of the implants in an appropriate bony volume in concert with the proper trajectory of reconstruction of the maxillofacial prosthesis.

NASAL DEFECTS

Patients who undergo partial or total rhinectomy can be adequately rehabilitated using a removable prosthesis. A split-thickness skin graft should be placed in the defect to stabilize the borders of the defect and to maintain a normal lift position. The prosthesis can be attached using adhesive over the skin. These are usually for partial nasal defects (Figures 22.43 and 22.44). For patients who undergo near-total rhinectomy

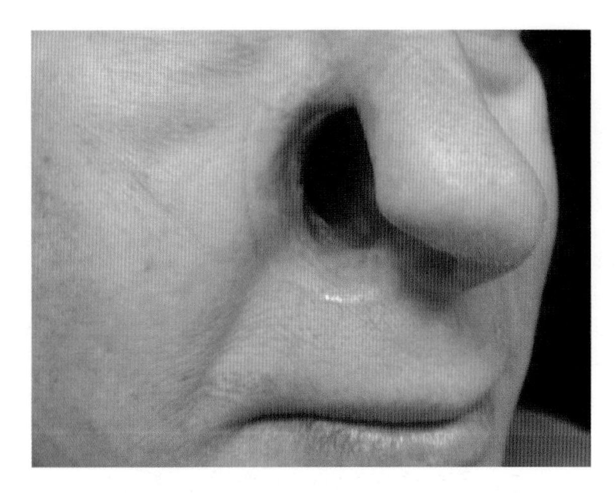

Figure 22.43 A patient with partial resection of the lower half of the nose.

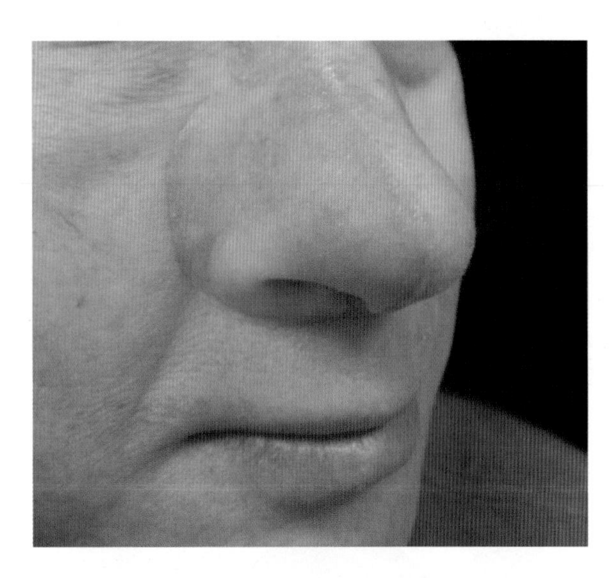

Figure 22.44 External prosthesis retained with glue on the patient shown in Figure 22.43.

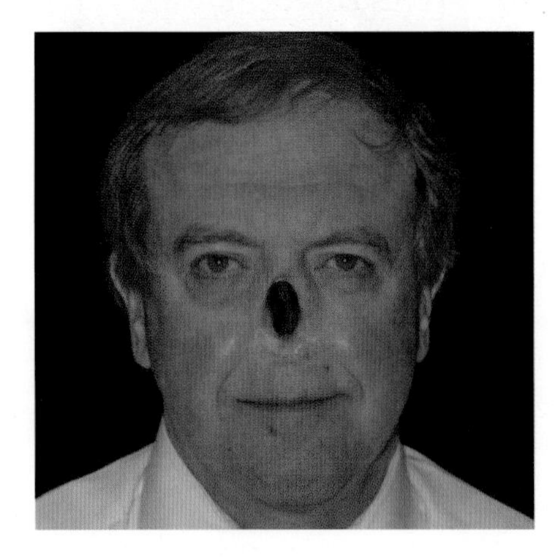

Figure 22.45 A patient with a partial rhinectomy defect lined with a split-thickness skin graft.

but in whom nasal bones are retained, a full nose prosthesis can be fabricated that will be retained with glue and eyeglasses (Figures 22.45 and 22.46). For patients undergoing total rhinectomy, it is especially important that the inferior border of the nasal defect be fixated. Placement of implants in the nasal region can be technically challenging because of the poor quality of bone. The available bone volumes that can support the implants are in the premaxilla and the frontal region. Placing two implants through the nasal floor at positions corresponding with the dental positions of teeth #7 and #10 is recommended. Vital structures, including the tooth sockets and nasopalatine canals, must be avoided during implant placement. The use of maxillofacial planning software allows visualization for avoiding such vital structures. Esthetic aspects of the final prosthesis must also be considered. The implants must be placed slightly within the nasal cavity to engage adequately with the bone and to provide satisfactory prosthetic thickness. After a 3–4-month osseointegration period, the implants are exposed and the prosthesis can be applied (Figures 22.47 and 22.48) (21).

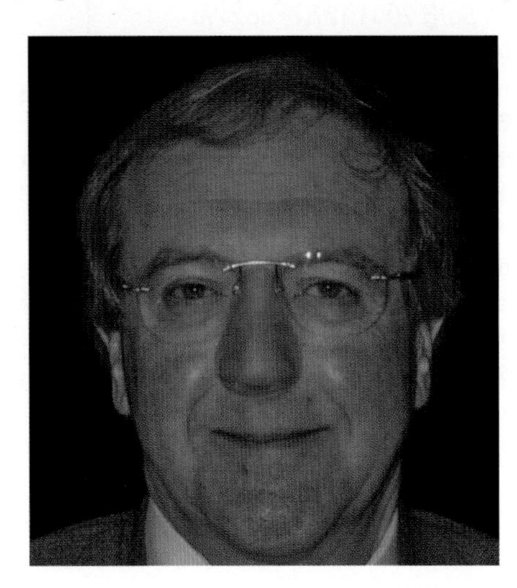

Figure 22.46 Nasal prosthesis retained with glue and eyeglasses on the patient shown in Figure 22.45.

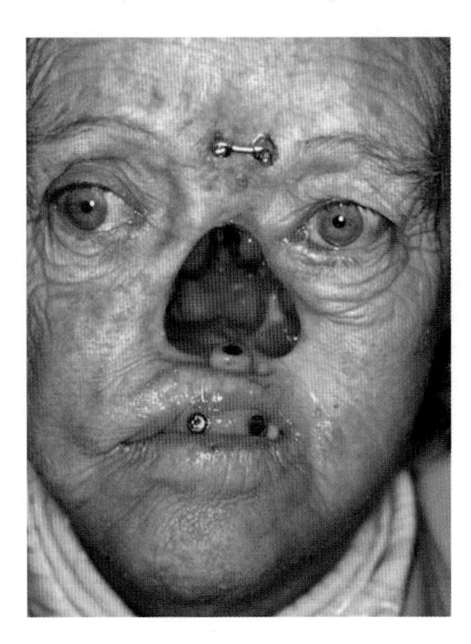

Figure 22.47 A patient with total rhinectomy, bilateral medial maxillectomies with resection of the hard palate and upper lip, rehabilitated with a double prosthesis to replace the hard palate and upper lip, with embedded magnets to support the nasal prosthesis. Note the placement of implants in the frontal bone for retention of the upper end of the nasal prosthesis.

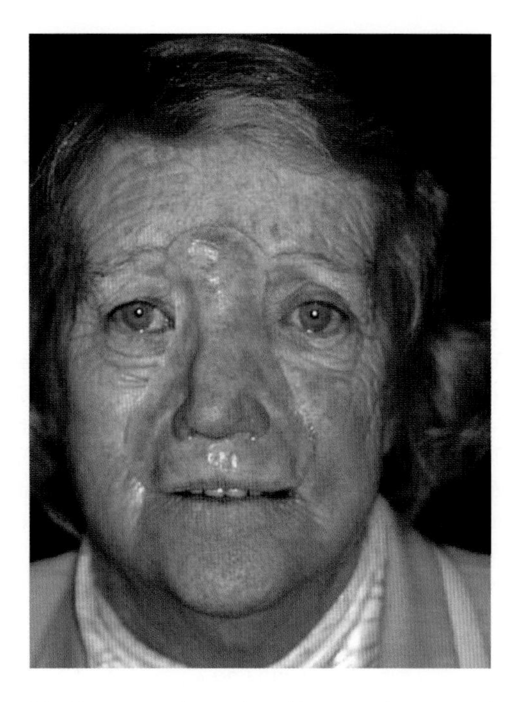

Figure 22.48 External nasal and lip prosthesis applied and retained with implants in the forehead and magnets in the palatal prosthesis of patient shown in Figure 22.47.

REFERENCES

1. Bohle GC, Huryn JM. Oncologic dentistry, maxillofacial prosthetics and Implants. In: Shah J, Patel S, Singh B, (eds). *Jatin Shah's Head and Neck Surgery and Oncology*. Philadelphia: Elsevier. 2012, 752–71.
2. Wood RE. Dental management of the head and neck patient. In: *Principles and Practice of Head and Neck Surgery and Oncology*, Montgomery, P. Q., Rhys Evans PH, Gullane PJ (Eds), (2nd Edition), CRC Press, Boca Raton, Florida, 2009, 139–50.
3. Lingeman RE, Singer MJ. Evaluation of the patient with head and neck cancer. In: Sven JY, Myers EN, (eds). *Cancer of the Head and Neck*. New York: Churchill Livingstone, 1981, 15.
4. Fleming TJ. Oral tissue changes of radiation-oncology and their management. *Dent Clin North Am* 1990;34(2):223–37.
5. Sonis S, Clark J. Prevention and management of oral mucositis induced by antineoplastic therapy. *Oncology (Williston Park)* 1991;5(12):11–8. discussion 18–22

6. Borowski B et al. Prevention of oral mucositis in patients treated with high-dose chemotherapy and bone marrow transplantation: a randomised controlled trial comparing two protocols of dental care. *Eur J Cancer B Oral Oncol* 1994;30(2):93–7.
7. Chambers MS et al. Oral and dental management of the cancer patient: prevention and treatment of complications. *Support Care Cancer* 1995;3(3):168–75.
8. Toth BB et al. Oral candidiasis: a morbid sequela of anticancer therapy. *Tex Dent J* 1998;115(6):24–29.
9. Peterson DE. Dental care of the cancer patient. *Compend Contin Educ Dent* 1983;4(2):115–120.
10. Muzyka BC, Glick M. A review of oral fungal infections and appropriate therapy. *J Am Dent Assoc* 1995;126(1):63–72.
11. Annane D et al. Hyperbaric oxygen therapy for radionecrosis of the jaw: a randomized: placebo-controlled, double-blind trial from the ORN96 Study Group. *J Clin Oncol* 2004;22:4893–900.
12. Maxymiw WG et al. Postradiation dental extractions without hyperbaric oxygen. *Oral Surg Oral Med Oral Pathol* 1991;72(3):270–4.
13. Myers RA, Marx RE. Use of hyperbaric oxygen in postradiation head and neck surgery. *NCI Monogr* 1990;9:151–7.
14. Marunick MT et al. Prosthodontic rehabilitation of midfacial defects. *J Prosthet Dent* 1985;54(4):553–60.
15. Martin JW et al. Postoperative care of the maxillectomy patient. *ORL Head Neck Nurs* 1994;12(3):15–20.
16. King GE et al. Patient appointments during interim obturation: Is it cost-effective? *J Prosthodont* 1995;4(3):168–172.
17. Martin JW, Austin JR, King GE. Oral and facial restoration after reconstruction. In: Kroll S (ed). *Reconstructive Plastic Surgery for Cancer.* St. Louis: Mosby, 1996, 130–8.
18. Beumer J 3rd et al. Prosthetic restoration of oral defects secondary to surgical removal of oral neoplasms. *CDA J* 1982;10(3):47–54.
19. Conley SF et al. Identification and assessment of velopharyngeal inadequacy. *Am J Otolaryngol* 1997;18(1):38–46.
20. Martin JW, Chambers MS, Lemon JC. Dental oncology and maxillofacial prosthetics. In: Harrison LB, Sessions RB, Hong WK, (eds). *Head and Neck Cancer: A Multidisciplinary Approach.* Philadelphia: Lippincott Williams & Wilkins; 2004, 115–29.
21. Spiro RH et al. Mandibulotomy approach to oropharyngeal tumors. *Am J Surg* 1985;150(4):466–9.
22. Teichgraeber J et al. Skin grafts in intraoral reconstruction. A new stenting method. *Arch Otolaryngol* 1984;110(7):463–7.
23. Urken ML et al. The scapular osteofasciocutaneous flap: A 12-year experience. *Arch Otolaryngol Head Neck Surg* 2001;127(7):862–9.
24. Hidalgo DA. Fibula free flap: a new method of mandible reconstruction. *Plast Reconstr Surg* 1989;84(1):71–9.
25. Urken ML et al. Oromandibular reconstruction using microvascular composite flaps: report of 210 cases. *Arch Otolaryngol Head Neck Surg* 1998;124(1):46–55.
26. Genden EM et al. Iliac crest internal oblique osteomusculocutaneous free-flap reconstruction of the post-ablative palatomaxillary defect. *Arch Otolaryngol Head Neck Surg* 2001;127:854–61.
27. Frodel JL Jr et al. Osseointegrated implants: a comparative study of bone thickness in four vascularized bone flaps. *Plast Reconstr Surg* 1993;92(3):449–55. discussion 456–448.
28. Okay DJ et al. Computer-assisted implant rehabilitation of maxillomandibular defects reconstructed with vascularized bone free flaps. *JAMA Otolaryngol Head Neck Surg* 2013;139(4):371–81.
29. Odin G et al. Immediate functional loading of an implant-supported fixed prosthesis at the time of ablative surgery and mandibular reconstruction for squamous cell carcinoma. *J Oral Implantol* 2010;36(3):225–30.
30. Bahr W et al. Use of the "double barrel" free vascularized fibula in mandibular reconstruction. *J Oral Maxillofac Surg* 1998;56(1):38–44.
31. Sinn DP et al. Craniofacial implant surgery. *Oral Maxillofac Surg Clin North Am* 2011;23(2):321–35. vi–vii.
32. Beumer J, Curtis TA, Marunick MT. *Maxillofacial Rehabilitation: Prosthesis and Surgical Consideration* (1st Edition). St Louis: Ishiyaku Euro America Inc, 1996.

23

Prevention of oral and oropharyngeal cancer

NEWELL W. JOHNSON, MUSHFIQ HASSAN SHAIKH, NIGEL ALAN JOHN McMILLAN, PANKAJ CHATURVEDI, AND SAMAN WARNAKULASURIYA

Firstly, some definitions. Approaches to disease prevention are often classified at three levels:

- *Primary prevention* is the approach that concentrates on minimizing risk factors in the community with the intention of minimizing the number of cases of the disease that arise in that community, namely reducing the incidence of disease. If effective at an affordable cost, this is clearly the best approach in terms of both public and personal health gain. It is reasonable to regard efforts to improve population health and resistance to disease (e.g., by healthy eating and physical exercise) as another form of primary prevention.
- *Secondary prevention* refers to the detection of cases of the disease in question at an early stage in its natural history at which intervention is likely to lead to cure or to minimize morbidity and reduce eventual mortality. This is the category that encompasses *screening*. Screening is a complex area of science and the risks and benefits need careful evaluation in every situation. It is also reasonable to regard the prescription of dietary supplements, particularly antioxidants and some anti-inflammatory agents, as a form of secondary prevention.
- *Tertiary prevention* refers to interventions designed to reduce recurrence of disease after treatment or to minimize the morbidity arising from treatment. Some of the approaches discussed under secondary prevention have application to patients already affected by the disease(s) in question.

PRIMARY PREVENTION OF ORAL AND OROPHARYNGEAL CANCER

The major risk factors for the most common types of these cancers are well understood and are exhaustively analyzed in Chapter 2. Taken together, the effects of tobacco use, heavy alcohol consumption and poor diet probably explain over 80% of cases. The preventive approach is therefore clear and all healthcare professionals have an obligation and excellent opportunities to contribute (1). Major international and national agencies are currently very active in this area (2–4). Many of these documents can be downloaded from the Internet (Table 23.1).

Table 23.1 Sources of information on tobacco cessation programs

- Action on Smoking and Health (ASH)
  www.ash.org
- Agency for Healthcare Research and Quality, Clinical Practice Guideline: *Treating Tobacco Use and Dependence* and supplements
  https://www.surgeongeneral.gov/library/reports/50-years-of-progress/index.html
- American Cancer Society
  https://www.cancer.org/healthy/stay-away-from-tobacco/
- American Dental Association
  www.ada.org
- American Dental Education Association
  http://www.adea.org/
- American Heart Association
  http://www.heart.org/HEARTORG/
- American Lung Association
  http://www.lung.org/stop-smoking/
- American Medical Association
  https://www.ama-assn.org/ama-strengthens-anti-tobacco-policies-further-protect-youth
- Breed's guide Tobacco Activism Guide
  http://archive.tobacco.org/Resources/lbguide.html
- British Dental Association
  https://bda.org/
- Campaign for Tobacco-Free Kids
  https://www.tobaccofreekids.org/
- Canadian Council for Tobacco Control
  https://www.canada.ca/en/health-canada.html
- Framework Convention on Tobacco Control
  http://www.who.int/fctc/en/
- FDI World Dental Federation
  https://www.fdiworlddental.org/
- Food and Drug Administration
  https://www.fda.gov/TobaccoProducts/default.htm
- Framework Convention on Tobacco Control Alliance (FCA)
  front page http://www.fctc.org/
- Institute for Global Tobacco Control
  http://globaltobaccocontrol.org/
- Journal of Tobacco Control
  http://tobaccocontrol.bmj.com/
- Make smoking history
  http://makesmokinghistory.org/quit-now/
- National Cancer Institute
  www.cancer.gov
- National Cancer Institute—publications locator
  www.smokefree.gov
  www.cancer.gov/publications
- National Center for Tobacco-Free Kids
  www.tobaccofreekids.org
- National Center for Tobacco-Free Older Persons
  http://www.tcsg.org/tobacco.htm

(*Continued*)

Table 23.1 (*Continued*) Sources of information on tobacco cessation programs

- National Institute of Drug Abuse
  www.drugabuse.gov
- National Oral Health Promotion Clearing House
  https://www.adelaide.edu.au/arcpoh/oral-health-promotion/
- National Spit Tobacco Education Program (NSTEP)
  https://oralhealthamerica.org/
- Office on Smoking and Health, CDC
  https://www.cdc.gov/tobacco/
- Oral Health America Foundation
  www.oralhealthamerica.org
- Program Against Teen Chewing
  http://kidshealth.org/en/teens/smokeless.html
- Society for Research on Nicotine and Tobacco
  www.srnt.org
- Tar wars: from the American Academy of Family Physicians
  https://www.aafp.org/patient-care/public-health/tobacco-nicotine/tar-wars.html
- Tobacco Control Research Branch
  https://cancercontrol.cancer.gov/brp/tcrb/
- Union for International Cancer Control
  https://www.uicc.org/
- World Health Organization, Tobacco or Health Program
  http://www.who.int/tobacco/en/

Disease prevention or health promotion messages can be directed at whole communities, targeted at sectors of the population such as youth, prepared specifically for defined populations such as employees of a business or factory or delivered to individual "clients" such as dental patients or those attending a school, workplace, health center, antenatal clinic, physician's office, etc. There will be much common ground in the material suitable for these approaches. Dentists and doctors can obtain literature suitable for use in their offices or hospitals from many sources including, in many cases, national medical and dental associations and national health promotion and cancer prevention agencies. Much excellent material is available on the Internet by inserting simple terms like "oral cancer," "tobacco control" or "alcoholism" into one of the common search engines. A number of suggestions are given in Table 23.1.

DEATHS THROUGH TOBACCO USE

One of the most valuable critical but concise analyses of the role of tobacco in health and disease, and of the approaches to prevention, is that produced by the Department of Health for England (5). Global Factsheets are regularly updated (e.g., http://www.who.int/mediacentre/factsheets/fs339/en/).

Table 23.2 Major cause of death from smoking tobacco

- Cancers of the lung, bladder, pancreas, mouth, esophagus, pharynx and larynx
- Chronic obstructive pulmonary and other respiratory diseases
- Vascular diseases, including coronary artery and peripheral arterial diseases
- Peptic ulceration

Every 10 seconds, another person dies somewhere in the world as a result of tobacco use. According to Doll et al. (6), who used data from the long-term study on male British doctors, about half of all regular smokers will be killed by their habit. The major causes of such deaths are listed in Table 23.2. Thus, tobacco kills more than 7 million people each year, about half its users, over 6 million from direct tobacco use while around 890,000 are deaths of non-smokers exposed to second-hand smoke. This has been calculated to represent an average loss of life for all cigarette smokers of 8 years and, for those whose deaths are directly attributed to tobacco, of 16 years (7). Tobacco users who die prematurely deprive their families of income, raise the cost of healthcare and hinder economic development. Surely such financial costs outweigh income from taxes on tobacco!

> ...for every 1,000 20-year-old smokers it is estimated that one will be murdered, six will die in road accidents and 250 will die in middle age from smoking.

Because nearly 80% of the world's more than 1 billion smokers live in low- and middle-income countries, more than 300 million in China alone, the burden of tobacco-related illness and death is heaviest there. However, smoking rates are highest in Eastern Europe and the former Soviet republics (271–273). Data from interactive maps are available at http://www.telegraph.co.uk/travel/maps-and-graphics/world-according-to-tobacco-consumption/ and http://www.telegraph.co.uk/travel/maps-and-graphics/Countries-according-to-alcohol-consumption/. Eastern European countries dominate the smoking statistics. Montenegro, where 4,124.53 cigarettes are smoked per adult per year, heads the list. Among men in industrialized countries, smoking is estimated to be the cause of 40%–45% of all cancer deaths, 90%–95% of lung cancer deaths, over 85% of oral cancer deaths, 75% of chronic obstructive lung disease deaths and 35% of cardiovascular disease deaths in those aged 35–69 years. Thus, while oral and pharyngeal cancer figure prominently, prevention of lung cancer, other pulmonary diseases and cardiovascular diseases should be the starting point for anti-tobacco counseling.

The proportions of cancer deaths attributed to smoking in developing countries as a whole are lower, being about 21% for men and only 4% for women. However, these figures are rising, with the fall in global tobacco consumption in the West being matched by growth in developing countries. Indeed, of the vast majority of the estimated 1,100 million smokers in the world, some 800 million are in developing countries. When the use of oral smokeless tobacco (ST) is added to these figures and the deaths it contributes through oral, pharyngeal and esophageal cancer, the seriousness of the global epidemic

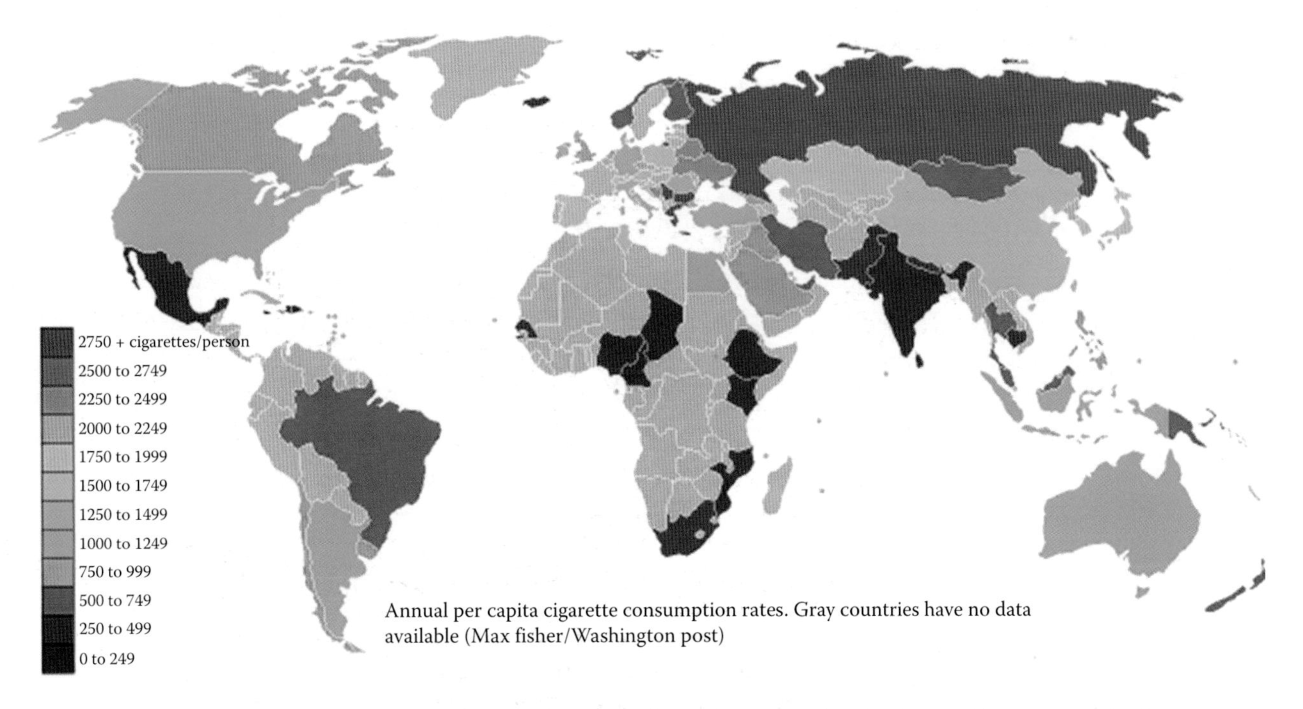

Figure 23.1 Annual per capita cigarette consumption. Note the serious situation in Eastern Europe and the former Soviet republics. Rates are general low in sub-Saharan Africa, most countries of which have generally low rates of oral and oropharyngeal cancer. https://www.washingtonpost.com/news/worldviews/wp/2012/10/19/who-smokes-most-a-surprising-map-of-smoking-rates-by-country/?utm_term=.6872b83f9e30

Table 23.3 A hierarchy of the cost-effectiveness of approaches to smoking cessation

- Imposition/raising of taxes
- Legislation against advertising and sponsorship
- Legislation for smoke-free areas in public places, transport, etc.
- Medical action: advice/intervention by healthcare professionals
- Education/health promotion at following levels:
  National
  State
  School
  Workplace, etc.
- Dedicated quitting group activities
- Dedicated individual quitting activities

Source: *Cost Effectiveness of Smoking Cessation Interventions.* London: Centre for Health Economics, University of York and Health Education Authority, 1997. https://cancercontrol.cancer.gov/brp/tcrb/monographs/21/docs/m21_9.pdf (9).

of tobacco-related diseases is even more staggering. We all share a responsibility to help quell this epidemic.

The World Health Organization (WHO) supplies extensive data on tobacco use and attempts at control around the globe (see Figure 23.1). The original World Tobacco Atlas produced in 2002 by the WHO is now produced and updated by the American Cancer Society and the World Lung Foundation, as well as an interactive version available at http://www.tobaccoatlas.org/.

There is a good deal of scientific evidence on the cost-effectiveness of approaches to tobacco (principally smoking) prevention/intervention. Table 23.3 ranks these: individual action by doctors and dentists is clearly important. The effectiveness of brief individual action by doctors and dentists is strikingly shown in the study from the UK Centre for Health Economics (Table 23.4) (8).

Adolescent smoking has been a concern in many countries, but rates are falling now in the West. For example, in Australia, the last decade has seen consistent falls in all age groups (Table 23.5). Personal, sociocultural and

Table 23.4 Life-years gained over age 45 for a Western population of about 500,000, smoking at a 27% prevalence, and estimated costs per life-year gained

Intervention	Effectiveness (%)	Population reached (%)	Life-years gained	Cost per life-year (undiscounted) (£)
Primary healthcare interventions				
Brief advice	2	80	3034	94
Additional gains and costs on top of brief advice from:				
Brief counseling	2	70	2665	545
Nicotine gum	8	50	7601	463
Community interventions				
Local "no smoking" days	0.15	90	284	21
Broader community-wide programs	0.50	100	948	54
	0.10	100	190	271
	0.05	100	95	541

Source: *Cost Effectiveness of Smoking Cessation Interventions.* London: Centre for Health Economics, University of York and Health Education Authority, 1997. https://cancercontrol.cancer.gov/brp/tcrb/monographs/21/docs/m21_9.pdf (9).

Table 23.5 Young adults: Percentage of regular[a] smokers[b] from 1995 to 2013—by age group and sex[c] (%)

Year	Males 18–24 years	Females 18–24 years	Total 18–24 years	Males 25–29 years	Females 25–29 years	Total 25–29 years	Males 30–39 years	Females 30–39 years	Total 30–39 years
1995	33	36	35	35	40	37	35	29	32
1998	38	36	37	38	34	36	31	27	29
2001	28	26	27	34	26	30	30	26	28
2004	24	23	23	31	27	29	26	24	25
2007	21	18	19	31	26	28	25	21	23
2010	20	17	19	25	20	22	23	18	20
2013	17	15	16	20	16	18	20	12	16

Source: Centre for Behavioural Research in Cancer analysis of National Drug Strategy Household Survey data from 1995 to 2013. Available from http://www.tobaccoinaustralia.org.au/chapter-1-prevalence/1-4-prevalence-of-smoking-young-adults (288).

[a] Includes those reporting that they smoke "daily" or "at least weekly."

[b] Includes persons smoking any combination of cigarettes, pipes or cigars.

[c] All data weighted to the Australian population appropriate for each survey year and may vary slightly from data presented in previous edition. Further, previous versions of this table used data from both the Anti-Cancer Council of Victoria and National Drug Strategy Household Survey (NDSHS), while this version uses NDSHS data only.

environmental factors all influence smoking uptake and interventions *via* schools, mass media, community-based programs and environmental measures covering controls on advertising, plain packaging, pricing, retailing and smoking policies have all had an effect. It is simply "not cool" to smoke in Australia anymore.

CLINICIANS AND TOBACCO CONTROL

Members of the health professions can be active in influencing politicians and community leaders to adopt appropriate legislative approaches. All professional associations are urged to adopt a policy on tobacco and health, and many have done so. That produced by the FDI World Dental Federation (FDI) might serve as a model (Table 23.6) (10).

Healthcare professionals can work within their clinical environment to great effect. There is ample evidence that general medical practitioner advice to quit tobacco use is respected by the majority of patients, and several recent studies show that dentists can be equally effective (Table 23.7). This is achieved by following the simple scheme of the 4As (expanded in Table 23.8 to the 5As), widely used around the world.

Dentists, and all clinicians involved in oral healthcare (17,18), have a natural entry to discussion of tobacco-related diseases with their patients because of the oral signs of tobacco use and its influence on many oral diseases and conditions (19). Many of these are covered in detail elsewhere in this book; they are summarized in Table 23.9. The malignant and potentially malignant lesions and disorders are of obvious importance; realistically, however, they are not common and do not give rise to many opportunities for true primary prevention in much of the world, although they must be the focus in those countries of South and Southeast Asia where head and neck malignancies are so prevalent. The socially important changes—bad breath and tooth staining—are often sufficient to focus clinicians and patients alike on the desirability of quitting. Because periodontal diseases are common in all populations, increased severity and extent of disease and poor response to periodontal treatment can be important "hooks" for involving an affected patient in tobacco control (see the American Academy of Periodontology) (21). The scientific evidence on the harm to general and oral health of tobacco use, with special emphasis on oral cancer and precancer, oral candidiasis, other mucosal diseases, periodontal diseases, salivary flow rate and composition, susceptibility to dental caries, impact on wound healing and the success or failure of dental implants is summarized in a report of the E.U. Working Group on Tobacco and Oral Health 1998 (22,23).

In the U.S.A., the National Cancer Institute, the American Medical Association and the American Dental Association have produced extensive literature to help train physicians, dentists and their teams in anti-tobacco counseling, as have a number of other countries (24). Almost all countries in the world have educational material designed for professionals and health promotion material designed for the public: these should be easily accessed by approaching the appropriate agencies, some of whom have been listed in Table 23.1 and can be download from the Web.

Table 23.6 FDI policy statement on tobacco

Tobacco in daily practice

The use of tobacco is harmful to general health, as it is a common cause of addiction, preventable illness, disability and death. The use of tobacco also causes an increased risk for oral cancer, periodontal disease and other deleterious oral conditions and it adversely affects the outcome of oral health care.

The FDI urges its Member Associations and all oral health professionals to take decisive actions to reduce tobacco use and nicotine addiction among the general public.

The FDI also urges all oral health professionals to integrate tobacco use prevention and cessation services into their routine and daily practice.

Tobacco in all education

Brief interactions, for example by identifying tobacco users, giving direct advice, supportive material and follow-up, all have a significant impact on the patients' use of tobacco products.

The FDI urges all oral health institutions and all continuing education providers to integrate tobacco-related subjects into their programs.

Protect the children

The adverse consequences of environmental tobacco smoke are particularly severe for children—and lifelong.

The FDI strongly endorses and promotes public and professional education and policies that prevent and/or reduce the exposure to tobacco smoke for infants, children and young people.

Prevent the initiation

More than 80% of adults who use tobacco started their use of tobacco before the age of 18. Use of tobacco among children and youths easily produces a nicotine dependency, the risk of which is vastly underestimated by the young people themselves.

The FDI vigorously supports all measures that endeavor to prevent the initiation of tobacco use.

Table 23.7 A selection of smoking cessation trials in primary care

References	Country	Year	Setting	n	Method	Period	Quit rate (%)
Cohen et al. (11)	U.S.A.	1989	Private dentists	374	Dentist training + brief advice (a)	1 year	7.7
					(a) + nicotine gum	1 year	16.3
					(a) + reminders on notes	1 year	8.6
					(a) + gum and reminders	1 year	16.9
Segnan et al. (12)	Italy	1991	GMP	923	Minimal intervention	1 year	4.8
					Repeated counseling	1 year	5.3
					Counseling + gum	1 year	7.5
					Counseling + spirometry	1 year	6.5
Russell et al. (13)	UK	1993	GMP	400	Brief advice + nicotine patches	1 year	9.3
			GMP	200	Brief advice + placebo patches	1 year	5.0
Stapleton et al. (14)	UK	1995	GMP	800	Nicotine patches	1 year	9.6
				400	Placebo patches	1 year	4.8
Macgregor (15)	UK	1996	Hospital periodontal	98	Dental health education + advice against smoking	3–6 months	13.3
			Clinic	98	Dental health education only	3–6 months	5.3
Smith et al. (16)	UK	1997	GDP	154	Brief advice + optional nicotine patches	9 months	11.0

Abbreviations: GMP: General Medical Practitioner; GDP: General Dental Practitioner.

Table 23.8 The five 'A's

- Ask patients about their tobacco habits
- Advise them on the importance of quitting
- Agree with them on a quit date
- Assist them in achieving this
- Arrange follow-up

Even in the absence of oral stigmata of tobacco use, dentists should *ask and advise* in order to detect new tobacco addicts and engage in early preventive activities. This is a particular challenge with young people. Surveys of dental practitioner knowledge, attitudes and behavior toward tobacco control have been conducted in a number of countries with, unsurprisingly, variable results. Encouragingly, a U.S. national survey showed that a quarter of tobacco users had been advised to quit by their dentist (25). However, in much of the world, a substantial proportion, often a majority, of colleagues are inhibited from asking and reluctant to advise. A large questionnaire survey of UK dentists in the mid-1990s found that half of the respondents did not routinely inquire about risk habits related to oral cancer; 30% inquired of their patients regarding smoking habits and 19% questioned on both smoking and alcohol use. (However, this sample is unrepresentative, as out of 2,532 dentists addressed, only 16% responded.) Of those inquiring into these risk habits, only 19.5% made appropriate notes in patients' records. Only 30% of dentists who inquired into smoking habits provided brief advice routinely to patients and a further 31% only to patients they regarded as being at high risk of oral cancer or another serious disease. A much smaller proportion (20%) of dentists in this study attempted to provide advice on alcohol moderation when patient histories suggested excess consumption. Dentists who were regular smokers themselves were less likely to inquire about the risk habits of their patients compared to those professionals who had either never smoked or were ex-smokers ($p < .05$). When asked whether dental practitioners should be involved in giving advice against tobacco use, 71% of respondents agreed that this was desirable, but many constraints were perceived, listed in Table 23.10. Understandably, dentists not already providing such advice felt constrained by a wider range of these items (26). Knowledge, attitudes and behavior surveys of U.S. dentists indicated similar gaps (27,28).

These results are similar to those reported from Texas (29). Educational efforts are thus required for both the public and for the profession in the hope of developing a growing awareness of the appropriateness of dentists addressing these issues. At present, it is likely that many practitioners will opt to refer interested dental patients to an individual specialist or group: the AA-R approach (Ask, Advise, Refer) rather than the 5As approach. Advice leaflets, which include telephone numbers and addresses of such resources, should be available in every healthcare setting (Figure 23.2).

Increasingly, dentists and other clinicians are willing to receive training in tobacco control methods *via* the many sources listed above. This may involve advice to clients on the use of nicotine replacement to help over the period of withdrawal. As an addictive substance, nicotine, on a milligram for milligram basis, is ten times more potent than heroin (30). An important study in the UK has shown that the use of nicotine skin patches can double the rate of smoking cessation handled through a medical practitioner, from around 5% to around 10% of recruits (31). This played a role in the comparable 11% quit rate we have demonstrated as

Table 23.9 Oral tobacco-induced and tobacco-associated conditions

Oral cancer
Leukoplakia
- Homogenous leukoplakia
- Non-homogeneous leukoplakia (precancer)
- Verrucous leukoplakia
- Nodular leukoplakia
- Erythroleukoplakia

Other tobacco-induced oral mucosal conditions
- Snuff dipper's lesion
- Tobacco pouch
- Smoker's palate (nicotine stomatitis)
- Smoker's melanosis

Tobacco-associated effects on the teeth and supporting tissues
- Tooth loss (premature mortality)
- Staining
- Abrasion
- Periodontal diseases
  - Destructive periodontitis
  - Focal recession
  - Acute necrotizing ulcerative gingivitis

Other tobacco-associated oral conditions
- Gingival bleeding
- Calculus
- Halitosis
- Leukoedema
- Chronic hyperplastic candidiasis (candidal leukoplakia)
- Median rhomboid glossitis
- Hairy tongue

Possible association with tobacco
- Oral clefts
- Dental caries
- Dental plaque
- Lichen planus
- Salivary changes
- Taste and smell

Source: Mecklenburg RE et al. *Tobacco Effects in the Mouth. NIH Publication No 96-3330.* Washington, DC: US Department of Health and Human Services, 1996 (20).

Table 23.10 Constraints felt by dental practitioners in the UK toward giving clients advice against tobacco use

	Those who feel dentists should give advice (71%) (%)	Those who feel dentists should not give advice (29%) (%)
It is frustrating	26	15
It is not important	3	6
It is not effective	9	22
It is not cost-effective	24	21
We are not trained	28	21
Other reasons	10	14

possible in dental practice (16). The California tobacco survey showed that such patches are significant aids to smokers who want to quit when used as an adjuvant to other forms of assistance (32). Nicotine replacement is available as skin patches, chewing gums, nasal sprays or as an inhaler fashioned like a cigarette (which then helps with the oral and tactile stimulation that is part of smoking addiction). The latter are forerunners of the explosive use of electronic cigarettes. All have a role to play in appropriate circumstances (33). These devices deliver nicotine with different pharmacokinetic consequences, as shown in Figure 23.3. Advice on their appropriate use, including dosages and contra-indications, is included in the training literature referred to above and from the manufacturers. In some countries, these products are available over the counter, with detailed instructions: pharmacists/drug stores can also be consulted by doctor, dentist or patient for advice.

E-cigarettes have simply not been in common use for sufficient time for their health effects, on the mouth and the whole body, to be assessed. Nicotine has significant cardiovascular effects and may induce Type II diabetes over time. An accessible summary with a bibliography is available on the website of the U.S. National Institute on Drug abuse (https://www.drugabuse.gov/pulications/drugfacts/electronic-cigarettes-e-cigarettes).

ORAL SMOKELESS TOBACCO (ST)

As shown in Chapter 2, there is no doubt that the addition of tobacco to areca nut (betel) quids, consumed by millions in South and Southeast Asia, confers a major increase in their carcinogenicity (34) and habitués must be encouraged to quit; indeed, the benefits of doing so are clear (35). Omitting tobacco from quids and washing the mouth well after use may be helpful intermediate steps. We have seen that the tobaccos used in mixtures such as *nass*, *niswar* or *toombak* in North Africa, the Middle East or northern parts of the Indian subcontinent also contain high levels of nitrosamines and are dangerous (36). A clear summary of the evidence for oral cancer associated with the various forms of tobacco use around the world is provided by Gupta et al. (37).

Controversy exists, however, as to the danger of moist, loose or portion bag-packed snuff in the West, notably Scandinavia and the U.S.A. It appears that the risk of oral cancer is low with these products (38), and the chemical, behavioral and risk differences associated with Swedish *snus* and Sudanese *toombak* have been compared in detail by Idris et al. (39). There is even the suggestion that smokers should be encouraged to take up oral ST as a less dangerous means of coping with nicotine addiction (40). However, this is an unproven and potentially dangerous approach; there are safer forms of nicotine replacement available and the cardiovascular effects and risks of cancer at other sites have not been fully evaluated.

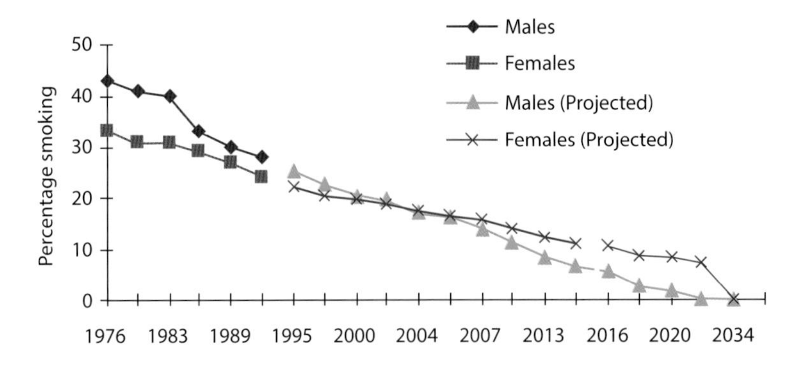

Figure 23.2 Projected male and female adult smoking rates in Australia. (Reproduced from Scollo MM, Winstanley MH. *Tobacco in Australia: Facts and Issues*. Melbourne: Cancer Council Victoria; 2016. Available from http://www.tobaccoinaustralia.org.au/ (289); Projections based on prevalence surveys by Hill et al. and Hill and White.)

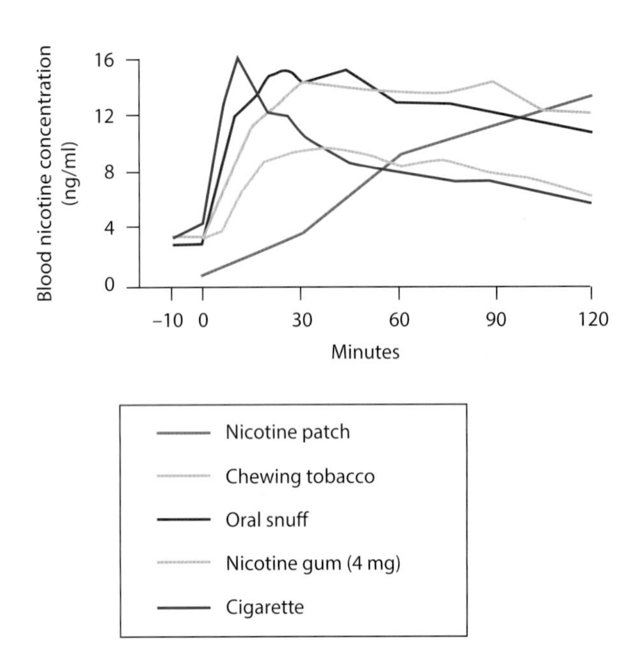

Figure 23.3 Blood nicotine concentration over time by method of administration.

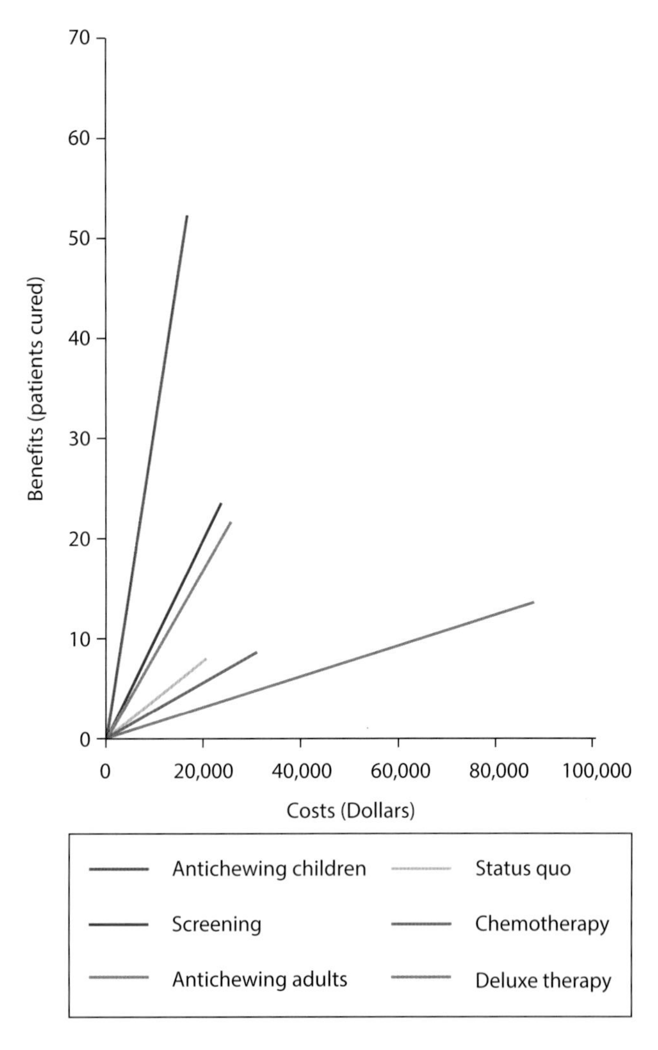

Figure 23.4 Cost–benefit analysis of managing oral cancer in Sri Lanka.

There is no doubt that primary prevention by habit intervention is the most cost-effective approach to the management of oral cancer. This is strikingly demonstrated in a model of the situation in Sri Lanka (Figure 23.4) (Stjernsward J., WHO, personal communication).

ARECA NUT WITH AND WITHOUT ST

DEATHS DUE TO ST AND ARECA NUT

Tobacco and areca nut are the second and fourth most common psychoactive substances used around the world, respectively (41). Tobacco is now the world's leading cause of death (42). Areca nut is used by over 600 million people or about 10% of the world's population (43). If current trends continue, it will lead to 1 billion premature deaths in this century. A third of the users of tobacco die due to its use, leading to health inequalities in low-income countries where its use is rampant (42). Areca nut and ST are used extensively in South and Southeast Asia, Asia-Pacific and parts of North America, Africa and Europe amongst migrants (42). ST products have been popular in the U.S.A. and Sweden since the 1960s. According to the Global Adult Tobacco Survey (GATS) of 2009, 25.9% adults use ST in India, comprising 32.9% males and 18.4% females out of the total adult population (44). In the U.S.A., 3.9% of the population was using it in 2010 and its use was more common among workers (45). Areca nut may be used with or without tobacco and is used in many forms like betel quid (BQ), with betel leaves, pan masala, supari, etc. (41). ST is used in many forms around the word like *khaini*, *mishri*, *zarda*, *mawa*, snuff, *shammah* and *toombak* (46).

ST and areca nut are proven carcinogens leading to cancers of the oral cavity, pharynx, esophagus and lungs and are also responsible for various systemic diseases like cardiovascular diseases, diabetes, hepatotoxicity, metabolic syndrome (47–50). A study done amongst Taiwanese men has shown that the relative risks (RR and 95% confidence intervals) of all-cause mortality and cardiovascular diseases amongst present users of BQ are 1.4 (1.16–1.70) and 2.02 (1.13–3.13), respectively, and amongst the past users the RRs are 1.40 (1.17–1.68) and 1.56 (1.02–2.38), respectively, when compared to people who had never chewed betel nut (48). A large cohort study in Mumbai involving 52,000 persons showed that there is an increased RR of death for ST (mainly *mishri* and BQ) users. The age-adjusted RRs for users are 1.22 and 1.35, respectively, for males and females when compared to non-users. The study also suggested a dose–response relationship when ST is used daily (51). Another cohort study involving 10,287 subjects done in Kerala, India, on ST (mainly betel leaf with tobacco) users showed that the RRs of death were 1.2 (not significant) and 1.3 ($p < .05$), respectively, for men and women (52). These studies show that, like smokers, the age-adjusted RRs of ST users are also elevated (47). After evaluating epidemiological studies on carcinogenic risks to humans due to tobacco habits the International Agency for Research on Cancer (IARC) concluded that there is enough evidence to show that chewing tobacco mixed with lime and BQ containing tobacco is carcinogenic (53). Six studies done in India have shown that RRs for oral cancer in current chewers of *pan* with tobacco varies from 1.8 (95% confidence interval [CI]: 1.2–2.7) to 5.8 (95% CI: 3.6–9.5) and 30.4 (95% CI: 12.6–73.4) to 45.9 (95% CI: 25–84.1) for men and women, respectively (47). A meta-analysis done by Guha et al. has shown that the meta-RR (mRR) for oral cancers in the Indian subcontinent was 7.74 (95% CI: 5.38–11.13) for BQ plus tobacco as compared to 2.56 (95% CI: 2.00–3.28) for BQ without tobacco (49). In China and Taiwan, the mRR for BQ without tobacco was 10.98 (95% CI: 4.86–24.84). The mRR was much higher in women as compared to men and was 14.56 (95% CI: 7.63–27.76) (49). The risk of oral cancer is elevated with increasing daily amount and duration of the habit. About half of oral cancer deaths in India, China and Taiwan could be prevented if BQ was not chewed (population attributable fraction = 53.7% for BQ without tobacco in Taiwan, China and 49.5% for BQ plus tobacco in India) (49). Studies have shown that the carcinogenic and genotoxic effects of ST and areca nut are due to reactive oxygen species (ROS) and tobacco- and areca nut-specific nitrosamines. Higher iron and copper content in these products adds to the ROS produced, increasing the damage to the cells. Areca nut chewing also leads to local trauma and injury that, on chronic exposure, lead to cancer. Areca nut-exposed cells show decreased activity of cellular antioxidant glutathione and glutathione S-transferase, leading to oxidative stress and DNA damage. The key step in initiating cancer is the formation of DNA adducts, which leads to miscoding, mutations and disturbance of mechanisms controlling cell growth (54).

APPROACH TO MANAGING ST AND ARECA NUT USE

ST and areca nut need equal attention in control as is given to other forms of tobacco as they are used by more than 10% of the world's population. Spitting leads to unhygienic conditions, encouraging the spread of serious diseases such as tuberculosis. ST is the preferred form of tobacco in rural and poor populations who may be relatively uneducated. It conflicts with the millennium development goals set by United Nations Organisation (44). For controlling the use of tobacco around the world, the WHO has formed the Framework Convention for Tobacco Control (FCTC), which is supported by countries comprising more than 80% of the world's population (55).

For application of the FCTC, the WHO has formed MPOWER*, which is a package of policies that have been proven to control tobacco use. It is designed to help countries in framing policies for tobacco control and to scale up of the WHO FCTC (55).

Monitor tobacco use and prevention policies

Countries need to determine patterns and prevalence rates of tobacco use to frame policies of tobacco control that are suitable to them. There is a need to assess effects of smuggling prevention, taxation, cessation interventions and knowledge about tobacco amongst the population (42,55).

Offering help with quitting tobacco

Many people addicted to tobacco want to quit, but very few get the help required. Only nine countries in the world provide full services to quit tobacco dependence (55). Offering

* MPOWER = M, Monitor tobacco use and prevention policies; P, Protect people from tobacco smoke; O, Offer help to quit tobacco use; W, Warn about the dangers of tobacco; E, Enforce bans on tobacco advertising, promotion and sponsorship; R, Raise taxes on tobacco.

tobacco users help to quit doubles their chances of quitting (42). A study done in rural parts of India has shown that 32.5% of users of tobacco intended to quit, but are unable to do so due to a lack of proper counseling and medical care (56). Medical professionals have a very big part to play by helping users to quit this habit *via* counseling and referral to de-addiction centers (42).

Warn about the dangers of tobacco

The use of tobacco is glorified by various forms of direct and indirect advertising methods. Countries need to counter this by hard-hitting anti-tobacco campaigns that make people aware of the harmful effects of tobacco, the benefits of quitting and industry tactics. A study done in India has shown that people who are exposed to anti-tobacco campaigns through different forms of media are more likely to quit (56). There is a need to educate children in schools about the harmful effects of this habit. This has been proven in Thailand, where anti-tobacco campaigns in primary schools brought down the incidence rate of oral cancer from 3.6% to 1.2% in males and 2.6% to 1.1% in females (44). The educational interventions are also helpful in decreasing relapse rates, providing higher rates of spontaneous regression of oral potentially malignant lesions amongst quitters (47). A successful anti-tobacco program must have clear long-term goals, be comprehensive by having active participation of the government and community and be implemented at all levels—local, regional and national (55).

All countries must unite and fight this menace together and with sustained efforts.

Raising taxes on tobacco

Raising the price of tobacco products by increasing taxes is the most effective ways to reduce tobacco use, especially amongst low-income groups and in youngsters and children (55). This has been proven all over the world by decreases in smoking prevalence following increased taxes on cigarettes (42,55). For every 10% increase in taxes, there is reduction in tobacco consumption by 2.5%–5.0% (42). A 70% increase in the price of tobacco could reduce the tobacco related deaths by 25% worldwide. Higher taxes will provide funds to the government to implement anti-tobacco polices more effectively and also finance social and public health programs (55).

Bans on sale, advertising, promotions and sponsorships

The tobacco industry spends billions of dollars all over the world on sponsorships, advertising and promotions. Such bans help in countering the false positive image of tobacco created by industry (42). Many countries have banned direct advertising by industry, which then bypasses such a ban by directing resources to non-regulated media like point-of-sale promotions, movies, the Internet and social media (55). A study in Maharashtra, India, has shown that after a ban on ST, 27.7% of the users quit this habit and agreed that this is a good step by the government to decrease consumption (57).

Protecting people from tobacco exposure

Many countries have enforced strict laws for bans on smoking in public places. Similar laws are required for the use of ST and areca nut, as many people openly spit these products in public places, exposing people to these toxic products and creating an unhygienic environment (42,47,55).

PASSIVE SMOKING

Two critical meta-analyses of the world literature from the Wolfson Institute of Preventive Medicine in London (58,59) and reviews from the California Environmental Protection Agency (60) and the U.S. Environmental Protection Agency (61) show conclusively that exposure to environmental tobacco smoke is a major cause of serious illness. In the U.S.A. alone, exposure to environmental tobacco smoke is calculated to be responsible for 3,000 deaths from lung cancer each year, 35,000–62,000 deaths from ischemic heart disease (tobacco smoke has a marked effect on platelet biology, even at low doses), 150,000–300,000 cases of bronchitis or pneumonia in infants and children up to 18 months of age (of whom a proportion die), 8,000–26,000 new cases of asthma and exacerbation of asthma in up to a million children, 9,700–18,600 cases of low birth weight and 1,900–2,700 sudden infant deaths (62).

Chapter 2 provides evidence for the role of environmental tobacco smoke in upper aerodigestive tract cancers. All health professionals should set an example by not smoking (or seeking help if they are current smokers) and by ensuring that the whole work environment is smoke free.

CLINICIANS AND THE MANAGEMENT OF HEAVY ALCOHOL CONSUMPTION

Excessive alcohol consumption is a major cause of individual morbidity and mortality and contributes much damage to society. In the U.S.A., it is estimated that alcohol-related diseases contribute 100,000 excess deaths each year. In this respect, tobacco and alcohol abuse are much more significant than hard drugs, when measured by outcomes such as person-years of life lost or bed days occupied in hospital. Figure 23.5 shows data from Australia that illustrate this dramatically. All healthcare clinicians have a responsibility, therefore, to help their clients (patients, colleagues and students) use alcohol sensibly. This is especially true in teaching and training centers, because students and staff in medical institutions are amongst the highest-risk groups for dangerous drinking (63).

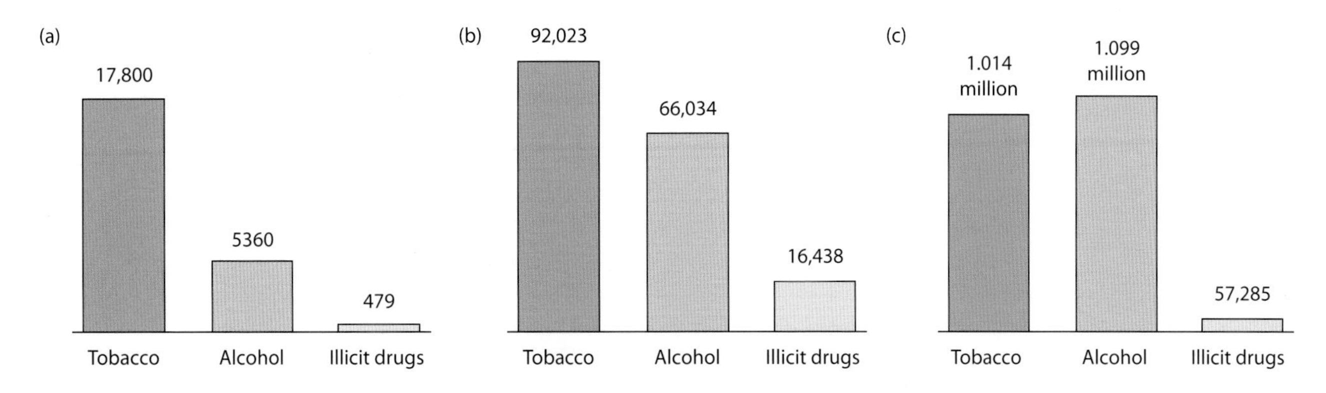

Figure 23.5 **(a)** Deaths (ages 0–69) due to tobacco, alcohol and illicit drugs, Australia 1996. **(b)** Person-years lost (ages 0–69) due to tobacco, alcohol and illicit drugs, Australia 1996. **(c)** Bed days (ages 0–69) due to tobacco, alcohol and illicit drugs, Australia 1996. (Courtesy of Dr. Nigel Gray, UICC and Anticancer Council of Victoria.)

Many primary care clinicians are inhibited from taking alcohol histories from their patients, but all should, with tact, be able to help their patients see that such questioning is directed at genuine concerns for their general health and that this is relevant to their oral health. Oral and other upper aerodigestive tract cancers and potentially malignant disorders are perhaps our major concerns as clinicians interested in diseases of the head and neck. As explained earlier, many epidemiologists believe that the rise in both the incidence and mortality of these cancers seen in a number of countries, particularly in Europe, is related to rising alcohol consumption over recent years. Differences in alcohol consumption (particularly amongst those who also smoke) explain most of the increasingly higher rates of oral cancer amongst blacks as compared to whites in the U.S.A. (64). Current disease levels were predicted by trends in alcohol consumption over the past three decades (Figure 23.6) (65). In addition, alcohol contributes to dental and maxillofacial injuries and, by secondary effects following liver damage and, often, undernutrition, compromises periodontal health, wound healing and resistance to infection (66).

All clinicians can see these facial and intraoral signs in their patients, and suspicion may be aroused because of patient behavior. There are a number of well-established tools for the estimation of problem drinking in our patients. These include the so-called CAGE* and AUDIT (Alcohol Use Disorders Identification Test) questionnaires, of which a recent study showed the AUDIT to be marginally superior (67). We have validated the AUDIT questionnaire, as developed by the WHO (68). In a study of 107 south London misusers, over half of whom consumed more than 200 units of alcohol per week and 80% of whom also smoked, eight subjects had oral mucosal lesions, including two previously treated carcinomas in one individual. Dental caries experience did not differ from an age-matched national sample, but periodontal disease was more severe and was related to both smoking and undernutrition as recorded by body mass index and mid-arm muscle circumference measurements. Clearly, such individuals, to be found in most societies worldwide, are a priority group for preventative counseling (69). A policy of "Ask, Advise" ought then to be followed, accepting that "Referral" is probably wise for patients with a suspected alcohol problem, given the complexity of the addictive process and the therapeutic challenges in this demanding, specialized field. A wide variety of dedicated groups, agencies and clinics exist in most countries, and practitioners are advised to be aware of what networks exist locally. Serious alcohol dependence often requires inpatient and/or day stay treatment, which is both demanding and expensive (70). Again, the Internet is a source of much professional advice and provides access to self-help and support groups for individuals with alcohol problems and their families.

It is clear that specific training can enhance the effectiveness of primary care physicians in detecting and managing hazardous drinking in their patients and that direct contact with trainers, face to face or on the telephone, is more effective than mailed training kits (71). In a study in Sydney, Australia, 36 trained general medical practitioners recruited 179 patients with an alcohol problem over 3 months, 32% of whom reported reduced drinking to the researchers (72). As with tobacco control, education and health promotion interventions need to be undertaken at all levels of society, and many governments around the world are working to improve their effectiveness and cost-effectiveness (73).

Moderate alcohol consumption has long been regarded as not especially harmful, even beneficial, particularly in reducing the risk of cardiovascular diseases. The so-called J-shaped curve relation between alcohol consumption and total mortality has been established for some years (74). This argues that lowest mortality occurs in those who consume one or two drinks per day. In teetotalers or very occasional drinkers, the mortality rate was interpreted as higher than in those who take one or two drinks per day. Importantly, in those who take three or more drinks per day, mortality

* The CAGE questionnaire asks the following questions:
Have you ever felt you needed to Cut down on your drinking?
Have people Annoyed you by criticizing your drinking?
Have you ever felt Guilty about drinking?
Have you ever felt you needed a drink first thing in the morning (Eye opener) to steady your nerves or to get rid of a hangover?

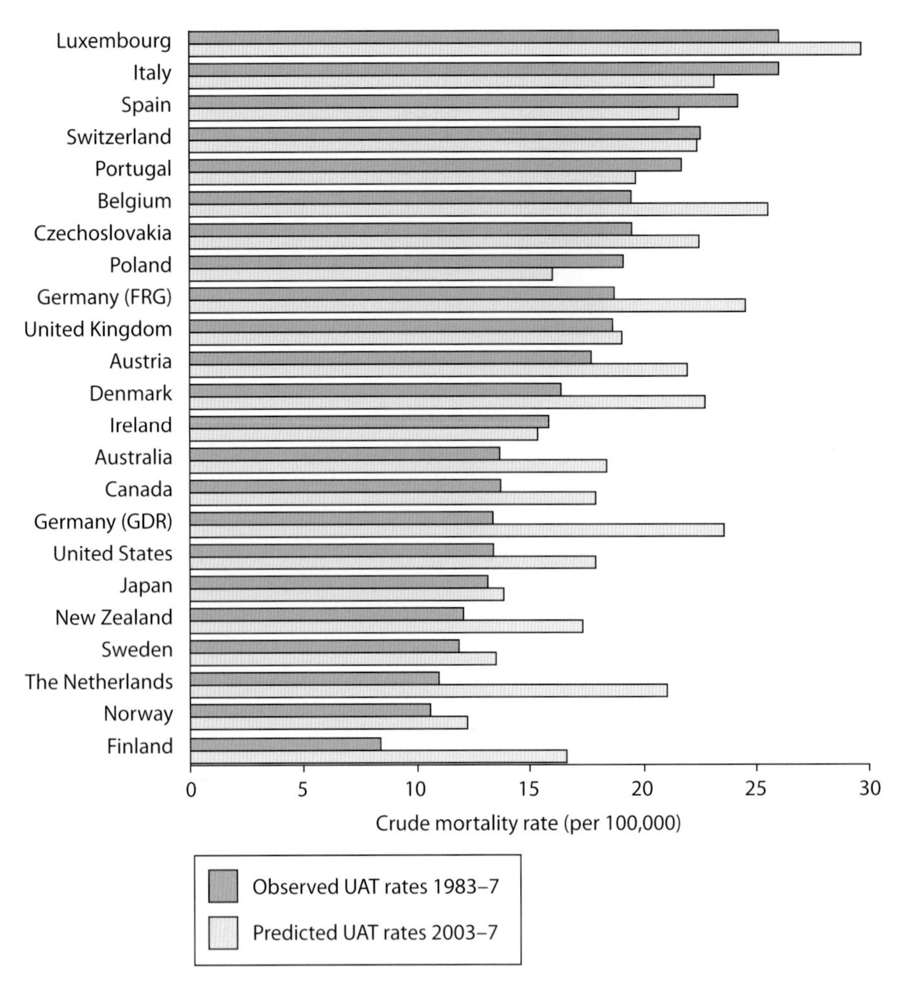

Figure 23.6 Observed mortality from upper aerodigestive tract (UAT) cancers in males in the countries listed, with projections for two decades later. (Data from Macfarlane GJ et al. *J Epidemiol Commun Health* 1996;50:636–9 (65).)

rises rapidly in a dose-dependent manner. The major causes of death are shown in Table 23.11.

The protection against coronary heart disease provided by one or two drinks per day has been reported as in the order of 30–50% (75), with less atherosclerosis in such moderate drinkers, visible at catheterization or at autopsy. In some studies, this effect seems to be independent of possible confounders such as smoking and poor diet. It is generally considered (76) that about half of the protective effect is mediated through increased levels of high-density lipoprotein cholesterol, which carries cholesterol from arterial walls back to the liver (77). Other beneficial effects may be mediated through reductions in clotting factors and platelet activity and/or clot lysis (78,79).

Table 23.11 Major causes of drink-related death

- Stroke
- Cardiomyopathy
- Cancer (several sites)
- Liver cirrhosis
- Pancreatitis
- Accidents
- Suicide
- Homicide

Other protective substances have been identified in several beverages, such as the antioxidants in wine derived from grape skins (resveratrol mainly) (80) and in dark beer. However, the available epidemiological evidence does not show any particular type of beverage to be consistently more effective in reducing coronary heart disease, perhaps because of considerable variability in confounding factors such as smoking, diet and age in the various studies (81). The frequency of alcohol consumption is also critically important: studies in Eastern Europe, where patterns of alcohol use and heart disease are different from the West, show binge drinking to be dangerous, without the raised high-density lipoproteins, indeed with raised low-density lipoproteins, and with a tendency to increased thrombosis after cessation of drinking (82).

What, therefore, constitutes potentially unhealthy levels of alcohol consumption? Many governments and agencies have long suggested a healthy limit of 21 units of alcohol a week for men and 14 for women, with at least two alcohol-free days per week. UK authorities now recommend that the limit for men be reduced to 14 units, the same as for women. A unit of alcohol is taken to be a single glass (approximately 284 mL) of average-strength beer or lager, a single measure (approximately 25 mL) of spirits or a single standard (approximately 113 mL) glass of wine or aperitif (50 mL) (83). Currently, most agencies are arguing that *any amount* of alcohol is risky. Precise limits and advice varies from country to country, and these have been helpfully set out by Wikipedia at https://en.wikipedia.org/wiki/Recommended_maximum_intake_of_alcoholic_beverages.

Very importantly, IARC (http://www.iarc.fr/) has declared alcohol carcinogenic. The last full version was published in 2010 and a revision published in 2012 (http://monographs.iarc.fr/ENG/Monographs/vol100E/mono100E-11.pdf). The World Cancer report of 2014 describes the dose response of the at-risk cancer sites (https://www.iarc.fr/en/media-centre/iarcnews/2016/WCR_2014_Chapter_2-3.pdf). The Alcohol Health Alliance UK is a valuable source of up-to-date factual and policy information (http://ahauk.org/alcohol-cancer-knowing-risks-2017/).

It is the ethanol within alcohol, once metabolized, that is carcinogenic, and it is impossible to differentiate between different risks associated with different alcoholic beverages. According to some studies, 10% of total cancers in men and 3% of total cancers in women could be attributable to alcohol consumption.

It is clear that national policies are needed to prevent tobacco use and to limit alcohol consumption in the young in order to reduce future morbidity and mortality from upper aero-digestive tract cancers cancers (84). Price, availability, trading hours, volume of containers, alcohol content of beverages and social norms are all important. A study in Switzerland suggests that it takes some years for alcohol cessation to have an effect on cancer risk (85). In addition, public recognition of the importance of alcohol as a risk factor for cancer, especially oral cancer, is poor (86,87).

HEALTHY EATING IN THE PREVENTION OF ORAL CANCER

Clinicians, it is hoped, routinely inquire about the dietary habits of their patients, usually because they are interested in their likely adverse effects on cardiovascular health or—particularly for dentists—in their possible cariogenicity. Adequate (neither under- nor over-) nutrition is essential to host resistance against all diseases and this is strongly true of cancer. Table 23.12 summarizes dietary measures suggested for the prevention of cancer based on a critical review by Sir Richard Doll, the epidemiologist who has made perhaps the biggest single contribution to knowledge of the causes and prevention of cancer over the past 100 years (88). He believed that the risk of cancer overall could be reduced by a third or more by modification of diet in a way that has already proved acceptable to many.

The protective role of diets adequate in trace elements, minerals and vitamins (particularly the antioxidant or free radical-scavenging vitamins A, C and E) has been emphasized in Chapter 2. An extensive literature in relation to head and neck cancer was reviewed by La Vecchia et al. (89). Two publications, produced with characteristic thoroughness by the International Agency for Research on Cancer, are strongly recommended (90,91). The benefits are apparent even in the case of such high-risk habits as reverse smoking (92).

Table 23.12 Dietary measures suggested for the prevention of cancer

Measure	Type of cancer affected
Reduce	
Calories (avoid obesity)	Gallbladder, body of uterus, possibly breast
Fat	Breast, colon and rectum, prostate and endometrium
Smoked and grilled food	Stomach, perhaps others
Salt-cured food	Stomach
Nitrates	Stomach, possibly others
Saccharin	Possibly bladder
Increase	
Fiber	Colon and rectum
Vegetables	Colon and rectum; many sites, including head and neck
Fruit	Colon and rectum; many sites, including head and neck
Vitamins A, C and E	Many sites, including head and neck
β-carotene	Many sites, including head and neck
Selenium	Many sites, including head and neck

Source: Doll R. The prevention of cancer: Opportunities and challenges. In: Heller T, Davey B, Bailey L (eds). *Reducing the Risk of Cancers*. London: Hodder and Stoughton, 1989 (88).

Many studies have shown that intake of protective nutrients is more effective when these are derived from natural foodstuffs rather than from synthetic food supplements (93). This is particularly important in smokers and drinkers (94). Thus, the advice that we should give to our patients, which is part of every nation's health promotion guidelines, is summarized in Table 23.13, developed from the American Cancer Society (95).

Most foods that are protective against cancer of the mouth and pharynx are from plant origin. Based on the evaluation published by the World Cancer Research Fund (96), there is convincing evidence that higher consumption of non-starchy vegetables (raw vegetables including cruciferous and green, leafy vegetables) and non-starchy tubers (e.g. carrots) may protect against cancers of the upper aerodigestive tract, including the mouth and pharynx (summary odds ratio [OR] 0.72, 95% CI: 0.63–0.82). There is published evidence that fruits (particularly citrus fruits) may also provide protection (summary OR 0.72, 95% CI: 0.59–0.87; per 100 g/day). A meta-analysis focusing on oral cancer alone that examined

Table 23.13 American Cancer Society guidelines on diet, nutrition and cancer prevention

1. Choose most of the foods you eat from plant sources
   - Eat five or more servings of fruits and vegetables every day
   - Eat other foods from plant sources, such as breads, cereals, grain products, rice, pasta or beans, several times each day
2. Limit your intake of high-fat foods, particularly from animal sources
   - Choose foods low in fat
   - Limit consumption of meats, especially high-fat meats
3. Be physically active: Achieve and maintain a healthy weight
   - Be at least moderately active for 30 minutes or more on most days of the week
   - Stay within your healthy weight range
4. Limit consumption of alcoholic beverages, if you drink at all
5. Do not smoke
6. Avoid sexually transmitted infections

Source: American Cancer Society. *CA Cancer J Clin* 1996;46: 325–41 (95).

15 case–control studies and one cohort study providing diet data from nearly 5,000 subjects estimated that each portion of fruit or vegetables consumed per day reduced the risk of oral cancer by around 50% (97). Their effect may be mediated through antioxidant vitamins. A critical appraisal of the chemopreventive diets can be found elsewhere (98).

Based on the above observations that suggest reductions in cancer risks from good diets, the World Cancer Research Fund International (2007) (96) has issued the following "healthy eating" messages:

- Public health recommendations
  - Population average consumption of non-starchy vegetables and of fruits to be at least 600 g (21 oz) daily
- Personal recommendations
  - Eat at least five portions/servings (at least 400 g or 14 oz) of a variety of non-starchy vegetables and of fruits every day

These health promotion messages on dietary interventions can be directed at whole communities or to individuals, particularly when opportunities arise in clinical practice.

CHEMOPREVENTION OF ORAL AND OROPHARYNGEAL CANCER

Chemoprevention refers to the appropriate selection and regular consumption of diets rich in anti-cancer agents or the use of medical therapies—either natural or synthetic products—to arrest or reverse the process of cancer development. Chemopreventive agents may be applied as topical therapies to the sites of the oral cavity showing an increased risk of cancer or through systemic administration. The scenarios in which chemoprevention may work extend right from primary to secondary and to tertiary prevention of cancer. Such matters are addressed again in the last section of the present chapter under the heading of tertiary prevention.

CHEMOPREVENTION AS SECONDARY PREVENTION

An approach for the prevention of oral cancer includes treatment of oral potentially malignant disorders once they are detected in primary care and confirmed by biopsy at a health facility. The focus on such interventions has so far been mostly on treating oral leukoplakia. The standard approach has been surgical or laser excision of the clinically visible patch or plaque in the mouth, but in a significant number treated by surgery, recurrences were common. Following surgery, cancer may arise at the site of excision mostly due to poor margin clearance or elsewhere in the oral cavity due to the process of field cancerization in the oral cavity. The administration of chemopreventive agents aims to address the challenges associated with surgery (99).

Different classes of agents have been evaluated so far, including some natural products listed below:

- Vitamin A and retinoids
- β-carotene and carotenoids
- Non-steroidal anti-inflammatory drugs (NSAIDs), such as ketorolac and celecoxib
- Tea components
- Chinese herbal mixtures
- Freeze-dried black raspberries
- Bowman–Birk inhibitor
- Curcumin—the active ingredient in turmeric
- Bleomycin

These agents may act through various mechanisms, mostly as antioxidants to reduce the oxidative DNA damage that has occurred due to specific carcinogenic agents, such as tobacco. One other mechanism of action of several retinoids is *via* inhibition of NF-κB activation (100).

The outcomes of these chemoprevention trials have been assessed in various ways including clinical or histological changes of oral leukoplakia or preventing cancer development over a follow-up period and by some authors using intermediate biomarkers (e.g. micronuclei). Though the primary purpose of chemoprevention is to prevent the development of a malignancy, most studies have not extended their follow-up long enough to include this as the endpoint of their trials.

In a review of 16 chemoprevention trials on oral leukoplakia, Ribeiro et al. (101) reported clinical responses that ranged from 4% to 55%: the definition of what is a meaningful response is, of course, critical. Retinoids have been the most investigated chemopreventive agent for oral leukoplakia, with a reported response of 45%–67%. However, the recently published Cochrane Review that strictly considered randomized clinical trials on oral leukoplakia (14 studies; 909 participants) provided a less favorable judgment on their effectiveness based on the authors' strict statistical evaluation of the reported studies (99). Limitations of most of the studies of retinoids and β-carotene for oral leukoplakia (OL) are that the primary endpoint focused on OL clinical and/or histological response, which only marginally correlates with long-term oral cancer-free survival, and molecular abnormalities may still persist despite the disappearance of the clinical lesion with the chemopreventive agent.

EFFICACY OF VITAMIN A, RETINOIDS AND CAROTENOIDS

Retinoids are naturally occurring and synthetic vitamin A (retinol) metabolites and analogues that bind to retinoid receptors of the RAR and RXR types and promote cell differentiation, decrease proliferation and assist in apoptosis. Ralhan's group have reported a significant increase in RARα immunopositivity in oral squamous cell carcinomas (SCCs) compared to normal tissue (102), which suggested that targeting the retinoid signaling pathway could have some merit as a chemopreventive strategy. 13-*cis* retinoic acid (1.0 mg/kg/day) has been shown to modulate TGF-α expression in dysplastic oral leukoplakia (103).

There has been an extensive evaluation of retinoids in chemoprevention of oral leukoplakia with mixed outcomes. However, the toxicity of the retinoids and the rapid reversal of their beneficial effects after stopping these agents has prevented them from being considered for routine use.

STUDIES ON ORAL LEUKOPLAKIA

Early studies on chemoprevention of oral leukoplakia using vitamin A, its derivatives, retinoids and carotenoids were conducted in the U.S.A. and India by Shah et al. (104–109) and Sankaranarayanan et al. (110). Due to high toxicities, their trial designs and dosages often required changes. Trials published up to the end of the last century have been reviewed earlier (98). Gorsky and Epstein (111) reviewed four studies using topical vitamin A for patients with oral leukoplakia reported up to 2000. A complete clinical response was achieved in 10%–27% of patients and a partial response was achieved in 54%–90% of patients; however, recurrence of leukoplakia was reported after withdrawing the medication in approximately 50% of patients. Clinical trials published since 2000 using retinoids and carotenoids hoping to prevent malignant transformation of oral leukoplakia are listed in Table 23.14. There are a number of valuable recent references (274–285).

Based on the published clinical trials on chemoprevention of oral leukoplakia, the Cochrane Group has summarized "Treatment with beta carotene, lycopene and Vitamin A or retinoids was associated with significant rates of clinical resolution, compared with placebo or absence of treatment. In most studies a high rate of relapse was a common finding. Side effects of variable severity were often described; however, interventions were well tolerated since dropout rates in intervention and control groups were similar. Useable data on malignant transformation was reported in

Table 23.14 Chemoprevention trials on oral leukoplakia using retinoids or carotenoids (data published since 2000)

References	Agent	Phase	*n*	Regimen	Outcome
Gaeta et al. (112)	Acitretin	111	21	Acitretin[a] 20 mg for 4 weeks	Positive
Chiesa et al. (253)	Fenretinide	111	170	Fenretinide 200 mg QDS for 1 year vs no treatment	Positive
Lippman et al. (207)	Fenretinide	11	35[b]	Fenretinide 200 mg/day for 3 months	Limited
Papadimitrakopoulou et al. (113)	13-cRA or BC + RP	111	162	13-cRA 0.25 mg (1 year)–0.5 mg (2 years)/kg/day or BC 50 mg/day + RP 25 kIU/D for 3 years or RP 25 kIU/day for 3 years	Negative
William et al. (114)	Fenretinide	11	15	Fenretinide 900 mg/m² twice daily days 1–7, repeated every 3 weeks with four 3-week cycles (trial closed early; 15 subjects out of 25)	Limited
Scardina et al. (115)	Isotretinoin	111	40	0.05% or 0.18% isotretinoin BD for 3 months	Positive
Singh et al. (116)	Lycopene	111	58	Lycopene 4 or 8 mg/day, placebo	Positive
Nagao et al. (280)	β-carotene	111	46	β-carotene 10 mg + vitamin C 500 mg versus vitamin C 50 mg (placebo)	Negative

Abbreviations: 13-cRA: 13-*cis*-retinoid acid; RP: retinyl palmitate; BC: beta carotene.
[a] Used as a mucoadhesive tablet.
[b] Used on natural retinoid resistant leukoplakia subjects.

just three studies. None of the studies showed any benefit to prevent cancer development."

Other agents used in clinical trials to halt the malignant transformation of oral leukoplakia include black raspberry extract, green tea extracts, Bowman–Birk inhibitor, COX inhibitors, curcumin and PPARγ agonists. The modes of action of these natural agents have been discussed recently (117–119). COX-2 expression is noted to increase progressively through the early stages of "premalignancy" (120). NSAIDs and selective COX-2 inhibitors have antiproliferative activity and promote apoptosis. Celecoxib (268), used in several chemopreventive trials, is a selective COX-2 inhibitor (283–285). COX inhibitors have been shown to be effective in colon cancer. Curcumin is a potent inhibitor of COX-2 (121), NF-κB and AP-1 transcription factors (122). Green tea extracts contain several plant polyphenols, the most abundant being epigallocatechin-3-gallate. Thiazolidinediones, along with other anti-diabetic agents given to diabetic patients, reduced the risk of head and neck cancers by 41%–55% in one study (123), which justifies further investigation. Their mode of action has been ascribed to activation of PPARγ ligands (124).

Outcomes from some of these trials are listed in Table 23.15. The results derived from these studies appear more encouraging compared with the retinoid and carotenoid trials.

STUDIES ON ORAL SUBMUCOUS FIBROSIS

Medical management of oral submucous fibrosis was reviewed by Kerr et al. (132) and Chole et al. (133). None of the agents tried in small trials until 2011 had any significant effect on disease control or malignant transformation. Multiple vitamin and mineral supplementations appear to give some symptomatic relief and improvement in mouth opening (e.g. (134)). More recent trials with curcumin (135,136) and aloe vera (137,138) also appear to give symptomatic relief, but have not been tested for long enough to examine their role in cancer prevention.

TERTIARY PREVENTION BY FOOD SUPPLEMENTS

Following successful treatment of the primary oral cancer, 20%–30% of patients may develop a second primary tumor

Table 23.15 Other agents used in chemoprevention trials on oral leukoplakia (data published since 2000)

Compound	References	Agent	Phase	*n*	Regimen	Outcome
COX inhibitors	Mulshine et al. (125)	NSAID	IIb	57	Ketorolac[a] 10 mL 0.1% oral rinse BD for 90 days	Negative
	Papadimitrakopoulou et al. (126)	NSAID	II	50	Celecoxib 100 mg or 200 mg BD versus placebo for 3 months	Negative
	Wirth et al. (213)	NSAID	I	22	Celecoxib 400 mg BD for 3–12 months	Improved biomarkers
Green tea extracts	Tsao et al. [127]	Green tea extract	II	41	GTE 500, 750 or 1000 mg/m^2 OD versus placebo for 12 weeks	Positive?
Black raspberry extract	Shumway et al. (114,128)	Black raspberry extract	II	29	0.5 g 10% gel[b] QDS for 6 weeks	Positive in a subset
	Mallery et al. (286)	FD black raspberries	II	40	FD BRE 0.5 g QDS versus placebo for 12 weeks	Positive
PPARγ agonists	Rhodus et al. (129)	PPARγ agonists	IIa	44	Pioglitazone 45 mg QDS for 3 months	Positive
Curcumin	Cheng et al. (130)	Curcumin	I	7	Curcumin 500–12,000 mg/day QDS for 3 months	2/7 improved
	Rai et al. (131)	Curcumin	I	100	Curcumin 1 g/day for 130–190 days	Positive
	Kuriakose et al. (276)	Curcumin	III	137	Curcumin 3.6 g/day for 6 months	Positive in some subgroups
Soya bean	Amstrong (287)	Bowman–Birk inhibitor	IIb	89	3 g Bowman–Birk inhibitor BD 6 months versus placebo	Negative

Abbreviations: GTE: green tea extract; FD: freeze-dried; BRE: black raspberry extract.

[a] As a mouthwash.

[b] As a bioadhesive gel.

Table 23.16 Chemoprevention trials for secondary prevention of head and neck cancer using retinoids or carotenoids (data published since 2000)

References	Agent	Phase	*n*	Regimen	Outcome
van Zandwijk et al. (142)	RP	III	2592 (60%)	RP 300 kIU/day for 1 year 150 kIU/day for 1 year versus none	Negative
Mayne et al. (2000)	BC	III	264	BC 50 mg/day versus placebo for 90 months	Negative
Toma et al. (143)	BC	III	214	BC 75 mg QDS versus no treatment for 3 years	Negative
Toma et al. (282)	13-cRA	III	267	13-cRA 0.5 mg/kg/day versus control for 3 years	Negative
Perry et al. (144)	13-cRA	III	151	13-cRA 1 mg/kg/day versus 0.5 mg/kg/day versus placebo for 1 year	Negative
Khuri et al. (145)	13-cRA	III	1190	13-cRA 30 mg/day versus placebo for 3 years	Negative

Abbreviations: 13-cRA: 13-*cis*-retinoid acid; RP: retinyl palmitate; BC: β-carotene.

(SPT) in the oral cavity, head and neck region or in the rest of aerodigestive track by 20 years (139). Close to 10% may develop an SPT in the first 5 years of follow-up (140). Occurrence of an SPT is an important cause of morbidity and mortality. Hong et al. (141) hypothesized that isotretinoin supplements (13-*cis*-retinoic acid—an analogue of vitamin A) would prevent a second cancer in head and neck cancer patients. Since their original work, several chemopreventive trials have attempted to reduce the occurrence of SPTs. Trials testing retinoids or β-carotene to prevent an SPT reported since the year 2000 are listed in Table 23.16. Other agents used include green tea extracts (146) and, more recently, one trial used fruit and vegetable concentrates (147). Although Hong et al. (141), with high doses of isotretinoin (50–100 mg/m^2/day), showed clinical benefit, none of these later reported randomized controlled trials showed any significant reduction in SPTs compared with no treatment or placebo agents. A phase III trial that used vitamin E (α-tocopherol 400 IU/day) versus placebo also reported negative results and worse outcomes than the placebo arm (148).

Poor locoregional control leads to significant morbidity and high mortality rates within the first 5 years following surgical treatment of oral SCC. Isotretinoin oral rinses, as a method of chemoprevention for recurrent oral cavity SCC, was recently reported by Kadakia et al. (149) and found to be associated with lower recurrence rates in two of the study groups.

FURTHER STUDIES ON CHEMOPREVENTION

Based on the data accrued from the many published trials summarized in this section, a range of new clinical trials are registered with one or other of the national and/or international clinical trials registers and are underway. Anti-diabetic agents, notably metformin, are being tested in multicenter clinical trials in the U.S.A. Due to the systemic toxicities of retinoids encountered in past trials, new approaches are being explored to deliver these agents topically. Instead of relying on clinical "improvements" and histology to assess outcomes, functional biomarkers are gradually being introduced, such as to explore reversal of genetic abnormalities (150).

PREVENTION OF HUMAN PAPILLOMAVIRUS-RELATED HEAD AND NECK CANCER

DETECTION OF HUMAN PAPILLOMAVIRUS-ASSOCIATED CANCERS

In recent times, it has been recommended to perform human papillomavirus (HPV) testing for all head and neck cancer patients, especially those with oropharyngeal SCCs (OPSCCs), as standard practice. HPV-associated Head and Neck Squamous Cell Carcinomas (HNSCC), especially OPSCCs, constitute a distinct tumor entity with distinct clinical features and, usually, better prognosis. Nevertheless, heterogeneity in both clinical and biological behaviors exists (151,152). Histopathological study using hematoxylin and eosin staining is the oldest and still most commonly practiced method for diagnosis and prognosis. A range of biomarkers has been used for the detection of biologically active HPV infection in SCC. Among these, p16^{INK4A} immunohistochemistry is used frequently as a surrogate marker (153). However, 10%–20% of p16-positive tumors do not show evidence of HPV when screened by polymerase chain reaction (PCR) (154–157). Ideally, p16 immunohistochemistry should not be used as a diagnostic tool alone, but rather in conjunction with a nucleic acid-based assay (158,159). The diagnostic assays available for screening for HPV-DNA in tissues vary considerably in sensitivity and specificity. It is important to select a technique that is highly sensitive, well standardized, easily accessible, economically viable and has a short turnaround time. Southern blot is one of the oldest and still most reliable techniques; it is highly sensitive and with the ability to identify specific HPV types (160). Unfortunately, it is not suitable for routine clinical use as it is time consuming and requires a large quantity of cellular DNA. *In situ* hybridization (ISH) has high specificity but is less sensitive than Southern blotting: Southern blotting has 76% sensitivity and 87% specificity, while ISH has shown 50% sensitivity and 93% specificity (161). Furthermore, sensitivity may vary in different disease categories: ISH is more sensitive when applied to condylomatous tissue, but less sensitive in invasive neoplasms (161). PCR can be used when only a small amount of sample is available and HPV loads are low. However, false-positive results may be an issue if strict control over contamination is not maintained (162,163).

For PCR, studies have shown that the combination of two sets of degenerate primers (MY09/11 and GP5+/6+) (164), amplifying fragments of the widely conserved HPV *L1* gene in "nested PCR," is more efficient for the detection of HPV in oropharyngeal cancer tissues with low viral load compared to conventional PCR (165,166). All of these methods detect the presence of the HPV genome, and show association, not causation; in other words, the presence of the virus does not prove that it is integrated into the host genome and is driving the cancer. Ideally, the gold standard for identifying clinically relevant HPV would be detecting transcriptionally active viral oncoprotein *E6* and *E7* mRNA in fresh or frozen tissue (Westra, 2014). Two commercial assays are available for this: the PreTect® Proofer assay and the APTIMA® assay (167,168). These function by transcription-mediated amplification of the full lengths of the *E6* and *E7* oncogenes. They require good-quality mRNA, which can be extracted from fresh materials or even tissues stored at −80°C for a short period, but which is not possible in formalin-fixed and paraffin-embedded tissue, as mRNA degrades during the fixation process. They are unlikely to be used for routine diagnosis (169).

Direct bi-directional sequencing of an amplicon of *L1* detects any HPV type present, but knowing whether and what high risk (hr) types are involved is important. To detect multiple HPV types in a mixed infection, the current U.S. Food and Drug Administration (FDA)-approved method, the Hybrid Capture® II system (Digene Corp.), is available. However, this can only detect hrHPV and lrHPV types as a group (170). The array-based HPV genotyping method or CAPH (Clinical Arrays Papillomavirus Humano) (170) has been shown to be capable of detecting single or mixed infections with up to 35 HPV types (20 hrHPVs and 15 lrHPVs). In future, next-generation sequencing will play a greater role in HPV genotyping as it examines the entire HPV genome and can detect any HPV type present, even in a mixed infection (171,172). This is currently costly and time consuming.

PROPHYLACTIC VACCINES

Since HPV-positive carcinomas are induced by a viral infection and the virus produces a range of foreign antigens, the host should be capable of mounting an immune response against the neoplasm. Humoral immune responses against viral antigens E6 and E7 are frequently found in HPV-positive cancer patients and can be correlated with increased survival, making both preventive vaccination and immunotherapy potentially effective. The concept behind the existing prophylactic vaccines is to stimulate the immune system to elicit an adequate neutralizing antibody response *prior to exposure* to hrHPVs, so that infection is less likely to take place. It is also expected that this effect would subsequently abolish the development of invasive cancers. Two *prophylactic* HPV vaccines have been available on the market for sometime with U.S. FDA approval. The first was the quadrivalent vaccine Gardasil introduced by Merk & Co. in 2006. This has shown 98% efficacy in protection against acquisition of HPV types 6,11,16 and 18 and a substantial reduction in the incidence of anal, cervical and vaginal "precancers" (173,174). The second HPV vaccine is Cervarix, a bivalent vaccine that has a protective effect against the hr types HPV-16 and HPV-18-associated pre-cancers with a high efficacy. In fact, both vaccines provide protection against ~70% of the cancer-causing virus types, while Gardasil also provides protection against genital warts. The other major difference is that while virus-like particles, which are the basis of both vaccines, are highly immunogenic, each vaccine uses different adjuvants to elicit immune responses. These vaccines have been adopted by most countries and have already proven to be highly successful in the prevention of HPV-associated cervical cancer. Things are moving rapidly in this area of science: a nine-valent vaccine was introduced in 2015 (GARDASIL®9) and is now being evaluated in several countries. Unfortunately, all HPV vaccines have lower efficacy when individuals already have an HPV-16 and/or HPV-18-associated cancer (174,175) and are not a viable treatment strategy. Encouraging impacts of the present prophylactic vaccines and vaccination programs around the world on the incidence of head and neck cancer are now emerging.

Currently, a two-dose schedule is recommended (176); however, vaccine coverage among all eligible groups remains low in most countries, with males representing the most under-vaccinated population, despite the increased risk for oropharyngeal cancers among all men (177–179). A comprehensive report from the U.S.A. suggests that ~40% of girls and ~22% of boys aged 13–17 years had received all doses in the series in 2014 (180). Among 10,663 participants, approximately 69% ($n = 7321$) were female. Among females, 56% had received at least one dose of the HPV vaccine. In contrast, only 8% of males had received at least one dose (180). This is well below the desired goal of 80% coverage of both girls and boys across the U.S.A. as specified by the Healthy Population 2020 program. The recommendation for HPV vaccination among men was not issued in the U.S.A. until 2011. Another study from the U.S.A. reports on the ten states that had completed the HPV vaccination module by 2013. Young men aged 18–26 were studied ($n = 1624$), of whom only 16.5% reported at least one dose of HPV vaccine (181). However, in Australia, the school-based HPV vaccination program has a good success rate. In 2013, female coverage for one or more dose was ~80%, with that for males aged 12–13 years being 74%–79%. In fact, the three-dose complete course of HPV vaccination in females around the age of 15 years has consistently been ~71% (182).

Apart from gay and bisexual men, to the disappointment of some, a senior advisory committee to the Government of the UK has recently recommended on grounds of cost-effectiveness that boys be not routinely vaccinated in that country. It is argued that the success of the existing policy is establishing effective herd immunity (Joint Committee on Vaccination and Immunisation: https://www.gov.uk/government/uploads/system/uploads/attachment_data/file/630125/Extending_HPV_Vaccination.pdf).

Awareness and knowledge of HPV are important to vaccine uptake (183,184). A higher perceived risk of acquiring HPV is associated with higher perceived benefits and intentions to vaccinate, both among individuals (185,186) and parents (187). However, knowledge and awareness are highly variable (188–190), and recently published research found that only 68% of respondents from a nationally representative sample of U.S. adults had heard of HPV and the HPV vaccine (189). Studies show that most individuals know little about the association between HPV and non-cervical cancers (191–194).

A large randomized study ($n = 4{,}055$) from Norway shows that prophylactic administration of a quadrivalent HPV vaccine was efficacious in preventing external genital lesions infected with HPV-6, -11, -16 and/or -18 in males aged 16–26 years (RR 0.33, 95% CI: 0.25–0.44) (https://www.fhi.no/en/publ/2015/effect-of-hpv-vaccination-of-boys/). Among the external genital lesions, the outcome that predominates is reduction in the incidence of genital warts: significant prevention by vaccination was observed (RR 0.39, 95% CI: 0.25–0.58). This shows that the vaccine is effective against several HPV types. However, the study was only conducted for 3 years and a longer follow-up is required to demonstrate efficacy on precancerous lesions, cancer prevalence and cancer-related mortality for penile, anal and oropharyngeal cancers. A similar study from England also showed a reduction in the rates of genital warts among young women and young men (aged 15–19 years) by 30.6% and 25.4%, respectively, when they were administered the bivalent vaccine (195).

Even though many countries have now started national vaccination programs for girls, and some such as Australia for boys, we will only have evidence on the true effect on cancer outcomes 20–30 years from now; long-term follow-up data for the vaccinated populations are essential. Other issues are costs of prophylactic vaccines, which are very expensive for developing parts of the world, and these vaccines have an as yet not fully determined protective effect against HPV-associated HNSCCs. The Centers for Disease Control and Prevention (CDC) website keeps the public well informed (https://www.cdc.gov/cancer/hpv/basic_info/hpv_oropharyngeal.htm).

THERAPEUTIC VACCINES

Therapeutic vaccines aim to treat HPV-infected cells, and this might be achieved by developing a T-cell immune response that can recognize and eliminate HPV-infected cells. Because the HPV-16 *E6* and *E7* genes are uniquely expressed by virus-infected cells, a specific therapeutic vaccine is theoretically feasible and desirable. High frequencies of T regulatory cells, which inhibit cellular immune responses, are often found in HPV-positive HNSCC tissues. Thus, using a low dose of cyclophosphamide (200 mg/m^2) with a therapeutic vaccine might effectively reduce T regulatory cell activity, as this has been demonstrated to increase the efficiency of Granulocyte-macrophage colony-stimulating factor (GM-CSF) tumor vaccines in breast cancer patients (197).

From current knowledge, although vaccines are very effective in the prevention of HPV infection, there is still limited evidence of an effect on reducing the incidence of HNSCC. Recently, some countries have started vaccinating young boys. The true efficacy of prophylactic vaccines against head and neck cancer will take several decades to become clear. Further, these vaccines are not likely to be effective in individuals who already have an HPV-associated cancer, although work is proceeding on therapeutic vaccines. New approaches are required.

Sequencing of the genome has identified areas that may be fruitful for the treatment of advanced cervical cancers. Targets in the PI3K/AKT pathway, EGFR- and HER2-directed therapy, immunotherapy and hormonal therapy are promising areas for future research. Most promising is the concept of targeting the driver oncogenes within cervical cancer and those HPV-driven HNSCC, namely the E6 and E7 proteins expressed by the virus itself. Promising research using peptides of these proteins to immunize patients have indicated a ~50% response rate (196). Could a promising approach be to suppress production of E6 and E7 proteins by siRNA (small interfering RNA) therapy? siRNAs can act as direct anti-virals by targeting the mRNA sequences of viral oncogenes. It is a highly specific therapy with few side effects and overcomes the non-specific toxicity to surrounding cells. siRNAs targeting HPV-infected cells lead to induction of Toll-like receptors, which in turn upregulate interferons, with consequent enhancement of innate immunity. Further the activation of T-cell immunity and an increased response to cytotoxic T cells ultimately induces apoptosis (197). The role of siRNAs in treating cervical cancer, effectively by knocking down *E6* and *E7* oncogenes, has already been demonstrated in *in vitro* and *in vivo* models (198,199). Recent DNA vaccines that express inactive versions of *E7* also have shown a 53% response rate (200). Such a therapy could be effective for HPV-associated head and neck cancer. Further, preclinical trials using siRNAs to silence *E6*/*E7* show profound loss of viability of these cells. Using new genome-editing technology to remove them is a promising approach for the future (Figures 23.7 and 23.8) (201).

SECONDARY PREVENTION: SCREENING FOR ORAL CANCER AND POTENTIALLY MALIGNANT LESIONS

Screening for disease is a very precise science (202) and must follow established principles (Table 23.17) (203). Oral cancer meets some, but not all, of these criteria and, although there are clear potential advantages (Table 23.18), there are also potential disadvantages (Table 23.19).

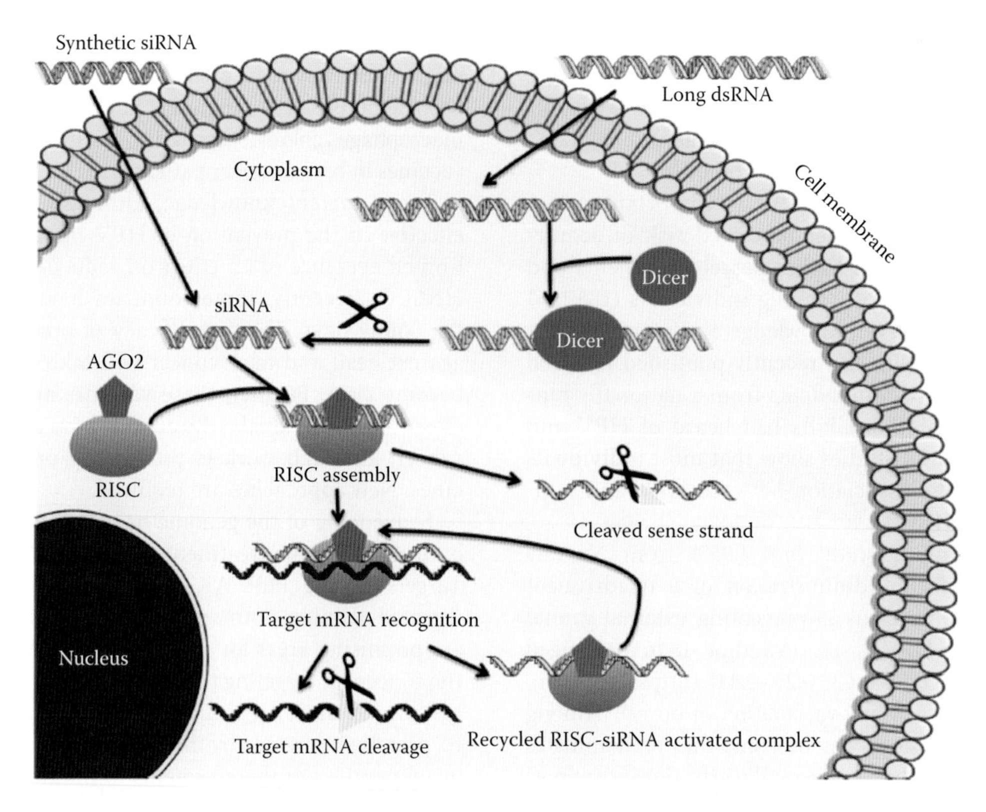

Figure 23.7 The gene silencing mechanism of siRNA. A synthetic siRNA and a long double-stranded RNA (dsRNA) are processed by Dicer to form siRNA in the cytoplasm. This activated siRNA associates with the RNA-inducing protein complex (RISC) and mediates target specificity for subsequent cleavage of mRNA. The RISC is recycled and induces multiple rounds of silencing. (Reproduced from Shaikh MH et al. *Oral Oncol* 2017;68:9–19, with permission (201).)

The rationale for screening for oral cancer is based on the fact that these malignancies are asymptomatic and localized for a period of their natural history and are often preceded by a potentially malignant disorder, often with recognizable lesions such as leukoplakia, erythroplakia and submucous fibrosis, when they can be detected by simple oral examination. This is important because habit intervention (204), dietary intervention (205) and surgical treatment (206,207) can result in their resolution or elimination.

However, *population screening* for oral cancer cannot be recommended (208,209), because there is inadequate understanding of the natural history of this group of disorders (210) and there is insufficient evidence for the utility (211) or cost-effectiveness of screening whole populations. Oral cancer screening programs have been carried out on several hundreds of thousands of individuals in developing countries (mostly Sri Lanka, India and Cuba) and several thousands of individuals in developed countries (mostly the U.S.A., the UK and Italy) and the evidence from these is reviewed by Warnakulasuriya and Johnson (212) (from which Table 23.20 is derived) and by Franceschi et al. (210). A meta-analysis of these studies has just been published (214). In the high-incidence parts of the world, a substantial proportion of suspicious lesions has been found (ranging from 2% to 16% in South Asia), but compliance of patients to attend follow-up was poor. In the West, the yield is substantially lower. For example, the largest group studied was in Minnesota and consisted of over 23,000 adults, over age 30, whose mouths were examined by dentists between 1957 and 1972. Although more than 10% of those screened had an oral lesion, these were mostly benign; "precancer" was encountered in 2.9% and cancer in less than 0.1%. A very large, community-based, controlled oral cancer screening trial in Kerala, southern India, has demonstrated that lives can be saved in this way (215). This study, and an update of the literature, can be accessed through the World Bank's Disease Control Program series (http://dcp-3.org/sites/default/files/chapters/DCP3 Cancer_Ch 5.pdf).

Logically, a stronger case can be made for *targeting screening* to at-risk populations—in the context of oral cancer, perhaps to smokers and heavy drinkers over the age of, say, 40. Such individuals can be identified from the records of family medical practitioners or occupational health records. Even so, studies of this kind conducted in the UK (216) and in Japan (217,218) have shown high non-attendance rates for the initial oral examination. This, together with the still low prevalence of lesions, makes even this type of screening of dubious utility. In a series of studies conducted by ear, nose and throat (ENT) specialists in Northern Italy between 1994 and 1998, the yield was substantially increased by adding inspections of the pharynx and larynx (with appropriate instrumentation) and aiming the program at smokers and/or heavy drinkers, relying on general practitioners for the identification of these high-risk

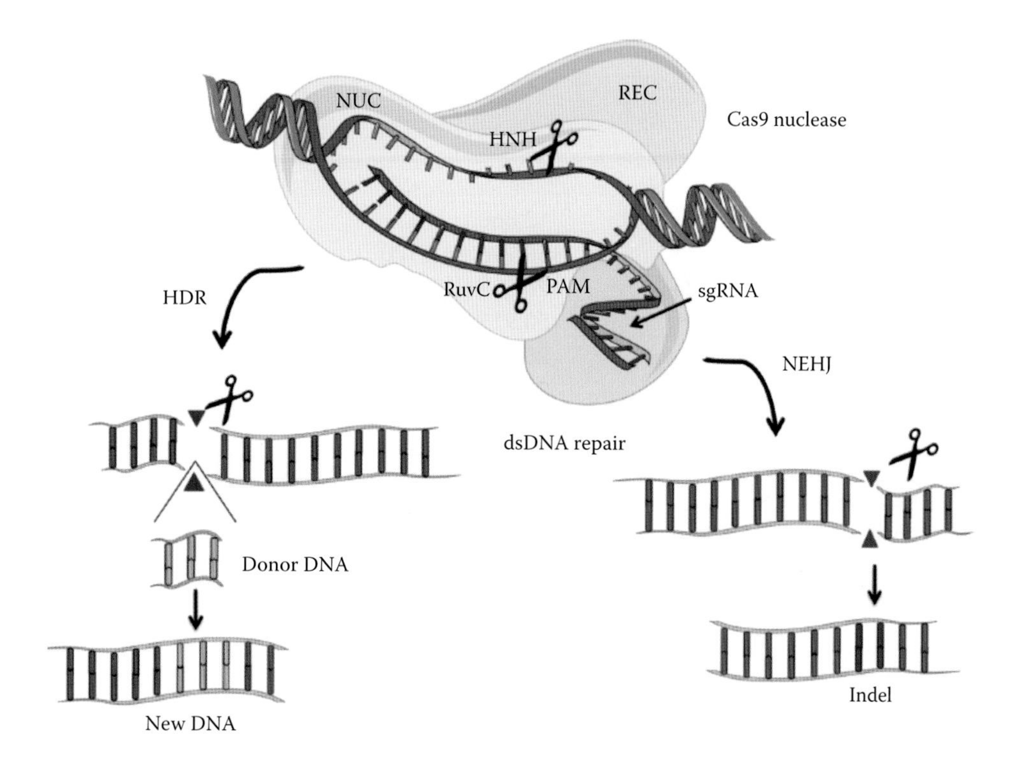

Figure 23.8 The mechanism of CRISPR/Cas9 gene editing, which is attracting enormous current interest. Single guided RNA (sgRNA, processed by tracrRNA-crRNA) directs the Cas9 nuclease to a target sequence that would consist of a short DNA sequence tag (protospacer adjunct motif [PAM]), where it unzips DNA complementary to the sgRNA. Concurrently, the recognition (REC) and nuclease lobes (NUC) enclose the DNA target sequence and the RuvC and HNH nuclease domains initiate site-specific double-strand breaks (DSBs). The DSBs are then repaired by either of two DNA repair mechanisms: non-homologous end joining (NHEJ), resulting in insertion of small deletions (indels) at the targeted site; or homologous directed repair (HDR), which creates precise mutations and knock-ins. (Reproduced from Shaikh MH et al. *Oral Oncol* 2017;68:9–19, with permission (201).)

Table 23.17 Screening for disease

The basic principles concerning screening for disease are:

- The condition should be an important health problem whose natural history is understood
- There should be an accepted and proven intervention
- There should be a suitable and accepted diagnostic test
- The cost of screening should be balanced in relation to other healthcare expenditures

Source: Wilson JMG, Jungner G. *Principles and Practice of Screening for Disease. Public Health Paper No. 34.* Geneva: WHO, 1968 (203).

Table 23.18 Potential advantages of screening for oral cancer and precancer

- Reduced mortality
- Reduced incidence of invasive cancers
- Improved prognosis for individual patients
- Reduced morbidity for cases treated at early stages
- Identification of high-risk groups and opportunities for intervention
- Reassurance for those screened negative
- Cost savings

Table 23.19 Potential disadvantages of screening for oral cancer and precancer

- Detection of cases that are already incurable may increase morbidity for some patients
- Unnecessary treatment of those potentially malignant lesions that may not have progressed
- Psychological trauma for those with a false-positive screen
- Reinforcement of bad habits among some individuals screened negative
- Costs

groups. Even so, only 1,564 out of 4,419 (35%) individuals complied with the examination. This yielded 152 (9.7%) "precancerous" lesions (mostly low-risk flat leukoplakias) and 20 (1.3%) cancers at any of these upper aerodigestive sites. A better participation rate can be obtained when oral screening is part of general health screening (219).

The Oral Cancer Screening Group at the Eastman Dental Institute, London, carried out an outstanding series of investigations several years ago. They have shown that the sensitivity and specificity of lesion detection is comparable to that of oral examination by the use of artificial intelligence

Table 23.20 Results of oral cancer/precancer screening programs

Investigators[a]	Year	Country	Sample	Cancer		Precancer	
				n	Rate (per 100,000)	*n*	Rate (%)
Ross and Gross	1971	U.S.A.	12,868	1	8	339	2.6
Folsom et al.	1972	U.S.A.	158,996	120	75	802	0.5
Axell et al.	1976	Sweden	20,333	1	5	732	3.6
Mehta et al.	1969	India	50,915	26	51	881	1.7
Warnakulasuriya et al.	1983	Sri Lanka	28,295	4	14	1,220	4.2
Bouquot and Gorlin	1986	U.S.A.	23,616	22	93	682	2.9
Ikeda et al.	1991	Japan	3,131	None		77	2.5
Banoczy et al.	1991	Hungary	7,820	1	13	104	1.3

Source: Warnakulasuriya KAAS, Johnson NW. *Eur J Cancer Prev* 1996;5:93–8 (212).
Note: Includes benign keratoses in some surveys.
[a] See source reference.

Table 23.21 Screening for oral cancer and potentially malignant lesions

Location	*n*	Lesion prevalence (%)	Sensitivity	Specificity
Dental hospital	1,042	3.00	0.81	0.99
Medical practice	985	2.22	0.64	0.99
Company headquarters	309	5.50	0.71	0.99
Neural network	365	2.74	0.80	0.77

Note: Based on clinical and digital examination of the oral mucosa by dentists, with confirmation by an oral medicine specialist. The first three studies provided the data for training the neural network.

systems to compute all known risk factors for oral cancer (Table 23.21) (220).

In a simulation model, estimates of quality-adjusted life-years and of lives gained from screening were obtained and compared with the status quo of no screening. Participants were a notional population of 100,000 adults of average age 55 years and 20 years' life expectancy. The basic assumptions were a 50% attendance of the eligible population, a prevalence of oral cancer of 0.098% and of precancer of 2.57%, a positive predictive value of the screening test of 0.67 and a negative predictive value of 0.99. The cancers were assumed to be 40% stage 1 and 60% stage 2+ without screening and 60% stage 1 and 40% stage 2+ with screening. Patients with oral precancer were assumed to have a survival of 19.2 years, with stage 1 cancer 14.6 years and with stage 2+ cancer 10.8 years. The public's perceived utilities were 0.92 for precancer and 0.88 and 0.68 for stage 1 and stage 2+ cancer, respectively, compared to a utility of 1.0 for health. One cycle of the program was modeled over 1 year in a dental practice setting. Under these circumstances, the costs and benefits obtained are shown in Table 23.22.

This estimate of a cost per life saved by screening a high-risk population for oral cancer, £8,333, compares very favorably with costs estimated for other, more common, cancers, for which population screening programs already exist in many countries (Table 23.23). Indeed, the longest-established cancer screening programs in the world—those for cancer of the uterine cervix—are extremely expensive and controversial. They have never been evaluated by means of a randomized controlled trial and, although changes in incidence make it difficult to estimate the effect of a screening program quantitatively, the impact on this disease is less than that which might be thought feasible. These observations apply to screening programs using traditional cytology on Papanicolaou stained smears. There is now widespread replacement of these by screening for high risk HPV in cervical specimens, which will improve utility greatly.

The use of the most powerful risk factors specific to the population concerned can produce simple models for the detection of subjects at risk, as we have recently shown in Sri Lanka (221) and in the Pune district in India (222) (see Table 23.24 and Figure 23.9). However individuals at high risk are

Table 23.22 Hypothetical costs and benefits of oral cancer screening programs (assuming the cost of a screening examination to be £5)

Screening of whole population

- Cost of screening 100,000 = £500,000
- Lives saved = 5.6
- Cost per life saved = £89,286

Screening a high-risk population

- Cost of screening 25,000 = £125,000
- Lives saved = 15
- Cost per life saved = £8,333

Table 23.23 Costs per life saved for cancer screening programs

Breast cancer	£80,000
Cervical cancer	£300,000
Colon cancer	£6,500
Oral cancer (high-risk)	£8,883

Source: Roberts CJ et al. *Lancet* 1985;i:89–91 (118).

identified, bringing them to early management remains challenging everywhere in the world.

Opportunistic screening, namely offering a screening test for an unsuspected disorder at a time when a person presents to a doctor—or a dentist or any other suitably trained primary healthcare professional (223)—for another reason, is rational and cost-effective. This is the basis of the screening examination of the oral soft tissues recommended at every dental visit, perhaps also at periodic visits to a family physician. We have the manpower available—ourselves as trained specialists in what constitutes normal and abnormal tissues—and it need take only 3 minutes for a thorough visual examination of the whole oral mucosa. This we have a duty to perform. The clinical identification of suspect lesions by visual observation and manual palpation is a skill that can be taught to any primary healthcare worker, even those with quite basic training such as the medical auxiliaries found in some developing countries (224). The most encouraging outcome of such studies so far published comes from the Oral Cancer Case Finding Program in Cuba. Between 1983 and 1990, 10,167,999 patients were examined nationwide when they attended stomatological clinics: only 8,259 out of 30,478 patients (27%) with suspect lesions complied with referral and, of these, there were 3,220 potentially malignant lesions, 581 SCCs and 127 other malignancies. However, although no doubt at considerable cost, the program was shown to be effective because there was "downstaging" of the cancers seen: stage I lesions rising from 22.8% to 48.2% and stages II, III and IV lesions falling from 77.2% to 51.8% (225). This study used specially trained stomatologists. In spite of their lower cost and comparable accuracy to dentists, use of auxiliaries for population screening still cannot be recommended because there is no evidence yet available of the efficacy of such an approach in reducing the incidence and mortality of oral cancer.

Table 23.24 Risk factors for oral cancer in Pune District of India, which give rise to the ROC curve in Figure 23.9

Risk factor	Adjusted OR[a]	Risk scores
Smoking		
Never	1.00 (Ref)	0
Ever	2.75	3
Chewing tobacco		
Never	1.00 (Ref)	0
Ever	7.81	8
Mishri use		
Never	1.00 (Ref)	0
Ever	1.69	2
Second hand exposure to tobacco smoke		
Never	1.00 (Ref)	0
Ever	2.84	3
Drinking alcohol		
Never	1.00 (Ref)	0
Ever	1.60	2
Spices in food		
Less spicy	1.00 (Ref)	0
Very spicy	1.69	2
Type of housing		
Pucca	1.00 (Ref)	0
Kutcha	3.22	3
Body Mass Index		
18.50–24.99: Normal	1.00 (Ref)	0
<18.50: Underweight	2.80	3

Source: From Gupta B, Kumar N, Johnson NW. *J Oral Pathol Med* 2017;46(6):465–71, with permission (222).

[a] OR, odds ratio.

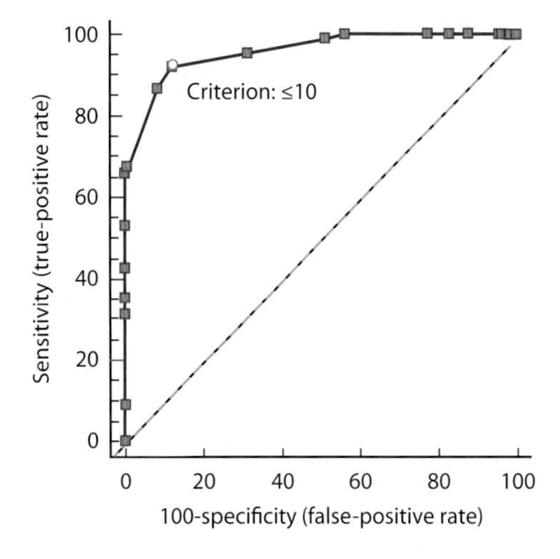

Figure 23.9 Receiver operator characteristics curve for our risk factor model in Pune, India. The criteria score is derived by adding the scores listed there for each individual subject. (From Gupta B, Kumar N, Johnson NW. *J Oral Pathol Med* 2017;46(6):465–71, with permission (222).)

DIAGNOSTIC AIDS FOR SCREENING STUDIES AND PRACTICE

These have been illustrated and evaluated in detail in Chapter 3. There are many optical and molecular methods under investigation. The following summary is retained from the first edition in order that important principles remain in context here.

Toluidine blue

The use of Toluidine blue (tolonium chloride) dye as a mouthwash or topical application continues to receive

Table 23.25 Evaluation of Toluidine blue staining as a screen for oral cancer

Study	Number of reported evaluations	Sensitivity (%)	Specificity (%)	False positives	False negatives
Trials involving a single application of stain					
Nibel and Chomet (1964)	11[a] (20 patients)	100	NR	NR	0/11
Shedd et al. (1965)	44[b] (50 patients)	100	85	2/13	0/31
Shedd et al. (1967)	62 (23 volunteers)	100	(a) 85[c]	3/20	0/42
			(b) 94	0/23	
Myers (1970)	71	98	100	0/19	1/52
	100L[d]	NR	75	18/71	NR
Srivastava and Mathus (1971)	100P	NR	94	6/97	NR
	Combined	NR	86	24/168	NR
Rosen et al. (1971)	45	50	50	20/39	3/6
Vahidy et al. (1972)	1,030	86	76	131/549	66/481
	(+160 cases[e] excluded)			(+106 doubtful)	(+54 doubtful)
Reddy et al. (1973)	490	99	83	6/37	2/453
Sigurdson and Willen (1975)	54	100	87	2/23	0/31
Barrellier et al. (1982)	115 (111 patients)	100	93	7/105	0/6
Silverman et al. (1984)	132	98	70	10/33	2/99
Epstein and Scully (1992)	59	93	63	7/19	3/40
Barellier et al. (1993)	235	95.7	85.9	30/212	1/23
Warnakulasuriya and Johnson (1996)	86 (102 patients)	100	62	11/29[f]	0/18
Portugal et al. (1996)	50	100	86	6/44	0/6
Epstein el al. (1997)	81 (46 patients)[g]	100	52[h]	26/53	0/28
Total	2,948				
Trials involving a second application of stain or a period for resolution of transient inflammatory lesions					
Pizer and Dubois (1979)	255	NR	99	3/248	0/7
Mashberg (1980)	235	93	92	11/130	7/105
Mashberg (1981, 1983)[i]	179, (a) rinse	89	91	9/98	9/81
	179, (b) direct application	98	88	12/98	2/81
Moyer et al. (1986)	76 (75 patients)	NR	92	7/76	NA
Total	924				

Note: NR: not reported; NA: not applicable.
[a] Malignant lesions only reported on.
[b] Results from 44 patients given.
[c] (a) Specificity with respect to negatively staining patients; (b) specificity including volunteers.
[d] 100 patients with lesions (L); 100 randomly selected patients (P).
[e] Excluded as stain reading doubtful.
[f] This includes precancer.
[g] Treated patients with a 33% prevalence rate of new lesions.
[h] Benign and all levels of dysplasia regarded as negative.
[i] Figures counted twice as two evaluations per patient were carried out.

much attention as an aid to the diagnosis of oral cancer and potentially malignant lesions. It has a place, with appropriate training, in screening of high-risk subjects and in helping to define the site for biopsy. There have been a number of clinical trials using Toluidine blue and these are summarized in Table 23.25 (226). The table shows that the method has good sensitivity, with a very low false-negative rate. However, it is important to realize that most of these studies have taken both overtly invasive carcinomas and severe (or even moderate) dysplasias as true-positive lesions under the umbrella "oral cancer." Although 100% of invasive lesions will stain, most studies show that only 50% or less of dysplasias are detected. The false-positive rate is likely to be very low in patients presenting with perfectly healthy mucosae, but areas of inflammation, ulceration or erosion stain positively whatever their cause. False positives may be as high as 48% following a single application. Repeating the stain 10–14 days later to allow for the healing of acute ulcerative or traumatic lesions has been shown to reduce the false-positive rate to 11%. The dorsum of the tongue always stains positively due to retention of dye in crevices between the papillae, making it of limited value for studying lesions

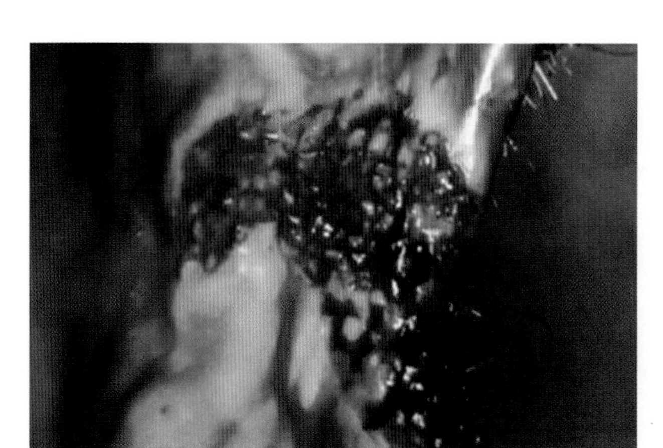

Figure 23.10 Speckled leukoplakia at the commissure heavily stained by Toluidine blue.

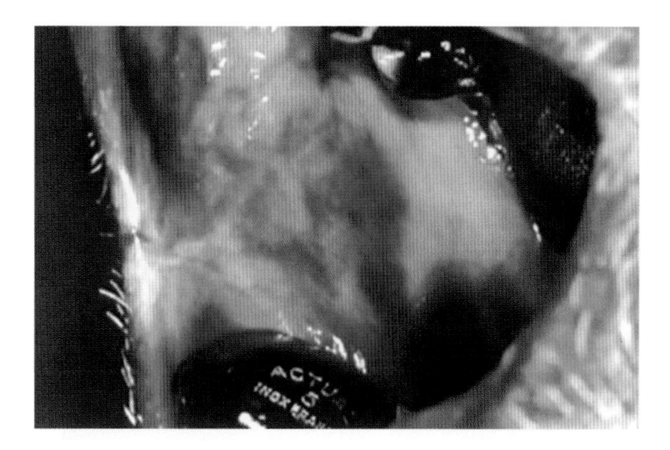

Figure 23.11 Area of atrophic mucosa stained by Toluidine blue. This, on biopsy, proved to show significant epithelial dysplasia.

at this site, unless the lesion arises out of an atrophic area. Likewise, crevices and cracks within thick keratotic plaques retain dye and produce a false-positive result.

Thus, good clinical judgment, training and experience in the use of Toluidine blue ensure rational use of this diagnostic aid. Biopsy remains the gold standard for the diagnosis of oral cancer and potentially malignant lesions. False positives are of less concern than false negatives. All positive stain reactions require biopsy, as do any suspicious lesions that do not stain.

Figure 23.10 shows a heavily stained speckled leukoplakia at the commissure. Figure 23.11 shows an area of atrophic mucosa without a distinctive lesion that took up the dye and proved, on biopsy, to show epithelial dysplasia, indicating an increased risk of progressing to malignancy if untreated. Figures 23.12 through 23.14 show pre- and post-stain results for an overt cancer, a severe dysplasia and a benign keratosis (Figure 23.15).

The FDI Commission, through its project on oral cancer, has recently agreed to a statement on the use of Toluidine blue, supporting its use in appropriately experienced hands and urging further research on its clinical utility in primary care settings. This states that the use of Toluidine blue, in expert and experienced hands, is recommended for:

- Monitoring of suspicious lesions over time
- Screening for oral mucosal malignancy and premalignancy in high-risk individuals and population groups
- Follow-up of patients already treated for upper aerodigestive tract cancer (228)
- Helping to determine an optimal site for biopsy when a suspicious lesion or condition is present
- Intraoperative use during surgery for upper aerodigestive tract malignancy as an application to help judge the borders of the neoplasm (229)

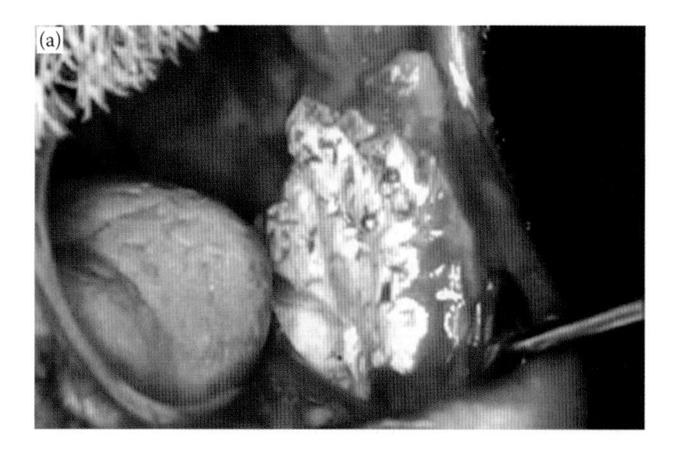

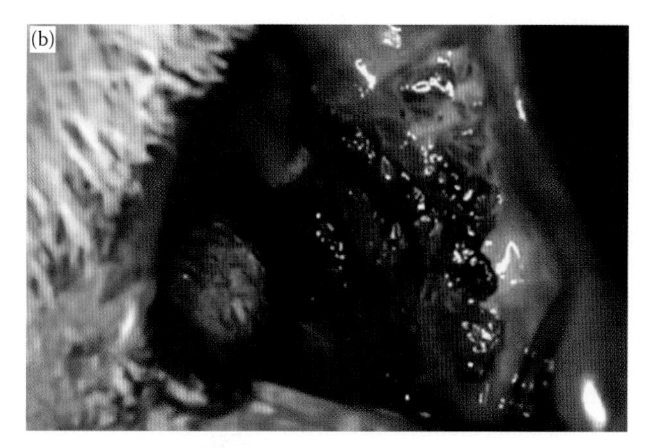

Figure 23.12 **(a)** A large exophytic tumor with a partly red, partly white surface. Clinically, this is almost certainly a carcinoma of the buccal mucosa, which nevertheless requires diagnostic confirmation by biopsy. Several biopsies from the junction between clinically normal and tumor tissue, including the deep invasive front, are desirable to provide details for treatment planning. **(b)** The tumor mass is stained a deep royal blue, with clearly defined borders. In this example, Toluidine blue has not contributed to the diagnosis because the lesion is so clinically obvious. It may, however, help to delineate the margins and thus indicate appropriate sites for biopsy.

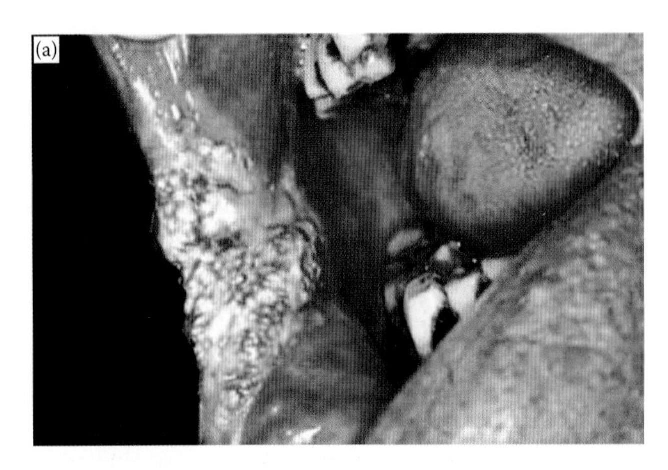

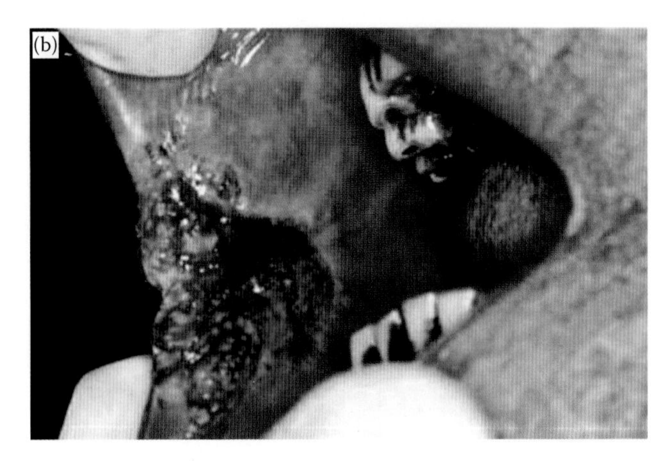

Figure 23.13 **(a)** A mixed nodular leukoplakia and erythroplakia at the commissure. **(b)** This also shows clearly demarcated, intense staining, including an area of ulceration in the upper posterior part of the lesion. Once again, biopsy would have been mandatory on the basis of clinical appearance alone. In this case, histology demonstrated severe epithelial dysplasia, short of overtly invasive carcinoma.

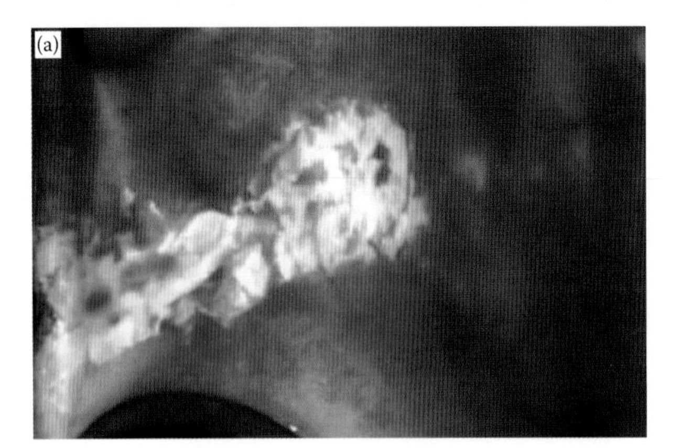

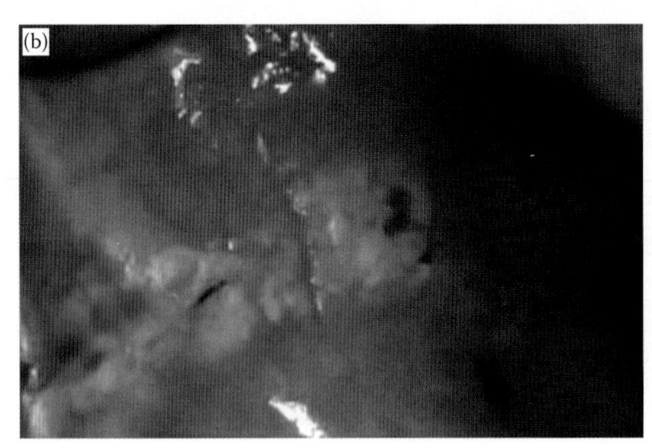

Figure 23.14 **(a)** A homogenous leukoplakia on the right commissure, with intervening areas of more normal mucosa. This appearance does not suggest a high-risk lesion. **(b)** Apart from retention of a little dye in creases in the surface keratin, this lesion is Toluidine blue negative. Nevertheless, biopsy is still required, on the basis of the initial clinical observations alone. No epithelial dysplasia was present histologically.

Other fluorescent dyes (23,230,231), direct microscopy (232,233) and image analysis of brush biopsies (234) are currently under study.

Molecular screening

It is possible to analyze tissue, and indeed a variety of body fluids, increasingly including saliva and exhaled air, for markers of aberrations in oncogenes, tumor suppressor genes or their protein products. It is also possible to screen chromosomes from oral epithelial cells in health, from potentially malignant lesions and from overt cancers, and to record abnormalities such as loss, amplification or transposition of parts of the genome thought to be important in carcinogenesis. Existing knowledge in the rapidly developing field is given in Chapter 5.

It is not known precisely how many "hits" or aberrations are necessary to render a clone of cells malignant, although a figure of around six is often quoted. There is continuing research seeking models of sequential mutations or other changes to the genome of pre- or potentially malignant clones of cells for the development of head and neck cancer. An early one, which followed the then famous Vogelstein model for the transformation of intestinal polyps into adenocarcinoma of the large bowel, is shown in Figure 23.14. Other molecular markers are discussed extensively in Chapter 5. A recent monograph (235) covers those with therapeutic potential comprehensively. Such models should not be taken to imply that precisely this series of abnormalities, in precisely that order, are necessary or sufficient for a cancer to develop: the number, type and order undoubtedly differ from patient to patient. Whilst common things occur commonly and there a similarities between the most common cancers, it is now argued that the number of driver gene mutations sufficient for malignant transformation is limited, and identifying these is the basis of personalized therapy (236). Understanding this can also be approached mathematically: mutations in DNA repair, replication or

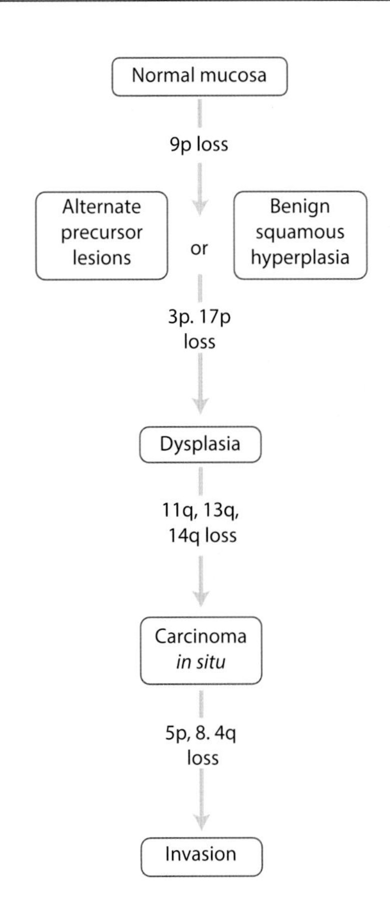

Figure 23.15 Genetic progression model for head and neck squamous cell carcinomas: implications for field cancerization. Not all patients may follow this sequence, as discussed in the text. (Adapted from Califano J et al. *Cancer Res* 1996;56:2488–92 (227).)

cell cycle checkpoints accumulate and many are fatal to the clones of cells involved, but a process of natural selection ensues and the fittest clones survive. The fact that the host also dies is counterintuitive to this Darwinian view, until one reflects that cancer is primarily a disease of people past reproductive age (237).

Thus, which genetic changes are necessary and how many are sufficient for malignant transformation remains debatable; nevertheless, accumulation of genetic aberrations indicates increasing risk, and this information will, in the future, be put to use in:

- Screening clinically normal patients, who are heavy smokers and drinkers, to determine their risk of a future cancer.
- Screening potentially malignant lesions and conditions in order to assess how far along the path to malignancy has been reached and thus to focus intervention for the individual patient.
- Determining completeness of excision/killing by radiotherapy/chemotherapy, by sampling tissue *in situ* after treatment for an overt cancer, in order to assess the risk of recurrence or second primary. This encompasses the concepts of "field change" and of "residual disease."
- Screening peripheral blood or bone marrow for malignant cells disseminated from the primary lesion.
- Screening blood or saliva (238) or scrapings/washings (239–241) for the presence of a marker indicative of the presence of neoplasm—residual or recurrent primary, new primary or metastatic disease (242).

TERTIARY PREVENTION: PREVENTING RECURRENCE OR FURTHER PRIMARY CANCERS AND MINIMIZING MORBIDITY

Chemoprevention as secondary prevention has been discussed above. When a patient treated for an oral cancer develops further cancer in the mouth months or years after apparently successful treatment, it is often not clear whether the new lesion is a recurrence, arising because of incomplete removal of the primary lesion, or a second primary lesion, arising in a field of altered mucosa. The concept of *field cancerization* states that the patient's genetic predisposition plus the lifelong accumulation of potentially carcinogenic insults from known and unknown risk factors renders the patient, and the anatomical area most affected, at increased risk of cancer. This applies whether the second cancer is synchronous with the first or arises later (metachronous). An alternative view is that a clone of genetically damaged and therefore "premalignant" cells migrates in the anatomical area and may give rise to second tumors (243). Either way, it is clear that with oral cancer the whole of the upper aerodigestive tract can be regarded as the susceptible field (244). Unsurprisingly, therefore, the risk of a further cancer is high once a patient has been treated for oral cancer, amounting to some 20% of patients over a 5-year period. This is especially so if the tobacco, alcohol and dietary risk factors continue to be present. All of the above primary prevention approaches are therefore especially important at this stage, including supplementation with antioxidants such as vitamin A (245) or retinoids (246,247).

Chemoprevention of malignant transformation of oral precancerous lesions (leukoplakia has been most extensively investigated, as it is the commonest, even if variably and loosely defined) and conditions by dietary supplementation is another exciting field under active investigation. Data from some selected trials are summarized in Table 23.26.

Synthetic retinoids (255) and curcumin (256) are currently attracting interest.

The current position was thoroughly evaluated by Sankaranarayanan et al. (257), from which the following summary is partly derived. Both the experimental animal evidence and the then published clinical trials were thoroughly analyzed by Tanaka in 1995 (258). Many of the field studies have been conducted in India on *pan* or other ST-associated lesions, with or without *beedi* smoking and alcohol as cofactors. Those from the West relate to smoking- and alcohol-related cancers.

Table 23.26 Selected chemoprevention trials in oral premalignancy

References	Year	Agent(s)	Patients (*n*)	Results
Hong et al. (248)	1986	13-cRA at 1–2 mg/kg per day for three months, followed for 6 months versus placebo	44	67% response (13-cRA) versus 10% response (placebo) ($p = .0002$)
Stich et al. (249)	1988	β-carotene retinol (100,000 IU/week; (180 mg/week) versus placebo	103	27.5% versus 14.8% versus 3.0% ($p < .001$)
Stich et al. (250)	1988	Vitamin A (200,000 IU/week) orally for 6 months versus placebo	64	57.1% complete remission (vitamin A) versus 30% (controls) ($p < .01$)
Han et al. (251)	1990	4-HCR (40 mg/day) versus placebo	61	87% complete remission versus 17% ($p < .01$)
Lippman et al. (252)	1993	13-cRA (1–5 mg/kg per day) for 3 months followed by 13-cRA (0.5 mg/kg per day) for 9 months versus β-carotene (30 mg/day) for 9 months	70	Initial response 55% to high-dose 13-cRA; continued response or stable disease 92% in 13-cRA maintenance versus 45% in β-carotene ($p < .001$)
Chiesa et al. (253)	1993	4-HPR (200 mg/day) for 52 weeks versus placebo	153	Failure in 6% (4-HPR) versus 30% (placebo) ($p < .05$)
Costa et al. (254)	1994			

Abbreviations: 13-cRA: 13-*cis*-restinoic acid; 4-HCR: 4-(hydroxycarbophenylretinamide); 4-HPR is Fenretinide or N-(4-hydroxyphenyl) retinamide, a synthetic vitamin A analogue.

CONCLUSION

- In the *primary prevention* of oral and other epithelial cancers, as discussed earlier, a substantial reduction in risk can be obtained by increasing fruit and vegetable consumption (259,260). This is quite distinct from the use of nutritional supplements in *secondary and tertiary prevention*.
- Retinoids and β-carotene have been shown to result in the regression of oral leukoplakia, but the lesions soon recur after the chemopreventive agents are stopped (261).
- Lower frequencies of malignant transformation have been observed in a small number of subjects with leukoplakia receiving retinoids compared to subjects receiving β-carotene (252).
- Supplementation has not been shown to reduce the risk of locoregional recurrence in treated head and neck cancer patients.
- A reduction in the frequency of second primaries has been observed with 13-*cis*-retinoic acid (262), but not with etretinate (263).
- Although retinoids seem to be effective at inhibiting head and neck carcinogenesis, compared with β-carotene, the synthetic retinoids are quite toxic, which limits their usefulness (252).
- Retinoids have the potential to enhance carcinogenesis under certain conditions, perhaps due to an angiogenic effect, so their use cannot yet be justified outside of clinical trials (264).
- There is insufficient evidence to evaluate the chemopreventive effects of vitamin E or of selenium in head and neck cancer. Some early results on combinations of vitamin E and β-carotene are encouraging (265).
- None of the potential intermediate biomarkers studied for the effect of chemopreventive regimes have yet been fully validated. Amongst these, micronucleated epithelial cells have received the most attention (266), and Sankaranarayanan et al. (257) concluded that this method has value in monitoring compliance amongst patients.
- Many other potential biomarkers, discussed in Chapter 6, are under investigation. These include DNA adducts (266), cell proliferation markers such as Ki67 and PCNA, EGFR and erbB expression, aberrations of the *p53* gene or its protein and HPV gene expression or integration. In respect to studies on retinoid chemoprevention, it may be possible to use nuclear retinoic acid receptors for this purpose (267).
- Attempts at chemoprevention of head and neck cancer should only be made in the context of well-planned, preferably multicenter, clinical trials. Many of these are ongoing.

Further secondary prevention (by screening) is also especially important. Treated patients should be monitored regularly in order to ensure that their mastication, swallowing, speaking, smiling and other functions, their physical appearance and their social integration are as good as the cancer care team can manage, and they should be screened for the possibility of new lesions. In this latter respect,

Toluidine blue application may have particular utility. The cost-effectiveness of regular upper aerodigestive tract endoscopy has yet to be established.

Nowhere is teamwork in cancer care more important than with treated patients, in order to maximize the quality of life for those afflicted and to ensure the best possible quality of death.

REFERENCES

1. Alfano MC, Horowitz AM. Professional and community efforts to prevent morbidity and mortality from oral cancer. *J Am Dent Assoc* 2001;132:24S–9S.
2. WHO. *Tobacco Control Initiative: Rationale, Update and Progress*. Geneva: World Health Organization, 1998.
3. Centres for Disease Control and Prevention. *Preventing and Controlling Oral and Pharyngeal Cancer, MMWR* 1998;47(14). Washington, DC: U.S. Department of Health and Human Services.
4. Kills S. *A White Paper on Tobacco*. London: The Stationery Office, 1998.
5. Department of Health. *Report of the Scientific Committee on Tobacco and Health*. London: HMSO, 1998.
6. Doll R, Peto R, Wheatley K et al. Mortality in relation to smoking: 40 years' observations on male British doctors. *Br Med J* 1994;309:901–911.
7. Peto R, Lopez AD, Boreham J et al. *Imperial Cancer Research Fund and World Health Organization. Mortality from Smoking in Developing Countries 1950–2000*. Oxford: Oxford University Press, 1994.
8. Stead M, Hastings G, Tudor-Smith C. Preventing adolescent smoking: a review of options. *Health Educ J* 1996;55:31–54.
9. *Cost effectiveness of smoking cessation interventions*. London: Centre for Health Economics, University of York and Health Education Authority, 1997. https://cancercontrol.cancer.gov/brp/tcrb/monographs/21/docs/m21_9.pdf.
10. FDI World Dental Federation. Position statement on tobacco. *FDI World* 1996;6:9.
11. Cohen SJ, Stookey GK, Katz BP et al. Helping smokers quit: a randomised controlled trial with private practice dentists. *J Am Dent Assoc* 1989;118:41–5.
12. Segnan N, Ponti A, Battista RN et al. A randomised trial of smoking cessation interventions in general practice in Italy. *Cancer Causes Control* 1991;2:239–246.
13. Russell MA, Stapleton JA, Feyeraband C et al. Targeting heavy smokers in general practice: randomised controlled trial of transdermal nicotine patches. *Br Med J* 1993;306:1308–12.
14. Stapleton JA, Russell MAH, Feyerabend C et al. Dose effects and predictors of outcome in a randomised trial of transdermal nicotine patches in general practice. *Addiction* 1995;90:31–42.
15. Macgregor IDM. Efficacy of dental health advice as an aid to reducing cigarette smoking. *Br Dent J* 1996;180:292–6.
16. Smith SE, Warnakulasuriya KAAS, Feyerabend C, Belcher M, Cooper DJ, Johnson NW. A smoking cessation programme conducted through dental practices in the UK. *Br Dent J* 1998;185:299–303.
17. Watt RG, Johnson NW, Warnakulasuriya KA. Action on smoking: opportunities for the dental team. *Br Dent J* 2001;190:227.
18. Tomar SL. Dentistry's role in tobacco control. *J Am Dent Assoc* 2001;132:30S–5S.
19. Johnson NW, Bain CA. Tobacco and oral disease. EU-Working Group on Tobacco and Oral Health. *Br Dent J* 2000;189:200–6.
20. Mecklenburg RE, Greenspan D, Kleinman DV et al. *Tobacco Effects in the Mouth. NIH Publication No 96-3330*. Washington, DC: U.S. Department of Health and Human Services, 1996.
21. Tobacco use and the periodontal patient. *J Periodontol* 1996;67:51–56.
22. EU Working Group on Tobacco and Oral Health Consensus Meeting. Copenhagen, 23–26 October 1997. Abstracts. *Oral Dis* 1998;4:48–67.
23. van Staveren HJ, van Veen RL, Speelman OC, Witjes MJ, Star WM, Roodenburg JL. Classification of clinical autofluorescence spectra of oral leukoplakia using an artificial neural network: a pilot study. *Oral Oncol* 2000;36:286–93.
24. Reibel J, Stoltze K, Pindborg JJ. *Tobakkens Skadelige Virkninger i Mundhulen*. Copenhagen: Danish Dental Association.
25. Martin LM, Bouquot JE, Wingo PA, Heath CW Jr. Cancer prevention in the dental practice: oral cancer screening and tobacco cessation advice. *J Public Health Dent* 1996;56:336–40.
26. Warnakulasuriya KAAS, Johnson NW. Dentists and oral cancer prevention in the UK: opinions, attitudes and practices to screening for mucosal lesions and to counselling patients on tobacco and alcohol use. *Baseline data from 1991. Oral Dis* 1999;5:10–4.
27. Horowitz AM, Drury TF, Goodman HS, Yellowitz JA. Oral pharyngeal cancer prevention and early detection. Dentist's opinions and practices. *J Am Dent Assoc* 2000;131:453–62.
28. Yellowitz JA, Horowitz AM, Drury TF, Goodman HS. Survey of U.S. dentists' knowledge and opinions about oral pharyngeal cancer. *J Am Dent Assoc* 2000;131:653–61.
29. Dodds AP, Rankin KV, Jones DL, Seals RR. What are you doing about oral cancer? Report of a survey of Texas dentists. *Texas Dent J* 1994;114:39–41.
30. Sachs DPL. Advances in smoking cessation treatment. In: Simmons DH (ed). *Current Pulmonology*, Vol 12. Chicago: Year Book Publishers, 1991, 139–98.

31. Russell MA. Targeting heavy smokers in general practice: randomised controlled trial of transdermal nicotine patches. *Br Med J* 1993;306:1308–12.
32. Pierce JP, Gilpin E, Farkas AJ. Nicotine patch use in the general population: results from the 1993 California Tobacco Survey. *JNCI* 1995;87:87–93.
33. Silagy C, Mant D, Fowler G, Lodge M. Meta-analysis on efficacy of nicotine replacement therapies in smoking cessation. *Lancet* 1994;343:139–42.
34. Johnson NW. A global view of the epidemiology of oral cancer. In: Johnson NW (ed). *Risk Markers for Oral Diseases*, Vol 2. Oral cancer: detection of patients and lesions at risk. Cambridge: Cambridge University Press, 1991, 3–26.
35. Gupta PC, Murti PR, Bhonsle RB et al. Effect of cessation of tobacco use on the incidence of oral mucosal lesions in a ten year follow up study of 12,212 users. *Oral Dis* 1995;1:54–8.
36. Idris AM, Warnakulasuriya, KAAS, Ibrahim YE et al. Toombak-associated oral mucosal lesions in Sudanese show a low prevalence of epithelial dysplasia. *J Oral Pathol Med* 1996;25:239–44.
37. Gupta PC, Murti PR, Bhonsle RB. Epidemiology of cancer by tobacco products and the significance of TSNA. *Crit Rev Toxicol* 1996;26:183–98.
38. Lewin F, Norell SE, Johansson H et al. Smoking tobacco, oral snuff and alcohol in the aetiology of squamous cell carcinoma of the head and neck. A population based case-referent study in Sweden. *Cancer* 1998;83:1367–75.
39. Idris AM, Ibrahim SO, Vasstrand EN et al. The Swedish snus and the Sudanese Toombak: are they different? *Oral Oncol* 1998;34:558–66.
40. Rodu B. *For Smokers Only: how Smokeless Tobacco Can Save Your Life*. New York: Sulzberger and Graham, 1995, 190.
41. Gupta PC, Ray CS. Epidemiology of betel quid uses. *Ann Acad Med Singapore* 2004;33(Suppl):31S–6S.
42. Frieden TR, Bloomberg MR. How to prevent 100 million deaths from tobacco. *Lancet* 2007;369:1758–61.
43. Gupta PC, Warnakulasuriya S. Global epidemiology of areca nut usage. *Addict Biol* 2002;7:77–83.
44. Gupta PC, Ray CS, Sinha DN, Singh PK. Smokeless tobacco: a major public health problem in the SEA region: a review. *Ind J Public Health* 2011;55(3):201–9.
45. Mazurek JM, Syamlal G, King BA, Castellan RM. Smokeless tobacco use amongst working adults—United States, 2005 and 2010. *MMWR Morb Mortal Wkly Rep* 2014;63(22):478–82.
46. Johnson NW. Tobacco use and oral cancer: a global perspective. *J Dent Educ* 2001;65(4):328–39.
47. Gupta PC, Ray CS. Smokeless Tobacco and health in India and South Asia. *Respirology* 2003;8:419–31.
48. Lin WY, Chiu TY, Lee LT, Lin CC, Huang CY, Huang KC. Betel nut chewing is associated with increased risk of cardiovascular disease and all-cause mortality in Taiwanese men. *Am J Clin Nutr* 2008;87:1204–11.
49. Guha N, Warnakulasuriya S, Vlaanderen J, Straif K. Betel quid chewing and the risk of oral and oropharyngeal cancers: a meta-analysis with implications for cancer control. *Int J Cancer* 2014;135(6):1433–43.
50. Garg A, Chaturvedi P, Gupta PC. A review of the systemic adverse effects of areca nut or betel nut. *Ind J Med Pediatr Oncol* 2014;35(1):3–9.
51. Gupta PC, Mehta HC. Cohort study of all-cause mortality among tobacco users in Mumbai, India. *Bull World Health Organ* 2000;78:877–83.
52. Gupta PC, Bhonsle RB, Mehta FS, Pindborg JJ. Mortality experience in relation to tobacco chewing and smoking habits from a 10-year follow-up study in Ernakulam District, Kerala. *Int J Epidemiol* 1984;13:184–7.
53. International Agency for Research on Cancer. Tobacco habits other than smoking; betel-quid and areca-nut chewing; and some related nitrosamines. In: *IARC Monographs on the Evaluation of the Carcinogenic Risk of Chemicals to Humans*, Vol. 89, Smokeless Tobacco and Some Tobacco-specific N-Nitrosamines. Lyon: IARC, 2007.
54. Nair U, Bartsch H, Nair J. Alert for epidemic of oral cancer due to use of the betel quid substitutes gutka and pan masala: a review of agents and causative mechanisms. *Mutagenesis* 2004;19(4):251–62.
55. Bettcher DW, Sanda LS. Clinical cancer control and prevention. Eliminating tobacco-induced cancers: a worldwide challenge. *Ann Oncol* 2008;19(Suppl 7): 230–33.
56. Gupta PC, Fong TG, Pednekar MS, Quak AC, Bansal-Travers M. Intention to quit among Indian tobacco users: findings from International tobacco control policy evaluation India pilot survey. *Ind J Cancer* 2012;49(4):431–7.
57. Dhumal GG, Gupta PC. Assessment of gutka ban in Maharashtra: findings from a focus group discussion. *Int J Head Neck Surg* 2013;4(3):115–8.
58. Hackshaw AK, Law MR, Wald NJ. The accumulated evidence on lung cancer and environmental tobacco smoke. *Br Med J* 1997;315:980–8.
59. Law MR, Morris JK, Wald NJ. Environmental tobacco smoke exposure and ischaemic heart disease: an evaluation of the evidence. *Br Med J* 1997;315:973–80.
60. California Environmental Protection Agency, Office of Environmental Health Hazard Assessment. Health effects of environmental exposure to tobacco smoke. https://www.arb.ca.gov/toxics/ets/factsheetets.pdf.
61. U.S. Environmental Protection Agency. *Respiratory Health Effects of Passive Smoking: lung Cancer and Other Disorders*. Publication EPA/600/6-90/006F. Washington, DC: US Environmental Protection Agency, 1992.

62. McGinnis JM, Foege WH. Actual causes of death in the United States. *JAMA* 1993;270:2207–12.
63. Gray JD, Bhopal RS, White M. Developing a medical school alcohol policy. *Med Educ* 1998;32:138–42.
64. Day GL, Blot WJ, Austin DF et al. Racial differences in risk of oral and pharyngeal cancer: alcohol, tobacco and other determinants. *J Natl Cancer Inst* 1993;85:465–473.
65. Macfarlane GJ, Macfarlane TV, Lowenfels AB. The influence of alcohol consumption on world wide trends in mortality from upper aerodigestive tract cancers in males. *J Epidemiol Comm Health* 1996;50:636–9.
66. Harris CK, Warnakulasuriya KAAS, Johnson NW, Gelbier S, Peters TJ. Oral health in alcohol misusers. *Comm Dent Health* 1996;13:199–203.
67. Bradley KA, Bush KR, McDonell MB, Malone T, Fihn SD. Screening for problem drinking: comparison of CAGE and AUDIT. Ambulatory care quality improvement project (ACQUIP). Alcohol use disorders identification test. *J Gen Intern Med* 1998;13:379–88.
68. Saunders JB, Aasland OG, Babor TF, De La Fuente JR, Grant M. Development of alcohol use disorders identification test (AUDIT): WHO collaborative project on early detection of persons with harmful alcohol consumption—11. *Addiction* 1993;88:791–804.
69. Harris C, Warnakulasuriya KAAS, Gelbier S, Johnson NW, Peters TJ. Oral and dental health in alcohol misusing patients. *Alcohol Clin Exp Res* 1997;21:1707–9.
70. Long CG, Williams M, Hollin CR. Treating alcohol problems: a study of programme effectiveness and cost effectiveness according to length and delivery of treatment. *Addiction.* 1998;93:561–71.
71. Gomel MK, Wutzke SE, Hardcastle DM, Lapsley H, Reznik RB. Cost-effectiveness of strategies to market and train primary health care physicians in brief intervention techniques for hazardous alcohol use. *Soc Sci Med* 1998;47:203–11.
72. Richmond RL, Novak K, Kehoe L, Calfas G, Mendelsohn CP, Wodak A. Effect of training on general practitioners' use of brief intervention for excessive drinkers. *Aust NZ J Public Health* 1998;22:206–9.
73. Subcommittee on Health Services Research, National Advisory Council on Alcohol Abuse and Alcoholism. *Improving the Delivery of Alcohol Treatment and Prevention Services: executive Summary.* NIH Publication No 4224. Bethesda: National Institute on Alcohol Abuse and Alcoholism, National Institutes of Health, Department of Health and Human Services, 1997.
74. Klatsky AL, Armstrong MA, Friedman GD. Alcohol and mortality. *Ann Intern Med* 1992;117:646–54.
75. Gazioano JM, Buring JE, Breslow JL et al. Moderate alcohol intake, increased levels of high-density lipoprotein and its sub-fractions, and decreased risk of myocardial infarction. *N Engl J Med* 1993;329:1829–34.
76. Pearson TA. Alcohol and heart disease. *Circulation* 1995;94:3023–25.
77. Suh I, Shaten BJ, Cutler JA, Kuller LH. for the Multiple Risk Factor Intervention Trial research group. Alcohol use and mortality from coronary heart disease: the role of high-density lipoprotein cholesterol. *Ann Int Med* 1993;116: 881–7.
78. Ridker PM, Vaughan DE, Stampfer MJ, Glynn RJ, Hennekens CH. Association of moderate alcohol consumption and plasma concentration of endogenous tissue-type plasminogen activator. *JAMA* 1994;272:929–33.
79. Renaud S, de Lorgeril M. Wine, alcohol, platelets, and the French paradox for coronary heart disease. *Lancet* 1992;339:1523–6.
80. Jang M, Cai L, Udeani GO et al. Cancer chemopreventive effect of resveratrol, a natural product derived from grapes. *Science* 1997;275:218–20.
81. Rimm EB, Klatsky A, Grobbee D, Stampfer MJ. Review of moderate alcohol consumption and reduced risk of coronary heart disease: is the effect due to beer, wine or spirits. *Br Med J* 1996;312:731–6.
82. McKee M, Britton A. The positive relationship between alcohol and heart disease in Eastern Europe: potential physiological mechanisms. *J R Soc Med* 1998;91:402–7.
83. UK Health Education Authority. *That's the Limit: a Guide to Sensible Drinking.* London: HEA.
84. Bray I, Brennan P, Boffetta P. Projections of alcohol- and tobacco-related cancer mortality in Central Europe. *Int J Cancer* 2000;87:122–8.
85. Franceschi S, Levi F, Dal Maso L et al. Cessation of alcohol drinking and risk of cancer of the oral cavity and pharynx. *Int J Cancer* 2000;85:787–90.
86. Warnakulasuriya KA, Harris CK, Scarrott DM et al. An alarming lack of public awareness towards oral cancer. *Br Dent J* 1999;187:319–22.
87. Hay JL, Ostroff JS, Cruz GD, LeGeros RZ, Kenigsberg H, Franklin DM. Oral cancer risk perception among participants in an oral cancer screening program. *Cancer Epidem Biomar Prev* 2002;11:155–8.
88. Doll R. The prevention of cancer: opportunities and challenges. In: Heller T, Davey B, Bailey L (eds). *Reducing the Risk of Cancers.* London: Hodder and Stoughton, 1989.
89. La Vecchia C, Tavani A, Franceschi S et al. Epidemiology and prevention of oral cancer. *Oral Oncol* 1997;33:303–12.
90. Hakama M, Beral V, Buiatti E, Faivre J, Parkin DM (eds). *Chemoprevention in Cancer Control.* IARC Scientific Publication No 136, Lyon: IARC, 1996.
91. Stewart BW, McGregor D, Kleihues P (eds). *Principles of chemoprevention.* IARC Scientific Publication No 139, Lyon: IARC, 1996.

92. Hebert JR, Gupta PC, Bhonsle RB et al. Dietary exposures and oral precancerous lesions in Srikakulam District, Andhra Pradesh. *India. Public Health Nutr* 2002;5:303–12.
93. Negri E, Franceshi S, Bosetti C et al. Selected micronutrients and oral and pharyngeal cancer. *Int J Cancer* 2000;86:122–7.
94. Morse DE, Pendrys DG, Katz RV et al. Food group intake and the risk of oral epithelial dysplasia in a United States population. *Cancer Causes Control* 2000;11:713–20.
95. American Cancer Society. Advisory Committee on Diet. Nutrition and Cancer Prevention; guidelines in diet,: nutrition and cancer prevention: reducing the risk of cancer with healthy food choices and physical activity. *CA Cancer J* 1996;46:325–41.
96. World Cancer Research Fund/American Institute for Cancer Research. *Food, Nutrition and Physical Activity and Prevention of Cancer. A Global Perspective.* Washington, DC: AIRC, 2007.
97. Pavia M, Pileggi C, Nobile CG, Angelilo F. Association between fruit and vegetable consumption and oral cancer; a meta-analysis of observational studies. *Am J Clin Nutr* 2006;83:1126–34.
98. Warnakulasuriya S. Food, nutrition and oral cancer. In: Wilson M (ed). *Food Constituents and Oral Health: Current status and Future Prospects.* Oxford: Woodhead Publishing Ltd., 2009, 273–95.
99. Lodi G, Franchini R, Warnakulasuriya S, Varoni EM, Sardella A, Kerr AR, Carrassi A, MacDonald LC, Worthington HV. Interventions for treating oral leukoplakia to prevent oral cancer. *Cochrane DB Syst Rev* 2016;7:CD001829.
100. Vander Broek R, Snow GE, Chen Z, Van Waes C. Chemoprevention of head and neck squamous cell carcinoma through inhibition of NF-κB signaling. *Oral Oncol* 2014;50(10):930–941.
101. Ribeiro AS, Salles PR, daSilva TA et al. Review of the nonsurgical treatment of oral leukoplakia. *Int J Dentistry* 2010;1155:1–10.
102. Chakravarti N, Mathur M, Bahadur S, Shukla NK, Rochette-Egly C, Ralhan R. Expression of RAR alpha and RAR beta in human oral potentially malignant and neoplastic lesions. *Int J Cancer* 2001;91(1):27–31.
103. Beenken SW, Hockett R Jr, Grizzle W et al. Topical application of a mucoadhesive freeze-dried black raspberry gel induces clinical and histologic regression and reduces loss of heterozygosity events in premalignant oral intraepithelial lesions: results from a multicentered, placebo-controlled clinical trial. *Clin Cancer Res* 2014;20(7):1910–24.
104. Shah JP, Strong EW, Decosse JJ, Itri LM, Sellers P. Effect of retinoids on oral leukoplakia. *Am J Surg* 1983;146:466–70.
105. Hong WK, Endicott J, Itri LM et al. 13 cis-retinoic acid in the treatment of oral leukoplakia. *N Eng J Med* 1986;315:1501–1505.
106. Stitch HF, Rosin MP, Hornby AP, Mathew B, Sanakaranarayanan R, Nair MK. Remission of oral leukoplakia and micronuclei in tobacco/betel quid chewers treated with beta-carotene and with beta-carotene plus vitamin A. *Int J Cancer* 1988;42:195–9.
107. Lippman SM, Lee JJ, Martin JW et al. Fenretinide activity in retinoid-resistant oral leukoplakia. *Clin Cancer Res* 2006;12(10):3109–14.
108. Toma S, Benso S, Albanese E et al. Treatment of oral leukoplakia with beta carotene. *Oncology* 1992b;49:77–81.
109. Chesia F, Tradati N, Marazza M et al. Prevention of local relapses and new localisation of oral leukoplakia with synthetic retinoid fenretinide (4-HPR). *Oral Oncol* 1992;28:97–102.
110. Sankaranarayanan R, Mathew B, Varghese C et al. Chemoprevention of oral leukoplakia with vitamin A and beta carotene: an assessment. *Oral Oncol* 1997;33:231–6.
111. Gorsky M, Epstein JB. The effect of retinoids on premalignant oral lesions: focus on topical therapy. *Cancer* 2002;95(6):1258–64.
112. Gaeta GM, Gombos F, Femiano F, Battista C, Minghetti P, Montanari L, Satriano RA, Argenziano G. Acitretin and treatment of the oral leucoplakias. A model to have an active molecules release. *J Eur Acad Dermatol Venereol* 2000;14(6):473–8.
113. Papadimitrakopoulou VA, Lee JJ, William WN Jr et al. Randomized trial of 13-cis retinoic acid compared with retinyl palmitate with or without beta-carotene in oral premalignancy. *J Clin Oncol* 2009;27(4):599–604.
114. William WN Jr, Lee JJ, Lippman SM et al. High-dose fenretinide in oral leukoplakia. *Cancer Prev Res (Phila)* 2009 Jan;2(1):22–6.
115. Scardina GA, Carini F, Maresi E, Valenza V, Messina P. Evaluation of the clinical and histological effectiveness of isotretinoin in the therapy of oral leukoplakia: ten years of experience: is management still up to date and effective? *Methods Find Exp Clin Pharmacol* 2006;28(2):115–9.
116. Singh M, Krishappa R, Bagewadi A, Keluskar V. Efficacy of oral leucopene in the treatment of oral leukoplakia. *Oral Oncol* 2004;40:591–6.
117. Foy JP, Bertolus C, William WN Jr, Saintigny P. Oral premalignancy: the roles of early detection and chemoprevention. *Otolaryngol Clin North Am* 2013;46(4):579–97.
118. Roberts CJ, Farrow SC, Charny MC. How much can the NHS afford to spend to save a life or avoid a severe disability? *Lancet* 1985;i:89–91.
119. Goodin S, Shiff SJ. NSAIDs for the chemoprevention of oral cancer: promise or pessimism? *Clin Cancer Res* 2004;10(5):1561–4.
120. Saba NF, Choi M, Muller S, Shin HJ, Tighiouart M, Papadimitrakopoulou VA, El-Naggar AK, Khuri FR, Chen ZG, Shin DM. Role of cyclooxygenase-2 in

tumor progression and survival of head and neck squamous cell carcinoma. *Cancer Prev Res (Phila)* 2009;2(9):823–9.

121. Goel A, Boland CR, Chauhan DP. Specific inhibition of cycloxygenase-2 (COX-2) expression by dietary curcumin in HT-29 human colon cancer cells. *Cancer Lett* 2001;172:111–8.
122. Duvoix A, Blasius R, Delhalle S et al. Chemoprevention and therapeutic effects of curcumin. *Cancer Lett* 2005;223;181–90.
123. Govindrarajan R, Siegel ER, Simmons DL, Lang NP. Thiazolidinedionne (TZD) exposure and risk of squamous cell carcinoma of the head and neck (SCCHN). *Clin Oncol* 2007;25:(18S):1511.
124. Burotto M, Szabo E. PPARγ in head and neck cancer prevention. *Oral Oncol* 2014;50(10):924–9.
125. Mulshine JL, Atkinson JC, Greer RO et al. Randomized, double-blind, placebo-controlled phase IIb trial of the cyclooxygenase inhibitor ketorolac as an oral rinse in oropharyngeal leukoplakia. *Clin Cancer Res* 2004;10(5):1565–73.
126. Papadimitrakopoulou VA, William WN Jr, Dannenberg AJ et al. Pilot randomized phase II study of celecoxib in oral premalignant lesions. *Clin Cancer Res* 2008;14(7):2095–101.
127. Tsao AS, Liu D, Martin J et al. Phase II randomized, placebo-controlled trial of green tea extract in patients with high-risk oral premalignant lesions. *Cancer Prev Res (Phila)* 2009;2(11):931–41.
128. Shumway BS, Kresty LA, Larsen PE, Zwick JC, Lu B, Fields HW, Mumper RJ, Stoner GD, Mallery SR. Effects of a topically applied bioadhesive berry gel on loss of heterozygosity indices in premalignant oral lesions. *Clin Cancer Res* 2008;14(8):2421–30.
129. Rhodus N, Rohrer M, Pambuccian S et al. Phase 11a chemoprevention clinical trial of pioglitazone for oral leukoplakia. *J Dent Res* 2011;90:945.
130. Cheng AL, Hsu CH, Lin JK et al. Phase I clinical trial of curcumin, a chemopreventive agent, in patients with high-risk or pre-malignant lesions. *Anticancer Res* 2001;21(4B):2895–900.
131. Rai B, Kaur J, Jacobs R, Singh J. Possible action mechanism for curcumin in pre-cancerous lesions based on serum and salivary markers of oxidative stress. *J Oral Sci* 2010;52(2):251–6.
132. Kerr AR, Warnakulasuriya S, Mighell AJ et al. A systematic review of medical interventions for oral submucous fibrosis and future research opportunities. *Oral Dis* 2011;17(Suppl 1):42–57.
133. Chole RH, Gondivkar SM, Gadbail AR et al. Review of drug treatment of oral submucous fibrosis. *Oral Oncol* 2012;48(5):393–8. doi:10.1016/j.oraloncology.2011.11.021. Epub December 27, 2011.
134. Maher R, Aga P, Johnson NW, Sankaranarayanan R, Warnakulasuriya K. Evaluation of multiple micronutrient supplementation of oral submucous fibrosis in Karachi, Pakistan. *Nutr Cancer* 1997;27:41–7.
135. Das DA, Balan A, Sreelatha KT. Comparative study of efficacy of curcumin and turmeric oil as chemopreventive agents in oral submucous fibrosis; a clinical and histopathological evaluation. *J Ind Acad Oral Med Radiol* 2010;22(2):88–92.
136. Yadav M, Aravinda K, Saxena VS, Srinivas K, Ratnakar P, Gupta J, Sachdev AS, Shivhare P. Comparison of curcumin with intralesional steroid injections in oral submucous fibrosis—a randomized, open-label interventional study. *J Oral Biol Craniofac Res* 2014;4(3):169–73.
137. Sudarshan R, Annigeri RG, Sree Vijayabala G. Aloe vera in the treatment for oral submucous fibrosis—a preliminary study. *J Oral Pathol Med* 2012;41(10):755–61.
138. Alam S, Ali I, Giri KY, Gokkulakrishnan S, Natu SS, Faisal M, Agarwal A, Sharma H. Efficacy of aloe vera gel as an adjuvant treatment of oral submucous fibrosis. *Oral Surg Oral Med Oral Pathol Oral Radiol* 2013;116(6):717–24.
139. Warnakulasuriya KA, Robinson D, Evans H. Multiple primary tumours following head and neck cancer in southern England during 1961–98. *J Oral Pathol Med* 2003;32(8):443–9.
140. Priante AV, Carvalho AL, Kowalski LP. Second primary tumor in patients with upper aerodigestive tract cancer. *Braz J Otorhinolaryngol* 2010;76(2):251–6.
141. Hong WK, Lippman SM, Itri LM et al. Prevention of second primary tumours with isotretinoin in squamous cell carcinoma of the head and neck. *New Eng J Med* 1990;323:795–801.
142. van Zandwijk N, Dalesio O, Pastorino U, de Vries N, van Tinteren H. EUROSCAN, a randomized trial of vitamin A and N-acetylcysteine in patients with head and neck cancer or lung cancer. For the EUropean Organization for Research and Treatment of Cancer Head and Neck and Lung Cancer Cooperative Groups. *J Natl Cancer Inst* 2000;92(12):977–86.
143. Toma S, Bonelli L, Sartoris A et al. Beta-carotene supplementation in patients radically treated for stage I-II head and neck cancer: results of a randomized trial. *Oncol Rep* 2003;10(6):1895–901.
144. Perry CF, Stevens M, Rabie I, Yarker ME, Cochrane J, Perry E, Traficante R, Coman W. Chemoprevention of head and neck cancer with retinoids: a negative result. *Arch Otolaryngol Head Neck Surg* 2005;131(3):198–203.
145. Khuri FR, Lee JJ, Lippman SM. Randomized phase III trial of low-dose isotretinoin for prevention of second primary tumors in stage I and II head and neck cancer patients. *J Natl Cancer Inst* 2006;98(7):441–50.
146. Pisters KM, Newman RA, Coldman B, Shin DM, Khuri FR, Hong WK, Glisson BS, Lee JS. Phase I trial of oral green tea extract in adult patients with solid tumors. *J Clin Oncol* 2001;19(6):1830–8.

147. Datta M, Shaw EG, Lesser GJ et al. A randomized double-blind placebo-controlled trial of fruit and vegetable concentrates on intermediate biomarkers in head and neck cancer. *Integr Cancer Ther* 2018;17(1):115–123.
148. Bairati I, Meyer F, Jobin E, Gélinas M, Fortin A, Nabid A, Brochet F, Têtu B. Antioxidant vitamins supplementation and mortality: a randomized trial in head and neck cancer patients. *Int J Cancer* 2006;119(9):2221–4.
149. Kadakia S, Badhey A, Milam M, Lee T, Ducic Y. Topical oral cavity chemoprophylaxis using isotretinoin rinse: a 15-year experience. *Laryngoscope* 2017;127(7):1595–1599. doi: 10.1002/lary.26463. Epub December 21, 2016.
150. Kelloff GJ, Lippman SM, Dannenberg AJ, Sigman CC, Pearce HL, Reid BJ et al. AACR Task Force on Cancer Prevention. Progress in chemoprevention drug development: the promise of molecular biomarkers for prevention of intraepithelial neoplasia and cancer—a plan to move forward. *Clin Cancer Res* 2006;12(12):3661–97.
151. Braakhuis BJ, Snijders PJ, Keune WJ, Meijer CJ, Ruijter-Schippers HJ, Leemans CR, Brakenhoff, RH. Genetic patterns in head and neck cancers that contain or lack transcriptionally active human papillomavirus. *J Natl Cancer Inst* 2004;96:998–1006.
152. Reimers N, Kasper HU, Weissenborn SJ et al. Combined analysis of HPV-DNA, p16 and EGFR expression to predict prognosis in oropharyngeal cancer. *Int J Cancer* 2007;120:1731–8.
153. Ang KK, Harris J, Wheeler R et al. Human papillomavirus and survival of patients with oropharyngeal cancer. *N Engl J Med* 2010;363:24–35.
154. Shah, NG, Trivedi TI, Tankshali RA, Goswami JV, Jetly DH, Shukla SN, Shah PM, Verma RJ. Prognostic significance of molecular markers in oral squamous cell carcinoma: a multivariate analysis. *Head Neck* 2009;31:1544–56.
155. Weinberger, PM, Yu, Z, Haffty, BG et al. Molecular classification identifies a subset of human papillomavirus-associated oropharyngeal cancers with favorable prognosis. *J Clin Oncol* 2006;24:736–47.
156. Harris SL, Thorne LB, Seaman WT, Hayes DN, Couch ME, Kimple RJ. Association of p16(INK4a) overexpression with improved outcomes in young patients with squamous cell cancers of the oral tongue. *Head Neck* 2011;33:1622–7.
157. Shaikh MH, Khan AI, Sadat A et al. Prevalence and Types of High-Risk Human Papillomaviruses in Head and Neck Cancers from Bangladesh. *BMC Cancer* 2017;17(1):792. doi: 10.1186/s12885-017-3789-0.
158. Smeets SJ, Brakenhoff RH, Ylstra B, Van Wieringen WN, Van De Wiel MA, Leemans CR, Braakhuis BJ. Genetic classification of oral and oropharyngeal carcinomas identifies subgroups with a different prognosis. *Cell Oncol* 2009;31:291–300.
159. Jordan RC, Lingen MW, Perez-ordonez B, He X, Pickard R, Koluder M, Jiang B, Wakely P, Xiao W, Gillison ML. Validation of methods for oropharyngeal cancer HPV status determination in U.S. cooperative group trials. *Am J Surg Pathol* 2012;36:945–54.
160. Singhi AD, Westra WH. Comparison of human papillomavirus *in situ* hybridization and p16 immunohistochemistry in the detection of human papillomavirus-associated head and neck cancer based on a prospective clinical experience. *Cancer* 2010;116:2166–73.
161. Caussy D, Orr W, Daya AD, Roth P, Reeves W, Rawls W. Evaluation of methods for detecting human papillomavirus deoxyribonucleotide sequences in clinical specimens. *J Clin Microbiol* 1988;26:236–43.
162. Kim CJ, Jeong JK, Park M, Park TS, Park TC, Namkoong SE, Park JS. HPV oligonucleotide microarray-based detection of HPV genotypes in cervical neoplastic lesions. *Gynecol Oncol* 2003;89:210–7.
163. Seo SS, Song YS, Kim JW, Park NH, Kang SB, Lee HP. Good correlation of HPV DNA test between self-collected vaginal and clinician-collected cervical samples by the oligonucleotide microarray. *Gynecol Oncol* 2006;102:67–73.
164. De Roda Husman AM, Walboomers JM, Van Den Brule AJ, Meijer CJ, Snijders PJ. The use of general primers GP5 and GP6 elongated at their 3′ ends with adjacent highly conserved sequences improves human papillomavirus detection by PCR. *J Gen Virol* 1995;76(Pt 4):1057–62.
165. Haws AL, Woeber S, Gomez M et al. Human papillomavirus infection and P53 codon 72 genotypes in a Hispanic population at high-risk for cervical cancer. *J Med Virol* 2005;77:265–72.
166. Winder DM, Ball SL, Vaughan K, Hanna N, Woo YL, Franzer JT, Sterling JC, Stanley MA, Sudhoff H, Goon PK. Sensitive HPV detection in oropharyngeal cancers. *BMC Cancer* 2009;9:440.
167. Cuschieri K, Wentzensen N. Human papillomavirus mRNA and p16 detection as biomarkers for the improved diagnosis of cervical neoplasia. *Cancer Epidem Biomar Prev* 2008;17:2536–45.
168. Dockter J, Schroder A, Eaton B, Wang A, Sikhamsay N, Morales L, Giachetti C. Analytical characterization of the APTIMA HPV assay. *J Clin Virol* 2009;1(45 Suppl):S39–47.
169. Marur S, D'souza G, Westra WH, Forastiere AA. HPV-associated head and neck cancer: a virus-related cancer epidemic. *Lancet Oncol* 2010;11:781–9.
170. Garcia-sierra N, Martro E, Castella E et al. Evaluation of an array-based method for human papillomavirus detection and genotyping in comparison with conventional methods used in cervical cancer screening. *J Clin Microbiol* 2009;47:2165–9.
171. Barzon L, Militello V, Lavezzo E et al. Human papillomavirus genotyping by 454 next generation sequencing technology. *J Clin Virol* 2011;52:93–7.

172. Conway C, Chalkley R, High A et al. Next-generation sequencing for simultaneous determination of human papillomavirus load, subtype, and associated genomic copy number changes in tumors. *J Mol Diagn* 2012;14:104–11.
173. Garland SM, Smith JS. Human papillomavirus vaccines: current status and future prospects. *Drugs* 2010;70:1079–98.
174. Lu B, Kumar A, Castellsague X, Giuliano AR. Efficacy and safety of prophylactic vaccines against cervical HPV infection and diseases among women: a systematic review & meta-analysis. *BMC Infect Dis* 2011;11:13.
175. D'souza G, Dempsey A. The role of HPV in head and neck cancer and review of the HPV vaccine. *Prev Med* 2011;53(Suppl 1):S5–11.
176. Meites E, Kempe A, Markowitz LE. Use of a 2-dose schedule for human papillomavirus vaccination–Updated recommendations of the Advisory Committee on Immunization Practices. *Morb Mortal Weekly Rep* 2016;65(49):1405–8.
177. Daniel-Ulloa J, Gilbert PA, Parker EA. Human papillomavirus vaccination in the United States: uneven uptake by gender, race/ethnicity, and sexual orientation. *Am J Public Health* 2016;106:746–7.
178. Prue G, Lawler M, Baker P, Warnakulasuriya S. Human papillomavirus (HPV): making the case for "immunisation for all." *Oral Dis* 2017;23(6):726–730. Epub August 29, 2016.
179. Wilkinson JR, Morris, EJA, Downing A, Finan PJ, Aravani A, Thomas JD, Sebag-Montefiore D. The rising incidence of anal cancer in England 1990–2010: a population based study. *Colorectal Dis* 2014;16(7):234–9.
180. Reagan-Steiner S, Yankey D, Jeyarajah J et al. National, regional, state, and selected local area vaccination coverage among adolescents aged 13–17 years—United States, 2014. *Morb Mortal Weekly Rep* 2015;64:784–92.
181. Fuller KM, Hinyard L. Factors associated with HPV vaccination in young males. *J Community Health* 2017;42(6):1127–32. doi: 10.1007/s10900-017-0361-4.
182. Brotherton JM, Batchelor MR, Bradley MO, Brown SA, Duncombe SM, Meijer D, Tracey LE, Watson M, Webby RJ. 2015. Interim estimates of male human papillomavirus vaccination coverage in the school-based program in Australia. *Commun Dis Intell Q Rep* 2015;39(2):E197–200.
183. Beavis AL, Levinson KL. Preventing cervical cancer in the United States: barriers and resolutions for HPV vaccination. *Front Oncol.* 2016;6:19.
184. Foley OW, Birrer N, Rauh-Hain JA, Clark RM, DiTavi E, Del Carmen MG. Effect of educational intervention on cervical cancer prevention and screening in Hispanic women. *J Commun Health* 2015;40:1178–84.
185. Donadiki EM, Jiménez-García R, Hernández-Barrera V et al. 2014. Health belief model applied to non-compliance with HPV vaccine among female university students. *Public Health* 2014;128:268–73. doi: 10.1016/j.puhe.2013.12.004. Epub February 13, 2014.
186. Fontenot HB, Fantasia HC, Charyk A, Sutherland MA. Human papillomavirus (HPV) risk factors, vaccination patterns, and vaccine perceptions among a sample of male college students. *J Am Coll Health* 2014;62(3):186–92.
187. Holman DM, Benard V, Roland KB, Watson M, Liddon N, Stokley S. Barriers to human papillomavirus vaccination among U.S. adolescents: a systematic review of the literature. *JAMA Pediatr* 2014;168(1):76–82.
188. Beshers SC, Murphy JM, Fix BV, Mahoney MC. Sex differences among college students in awareness of the human papillomavirus vaccine and vaccine options. *J Am Coll Health* 2015;63:144–7.
189. Blake KD, Ottenbacher AJ, Finney Rutten LJ, Grady MA, Korbrin SC, Jacobson RM, Hesse BW. Predictors of human papillomavirus awareness and knowledge 2013: gaps and opportunities for targeted communication strategies. *Am J Prev Med* 2015;48:402–10.
190. Reimer RA, Schommer JA, Houlihan AE, Gerrard M. Ethnic and gender differences in HPV knowledge, awareness, and vaccine acceptability among white and Hispanic men and women. *J Community Health* 2014;39:274–84.
191. Davlin SL, Berenson AB, Rahman M. Correlates of HPV knowledge among low-income minority mothers with a child 9–17 years of age. *J Pediatr Adolesc Gynecol* 2015;28(1):19–23.
192. Fenkl EA, Jones SG, Schochet E, Johnson P. HPV and anal cancer knowledge among HIV-infected and non-infected men who have sex with men. *LGBT Health* 2016;3(1):42–48.
193. Giuliani M, Vescio MF, Dona MG et al. Perceptions of human papillomavirus (HPV) infection and acceptability of HPV vaccine among men attending a sexual health clinic differ. *Hum Vaccin Immunother* 2016;12:1542–50.
194. Nadarzynski T, Smith H, Richardson D, Jones CJ, Llewellyn CD. Human papillomavirus and vaccine-related perceptions among men who have sex with men: a systematic review. *Sex Trans Infect* 2014;90:515–23.
195. Canvin M, Sinka K, Hughes G, Mesher D. Decline in genital warts diagnoses among young women and young men since the introduction of the bivalent HPV (16/18) vaccination programme in England: an ecological analysis. *Sex Transm Infect* 2017;93(2):125–8.
196. Kenter GG, Welters MJ, Valentijn AR et al. Vaccination against HPV-16 oncoproteins for vulvar intraepithelial neoplasia. *N Engl J Med* 2009;361(19):1838–47.

197. Kanzler H, Barrat FJ, Hessel EM, Coffman RL. Therapeutic targeting of innate immunity with Toll-like receptor agonists and antagonists. *Nat Med* 2007;13:552–9.
198. Gu W, Putral L, Hengst K, Minto K, Saunders NA, Leggatt G, Mcmillan NA. 2006. Inhibition of cervical cancer cell growth *in vitro* and *in vivo* with lentiviral-vector delivered short hairpin RNA targeting human papillomavirus E6 and E7 oncogenes. *Cancer Gene Ther* 2006;13:1023–32.
199. Niu XY, Peng ZL, Duan WQ, Wang H, Wang P. Inhibition of HPV 16 E6 oncogene expression by RNA interference *in vitro* and *in vivo*. *Int J Gynecol Cancer* 2006;16:743–51.
200. Trimble CL, Morrow MP, Kraynyak KA et al. Safety, efficacy, and immunogenicity of VGX-3100, a therapeutic synthetic DNA vaccine targeting human papillomavirus 16 and 18 E6 and E7 proteins for cervical intraepithelial neoplasia 2/3: a randomised, double-blind, placebo-controlled phase 2b trial. *Lancet* 2015;386(10008):2078–88.
201. Shaikh MH, Clarke DTW, Johnson NW, McMillan NAJ. Can gene editing and silencing technologies play a role in the treatment of head and neck cancer? *Oral Oncol* 2017;68:9–19.
202. Chamberlain J, Moss S. *Focus on Cancer: evaluation of Cancer Screening*. London: Springer, 1996.
203. Wilson JMG, Jungner G. *Principles and Practice of Screening for Disease*. Public Health Paper No 34. Geneva: WHO, 1968.
204. Gupta PC, Murti PR, Bhonsle RB et al. Effect of cessation of tobacco use on the incidence of oral lesions in a ten year follow up study of 12,212 users. *Oral Dis* 1995;1:54–8.
205. Sankaranarayanan R, Matthew B, Varghese PR et al. Chemoprevention of oral leukoplakia with vitamin A and beta carotene: an assessment. *Oral Oncol* 1977;33:231–6.
206. van der Waal I, Schepman KP, van der Meij EH et al. Oral leukoplakia: a clinicopathological review. *Oral Oncol* 1997;33:291–301.
207. Tradati N, Grigolat R, Calabrese L et al. Oral leukoplakias: to treat or not? *Oral Oncol* 1997;33:317–21.
208. Speight PM, Downer MC, Zakrzewska JM (eds). Screening for oral cancer and precancer: report of a UK working group. *Comm Dent Health* 1993;10(Suppl 1):1–89.
209. Rodrigues VC, Moss SM, Tuomainen H. Oral cancer in the UK: to screen or not to screen. *Oral Oncol* 1998;34:454–65.
210. Franceschi S, Barzan L, Talamini R. Screening for cancer of the head and neck: if not now, when? *Oral Oncol* 1997;33:313–6.
211. Downer MC, Jullien JA, Speight PM. An interim determination of health gain from oral cancer and precancer screening: 1. Obtaining health state utilities. *Comm Dent Health* 1997;14:139–42.
212. Warnakulasuriya KAAS, Johnson NW. Strengths and weaknesses of screening programmes for oral malignancies and potentially malignant lesions. *Eur J Cancer Prev* 1996;5:93–8.
213. Wirth LJ, Krane JF, Li Y et al. A pilot surrogate endpoint biomarker study of celecoxib in oral premalignant lesions. *Cancer Prev Res (Phila).* 2008;1(5):339–48. doi: 10.1158/1940-6207.CAPR-07-0003.
214. Moles DR, Downer MC, Speight PM. Meta-analysis of measures of performance reported in oral cancer and precancer screening studies. *Br Dent J* 2002;192:340–4.
215. Sankaranarayanan R, Mathew B, Jacob BJ et al. Early findings from a community-based, cluster-randomized, controlled oral cancer screening trial in Kerala, India. The Trivandrum Oral Cancer Screening Study Group. *Cancer* 2000;88:664–73.
216. Jullien JA, Zakrzewska JM, Downer MC et al. Attendance and compliance at an oral cancer screening programme in a general medical practice. *Oral Oncol, Eur J Cancer* 1995;31B:202–6.
217. Ikeda N, Downer MC, Ozowa Y et al. Characteristics of of participants and non-participants in annual mass screening for oral cancer in 60 year old residents of Tokoname city, Japan. *Comm Dent Health* 1995;12:83–8.
218. Nagao T, Ikeda N, Fukano H, Miyazaki H, Yano M, Warnakulasuriya S. Outcome following a population screening programme for oral cancer and precancer in Japan. *Oral Oncol* 2000;36:340–6.
219. Nagao T. Warnakulasuriya S, Ikeda N, Fukano H, Fujiwara K, Miyazaki H. Oral cancer screening as an integral part of general health screening in Tokoname City, Japan. *J Med Screen* 2000;7:203–8.
220. Speight PM, Elliott AE, Jullien JA et al. The use of artificial intelligence to identify people at risk of oral cancer and precancer. *Br Dent J* 1995;179:382–7.
221. Amarasinghe HK, Johnson NW, Lalloo R, Kumaraarachchi M, Warnakulasuriya S. Derivation and validation of a risk-factor model for detection of oral potentially malignant disorders in populations with high prevalence. *Br J Cancer* 2010;103(3):303–9.
222. Gupta B, Kumar N, Johnson NW. A risk factor-based model for upper aerodigestive tract cancers in India: predicting and validating the receiver operating characteristic curve. *J Oral Pathol Med* 2017;46(6):465–71.
223. Sankaranarayanan R. Health care auxiliaries in the detection and prevention of oral cancer. *Oral Oncol* 1997;33:149–54.
224. Warnakulasuriya KAAS, Pindborg JJ. Reliability of oral precancer screening by primary health care workers in Sri Lanka. *Comm Dent Health* 1990;7:73–79.

225. Santana JC, Delgado L, Miranda J et al. Oral cancer case finding programme (OCCFP). *Oral Oncol* 1997;33:10–2.
226. Onofre MA, Sposto MR, Navarro CM. Reliability of Toluidine blue application in the detection of oral epithelial dysplasia and *in situ* and invasive squamous cell carcinomas. *Oral Surg Oral Med Oral Pathol Oral Radiol Endod* 2001;91:535–40.
227. Califano J, van der Riet P, Westra W et al. Genetic progression model for head and neck cancer; implications for field cancerization. *Cancer Res* 1996;56:2488–92.
228. Guo Z. Yamaguchi K, Sanchez-Cespedes M, Westra WH, Koch WM, Sidransky D. Allelic losses in OraTest-directed biopsies of patients with prior upper aerodigestive tract malignancy. *Clin Cancer Res* 2001;7:1963–8.
229. Kerawala CJ, Beale V, Reed M, Martin IC. The role of vital tissue staining in the marginal control of oral squamous cell carcinoma. *Int J Oral Maxillofac Surg* 2000;29:32–5.
230. Leunig A, Mehlmann M, Betz C et al. Fluorescence staining of oral cancer using a topical application of 5-aminolevulinic acid: fluorescence microscopic studies. *J Photochem Photobiol B* 2001;60:44–9.
231. Leunig A, Betz CS, Mehlmann M et al. Detection of squamous cell carcinoma of the oral cavity by imaging 5-aminolevulinic acid-induced protoporphyrin IX fluorescence. *Laryngoscope* 2000;110:78–83.
232. Suhr MA, Hopper C, Jones L, George JG, Bown SG, MacRobert AJ. Optical biopsy systems for the diagnosis and monitoring of superficial cancer and precancer. *Int J Oral Maxillofac Surg* 2000;29:453–7.
233. Gynther GW, Rozell B, Heimdahl A. Direct oral microscopy and its value in diagnosing mucosal lesions: a pilot study. *Oral Surg Oral Med Oral Pathol Oral Radiol Endod* 2000:90:164–70.
234. Christian DC. Computer-assisted analysis of oral brush biopsies at an oral cancer screening program. *J Am Dent Assoc* 2002;133:357–62.
235. Warnakulasuriya, S, Khan, Z. *Squamous cell Carcinoma—Molecular Therapeutic Targets*. www.springer.com/gp/book/9789402410839.
236. Tomasetti C, Li L, Vogelstein B. Stem cell divisions, somatic mutations, cancer etiology, and cancer prevention. *Science* 2017;355(6331):1330–4.
237. Peterson LE, Kovyrshina T. Progression inference for somatic mutations in cancer. *Heliyon* 2017;3(4):e00277.
238. Warnakulasuriya S, Soussi T, Maher R, Johnson N, Tavassoli M. Expression of p53 in oral squamous cell carcinoma is associated with the presence of IgG and IgA p53 autoantibodies in sera and saliva of the patients. *J Pathol* 2000;192:52–7.
239. Califano J, Ahrendt SA, Meininger G et al. Detection of telomerase activity in oral rinses from head and neck squamous cell carcinoma patients. *Cancer Res* 1996;56:5720–2.
240. Nunes DN, Kowalski LP, Simpson AJ. Detection of oral and oropharyngeal cancer by microsatellite analysis in mouth washes and lesion brushings. *Oral Oncol* 2000;36:525–8.
241. Spafford MF, Koch WM, Reed AL et al. Detection of head and neck squamous cell carcinoma among exfoliated oral mucosal cells by microsatellite analysis. *Clin Cancer Res* 2001;7:607–12.
242. Forastiere A, Koch W, Trotti A, Sidransky D. Head and neck cancer. *N Eng J Med* 2001;345:1890–900.
243. Partridge M, Emilion G, Pateromichelakis S et al. Field cancerization of the oral cavity: comparison of the spectrum of molecular alterations in cases presenting with both dysplastic and malignant lesions. *Oral Oncol* 1997;33:332–7.
244. Ogden GR. Field cancerization in the head and neck. *Oral Dis* 1998;4:1–3.
245. Jyothirmayi R, Ramadas K, Varghese C et al. Efficacy of vitamin A in the prevention of loco-regional recurrence and second primaries in head and neck cancer. *Eur J Cancer B Oral Oncol* 1996;32B:373–6.
246. Lippmann SM, Spitz MR, Huber MH et al. Strategies for chemoprevention study of premalignancy and second primary tumours in the head and neck. *Curr Opin Oncol* 1995;7:234–41.
247. Anderson WF, Hawk E, Berg CD. Secondary chemoprevention of upper aerodigestive tract tumors. *Semin Oncol* 2001;28:106–20.
248. Hong W, Endicott J, Itri LM et al. 13-*cis* retinoic acid in the treatment of oral leukoplakia. *N Engl J Med* 1986;315:1501–5.
249. Stich HF, Hornby AP, Mathew B, Sankaranarayanan R, Nair MK. Response of oral leukoplakias to the administration of vitamin A. *Cancer Lett* 1988;40:93–101.
250. Stich HF, Rosin MP, Hornby P, Mathew B, Sankaranarayanan R, Nair MK. Remission of oral leukoplakias and micronuclei in tobacco/betel quid chewers treated with β-carotene and with β-carotene plus vitamin A. *Int J Cancer* 1998;42:195–9.
251. Han J, Jiao L, Lu Y, Sun Z, Gu QM, Scanlon KJ. Evaluation of N-4-(hydroxycarbophenyl) retinamide as a cancer prevention agent and as a cancer chemotherapeutic agent. *In Vivo* 1990;4:153–60.
252. Lippman SM, Batsakis JG, Toth BB et al. Comparison of low dose isotretinoin with beta carotene to prevent oral carcinogenesis. *N Engl J Med* 1993;328:15–20.
253. Chiesa F, Tradati N, Marazza M et al. Fenretinide (4-HPR) in chemoprevention of oral leukoplakia. *J Cell Biochem* 1993;17F(Suppl):255–61.
254. Costa A, Formelli F, Chiesa F, Decensi A, De Palo G, Veronesi U. Prospects of chemoprevention of human cancers with the synthetc retinoid fenretinide. *Cancer Res* 1994;54(Suppl):2023s–37s.
255. Femiano F, Gombos F, Scully C, Battista C, Belnome G, Esposito V. Oral leukoplaskia: open trial of topical therapy with calcipotriol compared with tretinoin. *Int J Oral Maxillofac Surg* 2001;30:402–6

256. Cheng AL, Hsu CH, Lin JK et al. Phase I clinical trial of curcumin, a chemopreventive agent, in patients with high-risk or pre-malignant lesions. *Anticancer Res* 2001;21:2895–900.
257. Sankaranarayanan R, Mathew B, Nair PP et al. Chemoprevention of cancers of the oral cavity and the head and neck. In: Stewart BW, McGregor D, Kleihues P. (eds). *Principles of Chemoprevention.* IARC Scientific Publication No 139. Lyon: IARC, 1996.
258. Tanaka T. Chemoprevention of oral carcinogenesis. *Oral Oncol* 1995;31B:3–15.
259. La Vecchia C, Tavani A. Fruit and vegetables and human cancer. *Eur J Cancer Prev* 1998;7:3–8.
260. De Stefani E, Deneo-Pelligrini H, Mendilaharsu M, Ronco A. Diet and risk of cancer of the upper aerodigestive tract—I. Foods; II. oral. *Oncology* 1999;35:17–21.
261. Stich HF, Mathew B, Sankaranarayanan R, Krishnan Nair M. Remission of oral precancerous lesions of tobacco/areca nut chewers following administration of β-carotene or vitamin A, and maintenance of the protective effect. *Cancer Detect Prev* 1991;15:93–8.
262. Benner SE, Pajak TF, Lippman SSM, Earley C, Hong WK. Prevention of second primary tumours with isoretinoin in patients with squamous cell carcinoma of the head and neck: long-term follow up. *J Natl Cancer Inst* 1994;86:140–1.
263. Bolla M, Lefur R, Ton Van J et al. Prevention of second primary tumours with etretinate in squamous cell carcinoma of the oral cavity and oropharynx. Results of a multicentric double blind randomised study. *Eur J Cancer* 1994;30(A):767–72.
264. Schwartz JL, Shklar G. Retinoid and carotenoid angiogenesis: a possible explanation for enhanced oral carcinogenesis. *Nutr Cancer* 1997;27:192–9.
265. Garewal H. Antioxidants in oral cancer prevention. *Am J Clin Nutr* 1995;62(Suppl):1410s–6s.
266. Prasad MPR, Mukundan MA, Krishnaswamy K. Micronuclei and carcinogen DNA adducts as intermediate end points in nutrient intervention trial of precancerous lesions in the oral cavity. *Oral Oncol* 1995;31B:155–9.
267. Khuri FR, Lippman SSM, Spitz MR. Lotan R, Hong WK. Molecular epidemiology and chemoprevention of head and neck cancer. *J Natl Cancer Inst* 1997;39:199–211.
268. Armstrong WB, Taylor TH, Kennedy AR, Melrose RJ, Messadi DV, Gu M, Le AD, Yueh B, Boyle JO. Pilot randomized phase II study of celecoxib in oral premalignant lesions. *Clin Cancer Res* 2008;14(7):2095–101.
269. Bland KI. Transforming growth factor-alpha: a surrogate endpoint biomarker? *J Am Coll Surg* 2002 Aug;195(2):149–58.
270. Chiesa F, Tradati N, Grigolato R et al. Review of drug treatment of oral submucous fibrosis. *Oral Oncol* 2012;48(5):393–8.
271. Peto R, Lopez AD, Boreham J, Thun M, Heath C Jr, Doll R. Mortality from smoking worldwide. *Br Med Bull* 1996;52:12–21.
272. WHO. *Tobacco or Health: a Global Status Report.* Geneva: World Health Organization, 1997.
273. Gupta PC, Mehta FS, Pindborg JJ. Mortality among reverse chutta smokers in south India. *Br Med J* 1984;289:865–6.
274. Formelli F, Costa L, Giardini R, Zurrida S, Costa A, De Palo G, Veronesi U. Randomized trial of fenretinide (4-HPR) to prevent recurrences, new localizations and carcinomas in patients operated on for oral leukoplakia: long-term results. *Int J Cancer* 2005;115(4):625–9.
275. Fritsche HA Jr, Zhou X, Papadimitrakopoulou V, Khuri FR, Tran H, Clayman GL. Future research opportunities. *Oral Dis* 2011;17(Suppl 1):42–57.
276. Kuriakose MA, Ramdas K, Dey B et al. A randomized double-blind placebo-controlled phase IIb trial of curcumin in oral leukoplakia. *Cancer Prev Res (Phila)* 2016;9(8):683–91.
277. Lee JJ, Hong WK, Hittelman WN et al. Predicting cancer development in oral leukoplakia: ten years of translational research. *Clin Cancer Res* 2000;6(5):1702–10.
278. Lippmann SM, Batsakis JG, Toth BB et al. Comparison of low dose isoretinoin with beta carotene to prevent oral carcinogenesis. *N Engl J Med* 1993;328:15–20.
279. Mallery SR, Tong M, Shumway BS et al. Randomized trial of supplemental beta-carotene to prevent second head and neck cancer. *Cancer Res* 2001;61(4):1457–63.
280. Nagao T, Warnakulasuriya S, Nakamura T et al. Treatment of oral leukoplakia with a low-dose of beta-carotene and vitamin C supplements: a randomized controlled trial. *Int J Cancer* 2015;136(7):1708–17.
281. Perloff M, Civantos F, Goodwin WJ, Wirth LJ, Kerr AR, Meyskens FL Jr. Bowman birk inhibitor concentrate and oral leukoplakia: a randomized phase IIb trial. *Cancer Prev Res (Phila)* 2013;6(5):410–8.
282. Toma S, Bonelli L, Sartoris A et al. 13-cis retinoic acid in head and neck cancer chemoprevention: results of a randomized trial from the Italian Head and Neck Chemoprevention Study Group. *Oncol Rep* 2004;11(6):1297–305.
283. Warnakulasuriya S, Kerr AR. Oral submucous fibrosis: a review of the current management and possible directions for novel therapies. *Oral Surg Oral Med Oral Pathol Oral Radiol* 2016;122(2):232–41.
284. Warnakulasuriya S. Squamous cell carcinoma and precursor lesions: prevention. *Periodontol 2000* 2011;57(1):38–50.
285. William WN Jr, Lee JJ, Lippman SM et al. A pilot surrogate endpoint biomarker study of celecoxib in oral premalignant lesions. *Cancer Prev Res (Phila)* 2008;1(5):339–48.

286. Mallery SR, Tong M, Shumway BS et al. Topical application of a mucoadhesive freeze-dried black raspberry gel induces clinical and histologic regression and reduces loss of heterozygosity events in premalignant oral intraepithelial lesions: results from a multicentered, placebo-controlled clinical trial. *Clin Cancer Res* 2014;20(7):1910–24. doi: 10.1158/1078-0432.CCR-13-3159. Epub January 31, 2014.
287. Armstrong WB, Taylor TH, Kennedy AR et al. Bowman birk inhibitor concentrate and oral leukoplakia: a randomized phase IIb trial. *Cancer Prev Res* (Phila) 2013;6(5):410–8. doi: 10.1158/1940-6207.CAPR-13-0004.
288. Centre for Behavioural Research in Cancer analysis of National Drug Strategy Household Survey data from 1995 to 2013. Available from http://www.tobaccoinaustralia.org.au/chapter-1-prevalence/1-4-prevalence-of-smoking-young-adults.
289. Scollo MM, Winstanley MH. *Tobacco in Australia: facts and Issues.* Melbourne: Cancer Council Victoria; 2016. Available from http://www.tobaccoinaustralia.org.au/.)

Index

Q

R

S

T

U

V

W

X